Parasitology and Vector Biology

SECOND EDITION

Parasitology and Vector Biology

SECOND EDITION

William C. Marquardt
Department of Biology
Colorado State University
Fort Collins, Colorado

Richard S. Demaree
Department of Biology
California State University, Chico
Chico, California

Robert B. Grieve
Heska Corporation
Fort Collins, Colorado;
and Department of Pathology
Colorado State University
Fort Collins, Colorado

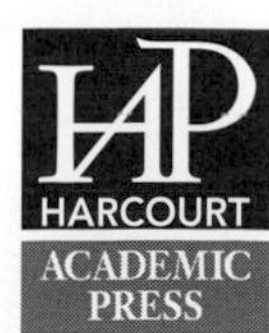

San Diego London Boston New York Sydney Tokyo Toronto

This book is printed on acid-free paper. 

Academic Press
A Harcourt Science and Technology Company
525 B Street, Suite 1900, San Diego, California 92101-4495, USA
http://www.apnet.com

Academic Press
24-28 Oval Road, London NW1 7DX, UK
http://www.hbuk.co.uk/ap/

Harcourt/Academic Press
A Harcourt Science and Technology Company
200 Wheeler Road, Burlington, MA 01803
http://www.harcourt-ap.com

Library of Congress Catalog Card Number: 99-60405

International Standard Book Number: 0-12-473275-5

PRINTED IN THE UNITED STATES OF AMERICA
99 00 01 02 03 04 MM 9 8 7 6 5 4 3 2 1

To Dr. Norman D. Levine

Teacher, Mentor, Colleague, Friend

Norman influenced many of my generation and,
in turn, those whom we taught and guided.
His intelligence, dedication to parasitology, integrity,
and equanimity under all circumstances were models
that few of us could hope to achieve.

William C. Marquardt

Contents

CHAPTER

6

Giardia and Giardiosis

CHAPTER

7

Amebas and Other Enteric Protists of Humans

CHAPTER

8

Free-Living Amebas as Pathogens

CHAPTER

9

Ciliates and Opalinids

CHAPTER

10

Introduction to the Apicomplexa

CHAPTER

11

The Gregarines

CHAPTER

12

The Intestinal Coccidia

CHAPTER

13

The Extraintestinal Coccidia

CHAPTER

14

Malaria in Humans and Related Organisms

CHAPTER

15

Piroplasmea and Piroplasmosis

CHAPTER

16

Myxozoa and Microspora

PART

2

PLATYHELMINTHES

CHAPTER

17

Introduction to the Flatworms and Aspidobothrea

CHAPTER

18

The Blood Flukes or Schistosomes

CHAPTER

19

Liver Flukes

CHAPTER

20

The Intestinal Flukes

CHAPTER

21

The Lung Flukes

CHAPTER

22

The Cercomeromorphae: The Monogeneans and the Cestodes, the Tapeworms

CHAPTER

23

Orders Pseudophyllidea and Proteocephala

CHAPTER

24

Order Cyclophyllidea

PART

3

NEMATODA

CHAPTER

25

Introduction to the Nematodes

CHAPTER

26

Strongyloides and Other Rhabditid Nematodes

CHAPTER

27

Introduction to the Strongyles and the Hookworms

CHAPTER

28

Strongyles of Horses

CHAPTER

29

Nodular Worms, Kidney Worms, and Other Strongyloidea

CHAPTER

30

Trichostrongyles of Cattle, Sheep, Goats, and Other Ruminants

CHAPTER

31

Strongylid Lungworms

CHAPTER

32

Ascarids of Humans and Other Hosts

CHAPTER

33

Pinworms

CHAPTER

34

Filarioid and Other Spirurid Nematodes

CHAPTER

35

Guinea Worm

CHAPTER

36

Trichinella, Trichuris, and *Capillaria*

PART

4

ACANTHOCEPHALA, NEMATOMORPHA, ANNELIDA, AND PENTASTOMIDA

CHAPTER

37

Acanthocephala: Spiny-Headed Worms

CHAPTER

38

Phylum Nematomorpha: Horsehair Worms

CHAPTER

39

Annelida

CHAPTER

40

Pentastomida

PART

5

ARTHROPODA

CHAPTER

41

Introduction to the Arthropods

CHAPTER

42

Crustacea

CHAPTER

43

Introduction to the Insects

CHAPTER

44

Mallophaga and Anoplura: The Lice; and Blattaria: The Cockroaches

CHAPTER

45

The Bugs: Order Hemiptera

CHAPTER

46

Fleas and Flea-Borne Diseases

CHAPTER

47

Diptera: Nematocera and Brachycera

CHAPTER

48

Diptera: Cyclorrapha

CHAPTER

49

Myiasis

CHAPTER

50

Introduction to the Arachnida and the Mites

CHAPTER

51

Ticks

Preface

Parasites have been known since antiquity when early medical writings described helminth parasites such as *Ascaris lumbricoides* and *Taenia* spp. in human excrement. The symptoms of parasitic infections were also written about in medical texts. Hippocrates described various fevers, and it is clear that he recognized the sequence of chills and fever associated with malaria. Among Egyptian hieroglyphs one symbol depicts male genitalia passing a small stream of urine, the translation of which is a cry of pain. This hieroglyph represents infection with *Schistosoma haematobium* and describes the symptom of painful urination experienced by infected individuals.

Despite such early beginnings, parasitology was not established as a distinct science until early in the 20th century. By this time, the germ theory of disease was accepted and many prokaryotic and eukaryotic disease agents were being described. A variety of techniques that allowed investigators to study both types of disease agents were developed, and as information accumulated, specialization became inevitable. Thus, those who worked with prokaryotes founded the disciplines of bacteriology and virology while those who worked with eukaryotic parasites established parasitology and medical entomology. This division between parasitology and microbiology is rather artificial, but it does, in general, represent the kinds of organisms in which specialities developed. The first journal in North America to recognize parasitology as a separate science was the *Journal of Parasitology*, established in 1914 by one of the pioneer parasitologists of the 20th century, Dr. Henry Baldwin Ward. Since then, perhaps 10 major journals have been founded to encompass ever more specialized aspects of parasitology and medical entomology.

All through the early years of the 20th century, basic information on eukaryotic parasites and parasitic diseases accumulated at an ever-increasing rate. The medical, veterinary, and zoological areas burgeoned, and by mid-century the life cycles, epidemiology, systematics, and pathology of the most important parasites were well described. Furthermore, parasitic and vector-borne diseases were recognized as limiting factors in raising developing countries from poverty to acceptable living standards. As knowledge progressed, more sophisticated concepts were formed in the epidemiology and physiology of parasitic agents and in their host–parasite interactions.

The mass of information that a neophyte parasitologist now faces is truly overwhelming. No one of us who has studied parasites can comprehend all of the basic information as well as the current approaches in immunology and molecular biology. There is too much of everything for the new person in the field to grasp and to gain a rounded view of parasitism.

What, then, is important for students to learn? Suffice it to say that there are a number of approaches to teaching parasitology and many of them do not reach, nor are likely to stimulate, the beginning students of parasitology. Some years ago, we reasoned that if students were to learn how to control parasitic diseases, they would then have a skill that could be put to use and also have a foundation in many aspects of parasitology on which they could build. Our courses have revolved around this theme, and so the first edition of this book also held that orientation.

We continue to emphasize control of parasitic diseases in this second edition of *Parasitology and Vector Biology*. But control is not implemented without knowledge of a number of aspects of the disease complex that one faces. To implement a control program, certain kinds of information are necessary, and we have built the written material around control of disease and how to implement control. Also, because we are writing for students, we have attempted to organize the material in a systematic way so that students can read a particular section and obtain whatever information is important at the moment. Where there are more than one or two approaches to be taken in control or diagnosis, we list the steps that can be taken and then discuss and evaluate them in turn. We hope that the readers will thereby readily find the salient facts needed, first for comprehension and second for testing—that dreaded occurrence in every student's life.

Since the publication of our first edition, parasitology has undergone the same revolution as other biological disciplines. Molecular biology and immunology have brought changes that affect every aspect of parasitology. The addition of Dr. Robert B. Grieve as a coauthor strengthens immunology and molecular biology throughout the book. We feel that increased emphasis in those areas and in certain aspects of applied parasitology provides a valuable contribution to the revision.

Significant changes have been made to this edition: 120 new halftones and diagrams have been added, the introductory chapter has been completely rewritten, 15 chapters have been significantly revised, and all chapters have been updated where appropriate. There have been revolutionary changes in the classification of and concepts of evolution among the protists and the platyhelminths that we have incorporated. In our first edition, discussion and evaluation of control methods were not much influenced by molecular biology and immunology, but in the intervening years this has changed. These advances are incorporated into our discussions of control wherever appropriate. Another area of recent major conceptual change in biology is in aspects of arthropod vectors. We have included a greatly expanded discussion of vector biology.

We three authors have accumulated many decades of combined experience in parasitology. Even for those of us who have been in the field for half a century, parasitology remains a continuing, intense interest. New host–parasite and ecological relationships have been uncovered, and new methods allow us to address questions that could not have even been approached a few years ago. Previously unknown parasitic diseases continue to emerge with regularity, and old ones are seen in new lights. The fascination with the parasitic relationship never wanes, and the problems that are presented for solution are challenging. What more can one ask for a life's work?

Acknowledgments

The Heska Corporation, Fort Collins, Colorado, provided clerical support in the preparation of some of the manuscript. We are grateful for this support.

Our illustrations have been gathered from many sources, and in a number of instances colleagues went out of their way to provide original halftones or line cuts. Among those to whom we are indebted are Dr. John F. Alderete, Dr. J. P. Dubey, Dr. Larry R. McDougald, Dr. Robert Mead, Dr. Harley Moon, Dr. Barbara A. Nichols, Dr. C. A. Speer, Dr. T. Bonner Stewart, Dr. Rex Thomas, Dr. J. P. Vanderberg, Dr. G. S. Visvesvara, Dr. Laurel L. Walters, and Dr. P. T. K. Woo.

New and refurbished drawings were prepared by Dave Carlson of Visible Productions, by Gary Raham, and by Kay Marquardt of Kay Marquardt Design, Fort Collins, Colorado.

W.C.M
R.S.D
R.B.G

CHAPTER

1

Introduction

Parasitic organisms include a spectrum of agents from 10-meter-long tapeworms (Fig. 1.1) down to the enigmatic prions, which seem to be comprised only of protein. In between is a bewildering array from molecules, prokaryotes, protists, and metazoa that are symbiotic in every ecologic niche imaginable (Fig. 1.2). These thousands upon thousands of organisms live in close association with their hosts, which are found in every taxonomic group of animals and plants. The ubiquity of parasites is perhaps exceeded only by their usual obscurity from human view, but we and all other organisms live every day with parasitic agents that sometimes cause disease and even death.

In the chapters that follow, we discuss primarily eukaryotic, symbiotic organisms, which have the potential of harming the animals with which they are associated. "Parasites" are traditionally considered to be protists, worms, and arthropods, a rather limited taxonomic array. Even so, we barely scratch the surface of all the organisms that could be discussed, and the sum of knowledge about them is beyond the capabilities of any one person. Of the approximate 35 animal phyla, nearly all have members that are parasitic. The exceptions are the echinoderms (starfish, sea urchins), the chordates (reptiles, birds, mammals, etc.), and a few of the minor phyla. Parasitism is both widespread and a common mode of existence.

Historically, metazoan parasites were the first transmissible agents to be seen and associated with disease in humans (Fig. 1.3). Tapeworms and large roundworms were known and described in early writings of the Middle East, but hundreds of years passed before their significance and association with disease were known. Since the 14th century, the beginning of the Renaissance, an ever increasing number of parasites have been described as well as their life cycles, damage to their hosts, their epidemiologies, and the plethora of interactions between host and parasite.

Protists, formerly called protozoa, were rather latecomers to our knowledge of infectious agents. Antony van Leeuwenhoek, a Dutch businessman and public servant, wrote letters to the Royal Society of London describing tiny organisms that he saw using the simple microscopes he had made. He wrote 200 letters over a period of nearly 50 years ending in the year of his death at 91 in 1732. Leeuwenhoek's observations were crucial in initiating and stimulating knowledge of microscopic organisms; he not only described more than 40 recognizable genera of eukarytoic protists, but he also described bacteria and even their flagella. This was truly a remarkable achievement that has set investigators on a 300-year quest for knowledge of microscopic (and submicroscopic) organisms. Leeuwenhoek opened up a whole world that had been unknown, and he was instrumental in establishing microbiology as a discipline.

Every practitioner of a profession undoubtedly has a somewhat peculiar view of the world. Those of us who study parasitic agents (of all taxonomic groups) look on the world as harboring a cloud of infectious agents. Potentially pathogenic organisms are all around us and able to move into our bodies and reproduce if given the opportunity. Just as the more obvious larger plants and animals continually move into diverse ecological niches, so also do the less obvious and hidden parasitic organisms move into niches in their hosts. They inhabit every organ system in the human (and other species) body: skin (Fig. 1.4A), intestinal tract, cardiovascular system (Fig. 1.4B), reproductive

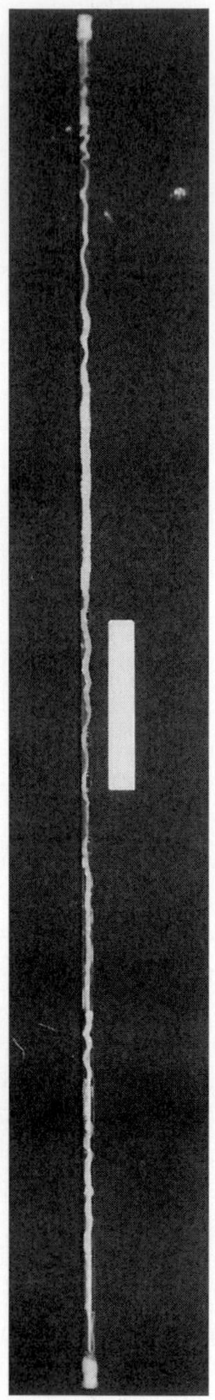

FIGURE 1.1 A taenioid tapeworm of humans; this worm can reach a length of more than 5 meters in the human intestine. The white bar represents 15 cm.

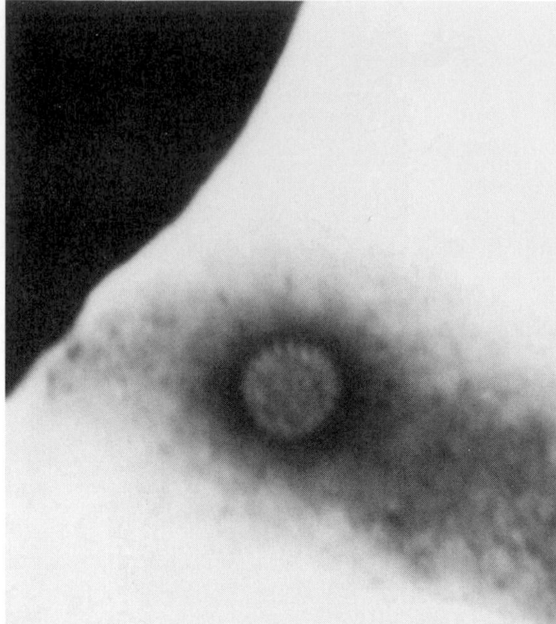

FIGURE 1.2 Transmission electron micrograph of a bovine rotavirus at 210,000 magnification. These organisms cause enteritis and diarrhea in humans.

system, nervous system (Fig. 1.4C), and the skeletal muscle system (Fig. 1.4D). But it should be kept in mind that parasitic agents are not purposely trying to kill their hosts; they move into an available niche and whatever damage they may do is coincidental. They are only trying to make a living and leave their DNA for posterity, the same things that the rest of us are trying to do.

WHAT IS PARASITISM?

A more or less permanent association of organisms of different species is referred to as *symbiosis*, and the participants are *symbionts*. Symbiosis can be subdivided into commensalism, mutualism, and parasitism. In *commensalism*, one partner may be benefited, but the other is neither harmed nor benefited. Those plants, which are called epiphytes (orchids and bromeliads) (Fig. 1.5), are provided a home by trees, but the epiphytes neither help nor harm the trees.

In *mutualism*, both partners derive benefit from the relationship. Lichens (Fig. 1.6) are formed from a union

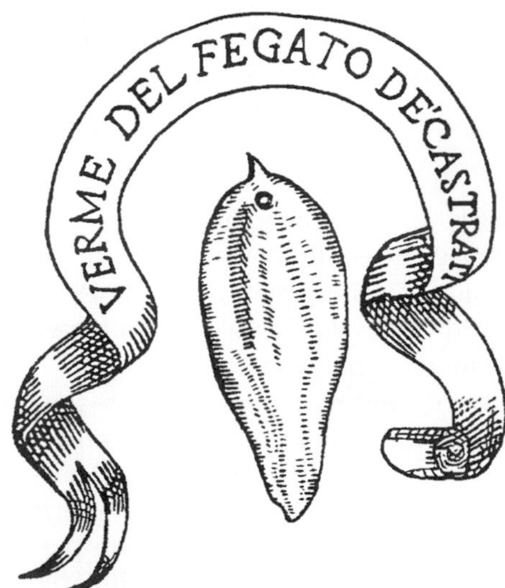

FIGURE 1.3 Illustration of *Fasciola hepatica*, from the liver of a sheep, dated 1668.

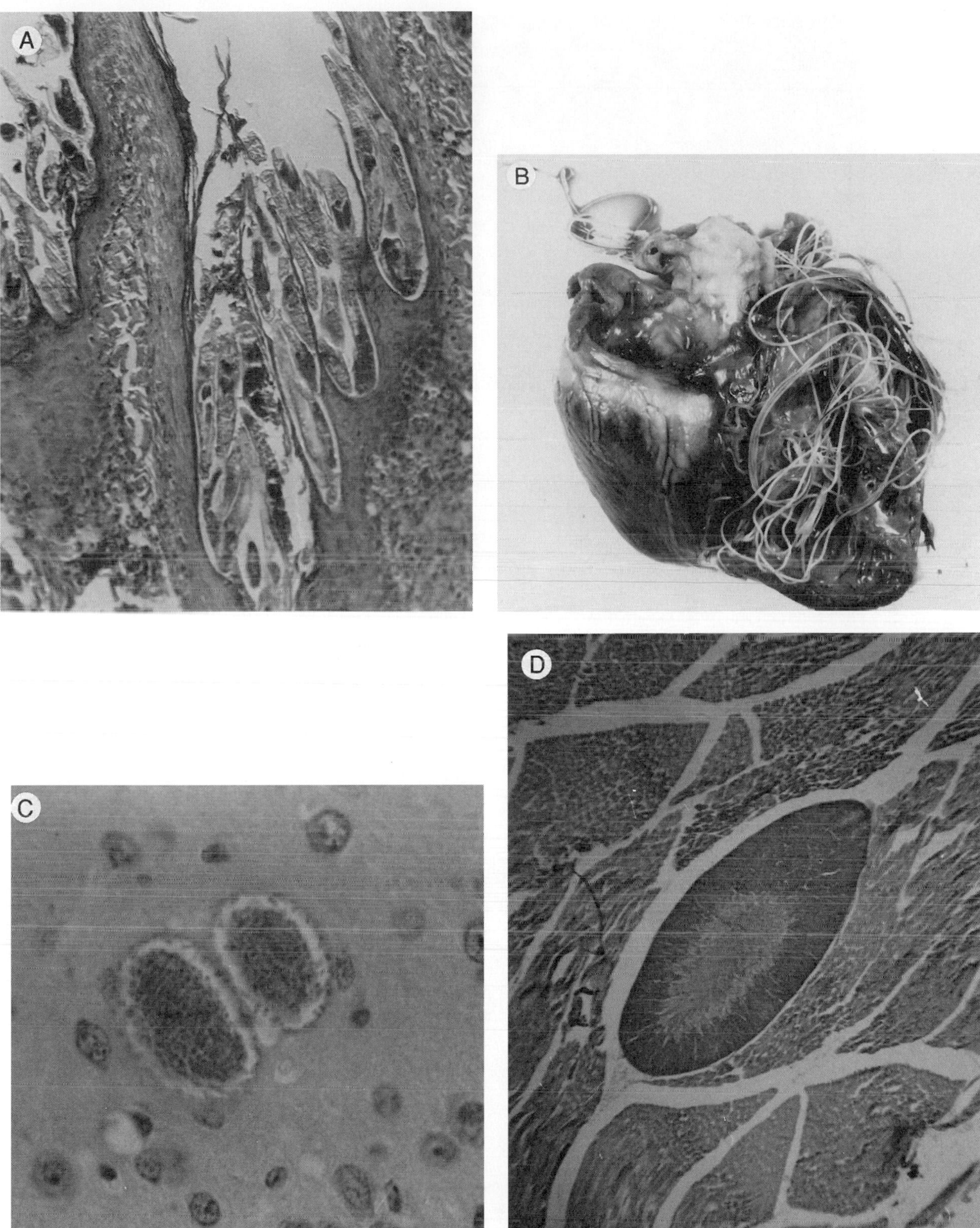

FIGURE 1.4 Photomicrographs of (A) the mite *Demodex* sp. in the skin of a dog (arrow). (B) *Dirofilaria immitis* in the heart of a dog. (C) *Toxoplasma gondii* in the brain of a mouse. (D) *Sarcocystis tenella* cyst in the somatic muscle of a sheep.

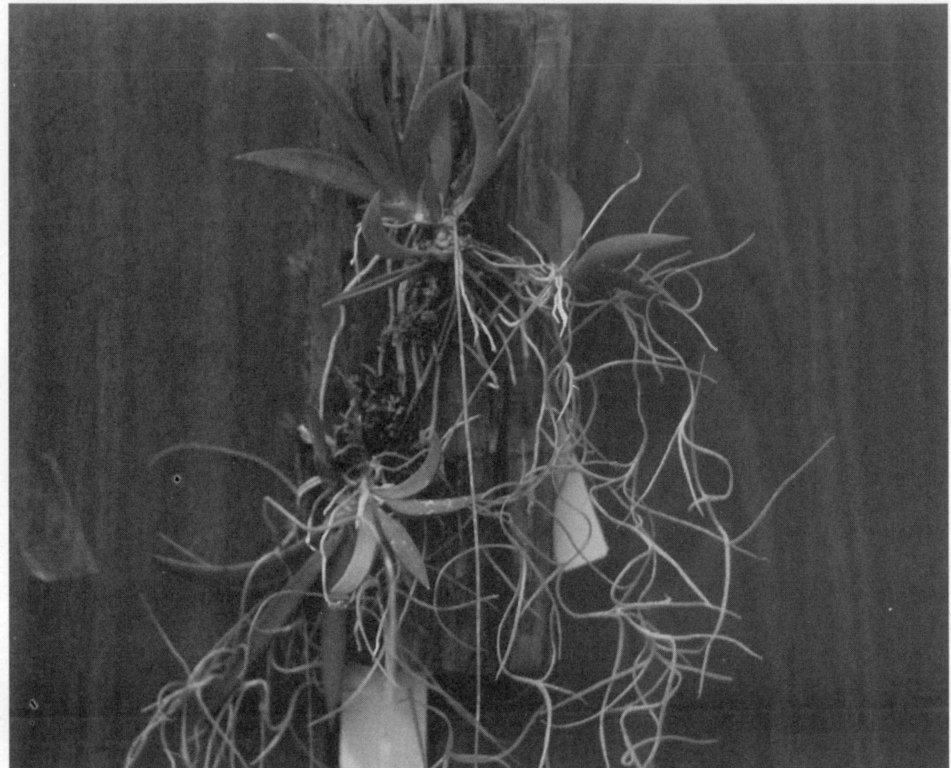

FIGURE 1.5 Photograph of an epiphyte, a commensal plant.

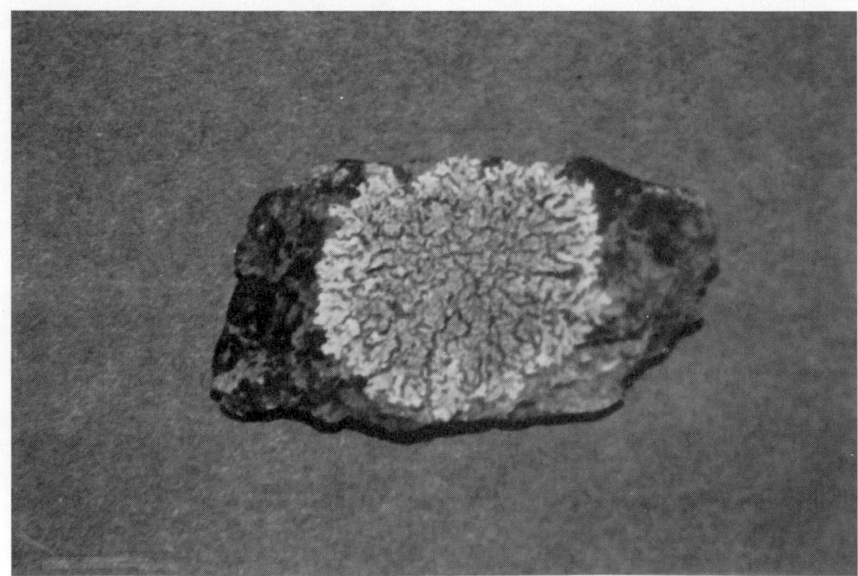

FIGURE 1.6 Photomicrograph of a lichen, *Xanthoparmelia* sp., a mutualistic association of an alga and a fungus.

of an alga and a fungus; both benefit from the relationship. Certain termites have flagellated protists (Fig. 1.7), which digest the cellulose that the termites eat; each is unable to exist without the other.

In *parasitism,* one partner is benefited while there can be harm to the other partner. That is the subject of this book, and what we do from here on describes "the parasitic relationship" and discusses how to alleviate the harmful aspects of it.

A number of approaches have been used in describing a parasite or parasitism. The situation is like some others—it is difficult to give an unequivocal definition, but we know it when we see it.

A straightforward definition of parasitism is a relationship of two organisms of different species in which the smaller (the parasite) has the potential of harming the larger (the host) and in which the parasite relies on the host for nutrient and for a place to live (often described as a niche). Usually, the parasite either reproduces in the host or produces many offspring that reach the outside by some means; the parasite has a greater reproductive potential than its host.

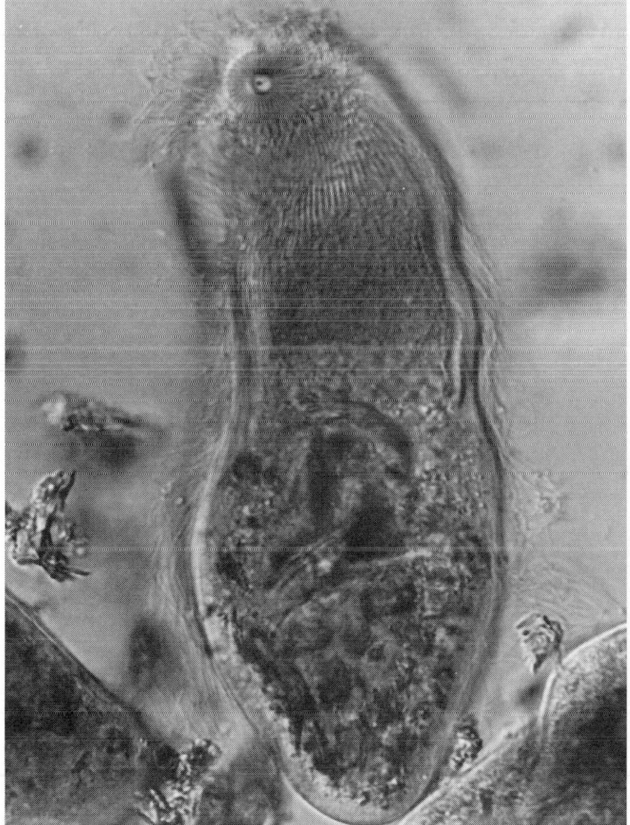

FIGURE 1.7 A photomicrograph of a mutualistic flagellated protist from the gut of a termite.

The parasitic relationship is a dynamic one and damage to the host may be influenced by the age of the host, the number of parasites present, and the ability of the host to respond by one means or another to invasion, among other factors. Thus, parasites may harm the host under some circumstances, but not others. It is emphasized that infection is not the same as disease; a host can be infected with any of a variety of disease agents and not show any signs or symptoms of the infection.

Even though there are situations in which the basic definition suffers from some strain, it works most of the time, but in some instances, the relationship is somewhat different. For example, a mosquito comes to feed on a vertebrate host, takes a blood meal, and departs. Certain mosquitoes are not completely dependent on a host since they can lay eggs without having taken a bood meal; this is referred to as *autogeny.* Also, since the relationship is temporary, some investigators prefer to call the mosquito a micropredator. Another example is the cluster fly, *Pollenia rudis,* which lives in an earthworm as a larva; it feeds on the earthworm tissue and finally kills the earthworm by eating nearly all of it. The cluster fly seems to be more of a predator than parasite. Likewise, certain wasps oviposit in insect larvae and the hymenopteran larvae feed on the tissues of their larval hosts until they emerge later as adult wasps. In both of these latter instances, the parasite is referred to as a *parasitoid* because it fails to reproduce in its host but merely eats it from the inside. Thus, the natural world always escapes the constrictions of neat definitions constructed by humans.

A parasite may live either on the surface of the host as an ectoparasite or within the body of the host as an endoparasite. Lice (Fig. 1.8) and ticks live on the skin of their vertebrate hosts, while a monogenean such as *Entobdella soleae* lives on the scales of its fish host. Certain other monogeneans, such as *Gyrodactylus,* live on the gills of fish, and are not exactly outside, but neither are they inside their hosts.

Parasites can also be *temporary* or *permanent, obligate* or *facultative.* Temporary parasites are those such as nest-inhabiting bedbugs that feed on nestling birds and then return to the nesting material until ready to feed again. Permanent parasites are those such as the enteric amebas of humans that exist outside of a host for only short time while in transition. Most of the organisms discussed in this book fall in that category. Likewise nearly all of the parasites we consider are obligate—they must have a host to complete the life cycle and to survive. Facultative parasites are represented by a few roundworms, such as *Pelodera strongyloides,* which are normally free living but can invade hosts under certain conditions. The same is true of many flesh flies;

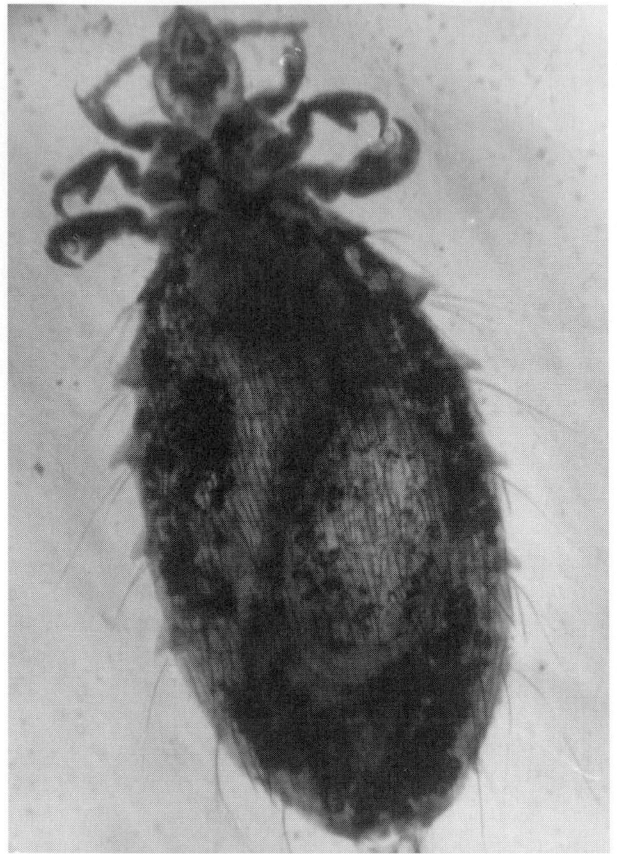

FIGURE 1.8 Photomicrograph of a sucking louse, *Solenopotes capillatus,* the little blue louse of cattle.

they normally are found in decaying carcasses but can invade the tissues of a living host if proper conditions are found by the ovipositing female flies.

Parasites have both *direct* and *indirect* life cycles. A direct life cycle is one in which the organism is passed from one host to the next through the air, by a fomite, or in contaminated food or water. Organisms such as enteric protists, which are transmitted with contaminated food or water, or those such as *Tritrichomonas foetus,* which are transmitted by sexual intercourse, are examples of direct life cycles.

In an indirect life cycle, the organism develops or multiplies in a *vector* or in an *intermediate host.* A vector is an invertebrate organism that transmits the parasitic agent from one vertebrate host to the next. The vector may either be a *mechanical vector,* in which no development or multiplication takes place, or a *biological vector,* in which either multiplication or development occurs. *Trypanosoma evansi,* a protistan parasite of large ruminants, is transmitted by flies in the family Tabanidae. These flies are restless feeders and they transmit *T. evansi* on their contaminated mouthparts. *Trypanosoma gambiense* on the other hand, is transmitted to humans by tsetse (Diptera, Glossinidae), in which both multiplication and development occur. The filarial worm, *Wuchereria bancrofti,* the cause of elephantiasis in humans, is transmitted by mosquitoes, in which development but no multiplication takes place.

An *intermediate host* is a type of biological vector. The term is used with eukaryotic parasites, which have sexual development in the life cycle. The host in which sexual development takes place is the *definitive host,* and the *intermediate host* is the one(s) in which asexual development or multiplication occurs. In the digenetic trematodes, the definitive host is a vertebrate, and the intermediate host is almost always a snail (Fig. 1.9). In the tissue coccidia such as *Sarcocystis* spp., the definitive host is an omnivore or carnivore, and the intermediate host is an herbivore.

Transport or *paratenic* hosts are those in which a parasite does not develop or multiply but is carried to the next host usually through ingestion of the transport host. In the life cycle of the broad fish tapeworm of humans, *Diphyllobothrium latum,* the first intermediate host is a copepod, and the second intermediate host is a planktonic-feeding fish. This fish, in turn, is eaten by a larger fish, a paratenic or transport host. Since large omnivores such as humans do not often eat tiny fish, transmission up the food chain takes place when a larger fish eats the small one. No development takes place in the second fish. Although a paratenic host may not be important for the development or

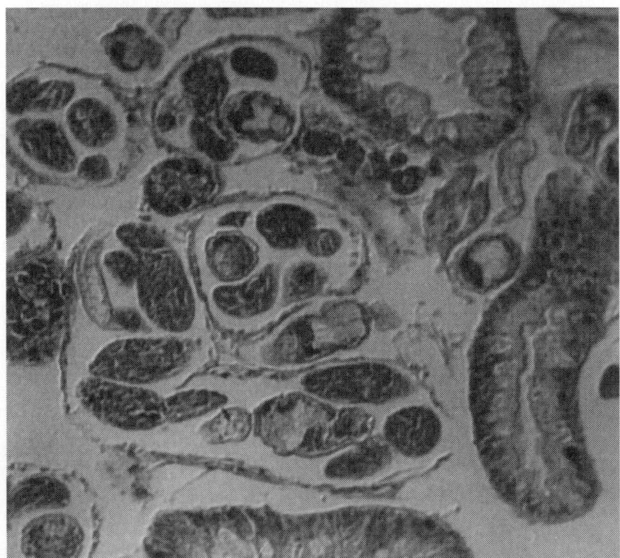

FIGURE 1.9 Photomicrograph of a histologic section of a snail infected with sporocysts of *Schistosoma mansoni.*

multiplication of parasites, it is usually important in dispersing the parasite and in accessing the definitive host.

Many parasites are found along with other species of parasites in the host. If a host is infected with a number of parasites at the same time, we refer to the situation as *polyparasitism.* In many circumstances in both humans and other mammals, a number of organisms, both prokaryotic and eukaryotic, contribute to bringing about the disease state. Children in developing countries often are infected with two or more species of nematodes and suffer from malaria as well. Livestock on pastures in warm, moist climates may harbor four or more species of intestinal nematodes, lungworms, and one or more species of flatworms. In Rocky Mountain bighorn sheep, a disease called "lungworm pneumonia" is actually caused by a virus, one or more species of bacteria, and, finally, the lungworm. On top of the disease agents, however, is laid the effect of poor nutrition, which predisposes the sheep to greater damage from the infections. Polyparasitism makes for a complex situation that often requires multiple approaches to intervene in and ameliorate the disease process.

The host range of a parasite is important in assessing its epidemiology and designing a control program. Only a few parasites have a narrow range of hosts in which they develop. The intestinal coccidia of livestock and poultry develop in only a single species of host or perhaps one or two additional closely related species. The beef tapeworm, *Taenia saginata,* probably has only humans as its definitive host. Many are like certain nematodes, which can have several species of hosts, or like the parasitic insects, which usually can develop in a wide range of hosts. Most mosquitoes feed either on birds or mammals, but some take blood from either group of hosts. A few parasites, such as ticks, are opportunistic and attach to any host that may happen to be in the vicinity.

Of particular concern are those parasitic agents which normally develop in hosts other than humans but which can infect humans if given the opportunity. These are so-called *zoonotic agents,* and they cause *zoonoses.* Many arboviruses (arthropod-borne viruses) cycle silently in the wild and become known only when humans are infected and show the signs and symptoms of disease. Among all kinds of parasitic agents, zoonotic ones are preponderant. Certain directly transmitted agents such as measles, chicken pox, trichomonad vaginitis (Fig. 1.10), and amebic dysentery do not have significant reservoirs other than humans, but many others, especially vector-borne agents, have reservoirs in other animal hosts.

The term *reservoir* has traditionally been reserved

EPIDEMIOLOGY

EPIDEMIOLOGICAL INVESTIGATIONS ARE IMPORTANT tools used by parasitologists to determine the source of infections. Epidemiology is the study of patterns of disease within populations. The epidemiologist attempts to determine what factors are responsible for the disease under investigation. Investigations may be retrospective (backward-looking) or prospective (forward-looking). There may be case control studies in which there is a "case group" whose members have contracted the disease and a "control group," those comparable individuals who have not contracted the disease. An attempt is made to correlate similarities and differences between the two groups. Many parasitological epidemiological investigations are of this type.

Another kind of epidemiological study is the convenience cohort study. Observed groups (cohorts) are selected with plans to test another hypothesis. Data which were collected are then utilized for another purpose (convenience). This type of study is not used frequently in parasitology.

An example which made newspaper headlines might be informative. A protistan, *Cyclospora cayatanensis,* was implicated as the cause of severe gastrointestinal disturbance in more than 1000 persons in 11 states. Early investigations implicated strawberries from California as the source of the parasite; most people who had become ill had eaten strawberries from California. A more thorough study revealed no trace of the parasite on fruit in California, nor reports of disease in that state, even though Californians ate similar strawberries. It was later determined that the real culprit was raspberries from Guatemala. The tracing and retracing of raspberries and related illness was a painstaking job in which many epidemiologists were involved. How the berries became contaminated remains a mystery.

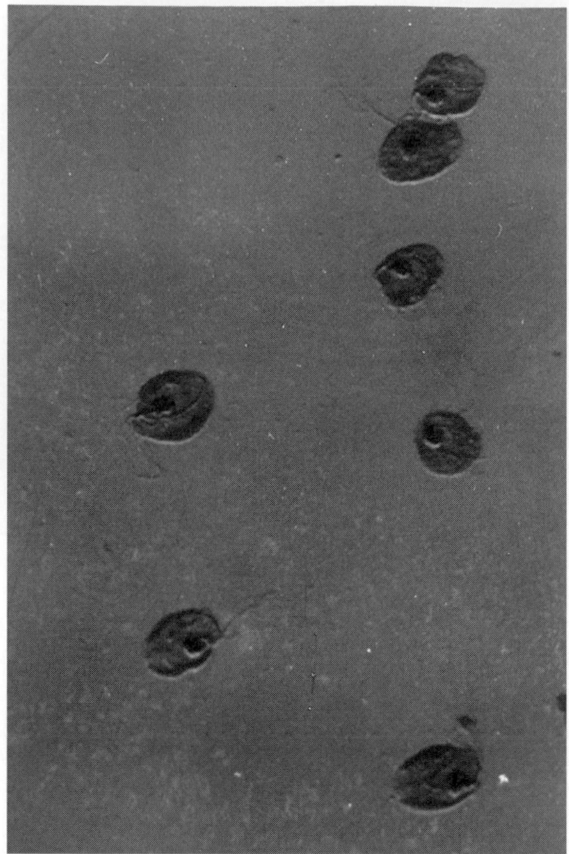

FIGURE 1.10 A photomicrograph of a trophozoite of *Trichomonas vaginalis,* the cause of vaginitis in women.

for a vertebrate host(s) other than humans that maintains the infectious agent. In recent years, the reservoir has come to include the whole complex of nonhuman vertebrate hosts, the vector(s), and the landscape itself. It seems better to maintain the term *reservoir* for the vertebrate host(s) and to use the term *nidus* to encompass the whole system. The term *nidus* was coined by the Russian epidemiologist Pavlovski and his coworkers to describe the whole complex of factors that interact to maintain an infectious agent in its natural habitat. A nidus is literally a nest and as such is a small ecosystem. In a nidus, all of the factors are present that are required to maintain the cycling of the parasitic agent. In Chapter 51 we discuss the Colorado tick fever ecosystem, and it is as good an example of a nidus as can be found.

HOW HAS PARASITISM EVOLVED?

There are tremendous variations in host–parasite associations and it is therefore difficult, even risky, to generalize about the way in which parasitism arose. It is assumed that symbioses arose through chance encounters between different species of free-living organisms. One of the species found the association to be beneficial and remained. The host can be viewed as an assemblage of ecological niches, which are available for exploitation by protoparasites.

One notion should be discarded early in this discussion—the "*preadaptation*" of an organism for a symbiotic life. Evolution is not "forward looking," it does not anticipate. Rather, various traits arise by chance, and some may prove to be useful in exploiting new ecological niches. If this happens to be one of the organs of another species of animal, symbiosis can begin.

No single trait allows a free-living organism to become a symbiont, but given the diversity of host–parasite associations, many factors would be useful:

1. Living in close proximity
2. Having a smaller size than the potential host
3. Having the ability to enter or associate with another species
4. Having a structure(s) at the gross or microscopic level allowing attachment to a substrate
5. Having the physiological capability to survive in or on another organism, including a means of feeding
6. Being able to reproduce in or on another species
7. Having a way for progeny to leave the host and to contact another potential host
8. Not eliciting a strong inflammatory and immune response that would be destructive to the protoparasite.

Parasites are frequently referred to as being "degenerate," and "*parasite*" is used as a perjorative of the strongest kind, particularly in political discourse. But nothing could be further from the truth. A tapeworm lacks eyes, a skeleton, and a respiratory system, but it has an exquisitely evolved interface with the host tissue and intestinal contents. It has no need for certain organ systems seen in other animals, and it therefore does not put its precious resources into unneeded structures. Surely, this is an economical approach that is to be acclaimed rather than deplored.

Today we can still see evolution in action. There are some groups such as the apicomplexans (e.g., malaria) that are entirely parasitic and probably have been for millions of years. Others, such as the flatworms (phylum Platyhelminthes), have members that are free-living, or obligate parasites, or every intergrade in between.

After a host–parasite association becomes well established, a number of alternatives are possible. Through coevolution the association can develop from parasitism to mutualism. For example, *Trypanosoma musculi* is a flagellated protist, which lives in the bloodstream of mice and fails to cause any detectable harm. Instead, mice actually benefit from nutrients such as B vitamins produced by the trypanosomes. In contrast, close relatives including *Trypanosoma cruzi* (Fig. 1.11) and the trypanosomes that cause African sleeping sickness are true parasites and cause millions of human deaths annually as well as losses in livestock. It is sometimes said that parasitic associations tend to evolve toward a benign state, and while there are some examples of this course of evolution, it is not possible to generalize. Many parasitic relationships have obviously been going on for eons, but there is no evidence of declining pathogenicity.

Certain host–parasite associations evolve into what John Rennie has called a "co-evolutionary arms race." Successful parasites reproduce prolifically and remove increasing amounts of nutrients from the host. At the same time, successful hosts develop mechanisms to eliminate their parasites or at least minimize their negative impact. Thus, if both host and parasite coevolve, a "biological detente" also evolves in which neither is destroyed but in which both retain vigilance and continue to maneuver.

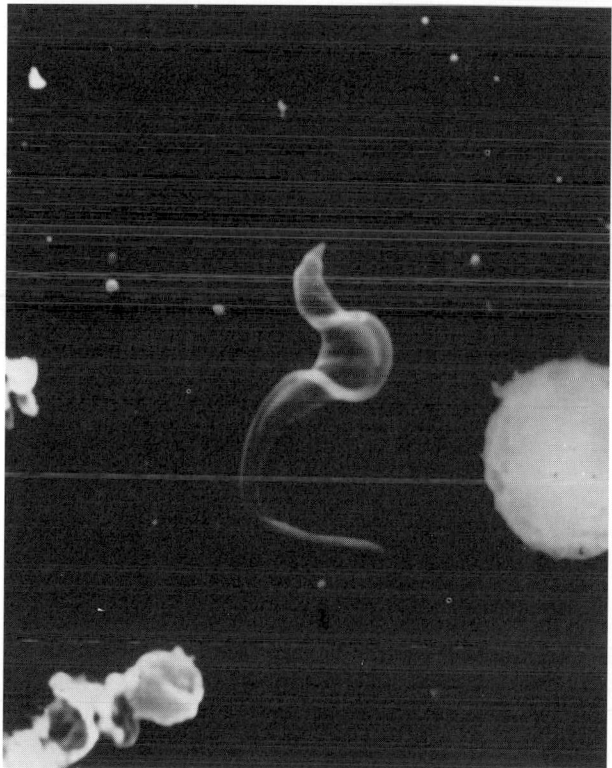

FIGURE 1.11 Scanning electron micrograph (SEM) of a trypomastigote of *Trypanosoma cruzi*, the cause of Chagas' disease or American trypanosomosis in humans.

HOW DOES THE PARASITIC RELATIONSHIP WORK?

With the exception of some kinds of interactions between the host and parasite, parasitism does not have unique features. The same general ecological principles apply to both free-living and parasitic organisms: Both need a physical place in the ecosystem, adequate food, and the ability to reproduce. In fact, parasites have been studied to elucidate certain ecological generalizations such as succession, island colonization, and niche diversification.

The life cycles of some parasites seem bizarre at first, but many parasites follow a course of development similar to those of their free-living counterparts. In those parasites that have direct life cycles, parallels can be seen among their free-living relatives. For example, all nematodes have five stages separated by four molts. In the strongylid nematodes, the infective stage is the third stage larva (L_3), which waits until it is ingested and can continue its development. In the free-living nematodes, development proceeds at a more or less fixed rate, given proper temperature and moisture in the environment. The parasitic species reach a certain point in the life cycle and then stop to await proper conditions for continuing toward the adult stage.

Another example comes from the dysentery ameba, *Entamoeba histolytica*, which forms cysts that transmit the organism from one host to another. Many free-living amebas form cysts to protect themselves from adverse environmental conditions or for reproduction. In the case of the dysentery ameba, the cyst has evolved in such a way that it is hardy enough to survive in the environment, pass through the stomach, and then excyst in the intestine where it can begin to feed and reproduce.

A host can be looked on as a collection of potential niches. In an animal as anatomically complex as a vertebrate, there are probably hundreds of niches that could be identified. These range from a dozen possible niches in the intestinal tract to at least three in the bloodstream (serum, red blood cells, white blood cells). Even considering somatic muscle cells there are differences that parasites recognize. *Trichinella pseudospiralis* enters only slow-twitch fibers, whereas *T. spiralis* (Fig. 1.12) enters and develops in either slow- or fast-twitch fibers.

With relation to intestinal parasites, the *paramucosal lumen* is a concept that is important for understanding the host–parasite interface. We tend to think of parasites as living in the lumen of the intestine where they are subject to enzymes, bacterial action, and an anaerobic or near-anaerobic environment. In fact, few parasites, live in the lumen; instead they are found under

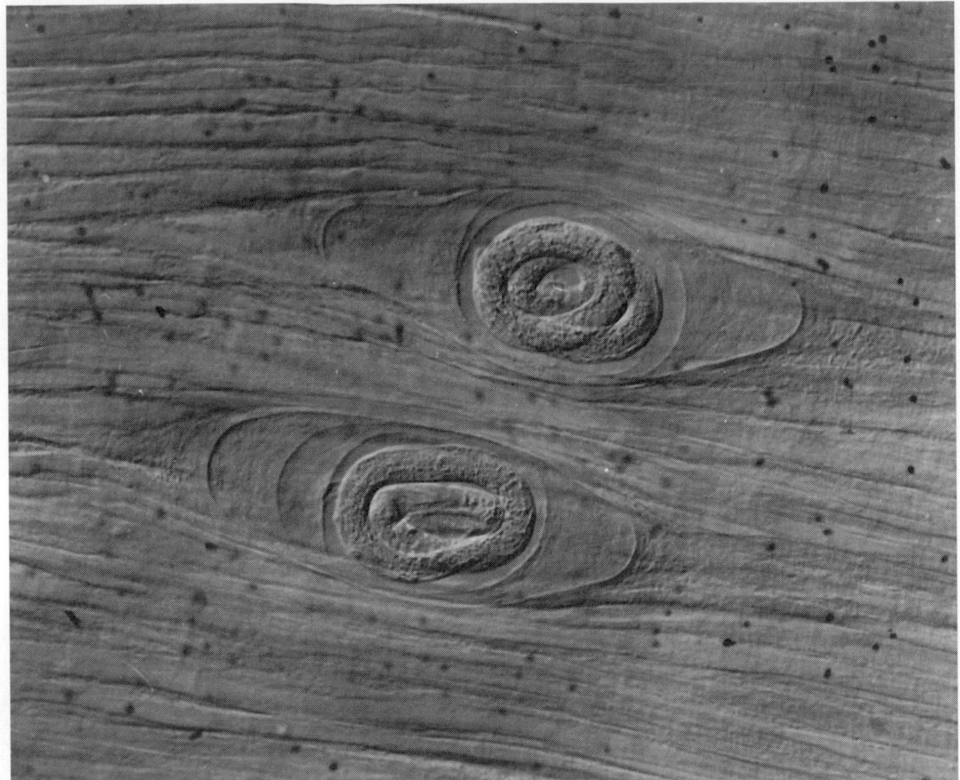

FIGURE 1.12 *Trichinella spiralis* larvae encysted in the somatic muscle of a mammal.

the layer of intestinal mucus or in the crypts of Lieberkeuhn. In this area the oxygen tension is nearly the same as in blood or tissue, it is probably free of bacteria and the parasites are in a location where they cannot only feed but also elicit a host immune response. This is the paramucosal lumen.

Parasites are not typically distributed randomly through a population of available hosts. Taking worms as an example, a large proportion of hosts have a few parasites, or none at all, but a few have large numbers (Fig. 1.13). This kind of distribution is referred to as "overdispersed" or "nonrandom." The concept can be applied to other organisms that reproduce within the host. For example, *Entamoeba histolytica* is typically found in about 4% of persons in temperate climates, but only about a fifth of those individuals show clinical signs and symptoms of amebic dysentery. So two factors are at work here, only a small proportion of the population becomes infected, and a smaller proportion of those become ill. The concept of overdispersion is much more than an academic exercise because it leads to the conclusion that only a small proportion of the members of a population provide the greatest probability of passing on an infection. If they can be identified, only those members of the population that are most heavily infected might be treated with a therapeutic

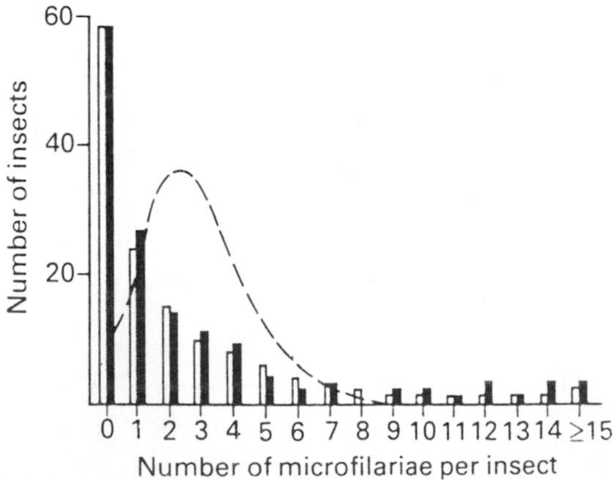

FIGURE 1.13 A graph showing the overdispersed distribution of microfilariae in the biting midge vector of *Chandlerella qiscali*. It is generally seen that most potential hosts in a population have few parasites, but a few harbor a large number. The reasons for this nonrandom or overdispersed distribution are not known except in a few instances, but it may relate to behavior, innate susceptibility, or the immune state of the host. [From Schmid *et al.*, 1972.]

compound thus reducing the parasite population in an entire community of hosts.

The large reproductive potential of many parasites is sometimes thought of as being characteristic of parasites, implying that free-living organisms do not have such a large potential. For example, the large ascarid of humans and swine may produce as many as 500,000 eggs per day and continue such production for many months. The common liver fluke of sheep and cattle, *Fasciola hepatica,* lays about 20,000 eggs a day and can live in a sheep for as long as 10 years. The question is whether this reproduction is different from free-living organisms. In Chapter 47 we refer to the reproduction of the housefly, *Musca domestica,* which, if left unchecked, could cover the earth 47 feet deep in one summer season. A single oyster produces tens of thousands of eggs in a season, and bacteria often have generation times as short as 20 minutes. Parasites probably do not reproduce any more rapidly than free-living animals, but nearly all parasites are opportunistic. Given the chance, they will increase in number dramatically in a short period of time.

In considering opportunistic parasites, two useful concepts are the *r*- and *K*-strategies, and the equations expressing the dynamics of parasite populations. In the former, the term *strategy* refers to an inherited characteristic that is shaped by the pressures of natural selection. Parasites that are *r*-selected put their energies into producing large numbers of offspring, usually within a short period of time. In this type of strategy, there are essentially no density-dependent effects and little or no competition. The opposite strategy are those species that are *K*-selected, which produce only a few extremely fit offspring because density effects are maximal and the environment is nearly saturated with organisms.

Most parasites, and vectors fall into the *r*-selected category, because they are nearly all opportunists. We have given some examples of *r*-selected organisms, but a few *K*-selected species might be mentioned. Most prominent are the tsetse, which transmit the causative agent of African sleeping sickness and nagana. Tsetse females nurture only a single larva at a time and produce only an average of nine offspring during a lifetime. Kissing bugs are the vectors of *Trypanosoma cruzi,* the cause of Chagas' disease. A female *Rhodnius prolixus* may lay as many as 300 eggs in a lifetime, but she lays them over a period of about six months. Female lice typically develop only a single egg at a time thereby investing a great deal of energy into one offspring.

A common aspect of reproduction in parasites is alternation of generation. An asexual cycle is alternated with a sexual cycle. Although such a mode of development is not unknown in free-living organisms (ferns and aphids are examples), it is a theme seen in a number of taxa of parasites. Members of the Apicomplexa (malaria, coccidia) alternate sexual and asexual development. Some nematodes such as *Strongyloides* alternate parthenogenetic reproduction with sexual development (Fig. 1.14). The digenetic trematodes have asexual reproduction in the snail intermediate host and sexual reproduction in the vertebrate host. Most tapeworms have evolved methods of both asexual and sexual reproduction, the most striking being the replication of sexual organs in each segment (Fig. 1.15). A few tapeworms replicate as larvae, thus providing additional infective units to complete the life cycle.

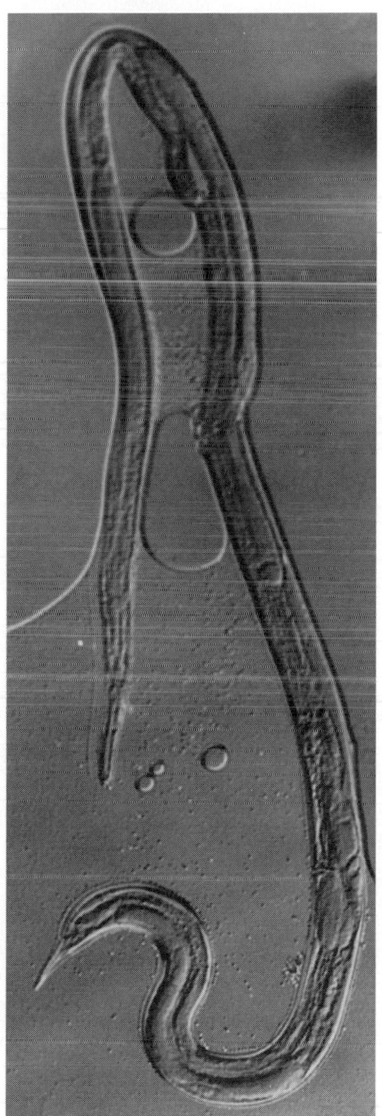

FIGURE 1.14 A photomicrograph of an adult female of *Strongyloides stercoralis,* a pathogenic intestinal helminth of humans and canids.

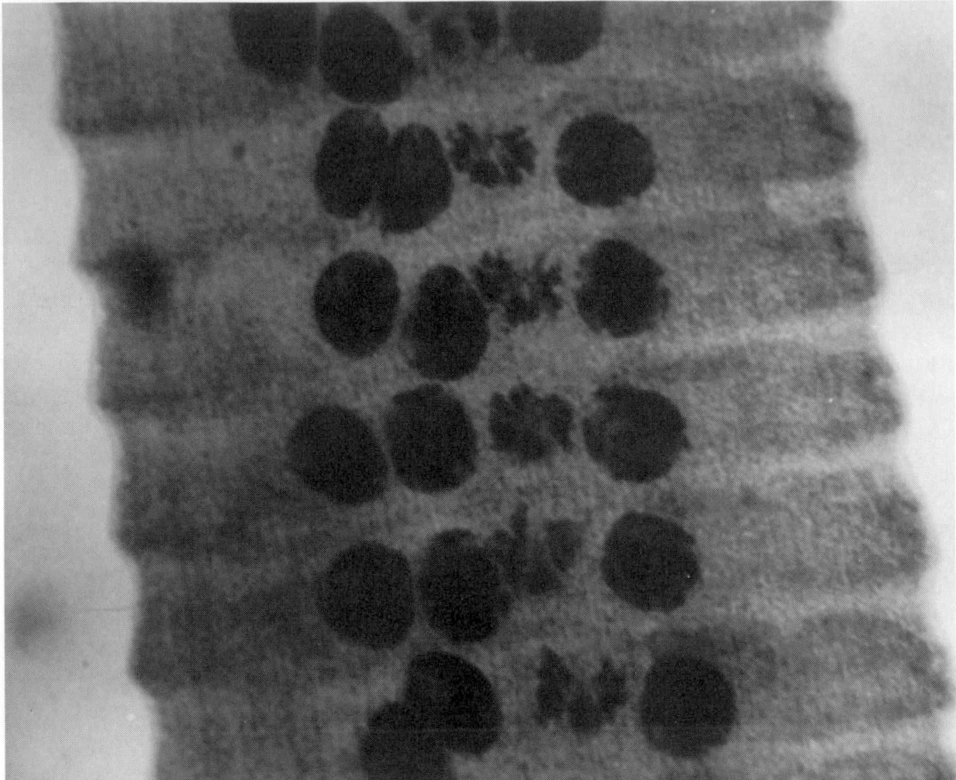

FIGURE 1.15 Photomicrograph of mature proglottids or segments of the tapeworm *Hymenolepis diminuta* of the rat. The large round structures are testes, and the bilobed ovary is in the center of the proglottid. The genital atrium is on the right margin seen as a rectangular indentation; the vagina extends from the genital atrium to the ootype about in the center of the ovary.

The life cycles of parasites are often complex and offer an opportunity to examine programming and genetic control of development. An organism such as a digenetic fluke may have three obligate hosts in its life cycle and five or more recognizable stages. Each of these stages requires control of development and each has a particular niche in the environment. Some stages pass through the external environment for development or exist as free-swimming stages; others have an intimate association with two hosts, and sometimes three. In the Digenea, as well as other parasites, the life cycle is truly a cycle, it runs only one direction and we do not have the means of causing it to return to an early stage.

In a seminal theoretical paper, Fairbairn (1970) considered the issue of whether those parasites that are so exquisitely dependent on a host that they have lost the capacity to live elsewhere have also lost genetic capacity. He concluded that, in general, parasites have retained the genome to survive and develop in other niches but do not use it. His examples come principally from helminths, which have complex life cycles, and show that they have the capacity for development and survival in a wide spectrum of niches as they pass from one stage of the life cycle to the next. Hence, different areas of the genome are in all likelihood employed at different life stages, which often exist in different niches.

Further evidence can be drawn from *Plasmodium*, the cause of malaria. This organism is generally said to be an obligate intracellular organism, but it has maintained the capacity to develop extracellularly in the oocyst stage (Fig. 1.16) in the mosquito. Thus, we see that parasites are not degenerate genetically, but rather they maintain a genome of which only a portion is used at any specific stage of the life cycle.

Nearly all parasites must contend with the external environment at some stage of their life cycles. Many nematodes with direct life cycles feed, grow, and develop as free-living organisms before entering a host to become sexually mature. The free-living stages have certain requirements and certain limitations that limit their geographic distribution. Studies of the limits and optima for development and survival of a particular

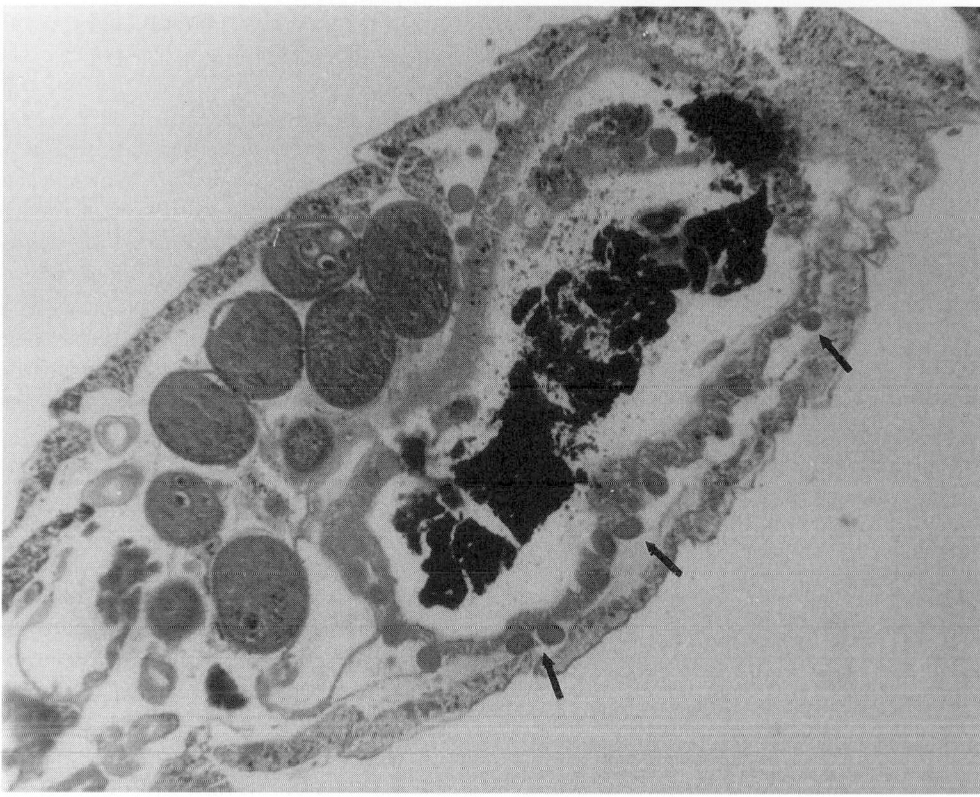

FIGURE 1.16 Oocyst of *Plasmodium* sp. on the midgut of a mosquito, a histologic section cutting across the whole abdomen of the insect. The black material represents a partially digested blood meal in the lumen of the midgut. The oocysts (arrows) are seen as small spheres on the hemocoel side of the gut. The gray spheres at the left of the midgut are cross-sections of ovary.

parasite represent the kind of basic biological data required for structuring a control program.

When a parasite enters a host it reaches the stage of physiological dependence, which defines the unique nature of parasitism. The pattern of development for eukaryotic (and some prokaryotic) parasites is to proceed with development in a particular environment (host or external) and then stop and wait. When the proper host is contacted, development then proceeds. We speak of the organism being "triggered" by the environment in the host, and usually specific signals of temperature of 37°C or higher, pH, redox potential, and organic chemicals are sensed by the parasite. It is thereby stimulated to proceed to the next stage of the life cycle. In many cases, we know what the stimuli are for triggering, but the exact mechanisms are not known in most cases. It is likely that the triggers turn on a set of genes that were previously unexpressed.

How a parasite depends on the host is often unknown. The host provides a physical space, food, and a place to reproduce, but that is no different from the free-living environment. In homeothermic hosts, parasites usually have adapted to 37°C or higher and do not do well at lower temperatures. Nutrient requirements have been described for both free-living and parasitic nematodes, but they are little different from one another. Some parasites feed on blood, but it is not a perfect food, and usually some metabolic acrobatics or symbiotic bacteria are required to make up for blood's nutritional deficits. In cell-free studies on *Plasmodium* in culture, it was found that ATP was indispensable, so it appears that this organism depends on the host for high energy phosphate.

In those helminths that lack a digestive tract, we can see that the host–parasite interface is complex. Studies in culture indicate that tapeworms require contact with a surface in order to grow and develop. Parasites such as digenetic flukes, tapeworms, and acanthocephalans obtain their food across the surface tegument. Energy is required, and it is a selective process. There are also tantalizing data indicating that the amino acid constituency in the intestine of the host may determine whether a species of tapeworm can live in a particular species of host.

Parasites are often profligate with nutrients, especially energy sources. Nematodes such as *Ascaris* undergo aerobic glycolysis and discard Krebs cycle intermediates without utilizing their full energy potential, and they employ the same pathway in aerobic or anaerobic conditions. Trypanosomes utilize only a small portion of the energy contained in blood glucose.

HOW DO THE HOST AND PARASITE RESPOND TO ONE ANOTHER?

When two organisms live in intimate association, each responds to the presence and activities of the other. This is especially true of the host–parasite relationship. First, we discuss how vertebrate hosts respond to parasites and then how parasites respond to hosts.

Vertebrates respond to the presence of nonself material (i.e., parasite) in two ways. First, there are nonspecific responses. The host is able to differentiate "self" from "nonself," but these responses are not dependent on specific recognition of a nonself molecule. Most invertebrates respond in this way, and it is a first line of defense in vertebrates. The second type of response is a specific recognition of foreign or nonself molecules.

Nonspecific Responses

A first line of defense against small foreign invaders, be they bacteria or parasitic protists, is *endocytosis*, the process of ingesting particulate bodies. Endocytosis is also referred to as *phagocytosis* when particulates are ingested or *pinocytosis* when liquid is ingested, but it is often not possible to differentiate between the two, and endocytosis is the preferred term. Several cell types are endocytotic including monocytes, polymorphonuclear leucocytes (PMNs), histiocytes in tissues, and sinus-lining reticuloendothelial cells in the liver and spleen.

The function of endocytosis is to engulf foreign material and digest it through lysosomal action. Lysosomes are organelles in phagocytic cells that release enzymes, have a low pH, and cause the breakdown of the foreign cell. Endocytosis can occur independently of specific responses, but it is greatly facilitated by certain specific responses such as *opsonizing antibodies* and indirectly by serum proteins called *complement.*

If the foreign invader is small, it may be surrounded by endocytotic cells and immobilized by the deposition of collagen around it. If the invader is large, a second type of nonspecific reaction takes place—*inflammation.* Inflammation is characterized by reddness, heat, swelling, and pain.

Acute inflammation, the first phase, lasts for about three days and is characterized by capillary dilatation leading to fluid accumulation or *edema* and an accumulation of PMN's in the tissues at the site of the insult. The second phase, *subacute inflammation,* lasts from three days to more than a week and is characterized by the presence of mononuculear cells (monocytes and lymphocytes) in the perivascular spaces and by fibrocytes, which secrete collagen. Collagen secretion leads to the production of a fibrous capsule commonly known as a *scar.*

The third phase is *chronic inflammation,* in which the tissue involved has not only the monocytic cells of the second phase but also plasma cells come into the area. Where there is a persistent object such as a schistosome egg or an ascarid larva, a granuloma forms (Fig. 1.17) This is an aggregation of mononuclear cells surrounded by fibrous connective tissue and the cells that secrete it. In many instances, these granulomas that form in response to a parasite also contain eosinophils, a subset of PMNs.

Another nonspecific response to parasites is *abnormal growth responses.* These include *hyperplasia,* in which

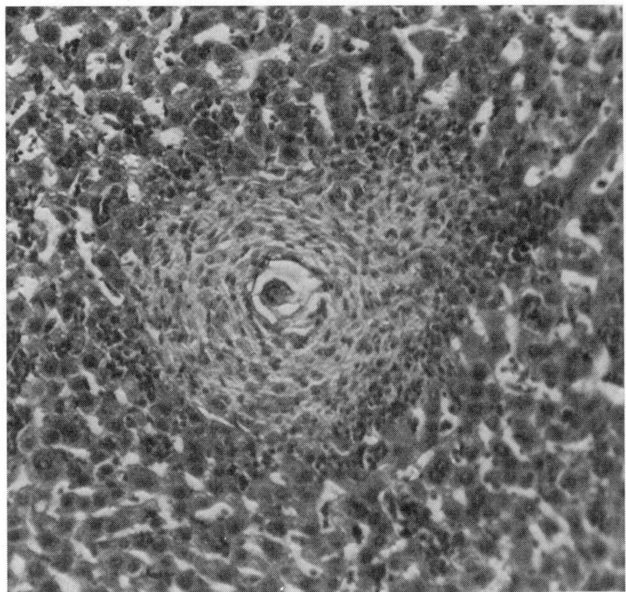

FIGURE 1.17 A photomicrograph of a granuloma, or foreign-body reaction, formed in response to the presence of the egg of *Schistosoma mansoni* in the liver of its vertebrate host. The remains of the egg lie in the center of clear area. Surrounding the egg are many layers of connective tissue cells indicating a long-standing inflammatory process. Some white blood cells lie at the periphery of the connective tissue.

the parasite stimulates the host to produce an increased number of cells. For example, when the adult liver fluke, *Fasciola hepatica,* reaches a bile duct, it induces the enlargement of the epithelium of the bile ducts. The fluke then grazes on these cells. The liver coccidium, *Eimeria stiedai,* of the domestic rabbit causes an exuberant growth of the bile duct epithelium, which appears microscopically to be much like neoplasia. However, much of the growth of the epithelium is resorbed when the infection is terminated. *Dirofilaria immitis,* the cause of heartworm disease in dogs, produces a soluble substance that causes endothelial proliferation in the lining of blood vessels.

Neoplasia (loosely, cancer) is also an abnormal growth response and there are a number of examples in which parasites are associated with this response. The larva of the tapeworm *Taenia taeniaformis* develops in the liver of the rat and causes sarcomas of the liver. *Spirocerca lupi* is a nematode located most often in the esophageal region of its definitive host, the dog. It gives rise to sarcomas of the esophagus upon long-standing infection. There is also a correlation between the presence of *Schistosoma mansoni* in the large intestine and the occurrence of colonic carcinoma. Even though these associations are clear, the mechanisms associated with the induction of neoplasia are yet to be elucidated.

Specific Responses

The surfaces of parasites have characteristic macromolecules such as proteins and polysaccharides, which the host recognizes as nonself. In other instances, parasites excrete or secrete characteristic large proteinaceous molecules. These substances are referred to as *antigens* (Ag), because they elicit either a specific immune response through the formation of protein *antibodies* (Ab) or the expansion of specific T-lymphocyte populations through Ag-specific T-cell receptor interactions. Antibodies or immunoglobulins (Ig) are secreted by B-lymphocytes (plasma cells) and they attach to specific sites on the antigen by molecular recognition. This attachment usually triggers additional host responses. There are five classes or isotypes of Ig—IgA, IgD, IgE, IgG, and IgM—all of which have different polypeptide structures and specialized functions.

The basic Ig molecule has a Y-shaped structure (Fig. 1.18) with antigen-binding sites at the ends of the arms of the Y. Production and secretion of Igs is called the *humoral response,* and it is manifested in a number of different ways.

Each of the Ig molecules listed here has particular functions. IgE responses are often elevated in helminth infections. IgE Abs bind to mast cells and basophils; the subsequent binding of Ag to cell-bound IgE induces the cells to release vasoactive substances, such as histamines, which increase capillary permeability. In addition to being commonly associated with helminth infections, IgE is most associated with hypersensitivity or allergy.

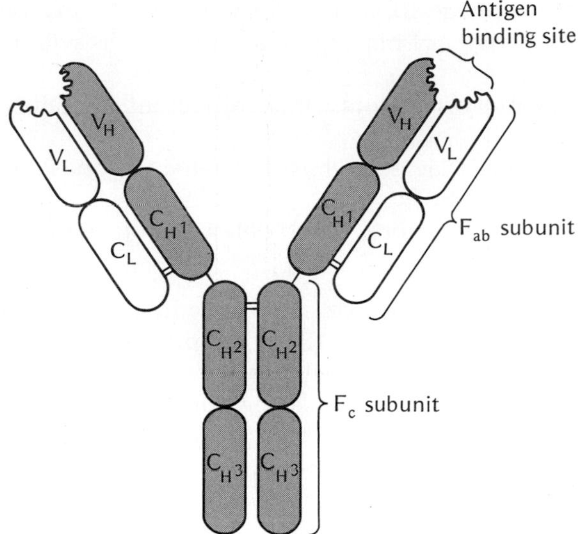

FIGURE 1.18 The structure of immunoglobulin G (IgG).

IgM and IgG are often considered to be most important in protistan infections, because they activate the complement system. This system consists of nine protein complexes that combine with many different Ag-IgM or Ag-IgG complexes. The first component of the complement system binds to Ag-bound IgM or IgG thereby initiating a cascade of reactions involving the components of the complement system. This series of reactions triggers a number of biological activities; one of the most important in parasitic infections is the damage to cell membranes leading to lysis of the cell.

In addition to the humoral response, the immune system also expresses *cell mediated immunity* (CMI), which classically involves the T-lymphocytes. When bound to Ags, T-lymphocytes release proteinaceous substances called *cytokines,* which, in turn, induce nonspecific reactions on other cells often leading to inflammation or to the release of other cytokines. Cytokines may also directly damage parasites.

Cytokines that are most relevant to parasitic infections include those with the following effects:

1. Migratory-inhibitory factors, which prevent the migration of white blood cells (wbcs)

2. Macrophage stimulating factors, which enhance the activity of macrophages against cells with the target Ag
3. Chemotactic factors, which attract inflammatory cells
4. Mitogenic factors, which stimulate the division of lymphocytes
5. Cytostatic factors, which delay or stop cell proliferation

Both B-cells and T-cells originate from stem cells in the bone marrow (Fig. 1.19). The processing of these cells in the thymus (T-cells) or in an organ equivalent, the bursa of birds (B-cells) determines which of the two immune responses will predominate. Although humoral and cell-mediated immunity are spoken of as two systems, they are intertwined and neither is ever the sole response. In addition, nonspecific resistance factors such as inflammation are often critical in both disease and immunity.

In general terms, macrophages (endocytotic cells) ingest and process parasite antigens. These processed Ags are then distributed on the surface of the macrophage and are said to be "presented." Both B- and T-cells contact the surface of the macrophage or the parasite directly and are primed against the specific Ag presented. Both types of lymphocytes are stimulated to divide and then to produce either Abs or cytokines. Ag combines with IgE bound to mast cells and basophils causing these cells to release pharmacologically active molecules such as histamine. The subsequent increase in capillary permeability allows lymphocytes and other white cells to reach the parasite. T-cells combine with parasite Ags and release cytokines, which may attract more endocytotic cells and keep them there to release their cytotoxic products. The final result is tissue injury by the cytotoxic products and nonspecific inflammation, which changes the parasite's immediate environment, often to its disadvantage.

Countermeasures by Parasites to Host Immunity

The immune responses to invasion by eukaryotic parasites is countered in a number of ways. Ingenious

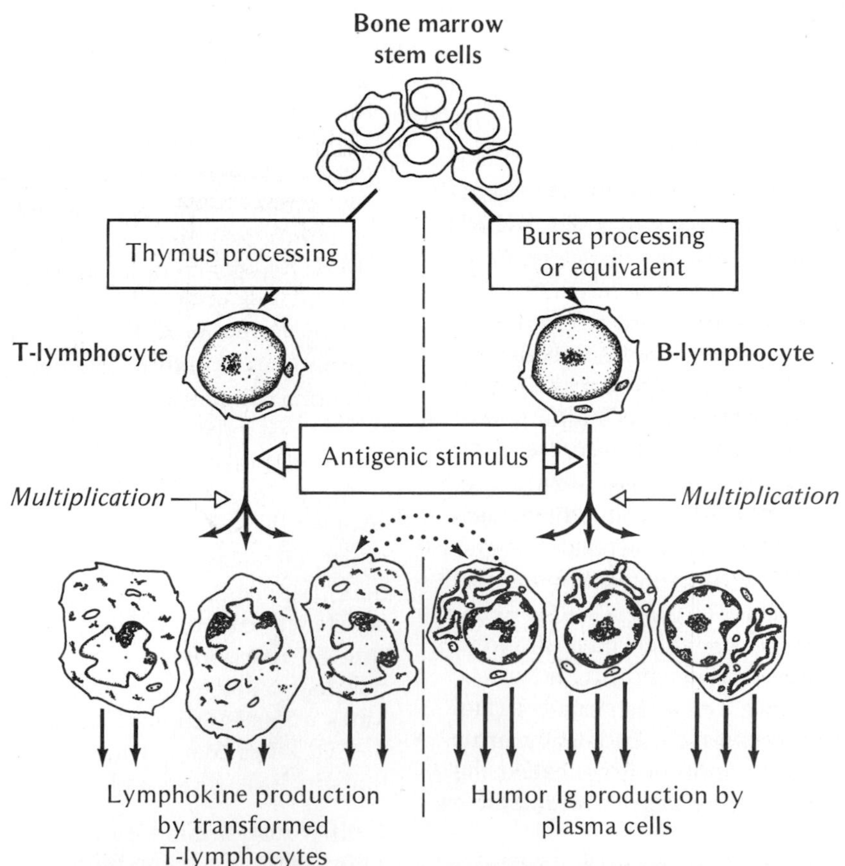

FIGURE 1.19 The origin, processing, and activities of T- and B-lymphocytes.

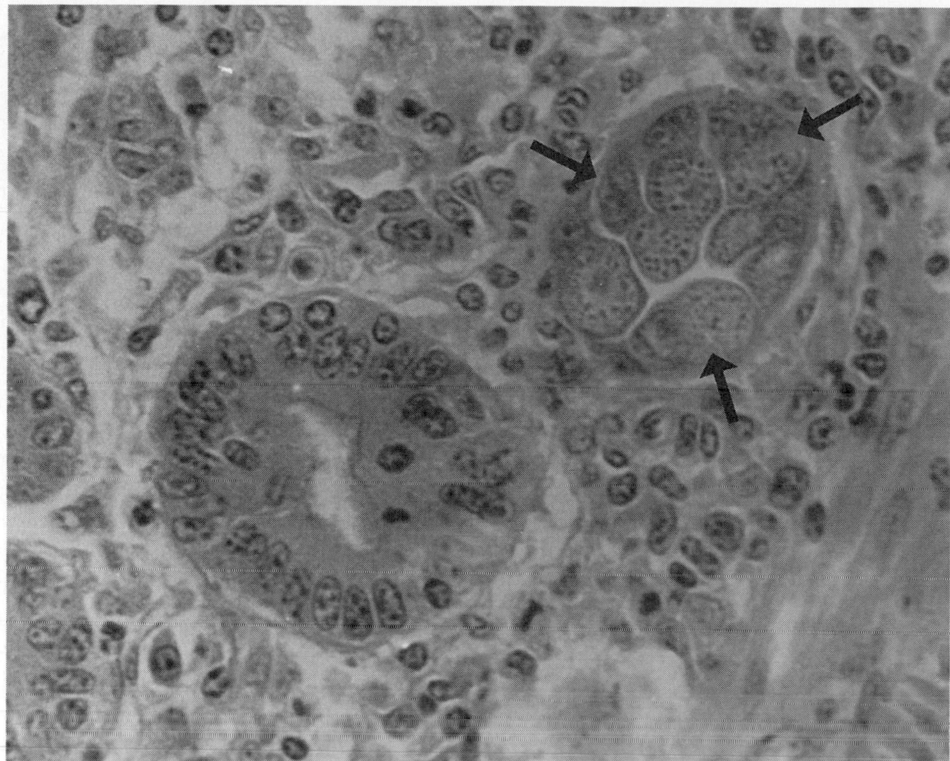

FIGURE 1.20 A photomicrograph of a histologic section of the colon of an ox showing intestinal cells infected with *Eimeria bovis*, a pathogenic coccidium of cattle. At the left is an uninfected gland or crypt of Lieberkühn. At the right is an infected crypt with macrogamonts (arrows) of the coccidium; the macrogamonts will become oocysts, which are then passed with the feces.

methods have evolved in order to escape the immune response. *Trypanosoma brucei,* the cause of African sleeping sickness, undergoes a continual change in its surface glycoproteins, called antigenic variation, so that the immune response must continually adjust in attempting to eliminate the trypomastigotes from the bloodstream. The immune system never catches up and trypansomes continue to produce new antigens.

Plasmodium spp., the cause of malaria, also changes its surface antigens, but *Plasmodium* has another tactic, namely being poorly antigenic. Malaria may continue for several months in a person before the immune response is sufficiently strong to reduce the numbers of the parasites. Then, within several months, the immunity wanes and the person is again susceptible to clinical disease.

Many protists, and some helminths, live within cells where they can escape the immune response. *Toxoplasma gondii, Leishmania* spp., *Trypanosoma cruzi, Eimeria* spp. (Fig. 1.20), and *Trichinella spiralis* are all examples of organisms that develop or multiply within cells.

The blood fluke of humans, *Schistosoma* spp., adsorbs host-produced molecules onto its surface so that the host fails to recognize the worm as nonself. The blood flukes can remain alive in the blood vessels of the human host for more than 10 years at least in part by utilizing this mechanism.

Many eukaryotic parasites reduce the immune response of the host. *Leishmania,* for example, modulates the production of certain T-cells so that the immune response is effectively depressed. Persons affected with malaria also have depressed immune systems, but the mechanisms are appear to be complex and are incompletely described. Arthropods that feed for a long time, such as ticks, also suppress the immune response, at least at the site where the tick feeds.

All of these escape mechanisms have made the production of vaccines against eukaryotic parasites extremely difficult. Immunologists have sought means of circumventing the parasites' evasive tactics and are beginning to succeed. Experimental or commercial vaccines are available for lungworms of cattle, haemonchosis of sheep, toxoplasmosis in cats, malaria in humans, and ticks on cattle as examples. As time passes, these vaccines will be improved and others developed for a wide range of parasites.

MAGIC BULLETS

THE GERMAN SCIENTIST Paul Ehrlich (1854–1915) had a unique background because he was a physician, chemist, and hematologist. He developed histologic stains for blood and other tissues that are still in use, and he made significant advances in theoretical aspects of chemotherapy that were remarkable for the time.

Arsenical compounds had been used to treat nagana in cattle, and Ehrlich's associate, Robert Koch, had treated several hundred Africans for sleeping sickness with an inorganic arsenical. The treatment was at best only partially successful, and worse, it had toxic side effects that were catastrophic for some patients.

Ehrlich felt that the toxicity of arsenic could be reduced by attaching it to an organic molecule, and he began testing organic arsenicals against *Treponema pallidum,* the cause of syphilis in humans. A treatment for syphilis was sorely needed; however, it was not, in Victorian times, a subject that was discussed in polite society. But Ehrlich was not only a determined man, but also a brilliant one.

The 606th arsenical that he and his coworkers tested was Salvarsan and it was effective in treating syphilis. He finally had what he had been searching for, a "magic bullet." Salvarsan was given by injection, and while it cured some people, most were rendered noninfectious. It was clearly an advance for use against a difficult disease such as syphilis, but because of its toxicity patients who received it probably felt that the "magic" part of the bullet was overstated. But it was almost the sole drug available for treating syphilis for more than 30 years.

With the development of penicillin in the early 1940s, the treatment of syphilis advanced tremendously. Penicillin was both effective against *Treponema pallidum* and nontoxic for the patient. But still, there were individuals who became allergic to penicillin and could not tolerate even a tiny amount of the drug.

Thus we have two compounds that are effective against syphilis, but each has its shortcomings. The pattern is seen again and again in chemotherapy for all kinds of infectious agents and for diseases such as cancer.

The objective in finding, say, an anthelmintic is that it have high toxicity against the parasitic helminth, but little or none for the mammalian host. Early anthelmintics used in livestock were copper sulfate and carbon tetrachloride. Both are toxic, and the latter is a liver poison. Phenothiazine, used in the 1930s to 1950s, was relatively nontoxic, but some animals suffered from skin problems when exposed to the sun after treatment. Organophosphate compounds walk a fine line between efficacy and toxicity, especially to the nervous system; acetylcholine accumulates at the synaptic junctions in treated animals, and they may suffer seizures and even die from the treatment. A number of anthelmintics now in use in domestic and companion animals are both nontoxic and efficacious, but vomiting and depression are not uncommon. Some leave residues in meat that require long holding periods before slaughter.

In human medicine, drugs have been developed for parasitic infections, and many are highly effective. But nearly all have side effects of greater or lesser severity. Some upset the digestive tract, and one or two cause nervous system abnormalities including psychotic episodes. Quinine, used for 300 years to treat and prevent malaria, causes deafness upon long intake. Aureomycin permanently discolors the teeth of children. Tartar emetic causes vomiting. Niridazole causes psychological changes that may last for weeks. Certain antibiotics destroy the intestinal flora. The list goes on and on.

Do we ever get something for nothing? Probably not. Even aspirin, which is a billion-dollar industry in itself, can sometimes have adverse effects. Alcohol, social drugs, over-the-counter drugs, prescription drugs, legal drugs, and illegal drugs all have their side effects that may be short term but also may be long term. There are bullets that come close to the center of the target, but there is no magic bullet. We must all look at the benefits and risks and make a judgment on what to take and what to avoid.

HOW ARE PARASITIC DISEASES CONTROLLED?

The ultimate goal of this book is to describe how parasitic diseases may be controlled. The general actions at our disposal are to:

1. Administer or apply toxicants
2. Reduce populations of reservoir hosts
3. Reduce populations of vectors
4. Induce immunity either naturally or artificially to a pathogen or vector
5. Modify the environment through a physical change in it
6. Avoid areas or activities of high risk; that is, change behavior
7. Protect the individual or group by a barrier, either a quarantine or a physical barrier
8. Alter the genome of the vector or of the vertebrate host
9. Separate age classes of potential hosts
10. Test for the presence of the disease agent and remove the infected hosts.

Toxicants

This broad category includes drugs to prevent or cure diseases, insecticides used to reduce populations of vectors, and inorganic substances that are toxic to either reservoir hosts or parasites. Basically these chemicals interfere with the normal physiology of the target organism. The ultimate effect is at the cellular level and may interfere with such processes as nucleic acid synthesis, membrane structure, neuromuscular transmission, or mitochondrial function.

In Western medicine, quinine was probably the first chemical used to treat a specific transmissible disease, malaria. During the past 60 years or so, a whole new armamentarium has been developed to treat and prevent transmissible diseases: sulfonamide drugs, antibiotics, antimalarials, anthelmintics, and antiviral agents, among others.

The chemical/pharmaceutical industry has made enormous strides not only in developing new drugs and insecticides but also in designing molecules to have specific physiological effects.

Reduce Populations of Reservoir Hosts or of Vectors

Many disease agents often cycle silently in populations of wild animals and move over to the human population or domestic animals under special circumstances. The system can often be manipulated so that the risk to human or animal health is held at an acceptable level by reducing the probability of contact with the reservoir host(s) or the vector(s).

Immunity

Immunity generally develops when a host is naturally exposed to a parasite. In many instances, the host becomes ill, but if it survives, it is usually immune for a period of time, sometimes for life. Of course, immunity is not always manifested as a sterile or complete immunity but rather as an immune response that controls the infection at a level below the threshold of disease. Artificial immunity is induced through vaccination. A living agent or part of an agent is injected into a host and elicits immunity so that the host does not become ill upon challenge.

Immunity can be used to protect individuals against an infectious agent, but it is often used to protect a population. At a certain level of immunity in a population, transmission is broken; an insufficient number of susceptibles prevents continued transmission. Populations are generally protected against a directly transmitted agent when at least 80% of the potential hosts have been immunized against the specific agent; however, with some vector-borne diseases, such as malaria, more than 99% of the population must have protective immunity in order to prevent transmission.

Environmental Modification or Management

A physical change can be made in the environment so that the survival of the parasite or its vector is unlikely. Eliminating domestic garbage reduces populations of houseflies. In the case of mosquitoes, various environmental modifications, such as draining areas that hold water, can reduce the habitat of the larvae.

In working with vectors, we also speak of *source reduction,* which is some kind of physical change in the environment that makes it unsuitable for the survival or multiplicaton of the vector.

Avoid Areas or Activities of High Risk

The method involves changing behavior so that the probability of coming into contact with the disease agent or vector is reduced. River blindness is a disease caused by a nematode that is transmitted by black flies. The black fly larvae live in well-oxygenated streams and as adults migrate out from them to spread the infection. When the risk becomes too great, people living near streams leave the area. In protecting live-

DRUGS, VACCINES, AND ANTIBIOTICS

A NUMBER OF KINDS OF products are given to humans and other animals for preventing and treating parasitic and microbial infections. It must be kept in mind that each kind of product is different in its mode of action and in the way in which it is manufactured. People often go to the doctor with an ailment and want a "shot" to alleviate whatever ails them. "Shots" may be any one of a number of things.

The following is a primer on the kinds of products that can be given by mouth, injected, or spread on the skin. It excludes those products that are used against vectors of disease agents such as mosquitoes and ticks; those are insecticides and acaricides, for the most part.

Drugs

These are natural or manufactured molecules that affect physiologic or metabolic processes in the body. Aspirin is a drug because it reduces inflammation through inhibition of production of a prostaglandin. Corticosteroids such as prednisone reduce the inflammatory process and thereby reduce the effectiveness of the immune system in mammals. Taxol is a compound isolated from the yew tree in the Pacific Northwest of the United States; it is used against some kinds of ovarian cancer. Oxmaniquine is a manufactured molecule that is effective against the blood flukes. Quinine was first obtained from the *Cinchona* tree for use against malaria. By the mid-20th century, atabrine, chloroquine, and other quinoline compounds had been synthesized using the quinine molecule as a model for making variations of it.

Antibiotics

Antibiotics are produced by living microorganisms; the substances are excreted by an organism into the medium in which it grows. The first antibiotic was penicillin, which is produced from the fungus *Penicillium notatum*. Ivermectin is an antibiotic, a molecule produced by the bacterium *Streptomyces avermitilis*. It acts by suppressing the action of a neurotransmitter, GABA (gamma amino butyric acid). An earlier antibiotic produced by members of the genus *Streptomyces* is streptomycin.

Vaccines

Vaccines stimulate the immune system of a human or animal to ward off an infectious agent when it enters the body. They can be made from living organisms, killed organisms, or specific molecular components of organisms.

These so-called antigens are protein, glycoprotein, or lipoprotein molecules that induce an immune response in a vertebrate, usually a mammal. Under natural conditions, a microorganism or a eukaryotic parasite bears proteins that stimulate the immune system to produce antibodies that act against the invader and immobilize or kill it.

Vaccines are derived from living infectious agents or, nowadays, produced by recombinant DNA methods in living cells such as bacteria or yeasts. Proteins are harvested, purified, or modified in some way and injected into the body of a potential host to stimulate the immune system to protect the individual from a specific invader. Recombinant DNA methods allow the mass production of single proteins that can be used as vaccines; these are monoclonal antibodies, or MABs.

The most effective vaccines are those that are living. The first vaccine ever developed was by Edward Jenner in 1792 for protection against smallpox. He infected a boy with material from a scab from a cowpox infection, and the boy was protected when exposed to smallpox virus. The first poliomyelitis vaccine was a killed poliovirus preparation; it worked well enough but required multiple inoculations to maintain a protective level of antibody. The Sabin vaccine came a few years later and it was a living, attenuated (nonvirulent) virus that multiplied in the intestinal tract and produced a high level of long-lasting immunity.

In parasitology, the first effective vaccine was a so-called attenuated larval vaccine against the lungworm *Dictyocaulus viviparus* (Chapter 31). The worms are injected into an ox and develop for a period of time, but they die about the time that immunity has developed.

A living vaccine has been produced against infection with *Toxoplasma gondii* in cats (Chapter 13). The vaccine has been attenuated by selecting a genetic mutant that grows for a period of time in the cat, but does not maintain an infection for a long period, nor does the cat show oocysts in the feces. On challenge, the cat fails to show oocysts in the feces. Human infections from contaminated cat feces are thereby prevented.

Blood Products

Portions of blood are used in preventing and treating some infectious diseases. Red blood cells (rbcs) are transfused into persons who are anemic. This anemia may develop by reason of surgery, nutritional anemia, or an infection such as malaria, which destroys rbcs.

The protein portion of the blood such as the gamma globulin fraction is often injected into persons who travel to areas of the world where viral hepatitis is prevalent. Gamma globulin is only a temporary protectant against hepatitis and must be renewed about every six months. It is not a drug, it is not a vaccine; instead it provides temporary, nonspecific protection against a viral disease.

Plasma is the protein and inorganic portion of the blood, and it is given to persons whose blood volume is low by reason, usually, of a serious physical trauma.

stock against liver flukes, contaminated pastures can be avoided at certain times of the year.

Quarantine and Barriers

The term *quarantine* is derived from the Italian word for *forty*. Quarantine was practiced as early as 1374 in Venice in an effort to prevent the introduction of plague. Persons disembarking from ships were held in designated areas for 40 days before they could mix with the citizens of Venice. At present, modified quarantine is used in cases of persons who have especially virulent infections that may be readily transmitted to others.

In control of African trypanosomosis in cattle, barriers are established to prevent the migration of the vectors, tsetse. Since tsetse migrate slowly and do not pass large open areas, brush and trees are cleared from an area 2 km (1 mile) in width, and one can be confident that the flies will not traverse the barrier.

Another disease of livestock, Texas cattle fever, caused by the protistan *Babesia bigemina*, was controlled in the United States by a quarantine program. Animals raised in an enzootic area could not be shipped from it until they were treated for the tick vector and declared to be tick-free.

Another barrier is the use of bed nets to prevent blood-sucking flies such as mosquitoes from reaching people as they sleep. If they are properly and diligently used, bed nets are an effective means of preventing mosquito-borne diseases such as malaria.

A novel barrier is the use of so-called *zooprophylaxis*. In instances where mosquitoes prefer to feed on livestock rather than people, keeping cattle near a house reduces the probability of the mosquitoes feeding on people. There are instances on record in which the introduction of tractors as a replacement for draft animals allowed the increase in vector-borne diseases of humans. Since the preferred hosts, domestic animals, were not present, the vectors fed on humans, a less desirable but acceptable host.

Biological Control

Biological control is defined as the use of parasites and predators to control vectors of disease agents. In nature, a whole array of biological entities regulate populations of organisms of all kinds. Biocontrol merely attempts to bring back these modulating factors when they get out of balance in the first place through human intervention.

Control of mosquitoes can be accomplished by introducing predators such as *Toxorhynchites*, a predaceous mosquito larva, or *Gambusia*, a fish that feeds on mosquito larvae. Certain species of Microspora have been used to control various insects, with mixed success. Mixed results have been obtained using nematodes to control arthropods or fungi to control nematodes.

Genetic Alteration of a Host

A genetic change may be induced in either the vertebrate host or the vector. Looking broadly at all kinds of transmissible diseases, there have been successful genetic changes induced in both vertebrates and invertebrates both naturally and artificially. Humans who are negative for the Duffy blood group are resistant to vivax malaria. Mosquitoes have become resistant to insecticides. The malaria parasite has become resistant to antimalarial drugs such as chloroquine, and various nematodes have become resistant to certain anthelmintics.

In the context of bringing about changes in vectors to control vector-borne diseases, only modest success has been achieved. The great success in genetic control is the sterile male technique as it applies to screwworms (*Cochliomyia hominovorax*) in the Western Hemisphere. A vaccine to prevent *Toxoplasma*-induced abortion in sheep uses a mutant of the organism, which provides the immunity associated with infection without the invasive properties of the wild-type organism.

Separate Age Classes

Although we use this method implicitly in some cases of human infectious diseases, it applies most often in diseases of livestock. Since all of us, humans and animals alike, live in a cloud of infectious agents, one means of lessening their detrimental effects is to reduce exposure in young animals until they can benefit from exposure-related immunity. Young animals are usually susceptible to nearly all parasites, and may succumb if they are exposed to many agents at one time. On the other hand, if their exposure can be limited both in the numbers and kinds of infectious organisms, they have the opportunity of developing immunity. Thus, newborn animals are kept separate from those that are, say, three months of age or older.

Test and Remove

This method is used solely with livestock. One determines whether an individual animal is infected or ill with a specific disease; if positive, the animal is removed from the herd and disposed of. Tuberculosis in dairy cattle was controlled in North America and western Europe by a test and slaughter program. On occasion, hoof and mouth disease has been introduced into North America and the control method used is to destroy all of the animals that have been exposed, whether they show signs or not. Prior to the development of second-generation insecticides such as DDT, scabies was controlled in sheep solely by a test and slaughter program. Many financial and political issues must be addressed if this method is to be employed.

HOW ARE HOST–PARASITE RELATIONSHIPS INVESTIGATED?

By the very nature of the discipline, parasitologists must be among the most broadly trained of all investigators in the biological sciences. Virtually every aspect of biology from the molecular to the ecosystem are exploited in parasitology. A successful generalist in parasitology must have a wide knowledge of both vertebrate and invertebrate biology as well as other transmissible agents, immunology, and cellular and molecular biology. Parasites exist and thrive in a particular set of climatic, topographic, and biotic factors all of which impinge on the way the system works and how it can be controlled. This is what makes the field so interesting and challenging.

As is true for all sciences, parasitology began with descriptions of various protists, worms, and arthropods. Histologic and cytologic techniques were developed so that basic structures could be described and evolutionary relationships established. These areas continue to be relevant with investigators using long-established methods as well as newer techniques such as electron microscopy, cladistic analyses (see Box), and molecular techniques that employ genes that code for ribosomal RNA and tubulins, for example. The relationship of the Myxozoa to the Cnidaria is discussed in Chapter 16, and their relationship was shown through a computer-generated tree (Fig. 1.21). The distance laterally (not vertically) shows relative closeness of various genera and these analyses have been instrumental in confirming previously established classifications or showing that earlier constructions were based on insufficient evidence.

In the late 19th century, life cycles began to be investigated with increasing frequency. In 1878 Patrick Manson showed that *Wuchereria bancrofti* is transmitted by mosquitoes; this was a landmark in our knowledge of what became known as vector-borne diseases. In 1881

CLADISTICS

Development of powerful computers and technology in molecular biology have allowed studies showing evolutionary relationships that were previously unforeseen. Until recently, there was no way to approach evolution except by comparing morphologies at a gross level and using some techniques now considered rather elementary. One breakthrough was the discovery of isozymes—enzymes that have the same function, but different molecular structures. That cracked the door so that we could begin to see what was inside. Since the mid-1980s molecular techniques have allowed gene sequencing. In the early 1990s, personal computers gained power undreamt of just a few years earlier.

Phylogenetic systematics, or cladistics, bloomed with computer and molecular power to support researchers. A clade is a group of species related by direct descent. Cladistics attempts to distinguish between apomorphic characters (advanced or derived) and plesiomorphic (primitive) characters.

Relationships can be determined by compiling unique or advanced characters (autapomorphies) which are key features in distinguishing that group. For example, the radula of members of the Mollusca does not appear in any other major taxon. Shared, advanced characters (synapomorphies) are important in linking taxa. For example, certain larvae in the phylum Platyhelminthes have cercomers (hooks) which define a major taxon, the Cercomeromorphae.

In order to complete an analysis, advanced and primitive features of the taxa in question are compared with that of a closely related "out group." The computer program then creates a best-fit cladogram or branching diagram. A recent study compared Cnidaria and Myxozoa and showed that these seemingly disparate groups are related (Fig. 1.21).

KOCH'S POSTULATES

Koch's postulates were formulated by Robert Koch (1843–1910), the great German microbiologist. The postulates, which rather should be "Koch's Dictum," were elucidated to ensure that the proper infectious agent was associated with a particular disease entity. They are as follows:

1. The infectious organism must be isolated in pure culture from a host having the disease.
2. The cultivated organism must be transmitted back to a susceptible host and cause the original disease.
3. The organism must again be isolated in pure culture and properly identified.

The postulates were set forth at a time when there was immense activity in bacteriology. Organisms were continually being found and identified as causing a large number of diseases in both humans and domesticated animals. Vaccination was in its infancy, but growing rapidly. Attempts were being made to develop treatments for infectious diseases. With a few exceptions, such as rabies, nearly all of these diseases were caused by bacteria. Assuming that the bacterial species in question can be readily cultivated, fulfilling Koch's postulates is fairly straightforward.

But other organisms such as viruses, protists, and helminths often could not at that time be made to conform to the neat system set forth by Koch. Viruses could not yet be cultivated nor, in fact, isolated. Some protists could be cultivated, but not cloned in the sense of a bacterial colony. Helminths could not be cultivated at all.

Because all pathogens could not be fit into Koch's postulates, it was a slow process to associate certain organisms with a disease. Even today, when a new disease is recognized such as HIV infection (AIDS), it is a long process until there is agreement on the nature of the causative agent.

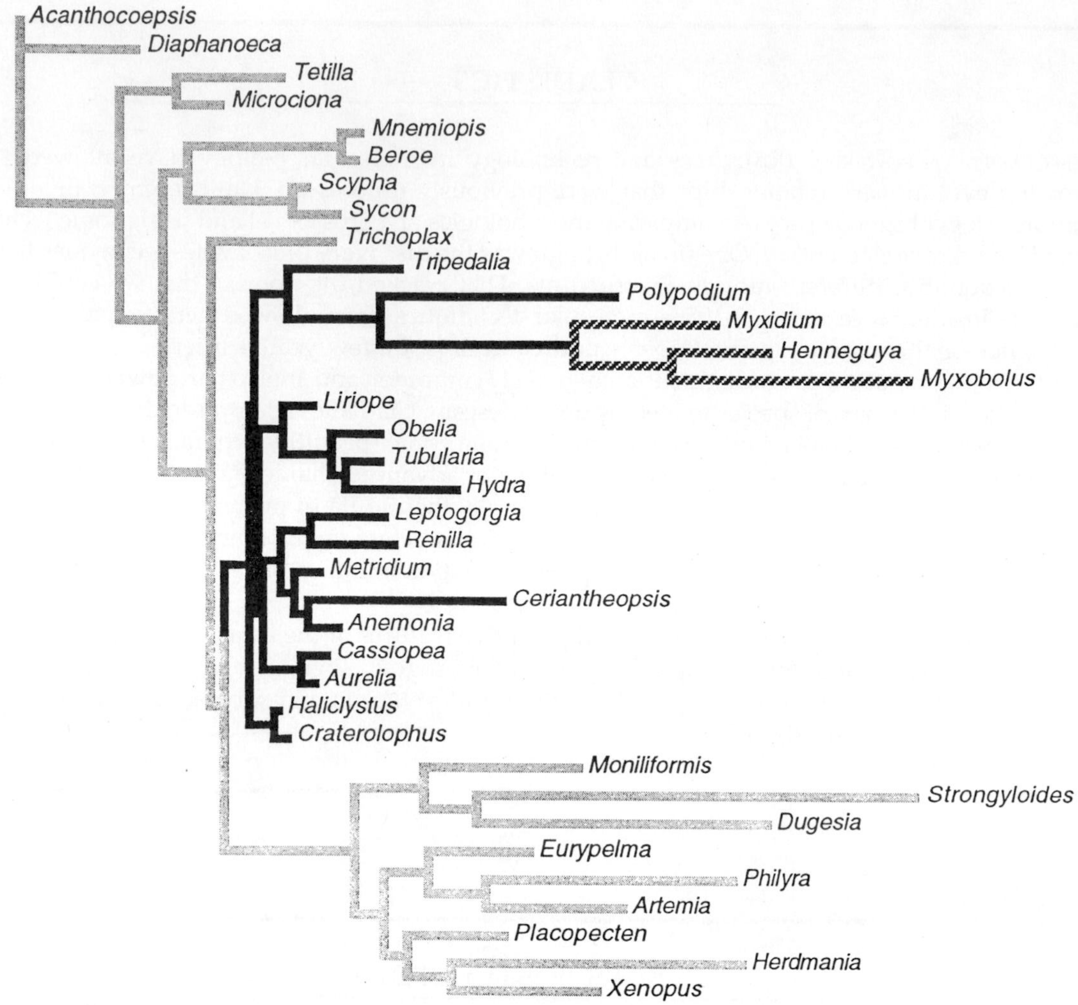

FIGURE 1.21 A phylogenetic tree based on molecular characteristics of various animals. In interpreting the cladogram, it is important to recognize that vertical distances are not important; it is the lateral distances that indicate relationships. In this study it was shown that members of the phylum Cnidaria (black lines) are closely related to the members of the phylum Myxozoa (diagonally hatched lines).The characteristics of three myxozoans, *Myxidium, Henneguy,a* and *Myxobolus* all lie close together and they are close to those of two cnidarians, *Myxidium* and *Polypodium* (further discussed in Chapter 16). [From Siddall, M. E., et al., 1995.]

Rudolph Leuckart in Germany and A. P. W. Thomas in Britain independently worked out the life cycle of *Fasciola hepatica,* the common liver fluke of sheep and cattle. The life cycle of *Schistosoma* spp. was made known in 1912. Certain parasites have been refractory to investigations on transmission. For example, *Sarcocystis* was first described in the somatic muscles of mammals in 1865, but a full century was required before Dr. Ronald Fayer associated sarcocysts with isosporoid oocysts in material grown in cell culture. The life cycles of parasites have been the subject of hundreds, perhaps thousands, of graduate theses and dissertations and we now have a bewildering array of stages and hosts and ecologies for all kinds of eukaryotic parasites.

Edward Jenner, a British physician, began the study of protective immunity against infectious diseases in 1796 by inoculating a boy with material from cowpox lesions and showing later that the boy was protected against smallpox. Jenner was an astute observer, but he had little conception of what was going on in the body of his human subject. A century later, the great Russian biologist, Metchnikoff, brought into being what was to become the science of immunology in 1882 by observing phagocytosis in the tiny crustacean, *Cyclops.* Early studies were directed toward microbial diseases, but by the third decade of the 20th century parasite immunology became an exciting field with studies such as those of William Talliaferro at the University of Chicago on the rat trypanosome *Trypanosoma lewisi.* Talliaferro and those who followed him began to pick apart aspects of immunity to the malaria organisms, *Plasmodium* spp., with the objective of producing a vaccine. Scores of investigators, too many to mention here, each added to the fund of knowledge, but an efficient, practical vaccine continues to be elusive.

Studies on immunity to parasites along with the exquisite methods of molecular biology promise the development of further vaccines for a variety of eukaryote parasites such as *Toxoplasma gondii,* various arthropods, and some helminths, as mentioned earlier.

Biochemical and molecular investigations have also shown the metabolic pathways of eukaryotic parasites and pointed the way toward new chemotherapies. Although most parasites have rather common metabolic patterns, in a few instances it seems possible to develop drugs that will affect the parasite and have little side effect in the host. Furthermore, increasingly exquisite technologies such as targeting gene expression through the use of antisense ribozymes, as well as highly focused combinatorial chemistry, have opened entirely new fields of therapeutic intervention possibilities that have gone well beyond conventional hit-and-miss chemical screening approaches.

CONCLUSION

Eukaroytic parasites (protists, helminths, and arthropods) have had impacts on human welfare that are almost beyond comprehension. They have direct effects on human health and indirectly affect humankind by losses to disease in domestic animals and in wildlife. Many diseases have been exacerbated by overpopulation, changes in the environment, and monoculture or inbreeding.

In a complex, ever-changing world, parasites remain with us and are a part of the ecosystem in which we live. The parasitic relationship, and all that it entails, is a fascinating subject in itself, but the needs of applied parasitology remain crucial. We look upon parasitology as an applied science in which a basic comprehension is essential to reduce significantly the detrimental effects of parasitic diseases on humankind. This theme recurs throughout the rest of the book.

Resources

A. Books. The following books provide a general entreé to parasitology and vector biology, but do not include specialized monographs or compilations. The latter are cited in the appropriate chapters.

Brooks, D. R., and McLennan, D. A. (1993). *Parascript;. Parasites and Their Language of Evolution.* Smithsonian Inst. Press, Washington, DC.

Bogitsch, B. J., and Cheng, T. C. (1999). *Human Parasitology,* 2nd Ed. Academic Press, San Diego.

Markell, E. K., John, D. T., and Krotoski, W. A. (1998). *Markell and Voge's Medical Parasitology,* 8th ed. Saunders, Philadelphia.

Roberts, L., and Janovy, J. (1999). *Foundations of Parasitology,* 6th ed. McGraw/Hill-W.C. Brown: New York.

Smyth, J. D. (1995). *Introduction to Animal Parasitology,* 3rd ed. Cambridge Univ. Press, New York.

B. Journals. These journals and review publications have half or more of their papers in the area of parasitology or vector biology.

Advances in Disease Vector Research
Advances in Parasitology
American Journal of Tropical Medicine and Hygiene
Annals of Tropical Medicine
Annual Review of Entomology
Annual Review of Tropical Medicine
Bulletin of the Society for Vector Ecology
European Journal of Protistology
Experimental and Applied Acarology
Experimental Parasitology
Folia Parasitologica
International Journal for Parasitology
Journal of Applied Entomology
Journal of Eukaryotic Microbiology (formerly Journal of Protozoology)
Journal of Helminthology
Journal of Medical Entomology
Journal of Parasitology
Journal of the American Mosquito Control Association
Journal of Wildlife Diseases
Medical and Veterinary Entomology
Molecular and Biochemical Parasitology
Mosquito News
Parasite (formerly Zeitschr. f. Parasitenkunde)
Parasite Immunology
Parasitology
Parasitology Research
Parasitology Today
Systematic Parasitology
Transactions of the Royal Society of Tropical Medicine and Hygiene
Veterinary Parasitology

These journals and review publications have some articles in parasitology and vector biology

Acta Tropica
Acarologia
American Journal of Epidemiology
Annals of the Entomological Society of America
Annual Review of Ecology and Systematics
Biological Bulletin
Biological Reviews
Biology of the Cell
Bulletin de l'Institut Pasteur
Bulletin of Entomological Research
Bulletin of the Pan-American Health Organization

Bulletin of the World Health Organization
Cell
Clinical Microbiological Reviews
Entomology Experimental and Applied
Experientia
FEBS
Infection and Immunology
International Review of Cytology
Invertebrate Biology (formerly Transactions of the American Microscopical Society)
Journal of Biological Chemistry
Journal of Cell Science
Journal of Clinical Microbiology
Journal of Economic Entomology
Journal of Environmental Health
Journal of Experimental Medicine
Journal of Experimental Zoology
Journal of Immunology
Journal of Infectious Diseases
Journal of Insect Physiology
Journal of Structural Biology
Molecular Microbiology
Nature
Philosophical Transactions of the Royal Society of London Part B.
Physiological Entomology
Proceedings of the National Academy of Science U. S. A.
Protoplasma
Research in Immunology
Science
Symposia of the Zoological Society of London
Tropical Medicine and International Health (first issued in 1996). Combines: Annales de la Societé Belge de Médecine Tropicale; Journal of Tropical Medicine and Hygiene; Tropical and Geographical Medicine; Tropical Medicine and Parasitology
Veterinary Record

C. Internet

A wealth of information is currently available on the "net" and items are continually being added. The following guide provides a beginning, but it changes frequently.

American Society of Parasitologists
hhttp://www.museum. unl.edu/asp_image/links.html
Bionet
http://www.bionet:80/hypermail/PARASITOLOGY
Communicable Disease Center
http://www.cdc.gov/
Medical Entomology
http://www.ent.iastate.edu/List/mosquito_1.html
World Health Organization (WHO)
http://www/who/ch
Worms on the Web, Nematode Links
http://helios.bto.ed.uk/mbx/fgn/wow/webworm.html
Parasite Genome Projects
http://woodland.bio.ic.ac.uk/fgn parasite-genome/parasite-genome.html
Pasteur Institute (Paris, France)
http.//www.pasteur.fr/Bio/parasite/Parasites/html

Readings

Anderson, R. M. (1976). Dynamic aspects of parasite population ecology. In *Ecological Aspects of Parasitology* (C. R. Kennedy, Ed.). North Holland, Amsterdam.

Barnard, C. J., and Behnke, J. M. (1990). *Parasitism and Host Behaviour.* Taylor & Francis, Bristol, PA.

Binford, C. H., and Connor, D. H. (Eds.) (1976). *Pathology of Tropical and Extraordinary Diseases,* 2 Vols. Armed Forces Institute of Pathology, Washington, DC.

Bloom, B. R. (1979). Games parasites play: How parasites evade immune surveillance. *Nature* **279,** 21–26.

Clayton, D. H., and Moore, J. (Eds.) (1997). *Host–Parasite Evolution. General Principles and Avian Models.* Oxford Univ. Press, New York.

Cox, F. E. G. (Ed.) (1996). *The Wellcome Trust Illustrated History of Tropical Diseases.* Wellcome Trust, London.

Esch, G. W., Hazen, T. C., and Aho, J. M. (1977). Parasitism and *r*- and *K*-selection. In *Regulation of Parasite Populations* (G. W. Esch, Ed.). Academic Press, New York.

Fairbairn, D. (1970). Biochemical adaptation and loss of genetic capacity in helminth parasites. *Biol. Rev.* **45,** 29–72.

Kim, K. C. (Ed.) (1985). *Coevolution of Parasitic Arthropods and Mammals.* Wiley, New York.

Macpherson, C. (1990). *Parasitic Helminths and Zoonoses in Africa.* HarperCollins Academic, New York.

Mayberry, L. F. (1996). The infectious nature of parasitology. *J. Parasitol.* **82,** 856–864.

McAdam, K. P. W. J. (Ed.) (1989). *New Strategies in Parasitology.* Churchill-Livingstone, Edinburgh, UK.

Mehlhorn, H. (Ed.) (1988). *Parasitology in Focus: Facts and Trends.* Springer-Verlag, New York.

Pianka, E. R. (1970). On *r*- and *K*-selection. *Am. Nat.* **104,** 592–597.

Schmid, W. D., and Robinson, E. J. (1972). The Pattern of a Host–Parasite Distribution. *J. Parasitol.* **57,** 907–910.

Siddall, M. E., *et al.* (1995). The Demise of a Phylum of Protists: Phylogeny of Myxozoa and Other Parasitic Cnidaria. *J. Parasitol.* **81,** 967–967.

Strickland, G. T. (Ed.) (1991). *Hunter's Tropical Medicine,* 7th ed. Saunders, Philadelphia.

Wakelin, D. (Ed.) (1996). *Immunity to Parasites: How Parasitic Infections Are Controlled,* 2nd ed. Cambridge Univ. Press, Cambridge, UK.

Warren, K. S. (Ed.) (1993). *Immunopathology and Molecular Biology of Parasitic Infections.* Blackwell, Boston.

Webber, R. (1996). *Communicable Disease Epidemiology and Control.* CAB International, Wallingford, UK.

Whitfield, P. J. (1979). *The Biology of Parasitism.* University Park Press, Baltimore.

Woo, P. T. K. (1995). *Fish Diseases and Disorders. Vol. 1. Protozoan and Metazoan Infections.* CAB International, Wallingford, UK.

Wyler, D. J. (Ed.) (1990). *Modern Parasite Biology. Cellular, Immunological, and Molecular Aspects.* Freeman, New York.

PART

1

EUKARYOTIC PROTISTA

CHAPTER

2

Introduction to the Parasitic Protists

Among living organisms, the principle line of division is between the prokaryotes and the eukaryotes (viruses, viroids, and prions excepted). The former category encompasses the bacteria while the latter category refers to all other organisms, unicellular and multicellular, which have their DNA enclosed by a membrane and the DNA most often divided among discrete chromosomes. The second major division, then, splits the eukaryotes into single-celled organisms and multicellular organisms. The single-celled organisms are the protists or protistans (traditionally protozoa and protophyta), and the multicellular organisms are the fungi, plants, and animals.

The protists have traditionally been classified at the higher taxonomic levels using their organelles of locomotion, nuclear structure, sexuality, and certain features seen only at the electron microscope (EM) level. But evidence now allows the conclusion that the group is polyphyletic and the so-called single-celled eukaryotes are distributed among three kingdoms. The protists range in size from 2 to about 2000 μm; most of them lie in a size range of 5 to 250 μm. Only some of the larger ones can be seen with the naked eye, so it was not until the time of the Dutch microscopist Anton van Leeuwenhoek (1632–1723) that the protists became known.

Van Leeuwenhoek wrote a series of papers published in the *Philosophical Transactions of the Royal Society* in London and the *Memoirs of the Paris Academy of Science* between 1674 and 1716. He described a number of microorganisms that he saw in his simple microscopes and is considered to be the first person to have seen and described both free-living and parasitic protists. Among the parasitic protists that he saw were the oocysts of *Eimeria stiedai* in rabbit bile and *Giardia* trophozoites from human feces.

The technology of the microscopes that Van Leeuwenhoek, and those who followed him, made are blushingly simple by today's standards, but they opened up a whole world that had hardly been suspected. In the ensuing 300 years, investigators have found organisms of extraordinary beauty and complexity and have described phenomena that belie the term *simple* as applied to these lovely creatures.

Protists are generally thought of as being composed of a nucleus with an outer limiting membrane, cytoplasm, and a plasma membrane (Fig. 2.1). By and large this is true, but many protists are multinucleate (ciliates and amebas) (Fig. 2.1B), and some have more than one cell (colonial phytoflagellates and ciliates) (Fig. 2.1C). The outer covering is also often much more complex than the plasma membrane of metazoan cells.

Certain of the protists may represent the earliest forms that came together with the symbiosis of primitive bacteria to form mitochondria, flagella, and other structures in the theory promulgated by Dr. Lynn Margulis. Despite this seemingly primitive state, the protists have evolved as long as other organisms and are highly adapted for each of their habitats.

The protists represent a unique type of evolution. Instead of the tissues and organ systems that have evolved in the multicellular organisms, the protists have developed *organelles*, which are cellular elaborations that perform the same functions as tissues and organs in the so-called higher organisms. The organelles that most biology students know are *cilia, flagella,* and *pseudopodia,* which occur in the protists studied in general biology courses. These organelles function in locomotion and feeding.

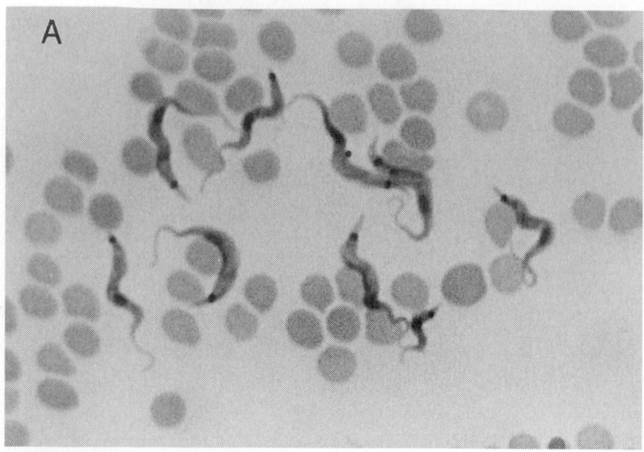

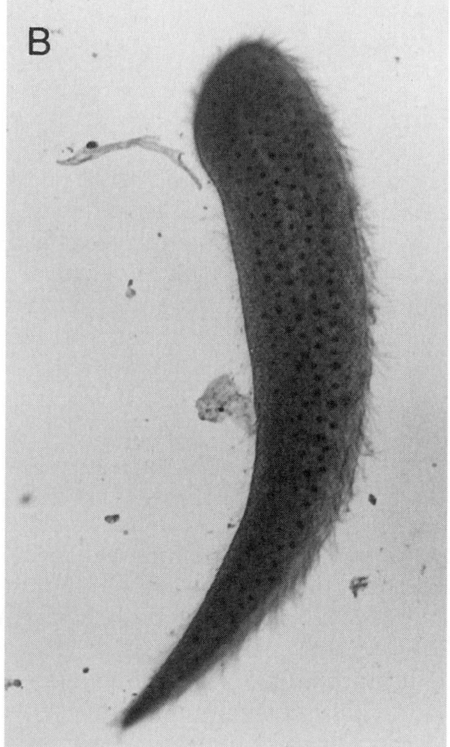

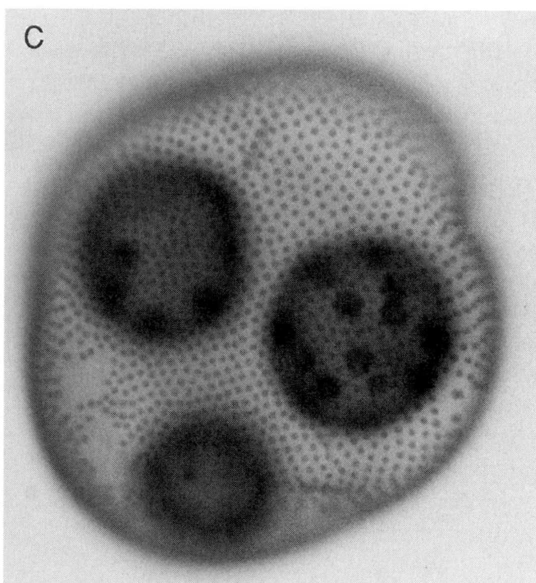

FIGURE 2.1 Variation in the morphology of some protists. (A) A uninucleate species, *Trypanosoma lewisi*, a blood parasite of the rat; this organism has a single nucleus and an outer limiting membrane. (B) *Opalina* sp., a protist that inhabits the colon of amphibia; this organism has a single outer limiting membrane but is multinucleated. (C) *Volvox* sp., a free-living protist comprised in many individuals united into a colony; even though there are many cells in the colony, they have not differentiated into expressing separate functions.

Some other organelles are the *pulsatory vesicle,* or *contractile vacuole,* which maintains proper osmotic concentration in the cytoplasm. The *infraciliature* lies just under the pellicle of ciliates and probably serves as a coordinating system for the cilia (Fig. 2.2). *Rhoptries* are found in members of the phylum Apicomplexa and are one kind of organelle in the group that aids in penetration of cells. Additional organelles are discussed along with various groups of protists in subsequent chapters.

Protists are strictly aquatic organisms. They must have an aqueous medium for feeding, locomotion, and reproduction. Many protists form cysts that may be protective or may function in some phases of the reproductive cycle. But the fact remains that the bulk of protistan activities occur in a fluid. Within this one limitation, protists have been a huge success. Members of the group have invaded every ecologic niche imaginable. The free-living forms are found in all marine and fresh waters, as well as in all soils, and they have been successful in both hot and cold waters.

When one looks at hosts of the parasitic protists, we find that nearly every species of metazoan has a complement of protists living in it; astonishingly, a few protists have parasitic protists themselves. Among the members of the invertebrate phyla, there is almost no species lacking protistan parasites, and vertebrate species are likely to be veritable zoological gardens when we look for protists.

Within the body of an animal host, protistan parasites are often found in all of its organ systems, and sometimes, such as in the intestinal tract, a dozen or

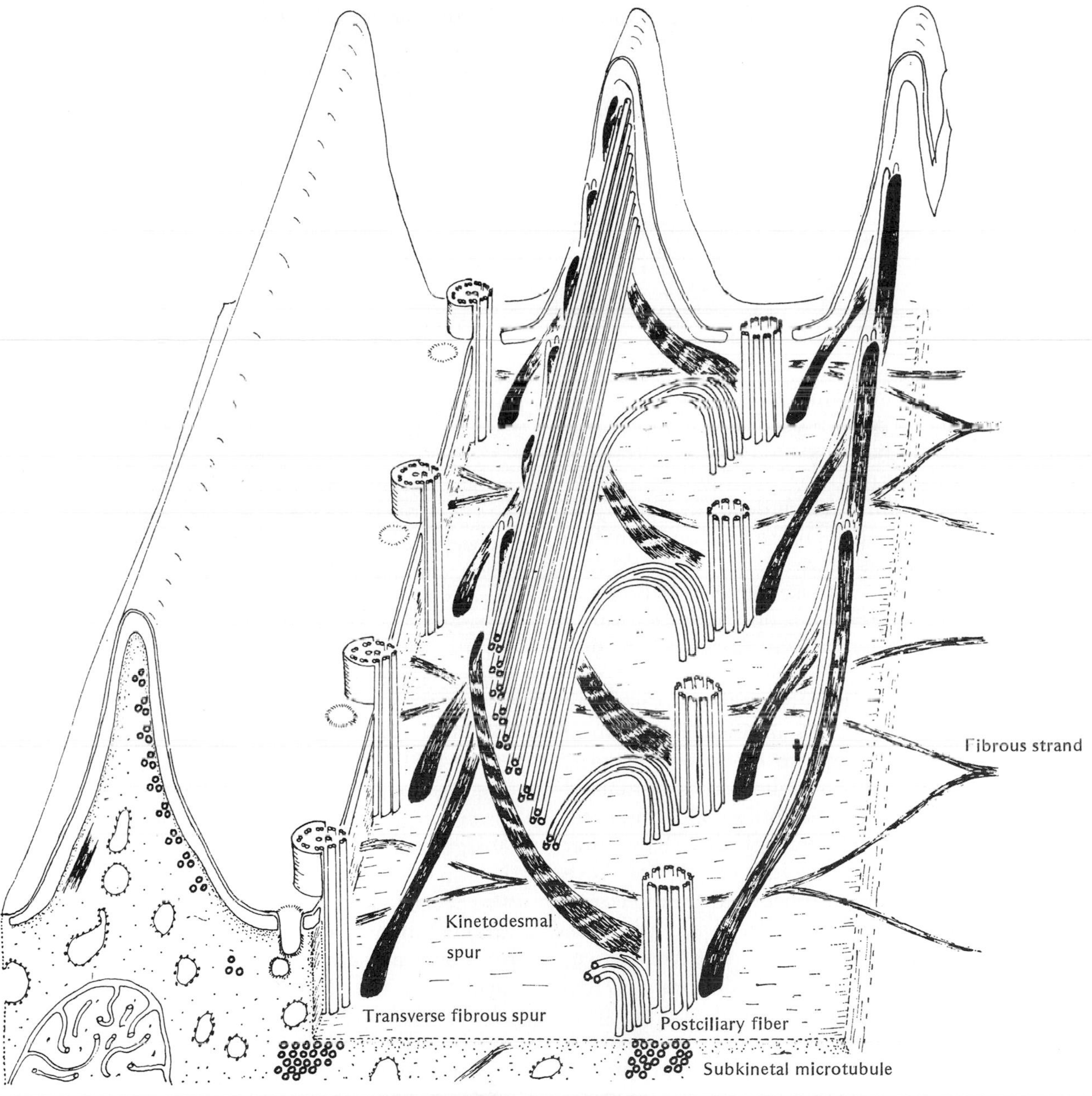

FIGURE 2.2 A diagrammatic representation of the infraciliature of a ciliate, *Brooklynella.* sp., as seen in TEM. Each cilium originates in a basal body that lies below the cortex of the organism. Fibers that are rung both longitudinally and laterally comprise the silverline system or infraciliature as seen in silver nitrate preparations at the LM level. [From Lom, J., and Corliss J. O. 1971.]

more species may live side by side. To illustrate the tissues and organ system that may serves as residences for parasitic protists of humans, the following listing gives an example of protists from each of a variety of tissues and organs.

Tissue or organ protozoan	
Skin	*Leishmania tropica*
Eye	*Encephalitozoon hellum*
Brain	*Naegleria fowleri*
Mouth	*Trichomonas tenax*
Small intestine, anterior	*Giardia lamblia*
Small intestine, posterior	*Pentatrichomonas hominis*
Large intestine	*Entamoeba histolytica*
Lungs	*Trichomonas* sp.
Reproductive tract	*Trichomonas vaginalis*
Liver	*Plasmodium vivax*
Spleen	*Leishmania donovani*
Skeletal muscle	*Sarcocystis* spp.
Cardiac muscle	*Trypanosoma cruzi*
Lymphoid cells	*Toxoplasma gondii*
Red blood cells	*Plasmodium falciparum*
Blood serum	*Trypanosoma gambiense*
Kidney	*Nosema* sp.

Of these organisms, all but two or three are medically important—and bear in mind that the list is not exhaustive.

Given that there are many parasitic protists, the question that needs to be addressed is their importance in causing disease in humans and economic losses in domestic animals and reducing wildlife populations. Losses may come about through death, debility, production losses, reproductive failures, or condemnation of food because of disease hazard or for aesthetic considerations. As emphasized elsewhere, infection and disease are not synonymous; a host infected with a particular pathogen may or may not become clinically ill.

Two examples from human infections, malaria and African sleeping sickness, give some idea of losses from human and animal infections. In the case of malaria, there were an estimated 350 million cases of malaria annually throughout the world in the 1930s and early 1940s. Of these about 3 million people died. Now, after more than 60 years of both extensive and intensive control programs, there are probably 489 million cases of malaria annually and 2.5 million deaths per year. While it appears that all of the efforts at control over the past century appear to have been for naught, it is well to consider that the earth's population has doubled in the past 50 years and that eradication of malaria has been achieved in the United States, Australia, and several western European countries. Reduction in the prevalence of malaria has been experienced in many countries in both the subtropics and tropics. Clearly, some battles have been won; however the war is not over.

African sleeping sickness has an impact on both human and animal health. The causative agent, *Trypanosoma brucei,* has subspecies that infect either humans or large herbivores (Chapter 3). The disease complex is distributed in sub-Saharan Africa over an area of 4 million square miles, an area approaching in size that of the 48 contiguous United States. Historically, sleeping sickness limited human colonization of that huge land mass affecting the ability of humans to survive or, alternatively, to raise livestock. Although progress has been made in achieving control of trypanosomiasis, efforts have by no means been completely successful.

Microspora (Chap. 16) are ubiquitous parasites of insects and they undoubtedly affect insect populations. Certain of them, such as *Nosema algerae,* infect mosquito larvae and prevent their emergence as adults. Under confined conditions such as where mosquitoes are raised in the laboratory, *N. algerae* can wipe out a colony, but in nature, it is one of the many parasites and predators that modulate mosquito populations.

CLASSIFICATION

The advent of thin-sectioning techniques for EM in the early 1960s set off ever-accelerating changes in the concepts of affinities among protists. There had been some anomalies that protozoologists and phycologists recognized but generally avoided facing. As time passed, data from EM, biochemical, and molecular studies accumulated, and classification schemes such as that of Levine et al. (1980) were found to be inadequate. Since about the mid-1980s, protistan classification has been in a state of flux, even chaos, with various groups being pushed into higher and higher taxa such that Corliss (1984) proposed that there are 45 phyla of protists, Cavalier-Smith (1993) proposed 19 phyla, and Margulis et al. (1990) yet another grouping. We have chosen the more recent Corliss (1994) scheme and feel that it recognizes what is currently understood to be the evolutionary relationships among protists and yet maintains a relatively simple structure for students to deal with. The classification presented here is quite abbreviated and includes only those taxa that have symbiotic or parasitic protists.

Corliss has established two *Empires* to contain pro- and eukaryotic organisms, respectively; his *Empires* are at about the same taxonomic level as the *Domains* proposed by Carl R. Woese. These proposals for a taxon above the level of *Kingdom* recognize fundamental differences among organisms and do explain well the divergence among the groups. However, neither Corliss nor Woese included two other groups of living agents, the prions and the viruses. Other workers have proposed that the viruses be placed in their own taxon and it seems approporiate to place them in their own *Empire.* Likewise, the prions, which cause a variety of central nervous system diseases lumped under the term *spongiform encephalopathies,* are unique insofar as they contain only protein, are heat stable, and can be transmitted either horizontally or vertically; they seem to integrate into the host genome in some hosts. It is likely that a classification with separate empires or domains for the prions, viruses, archaea, eubacteria, and eukarya will be accepted in the near future.

Of the six eukaryotic **kingdoms,** three are protistan and the other three are the traditional fungi, plants, and animals that have been accepted for many years. The erection of three kingdoms emphasizes the diversity among protists, and the fact that, while superficially simple, they have undergone evolution longer than the plants, animals, and fungi. It should also be noted that the terms **protozoa** and **protophyta** are no longer relevant considering current classification. All of these organisms are **protists,** neither plant nor animal, but simply what they are—a separate line of evolution with likely more than a single origin.

The three protistan kingdoms recognize that the Archetista have affinities to the prokaryotes, because of their lack of the usual eukaryotic organelles such as Golgi, mitochondria, and so on and their prokaryotic-like ribosomes and rRNA genes. These characters, or lack thereof, place them close to the prokaryotes. The kingdom Protista encompasses those protists that have traditionally been called protozoa and some protophyta. The third kingdom, the Chromista, are photosynthetic and have other characteristics that set them apart, but they are not symbiotic.

With respect to parasitic protists, at the taxonomic level of phylum and lower, the classifications remain rather traditional, with a few exceptions. For example, organisms that move and feed by pseudopodia, the amebas, are now split into the Archetista and several other phyla and classes in the Protista. Likewise, certain flagellated organisms are now in different Kingdoms rather than being placed close together as in former schemes. Little of this affects the way in which we deal with protists as parasites, but it is well to keep in mind that different evolutionary histories are likely to affect many aspects of biology as well as the host–parasite relationship.

PROTISTAN CLASSIFICATION

Kingdom I. Archetista (Archezoa)* (3 phyla)

Unicellular protists, lacking mitochondria, plastids, typical Golgi, hydrogenosomes, and peroxisomes; ribosomes and rRNA have prokaryotic features; energy obtained by anaerobic glycolysis; movement by a small number of flagella, pseudopodia, or no organelles; the majority is symbiotic.

Phylum **Metamonada**

Two to many flagella; 70s ribosomes and 16s rRNA; mostly symbiotic.

Giardia, Hexamita, Octomitus, Spironucleus, Trepomonas, Caviomonas, Enteromonas, Trimitus, Chilomastix, Retortamonas, Monocercomonoides, Oxymonas, Pyrsonympha, Saccinobaculus

Phylum **Microspora**

Minute unicellular, intracellular symbionts; 70s ribosomes; sporoplasm 1- or 2-nucleate; lack flagella; Golgi perhaps present; resistant spores contain a complex extrusosome with cap and polar tube; 1 layer of the spore wall is chitinous.

Amphiacantha, Metchnikovella, Burkea, Hessea, Encephalitzozoon, Culicospora, Enterocytozoon, Glugea, Nosema, Pleistophora, Stempellia, Thelohania, Vairimorpha

Kingdom II Euprotista (Protozoa) (7 phyla)

Protists which are unicellular, plasmodial, or colonial phagotrophic, colorless; lack walls in the trophic form; some capable of photosynthesis typically with cytosolic chloroplasts with stacked thylakoids, which lack starch and are usually surrounded by 3 membranes; mitochondria with tubular cristae (with a few exceptions); Golgi and peroxisomes present; flagellar mastigonemes, if present, never rigid or tubular; free-living and symbiotic.

Phylum **Percolotista (Percolozoa)**

Unicellular, non-pigmented; perhaps primitive; lacking Golgi; peroxisomes usually present; mitochondria with flat or discoidal cristae, or more rarely, hydrogenosomes present; 1–4 or sometimes more flagella but lacking mastigonemes; some species with both amoeboid and flagellated forms; fresh-water and marine, some facultative parasites.

Naegleria, Tetramitus, Vahlkampfia

*Taxa in parentheses are terms used by Corliss, 1994.

Phylum **Parabasala**

Unicellular, symbiotic; flagellates with mastigont system typically having 3 or more flagella; 70s ribosomes; no mitochondria but hydrogenosomes with a double envelope; parabasal body is the Golgi; many hosts including vertebrates and invertebrates, many species in termites.

Dientamoeba, Ditrichomonas, Hexamastix, Histomonas, Monocercomonas, Pseudotrichomonas, Trichomonas, Barbulanympha, Trichonympha, Tritrichomonas, Pentatrichomonas

Phylum **Euglenista (Euglenozoa)**

Species have 1–4 flagella with paraxial rods and non-tubular mastigonemes; peroxisomes present, mitochondria with discoidal cristae; microtubular cytoskeleton reinforcing the cortex; well developed Golgi; nuclear division with persistent nucleolus; fresh water and symbiotic.

Cryptobia, Ichthyobodo, Procryptobia, Rhynchomonas, Blastocrithidia, Crithidia, Herpetomonas, Leishmania, Leptomonas, Phytomonas, Trypanosoma, Proteromonas

Phylum **Opalotista (Opalozoa)**

Mostly small, free-living, unicellular, uninucleate, biflagellated (but with distinct exceptions); mitochondria with tubular cristae; symbiotic forms in amphibia. [This group seems to be a marriage of inconvenience and divorce seems inevitable]

Cepedea, Opalina, Protoopalina, Zelleriella, Protozellerellia

Phylum **Dinoflagellata (Dinozoa)**

Biflagellated, uninucleate; amphiesmal vesicles or cortical alveoli containing cellulosic plates in some groups; mitochondria with tubular cristae; peroxisomes present; single flagellum typically with paraxial rod; about one-half of extant species with chloroplasts containing chlorophylls *a* and *c* enveloped with 3 (rarely 2) membranes; chloroplasts lacking phycobilisomes and located in the cytosol; non-pigmented species are phagotrophic as are some pigmented species; nucleus haploid typically with distinct chromosomes on non-protein complexed DNA. (Includes dinoflagellates) [Again, this phylum may not survive partly because DNA of dinoflagellates has histones]

Hochbergia (a large parasite of cephalopods)

Phylum **Ciliophora**

Distinctive infraciliature usually associated with numerous longitudinal rows of cilia; with perkinetal (as opposed to symmetrogenic) division; many with complex oral ciliature; cortical alveoli characteristic of most groups; mitochondria with tubular, often curved, cristae; in anaerobic species, mitochondria may be replaced by hydrogenosomes; heterokaryotic, with 1 or more diploid micronuclei and 1 or more polyploid macronuclei; conjugation, or related process, the sexual phenomenon; heterotrophic with a few forms having algal symbionts; mostly free-living, but a few are symbiotic.

Balantidium, Tetrahymena, Ichthyophthirius

Phylum **Apicomplexa**

Apical complex, of which one or more elements are present at some stage of the life cycle, consisting of polar ring(s), rhoptries, micronemes, and a conoid; uninucleate or multinucleate; highly compressed, smooth-membraned cisternae (alveoli) usually present in cell cortex of infective stage; subpellicular tubules and cytostomes often present; syngamy the form of sexual reproduction; flagella only in microgametes, except in Perkinsidea; mitochondria with tubular cristae, but may be much reduced; all symbiotic.

Sarcocystis, Toxoplasma, Haemoproteus, Hepatocystis, Leucocytozoon, Plasmodium, Babesia, Dactylosoma, Theileria, Eimeria, Perkinsea

Phylum **Rhizopoda**

Pseudopodia serve both for feeding and locomotion; no flagella except in Granuloreticulosea (mostly Foraminifera); heterotrophic except for species with endosymbiotic algae; Golgi and mitochondria present except in Entamoebidea where mitochondria may have been lost secondarily; mostly uninucleate; free-living except for Entamoebidea and a few other forms;

Entamoeba, Iodamoeba, Endolimax, Endamoeba

Phylum **Acetospora**

Endosymbionts mainly of marine invertebrates; unicellular spores or production of sporoplasms within cells; unique haplosporosomes characteristic of most species; lacking polar capsules, filaments, flagellated stages; mitochondria with tubulo-vesicular cristae; perhaps polyphyletic.

Haplosporidium, Marteilia, Minchinia, Paramarteilia, Paramyxa, Urosporidium

Kingdom III. Chromista

Predominantly phototrophic; unicellular, filamentous, or colonial; chloroplasts in the lumen of the rough or smooth ER, lack starch and phycobilisomes and have a 2-membraned envelope inside a periplastid membrane; mitochondria usually with tubular cristae; Golgi, and peroxisomes always present; flagella (when present) at least one bears rigid, tubular, and usually tripartite hairs or mastigonemes (except in the haptophytes); majority with plastids; free-living.

Readings

Cavalier-Smith, T. (1993). Kingdom Protozoa and its 18 phyla. *Microbiol. Rev.* **57,** 609–615.

Coombs, G. H., and North, M. J. (Eds.) (1991). *Biochemical Protozoology.* Taylor & Francis, Bristol, PA.

Corliss, J. O. (1984). The kingdom Protista and its 45 phyla. *Biol. System* **17,** 87–126.

Corliss, J. O. (1994). An interim utilitarian (''user-friendly'') hierarchical classification and characterization of the protists. *Acta Protozool.* **33,** 1–51.

Grassé, P.-P. (Ed.) (1952/1953). *Traité de Zoologie,* Vol. 1, Fasc. 1 & 2. Masson, Paris.

Lee, J. J., Hutner, S. H., and Bovee, E. C. (1985). *An Illustrated Guide to the Protozoa.* Society of Protozoologists, Lawrence, KS.

Levine, N. D. (1985). *Veterinary Protozoology.* Iowa State Univ. Press, Ames.

Levine, N. D., *et al.* (1980). A newly revised classification of the protozoa. *J. Protozool.* **27,** 37–58.

Lom, J., and Corliss, J. O. (1971). Morphogenesis and Cortical Ultrastructure of *Brooklynella hostilis,* a Dysteriid Ciliate Ectoparasitic on Marine Fishes. *J. Protozool.* **18,** 261–281.

Margulis, L., Corliss, J. O., Melkonian, M., and Chapman, D. J. (1990). *Handbook of Protoctista.* Jones & Bartlett, Boston.

Mehlhorn, H. (1997). Cellular organization of parasitic protozoa. In *Microbiology. Vol. 5. Parasitology* In *Topley and Wilson's Microbiology. Vol. 5. Parasitology.* (A. Balows and M. Sussman, Eds.). Arnold, New York.

Sleigh, M. A. (1989). *Protozoa and Other Protists,* 2nd ed. Arnold, London.

CHAPTER

3

TRYPANOSOMES AND TRYPANOSOMOSIS

In this and subsequent chapters (Chapters 3 through 6) we consider flagellated protists which cause diseases in humans and other animals. None of these organisms obtains energy from sunlight, and they take food either by ingesting particulates or by absorbing nutrients through the plasma membrane.

The trypanosomes are members of the order Kinetoplastida, which are principally parasitic, but there is one suborder, the Bodonina that has a few free-living species. As indicated by its name, members have a kinetoplast, a conspicuous DNA-containing organelle from which a mitochondrion arises. The kinetoplast is self-replicating and contains genomic material in addition to that which is in the nucleus. Various members have from one to four flagella, and there is often a barren basal body oriented at a right angle to the basal body that bears the flagellum.

The family Trypanosomatidae is defined as having a single nucleus, a single flagellum, and a leaflike or rounded body. The family contains nine genera, two of which are of major medical and economic importance in humans and domestic animals. Members cause African sleeping sickness, Chagas' disease, oriental sore, and visceral leishmaniasis in humans and several related diseases in domestic animals.

Some trypanosomatids, members of the genus *Phytomonas,* are parasites of plants. Those best known are in latex-bearing plants such as milkweed; *P. elmassiani* is transmitted by *Oncopeltus* (Hemiptera, Lygaeidae). Two pathogenic *Phytomonas* spp. are known, *P. leptovasorum* of coffee plants, and *P. staheli,* which infects coconut palms in Surinam, South America. A few trypanosomatids have been found as intranuclear parasites of other protists.

Trypanosomatids range in size from about 2 to 80 μm, with most of them being between 5 and 30 μm. During their life cycles most of the trypanosomatids change body form depending on the host or the organ in which they are located. Often they undergo cyclic development as they pass from one host to the next. The terminology for the various forms has been standardized for a good many years (Fig. 3.1) and is useful in describing aspects of the life cycle.

Although trypanosomatids may shift back and forth between forms during their life cycles, the basic structure remains much the same. The trypomastigote form is common in the blood of infected vertebrates, and it serves as a type for reference. Trypomastigotes range in size from about 15 to 80 μm. The larger ones are found in some fish; one from a ray reaches 130 μm in length. Most of the trypomastigotes in the blood of mammals particularly the pathogenic ones range from 15 to 30 μm. These are the species on which a great deal of morphologic work has been done and we will use one as a type trypomastigote. *Trypanosoma brucei* is 15 to 30 μm long by 6 to 8 μm wide (Fig. 3.2). The body is sinuous and has a single flagellum that arises from the basal body or kinetosome in the flagellar pocket. Near the flagellar basal body and oriented at a right angle to it is the so-called barren basal body. The flagellar pocket is significant for our purposes because surface antigens seem to be produced there and move out over the surface of the organism.

In the slender bloodstream forms, the flagellum extends anteriorly beyond the body as a free flagellum. The flagellum has a typical "9 + 2" arrangement. A paraxial rod (Fig. 3.3) is associated with it, and both are enclosed by a sheath that represents the undulating

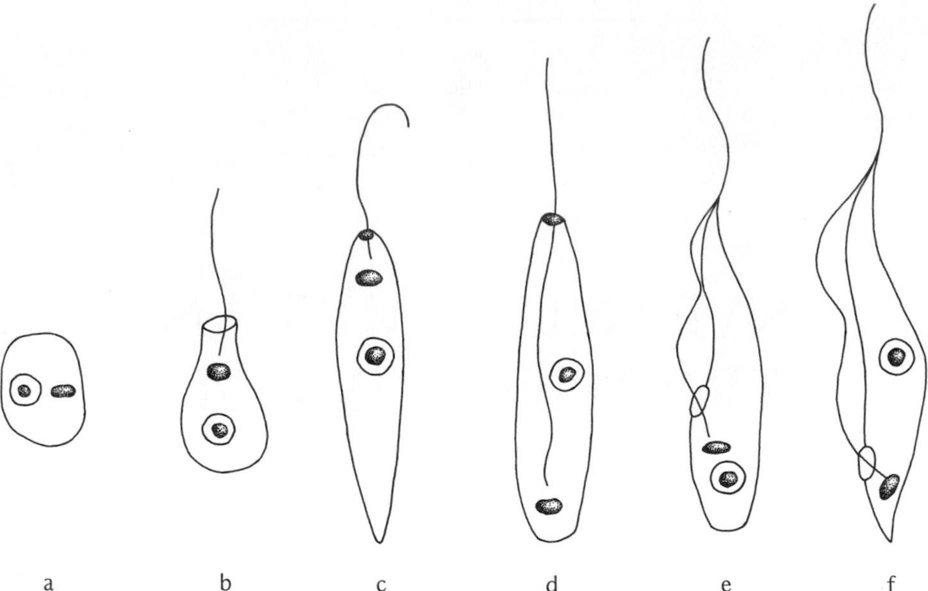

FIGURE 3.1 Forms of trypanosomatid flagellates. (a) amastigote; (b) choanomastigote; (c) promastigote; (d) opisthomastigote; (e) epimastigote; (f) trypomastigote.

membrane. Subpellicular tubules lie just beneath the outer limiting membrane and extend lengthwise through the organism; their number is variable. There is a single, centrally located nucleus. The kinetoplast lies near the basal body, but it is not attached to it. The basal body and the kinetoplast retain their association even during transformation to another form. The kinetoplast is less than 1 μm in length and perhaps half that in width; it is surrounded by a double membrane. At one or both corners of the kinetoplast the mitochondrion arises and extends through much of the body of the organism. While in the bloodstream of the vertebrate host, the surface area of the mitochondrion is relatively low indicating that it is not highly functional. Within the kinetoplast are numerous strands of DNA, which extend across the short dimension. Under appropriate treatment, these strands can be seen to be circles. Other cytoplasmic organelles or inclusions are Golgi, endoplasmic reticulum, lysosomes, glycosomes, and volutin granules.

Division in trypanosomatids is essentially like that of other flagellates such as euglenoids—; it is longitudinal (symmetrogenic). The nucleus divides by an amitotic process in which the nuclear envelope is retained. The kinetoplast-mitochondrion replicates just prior to nuclear division.

GENUS *TRYPANOSOMA*—GENERAL

Members of the genus *Trypanosoma* are widespread as trypomastigotes in the blood of vertebrates. Most remain in tissue fluids, but a few (*T. cruzi*) replicate within cells. All but a few members of the genus (e.g., *T. evansi, T. equiperdum)* are transmitted from one vertebrate to another through biological vectors. Transmission to the invertebrate vector takes place through blood feeding. Transmission back to the vertebrate host takes place through one of two routes: injection during feeding or fecal contamination of the site where the insect vector has been feeding. There is still no satisfactory scheme for classifying all of the trypanosomes of vertebrates, but one system for trypanosomes of mammals shows patterns within the genus (Tab. 3.1).

The trypanosomes make sense as mammalian parasites if it is assumed that they were originally parasites of insects. We know, for example, that there are kinetoplastids in a variety of true bugs (order Hemiptera). Since the Hemiptera have sucking mouthparts, it is logical that they would themselves have become infected when preying on other insects. Some of the Hemiptera have become blood feeders, and the step of injecting kinetoplastids into the skin of a mammal reasonably follows.

The genus *Trypanosoma* has been split into two "*Sections*" (not a recognized taxonomic term), the Stercoraria and Salivaria (Tab. 3.1) The root *sterc-* refers to feces and transmission from the invertebrate vector to the vertebrate host is through fecal contamination; these organisms are spoken of as developing in the "posterior station." In contrast, the Salivaria encompasses those trypanosomes that develop in the "ante-

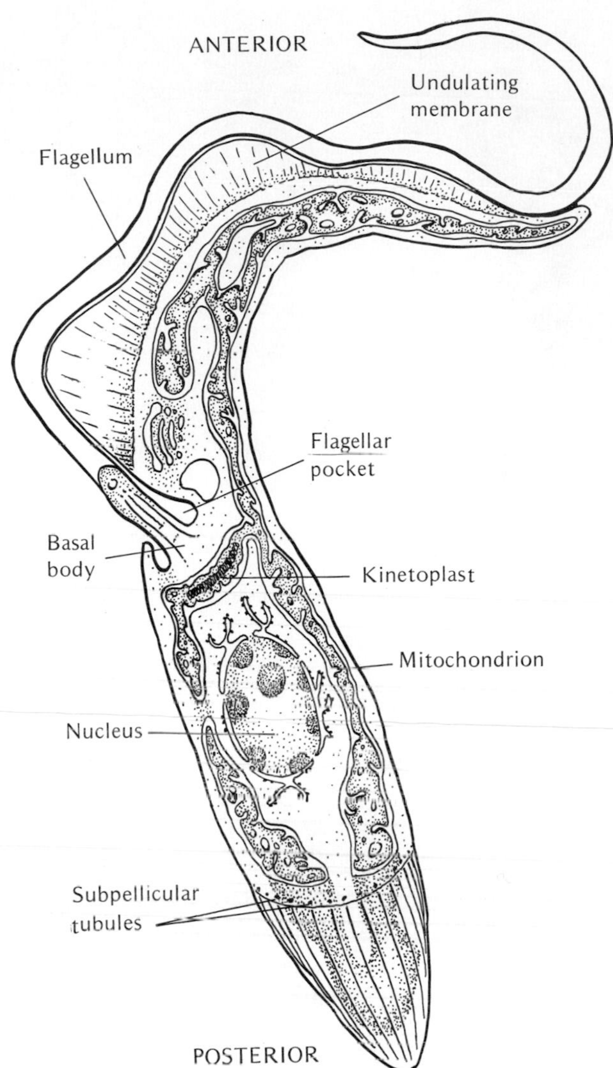

FIGURE 3.2 Diagram of *Trypanosoma brucei rhodesiense* as created from studies in the transmission electron microscope.

rior station" and are transmitted from the vector to the vertebrate host by injection during the act of blood feeding.

The classification of trypanosomes is useful in showing the patterns of development, structure, and metabolism within the genus, but it is of little help in identifying an organism in a stained blood film taken from a vertebrate. Trypomastigotes have characteristics that are fairly consistent, and an identification or description can usually be made if there are sufficient organisms in the blood. Protists, perhaps more than any other group of organisms, are best defined statistically, because any one organism may not represent the species adequately.

The following characteristics are used in identification:

1. Size—; length and width in micrometers
2. Location of the nucleus—; central or toward one end
3. Shape of body—; straight, sinuous, C-shaped
4. Kinetoplast—; present or absent (a few species), size, terminal or subterminal
5. Flagellum—; free (extending beyond the anterior of the body) or not
6. Undulating membrane—; high or low, number of loops
7. Staining quality of cytoplasm—; stains lightly or darkly, has granular inclusions or not

Representative trypomastigotes are illustrated in Figure 3.4.

The first part of this chapter concerns African sleeping sickness in humans with some attention paid to nagana in domestic cattle. A number of species in addition to *Trypanosoma brucei* are tsetse borne and a few are not; these pathogenic trypanosomes are of considerable economic importance in Africa and elsewhere in the world (Tab. 3.1).

Trypanosoma evansi is transmitted by blood-sucking flies in the suborder Brachycera, Family Tabanidae (Chapter 47). Transmission is mechanical in that there is no development inside the fly. Tabanids are restless feeders, and if one is disturbed while feeding, it may transmit *T. evansi* to an uninfected animal through its contaminated mouthparts. The disease, surra, occurs north of the tsetse belt in Africa but has also spread widely through the Eastern Hemisphere.

Dourine is a disease of horses and other equids caused by *T. equiperdum* and transmitted through sexual intercourse. It has been spread worldwide through trade, exploration, and military action. Dourine was a serious disease of horses in the United States but was eradicated through a test and slaughter program during the 1920s and 1930s. Dourine is occasionally reintroduced into the United States, and then a localized eradication program is instituted.

Both *T. evansi* and *T. equiperdum* have probably been derived from tsetse-borne trypanosomes of subsaharan Africa. They are structurally similar to *T. brucei* and the diseases they cause are similar to nagana. The principal difference is that these species have taken a step or two away from dependence on tsetse as vectors.

AFRICAN SLEEPING SICKNESS AND NAGANA

Names of Organisms and Disease Associations

Trypanosoma brucei causes African sleeping sickness (in humans), nagana (in cattle), trypanosomosis, and

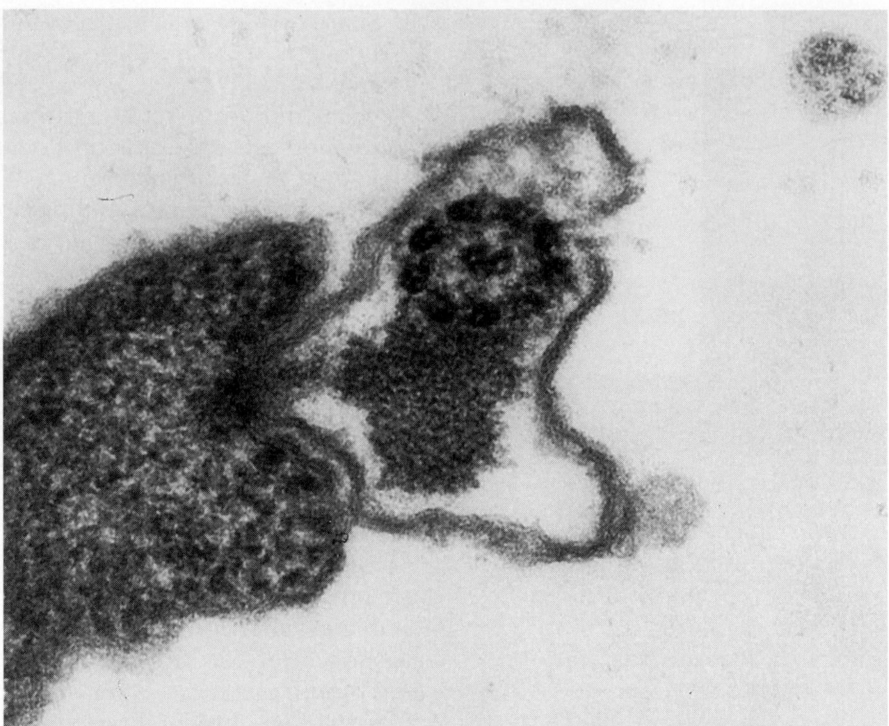

FIGURE 3.3 Flagellum and paraxial rod of *Trypanosoma avium* as shown by transmission electron microscopy. The flagellum shows the typical 9 + 2 arrangement of many flagella, and below it is the paraxial rod; both are surrounded by the pellicle of the trypomastigote.

trypanosomiasis. *T. brucei,* its subspecies, and some related species form a complex of organisms that cause the African trypanosomoses. Most of them are transmitted by tsetse, members of the genus *Glossina* (Diptera, Muscidae) (Chapter 48). The term *tsetse* means fly destructive to cattle in the Sechuana language of Botswana; thus the term *tsetse fly* is redundant (but nevertheless is still used).

Hosts and Host Range

T. brucei shows a moderate degree of host specificity with each of the subspecies infecting two or three species of natural hosts and some laboratory animals. For example, *T. b. gambiense* infects humans, probably some domesticated animals, and laboratory rats. The host preferences of tsetse are also somewhat limited, and usually a single species of fly serves as the vector in one locality, but others serve as vectors elsewhere. Often the specificity in transmission is based on feeding preferences, not physiological parameters.

Geographic Distribution and Importance

T. brucei is distributed over tropical Africa south of the Sahara Desert from 15° N latitude to 25° S latitude. The area encompasses more than 4 million square miles, about the same as the 48 continental United States. Until recent years, the three subspecies of *T. brucei—T. b. brucei, T. b. gambiense,* and *T. b. rhodesiense* and *T. congolense* effectively denied humans the use of this region for raising cattle and horses, and there was considerable hazard to humans directly from sleeping sickness.

In areas where *T. b. brucei* and *T. congolense,* the causes of nagana in cattle, were enzootic, it was not possible to raise large domestic mammals. The effect was to prevent human use of cattle, horses, and swine. The impact of not having oxen or horses was severe. Farming tasks performed for thousands of years in other parts of the world by oxen were still done by hand in large parts of Africa. The soil was tilled by hand, and even at the present time, programs to employ cattle in farm work are just now being introduced. Communication, travel, and war were all dependent on the horse in Asia, Europe, and North Africa, but in tropical Africa, all had to be done on foot or by boats on waterways. Invasions by Arab peoples from the Sahara southward were prevented because of the probability of epidemic deaths in their horses, and the Boers of South Africa in more recent times were prevented from migrating northward because of livestock deaths.

TABLE 3.1 Classification of the Genus *Trypanosoma*

Stercoraria	
Kinetoplast large, not terminal; posterior end of body pointed; typically, but not always, nonpathogenic; development in vector in posterior station; transmission contaminative.	
Subgenus *Megatrypanum*	Kinetoplast typically near nucleus, far from posterior end of body; includes *T. (M.) theileri, T. (M.) tragelaphi, T. (M.) melophagium, T. (M.) ingens*
Subgenus *Herpetomonas*	Kinetoplast subterminal, close to posterior end of body; includes *T. (H.) lewisi, T. (H.) duttoni, T. (H.) nabiasi,* and others
Subgenus *Schizotrypanum*	Typically curved, kinetoplast close to posterior end of body; includes *T. (S) cruzi, T. (S.) vespertilionis, T. (S.) pipistrelli* and others.
Subgenus *Endotrypanum*	Endoglobular forms. *T. (E). schaudinni*
Salivaria	
Kinetoplast terminal or subterminal; posterior end of body usually blunt; typically pathogenic; development in vector in anterior station; transmission inoculative	
Subgenus *Duttonella*	Posterior end of body rounded; kinetoplast large, terminal; includes *T. (D) vivax, T. (D). uniforme*
Subgenus *Nannomonas*	Kinetoplast typically marginal, includes *T. (N.) dimorphon, T. (N.) congolense, T. (N.) simiae*
Subgenus *Pyncnomonas*	Kinetoplast small, subterminal; *T. (P.) suis.*

Thus, trypanosomosis left people in central Africa with a risk of only sporadic incursions, but also with primitive farming methods and no beasts of burden nor means of easy transport, except by water.

In western Africa, sleeping sickness in humans was originally present in endemic foci with epidemics probably occurring at fairly regular intervals. Despite these episodes, it was a disease to which humans had adjusted insofar as the population was able to survive and generally avoid infection. During the later 1800s, European efforts at colonization of Africa increased resulting in greater movement of peoples and introduction of Western technologies. Steamers plied the Congo River and its tributaries, and persons living in endemic areas of sleeping sickness near the mouth of the Congo were transported hundreds of miles upstream as laborers or soldiers. By the turn of the century, it was clear that a disaster was in progress. In the Congo basin alone, it is estimated that half a million persons died of sleeping sickness between 1896 and 1906.

The disease spread not only through western Africa but was carried over into East Africa, probably by Emin Pasha's army. Sleeping sickness broke out on the shores of Lake Victoria in 1896, and by 1908 the original population of about 300,000 had been reduced to about 100,000 persons.

The result of these and other epidemics was that European countries with economic interests in Africa instituted research and control programs that ultimately reduced the prevalence of sleeping sickness (Fig. 3.5).

Even today, after extensive control programs, raising livestock is difficult or even impossible in areas that would otherwise be eminently suitable for it. It is estimated the 3 million cattle die annually from trypanosomosis. Ready sources of animal protein are often limited to poultry and goats. Cattle, on which people rely for milk, meat, and fiber, and swine and which can scavenge in marginal environments, are not available. Consequently, many people in tropical Africa, especially children, suffer from protein deficiencies. As has been well publicized in recent years, protein is essential for proper development of children's minds and bodies during their early years of rapid growth.

African sleeping sickness is on the rise in tropical Africa. In the late 1980s 5,000 to 10,000 persons were being treated each year for sleeping sickness. In 1994, after 4 years of little control, the caseload has increased to 150,000 with some villages reaching levels of 70% of persons infected, a level that is spoken of as being "unheard of." Part of the increase is probably due to more migration of infected persons taking the disease agent with them to new areas. Political unrest, and a reduction in governmental services have been the principal factors in the resurgence of sleeping sickness.

McKelvey's (1973) *Man against Tsetse: Struggle for Africa* sets forth in broad terms the scope of the trypanosomosis problem and details some of the events and people that have increased the problem of trypanosomoses and those who have developed the knowledge and techniques that have helped to control the diseases. The book is a microcosm of human ecology showing the kinds of forces that have impinged on Africa in the last two hundred years or so.

The three subspecies of *T. brucei* differ only in host preferences and the clinical course of the diseases that they cause. *T. b. gambiense* is the cause of Gambian fever in humans, the domiciliated form of sleeping sickness. *T. b. gambiense* is limited to humans, although some domestic animals may serve as minor reservoirs, and the disease is contracted at home. *T. b. rhodesiense*, the cause of Rhodesian fever, is more virulent and is usually contracted when a person leaves home and travels to another area for hunting or fishing. Gambian

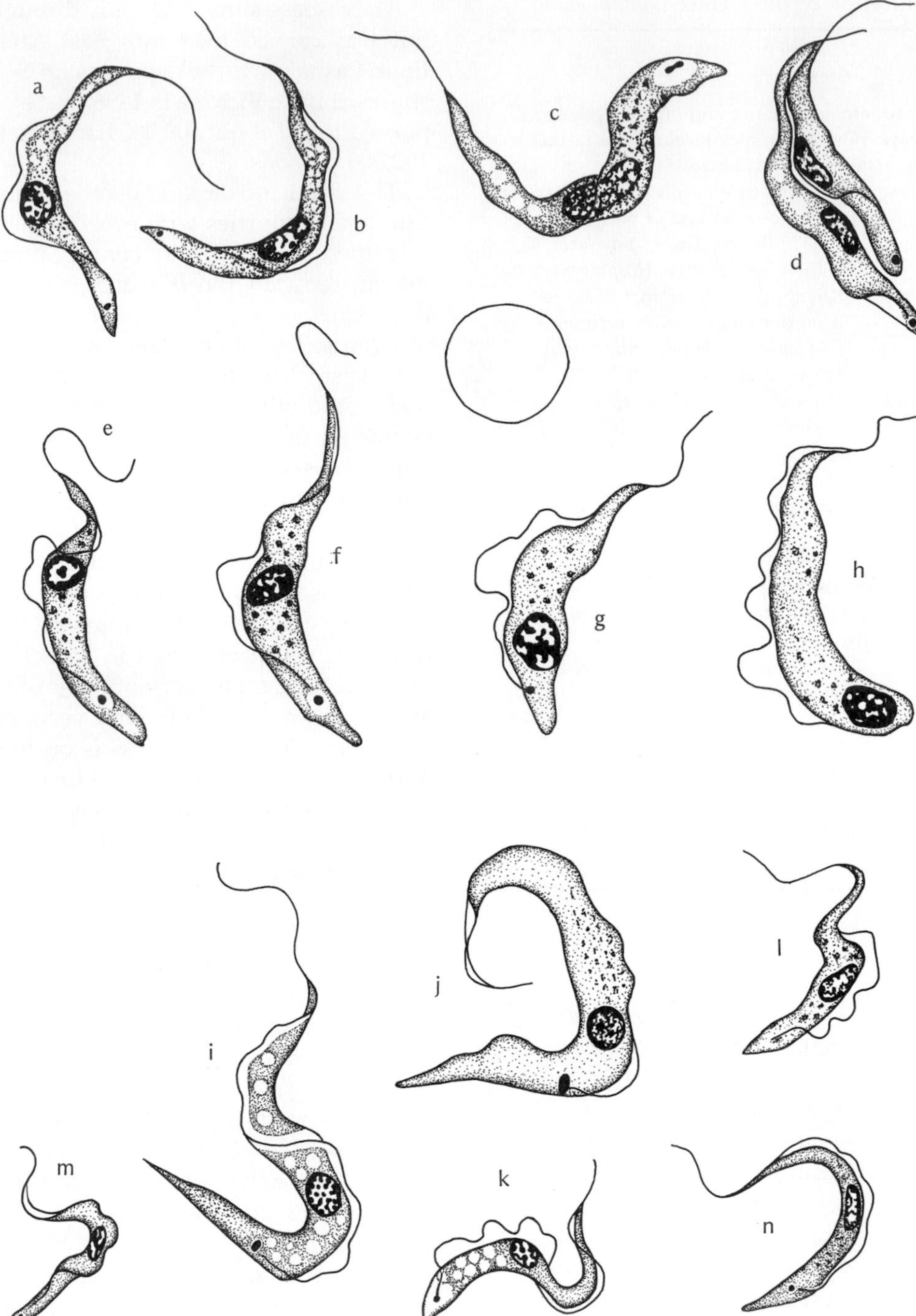

FIGURE 3.4 Trypomastigotes of some *Trypanosoma* spp. as seen in the light microscope in stained blood films: (a–d) *T. congolense;* (e–h) *T. brucei;* (i) *T. theileri;* (j) *T. melophagium;* (k) *T. evansi;* (m) *T. equiperdum;* (n) *T. lewisi.* The clear circle below *T. congolense* is a red blood cell of 7 to 8 μm in diameter for size reference.

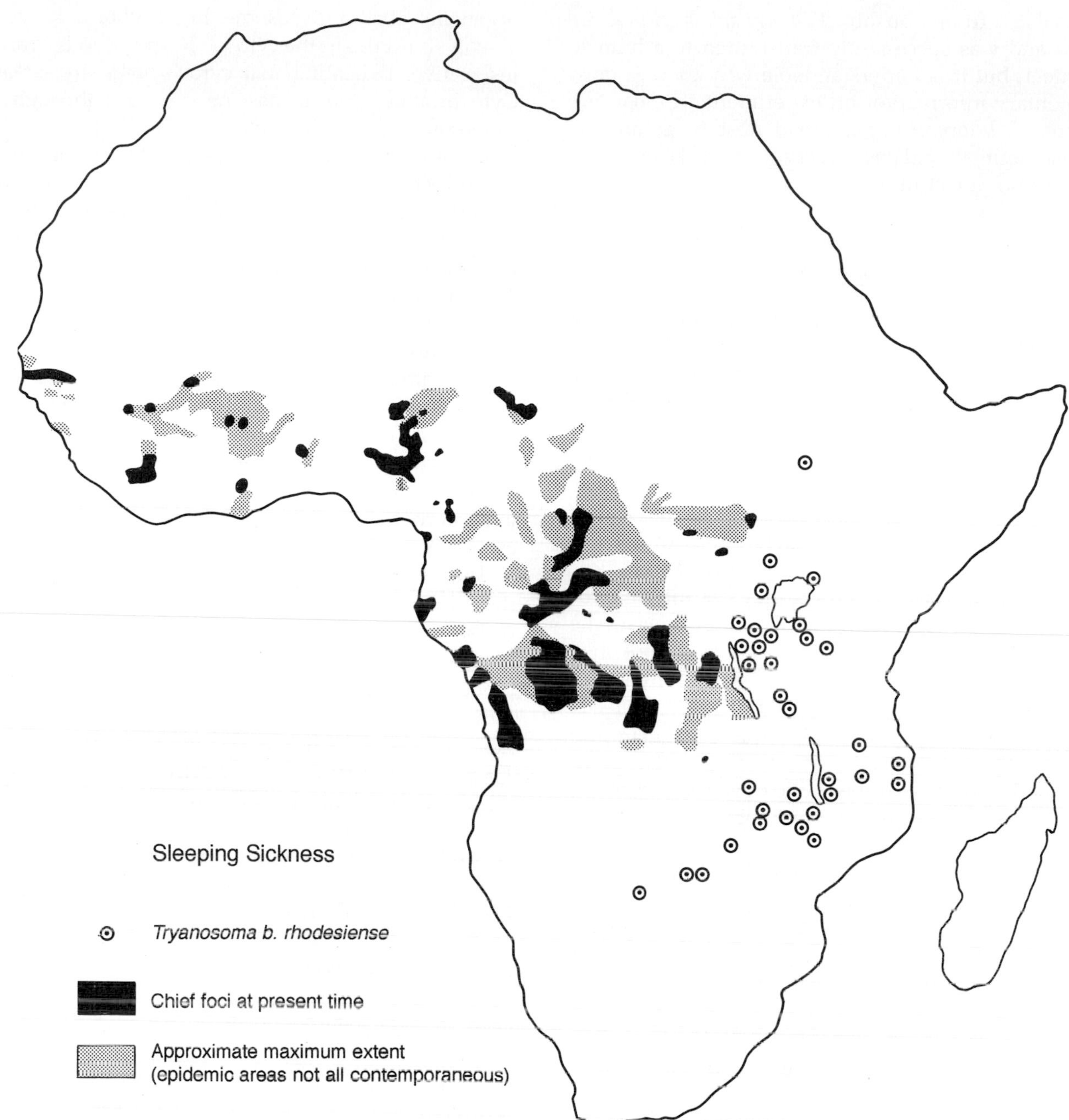

FIGURE 3.5 Map of the distribution of African sleeping sickness in humans.

fever is the more common and widespread form of sleeping sickness (Fig. 3.5). *T. b. brucei* is the cause of nagana in cattle, and the course of the disease is not unlike the infections in humans with the other subspecies.

Morphology

All members of the *T. brucei* complex are structurally alike. In the slender form they average 29 μm in length, and as stumpy forms they average 18 μm; the total size range is 12 to 42 μm (see Fig. 3.4 and, later, Fig. 3.9).

The difference among the subspecies is based mainly on the hosts that they infect. *T. b. gambiense* is a parasite of humans; the organism can be transmitted experimentally to other animals, including cattle, which may be a reservoir, but the evidence is still equivocal. *T. b. rhodesiense* is a parasite of wild herbivores, normally, but it has the capability of multiplying in humans if given the opportunity. *T. b. rhodesiense* was isolated from a bushbuck, *Tragelaphus scriptus,* in Kenya and was successfully transmitted to a human volunteer, but it is understandable why there is only fragmentary information on experimental human infections. *T. b. brucei* has a broad host range among domestic animals and has a reservoir in wild ruminants but does not infect humans.

Life Cycle

Trypomastigotes circulate in human blood and are taken up by tsetse (*Glossina* spp.) during feeding. They multiply as somewhat modified trypomastigotes in the midgut of the fly for about 10 days (Fig. 3.6) and then migrate toward the anterior portion of the gut. Upon reaching the salivary glands a few days later, the organisms transform into epimastigotes, attach to tissue by their flagella, and multiply. About 20 days after infection, the epimastigotes begin to transform back to the trypomastigote form. These are called *metacyclic trypomastigotes* and in this form they are infective for the human host. Prior to the appearance of metacyclic trypomastigotes, infection of a human is not possible. Mechanical transmission can occur when a fly is disturbed while feeding on an infected person and feeds on another susceptible person, but this is not an important type of transmission in Gambian fever. The point to be made here is that the cyclic development in the tsetse must be completed before transmission can occur.

Upon feeding, a fly carrying metacyclic trypomastigotes injects them with the salivary fluid into the skin of the person. The trypomastigotes remain in the serum and lymph where they multiply by binary fission. The slender forms in the bloodstream (Figs. 3.6, 3.9) multiply by binary fission; as time passes, stumpy forms begin to appear. The stumpy trypomastigotes do not divide and have prepared to enter the tsetse for transmission again.

The change in form from the trypomastigote to the epimastigotes and back in the vector seems due, in part, to changes in the mitochondrion. In the mammal, slender forms are seen early in infections; the slender forms are those that multiply by binary fission. Later, stumpy forms predominate (Figs. 3.6, 3.9) and they do not divide. The slender forms have what appear to be nonfunctional mitochondria (Fig. 3.7), and this is borne out by the fact that they have aerobic glycolysis, a type of respiration in which metabolism of glucose is incomplete. In the case of the slender trypomastigotes, glucose is broken down to pyruvate and no further; the rest of the Krebs cycle is lacking. A unique feature of kinetoplastids is that glycolysis takes place in an organelle called a glycosome. In all other eukaryotes, glycolysis occurs in the cytosol. Respiration is cyanide insensitive, indicating that cytochromes are lacking. Cytochromes serve in passing electrons through the elements of the Krebs cycle.

In culture forms, which correspond to epimastigotes in the vector, there is a well-developed mitochondrion extending posteriorly as well as anteriorly from the kinetoplast (Fig. 3.7). Epimastigotes have the complete Krebs cycle enzymes and oxidize glucose completely. They are also cyanide sensitive.

Two forms are intermediate between slender trypomastigotes and epimastigotes:stumpy trypomastigotes in the mammal and metacyclic trypomastigotes in the vector. The mitochondrion of the stumpy form develops tubular cristae seemingly in preparation for being picked up by a feeding tsetse. The metacyclic trypomastigote has a mitochondrion that is smaller and has less internal surface. The implication is that the metacyclic forms are preparing to reenter the mammal.

The change in the mitochondrion is a response to the environment in which the organism finds itself. In the mammal, the trypomastigotes have an almost inexhaustible source of energy and other nutrients. Blood is a rich, complex medium and its constituents remain fairly constant. In a sense, the trypomastigotes have no need to be frugal with their sources of energy. They can maintain only a relatively simple system, which allows them to split glucose to pyruvate and return the pyruvate to the bloodstream where it can be utilized by other body cells or recycled back to glucose. In the fly, on the other hand, the ecosystem is more limited. There is a need to be frugal with energy sources, and complete oxidation of carbohydrate, or other energy sources, is necessary.

The second issue relates to the ability of only metacyclic trypomastigotes to infect a mammal. The epimastigotes in the gut of the tsetse are incapable of establishing in the bloodstream of a mammal. Significantly, the stumpy bloodstream forms are also incapable of being passed by syringe from mammal to mammal as the slender forms can be. In the case of the metacyclic trypomastigotes in the vector, the crux of survival in the mammal is the production of a protective coat. The coat can clearly be seen as a layer 15 nm thick covering both the body and the flagellar sheath of the bloodstream forms (Fig. 3.7). The culture forms, on the other hand, are completely free of such a covering. There is a sequence of development in which the epimastigotes multiply and then begin to form nonmultiplying, metacyclic trypomastigotes, which prepare to reenter a mammal by producing a protective glycoprotein coat.

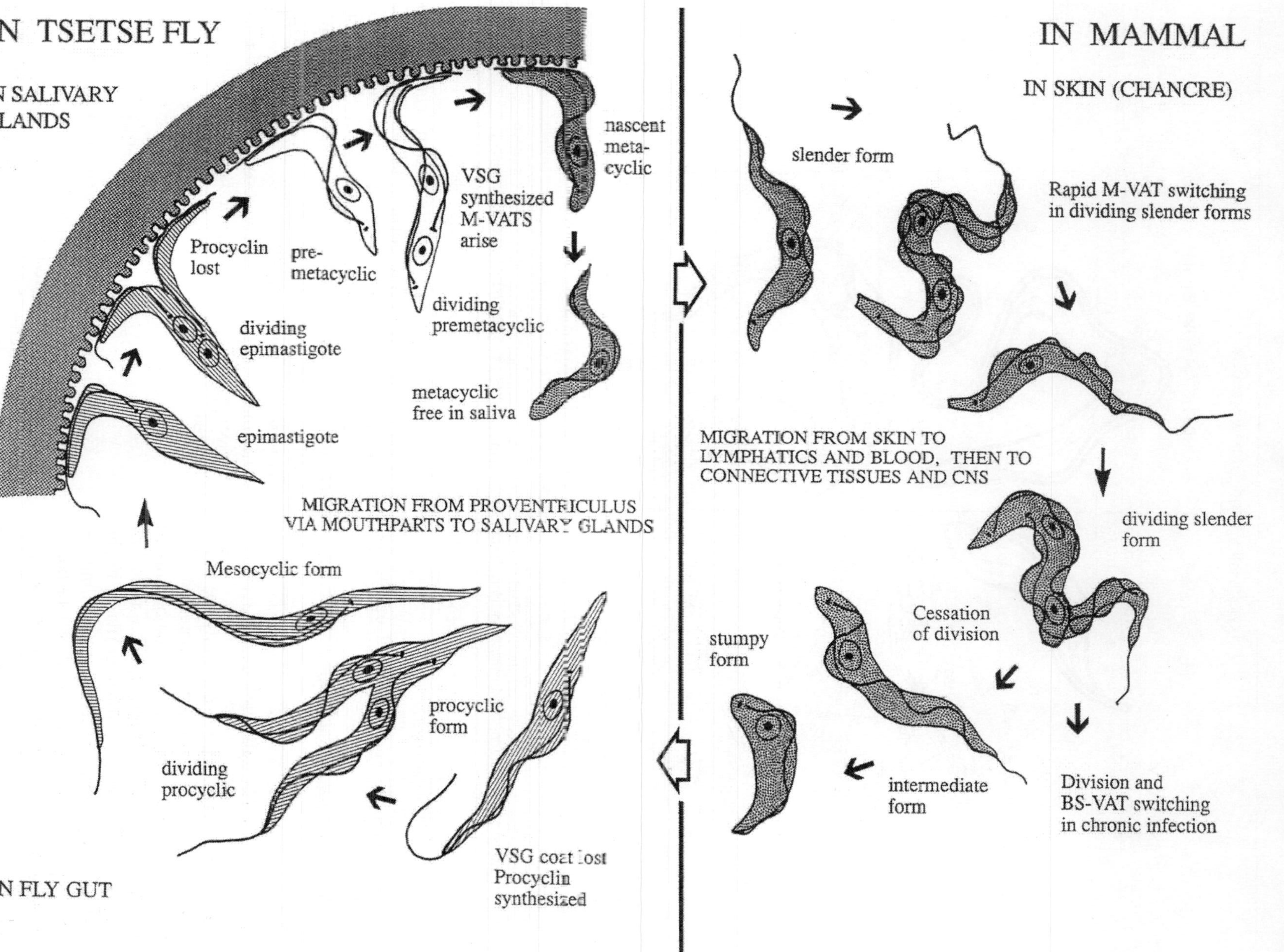

FIGURE 3.6 Change in the body form of *Trypanosoma brucei* during its life cycle. [From Vickerman, K., 1971. Morphological and physiological considerations of extracellular blood protozoa. In A. M. Fallis (ed.), Ecology and Physiology of Parasites. Univ. of Toronto Press, Toronto.]

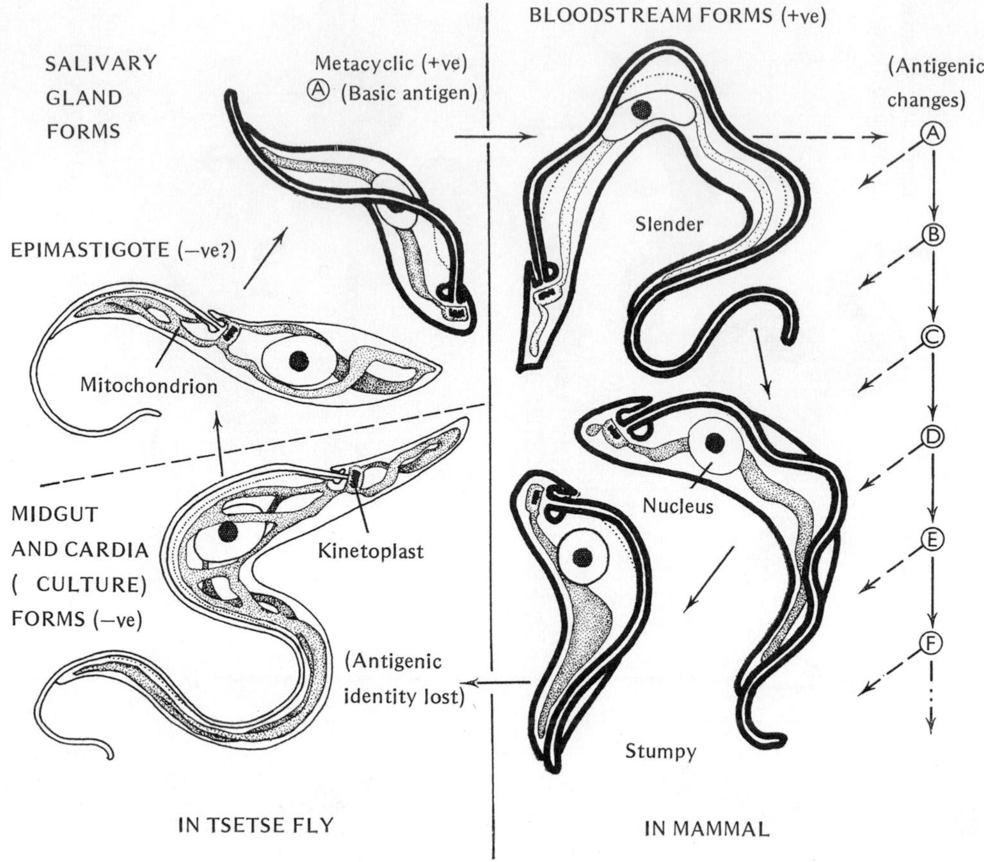

FIGURE 3.7 Diagram of the life cycle of *Trypanosoma brucei* showing cyclical changes in the surface coat, surface antigens, and mitochondrion. [From Vickerman, K., 1969. © The Company of Biologists.]

Diagnosis

Diagnosis of trypanosomosis is based on the following:

1. Clinical signs and symptoms
2. Medical history
3. Finding the organism
4. Finding antibodies through serology

In classroom exercises, students usually see blood films with large numbers of trypomastigotes on them and are likely to conclude that finding the organisms in a stained blood film is a simple, reliable means of determining whether a host is infected. Early in the disease, trypomastigotes are readily found in the peripheral blood, but later in the disease it may be necessary to examine lymph nodes, bone marrow, or cerebrospinal fluid.

Indirect means diagnosis include animal inoculation and cultivation. Laboratory rats are susceptible to infection, but other laboratory animals may also be used. Various culture media, both liquid and solid, can be used in cultivation of trypanosomes.

Once an organism has been found in a stained blood film or in culture, it is important to identify it. Because certain trypanosomes have broad host ranges, it should not be assumed that finding one in the blood of a person or animal means that it is a normal inhabitant of that host. The criteria given earlier in this chapter are used in identification.

Some serological tests have been developed for diagnosis of trypanosomosis, but they are of limited usefulness.

Host–Parasite Interactions

Gambian sleeping sickness is almost invariably fatal within two to about seven years after the disease is first seen if left untreated. The disease progresses intermittently in such a way that the affected person lapses into longer and longer periods of drowsiness or coma.

The first signs of infection are swelling at the site where the tsetse fed, fever, and swollen lymph nodes; this phase of the disease is sometimes absent in native Africans. These early signs, which may be seen starting a few days to several weeks after infection, are followed by a period of one to two years in which there is intermittent fever, headache, and swollen lymph nodes (Fig. 3.8), spleen, and liver. As time passes, muscular weakness and emaciation become evident. At two to three years after infection, drowsiness begins and there are longer and longer periods when the person is half awake, asleep, or actually unconscious. Irreversible coma and death ensue. During the latter stages of the disease, there may be psychopathologies and convulsions.

In Rhodesian sleeping sickness caused by *T. b. rhodesiense,* the reservoirs of infection are wild ruminants such as the bushbuck, and the organism is highly pathogenic for humans. Roughly the same sequence of events takes place as in Gambian fever, but the disease is acute rather than chronic; the person usually dies within six months to a year after onset.

T. b. gambiense is the cause of the peridomestic form of the disease and that it probably was derived from *T. b. rhodeiense* and has become less pathogenic through its association with humans. Although it still causes death, *T. b. gambiense* is said to be on its way toward developing a commensal relationship with its human host. For example, there is an instance in which an African woman was known to carry an infection of *T. b. gambiense* for seven years with little detrimental effect observed.

T. b. brucei and *T. congolense* cause nagana in cattle, and the pathogenesis is much the same as that caused by the related organisms in humans. Once an animal begins to show clinical signs, the disease progresses rapidly and the animal usually dies within a few weeks. Large ruminants that become seriously ill lie down and they must be gotten onto their feet and made to move around, or pooling of blood on the lower side of the animal causes collapse of the circulatory system within a day or so. Cattle therefore do not suffer the long course of disease seen in humans because once they are down for a day or two, death quickly follows.

During the early phase of infection, the trypanosomes remain in the skin of the host and reproduce there. Within a few weeks they reach the circulating blood and the lymph nodes. In the later stages, corresponding with the neurologic involvement, the organisms are found in the cerebrospinal fluid and other tissue spaces and between cells in the brain. The signs and symptoms of infections as well as the tissue changes seen in the disease have been well described for many years, but the mechanisms by which the organisms damage the host are just now coming to light.

Early in the disease most of the changes are seen in the lymph system. When the trypanosomes invade the central nervous system, there is evidence of inflammation of the central nervous system. How these changes are brought about has been the subject of considerable study. As is true with all scientific investigations, theories have been made and discarded several times.

The immunogenicity of the parasite and the response of the host are of considerable importance in various aspects of the disease complex in (1) pathogenesis, (2) in preparing the parasite to survive in the

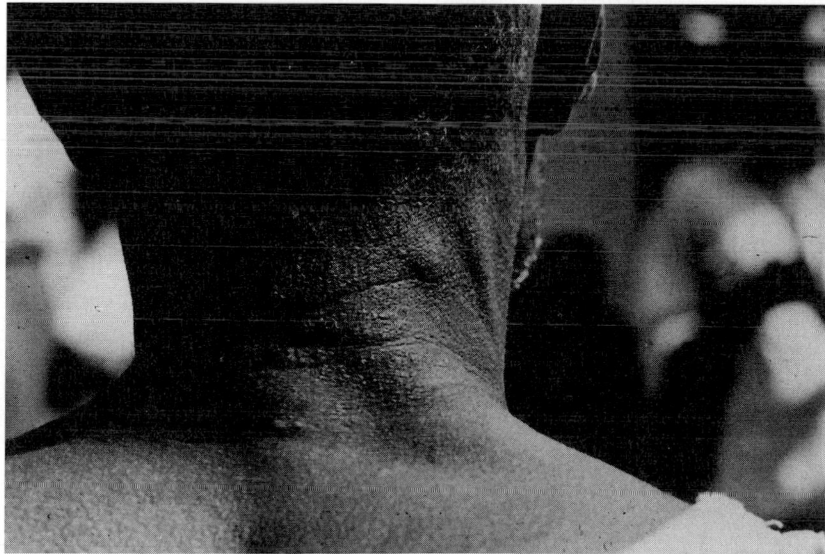

FIGURE 3.8 Winterbottom's sign, swelling of the cervical lymph nodes; an early sign of trypanosomosis in humans. [Courtesy U.S. Armed Forces Institute of Pathology, Negative No. 74-8337.]

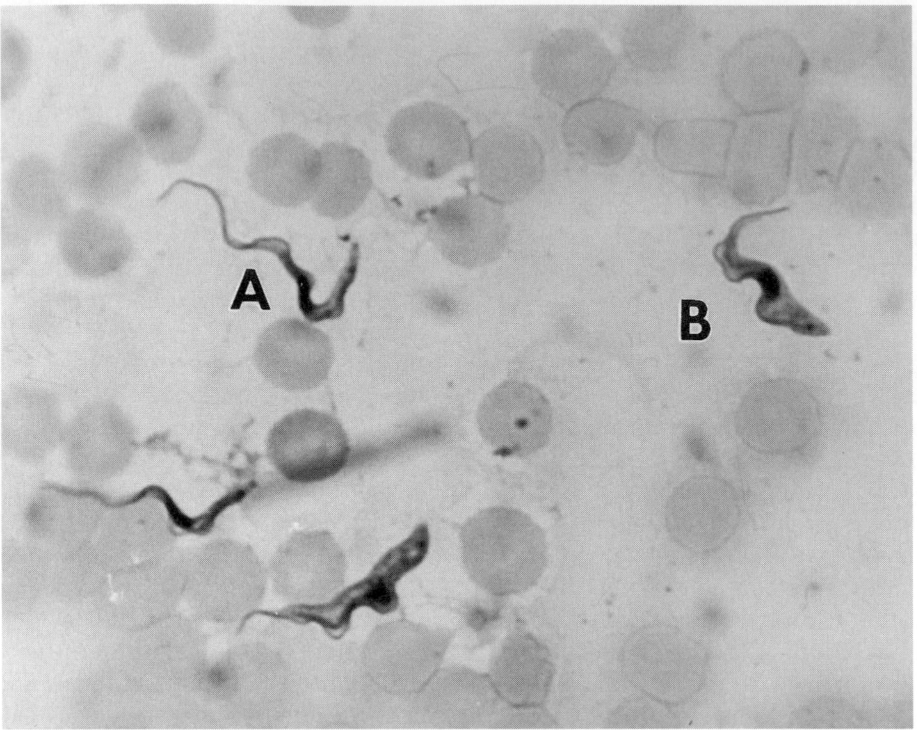

FIGURE 3.9 A stained blood film made from a person infected with *Trypanosoma brucei gambiense*. Note the slender form (A), which is the dividing stage, and the stumpy form (B), which is the stage which develops within the tsetse.

vertebrate, and (3) in the constant struggle of both the host and the parasite to survive.

As noted in the discussion of the life cycle, the metacyclic trypomastigote is the only form that is infective when a tsetse bites a mammal. The metacyclic trypomastigotes bear a glycoprotein coat that protects it from the immune response of the host. The parasite requires the glycoprotein coat for entrance and early survival in the mammal, but it has developed additional mechanisms for continued survival and reproduction in the long term. Superficially there is a fairly regular rise and fall in the parasitemia.

Each time there is a resurgence in the number of organisms, the protein coat is different (Fig. 3.7). In Figure 3.7, the sequence of A → B → C → D → E and so on, indicates that upon introduction of metacyclic trypomastigotes into a mammal by a tsetse the sequence of antigenic variants can be predicted with some degree of certainty. Passing the organism through a tsetse resets the sequence to type A, but if organisms are passed by syringe, they continue to produce different antigenic variants. Antigenic variaton is not unique to the kinetoplastids. It has been observed in *Borrelia* spp. that cause relapsing fever, and in malaria, to an extent.

Because the trypanosomes continually shift their surface antigens, natural immunity does little to control the infection. Likewise, producing an artificial vaccine has not yet been completely successful.

Epidemiology and Control

The tsetse-borne trypanosomoses can be discussed as a group whether one is concerned with human or animal infections. There are some differences between the details of the methods employed against human or animal infections, but the principles are the same.

Control programs are based on the following:

1. Tsetse control
2. Reservoir host control
3. Chemotherapy and chemoprophylaxis
4. Behavioral change in the vertebrate hosts

Bruce's report in 1895 showed the link between trypanosomes and tsetse. The transmission experiments that he performed in that year showed that tsetse transmitted trypanosomes to domestic animals, and this laid the basis for rational control of the trypanosomoses. Since that time, the greatest effort in control and eradication programs have been focused on reducing or eliminating populations of tsetse. Because of inadequate chemotherapeutic drugs and problems with immunity, as discussed earlier, the vector has been considered to be the best target for control.

The elements that must be coordinated are as follows:

1. Selective clearing of trees and brush
2. Application of insecticide
3. Control of land use—that is, farming and grazing practices

Because tsetse do not fly far nor migrate rapidly, a first step in a control program is containment. This is done by clearing all trees and brush in a band of 2 km (1 mile). Such a barrier prevents the flies from moving to a new area. Then, if a riverine species such as *G. morsitans* were the vector, the area would be cleared of brush and low-growing plants for a distance of about 10 m from the water's edge. This allows the ground to dry out so that pupae die and resting sites of the adults are eliminated. Finally, insecticides can be applied from a backpack sprayer to kill the remaining flies. In the early days of second generation insecticides, DDT was sprayed over wide areas from both the ground and the air; such an approach was wasteful and selective application to the areas where the adults rest is a more frugal and effective approach.

Land use is an important aspect of control in that once an area has been cleared of tsetse habitat, it should not be allowed to return to its former state. It should be kept in crops or grazed periodically by livestock so that it remains in grass and small forbs. Where all of these steps are taken and the area is monitored periodically to ensure that flies have not returned, the risk of infection to humans or livestock becomes minimal.

Where risk of infection remains, the human or livestock population must be monitored to detect new clinical cases and to institute treatment immediately. During the time of continued transmission, it may be necessary to administer drugs to either the human or animal populations on a prophylactic basis. If an area is made relatively safe, the major tasks are then to maintain surveillance and reporting systems and to exclude immigration of vectors or infected animals.

Chemotherapy has long been a part of the arsenal in control programs, but the toxicity and efficacy of drugs have not been satisfactory. Best current estimates are that about 200 persons die annually from sleeping sickness in Africa. Many areas have been made risk-free for human habitation. As far as livestock are concerned, the risks remain significant, but certain areas now utilized by cattle that were formerly too hazardous to occupy; however, surveillance must be maintained.

Finally, the question needs to be addressed whether eradication of the trypanosomoses of large ruminants is possible, or even desirable. If efforts were concentrated on eliminating all tsetse from the African continent, trypanosomosis would disappear. Even if it were possible, would eradication be a blessing? It has been proposed that control of trypanosomosis in cattle has allowed an increase in the population of cattle to the point where the Sahel of western Africa is overgrazed and contributed to drought conditions that have had catastrophic effects on millions of people in that area.

In another vein , Duggan (in Mulligan & Potts, 1970) put trypanosomosis in perspective on the dilemma and ethics of disease control:

> It is clear that the problem of trypanosomiasis in domesticated animals is now of far greater concern than human infection to the health and prosperity of Africa. Its biological complexity is vast, its physical extent is only vaguely defined and its significance is almost immeasurable. The burden of sleeping sickness in the 1930s was but thistledown in comparison the leaden weight of this gigantic land.
>
> It may seem necessary to change the face of rural Africa before the scourge is eliminated, yet as Barzun reminds us, there is no use struggling to save a world in which one would find it hell to live when saved. An Africa without game, tsetse and trypanosomes could turn a noble ambition to dust, for they are the guardians of the land. Overzealous guardians they may be, but their too peremptory dismissal from the scene could permit improvidence and exploitation on a ruinous scale.
>
> The biological complex of trypanosomiasis is in deep and mortal relationship with the life of Africa; to sever this relationship would be to change the bionomics of half a continent. It seems more commendable to leave the relationship alone, simply to thwart the undesirable effects of its progression by methods which anticipate its own beneficent destiny.

AMERICAN TRYPANOSOMOSIS—CHAGAS' DISEASE

Name of Organism and Disease Association

Trypanosoma cruzi (syn. *Schizotrypanum cruzi*), causes Chagas' disease or American trypanosomosis or trypanosomiasis. A person affected by the infection is referred to as a *chagasic patient.*

Hosts and Host Range

Humans are the primary concern here, but the normal hosts include many species of wild mammals. The armadillo, *Dasypus*, is the most important reservoir in some areas, and in other localities, rodents such as the wood rat, *Neotoma,* and carnivores such as the dog, cat, and raccoon serve as important reservoirs. The host range includes domestic animals.

Bugs (Hemiptera, Reduviidae, Triatominae) of the genera *Triatoma, Rhodnius,* and *Panstrongylus* are the vectors (Chapter 45). These insects are known as triatomins, kissing bugs, and cone-nosed bugs, among others.

Geographic Distribution and Importance

Chagas' disease or American trypanosomosis is a zoonosis that affects more than 15 million people in the Western Hemisphere, mostly in South America. The disease is enzootic throughout Latin America with the exception of Guyana and the Caribbean islands (Fig. 3.10). Almost 89 million people are at risk of infection, more than 24% of the total population. Only a few autochthonous cases are known from the United States, and the observed clinical effects have been milder than those seen in infections acquired farther south.

In the United States, *T. cruzi* is generally limited to the southern states, but it has been found as far north as Maryland on the east coast and a human case has been diagnosed in northern California. The organism is enzootic in woodrats in the Los Angeles area. A survey of 500 people in the lower Rio Grande Valley of Texas showed a prevalence of infection of 2.4% by serology.

The magnitude of the problem is seen in the areas of highest prevalence in South America. Of a population of 54 million in enzootic countries, 11.3 million (6.2%) are known to be infected. Many of these people live in poverty or near poverty, and their houses are constructed so as to become nests of the vectors. The greatest prevalences of infection are found in Chile (12.5%) and Paraguay (11.9%); Argentina and Bolivia are not far behind with prevalence rates exceeding 8%.

In urban areas, *T. cruzi* seems to be spread mainly

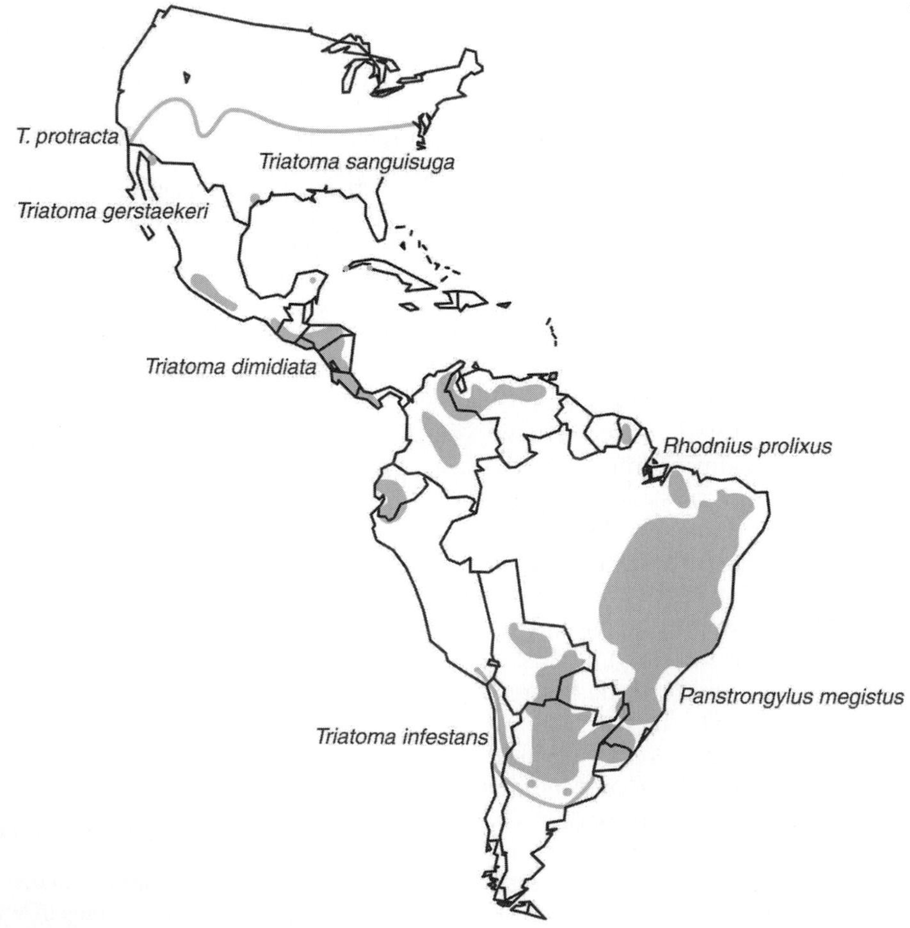

FIGURE 3.10 The distribution of *Trypanosoma cruzi* in the Western Hemisphere and of some of its vectors.

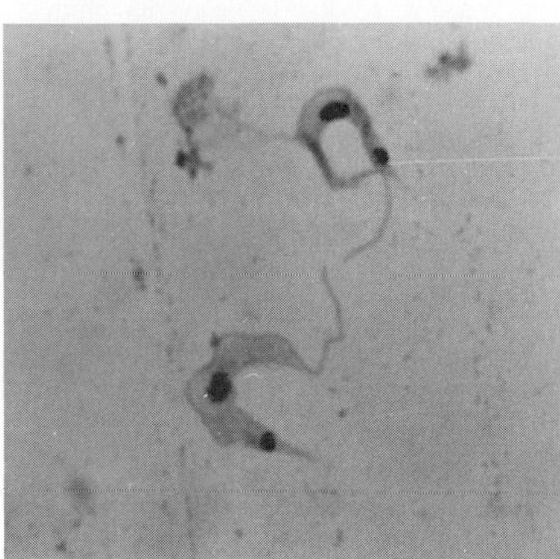

FIGURE 3.11 Trypomastigotes of *Trypanosoma cruzi* as seen in a stained film in the light microscope.

by blood transfusions. For example, in Argentina and Brazil, between 6 and 20% of blood donors are seropositive for the infection; more shocking is the figure of as many as 63% being seropositive in Bolivia. In 1989 it was found that at least three cases of Chagas' disease in the United States were caused by patients being given contaminated blood. There may be as many as 50,000 infected immigrants in the United States, but routine screening for antibodies to *T. cruzi* is not done.

Morphology

Trypomastigotes in the blood are 16 to 20 μm in length and generally they lie in a C-shape in a stained blood film. The kinetoplast is large and subterminal (Fig. 3.11). The amastigotes (Fig. 3.12) are from 1.5 to 4 μm but are generally toward the upper end of the size range. There is a large nucleus and a kinetoplast, but little else can be seen in LM.

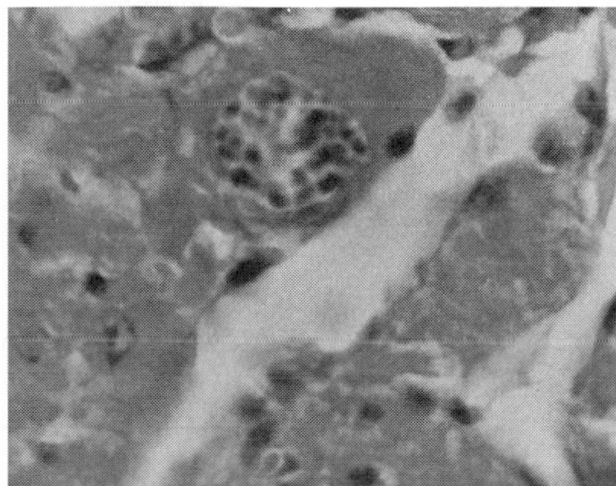

FIGURE 3.12 Amastigotes of *Trypanosoma cruzi* in the heart muscle as seen in a tissue section under LM.

Life Cycle

Small numbers of trypomastigotes circulate in the blood of the mammalian host. The organisms are picked up by kissing bugs (Fig. 45.2) during blood feeding. The organisms multiply as epimastigotes in the midgut and hindgut of the insect. One to two weeks after infection, depending on temperature, metacyclic trypomastigotes appear in the hindgut and the infection can then be transmitted back to another mammal (Fig. 3.13).

T. cruzi is a stercorarian trypanosome and is transmitted through fecal contamination. While taking a blood meal kissing bugs swell dramatically and tend to defecate; a species that is a good vector often defecates as feeding ends. The fecal droplet of an infected bug may contain thousands of metacyclic trypomastigotes. The trypomastigotes gain entry into the mammal when it scratches or rubs them into the skin, or they enter the mucous membranes of the eye, mouth, or nose. Studies in laboratory animals show that the organisms cannot enter the unbroken skin, but they readily establish when applied to a mucous membrane.

Upon regaining a mammalian host, the trypomastigotes may remain in the bloodstream for a time, but they do not multiply there. They invade cells of the reticuloendothelial system (RES or MPS) and skeletal and cardiac muscle cells, among other tissues. Multiplication is by binary fission in the amastigote form. As host cells break down, some organisms are released into the bloodstream. These free organisms transform into trypomastigotes in the bloodstream and are available to be picked up when a kissing bug feeds on the host. Trypomastigotes do not multiply in the bloodstream.

Diagnosis

Determining whether a persons is infected with *T. cruzi* is based on the following:

1. Examining a blood film or tissue fluid
2. Cultivating blood in a non-living medium or in cell culture
3. Performing xenodiagnosis
4. Inoculating laboratory animals
5. Conducting serologic tests for antibodies
6. Observing clinical signs and symptoms

Although trypomastigotes circulate in the bloodstream of the mammalian host, they occur in only small numbers except during the early, acute phase of the infection. The probability of finding *T. cruzi* by examining a stained blood film is quite low during the chronic phase of the infection in humans and in reservoir hosts.

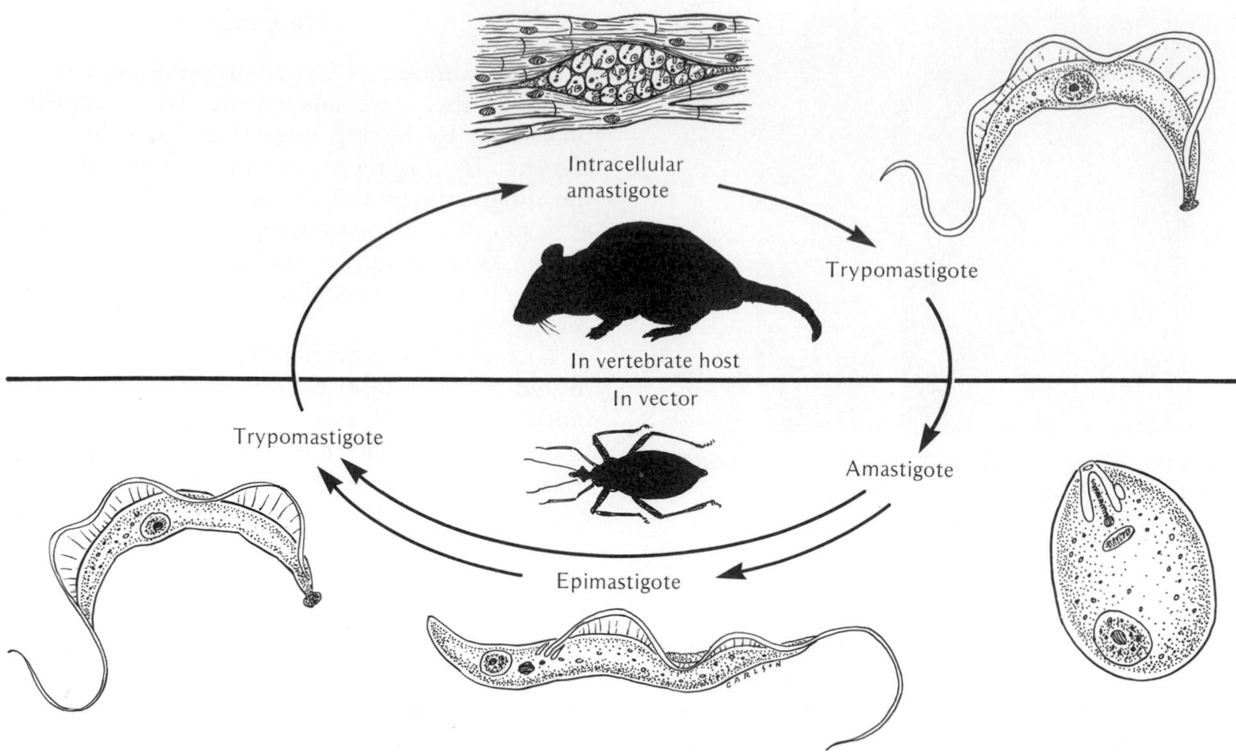

FIGURE 3.13 Diagram of the life cycle of *Trypanosoma cruzi.*

Other direct means of finding amastigotes are to examine the lesion at the site of entry, the juice of lymph nodes, or bone marrow.

T. cruzi grows in a variety of media and in tissue culture. Cultivation has a 35 to 50% probability of finding a positive patient. Xenodiagnosis has a 70% or greater probability of finding a positive infection. Laboratory-raised, uninfected triatomins are allowed to feed on a person suspected of being infected. The protocol calls for 40 3rd instar *Triatoma infestans* to feed simultaneously on the patient. After 30 to 60 days the bugs are squeezed gently and a droplet of feces is collected in physiological salt solution. The droplet is examined under a compound microscope for epimastigotes. The bugs can also be dissected and organisms looked for in the hindgut. Another kinetoplastid, *Blastocrithidia triatomae,* has been found in the intestine of *T. infestans,* and laboratory technicians need to be able to differentiate between the two species. It has been found that the vectors and disease agent from a particular location are adapted to one another and the probability of determining whether a person is positive is increased by using local bugs. Laboratory rodents such as mice and guinea pigs are susceptible to infection; puppies and kittens can also be used, but are costly.

As a general rule, *T. cruzi* elicits a high titer of antibodies that can be measured by a variety of tests. In some tests, up to 90% accuracy is achieved in determining whether an infection has taken place. Although the antibody titer is likely to be higher in the acute phase of the disease and shortly thereafter, it is not always possible to differentiate between a recent infection and one of long standing. Interpretation of positive tests also requires keeping in mind that other organisms such a *Leishmania* spp, *T. rangeli,* and *T. minasense* may cross-react with *T. cruzi* antigens.

A characteristic sign of early infection is swelling around the eye, Romaña's sign (Fig. 3.14). This swelling is not always seen, but is a good indication of Chagas' disease when it is.

Host–Parasite Interactions

T. cruzi multiplies within cells of the vertebrate host in the amastigote form. It forms nests of amastigotes (Fig. 3.12) that can be found in sections of tissue studied at the LM level. On occasion, infected cells break down releasing amastigotes, which then transform into trypomastigotes and they, in turn, infect additional cells.

Chagas' disease occurs in two forms, acute and chronic. The acute form is seen most often in children and it is a rapidly developing disease. Chronic disease

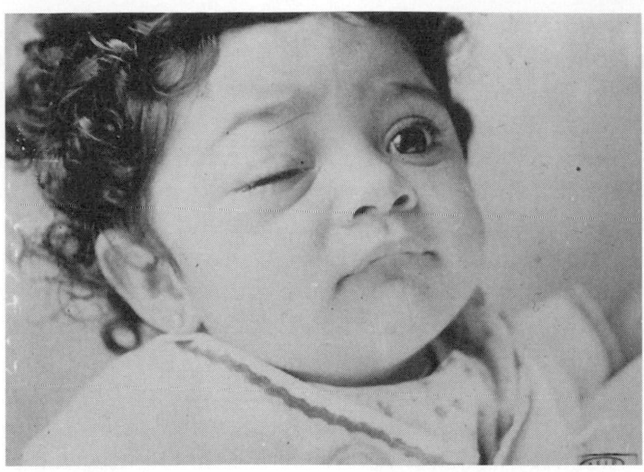

FIGURE 3.14 Romaña's sign; the girl's right eye is swollen shut probably from entrance of *T. cruzi* in or near the eye. [Courtesy of the U.S. Armed Forces Institute of Pathology. Negative No. 62-3934-6]

occurs in adults and is represented by a long-term decline in health.

In children, the organisms multiply in fat cells under the skin early in the infection, and then they spread to muscle cells and to leucocytes. As cells break down from distension with amastigotes, the organisms are carried throughout the body. A wide spectrum of cells is invaded: skeletal and cardiac muscle, lymphoid tissue, bone marrow, nervous tissue, intestine, and endocrine glands. Death occurs within a few weeks or months after onset.

Damage to the host in chronic Chagas' disease comes not so much from rupture of infected cells but rather by toxins that are produced by the amastigotes. Even though organs in many parts of the body are infected, two major systems are most affected: the intestinal tract and the heart. It appears that the organisms release a toxin that acts in the vicinity of a nest of amastigotes. It is a neurotoxin that affects the conducting systems in either the intestinal tract or the heart. The long-term effect, which may require many years to become a serious health problem, is that the muscle cells lose their ability to contract. In the intestinal tract, two conditions are most often seen: megesophagus and megacolon. The smooth muscle cells do not contract as they normally would in peristalsis and the intestinal contents are not moved along. There is difficulty in swallowing when the esophagus is affected and in evacuating the colon when the large intestine is affected. In the heart, the muscle fails to contract normally because of the effect on the bundle of His, and the cells become stretched. As a consequence, the heart becomes enlarged and increasingly less efficient in pumping blood. Heart failure is the eventual outcome.

An infected person develops antibodies to *T. cruzi*, and immunity seems to have some effect on the organism. However, the immunity is insufficient to clear the host of the organism although it does inhibit their multiplication and slows the course of the disease. Studies of immunity to *T. cruzi* have ultimately been directed toward the development of a vaccine, but one has not yet been found that is adequately efficient.

Epidemiology and Control

Control of Chagas' disease is based on the following:

1. Chemotherapy
2. Control of triatomins through source reduction and insecticides
3. Personal protection against triatomins
4. Reduction of populations of reservoir hosts

Two drugs are used with some efficacy early in an infection with *T. cruzi*, but they are ineffective later in the infection. The lack of effective chemotherapy or means of artificial immunization places the emphasis of control of Chagas' disease on prevention, and the major effort is directed toward vector control. Chagas' disease is primarily rural and associated with poverty. Where living standards are low, housing is poor, and given the opportunity, certain species of triatomins move into houses.

It is interesting to note that Chagas' disease was not known to the indigenous peoples of Central and South America. Triatomins have certainly been present in the Western Hemisphere for eons, and it seems likely that they have transmitted *T. cruzi* among animals for much of that time. However, in Brazil, it seems that the insects have colonized homes only during the past 100 years. Native peoples do not have names for the bugs, and there is no evidence of triatomins in primitive huts. Likewise, there is no evidence of infection with *T. cruzi* in these native people.

Carlos Chagas first described not only the organism and its natural cycle, but also the clinical aspects of the disease early in the 20th century. Brazilian scientists have been at the forefront of investigations on Chagas' disease, and their studies led to the conclusion that changes in land use and colonization of areas not previously occupied by many people caused an interface between the enzootic cycle and humans.

In the 19th century there was aggressive expansion of agriculture, especially coffee plantations. Expanding populations moved into these areas and established farms. Houses usually consist of clay and wattle,

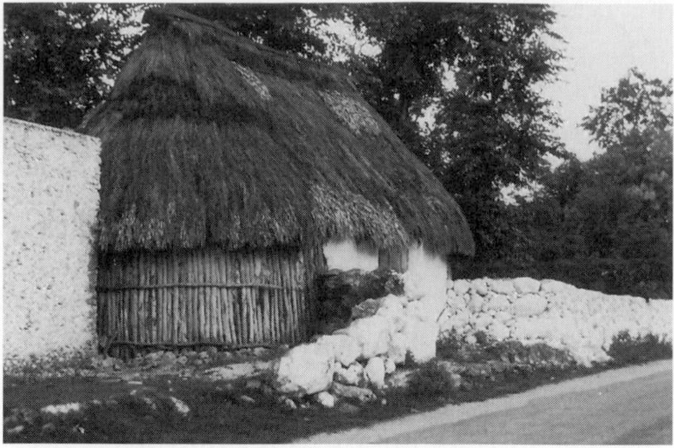

FIGURE 3.15 A Meso-American house typical of rural areas. The thatched roof and poorly plastered walls provide resting places for triatomins.

thatch, or adobe, or combinations thereof (Fig. 3.15). Many provide habitat for triatomins.

Triatomins live in a variety of habitats. Some live underground with burrowing rodents while others are associated with tree-dwelling vertebrates such as birds, bats, and small primates. Given the opportunity, certain species, as indicated, will move in with humans if suitable hiding places and a ready source of blood are available.

Kissing bugs typically remain in cracks, behind pictures, or in the thatched roof of the house during the day, and they come out at night to seek blood. Often animal enclosures are attached to rural houses; these structures are made of tightly woven sticks and brush or of rock. Both materials provide hiding places for bugs and they come out to feed when animals sleep lying next to the wall. Those that live inside the house are usually found in the bedrooms.

A relatively high percentage of bugs may be infected with *T. cruzi* in enzootic areas. In Central America, for example, the following rates of infection were found in more than 20,000 triatomins examined:

Country	*Species*	*% Positive*
Costa Rica	*Triatoma dimidiata*	30.9
El Salvador	*Rhodnius prolixus*	13.6
	T. dimidiata	30.8
Guatemala	*R. prolixus*	23.4
	T. dimidiata	34.7
Honduras	*T. dimidiata*	32.2
Nicaragua	*R. prolixus*	9.6
	T. dimidiata	39.0
Panama	*R. pallescens*	32.7

In a survey in Brazil in which more than 750,000 triatomins were examined, infections were found to be quite a bit lower than in Central America: *Triatoma infestans*, 8.7%, *T. brasiliensis*, 6.7%, *T. melanocephala*, 5.2%, *Panstrongylus lutzi*, 4.1%, *P. megistus*, 3.4%, *T. sordida*, 2.2%.

In several studies in Central America, more than 2400 rural houses were examined for triatomins and between 19.3% and 53.9% were found to be infested. In El Salvador from 2.0 to 5.4 bugs were found, on the average, in various kinds of rural houses. In another study in South America, 8500 bugs were found in a single mud house.

A serologic study done in rural areas of Brazil over the period of 1975 to 1981 showed that about 5 million persons are infected with *T. cruzi*; this figure was obtained by an average prevalence of all the states at 4.2%. The highest prevalences were in the southern coastal states of Mina Gerais and Rio Grande de Sul at 8.8%.

Some problems occur in urban areas as well as in rural ones. Two situations are of concern: (1) vectors carried to urban areas by migrants, and (2) blood donors. It has been found that small foci of triatomins occur in some poorer urban areas, and seemingly transmission of Chagas' disease takes place. However, these areas are not considered to be important in the overall epidemiology of the disease.

Blood donors are a potential source of infection, and perhaps 25% of donors in South America are infected. The migration of people from rural to urban areas has increased the risk of transmission through blood. Furthermore, migration of people from Latin America to North America raises the threat of Chagas' disease coming about through blood transfusions. It is known that three cases of the disease have been caused in the United States through blood transfusions.

The first steps, then are to eliminate, as best one can, the places where bugs rest during the daytime. Plastering walls, pouring concrete floors, and replacing thatch with metal roofs all reduce bug populations. Religious pictures and photographs from magazines are often tacked to walls, and these provide places for the bugs in the daytime; one might stick down the edges with cellophane tape to keep bugs out.

Screening doors and windows keep bugs out of the house. Nymphs walk in and adults fly in, so the windows and doors need to be tight. There are problems in this area, however, expense, and the discomfort of a tropical climate. Screening is expensive for those living as subsistence farmers, or day laborers. Also, a hot, humid climate leaves one wishing for a cool breeze at night, and screens are often avoided for that reason.

Various insecticides have been and are used to bug control. These are effective when sprayed in a dwelling.

Dogs, particularly, may be allowed the run of houses in rural areas, and they are often infected with *T. cruzi*. Cats are infected, too, but at a much lower rate than dogs and probably are much less important as reservoirs. Domestic animals kept near the house are also sources of infection, except for swine, which seem to have a consistently low prevalence of infection. It is difficult to know what to suggest for dogs and cats; they are important to the people and eliminating them is probably not feasible. In the case of animals kept in pens at the house, the type of enclosure can be altered so that it is less attractive as a place for bugs to rest during the daytime. Pens can also be sprayed with insecticide.

Since wild rodents are often sources of infection, rodent control in and near houses should reduce the probability of human contact with them through the vectors. The zoological garden that develops in a thatched roof has many members, rodents, birds, and reptiles that feed bugs. A metal roof removes that hazard.

Personal protection involves avoiding bugs through bed netting, and isolating the bed in other ways. Properly used bed nets protect the sleeper from triatomins and mosquitoes quite well. Again, netting reduces the circulation of air, and it may be difficult to institute them in a hot climate.

RELATED ORGANISMS

Trypanosomes of rodents have been studied by many investigators as models of host–parasite interactions in economically and medically important kinetoplastids. Two of those that have been investigated most are *Trypanosoma lewisi* of the rat and *T. duttoni* of the mouse. Both can be maintained in the laboratory by periodic passage to clean animals via syringe.

T. lewisi (Fig. 3.4n) is a stercorarian trypanosome, which is transmitted by the flea, *Ceratophyllus fasciatus*, among others. The protistan can be found frequently in wild rats, and is obtainable from a number of commercial sources for research or classroom purposes. The importance of *T. lewisi* lies in the elucidation of immune mechanisms that have significance not only for trypanosomes but for immunology in general. As early as the 1920s it was found that upon introduction into a clean rat, there was an increase in the number of trypomastigotes in the bloodstream for about ten days. At this time, the numbers dropped precipitously nearly to the baseline, and then in about another ten days, there was a second increase in parasitemia and then another drop to the point where organisms were difficult to find in the blood. William H. Taliaferro at the University of Chicago studied the mechanism of immunity and found that two different antibodies were involved. The first drop in parasitemia was brought about by an antibody that he called *ablastin*. Ablastin acts by preventing division in trypanosomes. The second increase and fall in parasitemia is brought about by a trypanocidal antibody thereby clearing the host of infection in three weeks or so after initial inoculation.

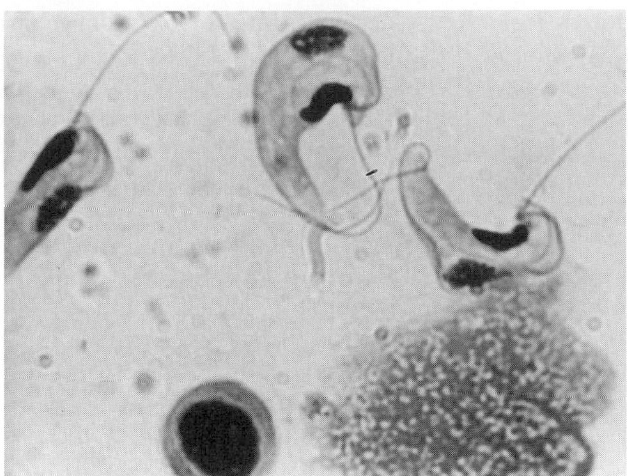

FIGURE 3.16 *Cryptobia salmostica*, a kinetoplastid which is found in the blood of fish. [Photomicrograph courtesy of Dr. P. T. K. Woo, University of Guelph.]

A series of provocative studies was done by Dr. David Lincicome on *T. duttoni* and *T. lewisi* in which he reasoned that a long association of host and parasite would bring about not only tolerance, but an advantage for the host to be infected. It would be advantageous for the parasite to keep its host in good physical condition so that both the host and parasite would live long and ensure their leaving progeny. He found, in fact, that a B vitamin was produced by the trypanosomes, which increased the well-being of the host when it was placed on a B vitamin–deficient diet.

Trypanosoma theileri (Fig. 3.4i) is a parasite of cattle and probably other large ruminants that is found worldwide. The organism occurs in about 20% of cattle in North America. It is transmitted by tabanids (Chapter 47) and may be important economically. There are several reports of cattle which seem to be affected by the infection, but Koch's Postulates have not yet been satisfactorily fulfilled.

Trypanosoma avium is an ill-defined species that is found in birds. Transmission takes place through flies of the dipteran family Hippoboscidae in which the organism replicates. It is interesting to note that replication does not take place in the bird. In fact, if log-phase organisms are inoculated into a bird, the trypanosomes are stopped in mid-division. The same phenomenon of failing to replicate in the vertebrate host is seen in *T. melophagium* of the sheep. This trypanosome is transmitted by *Melophagus ovinum*, also a hippoboscid fly.

Members of the genus *Cryptobia* (family Bodonidae) are found as parasites of many invertebrates and poikilothermic vertebrates. Some are transmitted directly from one host to the next, while others use vectors such as leeches. *Cryptobia salmostica* (Fig. 3.16) is a parasite of salmonid and other fishes and is transmitted by the leech *Piscicola*. It multiplies in the blood of the host and causes anemia, immunosuppression, and death in hosts with a high parasitemia.

Readings

Barry, J. D. (1997). The relative significance of antigenic variation in African trypanosomes. *Parasitol Today* **13,** 212–218.

Barry, J. D., and Turner, C. M. R. (1991). The dynamics of antigenic variation and growth of African trypanosomes. *Parasitol. Today* **7,** 207–211.

Bastin, R., Matthews, K. R., and Gull, K. (1996). The paraflagellar rod of Kinetoplastida: Solved and unsolved questions. *Parasitol. Today* **12,** 302–307.

Bloom, B. R. (1979). Games parasites play: How parasites evade immune surveillance. *Nature* **279,** 21–26.

Boothroyd, J. C. (1990). Molecular biology of trypanosomes. In *Modern Parasite Biology* (D. J. Wyler, Ed.). Freeman, New York.

Brenner, R. R., and de la Merced Stoka, A. (1988). *Chagas' Disease Vectors*, 3 Vols. CRC Press, Boca Raton, FL.

Brenner, Z., and Krettli, A. U. (1990). Immunology of Chagas' disease. In *Modern Parasite Biology* (D. J. Wyler, Ed.). Freeman, New York.

Donelson, J. E., and Turner, M. J. (1985). How the trypanosome changes its coat. *Sci. Am.* **252**(2), 44–51.

Ford, J. (1971). *The Role of Trypanosomiasis in African Ecology*. Clarendon, Oxford.

Hide, G., Mottram, J. C., Coombs, G. H., and Holmes, P. H. (Eds.) (1997). *Trypanosomiasis and Leishmaniasis: Biology and Control*. CAB International, Wallingford, UK.

Hoare, C. A. (1972). *The Trypanosomes of Mammals: A Zoological Monograph*. Blackwell, Oxford.

Imbuga, M. O., Osir, E. O., Labongo, V. L., and Orieno, L. H. (1992). Studies on tsetse midgut factors that induct differentiation of bloodstream *Trypanosoma brucei brucei* in vitro. *Parasitol. Res.* **78,** 10–15.

Jahnke, H. E. (1976). *Tsetse Flies and Livestock Development in East Africa. A Study of Environmental Economics*. Humanities Press, New York.

Jordan, A. M. (1986).*Trypanosomiasis Control and African Rural Development*. Longman, London.

Kingman, S. (1991, October 19). South America declares war on Chagas' disease. *New Scientist*, 16–17.

Mansfield, J. M. (1990). Immunology of African trypanosomes. In *Modern Parasitol Biology* (D. J. Wyler, Ed.). Freeman, New York.

McKelvey, J. J., Jr. (1973). *Man against Tsetse. Struggle for Africa*. Cornell Univ. Press, Ithaca, NY.

Michels, P. A. M., and Opperdoes, F. R. (1991). The evolutionary origin of glycosomes. *Parasitol Today* **7,** 105–109.

Mulligan, H. W., and Potts, W. H. (Eds.) (1970). *The African Trypanosomiases*. Wiley Interscience, New York.

Parthasarthy, M. W., van Slobbe, W. G., and Coudant, C. (1976). Trypanosomatid flagellate in the phloem of diseased coconut palms. *Science* **192,** 1346–1348.

Pereira, M. E. (1990). Cell biology of *Trypanosoma cruzi*. In *Modern Parasite Biology* (D. J. Wyler, Ed.). Freeman, New York.

Salazar-Schettino, P. M., I de Haro Artega, and Uribarren Berrueta, T. (1988). Chagas' disease in Mexico. *Parasitol. Today* **4,** 348–352.

Tait, A., and Turner, C. M. R. (1990). Genetic exchange in *Trypanosoma brucei*. *Parasitol. Today* **6**(3), 70–75.

Turner, M. J., and Donelson, J. E. (1990). Cell biology of African trypanosomes. In *Modern Parasite Biology* (D. J. Wyler, Ed.). Freeman, New York.

Vickerman, K. (1969). On the surface coat and flagellar adhesion in trypanosomes. *J. Cell. Sci.* **5,** 163–169.

Vickerman, K. (1971). Morphological and physiological considerations of extracellular blood protozoa. In *Ecology and Physiology of Parasites* (A. M. Fallis, Ed.). Univ. of Toronto Press, Toronto.

Wakelin, D. (1984). *Immunity to Parasites. How Animals Control Parasitic Infections*. Arnold, Baltimore.

Woo, P. T. K. (1991). Mammalian trypanosomiasis and piscine cryptobiosis in Canada and the United States. *Bull. Soc. Vector Ecol.* **16,** 25–42.

CHAPTER

4

Leishmania and the Leishmanioses

Leishmania spp. cause a complex of infections ranging from localized skin infections of relatively minor importance to generalized systemic disease with a high probability of mortality. Human infections occur worldwide in warm-temperate, subtropical, and tropical areas. Locations where leishmanial infections are important in humans are the Mediterranean, Middle East, Far East, tropical Africa, and Central and South America (Tab. 4.1 and, later, Fig. 4.3). A few infections are contracted in the United States.

The *Leishmania* spp. are kinetoplastids that develop intracellularly as amastigotes (Fig. 4.1) in many species of mammals; *Leishmania* of reptiles are mostly extracellular parasites of the intestinal tract. *Leishmania* occur both as amastigotes (in the vertebrate) and promastigotes (in the vector). Amastigotes are among the smallest parasitic protists; their size range is from 1 to 5 μm, but they usually are about 3 μm. Transmission takes place by blood-sucking insects in the dipteran family Psychodidae, so-called sand flies (Chapter 47).

About 22 species or subspecies of *Leishmania* have been described, half from mammals and half from reptiles. There is some doubt about the taxonomic status of the reptilian leishmanias since they are extracellular and form trypomastigotes in culture. The principal thrust of this chapter relates to leishmanias of mammals, especially those that have been implicated as disease agents of humans.

It is interesting to consider the development of knowledge on the *Leishmania* spp. so as to understand why certain species are currently accepted as valid. At the turn of the 20th century, many infectious diseases and their causative agents were being described; among those found were some protists causing both visceral (spleen and other internal organs) infections and cutaneous infections. These were named *Leishmania donovani* (Laveran and Mesnil, 1903; Ross, 1903), and *L. tropica* (Wright, 1903; Luehe, 1906), respectively. As knowledge progressed, it became clear that the visceral and cutaneous forms intergraded with one another and that there were perhaps 11 clinically distinguishable cutaneous and mucocutaneous forms as well as a number of epidemiologically distinct kinds of visceral leishmaniasis. There was a tendency to give a new name to each organism that caused a distinct clinical or epidemiologic entity; however, in a number of instances the clinical manifestations intergraded with one another. With the development of increasingly sophisticated and precise serological methods, it was shown that there were similarities among *Leishmania* spp., but differences among geographic isolates of what seemed to be the same species.

For a while it seemed appropriate to accept the original two species, but most workers now accept about 16 species. The organisms are nearly identical morphologically, and various characters of the organisms themselves and the diseases they cause have been the bases for establishing species. The basis of classification has moved from these criteria to biochemical characters. It is likely that molecular techniques will be used to further refine both evolution and classification; some of these methods are restriction fragment length poly-

TABLE 4.1 *Leishmania* spp. and the Leishmanioses

Type of Disease	Leishmania	Geographic Location
Visceral		
Kala azar	*L. donovani*	India, China, Russia, Iraq, Sudan, Kenya, Uganda
Infantile kala azar	*L. infantum*	France, Mediterannean Basin
Infantile visceral leishmaniosis	*L. chagasi*	Argentina, Bolivia, Brazil, Colombia, Ecuador, El Salvador, Guadeloupe, Guatemala, Honduras, Martinique, Mexico, Nicaragua, Paraguay, Suriname, United States
Old World Cutaneous Leishmaniosis		
	L. tropica tropica	Mediterannean, Middle East, India, Iran, Russia
Oriental sore	*L. major*	Iran, Russia
	L. tropica complex	Tanzania, Namibia, Senegal
Single sore and diffusa	*L. aethiopica*	Ethiopia, Kenya
New World Cutaneous and Mucocutaneous		
Cutaneous		
Single sore and diffusa	*L. mexicana*	Belize, Colombia, Costa Rica, Dominican Republ., Ecuador, Guatemala, Honduras, Mexico, Panama, United States, Venezuela
	L. amazonensis	Bolivia, Brazil, Colombia, Costa Rica, Ecuador, French Guiana, Panama, Peru, Venezuela
Mucocutaneous		
Espundia	*L. braziliensis*	Brazil, Peru, Ecuador, Bolivia, Venezuela, Paraguay, Colombia
Pian bois	*L. guyanensis*	Guyana, Brazil
Single sore, some lymphatic spread	*L. panamensis*	Panama, Central America, Columbia
Uta	*L. peruviana*	Peru (West of Andes)

morphisms (RFLPs), molecular karyotyping, rRNA gene sequences, and other gene sequences.

VISCERAL LEISHMANIOSIS

Name of Organisms and Disease Associations

Leishmania donovani is the causative agent of visceral leishmaniosis, leishmaniasis, kala azar, Dum-Dum fever, death fever, tropical splenomegaly, and ponos (in Greece).

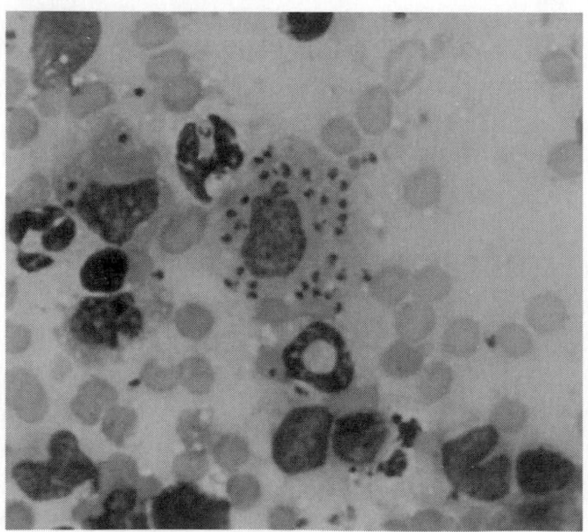

FIGURE 4.1 A light level photomicrograph of amastigotes of *Leishmania* in spleen cells.

Hosts and Host Range

The host range of *L. donovani*, as with most leishmanias, is quite broad including many mammals. With any of the geographic or epidemiologic forms, there is usually one or a few reservoir hosts (Chapter 47); canids (dog, fox, jackal) and sometimes felids (serval) are the principal reservoirs of infection. The sand fly vectors are *Phlebotomus perniciosus*, *P. major*, *P. papatasi*, and *P. longicuspis* in the Mediterranean area; *P. chinensis* and *P. sergenti* in China; *P. orientalis* and *P. martini* in East Africa; and *P. argentipes*. in India.

Geographic Distribution and Importance

Visceral leishmaniosis is widely distributed (Fig. 4.3); it occurs , or is suspected to occur, in 47 countries. Within a geographic area, there is often patchy distribution delimited by proper vector habitat and suitable reservoir hosts.

The World Health Organization (WHO) considers the leishmanioses to be among the six most important infectious diseases of humans worldwide. Despite its acknowledged importance, data on cases are often unreliable, probably on the low side. The reason is that leishmaniosis occurs mostly in rural areas of warm and tropical countries where public health infrastructures are inadequate. In urban endemic foci (Mediterranean, central Asia, Russia, and eastern China) there may be several hundred thousand cases annually.

Hundreds of thousand of cases are estimated to occur annually in India. In Bihar State 50,000 to 60,000 cases are recorded annually, but it is estimated that there are actually 250,000 cases. The disease is a significant problem in Central and South America; in Brazil, for example, of 47,000 persons examined postmortem in connection with a yellow fever study, 0.1% were positive for leishmaniosis.

A few examples how devastating visceral leishmaniosis can be show the impact of the disease. In Sudan a tribe of 3000 persons was reduced to about half from visceral leishmaniosis, the tribal unit was destroyed and the survivors scattered. Also, when the high dam at Aswan in Egypt began filling, persons were relocated from their village near the Egyptian border to a location about 500 km farther south; more than 50 of the 300 persons died because they were settled in an area where kala azar is prevalent. In a study conducted by the U.S. Navy's NAMRU-3, about 600 km south of Khartoum, a medical clinical treated from 1000 to 3000 patients each month when there were outbreaks of kala azar.

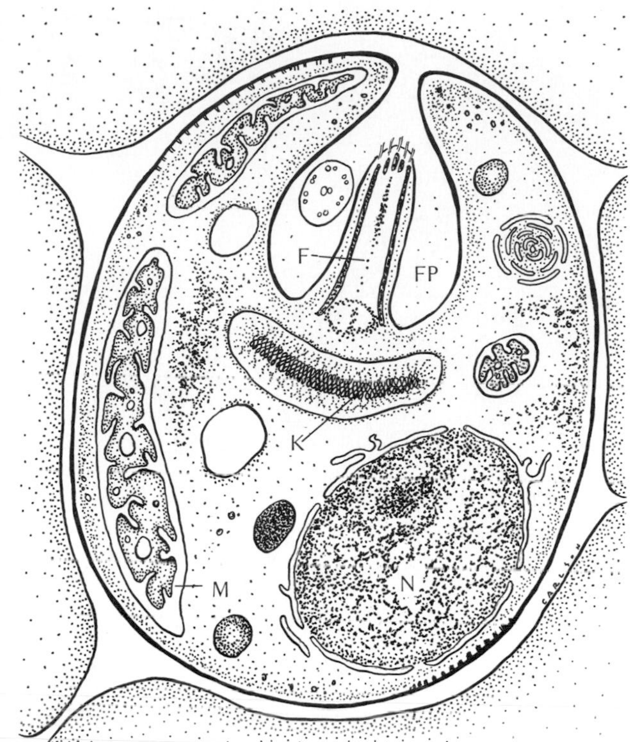

FIGURE 4.2 A diagram of an amastigote of *Leishmania* as seen in TEM.

Morphology

Amastigotes are intracellular, ellipsoid bodies 3.3 μm long by 2 μm wide. In Giemsa-stained material under the light microscope, the nucleus and kinetoplast are red and the cytoplasm is pale blue; the cell membrane can usually be seen (Fig. 4.1). The rudimentary flagellum can be seen in some preparations. In electron micrographs, additional structures can be seen (Fig. 4.2), such as the flagellar pocket, details of the kinetoplast, which is 0.3×0.7 μm, subpellicular tubules, and the mitochondrion.

In the sand fly a short promastigote has a rather stumpy or spatulate body form; the paramastigote is nearly globular and the kinetoplast lies alongside of the nucleus. The metacyclic promastigote is a slender form in which the flagellum is twice or more the length of the body (Fig. 4.4).

Life Cycle

All of the leishmanioses are vector-borne diseases in which the vectors are sand flies (Psychodidae, Phlebotominae, (Chapter 47) in the genera *Phlebotomus* and *Lutzomyia* in the Old and New Worlds, respectively. The development and transmission are much the same regardless of the species or clinical effects.

In the case of Old World visceral leishmaniosis, the principal vectors are *Phlebotomus papatasi,* and *P. perniciosis.* A fly becomes infected by taking a blood meal from an infected animal, or less often, a person who has amastigotes in circulating white blood cells (Fig. 4.5). Once in the midgut of the fly, the host cell breaks down releasing the amastigotes, which then transform into promastigotes (Fig. 4.4) within 24 hours.

There has been some proliferation of terms used to describe different morphotypes of the promastigote. When an amastigote is taken into the fly with the blood meal, it transforms into a stumpy promastigote and it, in turn transforms into a relatively slender promastigote, which is called a nectomonad (free-swimming form). As the organisms move forward in the gut, two other forms are seen: a pear-shaped haptomonad and a rather globular paramastigote. These forms may be free-swimming nectomonads, or haptomonads attached to the stomodeal valve by means of hemidesmosomes (Fig. 4.7). The metacyclic promastigote, most likely the infective form, is slender and has a flagellum about twice as long as the body (Fig. 4.5). The infective forms gain a thicker glycoccalyx reminiscent of the

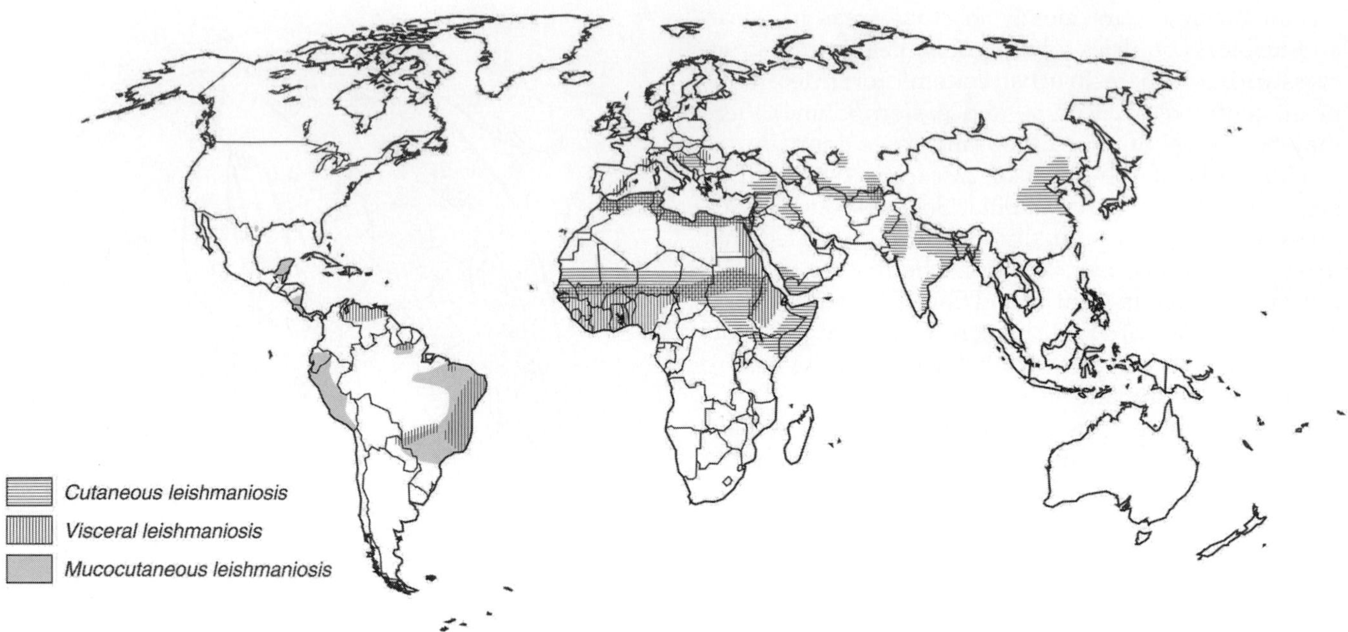

FIGURE 4.3 Most major areas of visceral, cutaneous, and mucocutaneous leishmaniosis.

changes that take place in the tsetse-borne African trypanosomes.

In a study of *L. donovani* in *Lutzomyia* multiplication took place in the stomach of the fly as nectomonads for the first three days and then they began to move anteriorly. By the fifth day the anterior midgut was packed with promastigotes and they were seen anterior to the proventricular, or cardiac, valve. The haptomonads attach to the proventriculus and the stomodeal valve area. They form a hemidesmosome with the host tissue.

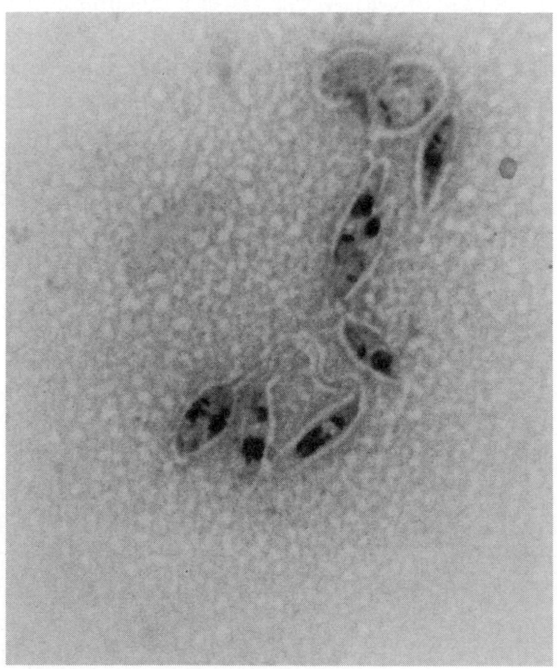

FIGURE 4.4 A light level photomicrograph of promastigotes taken from culture and stained with Giemsa.

Species of sand flies that serve as good vectors are those in which the promastigotes multiply well and in which the organisms move to the anterior part of the gut (Fig. 4.6). The interpretation for many years has been that the esophagus of the fly becomes partially blocked; when the fly takes another blood meal, it attempts to clear the obstruction and promastigotes are injected into the bite wound. Experiments have now shown that the nectomonads produce a protease in the anterior part of the peritrophic matrix, which breaks down the blood meal. The nectomonads then move forward and attach to cells where they produce a chitinase. This enzyme breaks down the cardiac valve which is located between the pharyngeal pump and the midgut. The result is that when the pharyngeal pump moves blood into the midgut, the valve does not then close and blood moves back into the mouthparts and into the wound carrying the infective leishmanias with it.

When promastigotes are reintroduced into a susceptible host, they are phagocytized by macrophages and begin to multiply by binary fission. Development first takes place where the vector has fed and usually a small lesion develops at that site. In some instances, the lesion becomes fairly large and it may appear to

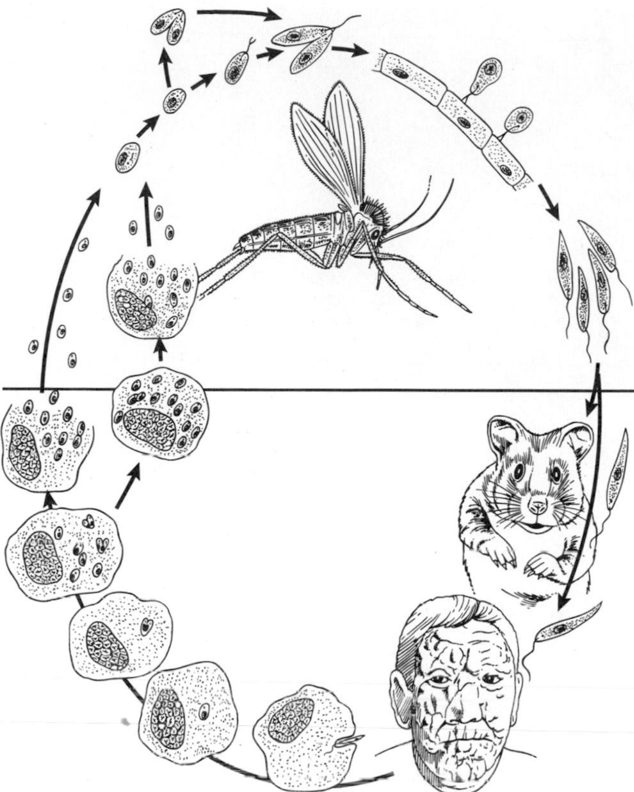

FIGURE 4.5 Life cycle of *Leishmania* spp. in the sand fly vector and the mammalian hosts. Amastigotes are ingested when the sand fly takes a blood meal; the amastigotes may either be in a macrophage or sometimes free in the blood. The amastigotes may or may not multiply in the blood meal, but within three to four days they transform into stumpy promastigotes. These promastigotes multiply further and transform into pear-shaped nectomonads or haptomonads; the haptomonad, or attached form, is shown. The paramastigote is the next form, and it may be either a haptomonad or nectomonad. The final stage, arising probably from the paramastigote, is the metacyclic promastigote, the infective form for the mammalian host. Multiplication of the asmastigotes takes place in macrophages in various places in the body, depending on the species of *Leishmania*.

be an infection with *L. tropica*. Within a matter of days, the organisms are carried to many parts of the body where the amastigotes are ingested by fixed phagocytic cells (histiocytes) and further multiplication takes place. Some of the amastigotes infect circulating phagocytic cells or those in the superficial layers of the skin, allowing them to be picked up by another sand fly during feeding.

Diagnosis

Determining whether an individual is infected with *Leishmania* spp. is based on the following:

1. Clinical signs and symptoms
2. Living in or visiting an endemic area
3. Serological tests
4. Finding the causative agent

Clinically, visceral leishmaniosis shows nonspecific signs and symptoms such as fever, prostration, and anemia. In endemic areas, leishmaniosis is usually seasonal, often coinciding with a wet season, and that should be taken into account. Also, persons traveling to enzootic areas for work or pleasure should let their physicians know where they have been when they show undefined illness upon return home.

Serologic tests reveal the presence of antibody and are useful in both individual diagnosis and epidemiologic surveys. There are a number of antibody-based tests:

1. High IgG level
2. Fluorescent antibody (FA) test
3. Enzyme-linked immunosorbent assay (ELISA)

Most important in diagnosis is finding the amastigotes in tissue; material is taken from spleen or bone marrow, or less often liver or lymph nodes. A tiny portion is processed by doing the following:

1. Examining a Giemsa-stained smear under a compound microscope
2. Examining the tissue after being processed for histology
3. Inoculating a culture medium and looking for promastigotes within a few days or as long as a month
4. Inoculating hamsters with the suspected material and looking for amastigotes in its tissues later
5. Increasing the amount of parasite DNA by PCR (polymerase chain reaction)

In the first four of the methods, skill and experience are required to determine the presence of the organisms. Promastigotes are fairly easy to recognize in culture, but amastigotes are about 3 μm in diameter and inconspicuous.

PCR has made an enormous difference in being able to detect leishmanial infections, both visceral and cutaneous. A small amount of biopsied material can be subjected to PCR and a nearly unequivocal answer obtained within a matter of a day. Specificity can also be obtained so that geographic isolates can be identified, or a more general answer that the organism is only a species of *Leishmania*.

Host–Parasite Interactions

Entrance into the host and establishment of infection by leishmanias is enhanced by saliva from the vector. Early experiments showed that the probability of infec-

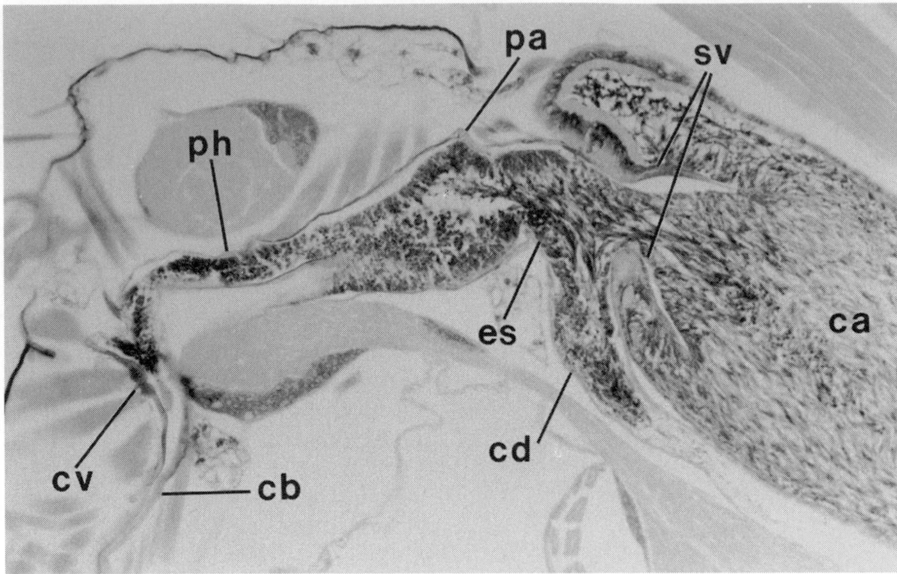

FIGURE 4.6 A parasaggital section of a sand fly infected with *Leishmania chagasi* as seen in LM. The head is at the left; essentially all of the darker material in the gut represents promastigotes of various kinds. Especially large numbers of organisms can be seen in the pharynx and in the region of the cibarium. Abbreviations: cv—cibarial valve; ca—cardia; sv—stomodeal valve; es—esophagus; cd—crop duct; pa—posterior armature region of the pharynx; ph—anterior tubular pharynx; cb—cibarium. [From Walters, L. L., *et al.*, 1989.]

tion as well as the increase in the numbers of amastigotes was many times greater when sand fly saliva was administered with the promastigotes. As a result of a series of investigations, it was found that two substances were involved, maxadilin, or maximum dilation molecule, and SIP, or salivary immunosuppressive protein. Maxadilin keeps the capillary bed open at the site of feeding for about 48 hours, and SIP restrains the immune system's early efforts to eliminate the parasites.

Leishmania spp. live in a most unlikely place in the vertebrate host—macrophages. Macrophages are a key element of the immune system. They engulf and destroy small invading organisms. They also present antigens from these destroyed organisms to other members of the immune system.

Infective promastigotes entering the blood of the vertebrate are covered by two key molecules: the protein gp 63 and a lipophosphoglycan (LPG). Both of these molecules mediate the uptake of promastigotes by interacting with components of the complement system and with surface molecules on the macrophages.

The promastigotes are engulfed by macrophages and contained in a so-called phagosome. The phagosome, in turn, fuses with a lysosome to form a phagolysosome. These organelles contain numerous enzymes, which normally break down organic compounds. As the promastigotes transform into amastigotes, they produce an arsenal of compounds to counter lysosomal enzymes such as catalase, superoxide dismutase, and glutathione peroxidase. The gp 63 molecule inactivates proteolytic enzymes and LPG protects against other enzymes.

Leishmanial organisms are able to survive the highly acidic environment of lysosomes by regulating their internal pH. In contrast, other intracellular pathogens such as *Toxoplasma* and *Legionella* block the formation of acid compounds in order to survive.

The infected sand fly must have a sugar meal for the leishmania to be infective for the vertebrate host, but the mechanism is not known.

Epidemiology and Control

The leishmanioses are zoonoses in all situations except one: in certain areas of India, animal reservoirs have dropped out of the epidemiologic picture of visceral leishmaniosis. In all other instances, various carnivores and rodents maintain the infection in nature. For example, in China the fox and probably the dog serve as reservoirs; in Iraq the jackal is the principal reservoir. In southern Sudan, the serval is the principal reservoir while in Kenya and Uganda, rodents maintain the cycle.

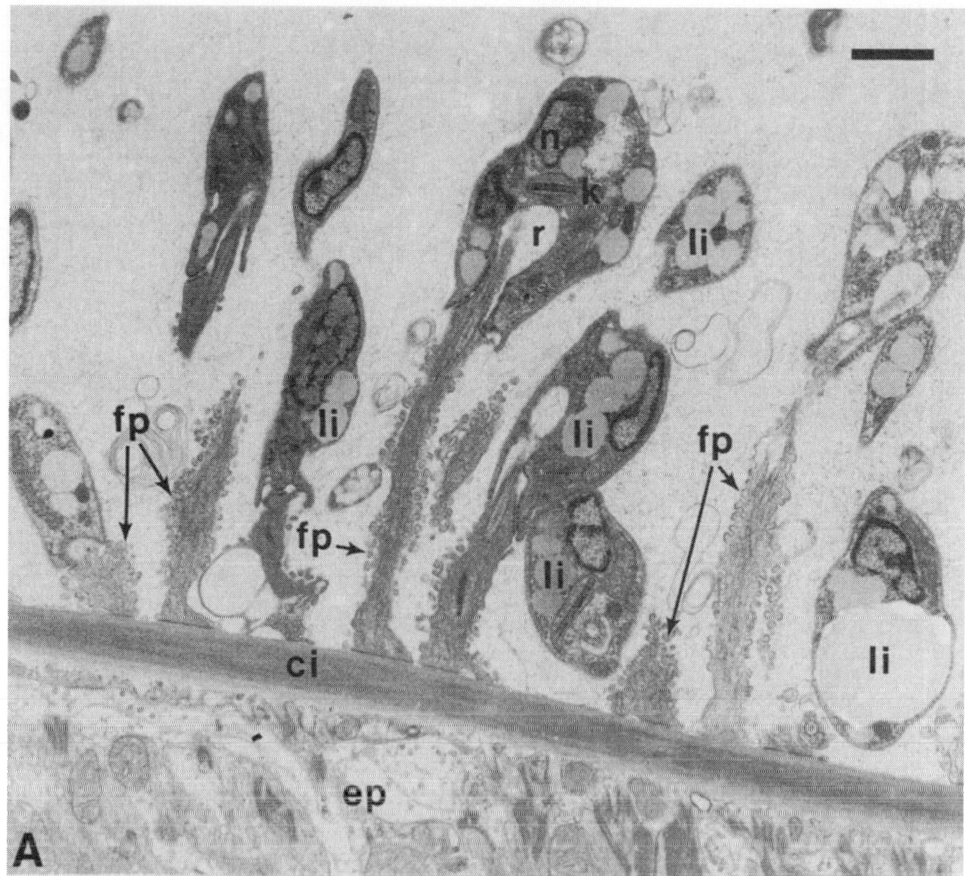

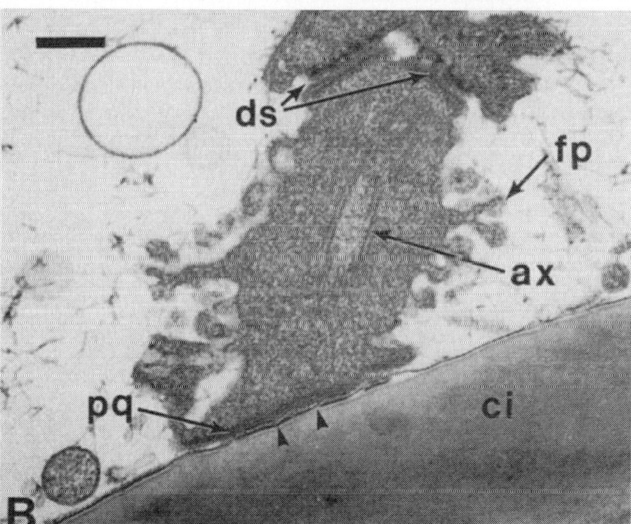

FIGURE 4.7 Attachment of paramastigotes of *Leishmania chagasi* to the gut of *Lutzomyia longipalpis* as seen in TEM. The attachment of each organism is by a hemidesmosome as seen in detail in (B). The paramastigotes extend into the lumen of the gut, and there is some modification of the flagellum during attachment; the plasmalemma becomes puckered in appearance. Arrowheads show the hemidesmosomal attachment of the flagellum to the cuticle of the pharynx. Abbreviations: n—nucleus; k—kinetoplast; f—flagellum; fp—puckering of plasmalemma of flagellum; ci—cuticular intima; ax—axoneme; ds—desmosomal attachment; ep—epithelium of pharynx; li—lipid inclusion; pq—plaque of hemidesmosome; r—flagellar reservoir. [From Walters, I. L., *et al.*, 1989.]

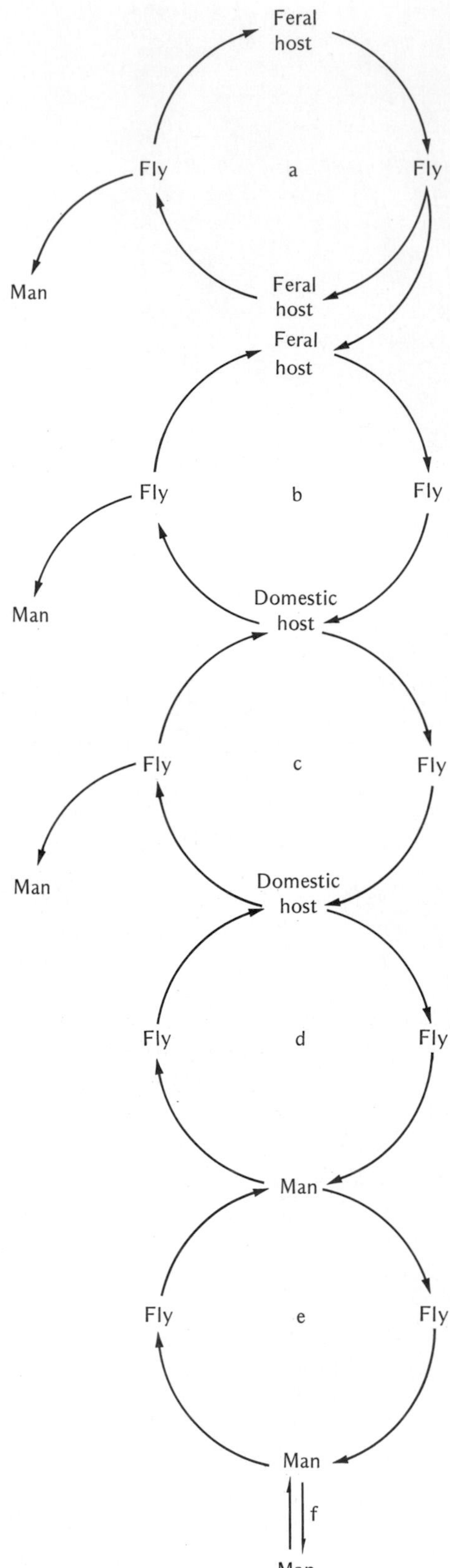

In establishing a control program, it is well to keep in mind that leishmaniosis is an evolving disease and the steps in its evolution can be discerned (Fig. 4.8).

1. *Enzootic foci in wild canids* (Fig. 4.8a). The primitive condition was one in which hosts such as the jackal in central Asia maintained the infection and human infections were rare or nonexistent.
2. *Rural endemic foci* (Fig. 4.8b). As humans colonized enzootic areas, infection began to include domestic canids, but with maintenance of enzootic foci in wild canids. Cases in humans are common. This type of cycle is seen in parts of Asia, Russia, China, and the area ringing the Mediterranean basin.
3. *Urban endemic foci* (Fig. 4.8c). Upon the expansion of the human population and the development of large, permanent towns, it was possible for the wild animal portion of the cycle to drop out (at least locally). Dogs became the reservoir and transmission to humans became frequent. This cycle occurs in central Asia and the eastern part of China.
4. *Endemic (sometimes epidemic) foci* (Fig. 4.8d). In this epidemiologic form, the reservoir may drop out and transmission can take place from person to person via sand flies. Foci in India are of this type, and probably more human cases occur than in any other type.

Each of these types of leishmaniosis requires a different emphasis in designing a control program, and regrettably all have been refractory to bringing the level of transmission down to an acceptable level.

Control efforts are directed principally at the following:

1. Control of the sand fly vectors
2. Protecting humans against the bites of sand flies
3. Treatment of infected individuals
4. Elimination of reservoir hosts
5. Vaccination of humans

FIGURE 4.8 Evolution of the epidemiologies of *Leishmania* spp. from feral cycles to peridomestic ones. (a) A feral cycle with humans as only a rare and dead-end host. (b) A cycle involving a feral host and an animal associated with humans such as the dog. Humans are an occasional and dead-end host. (c) A domiciliated cycle often with a peridomestic vector as well; humans are an occasional dead-end host. (d) A domiciliated cycle with animals such as the dog as the principal reservoir; humans are integrated into the cycle. (e) A cycle in which the reservoirs have dropped out and transmission takes place from person to person through phlebotomines. (f) Person-to-person transmission takes place through direct contact or by means of body fluids; the vector is no longer required.

Problems in implementing control lie in the following:

1. Finding and identifying the vectors
2. Developing feasible control methods for the vectors
3. Establishing barriers between the human population and the vectors
4. Inadequate chemotherapy
5. Lack of a vaccine
6. Identifying and reducing reservoir animal populations

In the evolution of the transmission cycles of leishmaniosis (Fig. 4.8) it can be seen that the hazard to human health increases as the cycle becomes more domiciliated or peridomestic, but the probability of succeeding at control becomes greater. If humans seldom penetrate the nidus of infection, control is not required, and even if it were, it would not be feasible.

Phlebotomines are tiny, have short flight ranges, and live in obscure places as larvae (Chapter 47). They are quite seasonal in both tropical and temperate climates, so finding adults requires knowing when they appear during the year. Often only a single species of sand fly is the vector in a region. In the NAMRU-3 study in southern Sudan, five years of intensive study showed that *Phlebotomus orientalis* was the most likely vector, but proof could not be obtained. Nor, for that matter, were the breeding sites of this putative vector ever found. Likewise, studies in the rain forest of Central America required several years of work to determine the species of the vector and where they are found.

In peridomestic transmission, it is easier to find flies and to determine which are the probable vectors. Flies can be collected at their resting sites or trapped if they cannot be seen. Sentinel animals and traps can be used to lure in flies that feed on mammals.

Only in the peridomestic situation is it feasible to develop programs that reduce fly populations. In the Indian foci of kala azar, flies, *P. argentipes,* breed in trash and garbage around houses; these can be eliminated. Spraying inside surfaces of houses with a residual insecticide is an effective method. In fact, where control programs for malaria have relied on spraying of houses, leishmaniosis has ceased to be a serious problem, also. As is true with most vector-borne diseases, the vectors become resistant to insecticides, and that occurred in India in the early 1990s.

In cases where there is an interface with the wild animal population, control becomes a possibility. In China and Russia, reduction of human infections has been observed following eradication of rodents in the vicinity of human habitation. Since burrowing rodents are the principal reservoirs in arid and semiarid foci, steps must be taken to destroy burrows and prevent their recolonization. Control by reducing populations of sand flies is not feasible in this situation.

As the infection moves into domestic animals such as the dog, it may be possible to effect control by a test and slaughter program. However the realities of the kinds of locations where leishmaniosis occurs militate against the licensing of dogs and the establishment of administrative structures that it would entail. Dogs are often visibly affected showing roughened skin, lesions on the muzzle, and hair loss; it would generally be within the powers of public health personnel to remove such animals from the community.

Personal protection is an important aspect of control for both the individual and the population. Because flies are small, a typical fly screen is inadequate to keep them out of buildings; a fly screen has openings of 1.3 to 1.5 mm, and phlebotomines are not kept out unless opening are 0.9 mm or smaller. An insecticide with a long residual activity can be painted on fly screens and give protection. Houses can also be sprayed with a residual or slow-release insecticide. Keeping plants, especially low-growing ones, away from houses also reduces the resting sites of adults. When it is necessary for a person to be in an area where flies are abundant, insect repellents provide protection.

Treatment of individuals is important not only for the well-being of the patient, but also to help prevent the spread of the disease among the human population where there are no mammalian reservoirs. Cases of leishmaniosis begin to appear about three months after the rainy and fly seasons begin. Since the signs and symptoms of disease appear seasonally, control methods can be employed strategically with the most economical use of resources. Drugs are important, but they have distinct disadvantages. Those in use are organic antimonials and diamidines, all of which require multiple doses. Even with a complete course of treatment, about 15% of persons retain the infection. More alarming are reports of failure of antimonials to cure the infection in a greater and greater numbers of cases. It appears that after more than 60 years of use, some leishmania are becoming drug resistant. Since there are no good replacements for this group of drugs, this is a potentially serious complication.

Related Organisms

In countries ringing the Mediterranean Sea such as Portugal, Spain, France, Italy, and North Africa, a childhood form of leishmanisis is caused by *L. infantum.* Although this species occasionally infects adults, about 80% of infections are seen in children.

The epidemiologic pattern is that of a peridomestic infection with the principal reservoir in dogs. The main vectors are *Phlebotomus ariasi* and *P. perniciosus.* The intimate interface between children and dogs in rural areas permits transmission to take place readily. Oddly enough, a small focus of leishmaniosis in dogs in Oklahoma seems to be caused by *L. infantum,* but no human cases have been seen.

L. chagasi, found in the Western Hemisphere and similar to *L. infantum,* is seen mostly in children. *Lutzomyia longipalpis* is one of the principal vectors in South America. This form of visceral leishmaniosis is much more prevalent in South America now than it was, say, 50 years ago.

OLD WORLD CUTANEOUS LEISHMANIOSIS

Three species of *Leishmania are* associated with cutaneous lesion of this disease complex (Tab. 4.1). The lesions are classified as being wet, dry, or diffuse, depending on the species.

Name of Organism and Disease Associations

Leishmania tropica (syns.: *L. l. tropica, L. t. minor*) causes cutaneous leishmaniosis, cutaneous leishmaniasis, oriental sore (Fig. 4.9), Aleppo button, and Delhi boil.

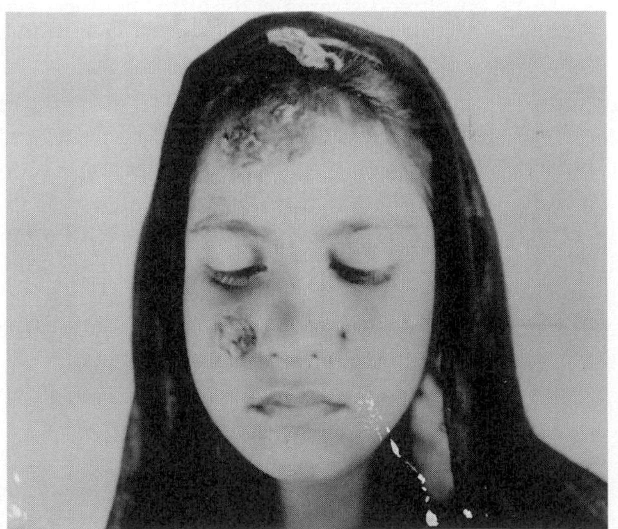

FIGURE 4.9 Typical cutaneous lesions on the cheek and forehead caused by *Leishmania* sp. [Courtesy of U.S. Armed Forces Institute of Pathology. Negative No. 80,717.]

Hosts and Host Range

The principal reservoirs are dogs, certain rodents including gerbils, and the vectors are *Phlebotomus sergenti, P. papatasi, P. ansarii,* and *P. mongolensis,* depending on the geographic area.

Geographic Distribution and Importance

This organism is found in India, the Mediterranean Basin, Iran, and southern Russia. It is common in hot, dry climates, and is mostly in urban areas.

Morphology

Same as *L. donovani.*

Life Cycle

Same as *L. donovani*

Diagnosis

The same principles apply to cutaneous leishmaniosis as to the visceral form when attempting a diagnosis, with two exceptions. Since the lesions are in the skin, a conclusion can be reached with some confidence in an enzootic area, but finding the organism is still important because of the side effects of treatment. Organisms are found in the lesion, but only at its margin; a needle biopsy is therefore taken from the area into which the lesion is advancing.

Host–Parasite Interactions

The lesion from infection with this organism is a so-called dry lesion, which is circumscribed with a depressed center. There is lymph node involvement in about 10% of cases. Healing is spontaneous in several months, and there is a solid immunity against reinfection.

Epidemiology and Control

The same principles of control apply in cutaneous and mucocutaneous leishmaniosis as in visceral leishmaniosis. The local pattern of transmission, the reservoirs, and the vectors must be determined before a control program is planned and implemented.

Name of Organism and Disease Associations

Leishmania major (syn. *L. tropica major*).

Geographic Distribution and Importance

This is the so-called wet Oriental sore and is found in Central Asia and southern Russia. It is found mostly in rural areas.

Hosts and Host Range

Gerbils and a few other rodents are the reservoirs, and *Phlebotomus papatasi* and *P. caucasicus* are the principal vectors.

Geographic Distribution

This organism is found in southern Russia and Iran principally in rural areas.

Host–Parasite Interactions

The lesions caused by *L. major* are wet and ulcerative but do not extend to the mucous membranes. The incubation period is one to six weeks, and healing is spontaneous. Individuals who recover from *L. major* infections are immune. The immunity is probably maintained through concomitant immunity (i.e., the person retains a small number of organism in the tissues). Immunity involves T-cells whose cytokines activate macrophages, which, in turn, identify and kill the parasites. There is some cross immunity between *L. tropica* and *L major;* persons immune to *L. major* are immune to *L. tropica* but not vice versa.

Name of Organism and Disease Associations

Leishmania aethiopica (syn. *L. tropica* in part). This organism causes both a single sore and a diffuse cutaneous infection.

Hosts and Host Range

The hyrax or cony (*Procavia*), a much smaller relative of the elephant, seems to be the principal reservoir and *Phlebotomus longipes* is the main vector.

Geographic Distribution

East Africa in Kenya and Ethiopia.

NEW WORLD CUTANEOUS AND MUCOCUTANEOUS LEISHMANIOSIS

The cutaneous and mucocutaneous leishmanioses of the Western Hemisphere or New World have presented enormous difficulties for those investigators that have tried to establish a coherent classification. As indicated earlier in this chapter, the organisms differ insignificantly in morphology, and clinical features also are inconsistent. Any one species may show a variety of clinical manifestations depending on the characters of both the organism and the vertebrate host, and, to make matters worse, the way the organisms develop in the vector sometimes affects the clinical course of the disease. *Leishmania* spp. have undoubtedly undergone rapid evolution in the New World and continue to evolve. Hosts change from sylvan mammals to dogs as forests are cut and colonized by humans. An increase in forest edge habitat may allow an increase in populations of the sand fly vectors.

The following discussion of cutaneous and mucocutaneous leishmaniosis simplifies the clinical features somewhat in favor of comprehensibility.

Certain species, *L. mexicana* and *L. amazonensis*, causes a *diffusa* type of lesion. In most instances, there is a single lesion at the site where the sand fly has injected the promastigotes. In the diffusa form, organisms are widespread in the skin and may cause general changes in the skin. This spread results from lack of a delayed type hypersensitivity (DTH) on the part of the patient. DTH seems to be essential for immunologic control of the infection.

All of the leishmanioses discussed in this section are zoonoses. A few have become peridomestic, such as *L. peruviana* whose reservoirs are dogs, but most have reservoirs in wild animals. In general, the options for control are as follows:

1. Vector control
2. Removal of reservoir hosts
3. Treatment of human cases
4. Personal protection
5. Immunization

Where the infection has become domiciliated, or peridomestic, control of either the vector or the reservoir hosts may be feasible. Since the flies do not venture far from their breeding and resting sites, both source reduction and insecticides can be used around houses. Likewise, dogs and other domestic animals such as horses may become reservoirs. Removal of these hosts may be undertaken in some circumstances.

Treatment of humans serves mostly to help the individual, not to reduce transmission. Humans seldom serve as reservoirs of infection.

Personal protection takes the form of bed nets, window and door screens, repellents, and avoiding places and times when sand flies are numerous. All of these can be effective if they are put into practice; however, tropical climates are not conducive to use of bed nets and screening since they reduce the flow of the cooling night air. Insect repellents are useful, but their cost may be prohibitive for persons living in straitened circumstances

Immunization has some distinct promise. In the Old World, cutaneous leishmanioses caused by *L. tropica* and *L. major*, purposeful infection of individuals with living organisms has been practiced. In the Mediterranean area, for example, parents may infect their children on a part of the body not ordinarily exposed to view so that they will not develop lesions on the face from a bite of an infected fly. Vaccines made from killed organisms have not been consistently effective. Success has been experienced in experimental animals such as mice using refined and recombinant antigens. A surface glycoprotein, gp 63, has been shown to have some effect in developing immunity.

Name of Organism and Disease Associations

Leishmania mexicana (syn. *L. m. mexicana, L. pifanoi*) causes cutaneous leishmaniosis and chiclero ulcer.

Hosts and Host Range

Forest rodents are the reservoirs of infection and *Lutzomyia olmeca* is the vector in Mesoamerica. *L. diabolica* and/or *L. anthophora* may be the vectors in the United States.

Geographic Distribution and Importance

Southeastern Mexico, much of Central America, the Dominican Republic, Venezuela, and Texas in the United States. This is epidemiologically a rain forest infection in most instances; however it is present in the Texas, in a relatively dry area. It has been found in four sites near San Antonio in addition to those in south central Texas.

Host–Parasite Interactions

Chiclero ulcer obtained its name from the fact that those persons who go into the forest to collect chicle, which is the principal ingredient of chewing gum, often are affected. Skin lesions typically heal spontaneously within weeks or months of their appearance. However, if the pinna of the ear is involved, the infection is likely to remain for years. Over time, the pinna is eroded and a good portion of it may eventually be lost.

Epidemiology and Control

Control programs are patterned after those established for visceral leishmaniosis.

Notable Features

Sporadic cases of cutaneous leishmaniosis have been reported in the United States for many years. A few have been seen in humans, but there have also been scattered reports in dogs (see also *L. infantum*). In most instances, the conclusion could be reached that the infection was contracted outside of the United States. However, by the mid-1980s it became clear that there was a focus of infection in south central Texas and that eight infections were contracted there. Further studies have indicated that as many as 29 human cases have been contracted in Texas, and *L. mexicana* has been isolated from wood rats. Control programs have not been established.

Name of Organism and Disease Associations

Leishmania amazonensis (syn. *L. m. amazonensis, L. garnhami*) is the cause usually of circumscribed skin lesions in humans.

Hosts and Host Range

A wide array of rodents, marsupials, edentates, carnivores, and primates have been implicated as reservoirs of infection, but a rodent, *Proechimys guyanensis*, is the only proven reservoir.

Geographic Distribution

This organism is found in parts of Central America and in the Amazon Basin (Tab. 4.1).

Host–Parasite Interactions

While *L. amazonensis* generally is associated with skin lesions, it has been isolated from patients with visceral leishmaniosis. It has also been found in persons suffering from post kala azar dermal leishmaniosis, a distressing disfiguring condition seen in a few patients after treatment for visceral leishmaniosis. This range of clinical manifestations emphasizes the diffi-

LEISHMANIOSIS IN TEXAS

THE UNITED STATES HAS long been considered to be free of enzootic leishmaniosis; only a few cases were imported now and again. A report of cutaneous leishmaniosis contracted by a resident of Texas in the 1940s was given short shrift, because the data were not definitive. Thirty years were to pass before a cluster of cases was reported in southern Texas in which the organism was unequivocally demonstrated. It was crucial, also, to demonstrate that the infected persons had not traveled to Mexico where there is a focus of *Leishmania mexicana.* The criteria were satisfied, and epidemiologic studies have been underway since 1976.

The epidemiologic pattern of maintenance and transmission of the agent, *L. mexicana,* has now been shown. Infections have all been located within the range of the southern wood rat, *Neotoma micropus,* and isolations of the causative agent have been made from this reservoir. Its habitat is a mesquite/prickly pear biotope, and in most instances this habitat has been close to the dwellings of infected persons. A total of 29 cases of leishmaniosis in humans in Texas have now been confirmed. Among humans, males and females have shown infections in about equal proportions, and any correlation with age and occupation has been negative.

As many as five species of sand flies are prevalent in this geographic area, but two of them seem to be most prevalent, *Lurzomyia anthophora* and *L. diabolica.* An isolation of *L. mexicana* has been made from the former, but it is not anthropophilic; *L. diabolica,* aptly named because it feeds avidly on humans and causes considerable pain while feeding, is prevalent, but no isolation of the causative agent has been made from it.

It is interesting to note that there was resistance to admitting that leishmaniosis occurred in the United States despite its prevalence in Mexico; it is as if the political border meant something to an infectious agent. Now, even though there is a rough outline of the nidus of infection, much remains to be done. The isolations from both reservoirs and vectors are fragmentary, only a few serologic studies have been done in the human population, and what other mammalian reservoirs may be involved is still unknown. Likewise, information on the bionomics of sand flies in the U.S. is woefully inadequate.

Knowledge often moves at a seeming snail's pace, and our understanding of leishmaniosis in the U.S. is a case in point. As time passes, it will be interesting to see whether it is an emerging disease or one which has been with us for a long time.

Reference: McHugh *et al.,* 1996. *Am. J. Trop. Med. Hyg.* **55,** 547–555.

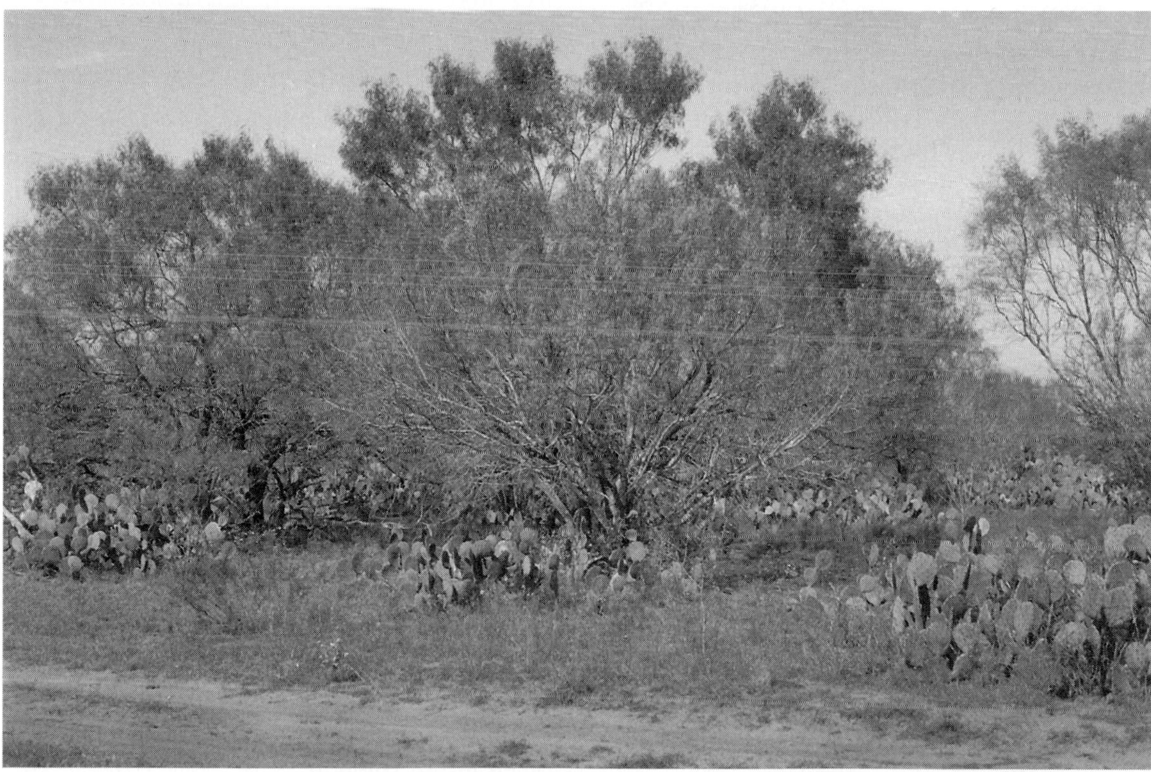

Picture of habitat courtesy of Dr. Chad P. McHugh, Armstrong Lab., Brooks, Air Force Base, Texas.

culties in reaching unequivocal conclusions about the leishmaniases and their causative agents.

Name of Organism and Disease Associations

Leishmania braziliensis (syn. *L. b. brasiliensis)* is the cause of espundia, a mucocutaneous form of leishmaniosis of humans.

Geographic Distribution

This disease entity is found in Central and South America in Argentina, Brazil, Peru, Ecuador, Bolivia, Venezuela, Paraguay, Colombia, Costa Rica, Guatemala, Honduras, Nicaragua, and Panama. It is transmitted principally in rain forests.

Hosts and Host Range

The reservoirs vary with the locality, but dogs have been found to be naturally infected, and various forest rodents serve as wild reservoirs. The rice rat, *Oryzomys*, may be the primary reservoir. Vectors are *Lutzomyia wellcomei, L. yucumensis, L. llanos martinsi, L. spinicrassa, L. whitmani,* and *L. carreri.*

Host–Parasite Interactions

Espundia is one of the most distressing of the mucocutaneous leishmaniases because it causes serious disfigurement and is often clinically intractable. Clinically the disease runs a long chronic course with the skin lesions spreading and invading the mucous membranes. The nose is affected in about 80% of cases. The result of long-standing infection is destruction of the facial cartilage so that the nose and soft palate are eroded and the patient suffers from severe disfigurement. Secondary infections of these tissues frequently occur.

The reason for the invasion of tissue and its destruction is not well known. Some parasites are resistant to elimination and there is persistence of a state of hypersensitivity so that there is an excessive inflammatory reaction. In addition there is an autoimmune response such that there is cross-reactivity between some antigens of the leishmania and host tissues. A reduced antigenic response is characteristic of many eukaryotic infections characterized by long chronic courses.

Name of Organism and Disease Associations

Leishmania guyanensis is the cause of American forest leishmaniosis, pian bois, or buba.

Hosts and Host Range

Reservoir hosts are the two-toed sloth, the lesser anteater, and probably both the opossum and small forest rodents. Vectors are *L. umbratilis, L. anduzei,* and *L. whitmani.*

Geographic Distribution

This organism is distributed in northern South America (Tab. 4.1) and is principally in rain forests.

Host–Parasite Interactions

The skin lesions are usually discrete and heal spontaneously. However, in some instances, where the nose is involved, for example, there may be invasion of the mucous membranes. Lymph nodes are involved in about 10% of cases.

Name of Organism and Disease Associations

Leishmania panamensis is the cause of cutaneous leishmaniosis that usually retains a discrete, circular lesion but may take other forms as well.

Hosts and Host Range

The reservoirs of infection are the two-toed and three-toed sloths, rodents and certain carnivore species. The vectors are *L. trapadoi, L. gomezi, L. ylephiletor,* and *L. panamensis.*

Geographic Distribution

Central America and northern South America (Tab. 4.1).

Name of Organism and Disease Associations

Leishmania peruviana causes a disease of humans called *uta*, which is characterized by skin lesions only.

Hosts and Host range

The dog is the reservoir. The vector is *Lutzomyia noguchii.* In some areas of Peru, *L. peruensis* seems to be the principal vector and may be more widespread; it enters houses readily and is found there in large numbers during the rainy season.

Host–Parasite Interactions

This may be the only leishmanial infection in the New World that is domiciliated and has the dogs as the principal reservoir. It is found on the western-facing slopes of the Andes Mountains in Peru.

Epidemiology and Control

In some localities of Peru such as the Purismas Valley, there is a high correlation between elevation and the occurrence of the disease. There was an increase in incidence with altitude and reached a peak between 2250 and 2750 m (7300 to 11,000 ft) above sea level.

Since this is a domiciliated infection, control has been effected through elimination of infected dogs, treatment of infected persons, and protection against the bites of the vectors.

Notable Features

Early explorers and settlers in Peru in the 17th century found that the indigenous people recognized uta as a disease entity. Of interest is the fact that they knew of the association of the vector with the disease, and the term *uta* is synonymous with both the fly and the disease.

RELATED ORGANISMS

Three agents causing cutaneous or mucocutaneous leishmanisis also occur in Latin America: *L. lainsoni, L. venezuelensis,* and *L. pifanoi.* They are not considered here in detail. *L. enriettii* is a parasite of the guinea pig, a South American native, and this organism has been useful as a laboratory model, especially in screening potential drugs for use against leishmaniosis. L. *hertigi* has been found only in the porcupine.

READINGS

Ashford, R. W., Desjeux, P., and deRaadt, P. (1992). Estimation of population risk of infection and number of cases of leishmaniasis. *Parasitol. Today* **8,** 104–105.

Bogdan, C., Rollinghoff, M., and Solbach, W. (1990). Evasion strategies of *Leishmania* parasites. *Parasitol. Today* **6,** 183–187.

Grimaldi, G., Jr., and Tesh, R. B. (1993). Leishmaniases of the New World: Current concepts and implications for future research. *Clin. Microbiol. Rev.* **6,** 230–250.

Handman, E. (1997). *Leishmania* vaccines: Old and new. *Parasitol. Today* **13,** 236–238.

Hoogstraal, H., and Heyneman, D. (1969). Leishmaniasis in the Sudan Republic. *Am. J. Trop. Med. Hyg.* **18,** 1090–1210.

McHugh, C. P., Melby, P. C., and LaFon, S. G. (1996). Leishmaniasis in Texas: Epidemiology and clinical aspects of human cases. *Am. J. Trop. Med. Hyg.* **55,** 547–555.

Peters, W., and Killick-Kendrick, R. (Eds.) (1987). *The Leishmaniases in Biology and Medicine,* 2 Vols. Academic Press, London.

Schlein, Y. (1993). *Leishmania* and sand flies: Interactions in the life cycle and transmission. *Parasitol. Today* **9,** 255–258.

Walters, L. L. (1993). *Leishmania* differentiation in natural and unnatural sand fly hosts. *J. Euk. Microbiol.* **40,** 196–206.

Walters, L. L., *et al.* (1989). Ultrastructural development of *Leishmania chagasi* in its vector, *Lutzomyia longipalpis* (Diptera: psychodidae. *Am. J. Trop. Med. Hyg.* **41,** 295–317.

World Health Organization (WHO) Expert Committee (1990). Control of the leishmaniases, Rep. Ser. No. 73. WHO, Geneva.

CHAPTER

5

Trichomonads and Trichomonosis

Members of the order Trichomonadida are all parasitic except for a few free-living forms that have been reported only infrequently. The organisms are small flagellates, generally less than 25 μm in length but structurally complex, that reproduce asexually and exist only as trophozoites. They do not form cysts and they reproduce by binary fission only.

A common structure underlies all trichomonads, but there is considerable variation on the theme. A generalized trichomonad (Fig. 5.1) seen at the LM level shows the structure of a trichomonad that might be found in nearly any vertebrate or many invertebrates. The organism is usually longer than wide, and has three or more anterior flagella, a recurrent flagellum usually attached to the body by an undulating membrane, an axostyle, a parabasal body, a costa underlying the undulating membrane, a pelta, and a single nucleus. All of these characteristic structures are referred to as the *karyomastigont apparatus.*

The axostyle serves as a central stiffening organelle and in life is quite flexible; the nucleus typically lies in a concavity near the anterior end of the axostyle. The parabasal body stains darkly with silver staining methods and is actually the Golgi apparatus found in other eukaryotic cells. The costa is a stiffening rod that lies just under the undulating membrane. It is composed of carbohydrate, probably a polysaccharide, and may also serve as a source of carbohydrate for energy needs.

At the EM level, additional detail can be seen (Fig. 5.2). The pelta, for example, appears to be a cap at the anterior tip of the organism at the LM level, but it is actually an extension of the axostyle. Likewise, what appears to be a single basal body at the LM level is a series of basal bodies, one for each flagellum. The parabasal body or Golgi shows as typical Golgi, it is made up of a series of lamellae.

Of interest is the fact that trichomonads lack mitochondria. At both the LM and EM levels, granules can be seen associated with the costa and the axostyle. These are double-membrane-bound bodies that are 0.5 to 3 μm in diameter. At the EM level, the interior structure consists simply of granular material. Biochemical studies have shown that these bodies serve roughly the same function as mitochondria since they contain certain enzymes of the Kreb's cycle. It is especially significant, however, that one of the end products of carbohydrate metabolism is hydrogen. These granules have therefore been termed *hydrogenosomes.* In nearly all eukaryotic cells, the end product of aerobic metabolism is water, but in this case, it is molecular hydrogen. The other end products of carbohydrate metabolism in trichomonads are malate and acetate (Fig. 5.3). This incomplete oxidation of pyruvate shuttles energy-yielding compounds back to the host for further utilization.

Trichomonads are found widely as parasites of both vertebrates and invertebrates. They are mostly in the intestinal tracts of their hosts, but those that are parasites of vertebrates are also found in the reproductive system, urinary tract, and the upper portions of the respiratory tract. Rodents, amphibia, and birds, all have at least one species of trichomonad in their intestinal tracts. *Trichomonas limacis* occurs in the gut and liver of slugs. Trichomonads also occur in the intestine of the large hog ascarid *Ascaris suum.*

Only a few species of trichomonads are pathogenic. Most live in the intestines of their hosts where they

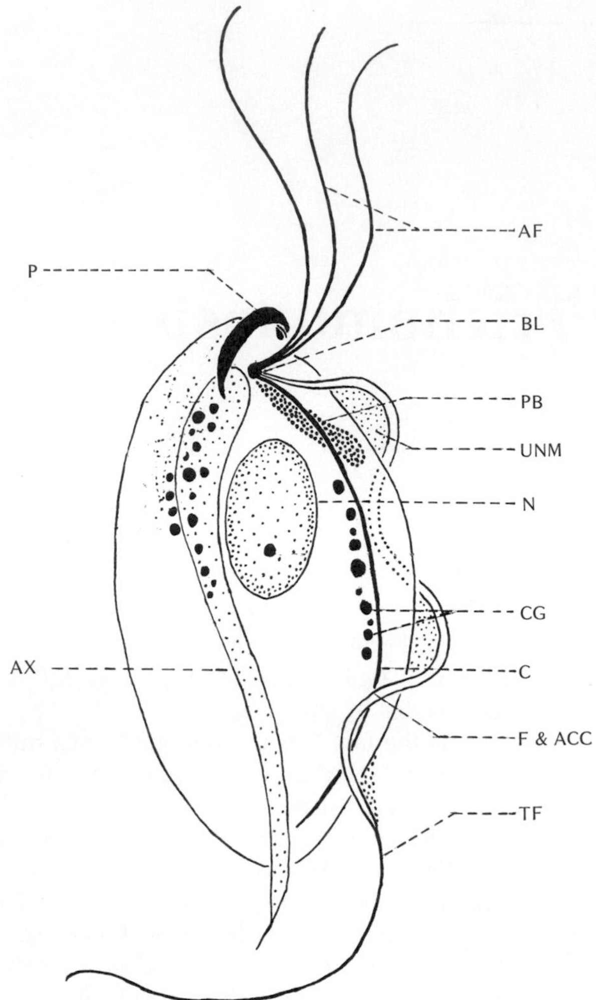

FIGURE 5.1 A generalized trichomonad showing structures used in identification and descriptions of species: P pelta; AX—axostyle; AF—anterior flagella; BL—basal body; PB—parabasal body or Golgi; UNM—undulating membrane; N—nucleus; CG—costal granules (hydrogenosomes); C—costa; F and ACC—flagellum and accessory filament; TF—trailing or recurrent flagellum.

may be readily found upon microscopic examination of gut contents. Under some conditions such the host experiencing enteritis, or eating a high carbohydrate diet, trichomonads may be found in large numbers. At various times, investigators have seen large numbers of trichomonads, or other protists, associated with a pathological condition and concluded that the organism was the cause of the disease. Such guilt by association is understandable but nevertheless to be deplored.

TRICHOMONAD ABORTION

Name of Organism and Disease Association

Tritrichomonas foetus causes trichomonad abortion, or bovine trichomonosis.

Hosts and Host Range

The principal host of *T. foetus* is the domestic ox where it infects the reproductive tracts of both cows and bulls. At one time, data supported the view that the ox was the only host of *T. foetus;* however, it is now known that *T. foetus*, or a closely related organism, also infects the horse and the pig. In horses, trichomonads have occasionally been found in association with abortion and infections of the reproductive tract. The organism from swine is usually referred to as *Tritrichomonas suis*, but the division between it and *T. foetus* is not as clear cut as once thought. Despite the presence of *T. foetus* in other hosts, the ox is the main host, and the one in which significant economic losses occur.

Geographic Distribution and Importance

Cosmopolitan. In surveys, infection rates in cattle have varied from 5 to 50% with the United States and Australia having relatively high prevalences of infection. Taking the lower level for the United States, it is calculated that there is an annual loss of $650 million to the cattle industry from trichomonosis.

Morphology

T. foetus is 10 to 26 μm long by 3 to 15 μm wide and has three anterior flagella. The recurrent flagellum is attached to the body by the undulating membrane and continues free beyond the body. There is a tubular axostyle that also extends beyond the body and the parabasal body is sausage shaped (Fig. 5.4). SEM shows the flagella emerging from a pocket as well as the undulating membrane and its associated filament (Fig. 5.5).

Life Cycle

Multiplication is by binary fission. Transmission takes place during sexual intercourse.

Diagnosis

There are three techniques used to determine whether an ox if infected with *T foetus*:

1. Direct examination of material from the reproductive tract
2. Inoculation of culture media to increase the number of trichomonads present
3. Amplifying the DNA in material from the reproductive tract by polymerase chain reaction (PCR)

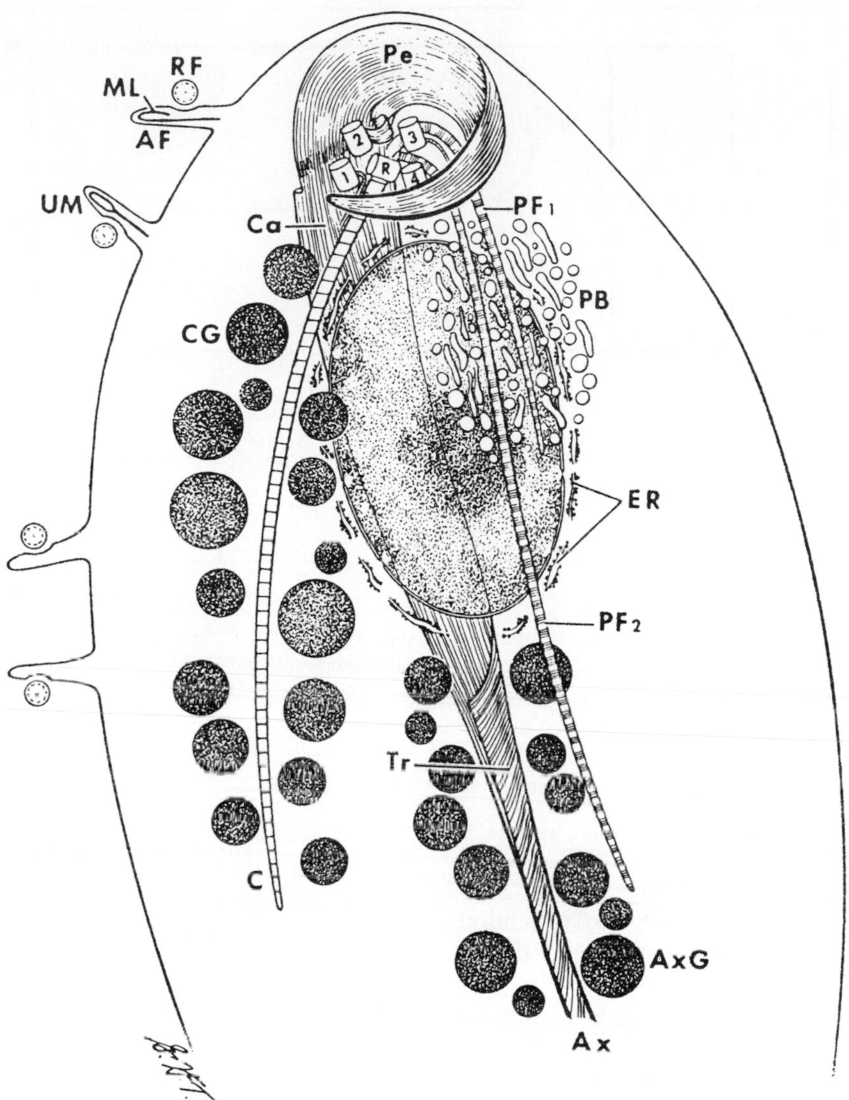

FIGURE 5.2 A composite diagram of *Trichomonas gallinae* as seen in the TEM. AX—axostyle; AXG—axostylar granules (hydrogenosomes); C—costa; CG—costal granules (hydrogenosomes); ER—endoplasmic reticulum; N—nucleus; PB—parabasal body or Golgi; PF—parabasal filament (two shown); Pe—pelta, a continuation of the axostyle; R—basal bodies 1 to 4 of the mastigont system; RF—trailing or recurrent flagellum; UM—undulating membrane. (Mattern, C. F. T., Honigberg, B. M., and Daniel, W. A., 1967.]

Determining whether a cow or bull is infected relies on finding the causative agent either directly or indirectly. Serologic tests have been developed, but they indicate only whether an animal has been infected, not whether there is an active infection at the time.

In the bull, organisms are found in the prepuce or sheath of the penis. A variety of techniques and instruments have been developed for obtaining material for direct examination or cultivation. Commonly, a plastic pipet about 10 mm in diameter and 50 cm long fitted with a rubber bulb on the free end is used with a small amount of balanced salt solution to aspirate material from the prepuce of the bull. This material can be examined in a wet mount under a compound microscope or inoculated into culture medium and organisms looked for 48 hours later.

Bulls remain infected for life if left untreated, and they readily transmit the infection to cows. Therefore it is important to determine whether a bull is infected. As a general rule, a bull is considered to be uninfected if microscopic examinations and cultures are negative on six different occasions.

In the cow, material may be aspirated from the vagina or uterus using a type of large pipet or similar

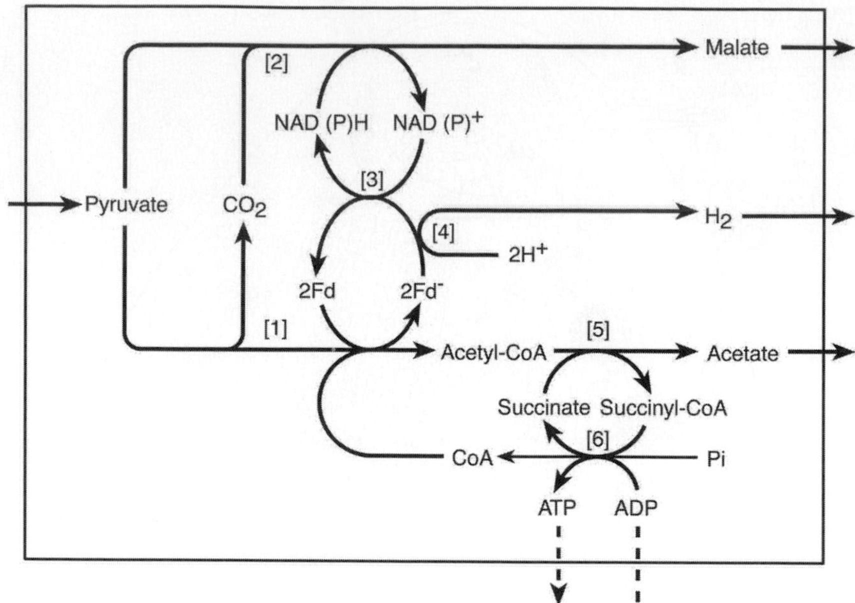

FIGURE 5.3 Metabolic pathways in the hydrogenosomes of trichomonads. The hyrogenosome has molecular hydrogen as its end-product rather than water as in other eukaryotic cells. [Redrawn from data provided by Dr. Miklós Müller, The Rockefeller University]

instrument. In most instances infected cows harbor large numbers of organisms and they can be seen readily on direct microscopic examination. Cultivation may be necessary if no organisms are found on direct examination.

When a cow has aborted, the fetus may be examined for trichomonads. The organisms may be found in the fetal membranes, amniotic fluid, digestive tract, or placenta. Direct examination and cultivation are used.

Molecular methods allow finding organisms when they are present in small numbers and in instances where large numbers of animals may need to be tested. A highly effective and specific method is based on unique nucleotide sequences in *T. foetus*. Material is collected from either a cow or bull as described earlier, the DNA is extracted, and deposited on a filter. The filter is then probed with the oligonucleotide. Results have shown a detection rate with 94.9% accuracy in infected animals. Direct examination and cultivation show about 50% of positives.

A variety of other agents may cause abortion in cattle, *Brucella abortus* and *Vibrio foetus* being among bacterial agents of importance. *Sarcocystis* spp. may also be involved in abortion (Chapter 13). When a breeding problem is recognized in a herd, it is usually important to consider a number of possible causes for it.

Host–Parasite Interactions

As a general rule, infections in bulls remain benign, but so far as is known, the infection does not clear up spontaneously. The organisms typically remain in the prepuce, but on occasion may infect the internal genitalia such as the seminal vesicles and the testicles.

Upon introduction into the reproductive tract of a cow during sexual intercourse, the trichomonads reproduce in the vagina where they may cause a vaginitis. If the animal is pregnant, the organisms may invade the uterus and infect the developing fetus. When this happens, the cow usually aborts during the first 16 weeks of pregnancy (gestation in cows is 37 weeks). If abortion does occur, the cow usually is free of infection after two estrus cycles (estrus in cows is 21 days). The infection in the cow is eliminated through the development of immunity.

In some instances, the fetus may die and be retained in the uterus, or a portion of the fetal membranes is retained after abortion. In these instances, uterine infections may ensue, which result in permanent sterility.

Where trichomonad abortion takes place in a herd, the owner usually perceives it as infertility. The calf is quite small early in pregnancy and the signs of abortion may be missed. Some other infectious agents cause abortion late in pregnancy and in those instances the owner becomes aware when an animal has aborted.

Epidemiology and Control

T. foetus is transmitted from cow to bull, and back, through sexual intercourse. Because trichomonads exist only as trophozoites, the probability of their being transmitted through contaminated bedding or from other species of animals is remote. Therefore, control programs revolve around eliminating the organism from a cattle herd and ensuring that it is not reintroduced.

When an outbreak of trichomonad abortion has been diagnosed in a herd, the first step is to determine which animals are infected and then to do the following:

1. Treat infected bulls
2. Isolate infected animals so that no further transmission can take place
3. Dispose of the animals that are economically marginal

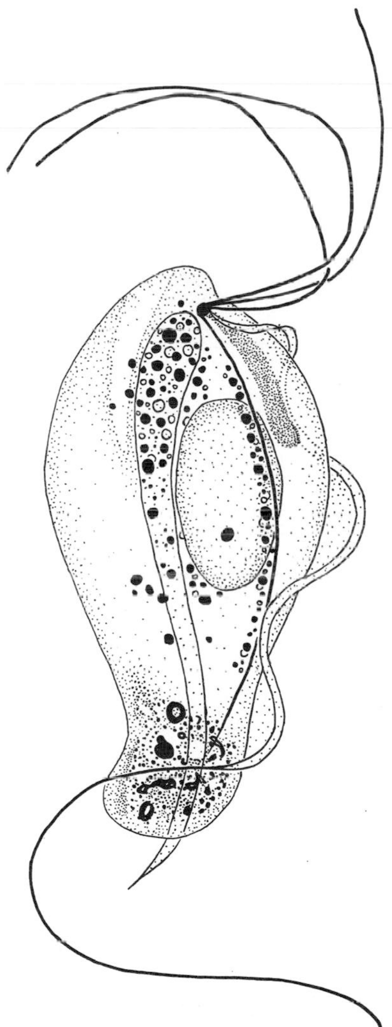

FIGURE 5.4 *Tritrichomonas foetus* as seen diagrammatically in the LM.

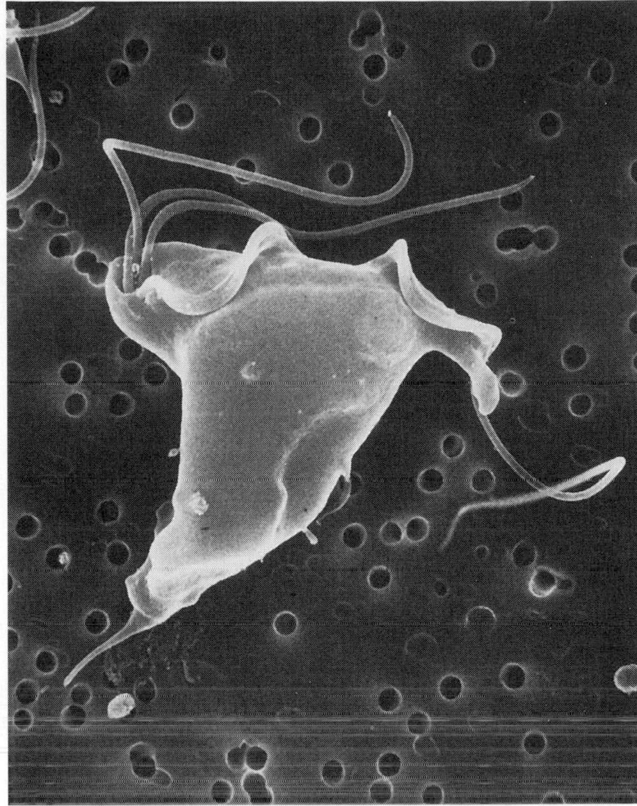

FIGURE 5.5 *Tritrichomonas foetus* as seen in SEM (magnification 6000X). Note the anterior flagella emerging as a pocket and the undulating membrane with its accessory filament. The axostyle protrudes from the posterior end, and the recurrent flagellum extends beyond the undulating membrane. [From Speer, C. A., and White, M. W., 1992.]

Cows usually eliminate the organism spontaneously after two estrus cycles or heat periods, about 42 days. Before returning them to the herd or allowing natural breeding, each one should be examined to ensure that they are free of infection.

Bulls present a particularly difficult dilemma. If left untreated, they retain infection for life. A drug not currently available in the United States, but probably is elsewhere, dimetridazole, provides almost 100% certainty that the bull will be free of infection after treatment. The question for the owner to answer is *almost* good enough? A good bull is worth tens of thousands of dollars and no owner wants to let that amount of money go to the slaughter house for minimal return. On the other hand, if the bull is not completely cleared of infection, it may infect, say, half a dozen cows who abort, are carried through the winter eating six pounds of hay each day and do not deliver a calf in the spring.

If treatment is *almost* perfect, and if the DNA-based diagnostic technique discussed earlier is *almost* perfect, the risk of keeping a bull in a herd is probably low enough to justify it. However, if the bull is not an especially good breeder, or lacks the best genetic qualities, or is nearing the end of his breeding life, it may be best to send him to slaughter.

Prevention is the watchword in bovine trichomonosis. Management should revolve around keeping this organism, and others that are passed during sexual intercourse, from entering a herd. Any bull that is to be introduced into a herd should be examined for infection with trichomonads. As a general rule, bulls to be sold on the open market are examined for fertility and for venereally transmitted infectious agents such as *Vibrio foetus* and *T. foetus.* A great deal of money is laid out for a quality bull, and the new owner should know that the purchase is a sound investment.

Artificial insemination (AI) is almost universal in the dairy industry in North America and it is being used more and more in the beef industry. Semen is collected from bulls, diluted and frozen in nitrogen in sealed ampoules for use months, or even years, later. The question is, does AI preclude infection with *T. foetus*? The answer is a qualified *yes*. In a properly run AI center, no infected bull would be allowed in. Second, semen collected from a bull is diluted with an extender and a chemical to protect the sperm from the effects of freezing. The fact of dilution serves to reduce the probability of trichomonads being transferred to a cow later. However, the conditions under which sperm are frozen are the same conditions under which trichomonads are successfully preserved. Freedom from venereally transmitted organisms requires vigilance on the part of buyers, sellers, and AI centers.

Progress is being made in developing one or more vaccines.

Related Organisms

Trichomonads are quite common in both the digestive and reproductive tracts of domestic animals. In swine, for example, they may be found in the nasal passages, the stomach and large intestine. In cattle there are forms in both the digestive and reproductive tracts that are morphologically similar. Horses have been infected with *T. foetus* and there is some observational evidence that this organism causes abortion in horses.

TRICHOMONAD VAGINITIS

Name of Organism and Disease Association

Trichomonas vaginalis is the cause of trichomonad vaginitis in women.

Hosts and Host Range

This is a parasite of humans, both men and women. It has been experimentally transmitted to some higher primates and to laboratory rodents.

Geographic Distribution and Importance

Cosmopolitan. Most surveys indicate a prevalence of infection of 10 to 25% among women. In some populations, the prevalence of infection has approached 90%. Presumably the prevalence of infection in men is about the same as in women, but data are fragmentary.

Trichomonad vaginitis causes considerable discomfort as well as mental distress. In a few reported instances, the infection has spread from the vagina to other parts of the urogenital system. Men remain asymptomatic.

Morphology

T. vaginalis ranges in size from 4 to 32 μm in length by 2 to 17 μm in width. The mean is about 10 x 7 μm. It has four anterior flagella and a recurrent flagellum attached to the body by an undulating membrane; the recurrent flagellum does not extend beyond the undulating membrane (Fig. 5.6 and 5.7). The axostyle is slender and extends beyond the posterior of the body. The parabasal body is single or V-shaped and has a filament associated with it.

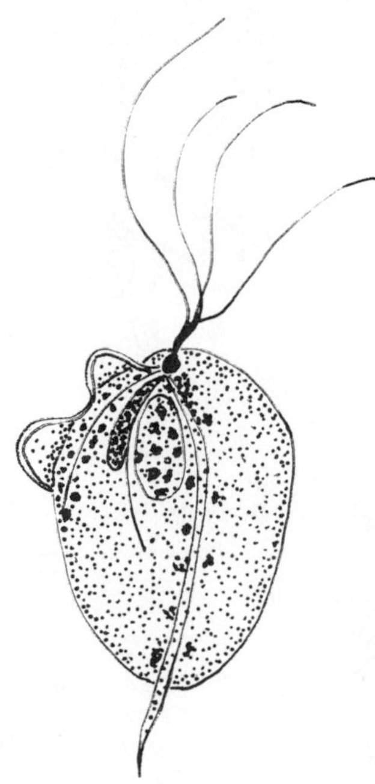

FIGURE 5.6 *Trichomonas vaginalis* as seen in a stained preparation from culture under the LM.

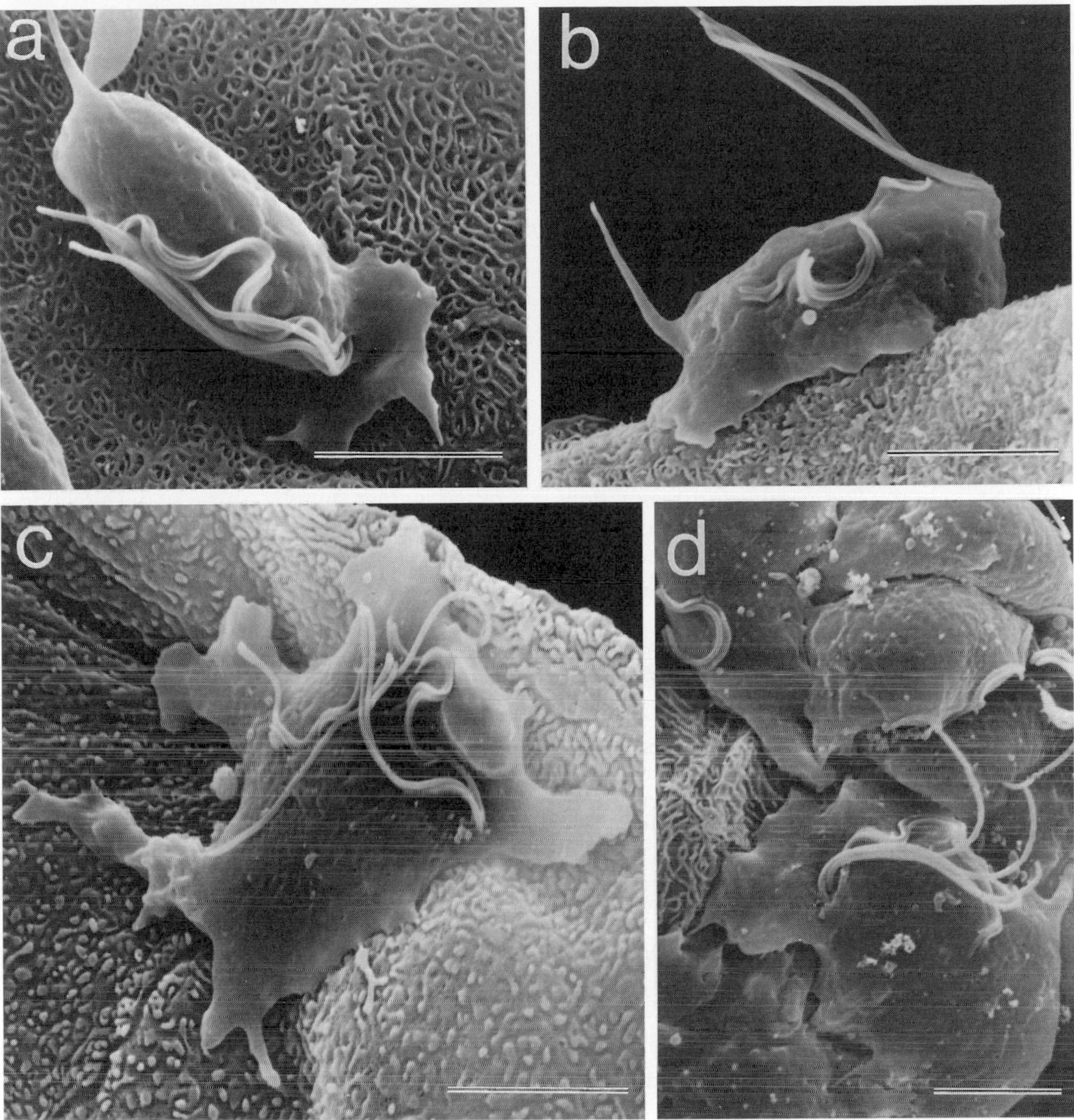

FIGURE 5.7 *Trichomonas vaginalis* as seen in SEM. (a) An organism just settling onto the surface; much of the normal morphology is retained. (b) An organism beginning to spread on the surface. (c) The organism has spread on the surface and interedigitated with the epithelial cells underneath. (d) A mat of *T. vaginalis* on the epithelial surface. [From Arroyo *et al.*, 1993.]

Life Cycle

This organism reproduces by binary fission. *T. vaginalis* is transmitted from one person to the next through sexual intercourse. There is some evidence that under unhygienic conditions, transmission may take place through soiled clothing or wash cloths, but such transmission is probably rare because trichomonads survive only a short time when exposed to the air. They also require physiological salt solution for survival, and they die immediately upon exposure to, say, tap water.

Diagnosis

Finding the living organisms in material taken from a person is the usual means of determining whether infection with *T. vaginalis* is present. In women, vaginal swabs are most commonly examined under a microscope. Trichomonads are sometimes an incidental finding in urine sediments or *Pap* smears taken for other diagnostic purposes. Vaginal discomfort and excessive production of mucus are reasons to suspect trichomonad vaginitis, but other infectious agents as well as noninfectious processes often cause such symptoms.

In men, urethral swabs or secretions obtained through prostatic massage are examined under a microscope to find the organisms.

Suspect material from either women or men may be cultivated in nonliving media as part of the diagnostic procedure if organisms are not found upon microscopic examination.

Host–Parasite Interactions

Although both men and women are equally infected with *T. vaginalis*, it causes disease almost exclusively in women. The organism usually remains confined to the vagina where it multiplies and causes an inflammation of the epithelium. The result of inflammation is tenderness, pain, itching, and excessive production of mucus. Intercourse may be painful.

It happens infrequently, but *T. vaginalis* can infect parts of the urogenital system other than the vagina. There are cases in which the organism has been found in the bladder, ureters, and even the kidneys. For example, there is a case of a woman having a large, tumorlike swelling in the body wall near the kidney; the swelling was found to have been caused by trichomonads, which had migrated to the kidney, broken out, and colonized the perirenal area.

Men usually remain asymptomatic, but infrequently there is inflammation of the urethra and the prostate gland.

Vaginal infections with *T. vaginalis* may take place prior to puberty, but they are only transient since they clear up spontaneously. At puberty, the bacterial flora change and increase the hydrogen ion concentration to about pH 4.5. This change leads to conditions in the vagina that allow *T. vaginalis* to flourish if the woman is exposed to the organism.

Despite the changes which take place in the vagina at sexual maturation, it remains a hostile environment for *T. vaginalis* and other potentially pathogenic organisms that live there. There is a continual turnover of epithelial cells and they probably vary physiologically with the stage of the menstrual cycle. The flow of mucus tends to carry the organisms toward the outside, and finally there are cytotoxic substances and antibody, which kill or immobilize the organisms.

In a series of elegant studies it has been shown that the trichomonad has evolved a number of mechanisms to remain in the vagina (Alderete et al., 1995). There are four different protein *adhesins* on the surface of trichomonad, which attach to receptors on the vaginal epithelial cells (VEC) allowing them to adhere tightly. Interestingly, these adhesins are covered with another protein, which must be removed enzymatically with a protease before attachment can occur. *T. vaginalis* adheres somewhat to other cells such as the HeLa cell line, but it is a rather tenuous association. Once attached to the VEC, the trichomonad flattens out within five minutes to form an extraordinarily intimate association (Fig. 5. 7b). It can be seen that the parasite interdigitates with the host cell (Fig. 5.7c) and that other trichomonads also cluster there (Fig. 5.7d). It may be that there is a taxis that draws a number of organism to the site once one of them has adhered. This exquisite interaction of parasite and host may allow the cytotoxicity of the parasite to be expressed giving rise, eventually, to the clinical signs and symptoms of trichomonosis.

No immunity per se has been demonstrated in infected women, but the course of the infection allows the inference that immunity does develop. Over a period of time, the severity of the clinical signs and symptoms decreases.

Epidemiology and Control

Control of trichomonad vaginitis involves the following:

1. Treatment of the infected woman
2. Treatment of her sexual partner(s)
3. Use of a condom during sexual intercourse

Among sexually transmitted diseases (STD), trichomonad vaginitis is not considered to be the serious problem that are gonorrhea, syphilis, chlamydial infections, or herpes. Although the infection may result in considerable discomfort, there are usually no catastrophic consequences for the infected woman. Consequently, trichomonad vaginitis is not a reportable disease and no effort is made by public health personnel to find and treat all sexual partners who may have been exposed as is done when gonorrhea or syphilis is diagnosed.

Control of infection is nearly always limited to individual treatment of a woman who has shown clinical signs and symptoms of infection. Since men nearly always remain asymptomatic, and many women, too, a relatively high level of infection can be achieved in a population in which sexual partners may be frequently changed.

When it has been determined that a woman is infected, it is essential to treat both her and her sexual partner(s), or nothing will be accomplished.

A variety of drugs have been used more or less successfully in the treatment of both men and women. Some of the drugs that have been used are quinolines, arsonic acid, and tetracyclines. These are usually administered topically—either vaginally in women or introduced into the urethra of men.

Metronidazole (Flagyl) is a highly effective drug that is administered by mouth. Metronidazole is an imidazole derivative and this moeity is known to have some carcinogenicity. The risk of cancer is sufficiently low, and the efficacy of the drug so high that the risk to the health of the patient is considered to be negligible. Metronidazole acts by inhibiting the enzymes in the hydrogenosomes.

Related Organisms

Two trichomonads other than *T. vaginalis* commonly occur in the humans. *Trichomonas tenax* is one of two protists that occur in the human mouth; *Entamoeba gingivalis* is the other. *T. tenax* has about a 10% prevalence in humans. It lies in the debris between the teeth and around the gum line. It has been accused of causing gum problems, but it is a commensal rather than a pathogen. It is structurally quite similar to *T. vaginalis* and the two species may well be closely related to one another.

Pentatrichomonas hominis is an inhabitant of the intestine of humans (Fig. 7.1 I) and a number of other species of hosts and sometimes occurs in large numbers. Again, it is an opportunist and does not cause any damage to the host. Its mode of transmission has remained a mystery.

AVIAN TRICHOMONOSIS

Name of Organism and Disease Associations

Trichomonas gallinae causes avian trichomonosis, avian trichomoniasis or canker.

Hosts and Host Range

Birds in the order Columbiformes (pigeons and doves) are considered to be the primary hosts of *T. gallinae*, but the organism is readily transmissible to birds in other orders as well. Infections have been seen in hawks, falcons, turkeys, and chickens, among others.

Geographic Distribution and Importance

Cosmopolitan. Economic losses are seen principally in doves and pigeons raised either for food or as a hobby. The infection probably is important in populations of wild doves, as well.

Figures on losses are sparse and difficult to evaluate. For example, in 1954 the USDA estimated that there is a $47,000 annual loss in the United States; later (1965) the same agency estimated that there is a $1.186 million annual loss in turkeys. The economic loss in chickens was estimated at more than $800,000.

Morphology

The body of *T. gallinae* averages 12 by 6 μm with four free flagella about 11 μm long. The recurrent flagellum terminates half to two-thirds down the length of the body; there is no free flagellum. The parabasal body is sausage-shaped in LM preparations and is roundish in EM. It has two filaments, one of which extends into the posterior portion of the body (Figs. 5. 2 and 5.8).

Life Cycle

T. gallinae is transmitted from one bird to another through close contact. Infection is most often seen in the upper part of the digestive tract such as the esophagus and crop, but other organs are infected as well. Young columbiform birds are infected when their parents feed them. In pigeons and doves, parents feed their young with a secretion of the crop called *pigeon's milk*, and in an infected parent this secretion becomes laden with trichomonads.

Transfer among other birds is by contamination of food and drinking water; fecal contamination seems

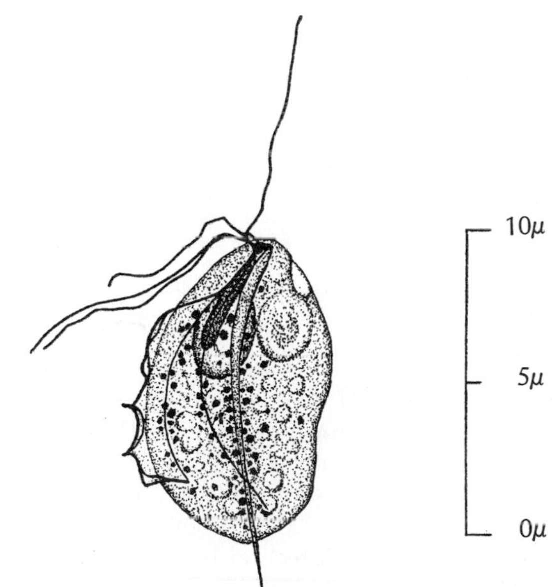

FIGURE 5.8 *Trichomonas gallinae*, a parasite of the upper digestive and respiratory tracts of columbiform birds. [From Stabler, R. M., 1947.]

not to be a mode of transmission. Falcons and hawks are infected through eating columbiform birds.

Diagnosis

The principal and most effective method of diagnosis is finding the organism in infected tissues. This may be done by direct microscopic examination of material or by cultivating swabs in appropriate nonliving media.

Postmortem examination of a bird shows yellow, caseous lesions of the intestinal tract, including mouth, crop, and esophagus, the lungs, and liver. Such lesions are helpful, but other microorganisms may cause similar gross changes.

Host–Parasite Interactions

Isolates of *T. gallinae* vary considerably in virulence, and the infection may range from benign in which there is uneventful recovery to an acute, rapidly fatal disease. The age of the bird also contributes to the pathologic effect: young birds are much more susceptible than adults. Thus, adult doves may carry the infection, but when it is transferred to their offspring, the young are likely to die. In young pigeons or doves (squab), the mortality may approach 90%.

T. gallinae infects the digestive tract, liver, and lungs. Early in the course of the infection, the organism remains in the upper part of the digestive tract, mouth, and crop. As the infection progresses, it moves farther down the digestive tract and then invades both the liver and the lungs. In this latter instance, death is likely.

Epidemiology and Control

A complete control program for avian trichomonosis should be based on:

1. Identifying infected birds
2. Treating or eliminating infected birds
3. Preventing reintroduction of the parasite

Trichomonosis presents a difficult problem for raisers of pigeons and doves. Death losses in squab are likely to be such that few survive. One means of control is to treat the adults with enheptin, a nitrofuran compound. Enheptin has some efficacy against *T. gallinae*, but it is not a panacea. The objective is to remove, or at least reduce, the infection in the adults so that they will not transmit the infection to their young.

In a dove cote or pigeon loft, it is often safest to remove the infected birds, and in some instances, it may be best to remove all of the birds and start with clean stock. Once having eliminated the infection, steps need to be taken to prevent reintroduction from wild birds that might contaminate the food or water. Construction of enclosures should be such that only the residents have access to the food and water that is provided.

Falconers sometimes use pigeons to train their birds to hunt. There are a number of instances on record in which the falcons were infected from their prey. The broad host range of *T. gallinae* makes control in any species of bird quite difficult.

Further complicating control is the immunity that surviving birds develop. Birds become immune but retain an infection that they are fully capable of transmitting. Worse, yet, infection with an isolate of low virulence confers immunity not only to that strain, but to virulent strains as well. A bird may become infected with a strain of low virulence, show little clinical effect, and then be infected with organisms that are highly lethal. This means that immune adults can pass the virulent organisms to their offspring with devastating results.

Based on these observations of immunity and virulence, it has been theorized that the extinction of the passenger pigeon in the early part of the 20th century was due not to human depredations but rather to these kinds of double infections coupled with nonsterile immunity. The two factors quickly reduced the fecundity of pigeons and led to their extinction. It is true that commercial hunting of the passenger pigeon was carried on at a scale that is almost unimaginable, but as populations of pigeons declined, commercial hunting became uneconomical. The population of pigeons should have stabilized, but it continued to decline. It is worth considering that this disease contributed to the inevitable elimination of the species.

BLACKHEAD OF TURKEYS

Name of Organism and Disease Association

Histomonas meleagridis causes blackhead, histomonosis, histomoniasis, and infectious enterohepatitis, principally in turkeys.

Hosts and Host Range

The principal host in which economic losses are seen is the turkey, *Meleagris gallopavo*, but the organism has a fairly broad host range among gallinaceous birds including the domestic chicken, pheasant, grouse, and quail.

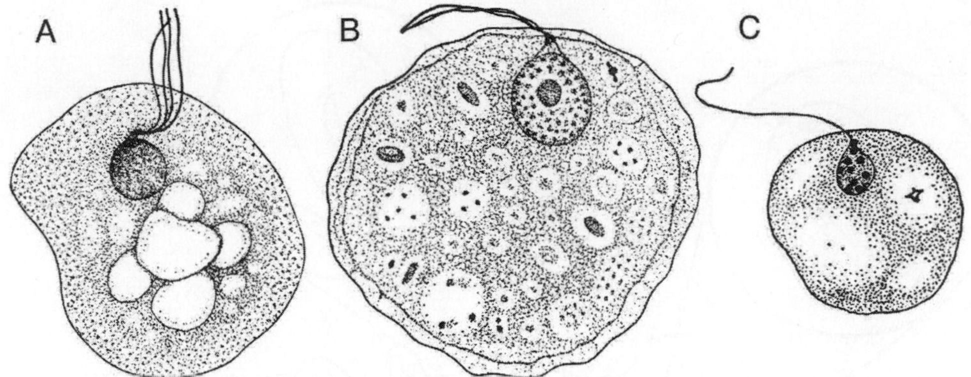

FIGURE 5.9 *Histomonas meleagridis*, a pathogen of turkeys and other gallinaceous birds as seen in stained smears under the LM. [From Wenrich, D., 1943.]

Geographic Distribution and Importance

Cosmopolitan. Estimates of economic loss due to histomonosis by the USDA in turkeys were $1.8 million and $2.7 million due to mortality and morbidity, respectively. Losses in chickens were estimated to be $1.9 million due to mortality and $2.9 million due to morbidity.

Morphology

This organism is referred to as being *pleomorphic*—that is, it does not have definite shape as do most of the other trichomonads (Fig. 5.9). The size ranges from 8 to 21 μm; there is a single nucleus and one to four flagella. In life, the organism often moves by ameboid movement.

H. meleagridis was originally classified in a group that is considered to be transitional between the amebas and flagellates. In the usual cytologic stains, such as hematoxylin, the organisms show little structure; usually only the nucleus, cytoplasm, and a plasma membrane can be seen. Studies at the LM level using silver stains, and EM studies have shown that *H. meleagridis* has affinities to the trichomonads (Fig. 5.10). The organism has basal bodies, a parabasal body and an associated filament, and an axostyle that continues anteriorly as the pelta. The structures are not as robust as in a typical trichomonad, but they are sufficient to show their affinity to the group. Serological studies that compared *H. meleagridis* to a number of other protists showed that it is closely related to the trichomonads.

Life Cycle

H. meleagridis reproduces by binary fission as do other trichomonads. Transmission from one bird to the next takes places through the cecal nematode, *Heterakis gallinarum* (Fig. 5.11). *Heterakis* serves as vector of *Histomonas*; the worm itself becomes infected with *Histomonas* by ingesting them with its food in the cecum of the bird. The trophozoites later infect the reproductive tract of the worm and become incorporated into the eggs as they are formed. When a bird ingests an infective egg of *H. gallinarum* containing *H. meleagridis*, it becomes infected with both parasites.

Diagnosis

Determining whether a bird is suffering from histomonosis is usually based on seeing the characteristic lesions in the ceca and liver. Finding the organisms themselves is possible, but they are so obscure that one does not usually look for them. *Parahistomonas wenrichi*, a nonpathogenic histomonad, may also be present, and it is not possible to tell the difference between the two organisms without special staining.

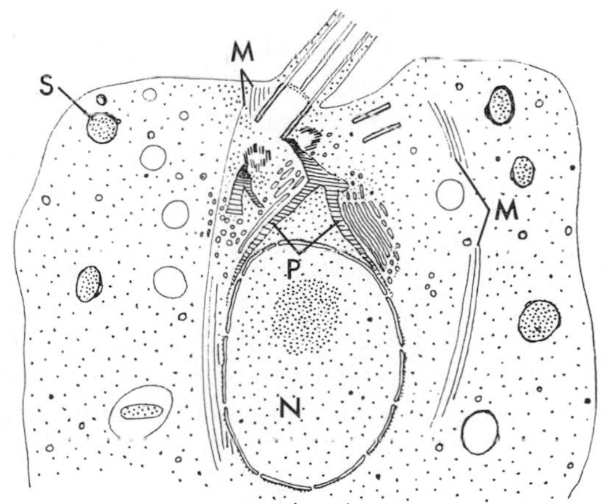

FIGURE 5.10 Fine structure of *Histomonas meleagridis* showing affinities to other trichomonads P—parabasal body and fibers (Golgi), M—microtubular elements; N—nucleus; S—cytoplasm-filled sacs. [From Schuster, F. L., 1968.]

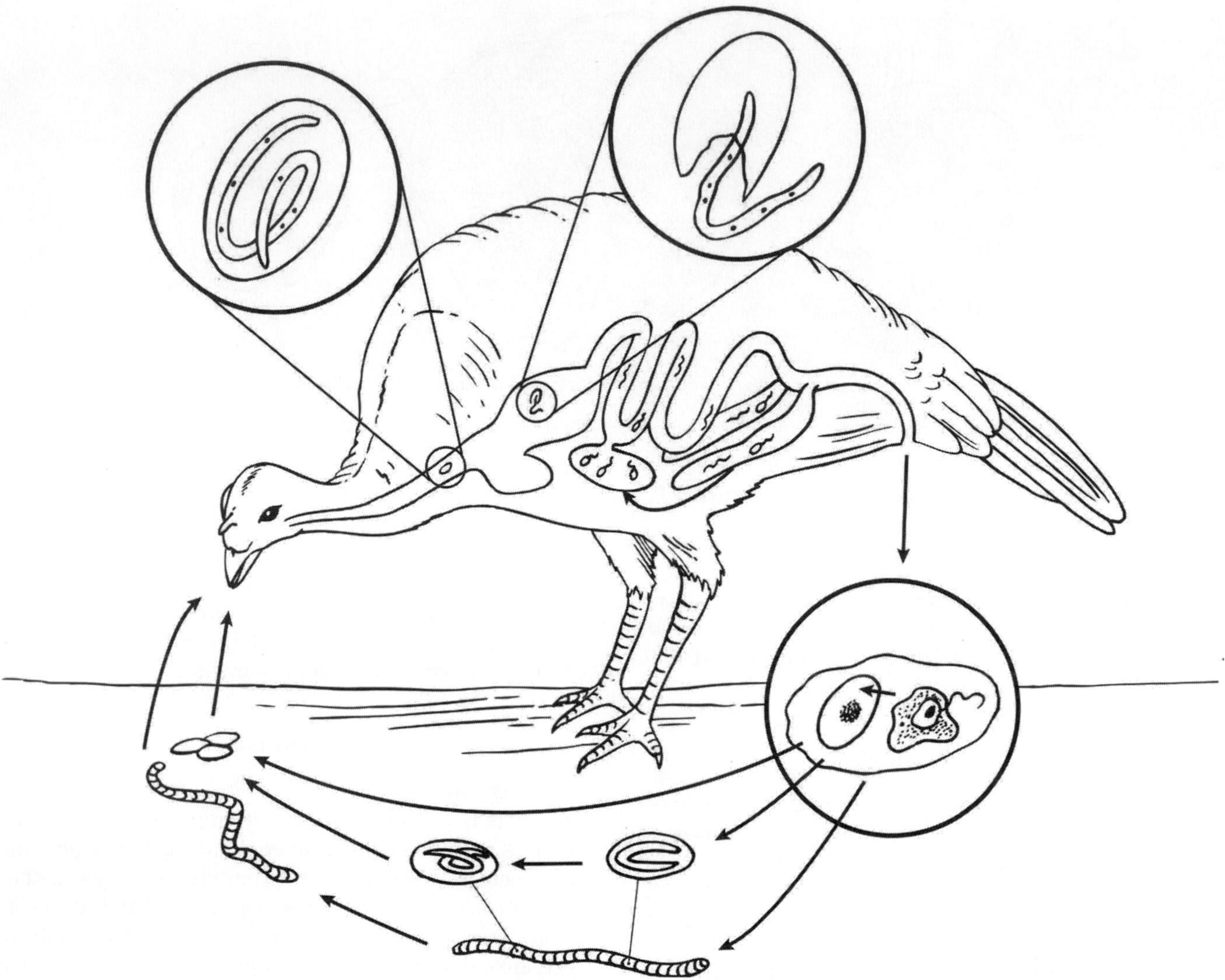

FIGURE 5.11 Life cycle of *Histomonas meleagridis*. The organisms involved in the life cycle are (1) the turkey, (2) the histomonads, (3) the cecal worm, *Heterakis gallinarum*, and (4) earthworms.

Lesions in the ceca, which may be seen early in infection, are small ulcers in the intestinal epithelium. Later, they become larger and tissue necrosis may be seen. The lumena of the ceca also become filled with a yellowish fluid, which is also evident as characteristic sulfur-colored droppings.

As infection continues, the histomonads move to the liver and cause characteristic lesions there. These are circular, depressed, yellowish areas; they may range in size from 1 to 2 mm to nearly 1 cm in diameter. These lesions are spoken of as being *pathognomic*, that is, they indicate with a high level of certainty that the disease is histomonosis.

Host–Parasite Interactions

The life cycle of *H. meleagridis* is an example of a helminth serving as a vector of another disease agent (see also *Dientamoeba fragilis* and *Nanophyetus salmincola*). Considering the fact that infecting birds with naked histomonads almost never occurs, and the intimate association that they have with the worms, it seems likely that the protists were first parasites of the worms and then later parasites of the avian hosts.

Two pioneer investigators in parasitic diseases, Smith and Graybill, first showed in 1920 that histomonosis is transmitted by *Heterakis gallinarum.* Since then, a number of studies have been done showing unequivocally that the histomonads are inside the egg capsules and that only embryonated eggs are capable of transmitting the infection. Only eggs containing the second stage infective larva hatch upon reaching the intestine of the bird; if unembryonated, they cannot respond to the stimuli and merely pass out with the egg capsules intact. Histomonads can also be seen in fixed and stained embryonated eggs.

Upon release from the egg capsules, the histomonads multiply in the cecum of the bird. Worms become infected by ingesting trophozoites with intestinal contents on which they feed.

Depending on the species of host, *H. meleagridis* may remain as a harmless commensal, or at the other extreme, it may invade the tissues of the gut, liver, and lung and cause the death of the host. Although there are sometimes losses in young chickens, histomonosis is not usually a problem in the domestic fowl.

The bird in which the greatest economic losses occur is the domestic turkey. In young birds, from a month to three months of age, death losses may approach 100% in a flock. Older turkeys are susceptible to infection, but death losses may reach only 25% in a flock.

Epidemiology and Control

Control of blackhead is based on the following:

1. Isolation of turkeys from chickens in both time and space
2. Chemoprophylaxis

Where the risk of infection of turkey poults is high, chemoprophylaxis may be practiced, but the side effects of drugs are such that they should be avoided if possible. A number of drugs have been recommended for use against histomonosis, but none is highly effective.

Chickens are relatively resistant to blackhead, but turkeys are highly susceptible. It seems likely that the organism was introduced into North America with colonization by Europeans. Chickens serve as a reservoir of infection for turkeys, and this is the basis of control through management.

Isolating turkeys from chickens is desirable, but may be difficult. Scrupulous washing of footwear, tools, and machinery is necessary to ensure that eggs of *Heterakis* are not transported from one place to another on a farm. The time and effort involved may be prohibitive.

The heterakid eggs that contain histomonads survive for an extraordinarily long time. It has been found that an area contaminated with *Heterakis* eggs was still capable of transmitting infections to clean birds 66 weeks later. In this study, plots were contaminated with nematode eggs, and then birds were put on for a short period of time every week. At the end of the experiment, birds were still becoming infected.

Earthworms serve as a means of helping both the histomonads and the heterakids to survive for long periods outside of the avian host. When earthworms ingest infective eggs of *Heterakis*, the worms hatch and invade the tissues of the earthworm. They remain there for two years or perhaps longer.

Isolation, then, means not only spatial isolation but also isolation in time. Obviously, the risks of infection are such that only ground not occupied by chickens for years should be used for raising turkeys.

Some additional control methods are to raise turkey poults on wire until they are old enough to resist the infection. Keeping age groups of turkeys separated from one another is also advisable. Lastly, in some areas, turkeys are herded, rather like sheep, and in this instance, the birds should be kept moving onto clean ground. Under ideal conditions, they should not return to the same pasture for at least one year.

If this all seems rather laborious, that is true. Consider the factors that require heroic measures to control blackhead. The organism has a broad host range and is relatively benign in most hosts, except the turkey. The causative agent has an extraordinary long survival time outside its hosts. Chemotherapy is not satisfactory. Natural immunity helps to protect turkeys but it is too slow in developing to expose young birds to heavily contaminated ground. Artificial immunity has not been successful yet. One is left with few choices, except to raise ducks.

Related Organisms

Parahistomonas wenrichi is a parasite of the intestinal tract of turkeys. It is closely related to *H. meleagridis*, but it is sufficiently different structurally to justify separate generic status. *P. wenrichi* is of interest because it has low pathogenicity but protects a bird against infection with *H. meleagridis*. It has been suggested that infection with *P. wenrichi* might provide protection from the effects of *H. meleagridis* and could be used as an artificial immunizing agent.

DIENTAMOEBA FRAGILIS

Name of Organism and Disease Associations

Dientamoeba fragilis is the cause of enteritis and diarrhea in humans.

Hosts and Host Range

The principal host is the human, but the organism has been found in some other higher primates such as baboon, macaque, and chimpanzee.

Geographic Distribution and Importance

Cosmopolitan. Estimates of prevalence in the human population worldwide vary from 4 to 20%. Of 65,444 fecal samples examined in Ontario, Canada, 4.1% were found to contain *D. fragilis*.

Morphology

The organisms have a broad size range varying from 3 to 22 μm in many reports. They average 9 μm. There are typically two vesicular nuclei which have a cluster of granules forming the endosome (Fig. 7.1 K), which may be the nucleolus. The granular cytoplasm contains bacterial inclusions. Cysts are unknown.

The binucleate condition occurs in more than half of organisms seen, for example, in a stained fecal smear. The two nuclei seems to be attached by a strand of material when examined at the LM level. At the EM level, it has been shown that the nuclei are in arrested telophase, thus the strand of material between them. Why the nuclei should remain in telophase most of the time has not been explained.

The taxonomic status of *D. fragilis* remained clouded for many years after it was first described. Since the organisms average only about 9 μm, it can be appreciated that some of its structures are so small that they approach the resolving power of the light microscope. The organism was originally described as an ameba, but more than 20 years after the original description, Clifford Dobell concluded that *D. fragilis* might be an aberrant flagellate closely related to *Histomonas meleagridis.* This was a highly intuitive, and correct, conclusion.

Studies using silver staining, electron microscopy, and serological analysis of proteins have allowed the conclusion that *D. fragilis* is a trichomonad. The generic name *Dientamoeba* implies that the organism is an ameba and it might appear to be appropriate to change it to something more descriptive. The rules of zoological nomenclature require that the original name be retained even though it seems to be the wrong taxon.

Life Cycle

D. fragilis multiplies by binary fission in the large intestine of the human host; there are neither cysts nor sexual stages. Transmission to a new host takes place by mouth. The human pinworm, *Enterobius vermicularis* (Chapter 33), serves as a vector of *Dientamoeba.* The protist is inside the egg of the pinworm; much the same mode of transmission as seen in the agent causing histomoniosis in turkeys, *Histomonas meleagridis.*

Diagnosis

Organisms may be found in freshly passed feces, but they die rather quickly outside of the host. The living trophozoites are active, move progressively, and show a clearly defined ectoplasm. In fixed and stained fecal smears, the organisms may well be missed by inexperienced persons. One needs to look for the smooth, membrane-bound outline of a protistan and the two small nuclei. Small bits of a fecal sample may be placed in culture media to encourage growth of the organisms.

Host–Parasite Interactions

D. fragilis is mildly pathogenic. The principal signs of infection are enteritis with diarrhea, abdominal pain, fever, vomiting, flatulence, general weakness, and weight loss. About 25% of infected persons experience symptoms.

Epidemiology and Control

Control of infection with *D. fragilis* takes two routes:

1. Treating infected persons
2. Preventing and treating pinworm infections

As is true with other trichomonads, *D. fragilis* exists only as a trophozoite, and transmission from one host to the next presents a problem to the organism. The great British protozoologist, Clifford Dobell, was the coauthor of the original description of the organism, and in his later studies on it, infected himself with organisms in culture. Despite numerous attempts and having drunk large numbers of organisms, he never experienced infection. His frustration at these failures shines through the bland prose of his scientific writing.

A breakthrough in the knowledge of how transmission takes place came in 1956, 38 years after the original description, when Burrows and Swerdlow presented epidemiologic and cytologic evidence that *D. fragilis* is transmitted in the egg of the human pinworm, *Enterobius vermicularis.* Additional studies by other investigators have shown good, though circumstantial, evidence that the pinworm does serve as the vector. For example, there is about a 20 times greater association of pinworms and *Dientamoeba* infection in the same person than would be expected by chance.

As a general rule, proper disposal of human feces is recommended as the principal means of controlling human infections with enteric protists. With *D. fragilis,* however, the principle does not apply. The emphasis comes back to the vector and treating affected persons. Several chemotherapeutic agents are effective in eliminating the organism from the human colon. Pinworms are intestinal parasites of humans, but they are not generally transmitted through contaminated food and water (Chapter 33). Pinworm eggs containing infective larvae are usually transmitted from one person to another through contaminated clothing and bed linens. An individual may also infect himself or herself directly by scratching the perianal region and then transferring eggs to the mouth on the fingers.

Readings

Alderete, J. F., Lehker, M. W., and Arroyo, R. (1995). The mechanisms and molecules involved in the cytoadherence and pathogenesis of *Trichomonas vaginalis*. *Parasitol. Today* **11,** 70–74.

Arroyo, R., *et al.* (1993). Signalling of *Trichomonas vaginalis* for amoeboid transformation and adhesin synthesis follows cytoadherence. *Mol. Microbiol.* **7,** 299–309.

Brooks, B., and Schuster, F. L. (1984). Oral protozoa: Survey, isolation and ultrastructure of *Trichomonas tenax* from clinical practice. *Trans. Am. Microsc. Soc.* **103,** 376–382.

Corbeil, L. B. (1994). Vaccination strategies against *Tritrichomonas foetus*. *Parasitol. Today* **10,** 103–106.

Dobell, C. C. (1940). Researches on the intestinal protozoa of monkeys and man. X. The life history of *Dientamoeba fragilis*—Observations, experiments, and speculations. *Parasitology* **32,** 417–461.

Honigberg, B. M. (Ed.) (1989). *Trichomonads Parasitic in Humans*. Springer-Verlag, New York.

Honigberg, B. M., and Kuldova, J. (1969). Structure of a nonpathogenic histomonad from the cecum of galliform birds and a revision of the trichomonad family Monocercomonadidae. *J. Protozool.* **16,** 526–535.

Jirovec, O., and Petr, M. (1968). *Trichomonas vaginalis* and trichomonosis. *Adv. Parasitol.* **6,** 117–188.

Lee, D. L. (1971). Helminths as vectors of micro-organisms. In *Ecology and Physiology of Parasites* (A. M. Fallis, Ed.), pp. 104–121. Univ. of Toronto Press, Toronto.

Mattern, C. F. T., Honigberg, B. M., and Daniel, W. A. (1967). Structure of *Pentatrichomonas hominis* (Davaine) as revealed by electron microscopy. *J. Protozol.* **14,** 320–339.

McDougald, L. R., and Reid, W. M. (1978). *Histomonas meleagridis* and its relatives. In *Parasitic Protozoa* (J. P. Kreir, Ed.), Vol. 3. Academic Press, New York.

Muller, M. (1997). Evolutionary origins of trichomonad hydrogenosomes. *Parasitol. Today* **13,** 166–167.

Schuster, F. L. (1968). Ultrastructure of *Histomonas meleagridis* (Smith) Tyzzer, a parasitic amoeboflagellate. *J. Parasitol.* **54,** 725–737.

Speer, C. A., and White, M. W. (1992). Bovine trichomonoasis. *Large Anim. Vet.* **46,** 18–20.

Speer, C. A., Severson, W. E., Crantson, H. J., Scollard, D., Thompson, J. R., and White, M. W. (1992). A diagnostic DNA assay for trichomonosis in cattle. Proceedings of the 1992 Livestock Conservation Institute.

Stabler, R. M. (1947). *Trichomonas gallinae*, pathogenic trichomonal of birds. *J. Parasitol.* **33,** 207–213.

Wenrich, D. (1943). Observations on the morphology of *Histomonas* from pheasants and chickens. *J. Morphol.* **72,** 279–303.

Yang, J., and Scholten, T. (1977). *Dientamoeba fragilis*: A review with notes on its epidemiology, pathogenicity, mode of transmission, and diagnosis. *Am. J. Trop. Med. Hyg.* **26,** 16–22.

CHAPTER

6

GIARDIA AND GIARDIOSIS

The order *Diplomonadida* contains the only protists that are bilaterally symmetrical. They have two nuclei and six or eight flagella. The members form cysts, and those that are parasitic are transmitted through food or water. Reproduction is by binary fission and there are no sexual stages in the life cycles.

A transition can be seen from the free-living *Trepomonas* to *Hexamita,* which has members that are ether free living or parasitic, to the parasitic *Octomitus, Spironucleus,* and *Giardia.* In this transition, the motility of the organisms is reduced as is their ability to ingest particulate food. *Giardia,* the final stage in the series moving toward parasitism, takes up nutrient across its external membrane and is adapted for attachment to the intestinal surface.

GIARDIA DUODENALIS

Giardia is recognized today as a cosmopolitan intestinal parasite of humans and other animals; infections range from inapparent to seriously debilitating. Human infections result from accidental ingestion of cysts from contaminated water, food, or poor sanitary practices in day care centers, or from sexual transmission. Contact with companion animals also is a source of infection.

Name of Organism and Disease Associations

Giardia duodenalis is the name most used for the parasite of humans, but *G. intestinalis* and *G. lamblia* are commonly seen in textbooks and periodical literature as well. European literature has often used *Lamblia intestinalis.* The following tabulation lists the organisms usually recognized as parasitizing common hosts.

For many years, new species of *Giardia* were named based on finding the organism in a host from which *Giardia* had not been reported. Thus, there is a whole litany of names such as *canis, cati, caprae, equi,* and so on that are all probably synonyms of *G. duodenalis.* Regrettably, giardiologists are not in agreement on the number of species of *Giardia* to accept. This issue is discussed at the end of the chapter under "Notable Features."

G. duodenalis is well known to be pathogenic giving rise to serious diarrhea. The disease should be referred to as giardiosis, although giardiasis is in common usage. It is also called back-packers diarrhea and beaver fever (a nice alliteration, but fever is not a sign of infection).

Hosts and Host Range

As indicated, early studies on *Giardia* allowed the conclusion that the organism has a narrow host range. The organism was not cultivated axenically until about 1975 and it was therefore difficult to carry out unequivocal cross-transmission experiments. In about 1970, however, Russian workers demonstrated cross-transmission between dogs and humans and it was then necessary to reassess the concept of host range. It is now known that *G. duodenalis* naturally infects humans, dog, cats, beaver, coyote, and cattle, and can experimentally infect a number of species of rodents and other mammals.

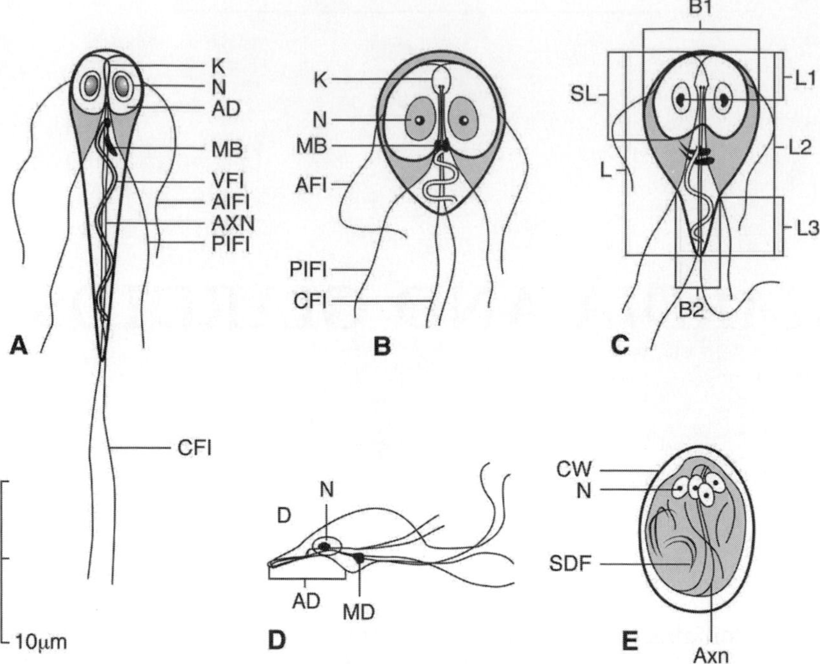

FIGURE 6.1 Types of *Giardia.* Diagrammatic representations of the three types of *Giardia* as seen at the light microscope level: A. *G. agilis* of amphibia; B. *G. muris* of mice and other rodents; and C. *G. duodenalis* of humans, other mammals, and some birds. Abbreviations: AD, adhesive disk; AIFL, anterior flagellum; Axn, axoneme, a bundle of microtubules; B1, width of trophozoite; B2, width of at the exit of the posterior flagella; CFL, caudal flagellum; CW, cyst wall; K, kinetosome or basal body; L, length of body not including the flagella; L1, length to the center of the nuclei; L2, length from the center of the nuclei to the exit of the posterior flagella; L3, length from the exit of the posterior flagella to the tip of the body; MB, median body; N, nucleus; PIFL, posterior flagellum; SDF, flagella; SL, length of adhesive disk; VFL, ventral flagellum. [Redrawn from Kulda & Nohynkova, 1978.]

Geographic Distribution and Importance

Cosmopolitan. Surveys indicate about a 7% prevalence in humans in temperate North America. In some populations as many as 67% of persons are infected. *Giardia* is said to be the most commonly reported human intestinal parasitic infection being responsible for more than 4000 hospital admissions and 100,000 to 1 million infections per year in the United States alone.

Giardiosis occurs in humans both as sporadic individual infections and in epidemic form. Epidemics are usually associated with drinking water. Those communities that obtain their drinking water from surface waters have had the highest risk of infection. *Giardia* was the agent most commonly implicated in waterborne disease outbreaks during the decade from 1978 to 1988. It has been found in 87% of untreated surface water from locations in the United States and Canada.

TABLE 6.1 Common Species of *Giardia* and Their Hosts

Species	Host range	Median body	Morphology
G. duodenalis	Humans, rodents, carnivores, ruminants	Clawlike	11–16 × 5–9 μm
G. agilis	Amphibia	Clubshaped	20 × 4.5 μm Elongated
G. muris	Rodents	Small, round	17–13 × 5–10 μm

Morphology

Three morphologic types of *Giardia* have been described (Fig. 6.1 and Tab. 6.1), and these characteristics are important in differentiating among organisms that might be seen in the intestinal contents of a host. The differences among them are based on length-width measurements and the median bodies. All have two nuclei and eight flagella. *G. duodenalis* trophozoites are pyriform and have an adhesive disk that is less than half of the body length. *G. agilis* is seen in amphibia, and it is long and narrow. The hosts of *G. muris* are the mouse and other rodents; it is nearly round with a large adhesive disk and small median bodies.

The trophozoites of *G. duodenalis* average 13 μm; the width averages 7 μm in length. The organisms are broadly rounded anteriorly and taper to a point posteriorly (Fig. 6.2A and 7.1E). When seen in stained fecal smears, the eight flagella appear only as wispy filaments at the margins of the organism. Each organism has two nuclei, which have a delicate envelope and a large, darkly staining central endosome. In the case of *G. duodenalis*, the median bodies are clawlike and they stain darkly with hematoxylin. Axial rods can often be seen faintly at the LM level.

Under a compound microscope, the cysts are ellipsoid in outline and usually 8–12 x 7–10 μm. Sometimes the sides of the cysts are almost straight, but usually they are rounded (Fig. 6.2B and Fig. 7.1F). Cysts have a double set of organelles; there are four nuclei and two sets of median bodies, but other organelles cannot be seen clearly. In living cysts, the organisms are often motile and can be seen to roll around with considerable vigor within the cyst wall.

Studies in EM have shown that the organisms lie closely applied to the microvilli of the enterocytes; they sink down a bit into the micromilli and leave rings where they have been. The trophozoites have flanges lateral to the adhesive disk (Figs. 6.3 and 6.4), and the body seems to be organized around the movement of fluid through the channel formed by the concave ventral surface and the flange distal to it.

The adhesive disk is supported by network of microtubules and the disk itself is not the absorptive surface. One might think that the movement of fluids across the ventral surface serves to place nutrient in contact with the membrane where uptake occurs; however, ferritin-tagged materials have been found to be taken up only on the dorsal surface.

Life Cycle

Giardia reproduces by binary fission; there are no sexual stages. Trophozoites live in the small intestinal lumen or paramucosal lumen. The trophozoites form cysts in the lower small intestine, usually in asymptomatic infections, and these pass out with the feces.

Cysts are generated under the influence of primary bile salts (tauro-glycochenodeoxycholate, and glycocholate), but not secondary bile salts (glycodeoxycholate). Cysts are infective to another host as soon as they are passed. Cysts are ingested with contaminated food or water, for the most part (Fig. 6.5).

Diagnosis

Determining whether an individual is infected with *Giardia* is based not only on finding the organism, but also on eliminating other protistan and microbial agents as the cause of the intestinal problem. The principal means are as follows:

1. Observing signs and symptoms
2. Finding motile trophozoites in a fresh fecal smear
3. Finding cysts in feces by a concentration technique

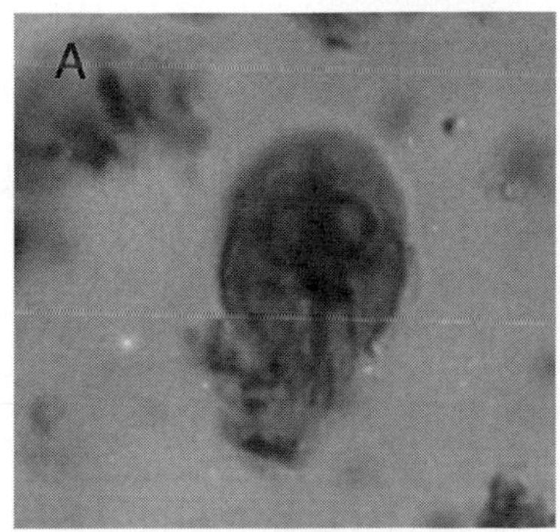

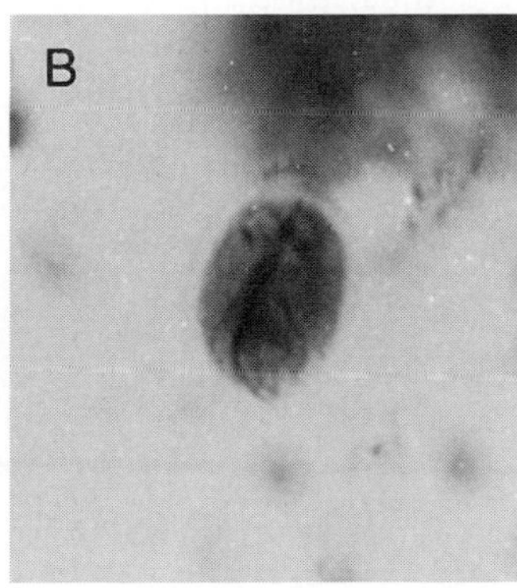

FIGURE 6.2 *Giardia duodenalis* trophozoite (A) and cyst (B) from stained fecal smears as seen in LM.

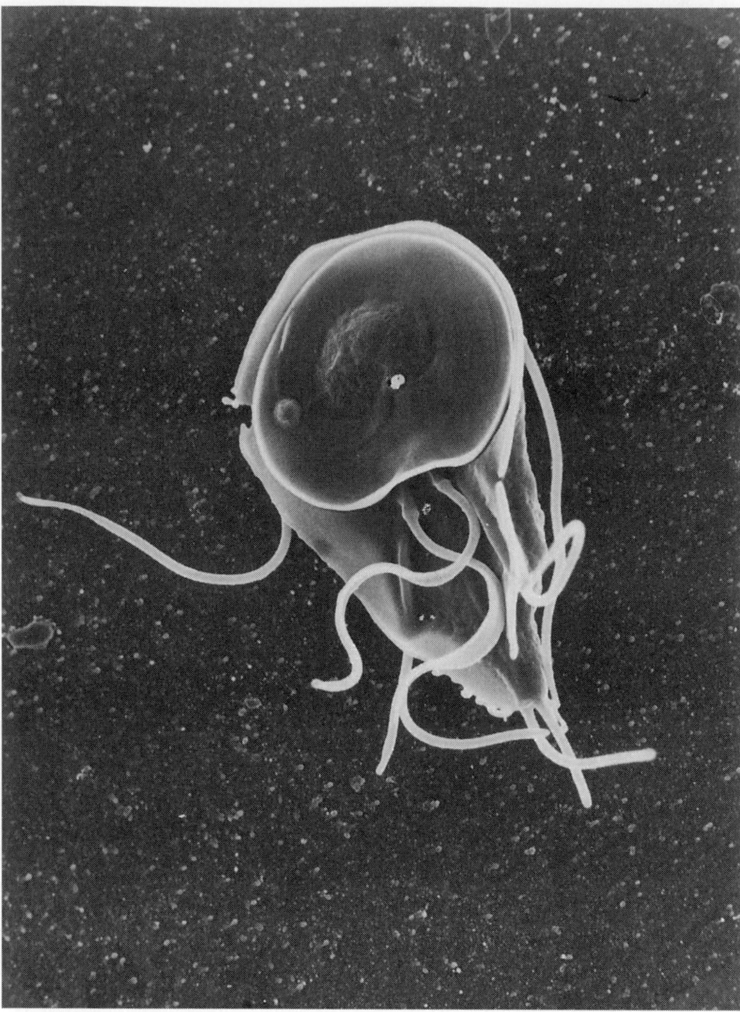

FIGURE 6.3 *Giardia duodenalis* trophozoite, ventral surface as seen in SEM. [Courtesy of Dr. David W. Dorward, Rocky Mountain Laboratory, Hamilton, Montana. NIH, USPHS, DHHS.]

4. Using fluorescent antibody to locate organisms in a fecal smear

The signs and symptoms most often seen in *Giardia* infections in humans are diarrhea, bloating or flatulence, nausea, and weight loss in the face of a good appetite (Tab. 6.2). *Entamoeba histolytica* infection (Chapter 7) as well as infection with a variety of prokaryotic organisms and viruses may also cause some of these symptoms. Generally, diarrhea lasting longer than seven days indicates *Giardia* infection while a shorter duration indicates something else (bacteria or viruses). Amoebic dysentery (Chapter 7) also shows a prolonged diarrhea.

Trophozoites of *G. duodenalis* (Fig. 6.2A) may be found in a freshly passed feces; especially if the person is showing diarrhea. In some instances it may be necessary to pass a tube by mouth through the stomach into the lumen of the small intestine to aspirate some of the contents.

Often a series of stools collected on alternate days is needed to find cysts or trophozoites. Since organisms are passed sporadically, even a series of six or more negative stools does not completely rule out a *Giardia* infection.

Since *Giardia* trophozoites are delicate creatures, it is essential to examine any specimen immediately upon obtaining it. The technique itself involves mixing a tiny portion of the sample with physiological salt solution on a microscope slide, adding a coverslip, and examining it for motile organisms under a compound microscope.

Cysts (Fig. 6.2B) may be concentrated by flotation or by sedimentation methods such as the formalin-

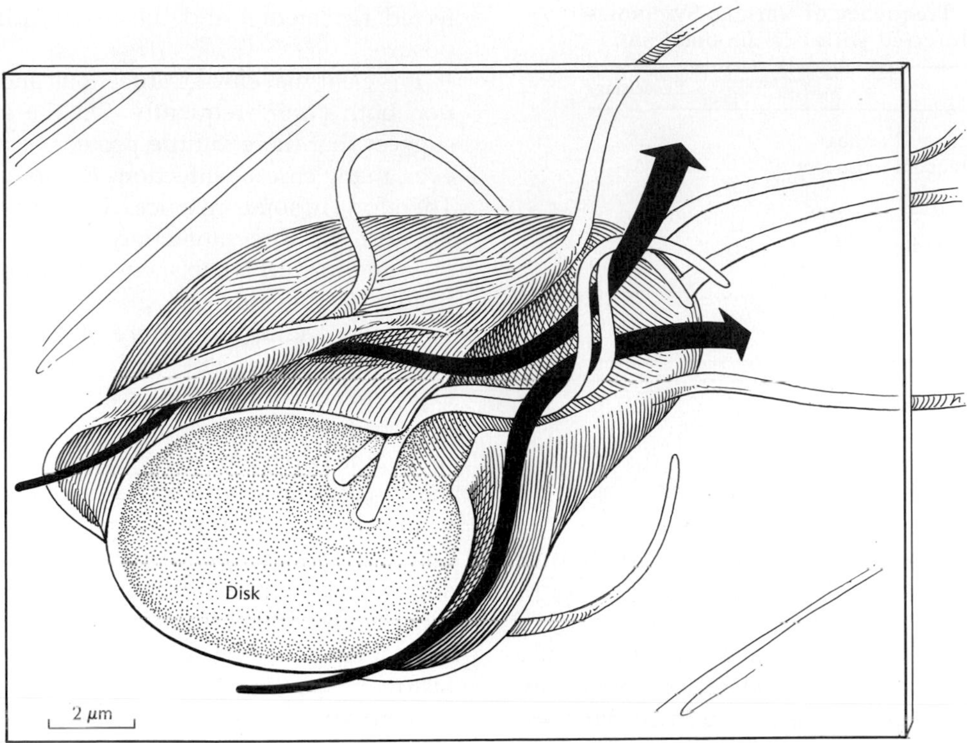

FIGURE 6.4 Ventral view of *Giardia* showing the movement of fluid through the action of the flagella. [Redrawn from Holberton, 1973. © The Company of Biologists.]

triton-ether (FTE) method and then looked for under a compound microscope.

A stained fecal smear should be made when it is not possible to examine a fecal specimen immediately or when a suspected *Giardia* has been found on a wet mount. The stained smear provides a permanent record that can be studied later should that be necessary.

Commercial monoclonal antibody (Mab) kits utilizing fluorescent microscopy are easy to use, and are reliable diagnostic tests.

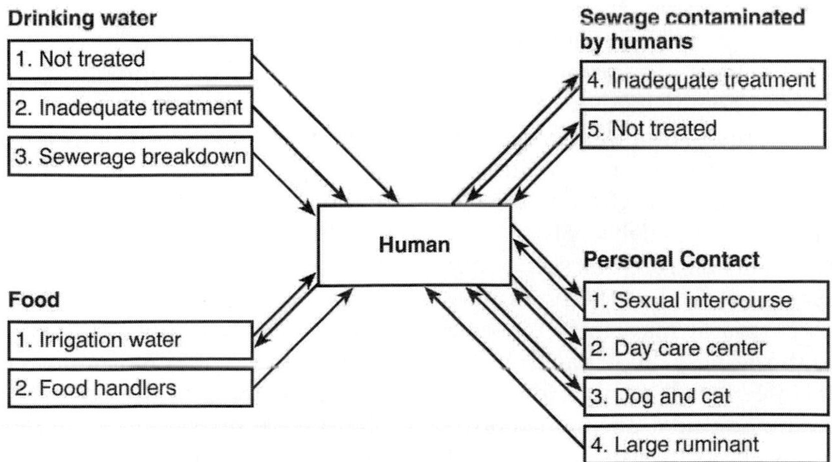

FIGURE 6.5 Pathways of transmission of *Giardia duodenalis* in humans and other hosts. Note that some modes of transmission are two-way and some are one-way.

TABLE 6.2 Frequency of Various Symptoms in Persons Infected with *Giardia duodenalis*

Symptoms	Percentage
Bloating, belching, diarrhea	97
Diarrhea or frequent loose stools	85
Nausea	79
Weight loss	56
Abdominal cramping	44
Loss of appetite	41
Vomiting	24
Fever	0

Host–Parasite Interactions

Giardia are located mostly in the upper portion of the small intestine. They adhere to the enterocytes and sink down into the microvilli.

The attachment to the surface of the small intestine results from an interaction between the trophozoite and the secretion of proteases by the intestinal cells. Under the influence of trypsin, *Giardia* trophozoites produce a lectin, which causes them to adhere to the surface of the enterocytes. This interesting interaction may give a clue to the mechanism for the organisms to locate in the upper part of the small intestine since that is where the trypsin is active.

It has been clearly established that *G. duodenalis* can be pathogenic in humans, although its pathogenic potential had been debated for many years. As with other infectious agents, infection results in a spectrum of responses from none at all to a severe, debilitating diarrhea and other symptoms (Tab. 6.2).

The ways in which *Giardia* damages the host are still uncertain. It is generally agreed that there is interference with absorption of nutrients from the small intestine in symptomatic infections. A frequent finding is the passage of fat with the feces (steatorrhea), which indicates that fat is either not emulsified or cannot be absorbed in the small intestine. Although there may be almost a solid mat of organisms on the epithelial surface of the gut, a mechanical obstruction of absorption is probably not the cause of malabsorption.

Signs and symptoms of infection are first seen about nine days after exposure to cysts, but the onset may vary from five to twenty days or may, in fact, not be experienced even though the host has a patent infection. Most experimental infections last only a few days, but of 409 men infected in one study, 2 remained positive for three months. Only about 10 cysts were needed to establish an infection, but 100 administered to an individual guaranteed infection. A person can be reinfected repeatedly, and the results differ at each exposure.

It is clear that chronic infections and repeated infection both occur frequently. On the surface it might suggest that there is little protective immunity; however, many chronic infections do not result in disease. Therefore, in some instances, immunity may modulate the host–parasite interaction so as to lead the clinical outcome toward a commensal relationship and away from a pathogenic one.

Understanding the nature of the protective immunity has been difficult. Apart from some interesting experiments in mice, the establishment of roles for either antibody, a cell-mediated response or a combination of the two has been largely dependent on correlating disease and the presence of some immune effector response. The difficulty in conducting interpretable research in this area is compounded by the presence of strains of parasites differing in virulence; in addition there is always considerable variation in nonspecific resistance in a population of seemingly susceptible hosts.

A provocative area of research on the immunology of *Giardia* infection is concerned with antigenic variation of the parasite. Although there are similarities to the variable surface antigens produced by *Trypanosoma brucei* (Chapter 3), there are fundamental differences in the mechanisms. In *Giardia,* there is likely to be a change in the surface coat about every 12 generations. There is always a small proportion of the population that shows different surface proteins. In laboratory experiments using Mabs, most of the trophozoites were killed when exposed to a specific antibody. However, some trophozoites survived the antibody exposure and their progeny no longer possessed that original surface antigen. Rather, the antigen was replaced by a distinctly different molecule. Unlike the African trypanosomes, the repertoire of surface antigens was limited in *Giardia* to 30 or so in one isolate and perhaps 150 in another. Although antigenic variation was first shown in culture, it has been demonstrated in vivo as well. In effect, the surface antigen of the parasites is a moving target that is difficult for the immune system to hit.

This phenomenon of antigenic variation appears to be under the control of a family of related genes, and it may be responsible for both persistent and repeated infection in immunologically competent hosts. Studies subsequent to the molecular cloning and expression of a gene that encodes two of the major proteins on the surface revealed that antibodies to these antigens should be important determinants of immunity. These antibodies reacted with the entire surface of the trophozoites and inhibited both the attachment and growth of the parasite. Again, regardless of this potentially effective parasitic-specific response, the ability of the parasite to undergo antigenic variation presumably limits the likelihood of a complete and permanent immunity.

Epidemiology and Control

Control of giardiosis falls into two main categories: public health and personal protection.

1. Public health
   a. Sewage treatment
   b. Adequate treatment of drinking water
   c. Proper location of intakes of surface waters
   d. Chemotherapeutic treatment of infected persons
   e. Surveillance and treatment of food handlers
2. Personal
   a. Treatment of drinking water to remove or kill cysts
   b. Avoidance of contaminated water
   c. Sanitary procedures to avoid contact with cysts
   d. Surveillance and treatment of companion animals in a household

Giardiosis occurs both sporadically and epidemically (Fig. 6.5). Sporadic infections seem to result from contact with contaminated food, other persons, or companion animals. On the other hand, epidemics take place when there is a breakdown at some level in a community's water delivery system.

In sporadic cases in humans, one of the difficulties associated with incriminating either a human or animal source has been distinguishing morphologically identical isolates of *G. duodenalis*. However, with the application of newly developed techniques, it has become feasible to identify sources of outbreaks and, of equal importance, to identify other populations of *Giardia* within a geographic region that are not responsible for the outbreak. These and related approaches should allow a more complete description of the epidemiology and differential pathogenicity of morphologically indistinguishable isolates of *Giardia*.

Epidemics occur in areas where there is breakdown in sewerage or where water treatment is inadequate. A classic example of a breakdown occurred in the ski resort town of Aspen, Colorado, where old sewer pipes leaked sewage into a well serving one part of the town. At least 25 persons suffered from clinical giardiosis. It is interesting to note that nearly all of the persons affected were visitors to Aspen; few local residents were affected.

Not all cysts of *Giardia* are killed by the levels of chlorine usually employed in municipal water treatment plants. Outbreaks have often occurred in water supplies that were chlorinated but not filtered. In these cases, surface waters have been used for drinking water, and despite chlorination, persons became infected and showed clinical signs and symptoms of giardiosis. In most instances, contamination of the water supply seemed not to come from human excreta.

In approaching the epidemiologic puzzle, it is known that *G. duodenalis* has a broad host range. In many localities, aquatic rodents such as beaver seem to be a major source of infection. Beaver can be infected with human isolates of *G. duodenalis* and they continue to produce millions of cysts per day for months. If water treatment is inadequate, cysts may reach the water delivery system and be spread throughout the community.

In the Aspen, Colorado, outbreak, the antique sewerage broke down and allowed sewage to leak into a nearby well. A good sewage treatment plant coupled to a tight sewer system should leave sewage effluents free of cysts of *Giardia* as well as other parasitic and microbial disease agents. The various elements of sewage treatment—anaerobic digestion, filtration, and the heat that is often generated in the process—all work together to kill the cysts. A few species of protistan cysts and helminth eggs (*Ascaris* and *Taenia*) can survive good sewage treatment, but cysts of *Giardia* are relatively susceptible to environmental insult. As a sewer system ages, it tends to lose integrity and leak. Raw drinking water for a typical city system undergoes flocculation and chlorination prior to distribution, but they are not adequate in eliminating cysts of *Giardia*. A number of outbreaks have occurred in communities that have taken their water from watersheds and provided those two types of treatment. The key to completely eliminating cysts of *Giardia* is to filter the water as well. Sand filtration is recommended as the most effective final step in preventing cysts from entering the water system.

Chemotherapy is generally successful and the risk of side effects is low. Three drugs are currently in use for treatment of giardiasis: quinacrine, metronidazole, and furazolidone. All are effective, but each has advantages and drawbacks. Usually a single course of treatment is effective against *Giardia*, but occasionally a second one is needed. A proviso for the use of quinacrine is that it may produce undesirable side effects, especially in children. Quinacrine is the drug recommended by the Centers for Disease Control and Prevention (CDC).

Metronidazole is probably the drug of choice for the general population in the developed world. Although it is used widely, it should be noted that the drug has not been approved for that use by the Food and Drug Administration (FDA). Also, the imidazole moiety on which the molecule is based is mildly carcinogenic.

Furazolidone, which is marketed as a liquid, is frequently favored for administration to children.

Debate continues on whether to treat persons that are infected with *Giardia* but not showing clinical signs and symptoms. Since ingesting only a few cysts can establish an infection, transmission can take place readily under some circumstances. Where the risk of transmission is judged to be high, treatment of asymptomatic individuals is justified. This would be especially true of food handlers who can serve as a source of infection where personal hygiene may not be at a high level.

In addition to treatment of infected persons, dogs and cats in a household should be examined and, if infected, treated also. Where there are sporadic cases of giardiosis, the source of the infection may be a companion animal, and treating only one of the infected parties may not be fruitful; as is true in human infections, dogs and cats may or may not be symptomatic.

Giardiosis has become rampant in some day care centers (as has cryptosporidiosis, Chapter 12). Stopping such an outbreak requires careful personal hygiene. Those persons responsible for taking care of children still in diapers must wash their hands after changing every child. Also, any procedure that sets up an aerosol should be avoided. For example, diapers should be removed in such a way that they are folded inward and disposed in whatever lidded container is used with as little shaking or other exposure as possible.

In the face of an epidemic, determining the source of the cysts is an essential part of a control program. The prime suspect should be the water supply, and it should be determined whether cysts appear in water used for domestic purposes. A large volume of water is pumped through a filter, the filter is washed and the residue is examined under a microscope for cysts. This technique has been used successfully in a large number of investigations to determine the source of cysts.

Assuming that cysts have been found in the water, a systematic determination of their source should be made. In a rural area, leakage from pit toilets or septic tank drainage fields into underground waters is a likely possibility. In small municipalities, a broken sewer leaking into a well should be looked for. In both of these instances, fluorescent dye can be used to determine whether there is movement of water from the waste disposal system into the water deliver system. Coliform bacteria counts can also be done to indicate whether there is fecal contamination of a water supply.

In communities that obtain their water from surface impoundments, the area should be searched for fecal contamination. The questions that need to be asked are whether humans have access to the watershed for recreation or whatever, and what susceptible animals are there. Contamination from human sources can usually be controlled, but that from animals may be difficult or impossible.

Individuals can protect themselves, and the first step in a control program is to ensure that all persons on the water system are informed as to the actions that they can take to prevent infection. This may not completely abort the epidemic, but it can do a great deal in the face of a difficult situation. It should be made clear that all water used for drinking, brushing teeth, cleaning fresh vegetables, and so on is boiled or treated with elemental iodine. Water used in cooking need not be boiled beforehand. In a home with a hot water heater, a temperature of 55°C (131°F) is sufficient to kill cysts. Water that has passed through the heater can be used for drinking and other such purposes.

The next step is to prevent cysts from reaching the tap water. Chlorination at the level used in most municipal water plants is insufficient to kill cysts of *Giardia*, and they can live in water for up to three months. Their hardiness is further shown by the fact that 2.5% (0.17M) phenol is required to kill them. The recommended treatment of water after chlorination is sand filtration. Such treatment virtually ensures that the cysts of *Giardia* as well as those of other protists and helminths eggs will be filtered out.

For those persons who enjoy the out-of-doors, a great deal can be done to prevent giardiosis. Hikers and backpackers are often exposed to infection when they take water from streams. As indicated previously, beaver and muskrat shed enormous numbers of cysts into the environment and probably present the greatest hazard to humans. A number of companies market filters for use in the field. Those that work well have a pore size less than 4μm; filters with larger pore sizes may remove some cysts, but not all. Filters are rather laborious to use since they require that water be pumped through them. An alternative is to heat water to 55°C (131°F), a temperature at which cysts are killed almost instantaneously. If a thermometer is not available, 55°C water is hot, but not so hot that you can not hold your hand in it. At 60°C, you can put your hand in the water but not hold it there. Iodine tablets at the recommended concentration kill cysts in 30 minutes at 15°C and in 15 minutes at 20°C.

Notable Features

The previous discussion implies that there is agreement on the species of *Giardia*. Such is not entirely the case, and some investigators take current evidence to mean that *G. duodenalis* is at least a species complex or a group of species. Also, we have stated that there is cross-transmission among various species of mammalian hosts in order to present a clear rationale for the development of control programs. However, many of the cross-transmission experiments can be criticized usually for failure to fulfill Koch's postulates. However, the authors feel that the evidence for cross-transmission is strong, but not airtight. If there is error in our position it is on the side of safety and fits with a conservative control program. Details can be found in Thompson et al., 1994.

SPIRONUCLEUS AND *HEXAMITA*

The organisms in these two genera are represented by both parasitic and free-living forms. *Hexamita* spp. are either free living or parasitic; *H. nelsoni*, for example, is a parasite of oysters, and *H. muris* is a parasite of rodents. Members of the genus *Spironucleus* are parasitic.

Name of Organisms and Disease Associations

Spironucleus meleagridis (syn. *Hexamita meleagridis*). The original description of the organism and the disease was such that the disease has been called hexamitiasis. With the change in the name of the organism, the disease should properly be called *spironucleosis*, but there may be some culture lag in terminology.

Hosts and Host Range

The organism is found in a wide range of gallinaceous birds including turkey, peafowl, quail, and pheasants. It has been transmitted experimentally to the chicken and duck, among others.

Geographic Distribution and Importance

Cosmopolitan. Information on economic losses in turkeys is fragmentary, but estimates are that there is about $1.8 million loss annually in the United States.

Morphology

The organisms are pyriform, bilaterally symmetrical and about 9 x 3 μm (Fig. 6.6) There are eight flagella, all arising from basal bodies in the anterior end; six exit anteriorly and two exit posteriorly. Axial rods (pseudoaxostyles) run the length of the organism in association with the posterior flagella. Two nuclei are located at the anterior end and are round or ellipsoid and have large endosomes. Cysts are ellipsoid and are about 8 μm long.

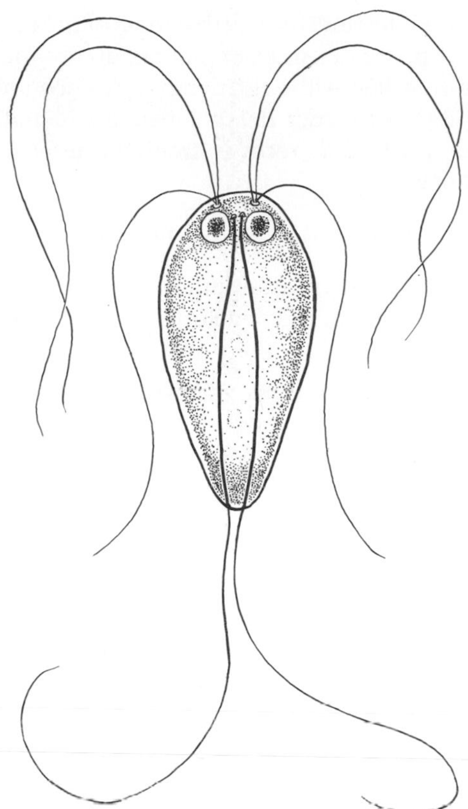

FIGURE 6.6 *Spironucleus meleagridis* trophozoite, a parasite of turkeys and other gallinaceous birds.

Life Cycle

Multiplication is by binary fission. Transmission from one bird to the next is through cysts ingested with contaminated food or water.

Diagnosis

Birds show a foamy diarrhea, fail to gain weight, and become listless. Clinical signs are suggestive, but finding the organisms in large numbers in the intestinal contents is the definitive diagnosis.

Host–Parasite Interactions

Infections with *S. meleagridis* are widespread, but disease is seen only sporadically, usually in birds 10 weeks of age or younger. The principal site of damage is the small intestine, the site that most of the organisms prefer. At postmortem examination, an obvious gross lesion is enteritis. Although deaths have been reported in 7 to 80% of birds, death losses are usually low; however, birds that recover from the infection may gain poorly.

Epidemiology and Control

Prevention of significant infection in young birds is the primary goal in the developing a control program for spironucleosis:

1. Separation of age classes of birds
2. Cleaning premises between batches of birds
3. Allowing time between housing birds in the same quarters
4. Making sure that workers and tools do not transfer infection between flocks of birds on the same premises
5. Administering drugs once an outbreak has begun

Keeping animals of different ages separate from one another is a general principle in control of diseases of domestic animals. Young animals are almost always highly susceptible to infectious agents, but they gain immunity as time passes. The older animals tend to shed organisms into the environment into which newborn animals may be introduced. Keeping them separated from one another allows the younger animals to gain immunity through being exposed to only a small number of infectious agents. A variation of this principle is separation in time. If a batch of birds has been raised and then sent to market, a two-week period is recommended before bringing in new poults.

In many infectious diseases, separating susceptible animals from older or infected animals by 50 to 100 m or keeping them in separate building may be adequate to prevent infections. One must then ensure that the infection is not carried on footwear, tools, or machinery from one place to another. Where risks of infection are high and profit margins low, a clear set of procedures must be established and to which all workers adhere. The poultry industry is based on large volume and low profit margin per bird, literally pennies. A slight reduction in weight gain or egg production may result in only breaking even or even a loss at the end of the growing period.

Name of Organism and Disease Associations

Hexamita salmoni causes hexamitiasis, hexamitosis.

Hosts and Host Range

Salmonid fish are the hosts and the infection develops in the intestinal tract, principally the pyloric ceca.

Geographic Distribution and Importance

Cosmopolitan. Economic losses are uncertain.

Morphology

Same as for *Spironucleus meleagridis*.

Life Cycle

Same as for *S. meleagridis*.

Diagnosis

Finding large numbers of organisms in the pyloric ceca of fish that fail to grow properly is indicative of hexamitosis.

Host–Parasite Interactions

Although there continues to be disagreement on the pathogenic potential of *H. salmonis*, the weight of the evidence favors the conclusion that the organism causes weight losses and deaths in salmonid fish in hatcheries. The uncertainty probably lies in the differences in susceptibility of different stocks of fish as well as differences in the virulence of isolates of the agent.

Epidemiology and Control

Outbreaks of hexamitosis probably occur when rearing raceways become contaminated with cysts and contamination reaches a critical level. Since outbreaks are sporadic, it seems likely that factors other than contamination of the environment bring about losses. Be that as it may, cleaning rearing facilities between batches of fish should be routine.

When an outbreak is recognized, chemotherapy should be applied immediately. In a hatchery, drugs are administered in the food or water, almost invariably the latter. Several drugs have been found to be effective; among them are dimetridazole, enhepten, cyzine, and carbasone oxide.

Name of Organism and Disease Associations

Hexamita muris causes hexamitosis or hexamitiasis.

Hosts and Host Range

H. muris has been reported from laboratory rats and mice and from other rodents. It is not known whether they are all the same species.

Host–Parasite Interactions

This organism is found frequently in the small intestines of laboratory rodents. It is often found in large numbers when an animal suffers from enteritis. These blooms indicate that *H. muris* is an opportunist, but there is some evidence that the organism may actually cause enteritis as well. Little else is known.

Readings

Belosevic, M., Faubert, G. M., Maclean, J. D., Law, C., and Croll, N. A. (1983). *Giardia lamblia* infections in Mongolian gerbils: An animal model. *J. Infect. Dis.* **147,** 222–226.

Brugerolle, G. (1975). Contribution a l'étude cytologique et phylétique des diplozoaires (Zoomastigophorea, Diplozoa, Dangéard, 1910) VI. Charactères généraux des diplozoaires. *Protistologica* **11,** 111–118.

Buret, A., den Hollander, N., Wallis, P. M., Befus, D., and Olson, M. E. (1990). Zoonotic potential of giardiasis in domestic ruminants. *J. Infect. Dis.* **162,** 231–237.

Collins, G. H., Pope, S. E., Griffin, D. L., Walker, J., and Connor, G. (1987). Diagnosis and prevalence of *Giardia* spp. in dogs and cats. *Aust. Vet. J.* **64,** 89–90.

Erlandsen, S. L., *et al.* (1988). Cross-species transmission of *Giardia* sp.: Inoculation of beavers and muskrats with cysts of human, beaver, mouse, and muskrat origin. *Appl. Environ. Microbiol.* **54,** 2777–2785.

Gillin, F. D., Reiner, D. S., Gault, M. J., Douglas, H., Das, S., Wunderlich, A., and Sauch, J. F. (1987). Encystation and expression of cyst antigens by *Giardia lamblia* in vitro. *Science* **235,** 1040–1043.

Gillin, F. D., Hagblom, P., Harwood, J., Aley, S. B., Reiner, D. S., McCaffery, M., So, M., and Guiney, D. G. (1990). Isolation and expression of a gene for a major surface protein of *Giardia lamblia. Proc. Natl. Acad. Sci. USA* **87,** 4463–4467.

Gillin, F. D., Reiner, D. S., and McCaffery, J. M. (1996). Cell biology of the primitive eukaryote *Giardia lamblia. Annu. Rev. Microbiol.* **50,** 697–705.

Hoffman, D. L., and Meyer, F. P. (1967). *Parasites of North American Fresh Water Fishes.* Univ. of California Press, Berkeley.

Holberton, D. V. (1973). Fine structure of the ventral disk apparatus and the mechanism of attachment in the flagellate *Giardia muris. J. Cell Sci.* **13,** 11–41

Kabnick, K. S., and Peattie, D. A. (1991). *Giardia:* A missing link between prokaryotes and eukaryotes. *Am. Sci.* **79,** 34–43.

Kirkpatrick, C. E. (1988). Giardiasis. In the veterinary clinics of North America. Small animal practice. *Parasitic Infect.* **17**(6), 1377–1387.

Kulda and Nohynkova (1978). Intestinal protozoa. In *Parasitic Protozoa* (J. P. Kreier, Ed.), Vol. 2. Academic Press, New York.

LeChevalier, M. W., Norton, W. D., and Lee, R. G. (1991a). Occurrence of *Giardia* and *Cryptosporidium* spp. in surface water supplies. *Appl. Environ. Microbiol.* **57,** 2610–2616.

LeChevalier, M. W., Norton, W. D., and Lee, R. G. (1991b). *Giardia* and *Cryptosporidium* spp. in filtered drinking water supplies. *Appl. Environ. Microbiol.* **57,** 2617–2621.

Lev, G., Ward, H., Keusch, G. T., and Pereira, M. E. A. (1986). Lectin activation in *Gioardia lamblia* by host protease: A novel host–parasite interaction. *Science* **232,** 171–173.

Levine, W. C., Stephenson, W. T., and Craun, G. F. (1990). Waterborne disease outbreaks, 1986–1988. *Morbidity Mortality Weekly Rep.* **39**(SS-1), 1–3.

Meyer, E. A. (Ed.) (1990). *Giardiasis.* Elsevier, Amsterdam.

Moore, G. T., Cross, W. M., McGuire, C. D., Mollohan, S. S., Gleason, N. N., and Newton, L. H. (1969). Epidemic giardiasis at a ski resort. *N. Engl. J. Med.* **281,** 402–407.

Nash, T. E. (1989). Antigenic variation in *Giardia lamblia. Exp. Parasitol.* **68,** 238–241.

Nash, T. E., and Mowatt, M. R. (1992). Characterization of *Giardia lamblia* variant-specific protein (VSP) gene from isolate GS/M and estimation of VSP gene repertoire size. *Mol. Biochem. Parasitol.* **51,** 219–228.

Nash, T. E., Herrington, D. A., Losonsky, G. A., and Levine, M. M. (1987). Experimental human infections with *Giardia lamblia. J. Infect. Dis.* **156,** 974–984.

Sarafis, K., and Isaac-Renton, J. (1993). Pulsed-field electrophoresis as a method of biotyping *Giardia duodenalis. Am. J. Trop. Med. Hyg.* **48,** 134–144.

Siddall, M. E., Hong, H., and Desser, S. S. (1992). Phylogenetic analysis of the Diplomonadida (Wenyon, 1926) Brugerolle, 1975: Evidence for heterochrony in protozoa and against *Giardia lamblia* as a "missing link." *J. Protozool.* **39,** 361–367.

Smith, H V., and Smith, P. G. (1990). Parasitic protozoa in drinking water. *Endeavor* **14,** 74–79.

Thompson, R. C. A., Reynoldson, J. A., and Lymbery, A. J. (Eds.) (1994). *Giardia: From Molecules to Disease.* CAB International, Wallingford, UK.

Warhurst, D. C., and Smith, H. (1992). Getting to the guts of the problem. *Parasitol. Today* **8,** 292–293.

Wolfe M. S. (1992). Giardiasis. *Clin. Microbiol. Rev.* **5,** 93–100.

CHAPTER

7

Amebas and Other Enteric Protists of Humans

The main objectives of this chapter are (1) to discuss the enteric amebas of humans as pathogens that may need to be controlled and (2) to use the protists of the human intestine as an example of the array of protists that may be found in the intestinal tract of almost any vertebrate.

Members of the phylum Rhizopoda in the Kingdom Protista are those protists that form pseudopodia, or temporary extensions of the cytoplasm, for feeding and locomotion; they are also called *Barcodines.*

Amebas feed on particulate or liquid food, which they capture by actively engulfing it, as in the free-living ameba, *Amoeba proteus.* In some cases, amebas feed on rapidly moving protists such as ciliates or flagellates. They are efficient predators despite their sluggish movement, and they immobilize their prey so that it can be ingested at leisure. The sarcodines have been successful, but they are not as conspicuous as other protists, because of their slow movement or small size.

Sarcodines are found most often in aquatic environments, but some species are found in soils where they constitute a significant part of the fauna. In the root zone of plants, even in xeric environments, interactions among protists and nematodes provide a mutualistic community of plant, animal, and protist.

Most amebas are free living, but a substantial number are associated with the intestinal tracts of various vertebrates and invertebrates. The free-living forms are usually in habitats that have at least a moderate amount of organic material, and some are found in situations where organic material is high and oxygen concentration is low. These are the conditions that apply to the intestinal tract of nearly any animal, and it is understandable that some have become symbiotic. A few, two or three in humans, for example, are pathogenic, but the bulk of amebas remain as commensals in the lumen or paramucosal lumen of the intestine.

In addition to amebas, the intestinal tract is home to many kinds of protists: flagellates, apicomplexans, and ciliates. The example used here is the veritable zoological garden contained in the human gut, but we could have chosen any of a number of other hosts to show the biological diversity found in this habitat.

There are perhaps 23 species of protists that are cosmopolitan parasites of the human digestive tract (Tab. 7.1, Fig. 7.1). A few additional species have been found on occasion, but they have not been included here because of their rarity, or their identity is doubtful.

Transmission of these intestinal parasites takes place through ingestion, but beyond that, there are some interesting adaptations allowing infection to occur. With two exceptions, the organisms that live in the region of the gut posterior to the stomach form cysts. A resistant covering, the cyst wall, allows the organisms to pass the rigors of the stomach and the upper part of the small intestine, which are replete with enzymes, wetting agents, and low pH in the stomach. Clearly, the cyst is an adaptation that provides protection so that the organism can leave its cloister and survive in the rigors of the outside world.

Pentatrichomonas hominis (Chapter 5) is an enigma since it enters the mouth of the host as a naked trophozoite. It is capable of passing through the low pH and pepsin of the stomach in order to establish in the lower part of the intestine, as has been shown in a number of species of hosts. The other is *Dientamoeba fragilis* (Chapter 5), which is also a trichomonad, and it enters the host while inside the egg of the human pinworm, *Enterobius vermicularis.*

TABLE 7.1 Some Enteric Protists of Humans

			Trophozoite					Cyst				
					Nucleus					Nucleus		
Name	Pathogenesis	Location in host	Size in μm	Flagella	Number	Chromatin	Remarks	Present	Size in μm	Number	Chromatin	Remarks
Retortomonas intestinalis	No	Large intestine	4–9 × 3–4	2	1	Central endosome		Yes	4.5–7 × 3–4.5	1	Central endosome	
Chilomastix mesnili	Perhaps	Large intestine	6–24 × 3–10	4	1	Small endosome	Flagella difficult to see	Yes	6–10 × 4–6 lemon shaped	1	Central endosome	Shepherd's crook as cytosomal fibril
Giardia duodenalis	Yes	Small intestine	9–21 × 5–15	8	2	Large central endosome	Barlike median body; bilaterally symmetrical	Yes	8–12 × 7–10 ovoid	4	Large endosome	Flagella and median bodies visible
Enteromonas hominis	No	Large intestine	4–10 × 3–6	4	1	Small endosome	Bacterial inclusions	Yes	6–8 × 4–6	2–4	Small endosome	
Pentatrichomonas hominis	No	Large intestine	8–20 × 3–14	6	1	Uneven distribution	Flagella difficult to see; post. flagellum attached by undulating membrane	No				
Trichomonas tenax	No	Mouth	4–16 × 2–15	5	1	Distributed	Post. flagellum attached by undulating membrane	No				
Dientamoeba fragilis	Yes, mild	Large intestine	5 × 12	0	2	Variable; in telophase	Bacterial inclusions	No				
Entamoeba histolytica and *E. dispar*	Yes and mildly, respectively	Large intestine	20–30	0	1	Central endosome and small peripheral granules	Rbc's ingested	Yes	10–16 (12)	4	Central endosome, small peripheral granules	Rounded chromatoid bodies
Entamoeba hartmanni	Probably not	Large intestine	3–10.5	0	1	Central endosome, chromatin unevenly distributed	Rbc's not ingested	Yes	4–10	4	Same as trophozoite	Rounded chromatoid bodies
Entamoeba coli	No	Large intestine	15–50 (27)	0	1	Eccentric endosome, chromatin granules clumped	Bacteria, cytoplasm vacuolated, no rbc's	Yes	10–33	8	Same as trophozoite	Splintered chromatoid bodies; cysts irregular in shape
Entamoeba gingivalis	No	Mouth	5–35	0	1	Central endosome; evenly distributed chromatin	Bacteria ingested	No				

Iodamoeba buetschlii	Occasionally (?)	Large intestine	4–20	0	1	Large endosome; no peripheral granules	Cytoplasm vacuolated	Yes	6–15	1	Same as trophozoite	Large glycogen vacuole
Endolimax nana	No	Large intestine	6–15 (10)	0	1	Large endosome of 4–6 granules; no peripheral granules	Cytoplasm vacuolated; and contains bacteria	Yes	5–14	4	Same as trophozoite	
Balantidium coli	Yes	Large intestine	30–150 × 25–120	Cilia	2	Macro- and micronuclei	Covered with cilia; mouth at anterior end	Yes	50–175	1	Same as trophozoite	
Isospora belli	Yes	Small intestine?	NA	0	NA	NA	NA	Yes	20–33 × 10–19 (30 × 12)	8	1/sporozoite; vesicular	Unsporulated oocyst in feces
Sarcocystis miescheriana	Yes	Intestine	NA	0	NA	NA		Yes	11.6–13.6 × 10.1–10.8 (13.5 × 10.5)	4	1/sporozoite; vesicular	Sporocysts in feces
Sarcocystis cruzi	No?	Intestine	NA	0	NA	NA		Yes	13.1–17.0 × 7.7–10.8 (14.7 × 9.3)	4	1/sporozoite	Sporocysts in feces
Cryptosporidium parvum	Yes	Intestine	NA	0	NA	NA		Yes	4.5–7.5 × 4.2–5.7	4	1/sporozoite	Oocysts in feces
Cyclospora caytanensis	Yes	Intestine	NA	0	NA	NA		Yes	7.7–9.9 (8.6)	4	1/sporozoite	Oocysts in feces; 2 sporocysts each with 2 sporozoites

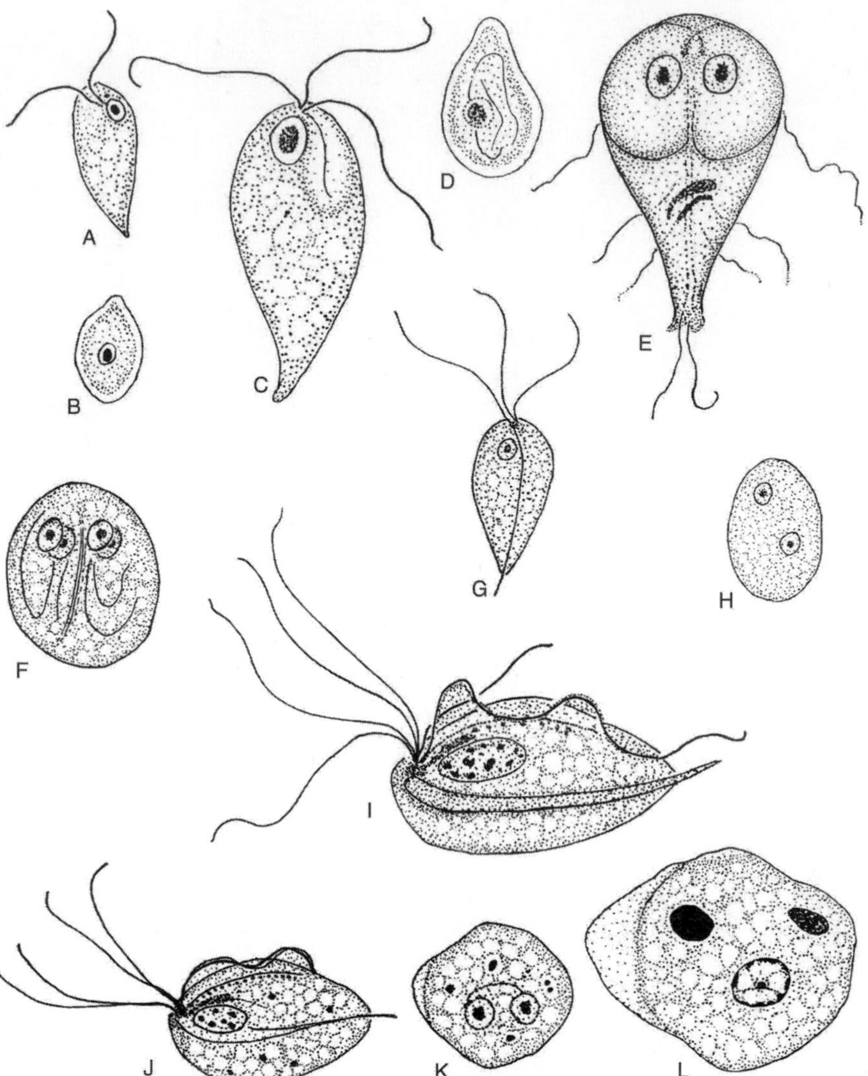

FIGURE 7.1 Some of the enteric protists of humans as seen in fecal smears and stained with iron hematoxylin. (A) *Retortamonas intestinalis* trophozoite; (B) cyst; (C) *Chilomastix mesnili* trophozoite; (D) cyst; (E) *Giardia duodenalis* trophozoite; (F) cyst; (G) *Enteromonas hominis* trophozoite; (H) cyst; (I) *Pentatrichomonas hominis* trophozoite; (J) *Trichomonas tenax* trophozoite; (K) *Dientamoeba fragilis* trophozoite; (L, M, N) *Entamoeba histolytica* and *Entamoeba dispar* trophozoites; (O) *Entamoeba histolytica* and *E. dispar* cyst; (P) *Entamoeba hartmanni* trophozoite; (Q) cyst; (R) *Entamoeba coli* trophozoite, (S) cyst; (T) *Entamoeba gingivalis* trophozoite; (U) *Iodamoeba buetschlii* trophozoite; (V) cyst; (W) *Endolimax nana* trophozoite; (X) cyst; (Y) *Balantidium coli* trophozoite; (Z) cyst. See the following figures for other protists seen in human feces: 12.8 *Cryptosporidium parva;* 12.9 *Cyclospora cayatanensis;* 13.1 *Sarcocystis* sp.; 13.5, 13.6, 13.7, and 13.8 *Toxopolasma gondii.*

Both of the organisms that live in the human mouth, *Entamoeba gingivalis* and *Trichomonas tenax* exist only as trophozoites and undoubtedly transfer from one host to the next takes place by oral contact or saliva.

A broad spectrum of pathogenicity is typical of infectious agents in general. Almost all of the various protists that are listed in Table 7.1 have been thought, at one time or another, to damage the host. Current evidence is quite good that the principal pathogens found in humans are *Entamoeba histolytica* and *Giardia duodenalis* (Chapter 6). *Dientamoeba fragilis* causes diarrhea of only moderate severity, and *Balantidium coli* is close behind in potential for damaging the gut of its host. *Entamoeba hartmanni* is doubtful as a pathogen. *Iodamoeba buetschlii* may occasionally cause damage, and *Chilomastix mesnili* has been implicated as causing diarrhea on a few occasions.

Five apicomplexans parasitize the human intestinal

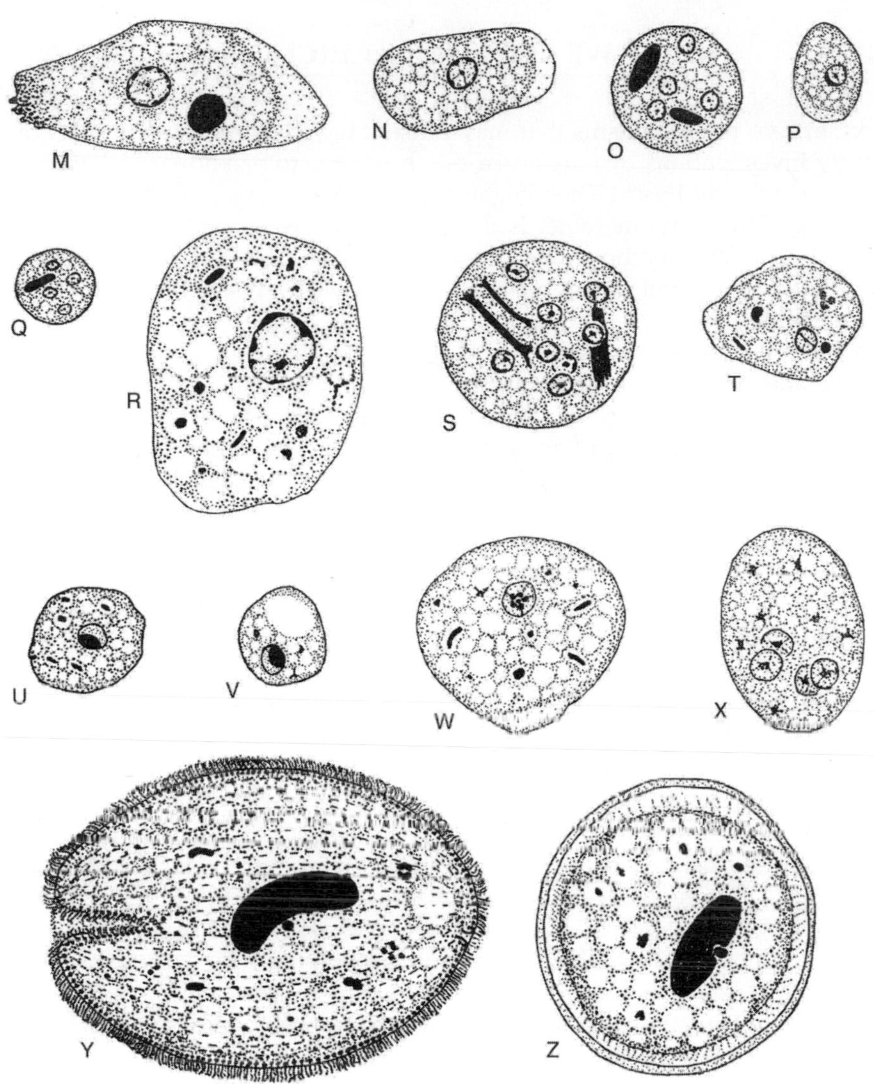

FIGURE 7.1 (*Continued*).

tract. Those that are strictly intestinal parasites are *Isospora belli, Cryptosporidium parva,* and *Cyclospora cayetanensis. Sarcocystis miescheriana* is a 2-host coccidium in which the sexual stages develop in the intestines of humans and the asexual stages (sarcocysts) are in swine (Chapter 13). *S. cruzi* has the same cycle, but the sarcocysts are in cattle.

ENTAMOEBA HISTOLYTICA

Name of Organism and Disease Associations

Entamoeba histolytica causes amebiosis, amebiasis, or amebic dysentery. In addition to infections of the large intestine, the organism may invade other internal organs such as the lung, liver, skin, and brain.

Hosts and Host Range

For most purposes, humans are the main host, but the organism is found naturally or experimentally in other hosts such as higher primates, dogs, cats, and a number of rodents.

Geographic Distribution and Importance

Cosmopolitan. Data on the prevalence of *E. histolytica* are confounded by the presence of the morphologically indistinguishable *E. dispar,* discussed later. On a worldwide basis, about 12% of people have been reported to be infected with *E. histolytica,* but in many early surveys, *Entamoeba hartmanni* was included, and the prevalence may be somewhat lower. Perhaps half of the identifications in surveys earlier than the 1960s are actually *E. hartmanni.* On a global basis, there are

WE COME FULL CIRCLE

AMEBIC DYSENTERY AND THE organisms that may cause it have been the subject of thousands of clinical and laboratory investigations. An organism that has come to be known as *Entamoeba histolytica* was described in Russia in 1875 by Lösch. Then began the troubles that extended over nearly 120 years. The questions posed were almost innumerable: Is this organism always pathogenic? Are the other several morphological types of amebas pathogenic or just commensals? Is there an organism morphologically identical to *E. histolytica* that is not pathogenic? Does *E. histolytica* lose its capacity to form cysts after it has invaded the intestinal mucosa?

In the early part of the 20th century, the accepted concept was that of a single species moving between a commensal phase and an invasive or pathogenic phase. The commensal was a small form and the invasive form was significantly larger. This was termed the "Unicistic hypothesis."

Fifty years after the original finding of an ameba in the feces of a person suffering from dysentery, the eminent parasitologist Emile Brumpt declared that there were two species: *E. histolytica*, which is invasive, and *E. dispar* which is benign; this was the so-called "Dualistic hypothesis." Brumpt's proposal in 1925 did not last long and was superseded by the "Neodualistic hypothesis," which stated that one of the small amebas was to be split off as a separate species, *E. hartmanni.* The remaining organisms were two versions of *E. histolytica,* an avirulent race and a virulent, or invasive, race. The latter could remain as a commensal or could invade the colonic tissue. All of this seemed overly elaborate and did not last long either in the hearts of protistologists.

The culmination seemed to come in the concept of *E. histolytica* having two races: a small, cyst-forming race that converted to a large, invasive, non-cyst-forming race. This "Neounicistic hypothesis" was greeted with shouts of enthusiasm in about 1968 ,and everyone felt that the solution had been achieved. Not to be. Reliable biochemical methods were becoming widespread and isozymes could be distinguished by electropohoresis. Immunologic methods became more precise and the weights and well as the antigenic characters of proteins could be measured more precisely. The polymerase chain reaction (PCR) allowed amplification of specific regions of DNA.

Now the fat was in the fire. As biochemical and immunologic studies accumulated on pathogenic and nonpathogenic isolates of what was called "*Entamoeba histolytica,*" they always fell into two groups. The pathogenic isolates were always different from the nonpathogenic ones. Diamond and Clark (1993) summarized all of these exquisite studies and concluded that there are two morphologically identical species of *Entamoeba*: a potentially pathogenic or invasive species, *E. histolytica,* and a species that can cause only slight damage to the colon, *E. dispar.*

Thus, it took just short of 70 years to return to Brumpt's proposal. Now, at least, the species and pathogenesis problems have been solved. Or have they? Stay tuned.

probably 50 million cases of invasive amebiasis annually with from 50 to 100 thousand deaths among them. Taking the United States as representative of the developed world, about 4% of the human population is infected with *E. histolytica.* In tropical areas, half or more of persons may be infected.

Data on the prevalence of *E. histolytica* in animals other than humans are fragmentary. Information on dogs is better than on any other species in which from 1 to 8% of animals have been found to be infected in various parts of the world. *E. histolytica* has been reported from primates, but most often captive primates, and these data are difficult to interpret. A high prevalence in such animals may indicate only that they are receiving less than adequate care.

The Centers for Disease Control and Prevention (CDC) recorded an annual average of 2892 human cases in the United States over the period 1962 through 1972. During the years 1962 to 1969 an average of 67 deaths due to amebiasis was reported. Amebiasis is not a reportable disease so the number of infections is undoubtedly low; however; the number of deaths per year may represent a fairly accurate figure. Although there are continuing sporadic cases of amebiasis in humans in the developed world, occasional severe outbreaks may represent a sporadic, acute problem for the community involved.

Morphology

The trophozoites of *E. histolytica* range from 20 to 40 μm in diameter; some have been reported as large as 60 μm (Fig. 7.1L, M, N). There is a thick, clear ectoplasm and a granular endoplasm that may contain ingested red blood cells and bacteria. The single nucleus is 4 to 7 μm in diameter(Fig. 7.2 A). The chromatin is located at the nuclear membrane and is generally evenly distributed around the periphery. A small endosome or nucleolus is usually located in the center of the nucleus. Red blood cells are often ingested and can be recognized in the cytoplasm.

The nucleus is not clearly seen in the living trophozoites, but the motility is distinctive. The trophozoites form "eruptive pseudopodia" in which there is rapid extrusion of a broad, ectoplasmic pseudopod formed in just a second or two before the endoplasm flows into it.

The cysts are 10 to 16 μm in diameter and average 12 μm (Fig 7.1 O). The cytoplasm is evenly granular and contains no food inclusions. When first passed, the cyst is uninucleate, but over about a 24-hour period, the nucleus divides twice and most cysts have four nuclei. The nuclei are 2 to 3 μm in diameter and have the same structure as the nuclei of the trophozoites. The chromatoid bodies have rounded ends.

At the level of TEM, trophozoites of *E. histolytica* lack practically all of the organelles that are associated with eukaryotic cells: mitochondria, Golgi, and rough endoplasmic reticulum. In the cyst, the chromatoid bodies are found to be clusters of ribosomes; they cannot be seen as individuals at the LM level, but do show when clustered.

Life Cycle

The trophozoites are located in the large intestine of the human host where they divide by binary fission.

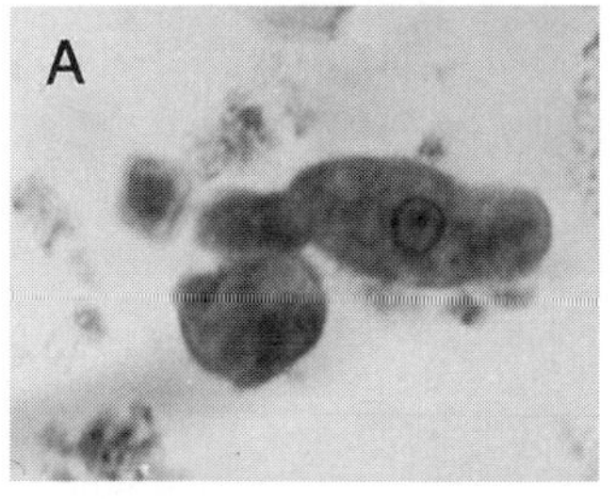

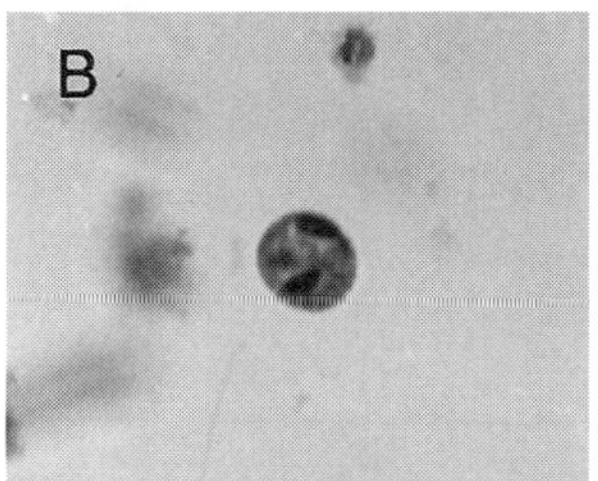

FIGURE 7.2 *Entamoeba histolytica* as seen in a stained fecal smear in LM. (A) trophozoite, (B) cyst.

Cysts are formed (Fig. 7.2 B) and pass out with the feces; they are infective when passed. Another host is infected by ingesting cysts, and excystation takes place in the small intestine. The prepatent period ranges from a few days to more than two months.

The stimuli to form cysts in the host are not known. In culture, trophozoites are transferred to culture media containing less and less nutrient and then are given rice starch in a larger than normal amount. Huge numbers of cysts are then formed within 24 hours.

The organism that leaves the cyst is a tetranucleate ameba; it divides almost immediately into four small amebas. These amebulae are carried to the large intestine where they establish.

Diagnosis

The means of determining whether a person is infected with *E. histolytica* are as follows:

1. Observing clinical signs and symptoms
2. Finding trophozoites or cysts in the feces
3. Cultivating the trophozoites from feces
4. Determining whether the person has antibodies through serology

Severe, usually intermittent, diarrhea or dysentery are the first signs that a person may be suffering from amebiasis. There is usually fever and abdominal discomfort, as well. It is well to note that other protists, helminths, bacteria, and viruses all may cause these generalized clinical features.

Determining whether a person or an animal is infected with *E. histolytica* or other intestinal protist must be approached with care in the laboratory procedures, and skill is required in identifying organisms that may be present. For example, if the host has received medication of any kind, the number of protists may be reduced to a point where they cannot be found for several days. If a fecal specimen cannot be examined within 30 minutes of being passed, it must be properly preserved for examination later.

Since the amebas live in the large intestine, it is often possible to find the living organisms in a freshly passed stool. The formation of explosive pseudopodia gives almost certainty to the diagnosis of *E. histolytica* being present. In any event, permanent stained slides should be made so that the organisms can be measured and nuclei examined for structural details.

When a person shows diarrhea, there are normally no cysts in the feces; trophozoites only are seen at this time. Cysts are seen at the times when the person passes a normal, formed stool.

Cysts are found by using either a sedimentation or a flotation procedure to separate them from the mass of fecal debris. In fecal examinations of cysts passers more than six specimens are required to reach a figure of 80% positives.

Cultivation techniques are used when more direct methods fail. A small amount of fecal material is placed in a culture medium, which contains antibiotics to suppress bacterial growth. When incubated at 37° C, the organisms usually multiply sufficiently by 48 hours that they can be found readily in the bottom of the culture tube.

Serological techniques are useful mostly in detecting extraintestinal amebiasis or in differentiating among species of amebas. Amebas are sometimes also carried from the colon to other sites in the body such as the liver and lung. The organisms multiply and form abscesses; a strong positive serological reaction gives a good indication that the problem may be extraintestinal amebiasis.

Host–Parasite Interactions

Entamoeba histolytica is, by definition, an invasive or pathogenic ameba. Different isolates have differing pathogenic potential, and there are probably a multitude of factors that contribute to the appearance of disease in any one person. These factors may include the isolate of ameba itself, the innate resistance of the host, bacterial associates, and food habits.

Zymodemes using several metabolic enzymes of *E. histolytica* have shown that there are certain patterns that show potential invasiveness. Eighteen zymodemes have been described in various parts of the world, and certain zymodemes in a locality indicate potential invasiveness.

When *E. histolytica* invades the tissue, there is a gradual onset of signs and symptoms. At the cellular level, there is a three-step process: (1) adherence to cells of the colon mediated by lectins, (2) cytolysis by secretion of enzymes, and (3) phagocytosis of cellular debris. When this process has gone on long enough to damage the tissues of the colon, clinical amebiasis may be seen. Usually abdominal tenderness and diarrhea are experienced about the same time. Diarrhea may progress to dysentery, in which there is passage of blood and mucus over a period of weeks. Diarrhea may be interspersed with periods of constipation. If the infection progresses so that there is increasing damage to the large intestine, there may be severe loss of blood and electrolytes. Finally, peritonitis may result if the intestinal wall is perforated thereby allowing bacteria to reach the abdominal cavity.

As they begin to invade the colon, the amebas form small ulcers at the surface of the intestinal epithelium. These ulcers become deeper and spread laterally as the colonies of amebas enlarge (Fig. 7.3). Portions of the intestinal mucosa or epithelium lack adequate circulation because of this undermining and sheets of tissue may slough off. There are two effects: bleeding occurs, and the gut loses its first line of defense, the intact epithelium. In severe invasion, the amebas reach the submucosal and muscular layers of the gut and cause the formation of large necrotic areas in the gut wall.

Human susceptibility to *E. histolytica* can be viewed as a continuum ranging from those few in the population who may be completely resistant to the many who will be moderately susceptible to those few at the other extreme who may succumb if exposed to the agent. A number of postmortem studies have shown that individuals 60 years and older in a population are unlikely to harbor amebas. It could be concluded that these older persons represent the resistant portion of the population and have survived longer than the more susceptible individuals. It has also been observed that British military personnel stationed in India suffered more frequently from amebiasis than their native counterparts. It is likely that the British population has not been subjected to the selective pressure of living in an endemic area where the risk of infection with *E. histolytica* is ever present. The Indian population was subjected to that selective pressure, and the highly susceptible persons in the population were removed

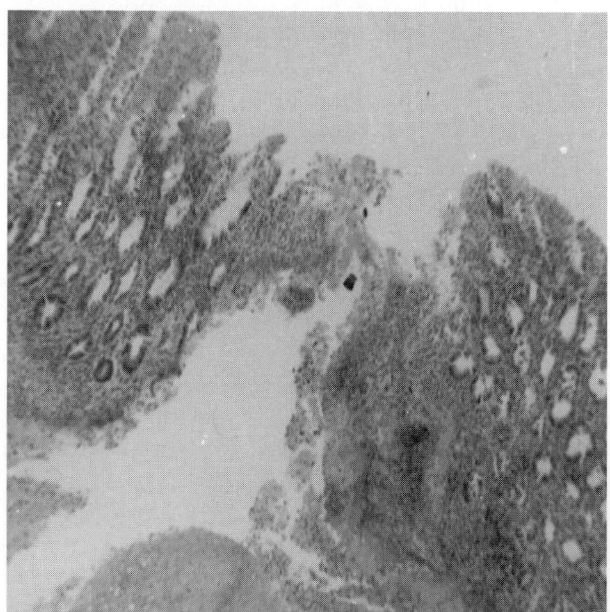

FIGURE 7.3 An ulcer in the colon of a person infected with *Entamoeba histolytica* as seen in a stained tissue section under the LM. The lumenal side of the colon is at the top, and it can be seen that the integrity of the epithelium has been breached and a flask-shaped ulcer extends down to the submucosa. The amebas are found at the margins of the ulcer.

thereby allowing the more resistant individuals to leave their resistant progeny. In experimental infection studies done in humans, the shortest prepatent periods have been a few days, but in some persons, amebas were not found for more than three months. Thus, the same isolate reproduced better in some persons than in others.

Bacterial associates play a role in the ability of amebas either to establish in a host and to cause damage once established. Amebas are not generally capable of infecting a gnotobiotic (germ free) animal. Likewise, those carried in monoxenic culture with the protistan, *Trypanosoma cruzi* were incapable of establishing in experimental animals without first being returned to cultures containing bacteria.

Some of the other factors that have been pointed to as providing conditions conducive to invasion by amebas are the following:

1. Temperature fluctuations in the host
2. Abnormal secretory function
3. Irritant foods
4. Inadequate diet (i.e., low protein)
5. Inflammatory or erosive processes

It should be kept in mind that many of these factors have been surmised from observations on individuals who were ill. Further, even if they are valid observations, a mechanism is not obvious, with one exception: in the case of erosive processes such as ulcerative colitis in which the integrity of the epithelium is lost and the amebas can readily gain access to the tissue. There are some tantalizing data on the role of bacteria in promoting invasiveness, but the mechanism(s) of what happens in the colon of an infected person is not at all clear.

An intriguing hypothesis has been set forth on invasiveness that states that amebas lie in a zone in the colon where there is a small mount of oxygen. The amebas are microaerophilic, and they move back and forth keeping in what might be called a comfort zone. If the amount of oxygen in the tissue declines, they move closer to it and sometimes become invasive.

Immunity traditionally has not been thought to play a role in resistance to invasion by *E. histolytica,* nor in clearing the host of infection. Until recently, serological techniques have not shown antibodies to amebas in the colon; however, if the amebas invade tissues other than the colon such as the liver or lung, antibody titers were generally observed to be high. Antibodies have not been observed to prevent infection. Some studies have indicated that immunity does at least modify the infection.

Epidemiology and Control

There are a number of steps to be taken to prevent infection with *E. histolytica* or that are useful in the face of an outbreak. It is well to note that other organisms causing enteric diseases are controlled by these methods.

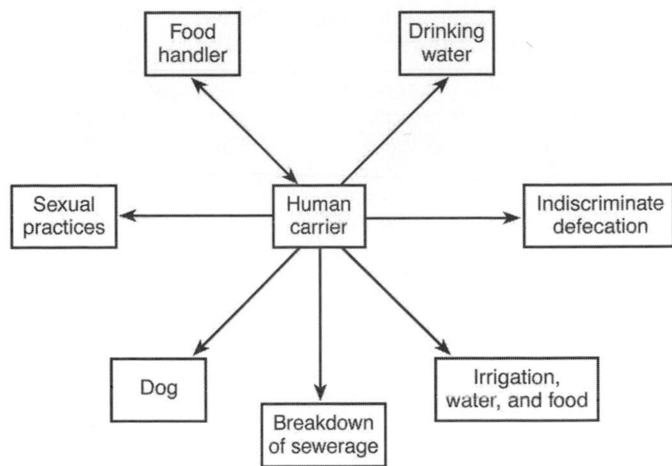

FIGURE 7.4 Pathways of transmission of *Entamoeba histolytica.*

1. Treating drinking water to kill or filter out cysts
2. Proper disposal and treatment of human excreta
3. Proper installation and maintenance of both water delivery and sewerage systems
4. Raising and preparing food free of contamination
5. Eliminating reservoir hosts
6. Treating infected individuals

Transmission of *E. histolytica* takes place most often by ingestion of contaminated food or water. In some instances, transmission may occur through close contact between infected and uninfected persons such as members of the same household, through food handlers, or through homosexual intercourse. However, the main culprits are faulty sewage disposal systems or fecal contamination of food and water (Fig. 7.4).

The cyst is the important stage in transmission. The trophozoite survives for only a short time outside of the host and cannot survive the low pH in the stomach.

Cysts are susceptible to freezing and to temperature above 50° C (Table 7.2). Cool temperatures are most conducive to long-term survival, and as the temperature exceeds 30° C, the death rate increases. It is clear also from the table that access to oxygen is important for survival; at comparable temperatures, survival is better in water than in feces. Soil is likely to have adequate oxygen, except where there is excessive moisture or organic material at the surface. Survival in soil has been good in the few studies reported.

When human excreta are used as fertilizer for crops, it appears that holding the material in a tank for two weeks would be sufficient to kill all of the cysts. All other infectious agents might not be killed however.

Knowledge of the resistance of *E. histolytica* cysts to

TABLE 7.2 Survival of Cysts of *Entamoeba histolytica* and/or *E. dispar* under Various Conditions

Temperature °C	Medium	Time exposed	Result
−28	Water	7.5 hr	Dead
−15	Water	24 hr	Dead
0	Feces	10 days	Dead
0	Water	17 days	Alive
2–6	Water	40 days	Alive
10	Water	30 days	Alive
16–20	Feces	10 days	Dead
16–20	Water	10 days	Alive
20	Water	10 days	Alive
27–30	Feces	9 days	Dead
27–30	Feces	4 days	50% alive
28–34	Soil	8 days	Alive
30	Water	3 days	Alive
37	Feces	3 days	Dead
46–47	Water	1 hr	Alive
52	Water	1 min	Dead
68	Water	5 min	Dead
100	Water	5–10 sec	Dead

(Adapted from several sources)

chemicals is of importance in treating drinking water and disinfection of objects and areas that may be contaminated. The objective of chlorination of water is to kill enteric bacteria; coliform bacteria are killed by concentrations of chlorine from 0.1 to 1.0 mg/l. On the other hand, *E. histolytica* requires 5 mg/l for an hour to kill the cysts. In another study, cysts remained alive after 30 minutes of exposure to 10 mg/l of chlorine. Therefore, the usual levels of chlorination of drinking water are insufficient to kill cysts of *E. histolytica.*

Certain common disinfectants are active against cysts of *E. histolytica*, but the concentrations required reveal the rather high resistance of the cysts to chemical insult. Cresol (isomers of methyl phenol) kills cysts at a concentration of 1:30 in 1 minute and at 1:100 in 30 minutes; the common disinfectant Lysol is a mixture of soap and cresol. Phenol at a dilution of 1:40 kills cysts in 15 minutes at 1:100 in 7 hours. A 50% solution of ethyl alcohol kills cysts within an hour, probably by desiccation, further showing the resistance of cysts to drying.

Food handlers have been implicated in the transmission of *E. histolytica*, and they are important in some circumstances. A 12-fold reduction in the prevalence of infection in Americans working in an oil camp in Venezuela was observed when infected food handlers were identified and treated. In another study, infected personnel in the U.S. Navy were not implicated in the transmission of amebiasis. Likewise, although 52.4% of workers in a factory in South Bend, Indiana, became infected through faulty plumbing, only 3.7% of their family contacts were found to be infected, a level no different from that of the population in general in that community. The crux of the matter with food handlers and transmission lies in their personal habits and sanitary practices, specifically hand washing. At the levels of the health department and kitchen manager, it is essential to enforce hand washing by persons after using the toilet. Transmission of other enteric agents will also be curtailed by this practice.

Certain peridomestic insects may play a role in the transmission of *E. histolytica* cysts. Both filth flies and flesh flies have been found to harbor cysts in their intestines for about two days when fed them experimentally. Also, flies harboring cysts have been caught in houses where infected persons lived. Cockroaches have also been fed cysts, and cultures were obtained from them as long as 48 hours after feeding.

There is a continual low-level transmission of *E. histolytica* in temperate climates that have good sewage disposal systems. The general level of 4% in North America and Western Europe supports this view. The levels of infection are considerably higher, 40 to 70%, in tropical climates and in warm climates where there may not be good sewage treatment. Under these conditions there are continual cases of amebiasis showing up in the population.

In temperate climates that have good sewage disposal systems, amebiasis occurs sporadically but often with serious effects. A case in point was an outbreak of amebic dysentery in a wood-working factory in South Bend, Indiana. The factory employed more than 1500 persons, and over the 2-year period of 1951 to 1953, 48 of them were diagnosed as having clinical amebiasis. Of 1542 employees examined, 52.4% were found to be infected.

When public health epidemiologists investigated the premises, they found that there were three sources of water: (1) a 40-ft (12-m) well used for a fire sprinkler system; (2) a 118-ft (36-m) well for potable, boiler, and industrial water; and (3) city water as a backup. Neither the sprinkler system nor the city water appeared to be the source of the infection. The remaining source of water came from a well situated 80 ft (25 m) from a pumping station and distribution point (Fig. 7.5). The water was pumped from the well to a 1300-gal (4900-l) holding tank. Water was then moved through a 6-in (15-cm) cast iron pipe by suction pumps to a pressure tank and then out through the distribution system. The sewer line roughly paralleled the suction line, but was thought to be separated from it by 5 ft (1.5 m). Some problems had been experienced earlier with bacterial contamination of the water, but they had been taken care of by chlorination.

Upon excavating the area, it was found that the water line and the sewer line were no more than 5 in (12 cm) apart and that the sewer line had leaked.

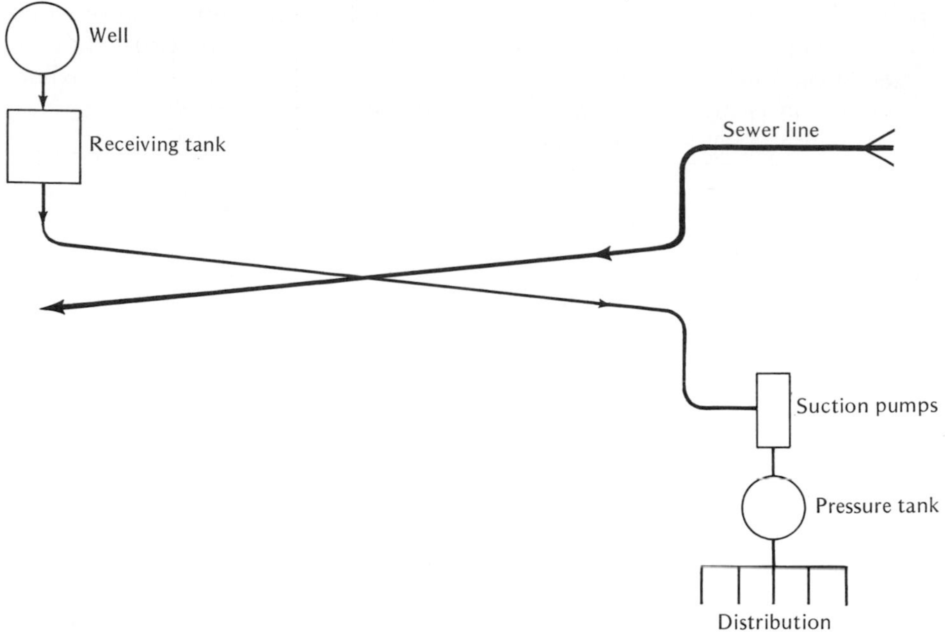

FIGURE 7.5 Relation of water lines and sewer lines in a woodworking factory where an outbreak of amebiasis occurred.

Although no break in the water line was found, fluorescent dye moved from the sewer into the water line when the suction pumps were operated.

In this case, the systems seemed to be well designed and were maintained within acceptable limits. The outbreak occurred because of a slight leak in the sewer, and a negative pressure as great as 15 in (381 mm) of mercury developed when moving water from the receiving tank at the well to the pumping station. It was generally felt that if the sewer and water lines had been separated by 6 ft (2 m), the filtering action of the soil would have been sufficient to prevent transfer of cysts from the sewer to the suction line.

Starting in 1933 there was an outbreak of amebic dysentery associated with two adjacent hotels in Chicago, Illinois. The Chicago Health Department was then headed by a great public health administrator and physician, Herman Bundeson. His report is the basis of the following brief summary.

From June 1, 1933 to June 30, 1934, there were 1409 confirmed cases of amebic dysentery originating in the city, and it was determined that 1209 had contact with one or both of the hotels. Among these persons, there were 62 deaths.

Investigation of the plumbing in the hotels showed that there were two major sources of potential contamination of the drinking water: (1) cross-connections between water and sewer pipes and (2) dripping from a faulty joint in a sewer into an uncovered tank of chilled water; minor sources were from (3) rusted sewerage, which allowed sewage to drip into food preparation areas, (4) back-siphonage from toilets into the water system; and (5) a sewer that ruptured during a heavy rainstorm.

The extent of the contamination in the hotels is exemplified by the fact that 37.8% and 47.4% of employees working in them were found to be infected.

Since cysts are not susceptible at the usual levels of chlorination used for domestic water supplies, water should be passed through a sand filter as well as being chlorinated. Filtration also removes cysts of other protists such as *Giardia* and helminth eggs. If such treatment is not carried out, water should be boiled for drinking, washing vegetables, and such things as brushing the teeth. Certain levels of iodine can also be used in washing vegetables.

Proper disposal of human excreta can range from a well designed pit toilet to a modern sewage treatment plants. Pit toilets, if properly designed, hold the material in an enclosed space and allow natural fermentation to act on whatever infectious agents may be in it. Promiscuous defecation or use of fresh night soil on crops should be curtailed.

In any community, water delivery and sewage systems tend to grow in a rather loosely controlled manner. Pipes do not last forever. Sewers leak at the joints in the pipes, and water mains rust through. But usually nothing is done unless the street caves in or water spews all over the neighborhood. The examples discussed here on outbreaks of amebiasis in a hotel and a factory show that location of pipes and maintenance of the systems are of utmost importance in preventing infection.

Keeping food free of direct or indirect contamination with feces is essential in protecting a community. This pertains at all steps from raising the crop to processing, cooking, serving, and cleaning utensils after serving it. The first step is in the field where workers must be provided with privies or other kinds of toilet facilities that prevent contamination of the crop. Irrigation water and human fertilizer are other sources of contamination of crops that must be controlled. Food handlers have been shown to be a source of infection, especially if personal habits of cleanliness are less than desirable; food handlers should be examined for infection and treated if necessary. Insects such as flies and cockroaches should be excluded from areas where food is stored or prepared. Proper cleaning, use, and storage of kitchen and serving utensils and dishes also keep infection to a minimum.

The only other host of *E. histolytica* considered to be of significance in the maintenance and transmission of it is the dog, even though a number of other species have been found to be infected. Dogs are known to be naturally infected with the organism, but there is still some disagreement on whether they play a role in the transmission of infection to humans. Until better data are developed, it is prudent to consider the dog to be a reservoir.

Amebiosis is widespread in all climates and living conditions, but the prevalence of infection and disease is higher in tropical than in temperate climates. The epidemics in the hotels in Chicago and the factory in South Bend, as discussed earlier, show how minor malfunctions in a high-technology society can have catastrophic results. Even so, greater public health effects of amebiasis occur in less developed countries and tropical countries. In those areas, the prevalence of infection may exceed 80% and the ratio of persons with clinical signs and symptoms is greater than in temperate climate countries. The construction and maintenance of water and sewerage systems require both capital and personnel training in sanitary engineering. Both are likely to be in short supply in developing countries, and it may be necessary to retreat to a level of appropriate technology.

At the public health level, prevention of indiscriminate defecation, tanking excrement before use as fertilizer, and requiring food handlers to wash their hands are all feasible in communities ranging in size from a village of a few hundred persons to a fairly large city.

At a personal level, boiling drinking water, not eating fresh fruits and vegetables than cannot be peeled, washing others in an iodine solution, and keeping insects out of the home can all be done by persons who recognize what the problem is and are motivated to carry these measures through. Therein lies the difficulty. Where amebiosis has a high prevalence, people are faced with a multitude of problems, perhaps the least of which is the prevention of disease. But the public health sector must do what it can to prevent this ubiquitous disease.

ENTAMOEBA DISPAR

Name of Organism and Disease Associations

Entamoeba dispar (in part, *E. histolytica)* is only mildly pathogenic. *E. dispar* can cause some superficial damage to the intestinal mucosa, but it does not invade the deeper tissues, nor does it infect organs other than the colon.

E. dispar is essentially identical to *E. histolytica.* It is morphologically identical at the LM and EM levels. It is consistently different from *E. histolytica* in its genetics, biochemistry, and at the molecular level. Various enzymes, many associated with pathogenesis, as well as antigens are significantly different between *E dispar* and *E. histolytica* that there is little doubt that they are different species. Diamond and Clark (1993) exhaustively reviewed the literature and concluded that there are two species, one potentially highly pathogenic and one only mildly pathogenic.

ENTAMOEBA HARTMANNI

Name of Organism and Disease Associations

Entamoeba hartmanni, (syn. in part, *E. histolytica)* is probably nonpathogenic or only mildly so.

Hosts and Host Range

Probably the same as for *E. histolytica.*

Geographic Distribution and Importance

Cosmopolitan. Its prevalence is rather difficult to determine since *E. hartmanni* was included in *E. histolytica* and *E. dispar* for many years, and its small size may also lead to its being overlooked. In an extensive tabulation of prevalence of infections, *E. hartmanni* was generally rated equal to *E. histolytica*: for example, of 14,744 military veterans, 2.0% were infected with *E. histolytica* and 1.6% with *E. hartmanni,* and in Tennessee, 6.2% of 2657 persons were infected with *E. histolytica* and 6.9% with *E. hartmanni.*

Morphology

This is a small ameba, 3 to 10.5 μm, and its nuclear structure is somewhat different from that of *E. histolyt-*

ica (Fig. 7.1P). The cysts are 4 to 10 μm (Fig. 7.1O); the division between cysts of *E. hartmanni* and *E. histolytica* is at 10 μm. Cytoplasmic inclusions include bacteria, but they do not ingest red blood cells

Life Cycle

The organism is transmitted as a cyst.

Diagnosis

The principal problem in diagnosis of this ameba is it small size, which causes it to be overlooked. When found, it must be differentiated principally from *E. histolytica.*

Host–Parasite Interactions

E. hartmanni is nonpathogenic, or at worst, causes only mild symptoms of enteritis. It is located in the large intestine.

Epidemiology and Control

Since it causes so little pathogenesis, if any, no programs of control are needed.

ENTAMOEBA COLI

Name of Organism and Disease Associations

Entamoeba coli is nonpathogenic.

Hosts and Host Range

Humans and other primates serve as hosts.

Geographic Distribution and Importance

Cosmopolitan. The prevalence of infection in the human population ranges from about 9 to 50%; the U.S. population has a 20 to 30% rate of infection. This ameba is nonpathogenic although it has at various times in the past been blamed for causing diarrhea and dysentery.

Morphology

This organism is somewhat larger than *E. histolytica*, and its nuclear structure (Fig. 7.1R) allows it to be differentiated from *E. histolytica* and other amebas, as well. The nucleus has large clumps of chromatin in a few locations at the nuclear envelope, and the large nucleolus is usually eccentric.

Life Cycle

Transmission from one host to the next takes place by mouth in the cyst form. The trophozoites live in the colon.

Diagnosis

Trophozoites and cysts are found in the feces, and it is important to differentiate this organism from *E. histolytica.* The trophozoites have many bacteria inclusions, and the cytoplasm is rather vacuolated. Nuclear structure is important in differentiating it from *E. histolytica*, as indicated earlier. The cysts are statistically larger than *E. histolytica*, and they typically have eight nuclei, as opposed to four in *E. histolytica. E. coli* cysts sometimes have fewer than eight nuclei, and *E. histolytica* cysts are sometimes seen with more than four nuclei. In life, the trophozoites move progressively but are sluggish, unlike *E. histolytica* which shows eruptive pseudopodia.

Host–Parasite Interactions

Nonpathogenic. As is true with other intestinal protists, *E. coli* may bloom when the host is on a high carbohydrate diet or has enteritis.

Epidemiology and Control

Since *E. coli* is nonpathogenic, control is not required. The prevalence of *E. coli* in a population has sometimes been used to determine the prevalence of *E. histolytica* indirectly since *E. coli* is easier to find in a stained fecal smear.

ENTAMOEBA MOSHKOVSKII

Name of Organism and Disease Associations

Entamoeba moshkovskii (syns. *E. histolytica*-like amebas, *E. histolytica* Laredo strain, *E. laredo*) is a complex of isolates of free-living amebas, some of which may be facultatively parasitic. These amebas can grow in culture at temperatures lower than mammalian body temperature, often at about 24°C.

E. moshkovskii and other isolates that have been made from free-living sources have been found to be a single species (except for one) on the basis of small subunit rRNA riboprints and RFLP analysis.

Morphology

Trophozoites are 9 to 29 μm, and average about 12 μm. The nuclear structure is almost identical to *E.*

histolytica. Cysts range from 7 to 17 μm and have four nuclei when mature, but the chromatoid body is rather diffuse.

Geographic Distribution and Importance

Probably cosmopolitan. *E. moshkovskii* was first isolated from sewage in Russia in 1941 and it has since been found as a free-living ameba in many parts of the world: Brazil, Britain, Canada, and the United States, for example. In 1956, an ameba was isolated from a patient suffering from cancer; this ameba was found to grow at 24°C and was originally called "*E. histolytica* Laredo strain" in honor of the Texas city where it was found. Isolates of these organisms grow poorly, or not at, all at 37°C. This organism is, in fact, *E. moshkovskii.*

Notable Features

The role of *E. moshkovskii* as an agent of disease remains clouded. The work of Clark and Diamond (1991) clarified the fact that nearly all isolates of free-living *Entamoba histolytica*-like organisms are, in fact, *E. moshkovskii* thus simplifying the view of the taxonomy of the amebas. Some workers have stated that *E. moshkovskii* is a human pathogen, but the data do not support such a conclusion at present.

ENDOLIMAX NANA

Name of Organism and Disease Associations

Endolimax nana is a small ameba that is nonpathogenic.

Hosts and Host Range

This organism is a parasite of humans, other primates, and probably the rat. It may also infect other mammals, but the data are unclear.

Geographic Distribution and Importance

Cosmopolitan. The organism is found in perhaps 20% of the human population, and it is important to differentiate it from *E. histolytica.*

Morphology

This is a small ameba 6 to 15 μm and averaging 10 μm. The cysts are 5 to 14 μm in diameter. The nucleus of the trophozoite has a thin envelope and a cluster of granules in the center. The cyst is oval and has four small nuclei that are similar to that in the trophozoite (Fig. 7.1W & X).

Life Cycle

This ameba is transmitted from one host to the next in the cyst form. It lives in the colon of its host.

Diagnosis

It is important to differentiate this ameba from *E. histolytica*. Both the trophozoite and the cyst are smaller than *E. histolytica*, and the nuclear structure is different.

IODAMOEBA BUETSCHLII

Name of Organism and Disease Associations

Iodamoeba buetschlii is considered to be a nonpathogenic ameba. It has been associated with diarrhea in humans on occasion, and the pathogenic potential of this organism may remain open.

Hosts and Host Range

Humans, other primates, and suids are the principal hosts.

Geographic Distribution and Importance

Cosmopolitan. The prevalence of infection is 5% or less, but it is probably higher in warm climates.

Morphology

The trophozoite is 4 to 10 μm and has a nucleus with a large endosome and a delicate nuclear envelope (Fig. 7.6). There are usually a number of inclusions in

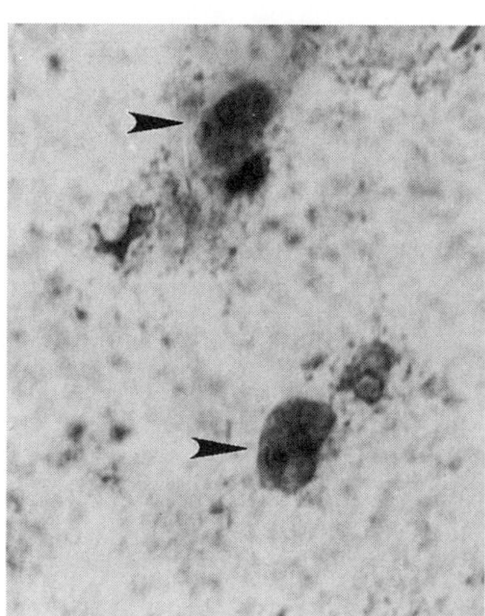

FIGURE 7.6 *Iodamoeba buetschlii* trophozoite as seen in a stained fecal smear.

the cytoplasm representing ingested food (Fig. 7.1U). The cyst is 6 to 15 μm, has a single nucleus similar to the trophozoite ,and usually has a large iodinophilous vacuole (Fig. 7.1V).

Life Cycle

Transmission from one host to the next takes place through ingestion of the cyst.

Diagnosis

The trophozoites and cysts are found in the feces. It is important to differentiate this ameba from *E. histolytica.*

Host–Parasite Interactions

Iodamoeba is usually considered to be nonpathogenic, and as long as it remains in the intestine, it may be. There are a few cases on record of organisms forming abscesses in organs other than the gut such as the liver, lung, and brain. The nuclear structure of *Iodamoeba* and that of *Naegleria* or *Acanthamoeba* are similar and a misidentification is possible (Chapter 8).

AMEBAS AS PARASITES OF HOSTS OTHER THAN HUMANS

Amebas are found as inhabitants of the intestinal tracts of a wide array of vertebrates and invertebrates. As a general rule, any one host usually harbors only one or two species of ameba, but the same host may have ten species of flagellates and apicomplexans, as well as one or two species of ciliates. With few exceptions, the amebas are not known to be pathogenic.

Entamoeba invadens is a cosmopolitan parasite of many reptiles: turtles, snakes, and lizards. The trophozoites are 9 to 38 μm averaging 16 μm. The cysts range in diameter from 11 to 20 μm and average 17μm. The nuclear morphology and formation of eruptive pseudopodia are quite similar to those of *E. histolytica.*

This is a pathogenic organism in some hosts. It remains as a commensal in herbivorous and omnivorous hosts such as turtles and some lizards. On the other hand, it is a serious pathogen in carnivorous lizards and snakes. The ameba infects not only all levels of the intestinal tract, but also the liver. Its effect on free-ranging reptiles is not known, but it is a significant problem in captive reptiles.

E. invadens is readily cultivated in nonliving media with bacteria, but has also been carried in bacteria-free culture and in defined media. *E. invadens* is much hardier outside of its host than is *E. histolytica*, and it therefore is used in experimental studies on locomotion, as an example. The mechanism of locomotion including the translocation of particles toward the rear of the moving ameba and the role of actin in the cytoskeleton of the organism have been particularly useful in developing theories on ameboid movement and invasion of tissue.

Some amebas found in domestic animals are *Entamoeba bovis* of cattle, and *E. gallinarum* of gallinaceous birds such as chickens and turkeys. Swine have two species, *E. debliecki* and *Iodamoeba buetschlii*, the latter a parasite of humans.

Among companion animals, dogs are naturally infected with *E. histolytica* and perhaps some of the other enteric amebas of humans. Cats do not have an ameba that they can call their own, but can be experimentally infected with *E. histolytica.*

Amebas of invertebrates are not prominent parasites, but they are present in many species of hosts such as the coelenterate *Hydra* and many insects. Cockroaches, for example, have two species of amebas, *Endamoeba blattae* and *Entamoeba thomsoni*, which can be studied alive under a microscope.

Readings

Bailey, G. B., Day, D. B., and McCoomer, N. E. (1992). *Entamoeba* motility: Dynamics of cytoplasmic streaming, locomotion and translocation of surface-bound particles, and organization of the actin skeleton in *Entamoeba invadens. J. Protozool.* **39,** 267–272.

Bruckner, D. A. (1992). Amebiasis. *Clin. Microbiol. Rev.* **5,** 356–369.

Campbell, D., and Chadee, K. (1997). Survival strategies of *Entamoeba histolytica*: Modulation of cell-mediated immune responses. *Parasitol. Today* **13,** 184–190.

Clark, C. G., and Diamond, L. S. (1991). The Laredo strain and other *Entamoeba histolytica* like amoebae are *Entamoeba moshkovskii. Mol. Biochem. Parasitol.* **46,** 11–18.

Diamond, L. S., and Clark, C. G. (1993). A redescription of *Entamoeba histolytica* Schaudinn, 1903 (Emend. Walker, 1911) separating it from *Entamoeba dispar* Brumpt, 1925. *J. Euk. Microbiol.* **40,** 340–344.

Guerrant, R. L. (1986). Amebiasis: Introduction, current status, and research questions. *Rev. Infect. Dis.* **8,** 218–227.

Kretschmer, R. R. (1990). *Amebiasis: Infection and Disease by Entamoeba histolytica.* CRC Press, Boca Raton, FL.

Martinez-Palomo, A. (1986). *Amebiasis. Human Parasitic Disease, Vol.* 2. Elsevier, Amsterdam.

Martinez-Palomo, A., and Espinoza-Catellano, M. (1998). Amoebiasis: New understanding and new goals. *Parasitol. Today* **14,** 1–3.

Meerovitch, E. (1982). The jigsaw puzzle of host–parasite relations in amoebiasis begins to take shape. In *Aspects of Parasitology* (E. Meerovitch, Ed.). Institute of Parasitology, McGill University, Montreal.

Ravdin, J. I. (Ed.) (1988). *Amebiasis.* Wiley, New York.

Ravdin, J. I. (1990). Cell biology of *Entamoeba histolytica* and immunobiology of amebiasis. In *Modern Parasite Biology* (D. J. Wyler, Ed.). Freeman, New York.

CHAPTER

8

Free-Living Amebas as Pathogens

Free-living aquatic and terrestrial amebas have always been considered merely to be elements in the microenvironment that cycle energy and prey on other small organisms without having any direct importance to mankind. In the late 1950s, it became necessary to reconsider whether these small amebas were as innocuous as they had been thought to be. At first, they were laboratory curiosities that appeared in primary monkey kidney tissue cultures grown for production of poliomyelitis virus. Some of these organisms were then found to produce disease in laboratory rodents inoculated experimentally. In the early 1960s, 19 isolates of amebas were made from human respiratory tracts as incidental findings in a study on respiratory viruses. Starting in 1965 a spate of fatalities caused by free-living amebas was seen in humans in Australia, Florida, Texas, and Czechoslovakia.

The question then arose as to the importance of these organisms in human and animal health. We now know that free-living amebas of a dozen or more species are facultative parasites of humans and other animals, and that a few can cause serious, even fatal, disease. There have been about 200 well-documented cases of fatal encephalitis in humans caused by free-living amebas worldwide. Of these, 144 have been caused by *Naegleria fowleri,* and the remainder were caused by *Acanthamoeba* spp., and *Balamuthia mandrillaris* divided about 40 and 16, respectively.

A number of organisms in three genera have been found to have the ability to live in the tissues of mammals and to have at least some pathogenic potential (Tab. 8.1) The very obscurity of these organisms coupled with the sporadic infections that have been seen in humans requires some detailed discussion of the organisms that are known to cause central nervous system (CNS) problems and infect other tissues as well.

Amebas have been classified and identified on the basis of (1) nuclear structure, (2) size of the trophozoite, (3) form of the pseudopodia, (4) number of nuclei, (5) cyst structure, (6) sexual reproduction , if any, and (7) formation of flagellated stages. In recent years, additional characters have been used such as (8) antigenic composition, (9) iosoenzyme migration patterns, (10) culture media that will support growth, and (11) temperature tolerance and preference.

NAEGLERIA FOWLERI

Name of Organism and Disease Associations

Naegleria fowleri is the cause of primary amebic meningoencephalitis (PAM) in humans and perhaps other hosts as well. This organism was originally identified as *N. gruberi*, a free-living ameba that is quite similar, but it fails to grow at mammalian body temperature.

Hosts and Host Range

Humans have been the hosts of greatest concern, but it seems likely that these amebas have little host specificity.

Geographic Distribution and Importance

Cosmopolitan. Human infections have been found in North America, Western Europe, Africa, Japan, and

TABLE 8.1 Some Prominent Signs and Symptoms of Infection in Humans with Facultatively Parasitic Free-Living Amebas

Symptoms	Signs
Headache	Coma
Seizures	Papilledema
Nausea and vomiting	Cranial nerve abnormalities
Vision problems	Nystagmus (rapid eyeball movement)
Mental problems such as hallucinations, drowsiness, confusion, irritability	Problems in walking
	Hemiparesis (Partial paralysis)

Australia. Infections are nearly always seen after people have swum in, or otherwise had contact with, warm to hot waters. Most human cases have been sporadic, but in a few instances there have been small epidemics of several people who have swum in a pool fed by a hot spring, for example.

Between 1965 and 1969 there were as number of documented fatalities: 4 in Australia, 3 in Florida, 1 in Texas, and 16 in Czechoslovakia. These outbreaks alerted public health workers to the fact that there was a new disease, and outbreaks were reported in several locations such as the state of Virginia.

Two retrospective studies using tissues saved for histologic examination from unexplained central nervous system deaths showed that a significant number of persons had died from PAM in the past. It was clear that this was not an emerging disease but more likely an unrecognized one.

In sum, central nervous system infections and deaths from free-living amebas are uncommon, but clusters of cases are often seen during the warm months of the year. Public health officials are faced with a dilemma in which the risk is small but the consequence of infection can be the death of the infected individual.

Morphology

These organism are typical of many small, free-living amebas that live in soil and water. Trophozoites are 10 to 20 μm, but sometimes smaller. They have a vesicular nucleus with a large, central nucleolus; the chromatin is scattered in small bodies near the nuclear membrane (Figs. 8.1 and 8.2). Cysts are usually about 11μm and they have pores that have mucoid plugs (Fig. 8.1).

Life Cycle

Multiplication is by binary fission; there are no sexual stages (Fig. 8.1). When mitosis occurs, the nuclear

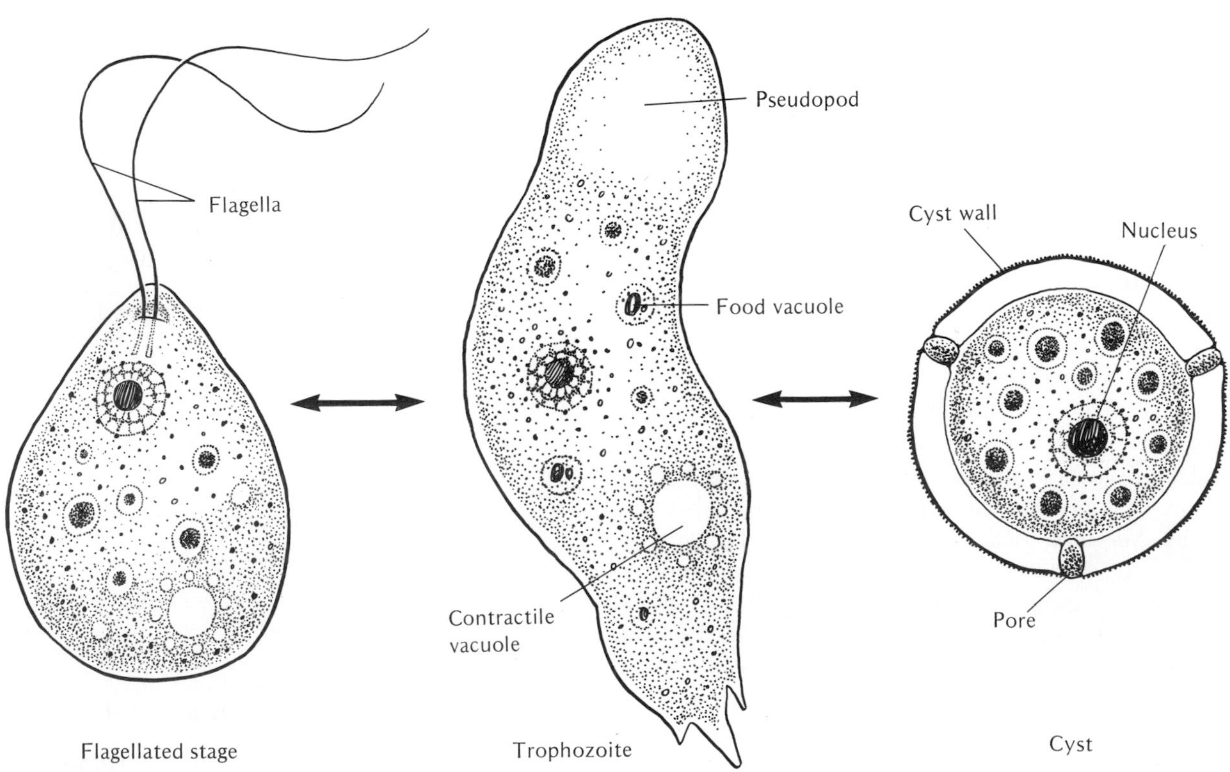

FIGURE 8.1 The life cycle and morphology of *Naegleria fowleri*: flagellated form, trophozoite, cyst.

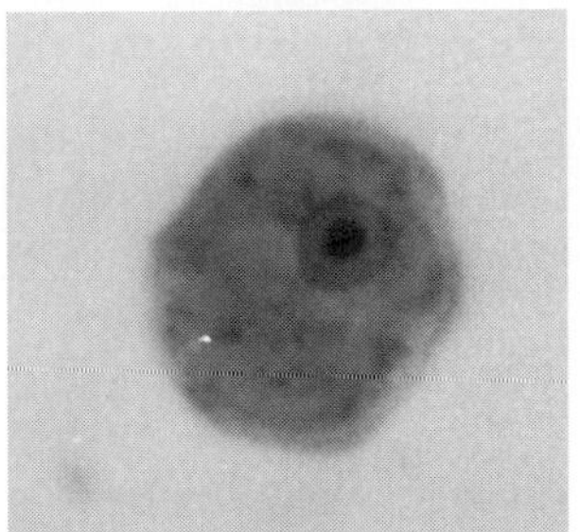

FIGURE 8.2 A fixed and stained specimen of *Naegleria fowleri* as seen in LM. Note the nucleus with a large nucleolus, characteristic of many free-living amebas.

membrane is retained, unlike some other free-living amebas. Encystment occurs frequently in culture. The exact stimuli have not been described, but cysts seem to be formed under unfavorable conditions. Cysts are seldom seen in clinical specimens.

The formation of flagella in *N. fowleri* and other members of the genus, allows for dispersal more quickly than by amoeboid movement. The most important factor in enflagellation is a reduction in nutrient. If *N. fowleri* trophozoites are transferred from culture medium to a non-nutrient buffer, enflagellation takes place. The best transformation to the flagellated form takes place when organism are cultivated at 37°C and when they have reached the stationary growth phase in culture.

It is not known what stage of the life cycle enters the potential mammalian host. Experimental infections have used trophozoites.

Diagnosis

The means of determining whether a person has PAM are as follows:

1. Clinical signs and symptoms
2. History of swimming in hot or warm water
3. Isolation of the amebas

Clinical signs and symptoms of a CNS disease are the first indications of PAM (Tab. 8.1). They are vague and rather general, and a number of infectious agents produce the same syndrome. Swimming in warm waters three to seven days prior to the onset of symptoms should raise the possibility of PAM. While it may be possible to isolate organisms from a person showing clinical signs of infection, they are most often found postmortem. The organisms can be cultivated and examined morphologically, as well as using biochemical markers, to determine their species.

Host–Parasite Interactions

Organisms probably enter the nasal passages when the person is swimming or otherwise has contact with warm waters. Once they have entered the nasal mucosa, the amebas follow the path of least resistance by moving along nerve tracts, principally the nasal nerve. They move through the cribriform plate into the cranial cavity. In the brain, the amebas remain associated mostly with the membranous coverings of the brain, the meninges, where they elicit an inflammatory response (Fig. 8.3).

In instances where exposure could be documented, signs and symptoms of infection appeared in less than a week following exposure. Although there may be some signs of inflammation in the upper respiratory tract early in the infection, usually the first symptoms are lethargy and headache (Tab. 8.1). Within two or three days the headache becomes more severe and there may be vomiting, stiff neck, and mental confusion. Alteration in normal sensations of taste and smell, double vision, incoordination of motor activity, and bizarre behavior may also be seen. Coma ensues as a result of intracranial pressure. Death usually occurs within 10 days of the onset of symptoms.

Epidemiology and Control

The crucial character of these amebas is their ability to multiply at mammalian body temperature, about 37°C; *N. fowleri* can grow at temperatures as high as 45°C. In epidemiologic studies, this is the first character that is tested.

N. fowleri can be found in natural hot waters such as springs, in cooling ponds for power generations stations, or in shallow ponds or lakes warmed by the

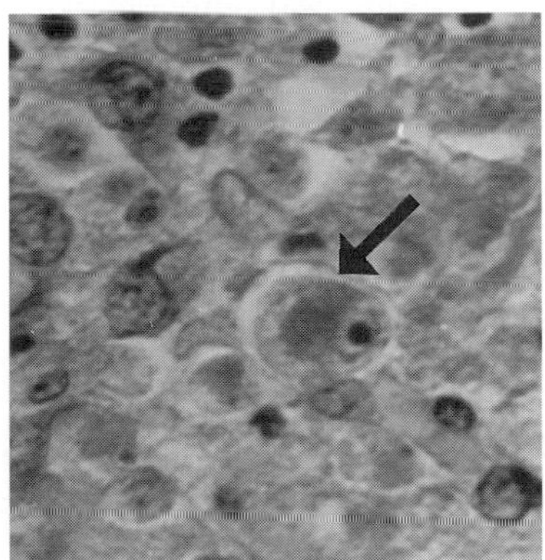

FIGURE 8.3 A histologic section of brain tissue infected with *Naegleria fowleri* (arrow) as seen in LM; the organism lies in a vacuole in the tissue and has a nucleus with a prominent endosome or nucleolus.

sun. In all cases, except one, the histories of affected individuals have included contact with warm or hot waters within the previous week or so. Typically an individual that is diagnosed with PAM has been swimming in a hot water pool from three to seven days earlier. Since swimming is a summertime activity, the warmer months are the times when cases are most often seen. The only case on record where the person had not contact with warm water and was that of an elderly woman in Texas who had not recent history of any such contact.

Special circumstances may also bring about PAM. For example, a farmer in Nigeria died from PAM. The history showed that he was a Moslem and had made his ablutions before prayer in puddles of water in or near his fields. In the tropics, shallow water becomes quite warm, and there was undoubtedly a bloom of thermotolerant amebas, which he splashed into his eyes, nose, and mouth.

Prevention of PAM has not been highly successful. The cysts are quite resistant and the usual chlorination of swimming pools may not kill them. In one report, 4.0 ppm chlorine killed both trophozites and cysts, but another stated that 10 ppm was ineffective. Some health departments have posted warnings at hot water swimming pools to the effect that swimmers should not get their heads into the water.

Treatment of PAM depends on an early diagnosis and use of antibiotics introduced directly into the central nervous system. Some success has been achieved with certain antibiotics, but better treatments are needed.

Related Organisms

A number if species of *Naegleria* have been described that can be cultivated at 37°C or higher and that are pathogenic in experimental animals.

ACANTHAMOEBA SPP.

Name of Organism and Disease Associations

Acanthamoeba castellanii, A. polyphaga, A. culbertsoni, and perhaps other species. These organisms cause granulomatous amebic encephalitis (GAE).

Hosts and Host Range

Nearly all infections have been reported from humans, but other known hosts are the dog and sheep.

Geographic Distribution and Importance

Cosmopolitan. Fewer than half of the cases of amebic encephalitis reported in the medical literature have been caused by *Acanthamoeba* spp.

Morphology

All of the species of *Acanthamoeba* have spikey pseudopods and a nucleus with a large, central nucleolus similar to that of *Naegleria* (Fig. 8.2). Group 1 consists of those trophozoites and cysts that are 18 μm or larger and includes *A. astronyxis, A. comandoni, A. echinulata,*and *A. tubiashi.* Group 2 has trophozoites and cysts that are 18 μm or less and includes *A. castellanii, A. polyphaga, A. rhysodes, A. mauaritaniensis, A. divionensis, A. griffini, A. lugdenensis, A. quina, A. hatchetti,* and *A. triangularis.* Members of Group 3 are the same size as those in Group 2, but the cysts are different morphologically. It includes *A. culbertsoni, A. lenticulata, A. palestinensis, A. pustulosa,* and *A. royreba.*

Life Cycle

There are two stages in the life cycles of these amebas: trophozoite and cyst. They do not enflagellate.

Diagnosis

Finding the amebas in tissue is the only sure method of diagnosis. Signs and symptoms are suggestive (Tab. 8.1).

Host–Parasite Interactions

The amebas probably enter the respiratory system, or perhaps the skin, and then migrate to the CNS via the blood. Once in the brain, the organisms cause a granulomatous encephalitis, which means that a more or less discrete mass of inflammatory cells and amebas are found in the meninges and superficial layers of the brain. The lesions develop slowly, perhaps a period of several weeks or months passes before clinical signs and symptoms are seen. If treatment is not administered, the progress of the disease is inexorable leading to death of the patient.

Most patients seen with GAE do not have normal immune systems. GAE has been seen in AIDS patients, as well as in hemophiliacs and alcoholics.

AMEBIC KERATITIS—INFECTIONS OF THE EYE

Name of Organism and Disease Associations

Acanthamoeba polyphaga A. castellanii, A. culberstoni, *A. hatchetti,* and *A. rhysodes* have all caused ulcers of the cornea of the eye in humans.

Hosts and Host Range

The clinical reports have been mostly in humans, but other animals should be considered as potential hosts.

Geographic Distributon and Importance

Cosmopolitan. About 250 infections of the cornea with *Acanthamoeba* spp. have been reported to or confirmed by the CDC.

Morphology and Life Cycle

These amebas are generally about 15 μm and they form spheroid cysts. The pseudopodia that they form are pointed and usually any one individual has a number of these filopodia extending a short distance. They divide by binary fission and have a cyst stage.

Diagnosis

Finding the amebas in a corneal ulcer is the only certain method of diagnosis.

Host–Parasite Interactions

The cornea is invaded when there is trauma to the eye or the presence of amebas in water contaminated with them. If the cornea is slightly damaged, it allows the amebas a place to colonize. In most instances, there is an association with wearing contact lenses and a failure to clean them properly.

In several documented instances, persons wearing contact lenses have used cleaning solutions that were not sterile,and seemingly brought the amebas into contact with the cornea thereby.

Either by close association with the cornea or an abrasion, the amebas invade the layers of the tissue and bring about inflammation and destruction of the cornea. The infections are stubborn but do respond to chemotherapy in many instances. In other cases, the infection progresses and a corneal transplant may be necessary.

Epidemiology and Control

Prevention of corneal infections is through the following:

1. Using sterile, commercially prepared cleaning solutions for contact lenses
2. Sterilizing contact lenses by heat
3. Following carefully the instructions of the manufacturer of the lenses with respect to the length of time the lenses can remain in the eyes and how the lenses should be cleaned

BALAMUTHIA MANDRILLARIS

Name of Organism and Disease Associations

Balamuthia mandrillaris is the cause of meningoencephalitis in higher primates such as the baboon, gorilla, and humans. It also has been found in the brain and lungs of a sheep.

Morphology

B. mandrillaris is distinctly different from the other amebas that have been associated with disease in humans and other animals. They belong to the order Leptomyxida, which is characterized as having members that are relatively large, often 50 μm or larger, uni- or multinucleate and forming complex, resistant cysts. These organisms have been considered to be solely free living, but the description of *B. mandrillaris* in 1993 changed, again, our view of potentially pathogenic amebas.

B. mandrillaris ranges in size from 10 to 60 μm with a mean of 30 μm (Fig. 8.4). It shows two forms of pseudopodia: broad, lobose pseudopodia or numerous, fingerlike pseudopodia, which it appears to use in a kind of walking movement. The cysts average 15 μm in diameter with a range of 6 to 30 μm. They have three walls: the outer layer is thin and irregular so that it gives a rough appearance; the middle layer consists of a layer of amorphous fibrils, while the inner layer is thick and electron dense in TEM.

Diagnosis

Determining whether a person has been infected with *B. mandrillaris* is based on the following:

1. Clinical signs and symptoms
2. Use of *in situ* immunofluorescence of the organisms in the CNS

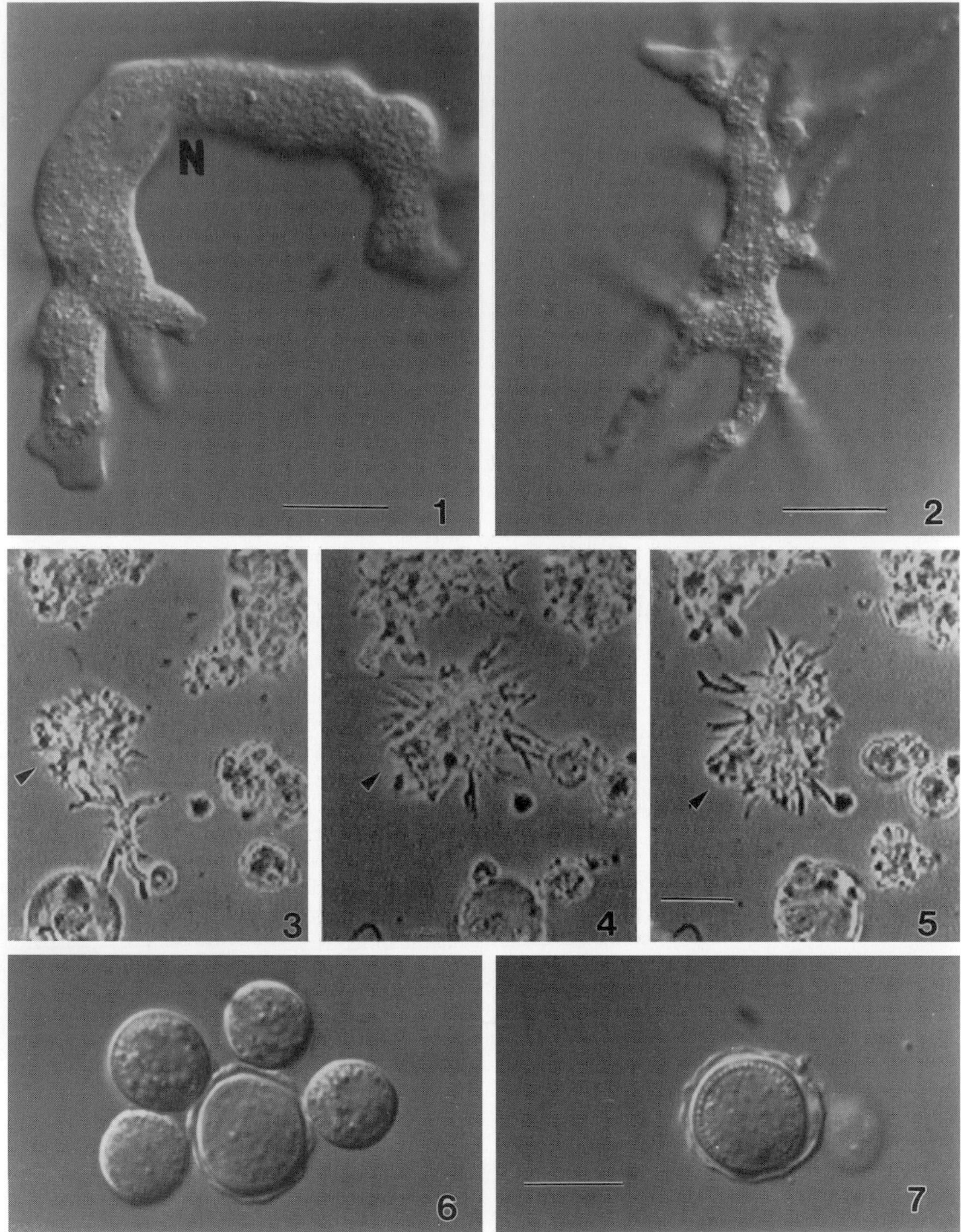

FIGURE 8.4 *Balamuthia mandrillaris* as seen alive under LM showing both trophozoite (1–5) stages and cysts (6, 7). The organism usually moves and feeds by using lobose pseudopodia (1, 2), but it occasionally forms many slender pseudopodia. The cysts are spheroidal with three layers best seen in 7. [From: Visvesvara, G. S., et al., 1993.

3. Finding typical organisms, trophozoites and cysts in tissue at postmortem examination

As is true with infections with *Naegleria fowleri*, the clinical signs and symptoms of infection with *B. mandrillaris* are not specific. Headache, vomiting, visual disturbances, fever, and neuromuscular dysfunctions are the most common signs. CAT scans may show dense areas in the brain where the organisms have multiplied. Most often, GAE has been seen in persons whose immune systems are compromised or who are otherwise in poor health.

Unfortunately, most diagnoses are made on persons who have died from GAE. Organisms are found in the tissues by common histologic examinations or by using a specific antibody that will fluoresce at the site of the amebas in the tissues. Organisms can also be cultivated from infected tissues. As indicated earlier, the organisms in culture are quite distinctive morphologically.

Host–Parasite Interactions

Parasitism by any leptomyxid ameba was unknown until *B. mandrillaris* was found in the brain of a mandrill, *Sphinx papio,* which died in the San Diego Zoo Wild Animal Park. Retrospective studies of tissues taken from humans and other higher primates showed that some previously identified cases of encephalitis were erroneously attributed to *Acanthamoeba.* Sixteen diagnoses of death in humans were determined to have been caused by a leptomyxid ameba, *B. mandrillaris,* or other closely related species.

B. mandrillaris causes GAE (granulomatous amebic encephalitis), which has a rather extended course compared to *N. fowleri.* It is not clear how long the mandrill was affected, but those persons in the retrospective study cited earlier had clinical signs and symptoms lasting from two weeks to more than six months before death ensued.

Epidemiology and Control

Little information is at hand on the natural route of infection. Laboratory mice were infected either by instilling amebas into the nasal passages or by intraperitoneal (IP) inoculation. Likewise, prevention of infection remains unknown.

It is interesting to note that *B. mandrillaris* has been cultivated only on living cells. The other facultatively parasitic amebas can be cultivated on bacteria seeded onto non-nutrient agar.

There is no effective chemotherapy for GAE.

Readings

Averner, M., and Fulton, C. (1966). Carbon dioxide: Signal for excystment of *Naegleria gruberi. J. Gen. Microbiol.* **42,** 245–255.

Cable, B. L., and John, D. T. (1986). Conditions for maximum enflagellation in *Naegleria fowleri. J. Protozool.* **33,** 467–472.

Dunnebacke, T. H., and Schuster, F. L. (1971). Infectious agent from a free-living soil ameba, *Naegleria gruberi. Science* **174,** 516–518.

de Jonckheere, J., and van de Voorde, H. (1977). The distribution of *Naegleria fowleri* in man-made thermal waters. *Am. J. Trop. Med. Hyg.* **26,** 10–15.

John, D. T., Cole, T. B., Jr., and Marciano-Cabral, F. M. (1984). Sucker-like structures on the pathogenic amoeba *Naegleria fowleri. Appl. Environ. Microbiol.* **47,** 12–14.

Lawande, R. V., Macfarlane, J. T., Weir, W. R. C., and Awunor-Renner, C. (1980). A case of primary amebic meningoencephalitis in a Nigerian farmer. *Am. J. Trop. Med. Hyg.* **29,** 21–25.

Ma, P., Visvesvara, G. S., Martinez, A. J., Theordore, F. H., Daggett, P.-M., and Sawyer, T. K. (1990). *Naegleria* and *Acanthamoeba* infections: Review. *Rev. Infect. Dis.* **12,** 490–513.

Moura, H., Wallace, S., and Visvesvara, G. S. (1992). *Acanthamoeba healyi* n. sp. and the isoenzyme and immunoblot profiles of *Acanthamoeba* spp. Groups 1 and 3. *J. Protozool.* **39,** 573–583.

Page, F. C. (1988). *A New Key to Freshwater and Soil Gymnamoebae.* Fresh Water Biological Assoc. Ableside, Cumbria, UK.

Riestra-Castenada, J. M., *et al.* (1997). Granulomatous amebic encephalitis due to *Balamuthia mandrillaris* (Leptomyxiidae); Report of four cases in Mexico. *Am. J. Trop. Med. Hyg.* **56,** 603–607.

Sawyer, T. K., Visvesvara, G. S., and Harke, B. A. (1977). Pathogenic amoebas from brackish and ocean sediments, with a description of *Acanthamoeba hatchetti,* n. sp. *Science* **196,** 1324–1325.

Visvesvara, G. S., and Stehr-Green, J. K. (1990). Epidemiology of free-living ameba infections. *J. Protozool.* **37,** 25S–33S.

Visvesvara, G. S., Schuster, F. L., and Martinez, J. J. (1993). *Balamuthia mandrillaris* n.g., n. sp., agent of amebic meningoencephalitis in humans and other animals. *J. Euk. Microbiol.* **40,** 504–514.

CHAPTER

9

Ciliates and Opalinids

Although this chapter combines the phyla Ciliophora and a few members of the Opalozoa, it is purely for convenience and does not imply any close taxonomic relationship of the two groups.

PHYLUM CILIOPHORA

The ciliates comprise a phylum of eukaryotic protists in which the three key characteristics are that they (1) are heterokaryotic (i.e., have two kinds of nuclei), (2) possess an infraciliature of complex structure that is the overriding feature of their structure, physiology, and evolution, and (3) have a sexual phenomenon, often seen as conjugation, in which there is a temporary union of two individuals for the exchange of nuclear material.

The general anatomy of ciliates can be illustrated by *Paramecium* (Fig. 9.1), a common free-living ciliate often studied in biology courses. In this genus, the whole body of the organism is covered with cilia by which it moves through the water. There is a macronucleus, which is polyploid and serves the metabolic activities of the organism while the micronucleus is the repository of the genome. The micronucleus seemingly does little except to participate in conjugation and, in many species, reforms the macronucleus following conjugation.

Food is ingested through the cytostome (Fig. 9.1), which has a complex structure of cilia designed to move small bits of detritus and bacteria into it (Fig. 9.2). Food is digested in vacuoles, which move around the cytoplasm of the organism, and the food residue is removed through a cytopyge or cell anus. The contractile vacuole has been given several names, but its function is osmoregulation.

The infraciliature is made evident at the LM level through the use of silver stains (Fig. 9.3), which deposit in the basal bodies and their fibrillar connections to one another. The cilia arise from basal bodies, which, in turn, are connected by fibrils that run anteriorly and laterally (Fig. 9.4). Depending on the species, a number of other organelles are associated with the infraciliature such as mucocysts and trichocysts.

The infraciliature is used in the identification and description of species of ciliates, but it has greater significance in describing pathways of evolution and in fundamental studies on cellular development and the genetics of development.

Division in ciliates is by a type of transverse division in which the longitudinal kinetids are severed and then reform after division is complete. This type of division is termed homothetogenic, as opposed to symmetrogenic, as seen in organisms such as the trypanosomes.

Classification dividing the phylum into 8 to 10 classes is based on the details of ciliation, structure of the kinetids, oral or buccal structures, and various pellicular structures such as mucocysts, trichocysts, and toxicysts.

Most ciliates are free living and feed on particulate food, some as small as bacteria; other ciliates are predaceous and feed on relatively large organisms. Some species obtain nutrient through a modified membrane uptake (endocytosis). Food is contained in vacuoles, digested in them, and then the residue is eliminated into the surrounding medium through the residual vacuole or cytopyge (Fig. 9.2).

Although most ciliophorans are free living, signifi-

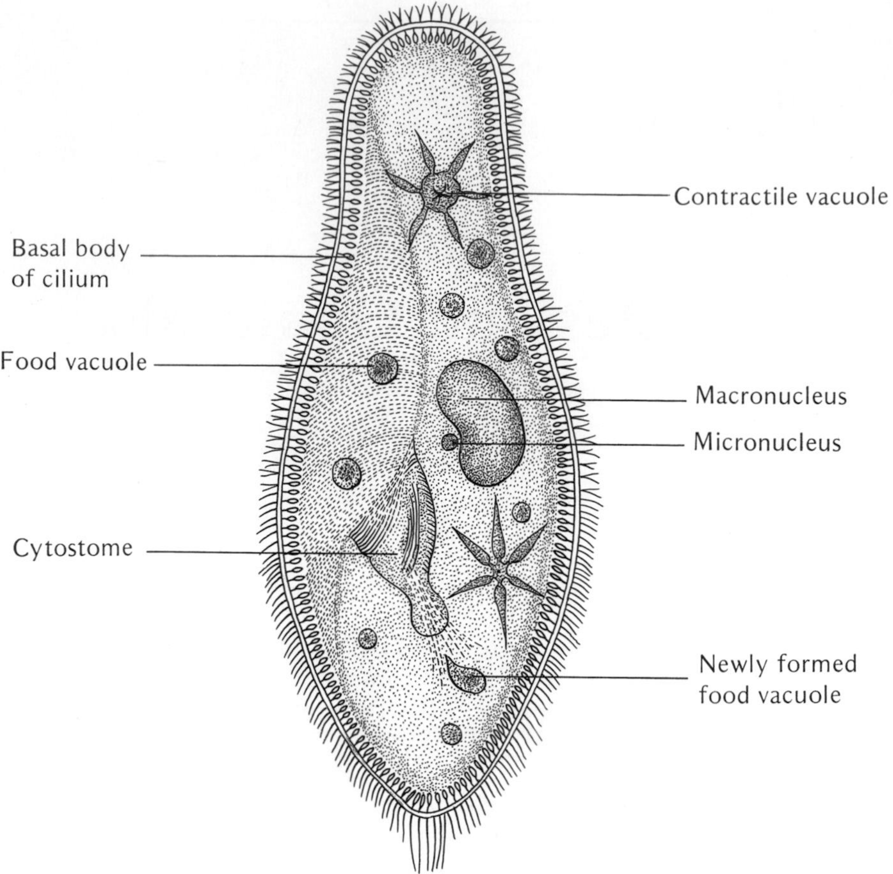

FIGURE 9.1 A diagram of the anatomy of a typical ciliate, *Paramecium*.

cant numbers are symbiotic in many invertebrate and vertebrates hosts. Fresh-water amphipods often have large numbers of ciliates in the hemocoel. Mosquito larvae are parasitized by *Tetrahymena*, and fresh water *Hydra* (Cnidaria) have a phoretic ciliate, *Kerona polyporum*, on the surface.

Ciliates play an important role in the digestion of cellulose by some herbivorous mammals. Ruminants and equids have an extraordinary array of ciliates in their intestinal tracts. Vertebrates cannot digest cellulose and rely on symbiotic organisms to break the molecule into smaller fragments. In ruminants and equids, both ciliates and bacteria are involved in digestion of cellulose. In studies on their role in ruminant nutrition, the results generally show that bacteria alone are sufficient to allow the digestion of cellulose, but that animals gain weight better when both bacteria and ciliates are present in the rumen. Both kind of microorganisms not only digest cellulose, but serve as part of the food of the host as well. It has been estimated that 20% of the protein in ruminant nutrition is derived from the ciliates, which pass from the rumen into the intestine.

BALANTIDIUM COLI

Name of Organism and Disease Associations

Balantidium coli is the cause of balantidiosis or balantidial dysentery.

Hosts and Host Range

Hosts include suids, humans, and other primates. Some animals such as rodents can be infected experimentally.

Geographic Distribution and Importance

Cosmopolitan. *B. coli* is common in pigs being found in from 20 to 100% of individuals in various populations. In humans the prevalence is spotty; some surveys indicate that the prevalence is less than 1%, but there are other populations where the organism is common. Not many surveys have been done for infections in

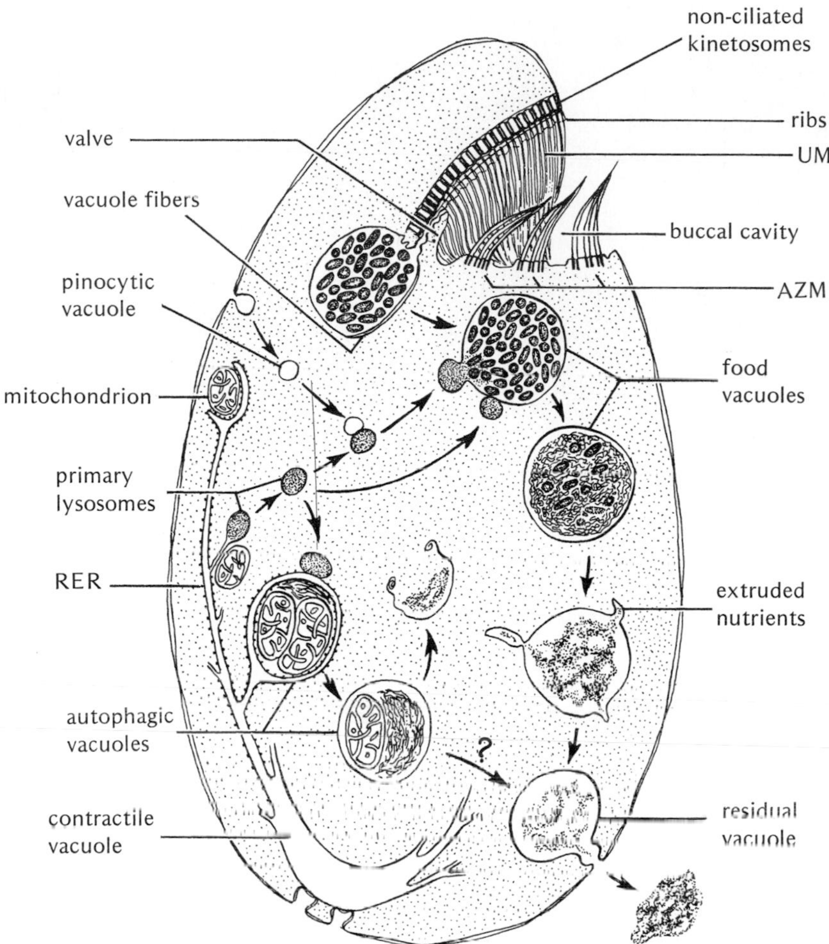

FIGURE 9.2 Ingestion and digestion of food in *Tetrahymena.* Abbreviations: UM—undulating membrane; AZM—adoral zone of membranelles; RER—rough endoplasmic reticulum. [From Elliot and Clemmons, 1966.]

humans. In primates other than humans, infections are common.

B. coli causes diarrhea and dysentery in both swine and humans, but the extent and importance of the disease are not well documented.

Morphology

The organisms are uniformly ciliated over the body and have about 60 kinetids; the mouth is at the anterior end and is of relatively simple structure (Fig. 7.1Y). There is a rather extreme size range extending from 30 to 150 μm but averaging 45 x 60 μm with an ovoid shape. There is a large macronucleus and a small micronucleus closely applied to the concave side of the former. *B. coli* has two contractile vacuoles, one anterior and one posterior. The cytopyge is near the posterior tip. Cysts are subspherical and 40 to 60 μm in size (Fig 7.1Z).

Life Cycle

B. coli is transferred from one host to the next usually in the cyst form, but the trophozoites are sufficiently resistant to pass through the stomach and reach the small intestine. The organism reproduces by binary fission in the large intestine of the host. Conjugation has been studied in culture.

Diagnosis

Since the parasite inhabits the large intestine and causes diarrhea, the trophozoites can be found by a direct microscopic examination of the feces using a wet mount preparation. Clinical signs and symptoms of balantidial dysentery in humans are much like those of amebic dysentery, and it is necessary to differentiate between the two infections.

Stained fecal smears can be made for examination

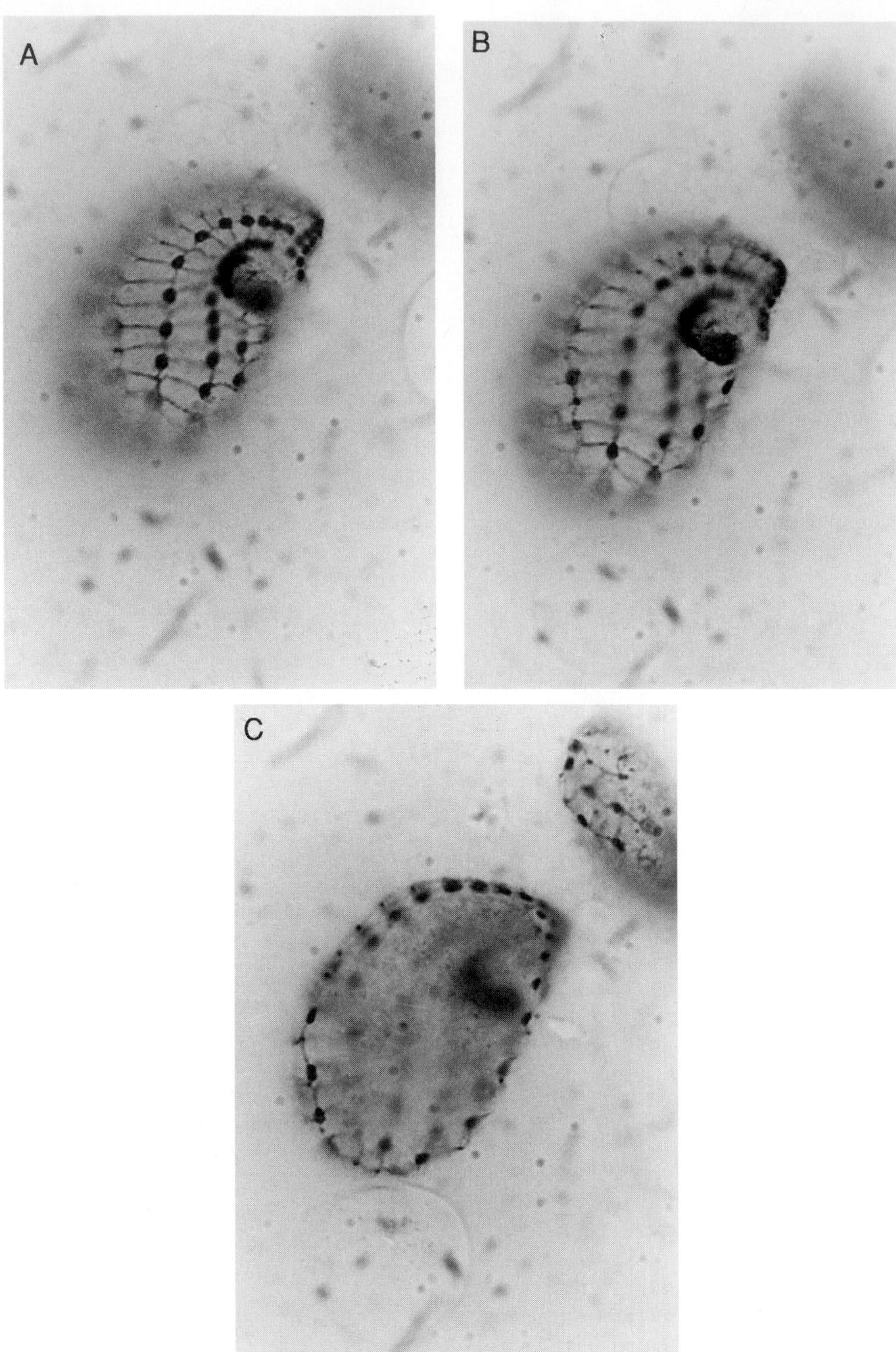

FIGURE 9.3 Infraciliature or silverline system of *Colpoda steinii* as seen under the LM The organism is suspended in gelatin, and the three views show basal bodies and kinetodesmata as seen when focusing down through the specimen.

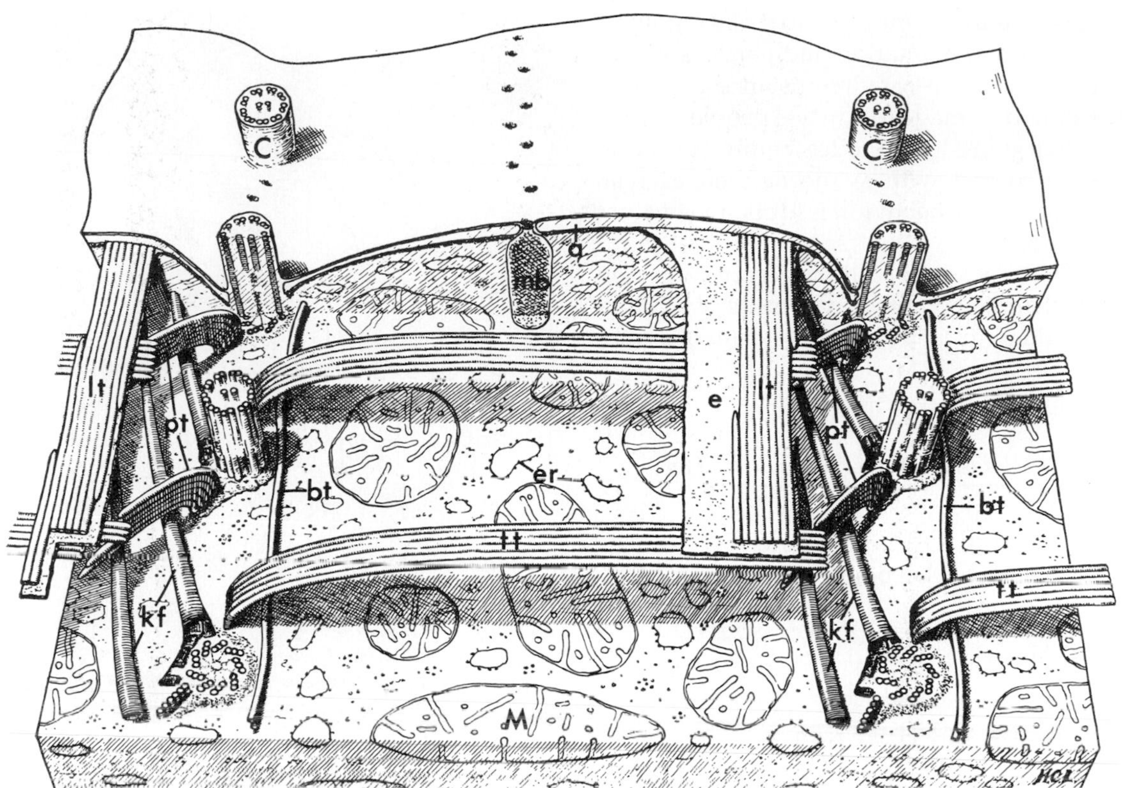

FIGURE 9.4 The somatic cortex of *Tetrahymena piriformis* as reconstructed from TEM studies. Abbreviations: C—cilium; mb—mucigenic body; pt—postciliary set; bt—basal microtubules; kf— kinetodesmal fiber; M—mitochondrion; er—endoplasmic reticulum; e—amorphous endoplasmic reticulum; a—alveoli. [From Allen, R. D., 1967.]

at a convenient time, and tissue sections of affected areas of the large intestine can also be made for study and identification of the organism.

Host–Parasite Interactions

The normal hosts of *B. coli* are suids, especially domestic swine. In swine, there is usually only slight damage at the sites of the organisms, but there are a few instances on record in which pigs have been seriously affected by the parasite.

In humans, the organism is invasive and damages the large intestine leading to diarrhea, dysentery, and ulceration of the tissue. There are a few case reports of finding *B. coli* in extraintestinal sites. Higher primates other than humans seem to have their own *B. coli* and probably do not become infected from suids. There is little information on the development of immunity in humans.

Epidemiology and Control

Control of *Balantidium coli* infection in humans should entail the following:

1. Establishment of a barrier of some sort between swine and humans
2. Careful hygienic practices by all individuals in a household
3. Treatment of human infections

There seems to be an relationship between human infection with *B. coli* and an association with swine. A high prevalence of infection in the human population generally correlates with close association with swine. Swine do not usually show signs of infection, but they may have enormous numbers of *B. coli* trophozoites in their intestines. It appears that swine shed large numbers of cysts, which are accidentally ingested by people with contaminated food or water. Person-to-person transmission is probably not important in maintaining and propagating the infection.

Reducing the incidence of infection in humans is difficult. Where balantidial dysentery is prevalent, the economic level is likely to be low, as is also the educational level. Swine are often an important protein source in the diet and raising them is nearly cost free since they scavenge on anything edible. Feces from domestic swine should somehow be kept away from areas where humans live. It might be that fencing swine out of areas of human habitation and gardens would break the contact under most circumstances.

Attempts should be made to educate people to wash their hands after going to the toilet, before preparing food, and after contact with swine or their excreta. Making this change in behavior is difficult, but not impossible, to do.

Although there seems to be little person-to-person transmission, treatment of infected persons, symptomatic or not, should upgrade the overall health of a community.

ICHTHYOPHTHIRIUS MULTIFILIIS

Name of Organism and Disease Associations

Ichthyophthirius multifiliis causes ichthyophthiriosis, ichthyophthiriasis, white spot, or ick.

Hosts and Host Range

I. multifiliis parasitizes a wide range of freshwater fish including carp, catfish, trout, and many tropical fish raised in tanks by hobbyists.

Geographic Distribution and Importance

Cosmopolitan. This organism is most important in small ponds or tanks where the water is warm. Losses to ick can be catastrophic for an individual fish fancier or raiser.

Morphology

The trophont or "adult" form on the fish varies from 100 μm to as large as 1 mm in length; the shape is ovoid, with the cystostome at the anterior tip (Fig. 9.5). Tomites or "swarmers" are 30 to 50 μm long and average 2 μm. Theronts, also known as "swarmers" are 10 × 40 μm. Tomites are surrounded by a gelatinous wall. There is a single large macronucleus and a micronucleus; the organism has numerous contractile vacuoles.

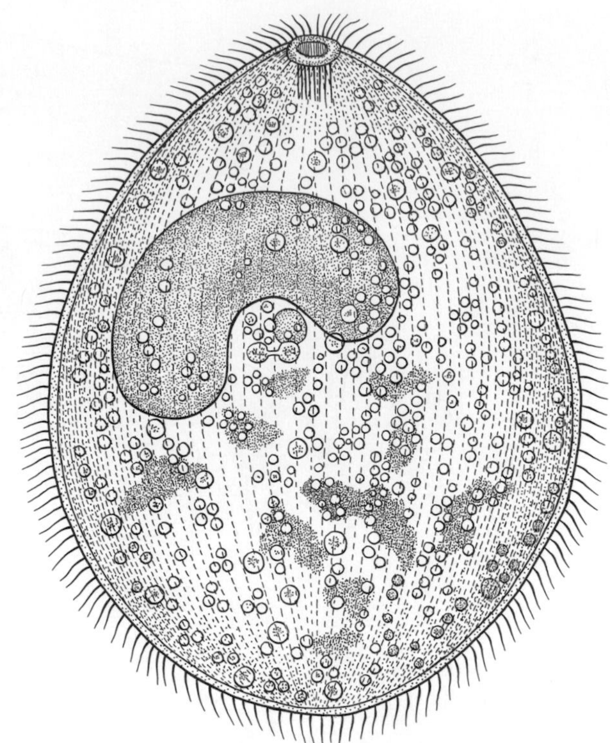

FIGURE 9.5 Trophont of *Ichthyophthirius mulltifiliis.*

Life Cycle

The theront is the infective form that transfers from the free-living phase of the cycle to the fish (Fig. 9.6). The theronts may live as long as 96 hours, but their infectivity decreases after 48 hours. Once having reached a fish, the theront enters its tissue by using a penetrating organelle at the anterior end; there is no mouth at this stage of the life cycle. Once inside the tissues of the fish, the organism is called a trophont; it grows without undergoing any division to produce an enormous uninucleated organism. During growth, the ciliate continually rotates in the cavity of the tissue. When full grown (i.e, at about three days and approaching 1 mm in length), the trophont drops off the host, forms a gelatinous envelope around itself and attaches to the substrate.

Nuclear and cytoplasmic division take place rapidly by a process referred to a palintomy. Within about eight hours, as many as 1000 theronts are formed these escape from the capsule to search for a fish.

Diagnosis

The trophonts are found on fish. The usual clinical signs of infection are pustules on the body of the fish.

Host–Parasite Interactions

I. multifiliis can be highly pathogenic and may even kill fish. If the parasites are on the body of the fish, the epidermal cells are destroyed and replaced by mucus-producing cells. If they are on the gills, they may be

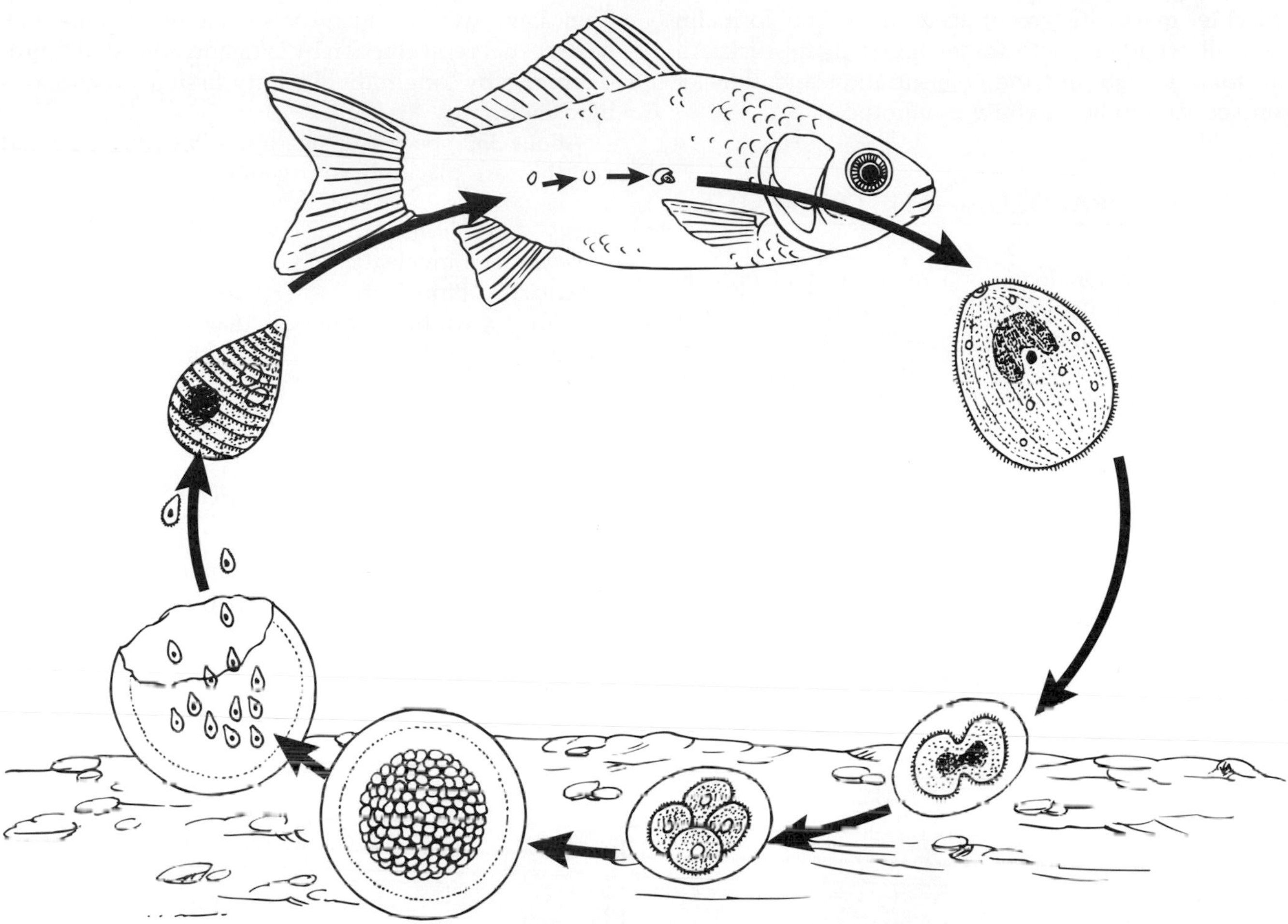

FIGURE 9.6 The life cycle of *Ichthyophthirius multifiliis*. The cycle begins with the small theront seeking a host. It attaches and penetrates a cell to become a trophont. The trophont increases in size without either nuclear or cytoplasmic division. It drops off, secretes a gelatinous covering, and attaches to the substrate where it undergoes many divisions (palintomy) to form theronts.

present in such large numbers that they interfere with gaseous exchange and may kill the host. On the eye, they cause corneal ulceration and blindness.

Epidemiology and Control

Control of ick is implemented by the following:

1. Keeping fish in running water
2. Quarantining fish before introducing them into an aquarium
3. Cleaning the tank or pond after an outbreak
4. Chemotherapy
5. Vaccination

I. multifiliis thrives when fish are concentrated. Ick usually is seen in farm ponds and fish tanks. Since one trophont can give rise to as many as a thousand theronts in eight hours, the infection can increase dramatically within a few days. Temperature is also a factor. A temperature of 25 to 27°C, a typical summertime temperature for carp ponds, is optimal for development.

For the fish fancier, prevention is the best means of control. Fish should be quarantined and monitored carefully before being placed in the same aquarium with clean fish. If a tank, pond, or raceway has been found to be contaminated, it should be drained, cleaned, and allowed to dry as completely as possible. The organisms are not resistant to drying and will be eliminated.

A vaccine has been developed that is placed in the water with the fish, and it is effective in preventing infection.

A variety of substances such as hypertonic sodium

chloride, malachite green, acetic acid, and formalin have all been used with some success against ick. All are toxic to fish and the concentration and time of contact need to be carefully monitored.

PHYLUM OPALOZOA—THE OPALINIDS

The phylum Opalozoa is a mixed bag of protists that more than likely will be separated or relocated into other taxa with time. The class Opalinatea contains those organisms that are usually called opalinids. These symbiotic protists are found in the intestinal tracts of amphibia and, occasionally, fish. None is known to be pathogenic, but they are ubiquitous in amphibia and are of zoological interest. Curiously enough, many species of opalinids are parasitized by *Entamoeba paulista*, whose trophozoites are 8 to 14 μm and the cysts are 8 to 12 μm.

Opalinids are covered with cilia, or short flagella, but they are not classified as ciliophorans. Except for their cilia, they have little in common with the ciliates. They have two too many vesicular nuclei and they have sexual reproduction by syngamy. Asexual reproduction is by longitudinal binary fission. Nutrition is by osmotrophy.

About 350 species of opalinids have been named and they are placed in four genera:

Genus	*Nuclei*	*Cross-Section*
Protoopalina	Binucleate	Circular
Zelleriella	Binucleate	Flattened
Cepedea	Multinucleate	Circular
Opalina	Multinucleate	Flattened

OPALINA RANARUM

Name of Organisms and Disease Associations

Opalina ranarum and *O. obtigonoidea.* Nonpathogenic.

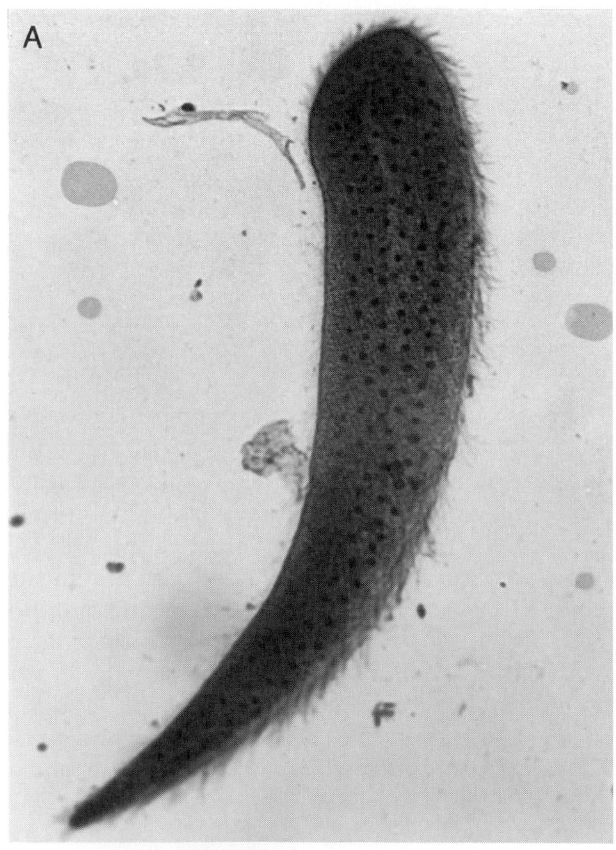

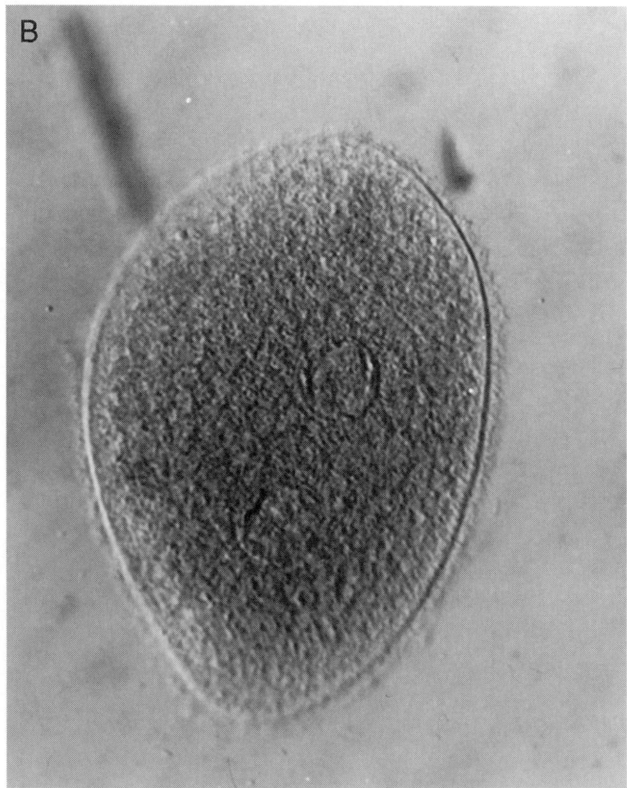

FIGURE 9.7 Trophozoites of *Opalina ranarum* (A) and *Zellerirella ellipticum* (B), both of anuran amphibians as seen in LM. *Opalina* is multinucleate—see the many small dark dots in the cytoplasm; *Zelleriella* is binucleate—note the spherical bodies in the center and somewhat posterior portion of the body.

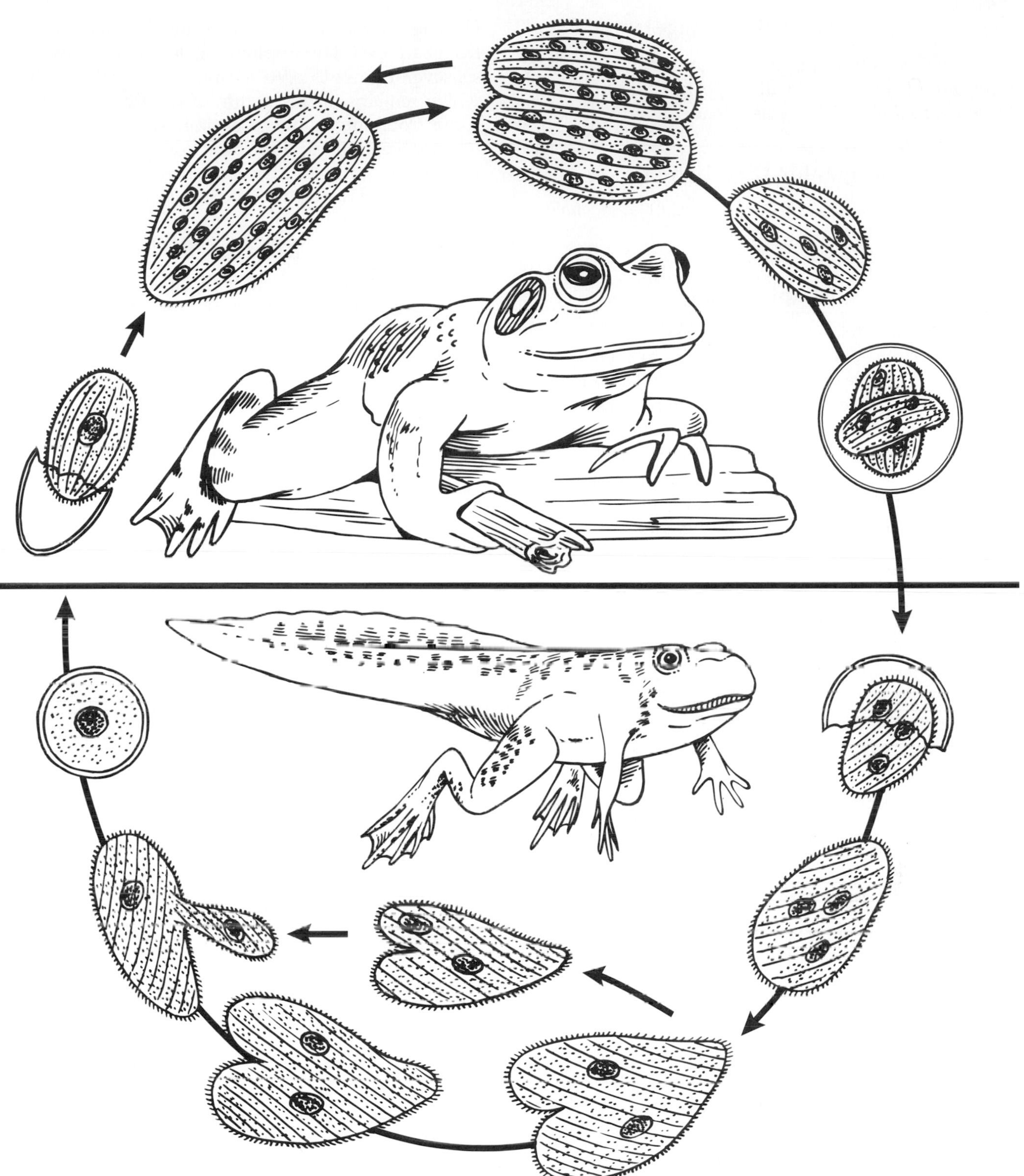

FIGURE 9.8 The life cycle of *Opalina*. Sexual reproduction occurs in tadpoles, and asexual reproduction occurs in frogs.

Hosts and Host Range

O. ranarum is found in the rectum of the frogs *Rana temporaria, Bufo bufo,* and in turtles and salamanders. *O. obtrigonoidea* is in frogs and toads.

Geographic Distribution

O. ranarum is found in Europe and *O. obtrigonoidea* is found in North America.

Morphology

O. ranarum trophonts are 190 to 385 by 160 to 200 μm. *O. obtrigonoidea* trophonts are 400 to 1300 by 170 to 270 μm. They are uniformly covered with cilia except at the blunt anterior end, which is more densely ciliated. This area along the anterior margin is called the falx, and the ciliary beat originates there. There is no cytostome. Kineties are present, and unusual folds in the pellicle separate them. Numerous nuclei are scattered throughout the cytoplasm (Fig. 9.7).

Life Cycle

Opalinid life cycles are synchronized with the life stage of their hosts. Host hormones apparently induce opalinid cyst aproduction, although temperature can also. Trophonts, in response to physiological changes in the host, divide repeatedly, producing many small infection cysts (Fig. 9.8). After ingestion by tadpoles, gamonts emerge from the cysts and divide by meiosis, producing macro- and microgametes. The gametes fuse to produce a zygocyst, which is passed in the tadpole feces. If zygocysts are ingested by young tadpoles, the sequence is repeated, and new zygocysts are produced. On the other hand, if metamorphosing tadpoles ingest zygocysts, a young trophont emerges from each cyst. The trophont nucleus divides by mitosis several times to produce a multinucleate trophont, which remains in the rectum of the frog. Apparently some trophonts undergo a similar sequence during the nonbreeding season, producing what are called dissemination cysts. These are identical morphologically and behaviorly to infection cysts.

READINGS

Allen, K. O., and Avaluit, Jr., J. W. (1970). Effects of brackish water on ichthyophthiriasis of channel catfish. *Prog. Fish Cult.* **32,** 227–230.

Allen, R. D. (1967). Fine structure, reconstruction and possible functions of the cortex of *Tetrahymena pyriformis. J. Protozool.* **32,** 227–230.

Ball, G. H. (1969). Organisms living on and in Protozoa. In *Research in Protozoology, Vol. 3* (T.-T. Chen, Ed.), pp. 565–718. Pergamon, New York.

Corliss, J. O. (1979). *The Ciliated Protozoa,* 2nd ed. Pergamon, New York.

Earl, P. R. (1979). Notes on the taxonomy of opalinids (Protozoa) including remarks on continental drift. *Trans. Am. Microsc. Soc.* **98,** 549–557.

Elliot and Clemmons (1966). An ultrastructural study of ingestion and digestion in *Tetrahymena pyriformis. J. Protozool.* **13,** 311–323.

Goven, G. A., Dawe, K. L., and Gratzek, J. B. (1980). Protection of channel catfish, *Ictalurus punctatus* Rafinesque, against *Ichthyophthirius multifiliis* Fouquet by immunization. *J. Fish. Biol.* **17,** 311–316.

Hausmann, K., and Bradbury, P. (Eds.) (1996). *Ciliates: Cells as Organisms.* Fischer-Verlag, Stuttgart.

Lynn, D. H., and Small, E. B. (1985). Subphylum Opalinata. In *An Illustrated Guide to the Protozoa* (J. J. Lee, S. H. Hutner, and E. C. Bovee, Eds.), pp. 156–157. Society of Protozoologists, Lawrence, KS.

Small, E. B., and Lynn, D. H. (1985). Phylum Ciliophora Doflein, 1901. In *An Illustrated Guide to the Protozoa* (J. J. Lee, S. H. Hutner, and E. C. Bovee, Eds.), pp. 393–575. Society of Protozoologists, Lawrence, KS.

Wessenberg, H. S. (1978). Opalinata. In *Parasitic Protozoa* (J. Kreier, Ed.), Vol. 2, pp. 551–581. Academic Press, New York.

CHAPTER

10

Introduction to the Apicomplexa

Those protists that make up the Apicomplexa are a diverse group all of which are parasitic. They have in common the elements of the apical complex (Fig. 10.1) and sexual reproduction characterized by syngamy. Many of the organisms in this group are of great medical and economic importance. Four species cause malaria in humans, while members of the genus *Eimeria* bring about millions of dollars in annual losses as the cause of intestinal coccidiosis in domestic animals. Piroplasmosis is a complex of diseases that probably cause a greater loss in domestic animals on a global basis than any other group of organisms.

Apicomplexans have undoubtedly been associated with their hosts through a long period of evolution, hundreds of millions of years, and have exquisite interactions with their hosts. Any one species may parasitize only a few closely related species of host indicating long co-evolution. Every bird and mammal that has been looked at has at least five species of apicomplexans parasitizing it, and many have ten or more species. The ubiquity of the group is arresting, and thousands of species remain to be described even in common animals.

As the name implies, the apical complex is located in one end of a zoites called the *anterior end* since the zoite moves with that end forward, and they usually enter cells by using elements of the apical complex. The complex consists of one or two polar rings at the anterior tip with associated subpellicular tubules that run most of the length of the zoite (Figs. 10.1–10.3), a conoid, rhoptries, and micronemes. Elements of the apical complex are instrumental in the penetration of host cells.

The organism illustrated in Figure 10.1 is a zoite of the genus *Eimeria*, and all of the elements are present in this genus. In some groups such as the gregarines (Chapter 11), some of the components are seen early in development but are then modified into holdfast organelles. In members of the Haemosporina, some of which cause malaria in humans (Chapter 14), the conoid is lacking, and in the piroplasms (Chapter 15), the elements are quite reduced. Likewise the Cryptosporina have elements of the apical complex, but the conoid is quite different from that seen, say, in *Toxoplasma gondii* (Fig. 10.2).

Life cycles of the apicomplexans include both asexual and sexual development. We can look on the basic life cycle as having three components (Fig. 10.4).

The stages of the diagram represent both sexual and asexual reproduction. Gamonts develop into either macro- (female) or microgamonts (male) in a number of groups. In some, such as the gregarines, isogamonts are seen (Chapter 11). When syngamy (fertilization) takes place, a new individual, the sporont, results.

The sporont, meront, and gamont multiply by an asexual process called *schizogony*. In schizogony nuclear replication occurs, and when the full complement of nuclei has been formed, daughter cells are formed all at one time. The process is the same in sporogony, merogony, and gamogony; only the product of this reproduction is different. When the sporont undergoes sporogony, the product is a large number of sporozoites. The sporozoite is the infective stage of the life cycle; it is always this stage that enters a new host, usually a vertebrate. In the meront, the product of merogony is the merozoite; the merozoite may either go through one or more additional generations of merogony or it may differentiate into a gamont. The cycle

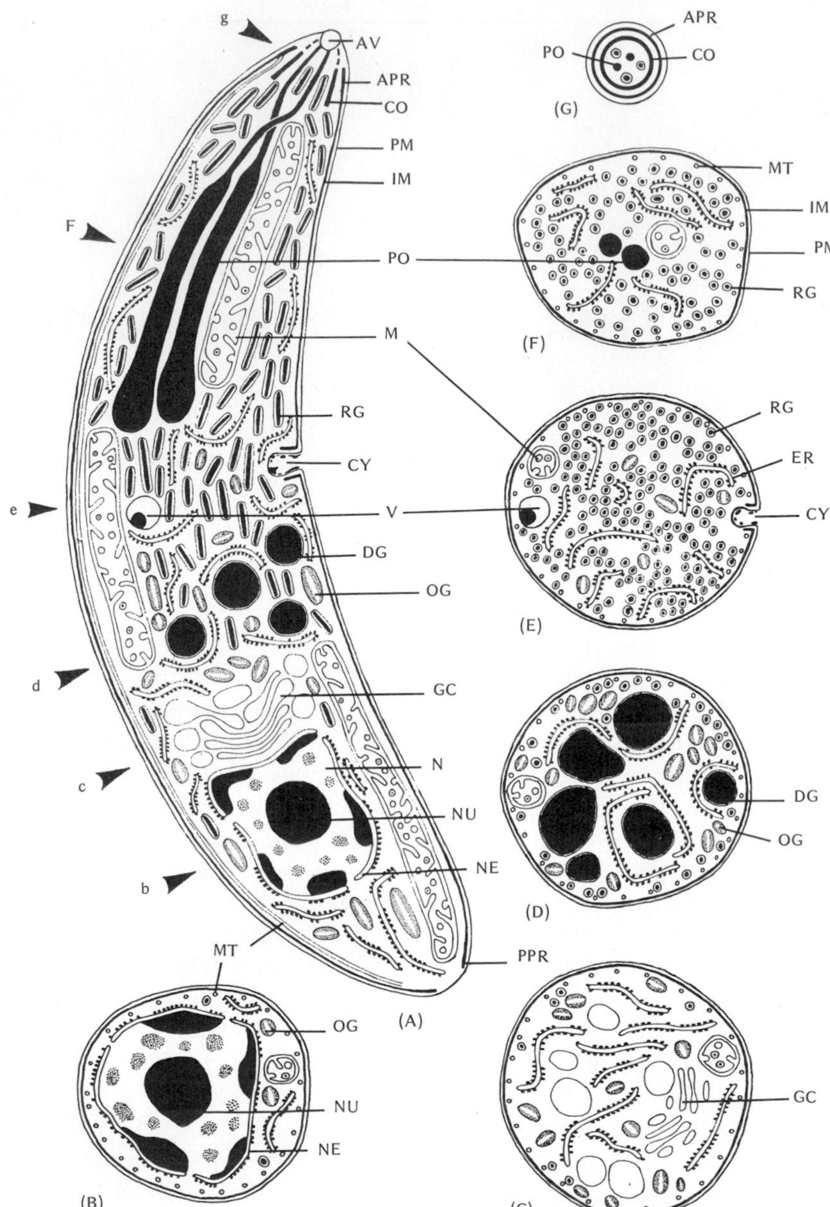

FIGURE 10.1 A zoite of an apicomplexan zoite showing structures revealed by electron microscopy. Abbreviations: APR—anterior polar ring; AV—anterior vacuole; PM—outer pellicular membrane; IM—inner pellicular membrane; PO—rhoptries; M - mitochondrion; RG—micronemes; CY—cytostome; V—unidentified body; DG—dark granule; GC—Golgi; N—nucleus; NU—nucleolus; NE—nuclear envelope; PPR—posterior polar ring; MT—microtubules; ER—endoplasmic reticulum. [From Andreassen and Behnke, 1968.]

always runs in the direction indicated in the diagram; sporogony, for example, never follows merogony.

As an example of a common life cycle of an intestinal coccidium, *Eimeria tenella* of the chicken shows a number of features common to most apicomplexans (Fig. 12.3). Development begins within intestinal cells of the cecum when an oocyst is ingested. The eight sporozoites are released in the intestine and invade enterocytes where they round up and begin to undergo nuclear replication. When there are 200 to 300 nuclei, merozoites are formed and released from the host cell.

The merozoites invade fresh enterocytes and again undergo a second round of nuclear replication. The second generation merozoites are released and they

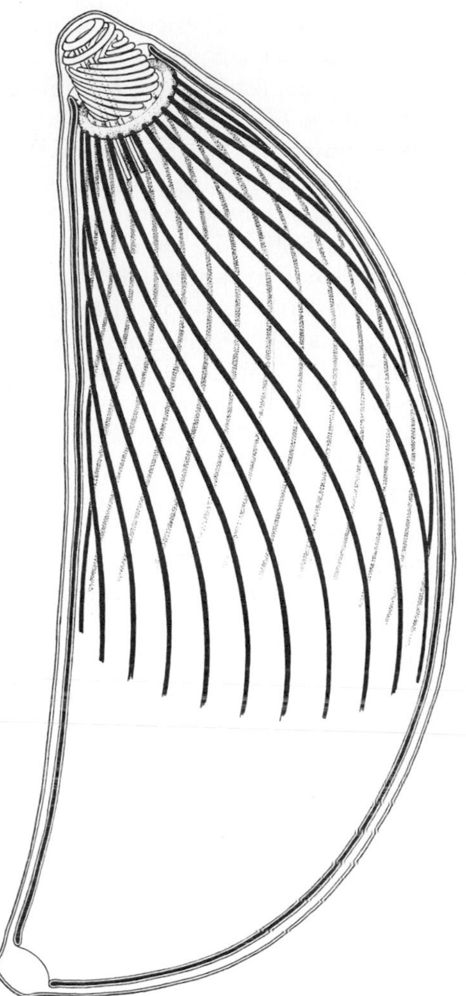

FIGURE 10.2 Cytoskeleton of *Toxoplasma gondii* showing the conoid at the apical end and the subpellicular tubules, which extend through most of the length of the zoite. [From Nichols, B. A., and Chiappino, M. L.,, 1987.]

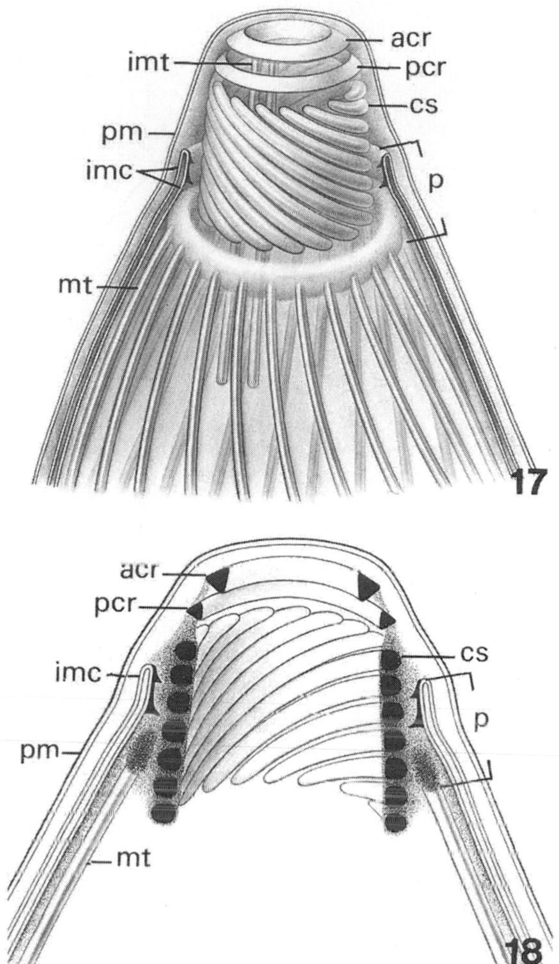

FIGURE 10.3 Detail of the conoid area of a zoite (*Toxoplasma gondii*). (A) Surface view; (B) Saggital section. Abbreviations: acr—anterior conoidal ring; cs—conoid subunit; imc—inner membrane complex; mt—microtubule; p—polar ring complex; pcr—posterior preconoidal ring; pm—plasma membrane) [From Nichols, B. A., and Chiappino, M. L., 1987.]

again enter enterocytes. After forming about ten nuclei, third-generation merozoites are formed and released from their host cells. At this point, the merozoites differentiate into micro- and macrogamonts. The microgamonts undergo nuclear replication and when nuclear replication is complete, microgametes are formed. The microgametes are released from their host cells and seek a macrogamont to fertilize. The zygote then develops into an oocyst by the formation of resistant walls around the living portion of the organism, the sporoplasm.

When the formation of the oocyst is complete, it is shed into the lumen of the intestine and passed out with the feces. In this kind of life cycle, sporogony, or sporulation, occurs outside of the host. Nuclear division takes place three times and eight sporozoites are formed. The oocyst is now infective and can establish an infection in another chicken if it is ingested.

Some life cycle variation are seen in organisms such as *Toxoplasma gondii* (Chapter 13), in which a number of mammalian species can support the development of the merogonous phase of the life cycle. In *Sarcocystis* two obligate hosts are involved: an herbivore in which merogony takes place and a carnivore in which gamogony and sporogony occur. Roughly the same pattern is seen in *Plasmodium* spp.(Chapter 14), which cause malaria; merogony and part of gamogony take place in the human host, and completion of gamogony and sporogony take place in the mosquito host.

Those life cycles in which the organism requires only a single host to complete the life cycle are said to

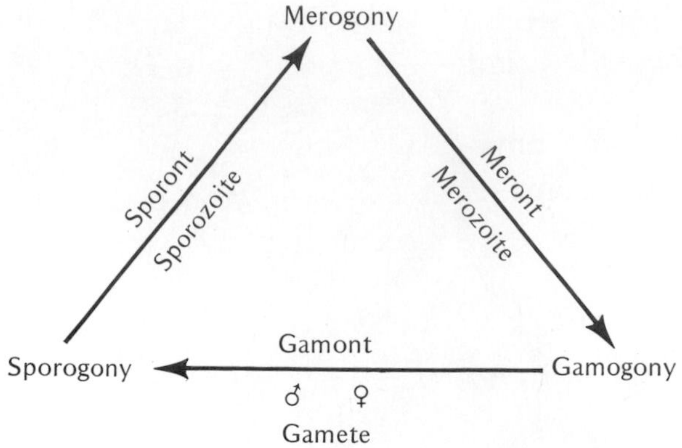

FIGURE 10.4 Processes and stages in the life cycle of members of the Apicomplexa. Schizogony occurs in all stages of the life cycle, but is referred to as sporogony, merogony, and gamogony at the particular stage. Note that the direction of the arrows indicates the direction of the cycle, which never runs backward.

have *direct life cycles,* or to be *homoxenous.* Members of the genus *Eimeria,* the cause of coccidiosis in domestic animals, are examples. Those organisms that require more than one host to complete the life cycle are said to have *indirect life cycles*, or to be *heteroxenous.* Members of the genus *Plasmodium,* the cause of malaria, are examples.

A consistent feature of development in apicomplexans is that they undergo schizogony within cells. Not all of them have all of their stages intracellularly, but merogony and gamogony nearly always are. The intracellular environment provides two important elements: (1) isolation from the immune reaction of the host and (2) proximity to the metabolic machinery of the host cell, which they probably parasitize.

Entry into host cells has been studied in a number of medically and economically important apicomplexans such as *Plasmodium, Toxoplasma,* and certain of the intestinal *Eimeria.* When the apical complex was first described, it was assumed that its elements were involved in penetration of potential host cells. At that point there was no experimental evidence to support the supposition; however, as time passed, some elegant experiments were performed. It is now clear in the organisms that cause malaria that the rhoptries empty when a red blood cell is invaded, but the role of the other elements of the apical complex is not clear. The conoid is seen to be protruded when cells are touched, but what exactly it does in penetration has not been described. In some organisms, such as *Plasmodium vivax,* the cause of benign tertian malaria, certain receptors must be present on the red blood cell for successful penetration; this relates to the so-called Duffy blood group, which is discussed in greater detail in Chapter 14. In other apicomplexans, penetration of cells is nonspecific (i.e., they are seen to penetrate almost any cell).

Once inside a suitable cell, an apicomplexan begins development. In the case of the eugregarines, the gamont develops outside of the host cell while the epimerite holds it in place by being embedded in the cell (Chapter 11). From a variety of studies it is clear that apicomplexans parasitize the metabolic machinery of the host cell. In some instances ATP has been found to be essential for multiplication of the organism. In other instances it is likely that genome is parasitized. It is important to note that the partners in these associations have evolved over millions of years and that each affects the other in ways that we are only beginning to describe. The data are fragmentary, but certain pathways in cells are up-regulated, and undoubtedly down-regulated in other instances.

In a few instances, apicomplexans develop extracellularly when one would have predicted that they would be within cells. An example is the oocyst of malaria, which develops on the surface of the midgut of the mosquito vector. The oocyst extends into the hemocoel of the mosquito and has been found by ultrastructural studies to be extracellular. If most of the organisms develop within cells, why should a few develop outside?

Nutrients are obtained either by osmotrophy or by endocytosis (sometimes called phagotrophy). In osmotrophy, substances are picked up across the plasma membrane. The process is undoubtedly selective and requires energy. Endocytosis is by a specific structure, the *cytostome* (Fig. 10.5); the cytostome is often called a *micropyle,* or *micropore*, but cytostome is more descriptive and is the preferred term. Endocytosis in *Toxoplasma gondii* takes two forms: (1) a receptor-mediated and (2) a fluid-phase endocytosis. In this species there appears to be ingestion of specific components and also there is recycling of degenerated organelles of other zoites in the parasitophorous vacuole. Because endocytosis is receptor-mediated, it has been suggested that the cytostome could be the target of chemotherapeutic agents and thereby interfere with the growth and development of the organisms.

Protistan phylogeny has been an extremely difficult subject to approach experimentally. With the advent of molecular techniques allowing the sequencing of DNA and RNA, new studies were possible. Some current studies show that the apicomplexans probably arose from dinoflagellates in a marine environment. The dinoflagellates are a distinct group of flagellates that have nuclear division and plasmotomy similar to the schizogony seen in apicomplexans. Other characters support the association, as well. Within the group, various studies support or contravene the present clas-

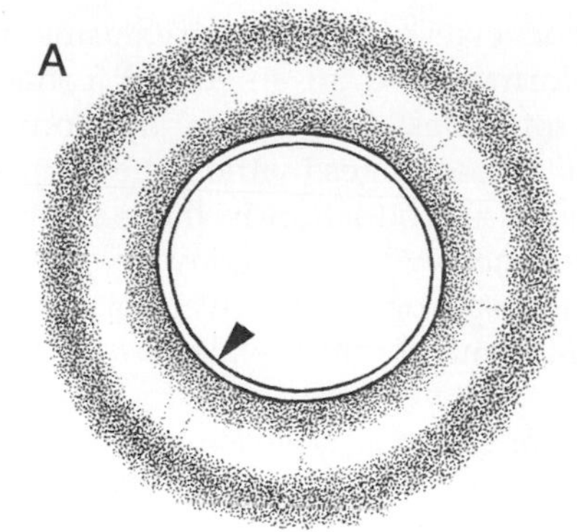

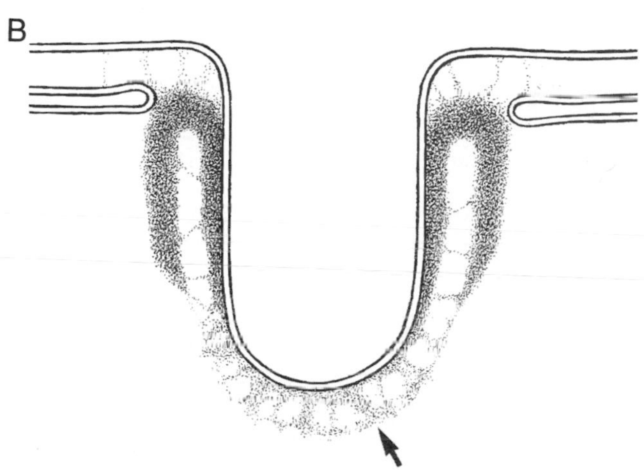

FIGURE 10.5 The structure of the cytostome of an apicomplexan, *Toxoplasma gondii.* The cytostome is often called a micropore or micropyle, but since it serves to ingest food, those terms are incorrect. (A) A sagittal section through the cytostome at a level just below the pellicle of the zoite. The plasmalemma continues as the inner surface of the cytostome (arrowhead). (B) A transverse section of the cytostome. The arrow indicates a clathrin-like layer at the margin of the cytostome. Receptors in the cavity of the cytostome probably serve to attract certain substances which are then internalized.

sification. For example, studies of the DNA sequences of the small RNA subunit place organisms together that have traditionally been considered to be separated some distance phylogenetically. Molecular and computer-based methods of determining phylogeny have brought an exciting era to studies of protists. The state of uncertainty will continue for some time, but eventually we will have a more rational way of dealing with these complex organisms. Until then, we will make do with adjusting the traditional classifications in ways that allow us to deal with them.

The classification of members of the phylum Apicomplexa at its higher taxonomic levels has been unsatisfactory and in a state of flux for some time. One proposal (Levine, 1988) was based on the presence or absence of a conoid and the form of the conoid. Three classes were established based on this character, but it was found that a number of the species purportedly lacking a conoid do, in fact, have a rudimentary one. Studies based on the 18s small subunit ribosomal RNA gene together with more traditional data on life cycles and ultrastructure generally confirm the classification presented next.

PHYLUM APICOMPLEXA

One or more elements of the apical complex present at some stage of the life cycle: polar ring, rhoptry, microneme, conoid; sexuality by syngamy; multiplication by schizogony, or endodyogeny; 9 + 2 flagella present in some gametes; locomotion by body flexion or gliding; subpellicular tubules present in most species; feeding by osmotrophy or phagotrophy; all species parasitic.

Class Perkinsea

Order Perkinsida

One family, one genus, *Perkinsus.* Conoid forms an incomplete truncated cone; sexuality absent; with flagellated zoospores that have an anterior vacuole; homoxenous. *Perkinsus marinus.*

Class Gregarinea

Conoid present in sporozoite for a period of time, converted to mucron upon entry into host cell; merogony absent except in one group; gamonts large, extracellular, usually found in syzygy; gametes usually similar (isogamous); parasites of the digestive tract or body cavity of invertebrates and some lower chordates; homoxenous. Three orders: Archigregarinida, Eugregarinida, Neogregarinida, *Gregarina, Monocystis, Selenidium, Mattesia.*

Class Coccidea

All elements of the apical complex present ; sporogony, merogony, and gamogony present in all except two obscure orders.

Order Adeleida

Macro- and microgamont usually associated in syzygy during development; one to four microgametes; sporozoites enclosed in an envelope, homoxenous or heteroxenous. *Adelea, Haemogregarina, Klossiella, Hepatozoon.*

Order Eimeriida

Macro- and microgamonts develop separately; large number of microgametes formed; zygote nonmotile; no syzygy; sporozoites typically enclosed in a sporocyst, which, in turn, is enclosed in an oocyst; large number of microgametes; homoxenous or heteroxenous. *Eimeria, Isospora, Tyzzeria, Sarcocystis, Toxoplasma, Frenkelia, Cyclospora.*

Order Cryptosporiida

Macro- and microgamonts develop separately; 16 or fewer merozoites and microgametes; sporozoites enclosed in a membrane, which is either single or double; rhoptry-like bodies in zoite, small conoid in some stages; no micronemes or polar ring; sporogony within the vertebrate host; retrofection an important part of the life cycle; endogenous forms usually about 5 μm and lying under the plasma membrane of enterocytes but extracytoplasmically; parasites of birds, reptiles, and mammals; homoxenous. *Cryptosporidium.*

Class Haemosporea

Zoites have rhoptries, micronemes, and polar ring but lack a conoid; macro- and microgamonts develop separately, microgamont produces eight flagellated microgametes; zygote motile (ookinete); sporozoite naked; heteroxenous with merogony in vertebrates and sporogony in invertebrates; transmission by blood-sucking insects. *Plasmodium, Leucocytozoon, Haemoproteus.*

Class Piroplasmea

Zoites have rhoptries, micronemes, and polar ring, and some species have a conoid; parasites of erythrocytes and leucocytes where the organisms are small rodlike, piriform, round, or amoeboid forms; usually lacking microtubules; locomotion by body flexion, gliding, or in sexual stages by the large axopodium or Strahlen; sexual reproduction in those studied intensively; heteroxenous with merogony in vertebrates and gamogony and sporogony in invertebrates; sporozoites with single-membraned wall; ticks are the only known vectors, but vectors of dactylosomatids are unknown. *Babesia, Theileria, Dactylosoma.*

READINGS

Andreassen, J. and Behnke, O. (1968). Fine structure of merozoites of a rat coccidium *Eimeria* miyairii, with a comparison of the fine structure of other Sporozoa. *J. Parasitol.* **54,** 150–163.

Barta, J. (1989). Phylogenetic analysis of the class Sporozoa (Phylum Apicomplexa Levine, 1970): Evidence for the independent evolution of heteroxenous life cycles. *J. Parasitol.* **75,** 195–206.

Carreno, R. A., Schnitzler, B. E., Jeffries, A. C., Tenter, A. M., Johnson, A. M., and Barta, J. R. (1998). Phylogenetic analysis of coccidia based on 18s rRNA sequence comparison indicates that *Isospora* is most closely related to *Toxoplasma* and *Neospora. J. Euk. Microbiol.* **45,** 184–188.

Levine, N. D. (1971). Uniform terminology for the protozoan subphylum Apicomplexa. *J. Protozool.* **18,** 352–355.

Levine, N. D. (1985). Apicomplexa. In *An Illustrated Guide to the Protozoa* (J. J. Lee, S. H. Hutner, and E. C. Bovee, Eds.). Society of Protozoologists, Lawrence, KS.

Levine, N. D. (1988). *The Protozoan Phylum Apicomplexa,* 2 Vols. CRC Press, Boca Raton, FL.

Long, P. L. (Ed.) (1981). *The Biology of the Coccidia.* University Park Press, Baltimore.

Nichols, B. A., and Chiappino, M. L. (1987). Cytoskeleton of *Toxoplasma gondii. J. Protozool.* **34,** 217–226.

Nichols, B. A., and Chiappino, M. L. (1994). Endocytosis at the micropore of *Toxoplasma gondii. Parasitol. Res.* **80,** 90–98.

Sam-Yellowe, T. Y. (1996). Rhoptry organelles of the Apicomplexa: Their role in host cell invasion and intracellular survival. *Parasitol. Today* **12,** 308–316.

CHAPTER

11

The Gregarines

As members of the Apicomplexa, the gregarines have some elements of the apical complex, and all are parasitic. They are mostly coelozoic parasites, although some groups are intracellular, and they are found widely spread through the invertebrate phyla, especially in insects. There is a single report of a gregarine in a vertebrate; it was found in the liver of the woodcock, *Scolopax*.

TEM studies showed that some of the elements of the apical complex (conoid, rhoptries, polar ring) are transiently present in the gregarines. These structures are converted into holdfast organelles (epimerite, mucron) (Fig. 11.1), but their presence in a part of the life cycle stages confirmed their membership in the phylum and helped to make the Apicomplexa a coherent group.

Members of the class Gregarinea seem primitively to have had all three phases of the apicomplexan life cycle: merogony, sporogony, and gamogony. In most species, merogony has dropped out and is replaced by a large (500μm or larger) uninucleated organism called a trophozoite, or (later in development) a sporodin. The trophozoite actually is converted into a gamont (Fig. 11.2).

Classification within the class Gregarinea is based on life cycle patterns and the morphology of the trophozoite. The members of the order Archigregarinida have merogony, but the Eugregarinida lack merogony, and the Neogregarinida seem to have acquired merogony secondarily. The features that are important in both identification and classification of the gregarines are as follows:

1. The large trophozoite (Fig. 11.2), which may begin life intracellularly but later becomes coelozoic and attached to the cell by a holdfast (Fig. 11.1). In the suborder Aseptatina, there is no differentiation within the trophozoite, but in the suborder Septatina there is a septum near the anterior end of the organism dividing it into an anterior protomerite and a posterior deutomerite (Fig. 11.2A); the deutomerite separates and the posterior portion becomes the gamont (Fig. 11.2B).

2. Gamogony takes place with the gamonts in syzygy, a union of two individuals during gamogony (Fig. 11.3). At the end of gamogony, there may be either isogametes (Fig. 11.3) or, less frequently, nonmotile macro- and motile microgametes. In either event, there is syngamy followed by sporogony.

3. The oocyst has a resistant outer wall and naked sporozoites within it (Fig. 11.3 and 11.4). The size, shape, and color of the oocyst as well as the number of sporozoites are useful in identification. It should be pointed out that the oocysts of gregarines are frequently seen in the feces of animals such as vermivorous and insectivorous birds.

4. The host range of most gregarines is limited to a few closely related genera or species.

5. Despite their widespread occurrence and often being found in large numbers in a host, gregarines seem to have only slightly detrimental effects on their hosts. Evidence of pathogenesis occurs in only a few instances such as *Gregarina locustae* of grasshoppers.

6. Nearly all gregarines have direct life cycles, but a few have two obligate hosts. For example, members of the family Porosporidae (Eugregarinea) have crusta-

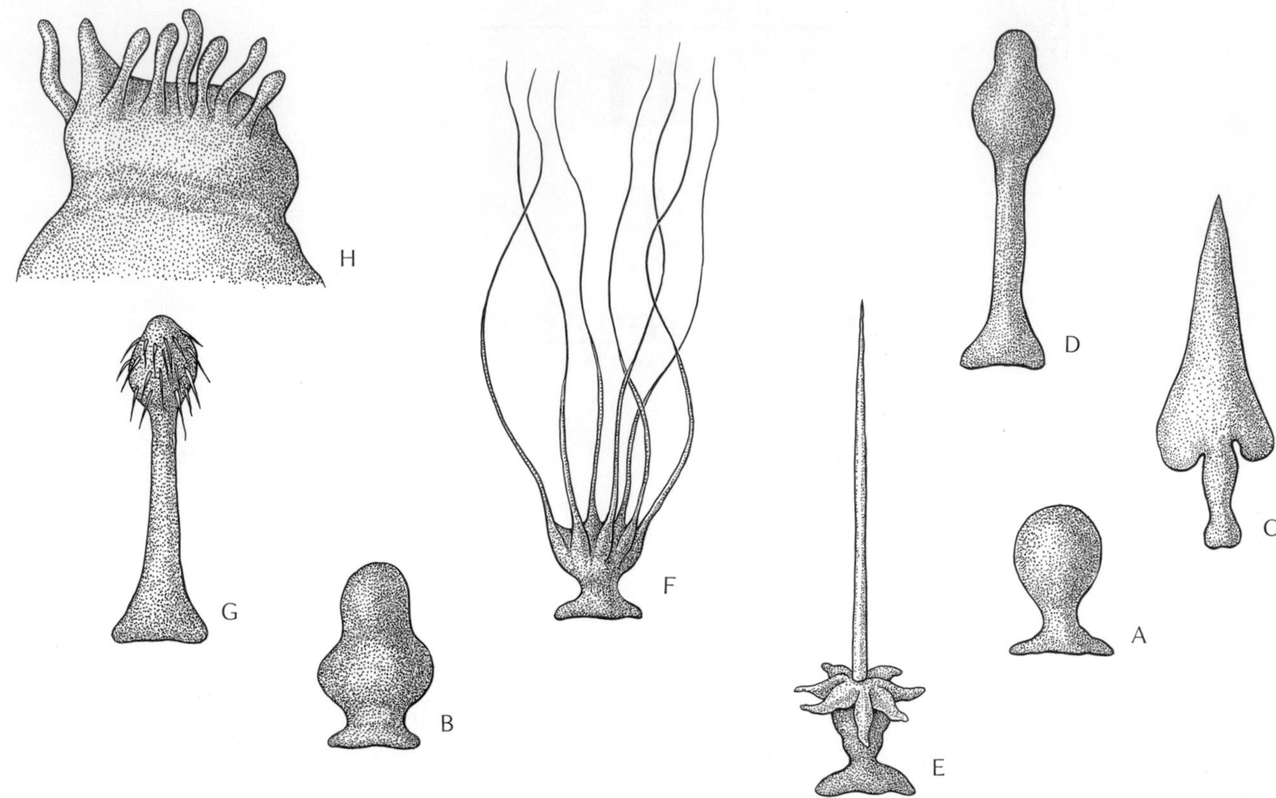

FIGURE 11.1 Structure of the epimerites of various gregarines. (A) *Gregarina longa;* (B) *Sycia inopinata;* (C) *Pileocephalus beeri;* (D) *Stylocephalus longicollis;* (E) *Beloides firmus;* (F) *Cometoides erinitus,* (G.) *Geniorhynchus monnieri;* (H) *Echinomera hispida.*

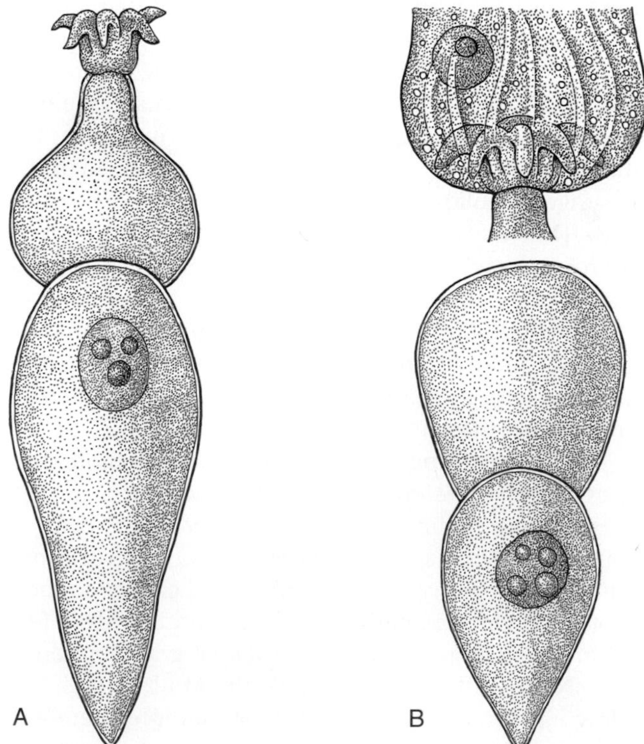

FIGURE 11.2 Trophozoite of *Corycella armata,* a septate gregarine., which parasitizes a whirligig beetle. (A) the intact trophozoite; (B) the organism separating and moving off to develop into a gamont in syzygy with another individual.

cea and mollusks as their hosts. *Nematopsis ostrearum* has gamogony in the crabs *Panopeus* and *Eurypanopeus* and sporogony in the oyster *Ostrea virginica.*

Three species of gregarines have been chosen as examples of the kind of variation that may be found in members of the class. *Lipocystis polyspora* of the scorpion fly has all three phases of the typical apicomplexan life cycle: sporogony, merogony, and gamogony. The sporozoite enters a cell and undergoes merogony, and there may be more than a single merogonous generation. The merozoites enter cells and two of them unite in syzygy and undergo gamogony. A large number of isogametes is formed and syngamy then takes place. An oocyst wall is laid down around the zygote and sporogony ensues (Fig. 11.3).

In *Monocystis lumbrici,* a common parasite of the large earthworm, *Lumbricus terrestris,* development

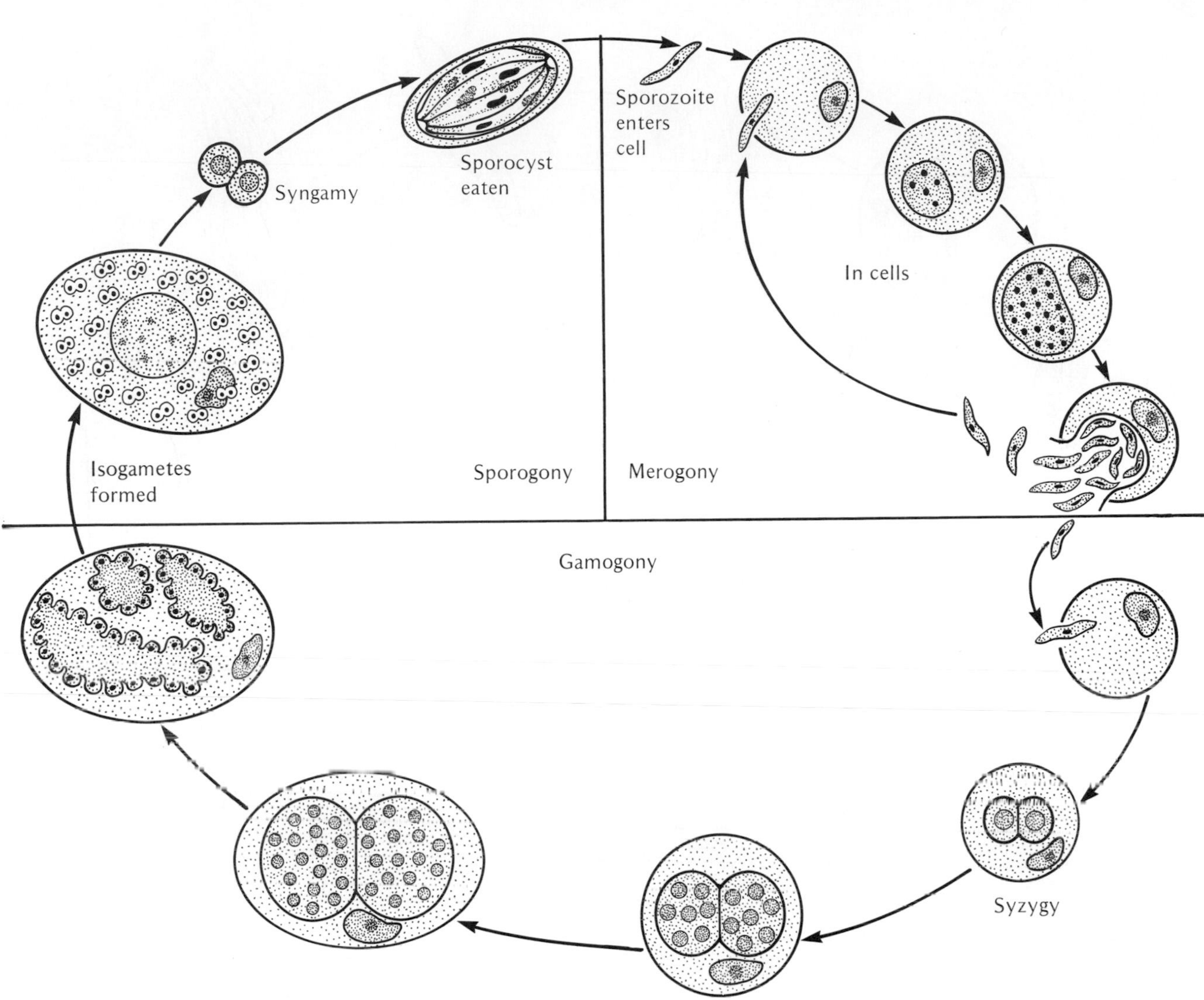

FIGURE 11.3 The structure and life cycle of *Lipocystis polyspora*, a member of the order Neogregarinida, which have merogony.

takes place in cells of the seminal vesicles. The sporozoite transforms into a large trophozoite, which unites with another in syzygy and forms a gametocyst. Isogametes are formed through schizogony, syngamy occurs, and an oocyst wall is laid down around the zygote. Two divisions take place in each oocyst with the formation of four sporozoites (Fig. 11.4).

Corycella armata is a septate gregarine, which is a parasite of the insect, *Gyrinus natator*. The sporozoite enters cells of the intestine and as the trophozoite grows, it becomes extracellular except for the complex holdfast or epimerite (Fig. 11.2A). The trophozoite later detaches as it becomes mature and enters into syzygy with another organism (Fig. 11.2B).

CLASSIFICATION

Class Gregarinea Dufour, 1928

Mature gamonts large, extracellular; mucron or epimerite present in some form as a cellular attachment; mucron formed from conoid; syzygy in gamonts; gametes usually similar (isogamous) or nearly so, with similar numbers of male and female gametes produced by gamonts; zygotes form oocysts within gametocysts; life cycle characteristically consisting of gamogony and sporogony; in digestive tract or body cavity of invertebrates or lower chordates; generally narrow host range.

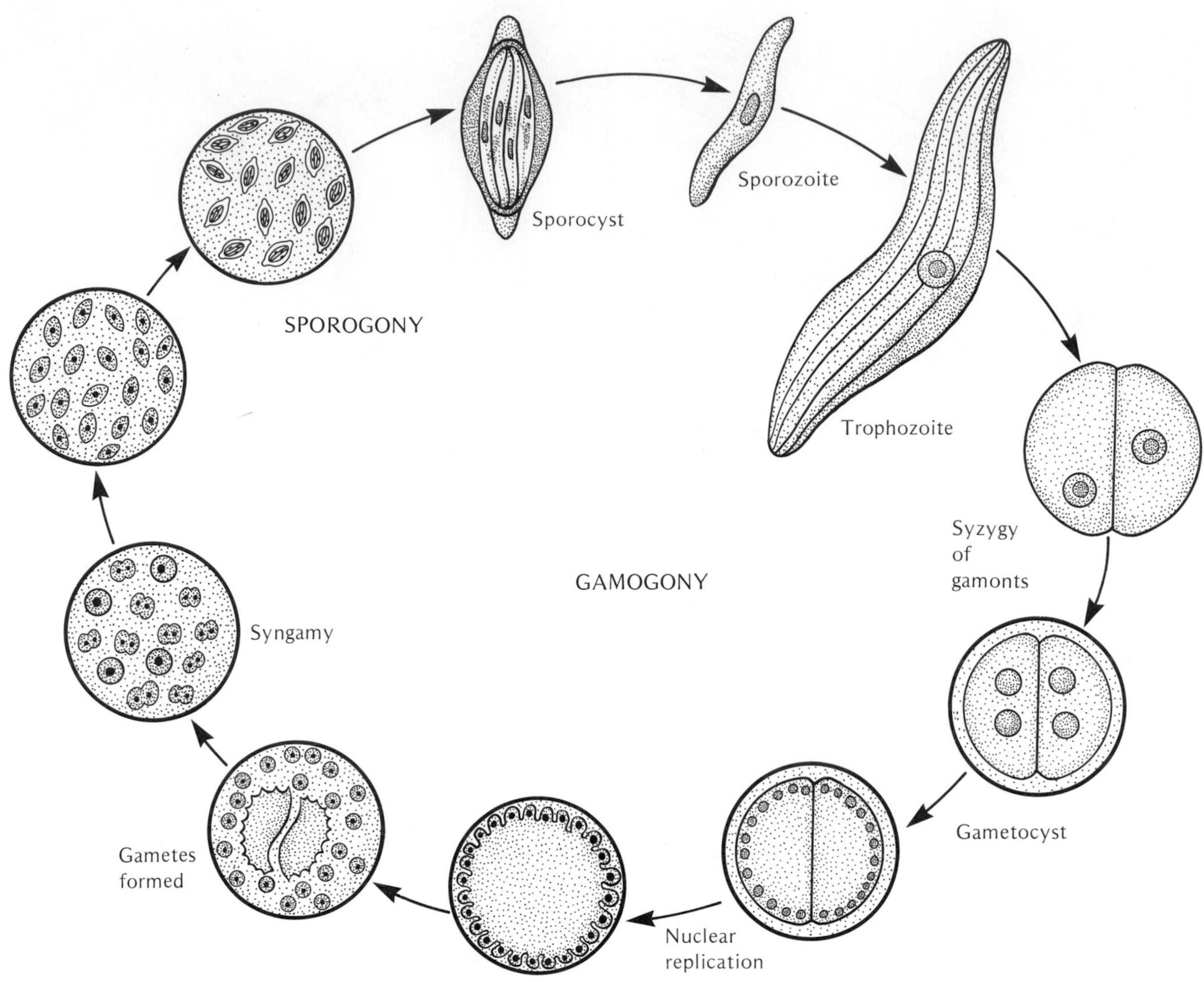

FIGURE 11.4 The structure and life cycle of *Monocystis lumbrici*, a eugregarine parasite of the earthworm, *Lumbricus terrestris*.

Order Archigregarinida Grassé, 1953

Life cycle apparently primitive, characteristically with merogony, gamogony, and sporogony; parasites of annelids, sipunculids, hemichordates, and ascidians. *Selenidioides, Exoschizon.*

Order Eugregarinida Léger, 1900

Merogony absent; typically parasites of annelids and arthropods; but some species in other invertebrates and lower chordates. *Siedleckia, Lecudina, Monocystis, Selenidium, Urospora, Stylocephalus, Gregarina, Stenophora., Corycella.*

Order Neogregarinida Grassé, 1953

Merogony present; presumably acquired secondarily; in Malpighian tubules, intestine, hemocoel, or fat body of insects. *Gigaductus, Mattesia, Lipocystis, Caullery ella.*

Readings

Grassé, P. P. (1953). Classe des grégarinomorphes (Grégarinomorpha n. nov. etc.). *Traité Zool.* **1**(2), 550–690.

King, C. A. (1988). Cell motility of sporozoan protozoa. *Parasitol. Today* **4**, 315–319.

Levine, N. D. (1985). Phylum II. Apicomplexa Levine, 1970. In *An Illustrated Guide to the Protozoa* (J. J. Lee, S. H. Hutner, and E. C. Bovee, Eds.). Society of Protozoologists, Lawrence, KS.

Mackenzie, C., and Walker, M. H. (1983). Substrate contact, mucus and eugregarine gliding. *J. Protozool.* **30,** 3–8.

Schrével, J. (1971). Observations biologique et ultrastructurales sur les Selenidiidae et leurs conséquences sur la systématique des Grégarinomorphes. *J. Protozool.* **18,** 448–470.

Walker, M. H., Mackenzie, C., Bainbridge, S. P., and Orme, C. (1979). A study of the structure and gliding movement of *Gregarina garnhami. J. Protozool.* **26,** 566–574.

CHAPTER

12

The Intestinal Coccidia

The coccidia are apicomplexans, most of which have all of the elements of the apical complex (Fig. 10.1) and, except for a few obscure species, have all three developmental portions of the life cycle: sporogony, merogony, and gamogony (Fig. 10.4). They are intracellular parasites principally of vertebrates, but some species are found in invertebrates as well. Transmission takes place from one host to the next by ingestion of a resistant form, the oocyst. In some instances, there is more than one host in the life cycle and transmission takes place also by carnivorism. This chapter concerns those coccidia that infect the intestinal tract of their hosts and that are transmitted from one host to the next by contaminated food or water. The genera most often involved in intestinal coccidiosis are *Eimeria, Isospora, Cyclospora,* and *Cryptosporidium.* Chapter 13 takes up those coccidia which invade organ systems in addition to the intestinal tract.

Geographic Distribution and Importance

Intestinal coccidiosis is a complex of diseases that are of great economic importance in domestic animals and of medical importance in humans in some circumstances in all parts of the world. Economic losses in domestic animals far exceed $100 million annually in the United States. A great deal of this loss is in chickens and secondarily in turkeys. Sheep, cattle, and goats are also subject to intestinal coccidiosis, and severe outbreaks result in both morbidity and mortality. Among companion animals, dogs and cats are subject to coccidiosis.

Intestinal coccidia are found in all birds and mammals as well as other vertebrates and some invertebrates, but not all of them cause medical or economic problems. Any species of bird or mammal has from two to a dozen species of coccidia. The domestic ox, for example, has about twelve species of *Eimeria,* but only three or four species are pathogenic. Any species of rodent has from two to perhaps six species of *Eimeria,* but few of them are seriously pathogenic. Birds, lizards, snakes, amphibia, fish, various insects, and even lower chordates such as sea squirts all have intestinal coccidia. More than 1200 species have been described, and many new species are described every year.

Life Cycle

All of the intestinal species have much the same pattern of transmission and development in the host. The oocysts are passed from the host with a uninucleated sporont. Sporogony or sporulation usually takes place outside of the host and infectivity is reached only after sporozoites have formed.

Sporulation requires moderate temperatures, between 15 and 32°C., and oxygen. Each species of coccidium can be characterized by the temperature and time over which its sporulation takes place and by its resistance to environmental stress. Many species are extraordinarily resistant to both physical and chemical agents. This resistance is best illustrated by the conditions under which oocysts are allowed to sporulate in the laboratory. Since oxygen is required for sporulation to take place and oocyst are most often recovered from feces, 2.5% potassium dichromate, 2% sulfuric acid, or 2% formalin are added to the suspension of oocysts to suppress bacterial growth.

If oocysts are kept cool (4–6°C) and bacterial growth is suppressed, oocysts of most species remain alive at least for a few months, and in some instances they have been found to survive for more than three years. Respiration at this time is at a level so low that it is not possible to measure it.

When oocysts are ingested by an appropriate host, the sporozoites become active within a few minutes to a few hours, leave the sporocyst and oocyst, and invade cells of the host (Fig. 12.3). The sporozoites respond to conditions in the intestine and become active quite quickly. In most species they respond to reducing conditions, enzymes (proteases), and wetting agents (bile), which signal the sporozoites to resume development.

Having exited the oocyst, the sporozoite seeks a proper host cell, most often an enterocyte but sometimes an endothelial cell. It is interesting to note that each species of coccidium seeks a preferred type of cell in a particular location of the intestines. How they sense the location and cell is not known.

The life cycle proceeds through a series of merogonous generations followed by gamogony and the formation of oocysts. The number of merogonous generations is fixed in almost all species. For example in *Eimeria tenella* of the chicken, there are three asexual generations. In *Eimeria bovis* of the ox, there are two, and in *Eimeria nieschulzi* of the rat, there are four. The organism is somehow programmed to run through a specific number of merogonies, and then it goes through a single generation of sexual development.

The coccidial life cycle is said to be *self-limiting* because after the merogonies and gamogony, the development in the host is terminated. Unlike *Cryptosporidium,* discussed later in this chapter, *Eimeria* and *Isospora* do not have the option of repeating an asexual generation once it has been completed.

Host–Parasite Interactions

Entry into a host cell is a nonspecific phenomenon. Sporozoites of *Eimeria* and *Isospora* spp. have been observed entering cells in vivo or in vitro that they would not normally contact. One might think *a priori* that there would be specific receptors on potential host cells to which the sporozoites would attach. Once inside the cell, the sporozoite may remain or it often exits only to enter another cell. It is not known what they respond to.

Nearly all of the intestinal coccidia have a narrow host range. They often infect only one or two species within a genus of host. Among *Eimeria* spp. of rodents, for example, most have been found to infect only a single species of host but a few are found in as many as four species within the same genus. *Eimeria citelli,* for example, has been reported from *Spermophilus tridecemlineatus, S. pygmaeus, S. citellus,* and *S. maximus.* Such a high degree of host specificity means that the parasite must derive something specific from its normal host cell that it cannot obtain from the cell of just any host or, for that matter, other cells in its normal host.

Upon infection and termination of the life cycle, the host becomes solidly immune. The greater part of immunologic studies have been done on *Eimeria* spp. of chickens, mostly *E. tenella.* Coccidiosis in cattle has been investigated in *E. bovis* although a few expose and challenge studies have been carried out with two other species. Coccidia of rodents have provided a laboratory model for the study of immunity to coccidia of mammals, and *E. nieschulzi* has been the primary organism studied.

When an oocyst is ingested by an immune host, excystation of sporozoites takes place normally and at least some of the sporozoites enter cells of the intestine. The immune response seems not to be directed toward the sporozoites but rather against the merogonous stages. The meronts (and possibly merozoites) are immunogenic, and the immune response is directed primarily toward them. Gamonts probably are poor antigens. Thus, the life cycle is affected in such a way that multiplication is reduced.

It has long been known that antibodies are present in the blood of animals after infection. It can also be shown in vitro that merozoites are detrimentally affected by exposure to immune serum. Their ability to infect cells may be reduced or they may even be lysed. The effect of antibody in the intact host is less clear. Transfer of serum to a naive host does not provide protection upon infection, for example. Functional immunity to the coccidia lies mainly in cell-mediated immunity (CMI).

Damage to the host takes place mainly through destruction of cells and the resulting inflammation, loss of fluid, and bleeding. Other factors are also involved, but they are beyond the scope of this discussion. Those species that are located deeply in the tissues of the intestine and that produce hundreds or thousands of merozoites in an asexual generation are most pathogenic.

Epidemiology and Control

Coccidiosis generally appears in a herd or flock when there is severe contamination of an area with infective oocysts. Even one oocyst ingested by a susceptible animal may result in tens of thousands of oocysts being shed at the end of the developmental period. These, in turn, are picked up and amplified by the other susceptible animals and move through the group causing a disease outbreak.

In nature, oocysts probably live for weeks or months unless they are subjected to drying, anaerobic conditions, heat, or freezing. It is insufficient to leave an area free of animals for a few weeks or to clean it half heartedly and expect it to be free of contamination. Oocysts can survive harsh disinfectants and heavy metals such as mercury or chromium that kill other organisms in short order.

Chemoprophylaxis, giving drugs before an outbreak is seen, is practiced in both poultry and large ruminant husbandry. Drugs are given in the food or water continuously so that the life cycle of the coccidium will be suppressed or stopped completely.

Notable Features

The oocyst stage is crucial in both the diagnosis of disease and the identification of species of coccidia. In a sporulated oocyst, the sporozoites are contained within the walls of the oocyst and usually the sporocyst (Tab. 12.1). The number of sporocysts and the number of sporozoites contained within them are the first characters that determine the genus one is dealing with. The genus that is most often seen and is of considerable economic importance is *Eimeria;* it has four sporocysts each of which contains two sporozoites. A second group are the so-called *isosporoid* oocysts, which encompass six or more genera including *Isospora, Toxoplasma,* and *Sarcocystis*; they have two sporocysts each of which has four sporozoites. The other genera are equally distinctive.

Going beyond the sporocysts and sporozoites numbers, the size of the oocyst and the sporocysts are next used quantitatively. Qualitative characters are the walls of the oocyst, oocyst and sporocyst residua, presence of a Stieda body, and the sporozoites themselves (Fig. 12.1).

TABLE 12.1 Generic Characteristics of the Oocysts of Some of the Coccidia

	Number of	
Genus	Sporocysts	Sporozoites/Oocyst
Cryptosporidium	0	4
Cyclospora	2	4
Pfeifferinella	0	8
Schellackia	0	8
Tyzzeria	0	8
Caryospora	1	8
Isospora	2	8
Toxoplasma	2	8
Besnoitia	2	8
Frenkelia	2	8
Hammondia	2	8
Sarcocystis	2	8
Dorisiella	2	16
Sivotashella	2	32
Eimeria	4	8
Wenyonella	4	16
Hoarella	8	12
Octosporella		

COCCIDIOSIS IN CHICKENS

The coccidia of poultry have been studied extensively, because coccidiosis is a cause of severe losses in chickens and turkeys. Since there is a great deal of information on the coccidia of chickens, they will be used here to illustrate many of the general principles in life cycles, development, host–parasite interactions, and control of coccidial infections.

Name of Organism and Disease Associations

All of the intestinal coccidia of chickens that are of economic importance are members of the genus *Eimeria.* Of the eight species listed in Fig. 12.2, the most pathogenic are: *E. tenella, E. necatrix, E. maxima, E. brunetti,* and *E. acervulina.* The others are only mildly pathogenic or benign.

Hosts and Host Range

Although certain of the species of coccidia of chickens are sometimes said to infect other hosts, well-controlled studies have shown that the domestic chicken, *Gallus gallus,* is the only host. Even closely related galliform birds have been shown to be refractory to infection. Birds farther removed taxonomically from the chicken such as turkeys, pheasant, or ducks do not support development of the coccidia of chickens.

Geographic Distribution and Importance

Poultry coccidia are cosmopolitan and ubiquitous. Wherever chickens are raised, there also will be coccidia. Laying hens continually pass a few oocysts, and eggs become contaminated when they are laid. Thus, newly hatched chicks become contaminated when sent to a raiser even though clean quarters are ready for the chicks.

Economic losses from coccidiosis come from a num-

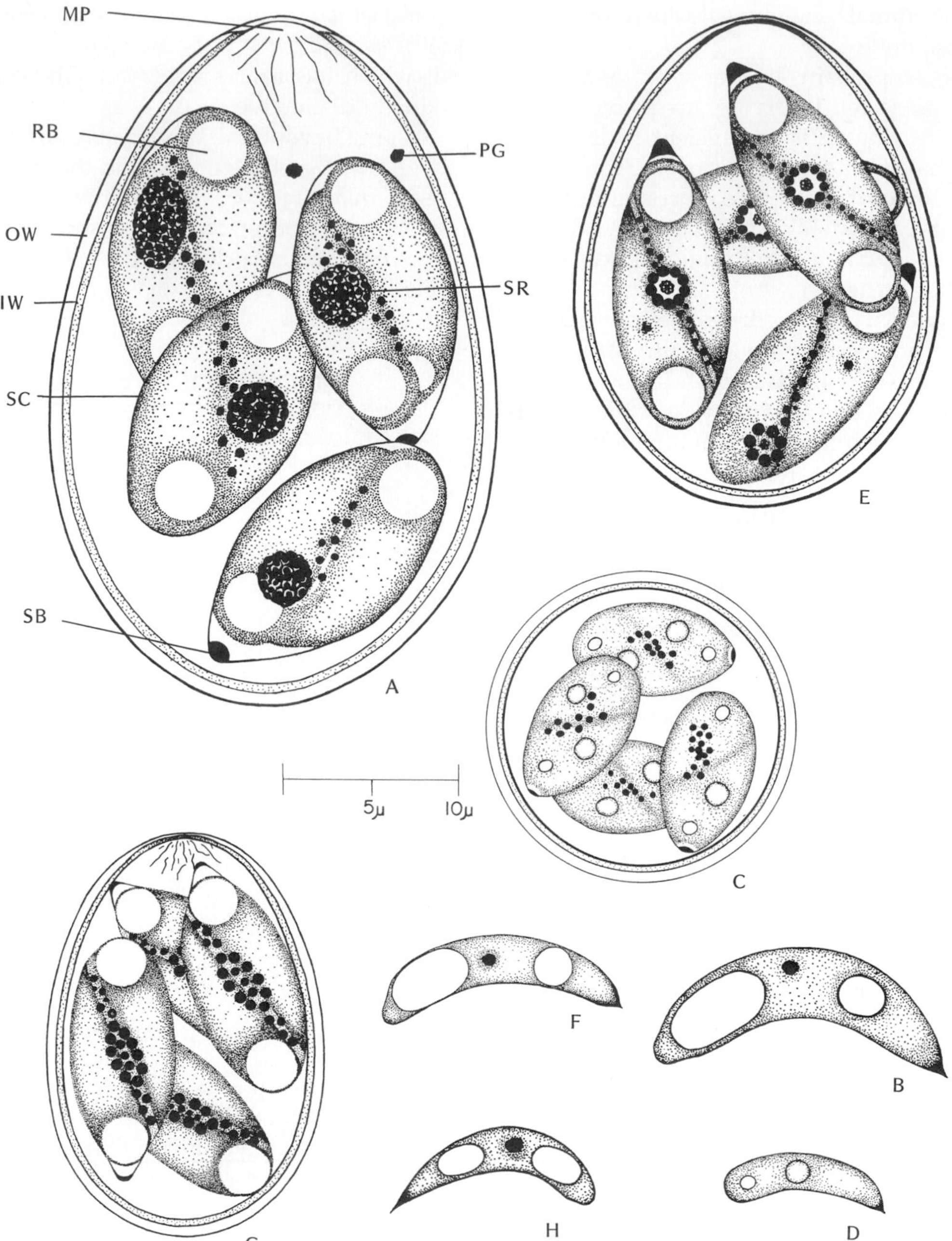

FIGURE 12.1 Oocysts of some coccidia of cattle. Oocyst (A) and sporozoite (B) of *Eimeria auburnensis;* oocyst (C) and sporozoite (D) of *E. zuernii;* oocyst (E) and sporozoite (F) of *E. bovis;* oocyst (G) and sporozoite (H) of *E. ellipsoidalis.* Abbreviations: IW—inner wall of oocyst, MP—micropyle, OW—outer wall of oocyst, PG—polar granule, RB—refractile globule of sporozoite, SB—Stieda body of sporocyst, SC—sporocyst, SR—sporocyst residuum. [From Nyberg and Hammond, 1965.]

ber of sources: weight losses, reduced feed efficiency, reduced egg production, and death. Additional losses lie in the costs of drugs, veterinary services, and overhead in labor and facilities to prevent clinical infections.

Estimates of economic losses have varied widely. The USDA estimated in 1965 that there is a $35 million loss annually in the United States, but others have estimated losses to be as high as $200 million. In two studies at veterinary diagnostic laboratories in poultry raising areas of the United States, 16 and 19% of birds submitted were found to be suffering from coccidiosis;

	Species of *Eimeria*							
Characteristics	***E. acervulina***	***E. brunetti***	***E. hagani***	***E. maxima***	***E. mitis***	***E. necatrix***	***E. praecox***	***E. tenella***
Oocyst size Average (μm) Length Width	 18.3x14.6 17.7–20.2 13.7–16.3	 24.6x18.8 20.7–30.3 18.1–24.2	 19.1x17.6 15.8–20.9 14.3–19.5	 39.5x20.7 21.5–42.5 16.5–29.8	 16.2x16.0 14.3–19.6 13.0–17.0	 20.4x17.2 13.2–22.7 11.3–18.3	 21.3x17.1 19.8–24.7 15.7–19.8	 22.0x19.0 19.5–26.0 16.5–22.8
Zone parasitized	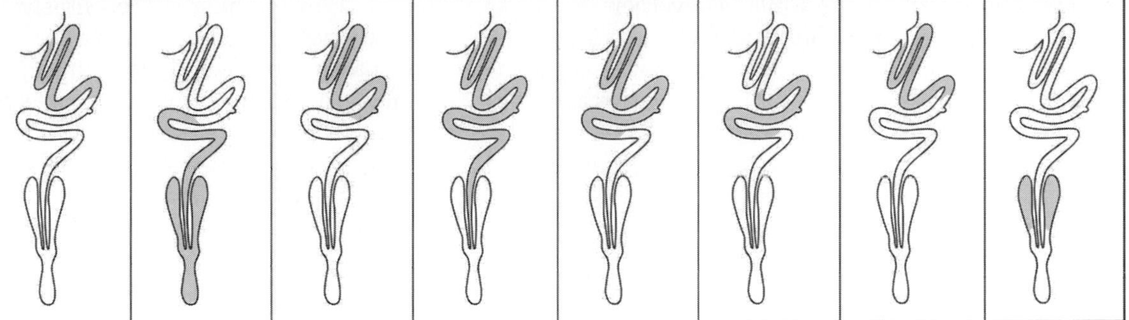							
Macroscopic lesions	White bands, thick wall, petechiae	Petechiae, catar, enteritis, blood, coagul. necrosis	Pinhead hemorrhages, petechiae	Petechiae pink, thick interior walls	None	Ballooning, white spots, hemorrhages	None	Hemorrhagic thickening of ceca
Intestinal contents	Creamy, mucoid	Mucoid, bloody	Mucoid	Mucoid, bloody	Mucoid	Mucoid, bloody	Mucoid casts	Bloody cores
Mortality	Low	Moderate	Low	Moderate	Low (young birds)	High	0	High
Morbidity	High	Low	Low	High	Low	High	Low	High
Sporulation minimum, in hours	17	18	18	30	18	18	12	18
Prepatent period, in hours	97	120	99	123	99	138	84	138
Immunity, speed of development	Prompt	"Sub-immediate"	"Prompt"	Prompt	Slow, little	Delayed	Prompt	Rapid
Immunity, duration	Moderate	Moderate	Unknown	Short	Moderate	Long	Moderate	Long
Schizont, max., in μm	10.3	30.0		9.4	11.3	65.9		54.0
Schizont, tissue location	Above epithelial nuclei	Second-generation subepithelium	Epithelial	Above epithelial nuclei	Below epithelial nuclei	Second-generation subepithelium	Below epithelial nuclei	Second-generation subepithelium
Gametocyte, tissue location	Above or below nuclei	Below epithelial nuclei	Unknown	Deep in epithelium	Above or below epithelial nuclei	Above or below epithelial nuclei	Above or below epithelial nuclei	Below epithelial nuclei

FIGURE 12.2 Characteristics of the chicken coccidia. [Redrawn with modifications from Reid and Long, 1979.]

thus, a fifth to a sixth of clinical diseases of all types were found to be coccidiosis.

Morphology

As a general rule, species of coccidia can be identified from the structure of the oocyst. In the chicken the oocysts of the various species are similar to one another, but some differentiation is possible (Fig. 12.2).

The location along the length of the intestines is a characteristic for each species, and this character is used effectively in diagnostic laboratories in determining the species present in an outbreak. In addition, the time required for sporulation of the oocysts, the location in the epithelial or subepithelial tissue, the type of lesions caused, and the prepatent period are all used in describing or identifying the species.

Life Cycle

Eimeria tenella is the most economically important of the poultry coccidia, and we will use it as an example of a coccidium of both birds and mammals. When sporulated oocysts are ingested, they experience a series of stimuli that trigger excystation of the sporozoites. The gizzard of birds is a specialized structure in the upper portion of the digestive tract that grinds food, and the oocysts require slight abrasion, which damages the outer oocyst walls. They then are subjected to reducing conditions and CO_2. Having been triggered by these conditions, the sporozoites are then activated by bile and trypsin. The sporozoites actively leave the oocysts and sporocysts in the lower part of the small intestine and then invade the tissue of the intestinal ceca of the large intestine (Fig. 12.3).

Sporozoites enter the tissue of the ceca through the tips of the villi. They migrate downward to the deeper parts of the tissue via the lacteals in the center of the villi. Having reached nearly the base of the cells forming the intestinal epithelium, the sporozoites enter cells in the crypts of Lieberkuehn and round up to form meronts.

The first merogony takes place in epithelial cells. Each sporozoite may produce as many as 900 merozoites and they are released from the host cell late on the second, or early on the third, day after infection.

The second merogony takes place in epithelial cells which round up and move away from their normal location. As many as 300 merozoites are produced by each meront, and they are released from the host cell late on the third, to early on the fourth, day of infection.

Third generation merogony also takes place in epithelial cells or enterocytes often near the tips of the villi. It is generally agreed that this generation is optional; when one studies tissue sections infected with *E. tenella,* these meronts are present in only small numbers. The merozoites are tiny, about 5 μm in length, and number about 16 per cell.

Second or third generation merozoites invade epithelial cells and develop into gamonts. Early gamonts are not distinguishable from early meronts, nor are the macro- and microgamonts different from one another at this time. When the microgamonts begin to undergo nuclear replication, the nuclei move to the periphery of the gamont, and their compact, darkly staining nuclei indicate that it is a microgamont. Late on the fifth day or early on the sixth, the flagellated microgametes have formed and they leave the host cell to seek a macrogamont (see Fig. 1.20).

Fertilization of the macrogamonts takes place within host cells. After fertilization, the oocysts walls are laid down. Two kinds of wall-forming bodies have been described in TEM, and they move peripherally in the gamont. As the bodies reach the margin of the fertilized gamete, they coalesce and form the outer walls of what is now an oocyst. During this time, the organism retains a single nucleus. Oocysts begin to appear in the feces late on the sixth day after infection and continue to be shed for about four days. Peak numbers of oocysts are seen in the feces during the seventh day.

The life cycle of *E. tenella* is self-limiting. When merogony has been completed, gamogony ensues, and the cycle in the host is then finished. In the coccidia, the number of merogonies is apparently programmed and, having completed them, the organisms commence gamogony. Such programming has been well demonstrated by experiments in which merozoites were transferred from infected animals to uninfected animals. The cycle continues as if it were still in the original host. Oocysts are produced at the same time in the recipients as would be expected if the parasites had remained in the same host. Thus, it is not immunity, or some other host influence, that causes the organisms to shift from merogony to gamogony.

Diagnosis

Diagnosis of coccidiosis in poultry is done by the following:

1. Clinical signs of diarrhea, often with blood
2. Weight loses, or reduced feed efficiency
3. Finding large numbers of oocysts in the feces
4. Finding characteristic lesions at postmortem examination

In a flock of birds, diarrhea typically shows in a few of them and then over a few days is seen in more and more of them. Birds become depressed and fail to eat normally. A bird that does not feel well sits on its haunches, ruffles its feathers, and usually closes it eyes. It looks depressed, but such demeanor is characteristic of many diseases of poultry, not only coccidiosis. The pattern of apparent rapid transmission through the flock is characteristic of coccidiosis; as explained earlier, the infection builds up through amplification of oocysts in the environment.

When death occurs, it usually slightly precedes or coincides with the production of oocysts. Where infections are exceedingly heavy, diarrhea may be seen, but the principal sign that something is wrong is a spate of dead birds with more dying each day.

The prepatent period, that is, the time from inoculation to production of oocysts of various species, ranges from four days to almost six days (Fig. 12.2). While useful in experimental studies, the prepatent period is not especially germane under field conditions. However, finding oocysts in the feces is important in obtaining a definitive diagnosis of coccidiosis.

In most instances, coccidiosis is diagnosed by examining dead or dying birds postmortem. A skilled pa-

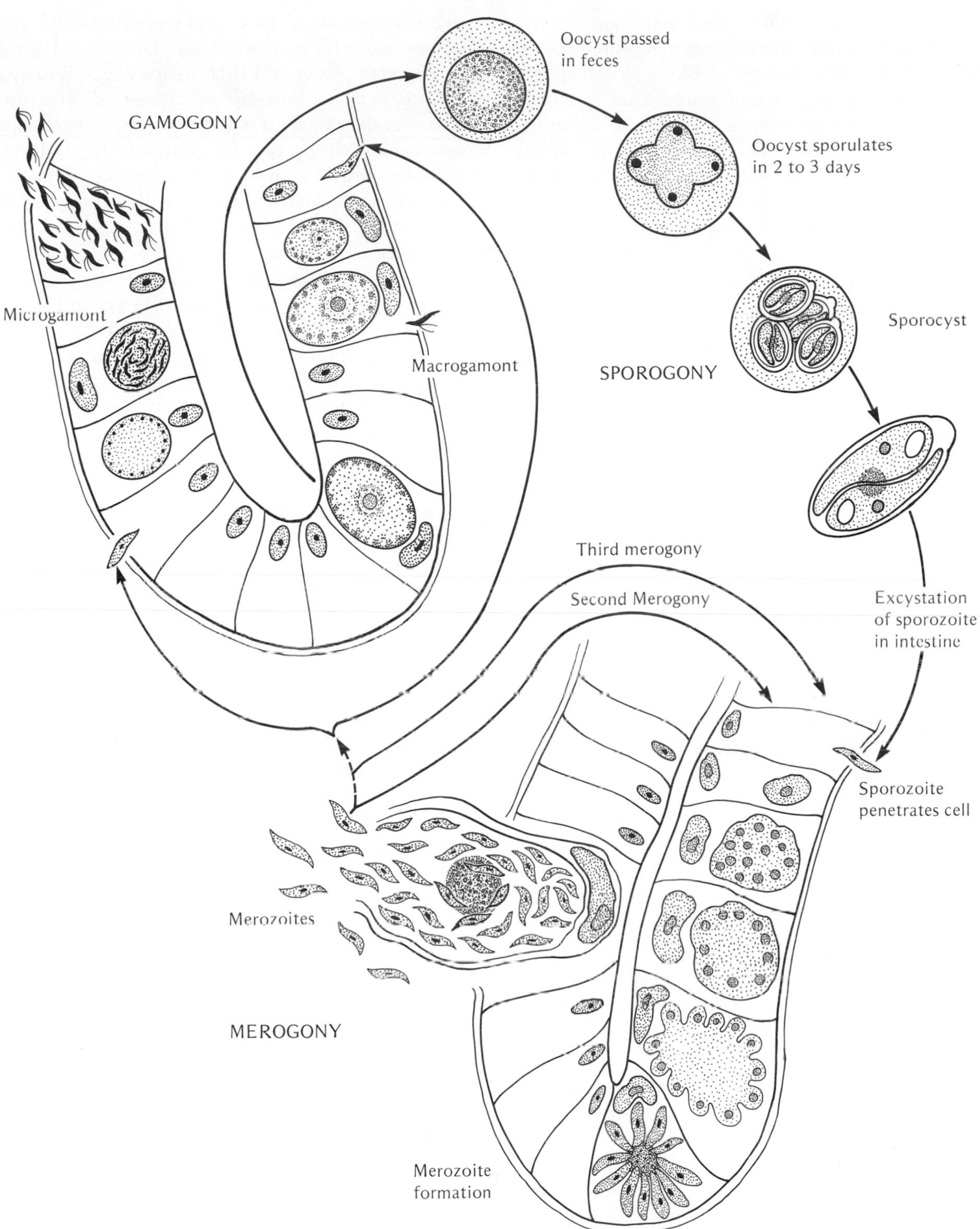

FIGURE 12.3 Life cycle of *Eimeria tenella.*

thologist can examine the intestinal tract and see the areas where the coccidia have developed and also see whether there is extravasation of blood. Microscopic examination of scrapings from the intestinal wall confirms that developmental stages are present. Other infectious agents may cause diarrhea, death, and blood in the intestine, but finding the coccidial stages is good confirmation of coccidiosis. Histologic examination of the intestinal tissue also allows the identification of the species present.

Host–Parasite Interactions

Different species of *Eimeria* cause differing levels of pathogenesis in chickens. The degree of pathogenesis is related to the following:

1. The number of merozoites produced at each asexual generation
2. The number of asexual generations
3. The depth in the tissue where development takes place

The term *reproductive index* (RI) is useful in showing how many cells may be parasitized in a single cycle of endogenous development of a coccidium. Each merogonous generation has a characteristic number of merozoites and the number of cells potentially destroyed can be estimated. In *E. tenella* there are 8 sporozoites in the oocyst, 900 first-generation merozoites, 350 second-generation merozoites, and 16 third-generation merozoites (all on average). Assuming that half of the gamonts are female, the number of oocysts potentially produced by ingestion of one oocyst can be calculated:

$$8 \times 900 \times 350 \times 16/2 = 20{,}160{,}000$$

These are useful working figures, but they assume that all of the merozoites succeed in entering new cells and developing there. Some RIs that have been obtained by experimental infections are the following:

tenella	60,000
acervulina	9,000
maxima	11,000
necatrix	50,000

The number of oocysts ingested is correlated with the amount of damage that occurs. The more cells that are infected, the greater the damage to the intestine. Ingestion of a few oocysts generally does not result in significant damage to the intestinal tract. However, if tens of thousands or millions are ingested, the result may be the death of the host.

In typical coccidial infections, a few oocysts are seen in the feces toward the end of gamogony and the number increases rapidly over about two days. The number in the feces peaks and then drops precipitously about four days or so, into the patent period. The intestinal tissue is damaged but then begins to heal as oocyst production drops off. In light infections, the gut is repaired within about a week after oocyst production has ceased. In heavy infections, there may be permanent changes in the gut and animals continue to be poor feed converters.

The depth in the tissue is also a factor in the degree of pathogenesis. In *E. tenella,* the second-generation meronts are subepithelial, and about the time when second-generation merozoites leave the cells, there is disruption of large areas of intestinal epithelium. Blood is lost, and the removal of the enterocytes removes the first line of defense; bacteria can then invade the tissue of the gut. In contrast, *E. debliecki* of swine inhabits only the epithelial cells of the intestinal villi; although a slight diarrhea may be seen in infected animals, the damage to the host is minor. In *Eimeria bovis* of the ox, the second-generation meronts and gamonts are deep in the crypts of Lieberkuehn and diarrhea coincides with the production of oocysts.

If the tissues of animals affected with coccidiosis are examined, characteristic changes can be seen grossly at postmortem examination and in tissues prepared for microscopic examination. The wall of the gut is thickened indicating retention of fluid (edema). There may be blood in the lumen of the gut indicating blood loss (hemorrhage), or merely retention of an excessive amount of blood in the tissue (hyperemia). There is also infiltration with various kinds of white cells (leukocytes) indicating a foreign body reaction and the development of the immune response.

For the poultry or livestock raiser, rapid weight gain and good feed conversion (amount of feed consumed/amount of gain) are important for adequate economic return. It is especially true in the poultry industry, where the profit margin on any one bird may only be pennies, that extra time to reach market weight or wasted feed through inefficient feed conversion may mean the difference between profit and loss on a flock. Most of the studies on weight gain and feed conversion have been done with chickens, and during the peak of coccidial infection, both are poor. The infected birds gain rapidly after the infection is over and they begin to approach the weights of the unaffected birds, but they never do as well as uninfected birds.

Immunity typically is seen following infection with coccidia. There are a few species in which several infections are required for immunity to develop, but they are rare. Immunity to coccidia is characterized by the following:

1. Clinical symptoms do not ensue following a challenge inoculation.
2. Immunity is almost completely sterile.
3. Immunity is not permanent.
4. Immunity is species specific.
5. The mechanism is principally cell mediated.

In a typical experiment designed to demonstrate immunity, a bird is inoculated with an initial dose of oocysts, perhaps a thousand oocysts. Usually a mild clinical episode is seen, but recovery ensues. About ten days or so after oocyst production has ceased, the bird is challenged with a large number of the same species of coccidium. The host will not show clinical signs of infection, nor will it produce many oocysts (perhaps 5 to10% of the number in the first infection). Obviously some of the sporozoites penetrate the host cells and develop through the whole cycle to produce oocysts, so the immunity is not completely sterile.

After four months, or so, if a bird can be kept from being reinfected through natural contamination of its quarters, immunity wanes. This can be demonstrated on challenge when large numbers of oocysts will again be produced, and clinical signs may be seen.

If a bird is immunized with *Eimeria tenella*, it is completely susceptible to another species such as *E. necatrix*. In a few instances, there is some cross immunity, but it is incomplete at best.

After an infection has run its course, serum antibodies can be measured in the blood of the host. Passive immunity cannot be demonstrated, however, by transfusing blood from one host to another. The mechanism of immunity is based principally in cell mediated immunity (CMI).

Epidemiology and Control

Control of coccidiosis in poultry is based on the following:

1. Chemoprophylaxis
2. Purposely exposing birds to infectious oocysts and controlling the infection with anticoccidial drugs

Because of the ubiquity and hardiness of oocysts, coccidiosis is difficult to control by management. In the developed world, and in certain countries of the developing world, poultry raising is integrated and intensive. Birds are confined and there may be as many as 40 thousand broilers in one building. From hatching till the chickens go to slaughter may be as few as six weeks. The whole flock starts together and goes to market together at two pounds. The broiler house is cleaned and then restocked with newly hatched chicks. Cleaning, at best, leaves the area contaminated with some oocysts, and other infectious agents. Left alone, the birds will inevitably suffer an outbreak of coccidiosis or other infectious diseases.

Egg production is also a high-tech industry. Hens are confined to batteries of wire cages such that eggs that are laid roll to the front of the cages where they may be harvested periodically. Feed and light are controlled by computer so as to maximize egg production.

The best solution to preventing coccidiosis in poultry has been to add chemicals to the food or water, mostly the former. The birds thereby self-medicate. In the late 1930s, drug treatment for infectious diseases began a revolution. The "sulfa" drugs (sulfanilamide, sulfaguanidine, etc) were developed for bacterial infections and within a short time order found to be effective against coccidial infections (Fig. 12.4). The rush was then on to develop additional *anticoccidials*, as they came to be called.

It is generally not feasible to await an outbreak before medicating the feed of birds. Medicating birds after the beginning of an outbreak does have the advantage of being more economical and chemicals are not used unless necessary. The disadvantage is that coccidiosis must be diagnosed early; a few hours' delay may mean excessive losses. Second, by the time the signs of coccidiosis appear, drug treatment may have little effect on the course of the disease. As discussed earlier, *Coccivac* can prevent economic losses by exposing birds to controlled dosages of oocysts and controlling the infection with an anticoccidial drug.

COCCIDIOSIS IN TURKEYS

Of the seven species of *Eimeria* in turkeys, *E. meleagrimitis* and *E. andenoeides* are pathogenic. The same principles apply to coccidiosis in turkeys as to the disease in chickens.

COCCIDIOSIS IN CATTLE

There are about a dozen species of *Eimeria* that are found in the domestic ox, *Bos taurus*. The same species are probably also found in the zebu, *Bos indicus*, and the water buffalo, *Bubalus bubalis*, as well. Some are also found in the bison, *Bison bison*, but the data are fragmentary. Of the dozen, or so, species, *E. bovis*, *E. zuernii*, and *E. alabamensis* are pathogenic. The others are nonpathogenic or cause only a transient diarrhea in calves.

Coccidiosis is seen in calves from a month of age

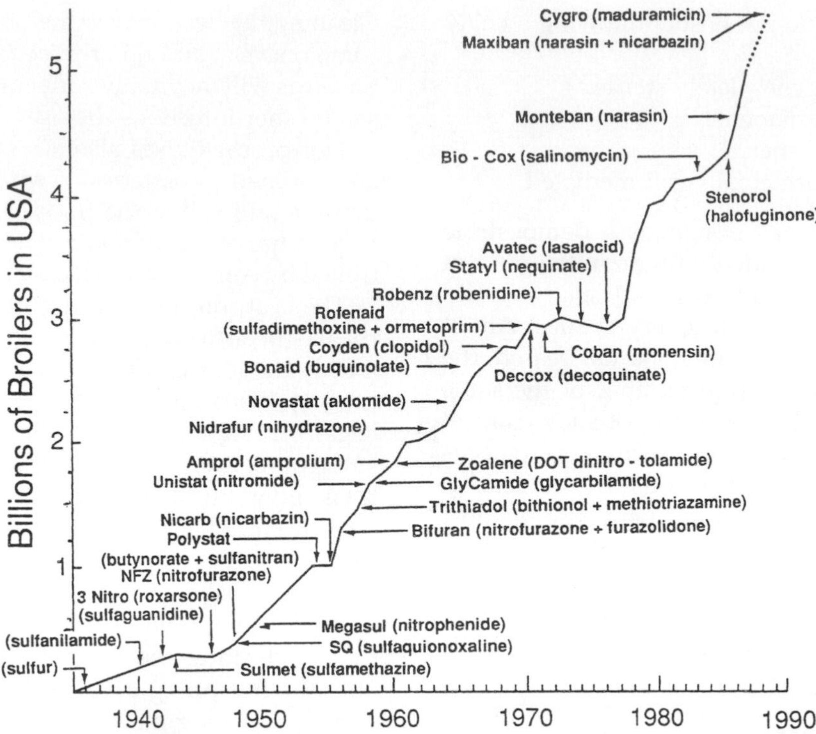

FIGURE 12.4 Broiler production in the United States and the introduction of new anticoccidials. [From McDougald, L. R., *in:* B. W. Calnek (ed.). 1997. As poultry raising became integrated and more of a mass-production enterprise, the need for anticoccidials also became greater. Over a 30 year period more than 30 compounds have been developed and marketed to prevent coccidiosis. Coccidia developed drug resistance to many of them within a few years after their introduction.

to about three months; after that time, they develop immunity because of exposure to infective oocysts or because of an age resistance. A young calf is not completely immunocompetent and may suffer from a variety of infections that cause diarrhea until the immune system is well developed; coccidiosis is only one diarrheal disease of importance (see also *Cryptosporidium).*

A number of methods have been developed to reduce losses from coccidiosis in calves. Where there is severe contamination of the premises, death losses may reach 50%. Separation of age classes is essential in a diary operation. Older calves develop immunity but still shed thousands of oocysts into the environment daily. Younger animals become infected and then contaminate the environment with billions of oocysts during a clinical infection. Each newborn calf also needs colostrum from its mother or from a frozen supply kept for that purpose. Colostrum provides essential immunoglobulins that allow the calf to survive during the first weeks of life. In some instances, calves can be fed anticoccidials, in the same way that chickens are, to prevent coccidiosis.

An innovation in calf-rearing was developed more than thirty years ago by Dr. Leonard Reid Davis of the USDA. His method has been adopted in a variety of forms by many dairy farmers. Calves are kept in small, portable pens measuring about 4 × 8 feet (1.5 × 3 m) in which there is a shelter at one end. Water and feed containers hang on the side of the pen. The kind of shelter varies with the climate so that in warm climates, the calf is protected from the sun and rain, and in cold climates, the animal has access to a small, warm house. The crucial part of the system is a regular, systematic movement of the pens. Calves are started at the bottom of a slope (which presumably has not had cattle on it for about a year). At intervals of three days, the pens are moved; the concept is to move the calves to clean ground in such a way that they leave any contamination behind. In about three months calves have adequate immunity and may placed with other older animals.

In addition to coccidiosis in young calves, another epidemiologic complex is seen in weaned calves or sometimes mature cattle. So-called winter coccidiosis occurs in temperate and cold climates when animals are on range and in feed lots where animals are stressed because of weaning, changes in feed, or severe winter weather. Animals typically begin to show diarrhea and then may pass large amounts of blood; perhaps a quarter of untreated animals die. The primary causative agent is *Eimeria zuernii,* but oocysts of a half a dozen or more species of *Eimeria* are usually present in the feces. Excessive contamination of pastures and corrals seems not to be important in the etiology of winter coccidiosis. Rather, some sort of stress may reduce the immunity of the animals. Morbidity and mortality can be reduced by making sure that the cattle are stressed as little as possible in shipping, change of feed, and weaning. Addition of anticoccidials such as monensin to the feed also seem to reduce losses.

COCCIDIOSIS IN SHEEP

Sheep have about twelve species of *Eimeria* in the intestinal tract. Of these, *Eimeria ahsata, E. ovinoidalis,* and *E. ovina* are pathogenic, and the others are nonpathogenic or only slightly so. These species are found in the domestic sheep, *Ovis aries,* the Rocky Mountain bighorn sheep, *Ovis canadensis,* the mouflon, and the argali. At one time it was thought that domestic sheep and goats have the same species of intestinal coccidia, but cross-transmission studies have shown that, even though the oocysts may be morphologically identical, isolates from sheep do not develop in goats, and vice versa.

Much the same pattern of coccidiosis occurs in sheep as in cattle. Lambs are susceptible, but by weaning age of five months or so, they are generally resistant to infection. Maintaining clean quarters is the key to avoiding coccidiosis in lambs.

Older animals are sometimes affected by coccidiosis under about the same circumstances as cattle. In the western United States, lambs are weaned in late summer or fall and moved to cut-over fields or feed lots. If the changes are too abrupt, the lambs are likely to show diarrhea, lose weight, and some of them will die. Also, pregnant ewes have been seen to develop diarrhea and die from coccidiosis. In these instances, the ewes pass only a few oocysts in the feces, but the intestinal tissues are massively infected with merogonous stages of coccidia, most likely *E. ovinoidalis.*

COCCIDIOSIS IN GOATS

Goats have about twelve species of *Eimeria* of which *E. arloingi, E. christenseni,* and *E. ninakohlyakimovae* are pathogenic. The others are nonpathogenic or only slightly so. The species found in the domestic goat probably also infect wild goats and the ibex.

COCCIDIOSIS IN CAMELS AND LLAMA

Nine species of *Eimeria* have been described from Eastern and Western Hemisphere camelids. In each instance the coccidia seem to cross-transmit among camelids within the hemisphere. For example, the Bactrian and dromedary have the same species, and the llama, guanaco, and alpaca all have the same species. It is interesting to note that at least two morphologically identical species, *E. cameli* and *E. macusaniensis,* occur in both Eastern and Western Hemisphere camelids, respectively. It appears that these species are pathogenic in their hosts. Cross transmission experiments have not been done. In fact, the life cycles of the coccidia of camelids are poorly known.

COCCIDIOSIS IN SWINE

The domestic and wild pig, *Sus scrofa,* are hosts to about twelve species of coccidia, ten species of *Eimeria* and two of *Isospora.* Among the *Eimeria, E. debliecki, E. polita, E. scabra,* and *E. spinosa* are mildly pathogenic. *Isospora suis* causes severe diarrhea and death in baby pigs. Maintaining a scrupulously clean environment in which pigs are born is essential to prevent isosporoid diarrhea, as well as other gastrointestinal infections.

COCCIDIOSIS IN HORSES

The only intestinal coccidium of horses of importance is *Eimeria leuckarti,* which has its endogenous stages in the small intestine. It is cosmopolitan, but seems to be rare. Whether this species is highly pathogenic remains a matter for further study.

COCCIDIOSIS IN RABBITS

The order Lagomorpha includes the European rabbit, *Oryctolagus cuniculi,* the cottontail, *Sylvilagus* spp., the jackrabbit, *Lepus* spp. and the coney or pika, *Ochotona* spp. The European rabbit or hare is the domesticated species raised for food and fiber and used as a laboratory animal. Coccidiosis in this animal can represent considerable economic loss and can confound laboratory experiments. Among the species that are important are *Eimeria magna, E. coecicola, E. flavescens, E. irresidua,* and *E. piriformis* in the intestine, and *E. stiedai* of the bile ducts of the liver. Raising rabbits on wire and otherwise keeping their quarters scrupulously clean are essential in preventing coccidiosis.

COCCIDIOSIS IN RODENTS

The coccidia of rodents have been studied from a number of standpoints such as endogenous life cycles, evolution, immunity, cross-transmission, and interaction of parasites with one another. Some species are pathogenic when studied in infections produced in the laboratory, but it is difficult to determine what effect these organisms have on their hosts in the wild.

These organisms provide an excellent model for experimentation in the laboratory. Rodents are inexpensive to purchase and to keep, they are readily infected, bled, and examined for parasites. *Eimeria nieschulzi* and *E. separata* of the rat have been studied extensively in the laboratory and continue to provide data on many aspects of coccidial infections.

COCCIDIOSIS IN DOGS

The domestic dog and other canids serve as hosts of two species of *Isospora, I canis,* and *I. ohioensis* and as the definitive hosts of several species of *Sarcocystis* (see Chapter 13). At one time it was assumed that dogs and cats harbored the same species of coccidia, and the literature prior to the 1960s is predicated on this error; thus, the names may be confusing.

Isospora in both dogs and cats can show both a traditional direct life cycle, and an indirect cycle by infection of animals such as small rodents in which some development may take place in extraintestinal tissues. Since little development seems to occur in these other hosts, they are usually referred to as paratenic host; transmission back to the canid takes place when an infected rodent is eaten.

Surveys have indicated that from 2.6 to 38.1% of dogs are infected with intestinal coccidia with most data being in the range of 4 to 8%. Intestinal infections with *Isospora* may cause severe, chronic diarrhea in the dog; this condition may cause as much distress to the owner as to the dog. Diarrhea has been reported to last for a week to nine weeks, but the sole cause may not be the coccidia and other contributing agents should also be suspected. Various sulfonamide drugs are effective. Prevention of infection is difficult because the oocysts are hardy and only a few may set off an infection in puppies who then contaminate the environment heavily. In a kennel, cleanliness is essential to prevent coccidiosis and other gastrointestinal infections.

COCCIDIOSIS IN CATS

Domestic cats serve as hosts for two species of *Isospora* , *I. felis,* and *I. rivolta,* and several species of two host coccidia (see *Toxoplasma* and *Sarcocystis* in Chapter 13). The comments on isosporoid infection in dogs applies as well to cats.

COCCIDIOSIS IN HUMANS

Isospora belli occurs commonly in humans globally. It most often causes a mild diarrhea, but infections in immunocompetant individuals are occasionally life threatening. In persons who are not immunocompetant, such as persons who are HIV positive, the infections is a severe, intractible one. *Sarcocystis suihominis,* which also has an isosporoid oocyst, is pathogenic in humans, but it has a two-host life cycle (Chapter 13). Cryptosporidiosis and cyclosporosis, both discussed later in the chapter, are serious intestinal infections of humans.

CYCLOSPOROSIS

The genus *Cyclospora* is defined as a coccidium having two sporocysts, each of which has two sporozoites. Prior to 1993 the *Cyclospora* that were known were from arthropods, moles, rodents, insectivores, and snakes. The identification of *C. cayetanensis* as a human pathogen has elicited research programs at a number of levels from the epidemiologic to the molecular. Studies on the rRNA gene of *C. cayetanensis* has shown that it is closely related to the genus *Eimeria.* Cyclosporosis is one of several emerging parasitic diseases. The emergence of cyclosporosis may hinge on rapid transport of food by air. The unraveling of this puzzle will be interesting to watch as time passes.

Name of Organism and Disease Associations

Cyclospora cayatanensis causes enteritis in humans and is referred to as cyclosporosis.

Hosts and Host Range

Human. Information on other hosts has not yet been developed.

Geographic Distribution and Importance

Peru, Mexico, Haiti, United States, Canada, Nepal, and possibly New Guinea and Guatemala. A number of outbreaks have been reported, but the importance of cyclosporosis is not yet clear.

Morphology

Members of the genus *Cyclospora* (family Eimeriidae) are characterized as having oocysts with two sporocysts, each of which has two sporozoites (Fig. 12.5). Oocysts are spheroidal 8.6 ± 0.6 μm (7.7–9.9 μm) with a bilayered wall that is 113 nm thick; the outer surface is rough. Sporocysts are ovoidal 4.0 ± 0.4 μm by 6.34 ± 0.63 μm (5.5–7.1 μm) with a sporocyst residuum and both Stieda and subStiedal bodies. The sporozoites are 1.2 by 9.0 μm (1.06–1.34 by 8–10 μm).

Life Cycle

Oocysts are passed in the feces, but other details of the life cycle are not known.

Diagnosis

Finding oocysts in the feces of a person showing a prolonged diarrhea is the current method of diagnosis. The oocysts are acid fast when stained by a Ziehl-Nielsen procedure, similar to those of *Cryptosporidium*, but *Cyclospora* are larger.

Host–Parasite Interactions

C. cayatanensis causes an intermittent diarrhea that lasts for an average of seven weeks.

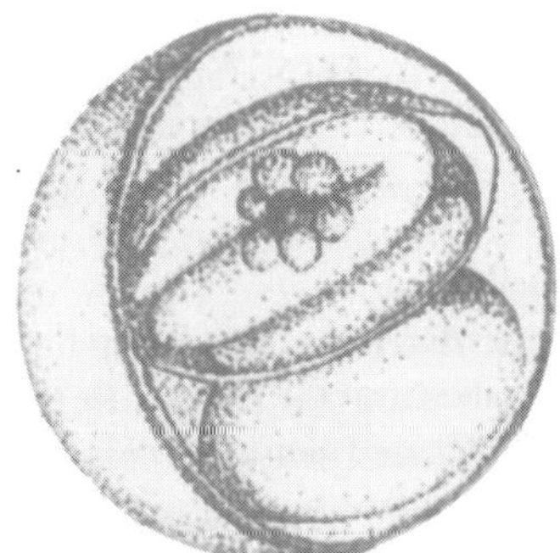

FIGURE 12.5 A diagram of the oocyst of *Cyclospora cayatanensis*, an enteric pathogen of humans. [From Ortega, et al., 1994]

Epidemiology and Control

Infections seem to be both food and water borne. The oocysts do not survive desiccation well, and it is likely that they must be kept moist for them to survive and infect a new host. Some infections were probably transmitted with fresh fruit, but it is not known how the fruit became contaminated. Because infections and outbreaks have been so sporadic, no control programs have been developed, but washing fresh fruit is always advisable. The drug co-trimoxazole has been shown to be effective in limited treatment trials.

CRYPTOSPORIDIUM AND CRYPTOSPORIDIOSIS

Cryptosporidium has been known since the great protozoologist Ernest E. Tyzzer described *Cryptosporidium muris* from the laboratory mouse in 1907. Tyzzer described an additional species from rodents, *C. parvum*, and he gave detailed descriptions of both species that have validity today.

It was not until the middle 1950s that *Cryptosporidium* was found to be other than an organism of obscure status. *C. meleagridis* was then described from the domestic turkey and shown to be the cause of economic losses. Still, the importance of the organisms was not clear, and even the occurrence of diarrhea in cattle caused by *Cryptosporidium* was only a minor ripple on the surface of our ignorance.

In 1976 cryptosporidiosis was reported in humans, but it was not known whether the disease was merely sporadic or only associated with persons whose immune systems were not normal. For example, cases were seen in children suffering from genetic agammaglobulinemia.

Cryptosporidiosis became an emerging disease in the early 1980s with the identification of AIDS as a clinical entity. AIDS patients suffer from a variety of infections not normally of great importance in humans. *Pneumocystis* pneumonia and diarrhea caused by *Cryptosporidium parvum* are among the most important infections of those persons whose immune systems are compromised by HIV infection. Infections have since been identified in large numbers of children in day care and in normal adults, as well. In livestock, cryptosporidiosis is an important disease of newborn calves.

Even though *Cryptosporidium* spp. are included with the other intestinal coccidia, the members are quite different from *Eimeria* and *Isospora*. Fine structural studies have shown that some of the elements of the apical complex are present, but some of them, such as the conoid, are in a different form. The life cycles are not programmed to move through a sequence of stages; instead, the same asexual stage may be repeated. Oocyst structure and the formation of the outer wall of the oocyst is somewhat different from other coccidia. Excystation of sporozoites occurs under rather general conditions such as mammalian body temperature and any bile salt. Studies on molecular evolution using the rRNA gene sequence indicate that *Cryptosporidium* is not closely related to other apicomplexans and certainly not to other intestinal coccidia. It is likely that the current placement of *Cryptosporidium* spp. in the family Cryptosporidiidae in the order Eimeriina will be changed so as to place them in their own taxonomic order; we have done so in placing them in the order Cryptosporiida (Chapter 10).

More than a thousand papers and monographs have been published on *Cryptosporidium* spp., most of them since the middle 1970s. The best single source of information is Dubey et al., 1990.

Name of Organism and Disease Associations

The organisms that are currently accepted as valid are the following:

Name	*Hosts*	*Pathogenesis*
Cryptosporidium muris Tyzzer, 1907	Rodents and some mammals	Mild
C. parvum Tyzzer, 1912	Many mammals including humans, companion animals, and domesticated ruminants	Severe
C. meleagridis Slavin, 1955	Turkey and other gallinaceous birds	Moderate
C. serpentis Levine, 1980	Snakes	Mild
C. nasorum Hoover et al., 1981	Fish	Possibly
C. baileyi Current et al., 1986	Domestic chicken and other gallinaceous birds	Moderate

Twenty-one species have been described over the years; all but six have now been synonymized to those listed here.

Hosts and Host Range

Each species of *Cryptosporidium* has a range of hosts in which it can develop; most seem to have at least a half a dozen species of hosts. *C. parvum* develops in the intestine and other tissues of a wide range of mammals. The usual site of infection is the intestinal tract, but certain species also develop in other organs such as the respiratory system.

Geographic Distribution and Importance

Cosmopolitan. Among the accepted species listed earlier, *C. parvum* is of greatest medical and economic importance. It affects the health not only of humans but also of domestic ruminants such as the ox, sheep, goat, pen-raised deer, and water buffalo. It has also been found in a variety of other ruminants throughout the world. Fifteen surveys of calves showing diarrhea gave prevalence rates of from 17 to 76% with most of the rates in the range of 21 to 27%.

The importance of *C. parvum* to human health has been recognized only in relatively recent times. Starting in about 1984, outbreaks of cryptosporidiosis were recognized in the human population of several urban areas:

Locality	*Date*	*Number of cases*
Braun Station, Texas	1984	59% of residents sampled were pos.
Sheffield, England	1986	
New Mexico	1986	78-Lab-confirmed cases
Carroll Co., Georgia	1987	13,000
Ayrshire, Scotland	1988	
Oxfordshire-Swindon, England	1989	
Milwaukee, Wisconsin	1992	400,000

Many other reports have involved children with genetic immunodeficiencies or adults suffering from AIDS. In these individuals, the clinical phase of the infection continues indefinitely, and is life threatening. Infections in normal immunocompetent persons have a clinical phase that is controlled by immunity.

Looking broadly at the prevalence of infection determined by fecal examination in humans, infants have the highest proportion infected with 5 to 30% of children in day care being infected. Adults usually show from 1 to 3% infection. Persons with AIDS show from 10 to 20% infection rates.

Seroprevalence is generally high indicating that many persons have been infected at some time in their lives. Infections in normal adults in the United States and Britain ranged from 25 to 35%, but blood donors in Edinburgh showed an 86% prevalence of infection. Persons having lived in the tropics had infection rates from 32 to 64%.

Morphology

The oocysts, which are shed in the feces, are smaller than any other intestinal coccidia. There is some variation from species to species, but the length ranges from 4.5 to 7.5 $\mu m \times$ 4.2 to 5.7 μm in width. The length/width ratio is 1.00 to 1.33, so the oocysts of most species are subspherical. Sporozoites are 4.5 to 7.5 μm long $\times$ 1.2 to 1.8 μm wide.

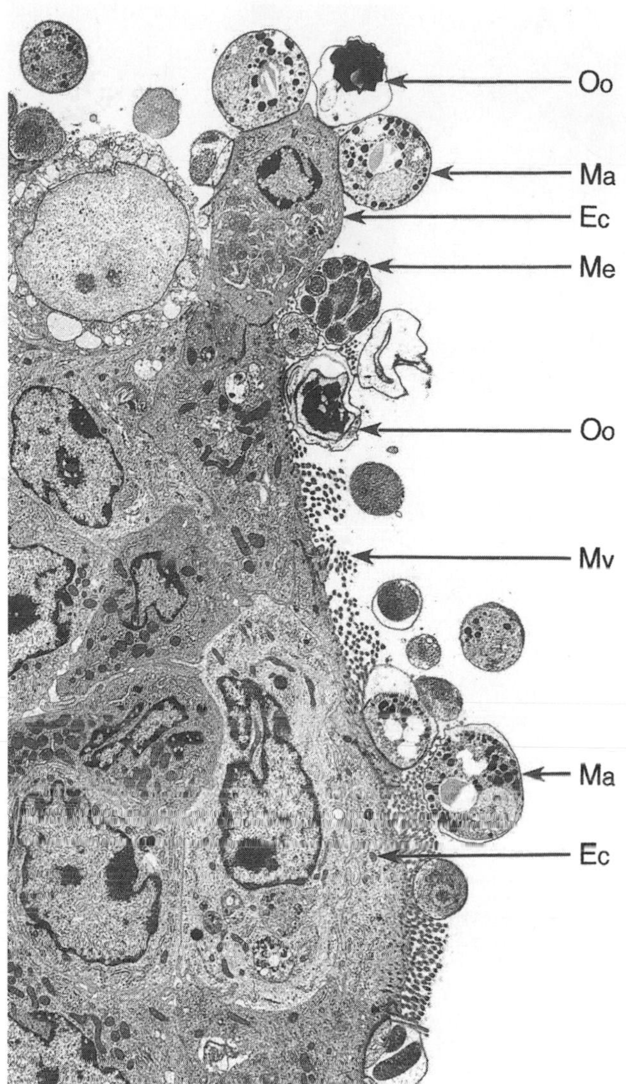

FIGURE 12.6 *C. parvum* in the small intestine of a calf as seen in a low power TEM. Endogenous stages protrude from the lumenal surface of the enterocytes. *Abbreviations:* Gc—goblet cell; Ma—macrogamaont, Mg—microgamont, Oo—oocyst, Sz—meront (schizont), Tz—early meront (trophozoite). [Courtesy of Dr. Harley Moon, National Animal Disease Center, ARS, USDA, Ames, Iowa.]

The endogenous stages in the intestinal tract are nearly spherical ranging in size from 4.0 μm to 6.9 μm in diameter (Figs. 12.6 and 12.7). Merozoites range in size from 3.6 $\times$ 1.1 μm to 5.0 $\times$ 1.1 μm. Microgametes are 1.7 μm in length.

At the EM level, the zoites of *Cryptosporidium* show some of the elements of the apical complex such as an electron dense collar similar to a conoid, micronemes, and electron-dense bodies that may be similar to rhoptries. Two apical rings can also be seen at the tip of the zoite. The pellicle is similar to that of other apicomplexans, and subpellicular tubules are present. They lack a true conoid, perhaps rhoptries, mitochondria, and a cytostome (micropore) (Fig. 12.8).

Life Cycle

C. parvum will serve as a model life cycle for this genus (Fig 12.9). The developing stages remain at the luminal surface of the enterocytes, but they are covered by the plasma membrane of the host cell; thus, they are spoken of as being intracellular but extracytoplasmic.

Type I meronts produce six to eight merozoites, which, in turn, invade epithelial cells and form the Type II meront. Four merozoites are produced by the Type II meront. Unlike other intestinal coccidia, *C. parvum* asexual stages have flexibility in their sequence of stages. Type I merozoites can either go to a Type II meront or return to form another generation of Type I. Type II meronts produce merozoites, which probably enter gamogony.

Upon fertilization, the oocyst is formed and sporulation takes place while it is still in the tissue. The oocyst may either pass out with the feces or excyst in the intestine and recommence infection.

The life cycle of *C. baileyi* of the chicken varies somewhat from the preceding description. It has three types of meronts and two types of oocysts. The thin-walled oocyst probably excysts in the intestine and reinitiates infection while the thick-walled oocyst passes out with the feces.

The prepatent period in experimental or accidental infections with *C. parvum* varies from 2 to 14 days in various animal hosts and from 5 to 28 days in humans. The patent period in domestic and companion animals varies from one day to two to four weeks. In humans, the patent period ranges from 18 to 31 days, but oocysts have been found in the feces up to three months later.

Diagnosis

Determining whether a host is affected by cryptosporidiosis is based on the following:

1. Observing typical clinical signs and symptoms
2. Finding the oocysts in the feces
3. Conducting serological tests that show antibodies

In a host showing a watery diarrhea, cryptosporidiosis should be suspected, but other infectious agents and some noninfectious processes can also cause such a condition. Even finding that *Cryptosporidium* is present does not necessarily mean that it is the cause of the disease; it may only be incidental or a minor contributing factor to the disease.

The clinical features seen in immunologically normal persons with cryptosporidiosis are diarrhea (73%),

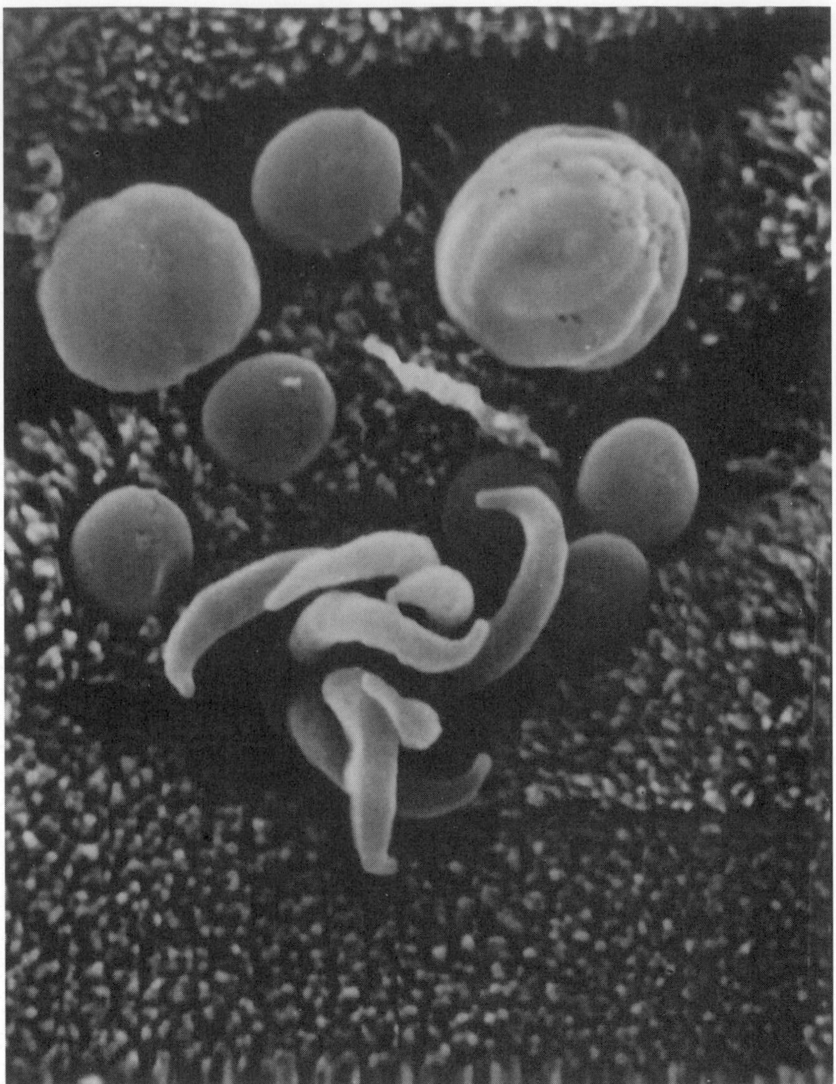

FIGURE 12.7 *Cryptosporidium* developing in the brush border of intestinal cells as seen in SEM. The smaller spherical bodies are developing meronts. The body at the upper right shows a meront with merozoites showing through the outer limiting membrane. At the lower portion of the picture are eight merozoites escaping from a meront. [From Dubey, J. P., Speer, C. A., and Fayer, R., 1990.]

abdominal pain (55%), vomition, nausea, not eating (29%), fever (22%), fatigue and so on (24%), respiratory problems (3%). Persons with immunodeficiencies, of whatever ilk, have about the same clinical signs, but respiratory problems appear more often (11–20%) than in normal persons.

The best method of diagnosis is finding oocysts in the feces of a person or animal showing diarrhea. The three principal methods are the following:

1. Stained fecal smear
2. Detection of antibodies expressed by oocysts
3. Fecal flotation

Large numbers of oocysts are shed in the feces during the clinical phase of the infection. A smear is made on a microscope slide, stained with an acid-fast stain such as is used to identify *Mycobacteria* spp., and then the red oocysts are looked for under a compound microscope (see color plate).

A number of commercial kits are available that are based on immunofluorescence or enzyme immunoassays. Such tests can be used on feces or on material collected by filtering suspect waters, but the results are the same being based on showing antigens in the oocysts. The tests are good for showing *C. parvum*, but with some there is a significant percentage of false positives where other species of *Cryptosporidium* are present.

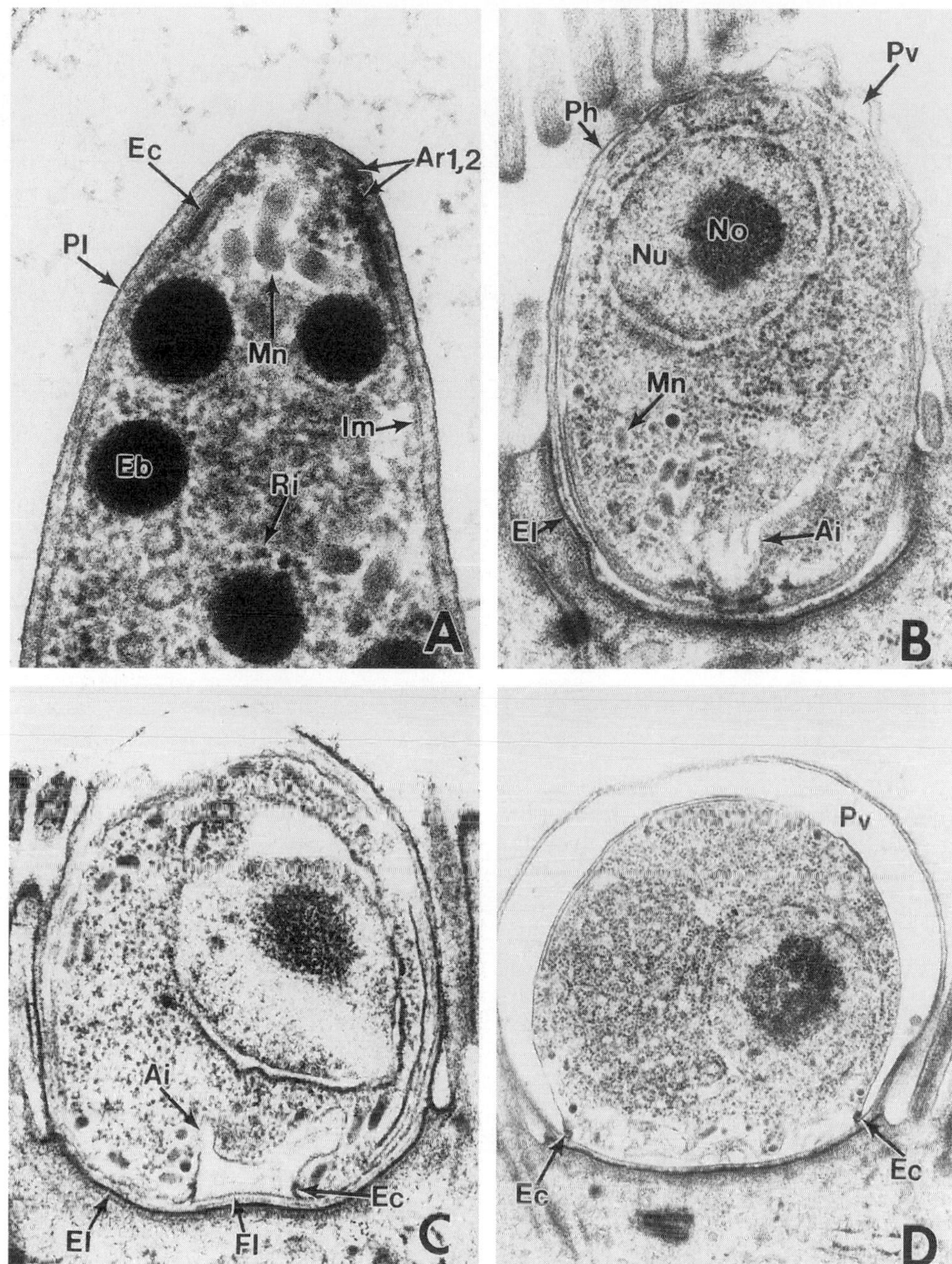

FIGURE 12.8 Transmission electron micrographs of *Cryptosporidium parvum* developing in enterocytes. (A) The apical complex shows anterior rings (Ar 1, 2), electron-dense bodies (Eb), an electron-dense collar, the inner membrane of the pellicle (lm), micronemes (mn), the plasmalemma of the pellicle I (PI). Ribosomes (Ri) can also be seen. (B) A merozoite in an early stage of attachment to its host cell and forming a meront. There is an anterior invagination (Ai), an electron-dense layer of the attachment zone (El). The nucleus (Nu), nucleolus (No), plasmalemma of the host cell (Ph), a newly formed parasitophorous vacuole (Pv), and micronemes (Mn) can be seen. (C) A slightly more advanced stage of attachment. There is an enlarged anterior invagination (Ai), an electron-dense collar (Ec), a fibrous layer (Fl) of the attachment organelle. (D) A meront (trophozoite) showing the electron-dense collar (Ec) at the margin of the attachment organelle. The fully developed parasitophorous vacuole (Pv) is readily seen. [From Dubey, et al., 1990.]

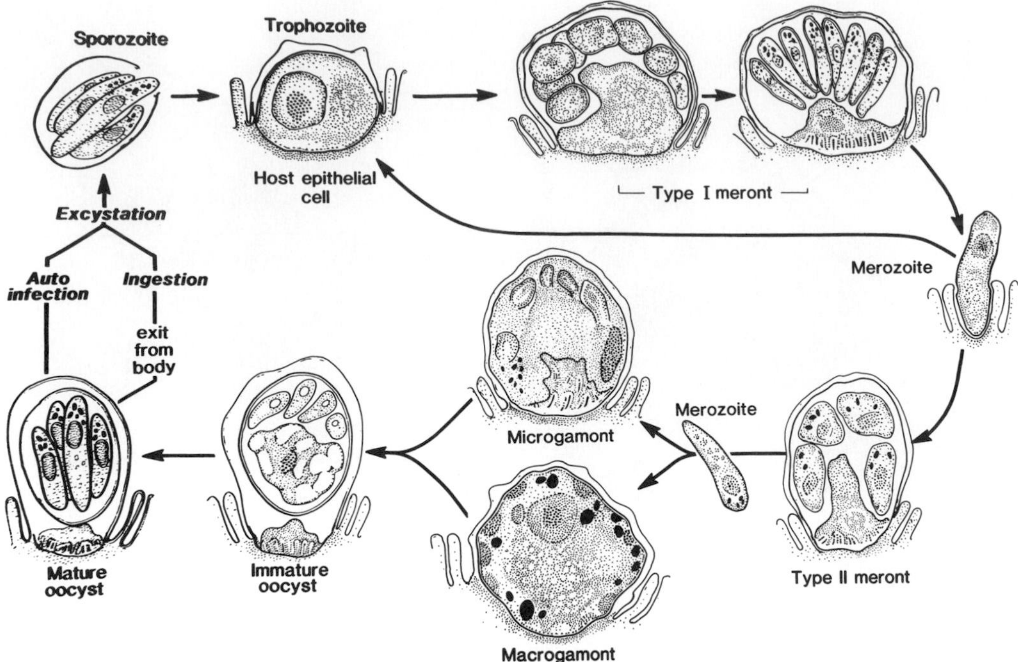

FIGURE 12.9 Life cycle of *Cryptosporidium.* [From Dubey, et al., 1990.]

Flotation techniques use a solution with a high specific gravity (sp.g. 1.18 to 1.27) in which protistan cysts or helminth eggs in the feces rise to the surface. Of the various flotation media, Sheather's sugar is the preferred one for *Cryptosporidium* oocysts. Since the oocysts are quite small, about 5 μm in diameter, one looks for them under a 40× objective. Phase-contrast or Nomarski interference contrast objectives are preferred.

In some instances, it may be necessary to perform a biopsy of host intestine to see whether endogenous stages are present. Tissue from the colon may be taken, fixed, and then stained with H & E and examined under a compound microscope. The various stages protrude slightly from the luminal tips of the enterocytes and, while small, may readily be seen (Fig. 12.6).

Since *Cryptosporidium* often develops in the respiratory system, one can look for oocysts in sputum or tracheal washings either directly or after concentration by flotation.

Circulating antibodies are found in the blood of normal persons following infection, and they may be present in detectable amounts for a year or more after infection. While seroantibodies are not useful in determining whether an active infection is present, they are useful in determining whether an individual or a population has experienced infection. A variety of techniques have been developed including ELISA and indirect immunofluorescent antibody tests.

Host–Parasite Interactions

The association of *Cryptosporidium* with its host cells has presented investigators with a challenge. In early studies, it was thought that the organisms merely sank into the brush border of the enterocytes and remained extracellular. Using thin-sectioning methods for TEM, it is clear the organisms are covered by the plasma membrane of the host cell, but do not actually lie in the cytoplasm (Figs. 12.5 and 12.6). Like most other apicomplexans, they are contained in a parasitophorous vacuole.

There is an intimate association with the cytoplasm of the host cell and apparently the means by which the organism obtains nutrient. There is an electron dense collar which lies at the organism-cytoplasm interface, and in the center of it is a fibrous layer (Fig. 12.6).

Because of the superficial relationship to the host cell, the pathogenesis of *Cryptosporidium* has presented a puzzle, but studies at the LM, TEM, and SEM levels give some hints as to the changes that cryptosporidia bring about. The absorptive surface is reduced through shortening of the microvilli, or brush border, of the enterocytes, and through a shortening in and loss of the number of villi. Physiologic evidence points to a lowered ability of the gut to absorb nutrients. Despite these observations, much remains to be learned about the mechanism of damage caused by this organism.

Depending on the host and its ability to launch an immune response, *C. parvum* may invade a number of organ systems. In uncomplicated cryptosporidiosis, the lower part of the small intestine, the jejunum and ileum, are infected. In hosts that are immuno-compromised, the whole intestinal tract from esophagus to rectum may be invaded. When the gut is extensively affected, the adjuncts to the intestine, the liver and pancreas, may also be sites of endogenous stages. Additionally, stages may be found in the respiratory system and kidney.

Newborns are generally susceptible to *C. parvum* infections. Calves within the first few weeks of life and humans less than two years of age are typically affected, for example. Oddly enough, *C. muris* affects older cattle, but the disease is usually quite mild.

Cryptosporidiosis seems to occur most severely in connection with other infections. Certain enteric viruses seem to exacerbate the disease. What mechanisms are involved are not known.

C. parvum infections in HIV patients presents a difficult problem for the clinician. Immunity does not develop, and there are no satisfactory drugs to terminate the infection. A person with AIDS shows a profuse diarrhea the volume of which may approach 20 liters per day. This is approximately 20 kg or 40 pounds of liquid passed, nearly 10% of an average person's body weight. The physician must not only attempt to maintain the patient's normal body water but also to replace inorganic salts that are lost as well.

Epidemiology and Control

Control of cryptosporidiosis is based principally on the following:

1. Breaking contact between infected and uninfected individuals of the same species
2. Breaking contact between infected and uninfected individuals of different species
3. Maintaining clean water supplies
4. Administering drugs to infected persons

Since the oocyst is the infective stage of the life cycle, it is important to recognize the following:

1. Oocysts are infective when they are passed from the infected host
2. Oocysts survive a relatively long time in the environment
3. The organism has a broad host range
4. Oocysts may be mechanically spread by fish, amphibia, reptiles, and birds

A specific treatment for cryptosporidiosis in humans or other hosts is not available. Some drugs are in development, such as nitazoxanide and paromomycin, and may presage drugs that will treat the infection successfully. Treatment remains largely symptomatic: maintaining proper water and inorganic balance in the patient and attempting to control the profuse diarrhea.

Outbreaks of cryptosporidiosis in day care centers illustrates the way in which the organism may be spread in a primary group. Since infants are highly susceptible to infection, the introduction of a few organisms from some source may set off an infection in one child that spreads epidemically to others in the group. Adults caring for the children often develop cryptosporidiosis as well. Likewise, persons who care for or have contact with cattle have come down with cryptosporidiosis; companion animals such as dogs and cats are less likely to serve as a source of infection, but the possibility exists of passing the infection among human and other hosts where sanitary disposal of human waste is inadequate.

A number of urban outbreaks since 1984 have been documented (see "Geographic Distribution and Importance"). All of these outbreaks were traced to contaminated water supplies. Differences were evident in each case, but inadequate treatment of drinking water was found in each case.

Cryptosporidial oocysts can live at least for weeks and sometimes months. Freezing and drying are likely to kill *C. parvum* oocysts within hours. High temperature, 65° for 30 minutes, kills all oocysts , and 45°C. for 5 to 20 minutes kills some of them. Autoclaving is certain to kill oocysts. Hydrogen peroxide, chlorine-producing molecules, and ammonia-producing molecules seem to be the most effective chemosterilants. As it true with bacteria, surfaces cleaned with a good detergent become sterile of cryptosporidia because of washing away the organisms, not because of the killing power of the detergent. In sum, eliminating oocysts from the environment is at least difficult and may be impossible in many instances.

A further complication in control concerns the observation that a number of species of animals have been found to transport cryptosporidial oocysts and may deposit them in water supplies or perhaps may contaminate food. For example, when *C. parvum* oocysts were fed to geese, oocysts were found in the feces for as long as nine days. The oocysts were infective for, and caused disease, in laboratory mice. Various cold-blooded vertebrates harbored oocysts after experimental inoculation but did not become infected; the oocysts from their feces were infective for laboratory mice. The full significance of these studies is not clear, but an epidemiologic study or the structure of a control program should be influenced by the possibility that certain vertebrates may contribute to the spread of infection without themselves becoming infected.

The host range of *C. parvum* implies that human association with animals passes the infection back and forth among species that live closely together. People who work with cattle may contract infections from calves. Since there may be several million oocysts in a gram of feces (from whatever host), a little bit of fecal contamination may represent a heavy inoculum. Epidemics among infants in day care centers have proved to be difficult to control once the organism has been introduced. Day care workers must be especially careful not to transfer infection to other children or themselves. But given the hazards of changing diapers and the need to take care of a number of children, containing the infection may be nearly impossible.

A published list of 11 steps that can be taken to prevent cryptosporidiosis in calves revolves principally around cleanliness of the environment and taking precautions to prevent transfer of infection from one animal or group of animals to another. Since there is no specific treatment and no vaccine, prevention is the only approach. While these general principles were developed for domestic animals, they apply equally well to infections in humans. Methods of providing a sanitary environment are the best we have, but they still may be difficult to put into effective practice.

Readings

Current, W. L., and Garcia, L. S. (1991). Cryptosporidiosis. *Clin. Microbiol. Rev.* **43,** 325–358.

Dubey, J. P., Speer, C. A., and Fayer, R. (1990). *Cryptosporidiosis of Man and Animals.* CRC Press, Boca Raton, FL.

Duombo, O., Rossignol, J. F., Pichard, F., Traore, H. A., Dembele, M., Diakite, M., Troare, F., and Diallo, D. A. (1997). Nitazoxanide in the treatment of cryptosporidial diarrhea and other intestinal parasitic infections associated with acquired immunodeficiency syndrome in tropical Africa. *Am. J. Trop. Med. Hyg.* **56,** 637–639.

Fayer, R. (1997). *Cryptosporidiosis.* CRC Press, Boca Raton, FL.

Graczyk, T. K., Cranfield, M. R., and Fayer, R. (1996). Evaluation of commercial enzyme immunoassay (EIA) and immunofluorescent antibody (IFA) test kits for detection of *Cryptosporidium* oocysts of species other than *Cryptosporidium parvum. Am. J. Trop. Med. Hyg.* **54,** 274–279.

Hammond, D. M., and Long, P. L. (Eds.) (1973). *The Coccidia. Eimeria, Isospora, Toxoplasma, and Related Genera.* University Park Press, Baltimore.

Kirkpatrick, C. E., and Dubey, J. P. (1987). Enteric coccidial infections. In: *Vet. Clin. North Am., Small Anim. Practice* **17**(6), 1405–1420.

Levine, N. D., and Ivens, V. (1965). The coccidian parasites of rodents. *Illinois Biol. Monogr.* **33.** Univ. of Illinois Press, Urbana.

Levine, N. D., and Ivens, V. (1970). The coccidian parasites of ruminants. *Illinois Biol. Monogr.* **44.** Univ. of Illinois Press, Urbana.

Levine, N. D., and Ivens, V. (1981). The coccidian parasites of carnivores. *Illinois Biol. Monogr.* **51.** Univ. of Illinois Press, Urbana.

Levine, N. D., and Ivens, V. (1986). The coccidian parasites of Artiodactyla. *Illinois Biol. Monogr.* **55.** Univ. of Illinois Press, Urbana.

Lindsay, D. S., Dubey, J. P., and Blagburn, B. L. (1997). Biology of *Isospora* spp. from humans, nonhuman primates, and domestic animals. *Clin. Microbiol. Rev.* **10,** 19–34.

Long, P. L. (Ed.) (1982). *The Biology of the Coccidia.* University Park Press, Baltimore.

Long, P. L. (Ed.) (1990). *Coccidiosis of Man and Domestic Animals.* CRC Press, Boca Raton, FL.

McDougald, L. R. (1997). In *Diseases of Poultry* (B. W. Calnek, Ed.), 10th ed. Iowa State Univ. Press, Ames.

Nyberg, P. A., and Hammond, D. M. (1967). Description of the sporulated oocysts and sporozoites of four species of bovine coccidia. *J. Parasitol.* **51,** 669–673.

Ortega, Y. R., Sterling, C. R., Gilman, R. H., Cama, V. A., and Diaz, F. (1993). *Cyclospora* species—A new protozoan pathogen of humans. *N. Engl. J. Med.* **328,** 1308–1312.

Ortega, Y. R., Gilman, R. H., and Sterling, C. R. (1994). A new coccidian parasite (Apicomplexa: Eimeriidae) from humans. *J. Parasitol.* **80,** 625–629.

Peiniazek, N. J., and Hewrwaldt, B. L. (1997). Reevaluating the molecular taxonomy: Is human-associated *Cyclospora* a mammalian *Eimeria* species? *Emerging Infect. Dis.* **3,** 381–383.

Petersen, C. (1993). Cellular biology of *Cryptosporidium parvum. Parasitol. Today* **9,** 87–91.

Reid, M. W., and Long, P. L. (1979). A diagnostic chart for nine species of fowl coccidia. Univ. of Georgia, Col. of Agric., Exp. Stat. Res. Rep., Athens.

Webster, K. A. (1993). Molecular methods for the detection and classification of *Cryptosporidium. Parasitol. Today* **9,** 87–91.

CHAPTER

13

The Extraintestinal Coccidia

The extraintestinal or tissue coccidia comprise a large group of organisms that are important to both human and animal health. New species are continually being described, and determining the identities and life cycles of those that are known has been a laborious and slow process. These organisms have so-called isosporoid oocysts because their oocysts have 2 sporocysts, each of which has 4 sporozoites (Fig. 13.1), similar to those of the genus *Isospora.* The sporocysts of various species are nearly identical to one another and therefore impossible to use in identification, unlike most of the intestinal coccidia in which the oocyst of a species is often readily characterized and identified. The cysts in extraintestinal tissue (Fig. 13.2 and 13.15) are often characteristic for a species and can be used for identification, or at least can be used in ruling out the presence of a particular species.

The life cycles of the tissue coccidia involve two hosts, usually a carnivore and an herbivore. The life cycle of *Toxoplasma* can be completed in one host, the cat, and its alternate (intermediate) hosts are not mandatory. Others, such as *Sarcocystis,* have two hosts in their life cycles and both are obligate. The hosts required to complete the life cycle are crucial in the identification of known species and the description of new species. Thus, identification of species relies on a microscopic examination (often at the EM level) of infected tissues and developmental stages, and in completing the life cycle in another host.

The terminology in describing the life cycle of a tissue coccidium is the same as that used in helminth life cycles. The definitive host is the one in which sexual reproduction takes place. Asexual reproduction takes place in the intermediate host. In nearly all instances, the definitive host is a carnivore or omnivore, and sexual reproduction occurs in the intestinal tract of the host. In the intermediate host, nearly always an herbivore, asexual reproduction takes place in small blood vessels, the liver, and in muscle or brain cells.

The typical pattern of development in the intermediate host is that of one to two generations of merogony before the organism enters a specific type of cell for its final generation of development. The early merogonous generations are referred to as *metrocytes* or mother cells and they produce tachyzoites ("tachy-" means fast) (Fig. 13.3A). The metrocytes multiply rapidly by endodyogeny, a process in which the organelles of the mother cell dedifferentiate and two daughter cells form within the body of the mother (Fig. 13.4). When the merozoites reach their final site, such as striated muscle cells in the case of *Sarcocystis*, there is a shift from the metrocyte/tachyzoite to the bradyzoite ("brady-" means slow) or slowly reproducing form (Fig. 13.3B). Multiplication by endodyogeny continues in the myocytes perhaps for many months, or years in some species.

As a general rule, there is greater host specificity in the definitive host than in the intermediate host, for any one species.

TOXOPLASMA AND TOXOPLASMOSIS

Name of Organism and Disease Associations

Toxoplasma gondii causes toxoplasmosis. Only a single species had been accepted until 1977 when Levine

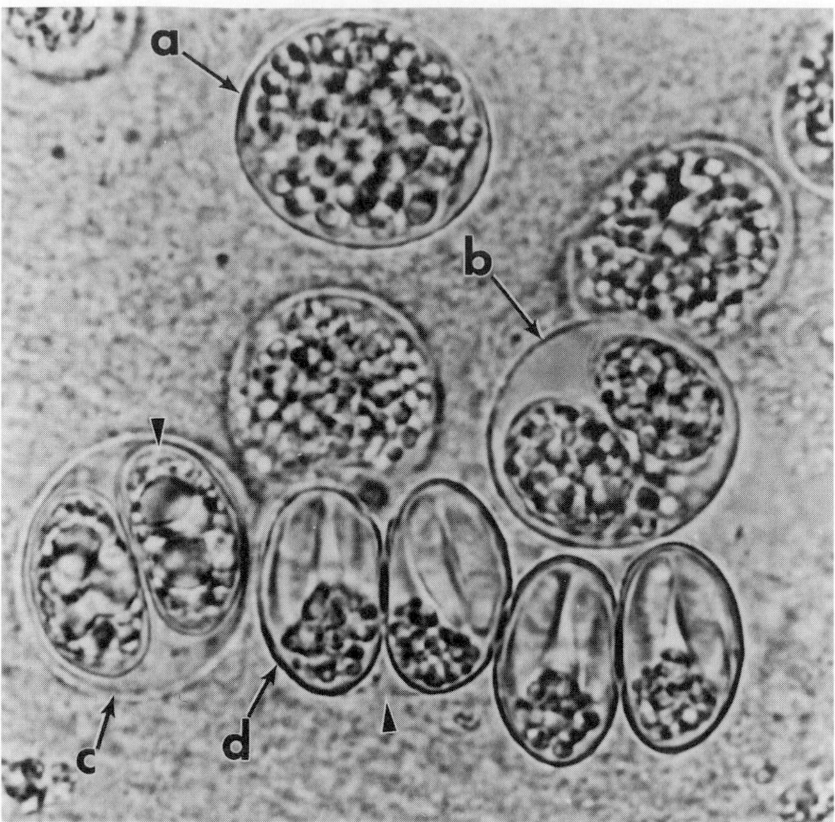

FIGURE 13.1 Isosporoid oocysts and sporocysts of *Sarcocystis cruzi* of the ox as seen in LM. Normally only sporocysts are seen in the feces of the definitive host, but these were taken from an experimentally infected coyote. (a) unsporulated oocyst, (b) formation of two sporoblasts, (c) sporocysts with their outer walls formed, but no sporozoites have yet formed, arrowhead at the nucleus of one sporocyst, (d) fully sporulated oocyst with two sporocysts each of which has four sporozoites and a mass of granules called the sporocyst residuum. [From Dubey, J. P., et al., 1989.]

divided the genus into 7 species. *T. gondii* is the species of most importance.

Toxoplasma hammondi is a closely related species that was originally placed in a new genus, *Hammondia,* but not all investigators accept this generic designation. The primary difference between *T. gondii* and *T. hammondi* is that the former has a facultative intermediate host and the latter has an obligate intermediate host. The difference of opinion revolves around whether this is sufficient to erect a separate genus.

Hosts and Host Range

About 200 species of mammals and birds have been found to be infected with the meronts or extraintestinal tissue stages of *T. gondii.* This wide array of hosts represents the facultative intermediate hosts of this organism.

The definitive host of most importance is the domestic cat, *Felis catus* (Fig. 13.5), but other felids are also infected. Some of the definitive hosts that have been shown to discharge oocysts are the mountain lion (puma, cougar, catamount,) (*Felis concolor*), ocelot (*F. pardalis*), margay (*F. wiedii*), jaguarundi (*F. jagouroundi*), bobcat (*Lynx rufus*) and the Bengal tiger (*F. bengalis*).

Geographic Distribution and Importance

T. gondii is a cosmopolitan organism that is found in all human communities except for a few isolated locales. The prevalence of infection in the human population ranges up to 90% as measured by serology (see Diagnosis). The greater prevalences are usually seen in warm, moist climates as opposed to cold, dry climates. For many years it was stated that the prevalence of infection in North America and Western Europe was about one-third of the adult population, but recent data indicate that more than half of the human population have been infected in those areas. About 47% of Africans show antibodies to *T. gondii.* In general, the

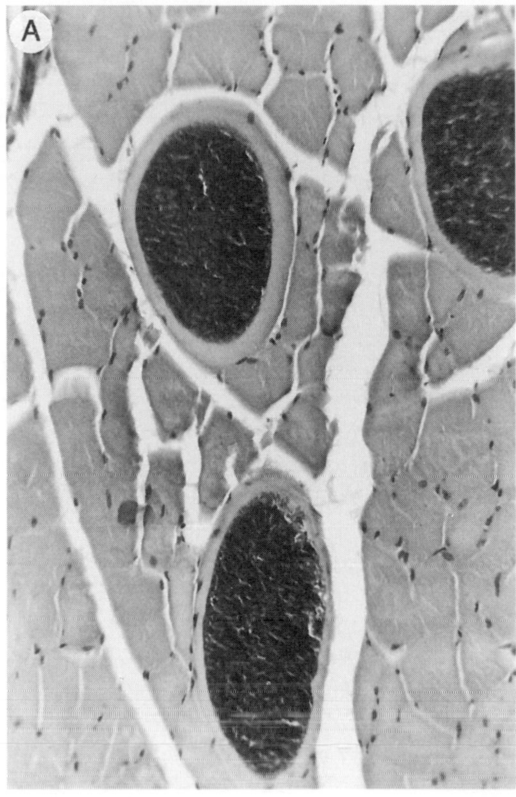

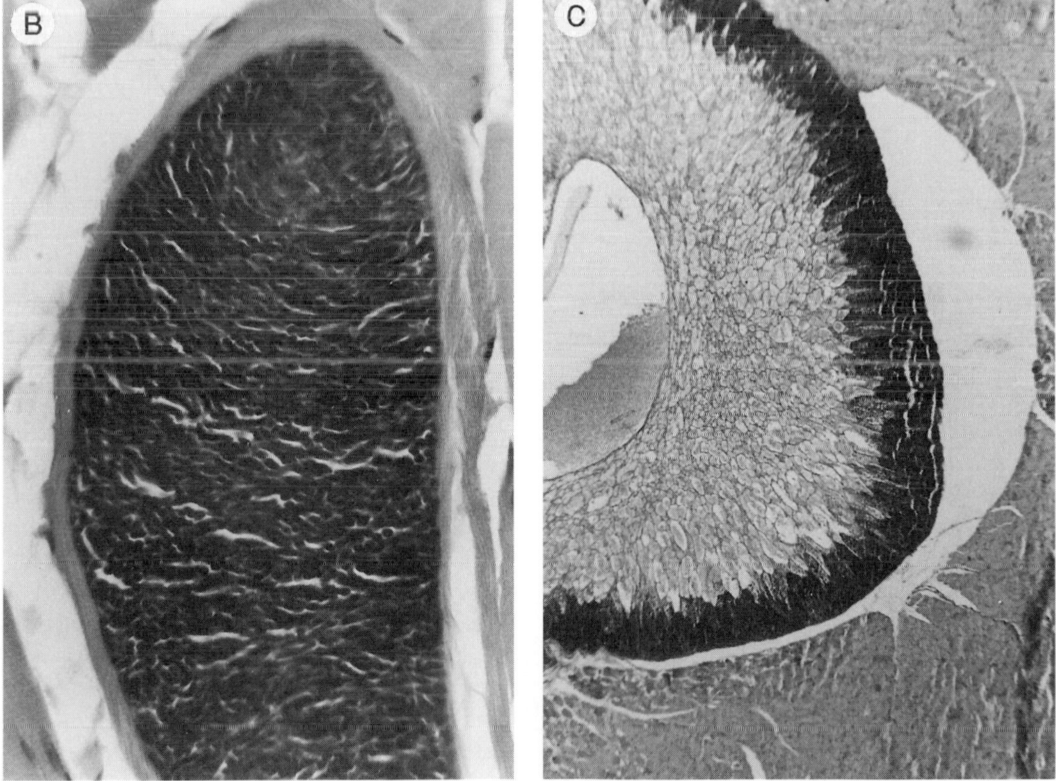

FIGURE 13.2 Sarcocysts of *Sarcocystis* spp. as seen in LM. Note that sizes vary as well as does the thickness (A and C) of the wall of the sarcocyst. In one shown here (C) there are septa partitioning the cyst and living zoites are found only at the margins of such a sarcocyst.

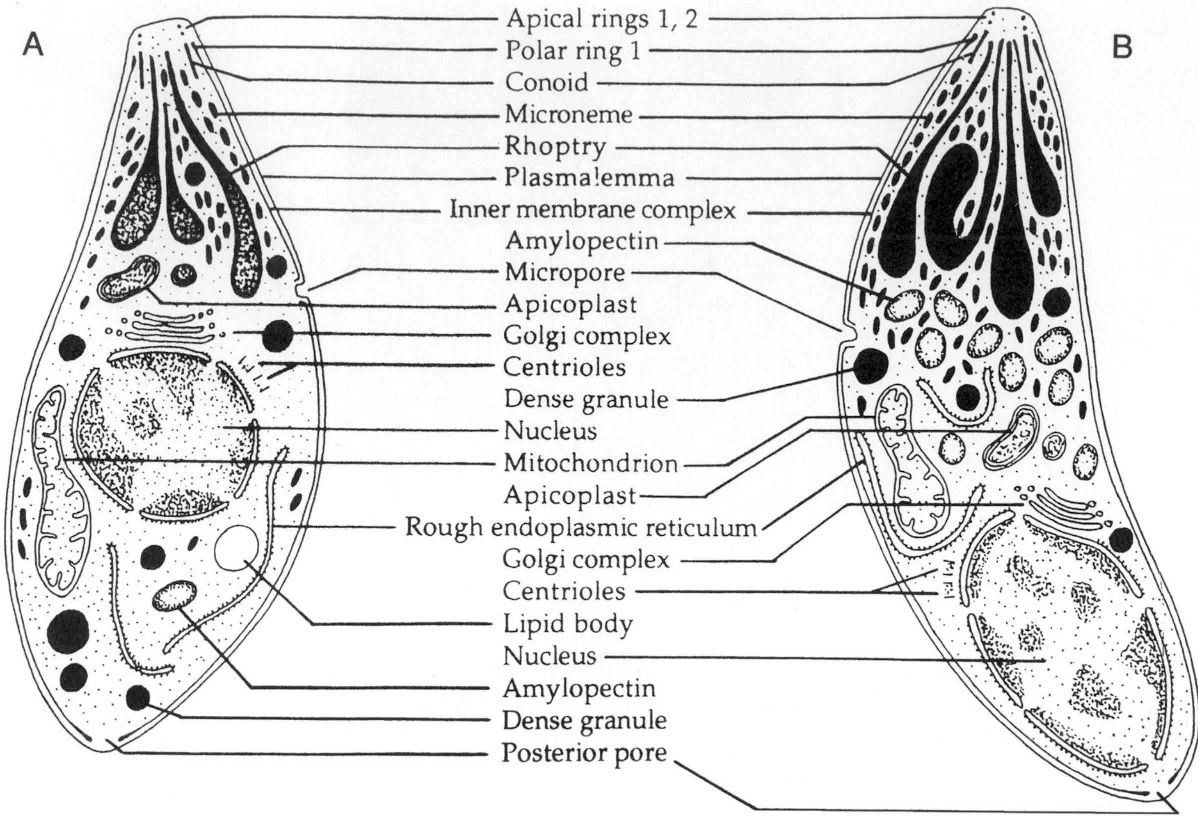

FIGURE 13.3 Comparison of a metrocyte (A) and a bradyzoite (B) of a tissue coccidium such as *Toxoplasma* or *Sarcocystis*. [From Dubey, J. P., et al, 1998.]

prevalence of infection in the human population rises with age so that peak percentages are seen in individuals 35 years of age and older.

Only about 1% of persons showing antibody to *T. gondii* have signs or symptoms of the disease. This observation is in keeping with nearly all infectious diseases in which a large proportion of the population may be infected, but only a small percentage shows clinical signs or symptoms. Having said that, it is important to recognize that clinical toxoplasmosis takes a serious toll on human health in the form of abortion, congenital defects in children, blindness, and both acute and chronic disease. In children who have been infected prenatally there are effects on the eyes and central nervous system that have long-term consequences. It has been estimated that the U.S. society bears an annual burden of from $400 million to $8.8 billion (1994 dollars) in caring for affected children.

Morphology

The sporulated oocyst has a thin outer wall and two sporocysts each having four sporozoites (Fig 13.5). The oocysts average 13×12 μm with a range of 12 to 15 × 10 to 13 μm. Sporocysts are 9×6.5 μm with a range of 6 to 10 × 6 to 8 μm. The sporozoites are 8×2 μm. At the EM level, it can be seen that the outer wall is further covered by a thin veil of unknown origin (Fig. 13.6), and that the oocyst wall has three layers (Fig. 13.7). The sporocyst walls are composed of four plates with sutures that break down when excystation of the sporozoites begins to occur (Fig. 13.8). In TEM, the plates have lip-like structures that extend toward the inner part of the sporocyst (Fig. 13.7). A micropyle can be seen on the surface of some sporocysts in favorable preparations (Fig. 13.6, upper left).

Five different merogonous generations have been described in the intestine of the cat. The meronts are designated as Types A through E and differ in their structure, mode of reproduction, and time of appearance after experimental infection (Fig. 13.9). Even compared to other species of coccidia, the endogenous stages of *T. gondii* are small; the details of their structure and number of merozoites are therefore quite tedious to work out. Also, there is overlap among the times when the generations are seen, and it is uncertain how these stages actually succeed one another. For example, Types D and E may both give rise to gamonts.

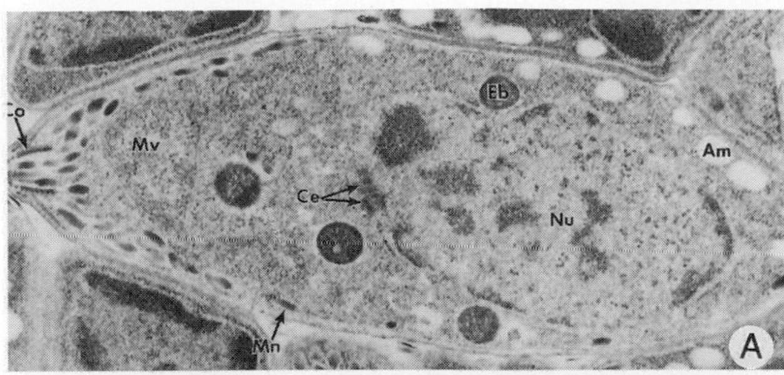

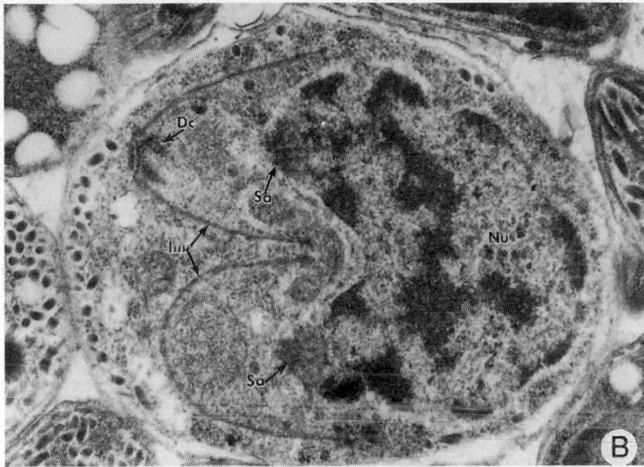

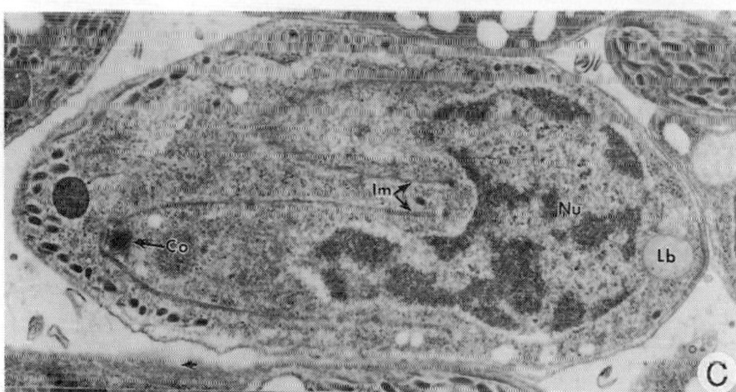

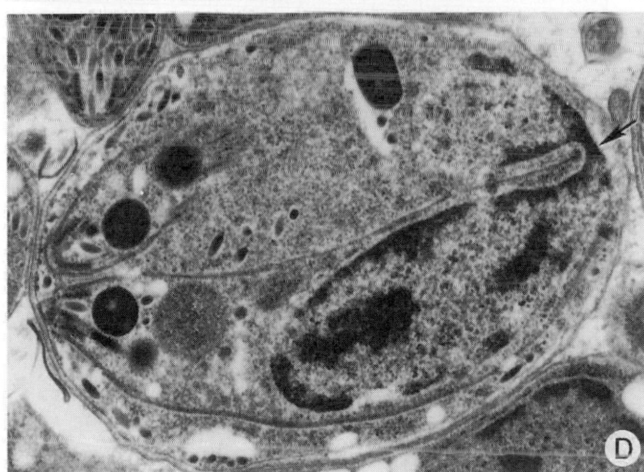

Life Cycle

The cat becomes infected through ingesting sporulated oocysts or sporocysts (Fig. 13.1). The sporozoites excyst in the small intestine and invade (Fig. 13.10) the epithelial cells (enterocytes) of the middle part (jejunum) of the small intestine. After asexual reproduction has been completed, gamonts form and oocysts are produced at 20 to 24 days. Oocyst production on initial infection extends over about 8 days. Sporulation of the oocysts occurs on the ground and sporulation takes place in 1 to 5 days, depending on temperature.

The cat also becomes infected through ingesting tissue cysts from a mouse. If tachyzoites are present, oocysts appear in the feces in 5 to 10 days. If bradyzoites are present, oocysts appear in 3 to 5 days. The implication is that there are additional merogonous generations after ingestion of tachyzoites, but only sexual development after ingestion of bradyzoites.

Interestingly, infection in the cat is not restricted to the intestine. The organisms leave the gut and multiply as tachyzoites in various tissues. The infection may remain in the cat in both the intestinal and other tissues for many months.

As indicated earlier, a wide range of mammals and birds serve as intermediate hosts of *T. gondii* (Fig. 13.9), and it is important to note again that sexual stages are seen only in the cat. When a rodent, or other susceptible intermediate host such as a human, ingests oocysts of *T. gondii*, the organisms excyst in the intestine, but leave it and develop in other tissues: lymph nodes, brain, eye, somatic muscle, diaphragm, and reproductive organs.

In the intermediate host, the meronts first develop quickly and produce tachyzoites. About 16 merozoites are formed by endodyogeny in each infected cell. The meronts containing tachyzoites are set off from the host cell only by a parasitophorous vacuole. After this acute infection is completed, meronts that form

FIGURE 13.4 Metrocytes in the process of endodyogeny in *Sarcocystis singaporensis* of the Norway rat, *Rattus norvegicus*. TEM photographs at 18,000 X magnification. (A) A metrocyte in an early stage of endodyogeny. A pair of centrioles (Ce) lie at the anterior margin of the nucleus of the parasite. There is a conoid (Co) and a few scattered micronemes. (B) Division of the nucleus (Nu) and the formation of two daughter zoites has begun. The apical complex (Dc) has begun to form. (C) A further stage in the formation of daughter cells with the conoid (Co) of one cell clearly visible. (D) The daughter cells are completely formed except for a slim band of cytoplasm at the posterior end (arrow). The structures of the daughter cells have formed and the organelles of the metrocyte have almost completely disappeared. [From Dubey, J. P., et al., 1989.]

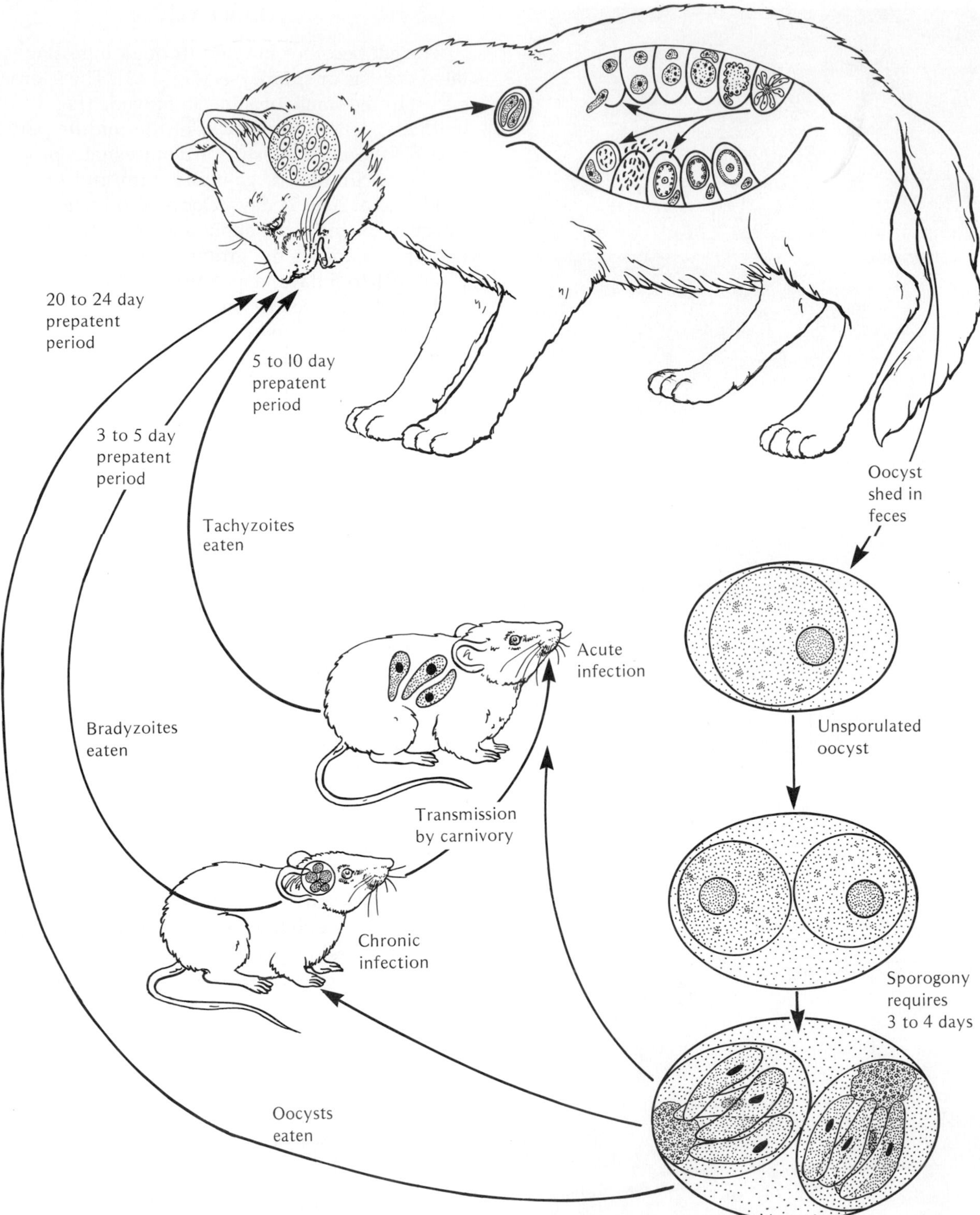

FIGURE 13.5 Diagram of the life cycle of *Toxoplasma gondii*. The normal hosts of *T. gondii* are cats and mice or other small rodents.

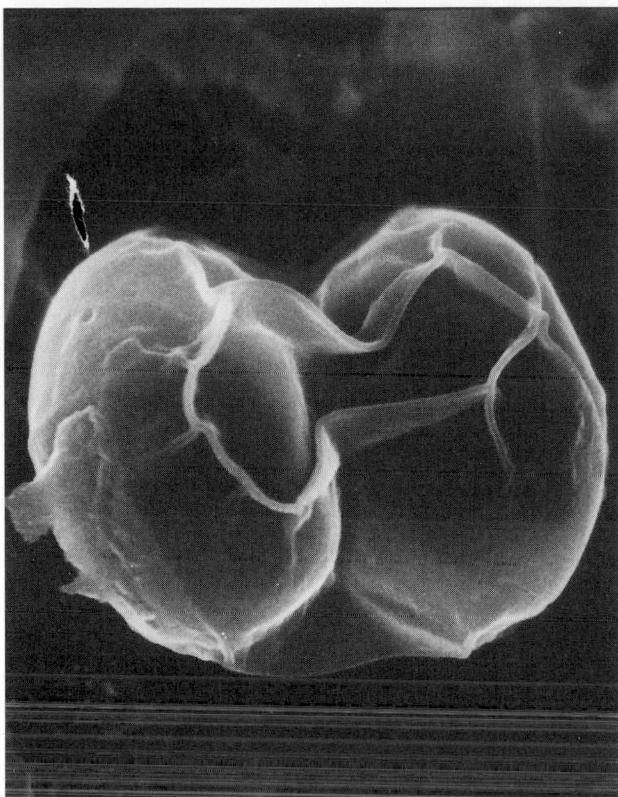

FIGURE 13.6 An oocyst of *Toxoplasma gondii* as seen in SEM. A thin "veil" covers the oocyst wall itself, which is thin and flexible. [From: Speer, Clark, and Dubey, 1998a.]

bradyzoites are seen. This meront is set off from the host cell by a distinct membrane and is referred to as a *tissue cyst* (see Fig. 13.15, presented later). Unless immunity in the host wanes, the bradyzoites are retained in the tissue cyst for months and even years. The bradyzoites are most often the stage that is transferred back to the cat.

Diagnosis

The means of determining whether a host is infected with *T. gondii* is by the following:

1. Finding the oocysts in the feces
2. Finding the zoites in the tissues
3. Observing clinical signs and symptoms
4. Finding antibodies in the blood

Only cats, many species in the family Felidae, serve as the definitive hosts of *T. gondii* and therefore are the only species that shed oocysts in the feces. Various concentration methods can be used to find oocysts, but those that are preferred use flotation of a water suspension of feces in a medium of high specific gravity such as sucrose or an inorganic salt (NaCl, ZnCl). Since cats shed oocysts for only about a week at a time, the probability of finding an infection is relatively low.

Zoites may occur in a number of tissues and these may be found either by direct or indirect means. Direct means involves digestion of tissues and looking for the zoites under a compound microscope after centrifugal concentration or by taking tissues for histologic examination at the LM level.

Indirect techniques involve blind passage of tissues in laboratory mice and looking for the zoites by the methods briefly described in the paragraph above. Tissues are fed to mice or injected parenterally and the zoites looked for a week or two later at postmortem examination.

Clinical signs and symptoms pertain almost exclusively to toxoplasmosis in the human host. In the newborn child, there may be hydrocephalus, partial or complete blindness and other neurological signs of infection. Even in a child with asymptomic infection, eye problems may arise several years later.

In the adult, infection often is manifested as a vague flu-like disease in which the lymph nodes are enlarged. As in African trypanosomosis, the posterior cervical lymph nodes are often enlarged (Fig. 3.8). These infections may persist for many months with the individual having fever, lassitude, headache, and other nondescript indications of infection.

The presence of *T. gondii* antibody in the blood is the usual sign that a physician looks for when suspecting toxoplasmosis. Serology is also used extensively in epidemiologic investigations where an investigator may be looking at broad patterns of infection in a population of humans or other hosts.

The following tests are in use:

1. Dye Test. DT. This is the Sabin-Feldman Dye Test, which was developed many years ago.
2. Indirect Hemagglutination Test. IHA.
3. Complement Fixation Test. CF.
4. Modified Agglutination Test. MAT.
5. Latex Agglutination Test. LA.
6. Indirect Fluorescent Antibody Test. IFA.
7. Enzyme-Linked Immunoabsorbent Assay. ELISA.
8. Immunoglobulin M Immunoabsorbent Agglutination Test. IgM-ISAGA.

The Dye Test has proven to be reliable and accurate in a range of hosts and is the preferred test in most circumstances. Each of the others may have certain advantages and all except the DT are available in kit form. The ELISA test can be automated and used in a large, central laboratory.

The disadvantage of the DT, despite its reliabililty, is that it uses living, infective zoites and it requires expertise in both the procedure and the reading of

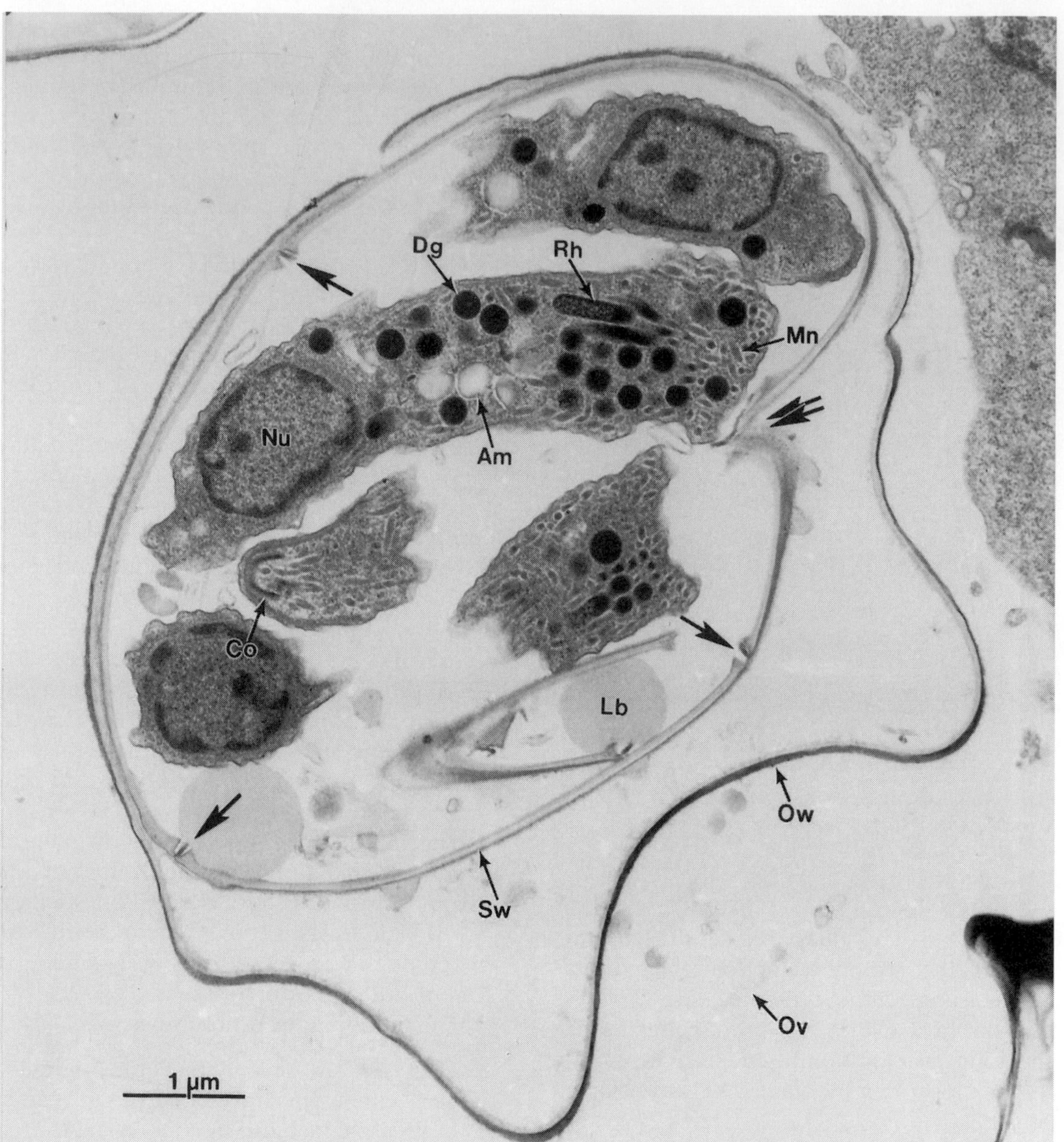

FIGURE 13.7 An oocyst of *Toxoplasma gondii* as seen in TEM. Both the oocyst wall and the sporocyst wall are three layered; joints in the plates of the sporocysts have lip-like structures that extend into the sporocyst. Abbreviations: Am, amyloid bodies; Dg, dark granule; Lb, lipid body; Mn, microneme; Sw, sporocyst wall; Ow, oocyst wall; Ov, oocyst veil; arrows, joints in the plates of the sporocyst. [From Speer, Clark, and Dubey, 1998b.]

the results. In performing the test, living tachyzoites, complement and the test serum are incubated at 37°C and then methylene blue is added. The living zoites are stained uniformly, but those that have been killed by immune serum lack cytoplasm and are seen as "ghosts." The proportion of living and dead zoites is determined and expressed as a titer. Thus, a dilution of the serum 1/16 in which 50% of the zoites are dead is given as a positive titer at 1/16. The higher the dilution at which 50% of the zoites are dead, the higher the level of antibody in the blood.

Host–Parasite Interactions

Among persons who become infected with *T gondii*, only a small percentage show clinical signs or symptoms of infection. It is estimated that perhaps 1% of those infected become ill. The prevalence of antibody

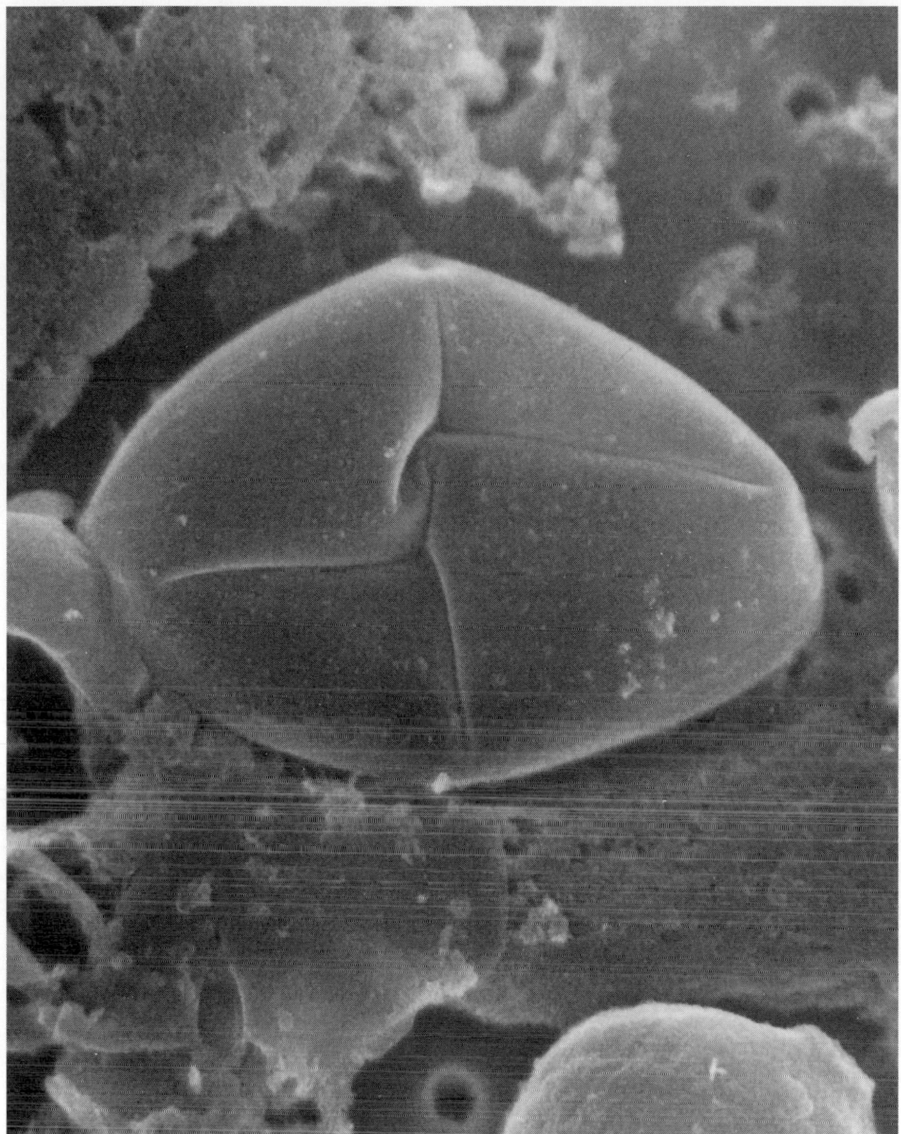

FIGURE 13.8 A sporocyst of *Toxoplasma gondii* as seen in SEM. Four plates make up the covering of the sporocyst; in this instance, excystation has just begun and the plates have curled slightly making the sutures between the plates visible. [From Speer, Clark, and Dubey, 1998b.]

in the human population does not represent the level of disease merely that this proportion of the population has responded to the agent.

The host is damaged by *T. gondii* by destruction of cells in which the meronts grow and by hypersensitivity to the organism. *T. gondii* does not produce a toxin. A tissue infected with *T. gondii* undergoes necrosis in direct proportion to the number of organisms multiplying in it. Thus, intestinal tissue, lymph nodes, or the brain may have lesser or greater damage depending on the number of organisms in them. In many instances, bradyzoites are an incidental finding in tissues taken routinely at postmortem examination. There is often little or no cellular response around the tissue cyst.

The most important infections in humans are those occurring in the developing fetus. The results of these infections range from quite mild to fatal. For example, 33% suffer from severe mental retardation, 53% moderate visual impairment, 23% slight mental retardation, 20% are cross-eyed, and 10% have hearing loss in one ear. Even children with only mild signs of toxoplasmosis at birth are likely to suffer further impairment as they mature.

In severely affected infants, the infection is dissem-

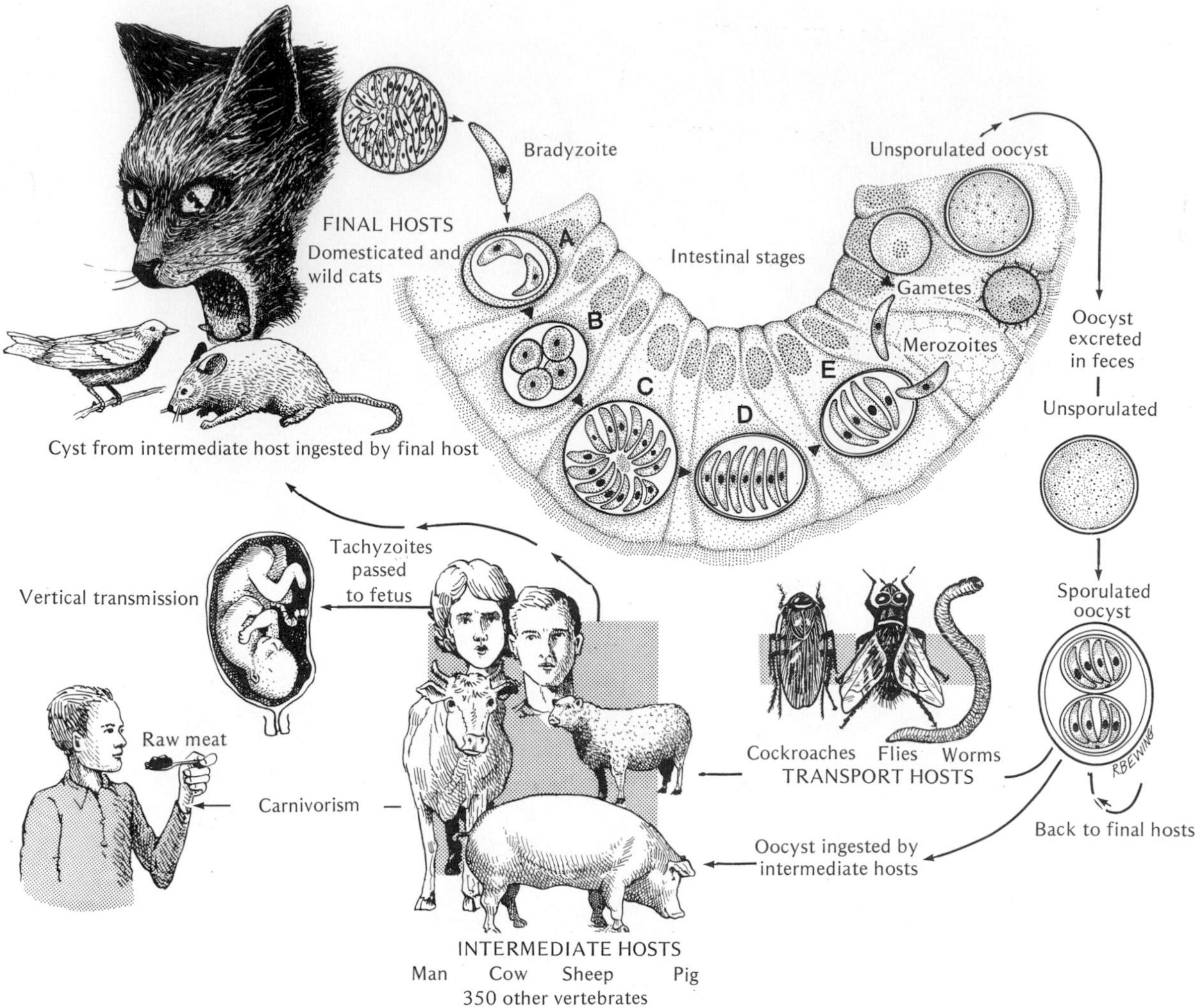

FIGURE 13.9. Life cycle and modes of transmission of *T. gondii.* [Courtesy of Agricultural Research Service, Beltsville, Maryland.]

inated widely in the tissues, but as the child gains ability to produce its own antibodies, the infection is likely to be controlled; however the infection may proceed in the central nervous system and the eye. Hydrocephalus is sometimes the result of prenatal infection of the central nervous system. This enlargement of the cranium is caused by blocking of the drainage system in the ventricles of the brain by cellular debris.

Acquired infections in humans take place after birth and result from the ingestion of infective oocysts or tissues infected with bradyzoites. Early in the infection, enterocytes and lymph nodes are commonly affected. The infection then spreads to other tissues such as somatic and cardiac muscle, nervous tissue, liver, pancreas, lymph nodes, and other organs. These types of infections show generalized signs and symptoms typical of a number of kinds of infection: fever, lassitude, headache, muscle and joint pain, and skin rash (seldom). As indicated earlier (Diagnosis), the posterior cervical (neck) lymph nodes are often enlarged. The disease may persist for weeks or months, or in a few cases years, before being controlled naturally or by chemotherapy.

Infections in humans that have been controlled by natural immunity may remain latent for many months or even years, because the thin-walled cysts containing bradyzoites are resistant to the effects of immunity. This is especially true in tissues such as the brain or eye that are somewhat removed from the immune response. When immunity wanes either naturally or through administering of certain drugs, the zoites become active and begin to multiply. Toxoplasmosis represents a difficult clinical problem in persons with AIDS, those who undergo chemotherapy for cancer, or those taking a corticosteroid drug for an inflammatory or autoimmune disease. The infection may break out and overwhelm the patient within a short time. Of AIDS patients seropositive for *T. gondii,* 30% will develop toxoplasmic encephalitis. Chemotherapy is poor (see Epidemiology and Control) and the prognosis is poor in these instances.

A crucial part of the life cycle of any parasite is the transition from one host to the next. The sporozoites of *T. gondii* leave the sporocyst under the influence of conditions in the small intestine (see Chapter 12 for details). The freed sporozoites then enter enterocytes by a process that has been described through TEM methods. The conoid is extended from the anterior tip of the zoite and somehow penetrates the plasma membrane. The contents of the rhoptries are then secreted into the cell and are seen as a cluster of vacuoles around the tip of the zoite (Fig. 13.10). The normally electron-dense rhoptries become less dense upon entry into a cell. In experiments with macrophages, full entry into the host cell requires about 15 seconds

Survival in a cell such as a macrophage and the ability to multiply there also presents an interesting problem for the parasite. Having entered a host cell, a parasitophorous vacuole (PV) is formed from both the plasmalemma of the host cell and tubules elaborated by the zoite. The membrane forming the interface between the cytoplasm of the host cell and the PV is altered in such a way that the PV and lysosomal vesicles do not fuse, and the vacuole is not acidified. This allows the parasite to remain alive and to multiply in the host cell.

Epidemiology and Control

There are three routes of transmission of *T. gondii*:

1. Fecal-oral
2. Congenital or vertical
3. Carnivorism

Each of these modes requires a different approach to preventing infection in humans or other animals. Much can be done by an individual to minimize the probability of transmission. For example, the fecal-oral route relates entirely to infections obtained from cats, and for most persons this means the house cat. If a cat is allowed to roam, it will hunt and can become infected either from small rodents or birds that it catches. It sheds oocysts some days later (Fig. 13.5) and contaminates the area. If there is a litter box in the home, oocysts may be thrown into the air and inhaled by people in the house. If there is a child's sandbox near the house, a cat will use it as a place to defecate. In both of these instances it is essential that steps be taken to prevent human infections. The litter box should be placed where the contaminated dust will not come into contact with people; the sandbox should have a cover that is in place when children are not playing in it.

Although the domestic cat is most often the culprit charged with infecting humans, wild cats may be part of the cycle in some circumstances. The cougar, *Felis concolor,* which is found in North America, becomes infected and passes oocysts. Nearly 100% of some populations of cougar are seropositive for *T. gondii.* They have been implicated in an outbreak of toxoplasmosis in humans in British Columbia as contaminating a water supply; the evidence, while circumstantial, is quite good.

Congenital transmission takes place when a pregnant woman inhales or ingests infective oocysts (Fig. 13.9). While the risk of infecting the developing fetus is low, the results (see Host–Parasite Interactions) can be catastrophic for the child. A pregnant woman should look on any cat as a potential source of infection and avoid it. Vaccination of cats is now possible and such immunized cats do not shed oocysts even if they do become infected.

Whether there should be a cat in the same house as a pregnant woman is a matter that is difficult to address. The risks are low, but significant. Each woman must make her own decision on whether the risk of infecting her child warrants keeping a cat.

Many infections in adults are contracted by eating uncooked or insufficiently cooked meat. Steak tartar is an example of uncooked meat that some persons enjoy, and there have been several outbreaks that have been described following meals of this type of food. Likewise, a wide range of hosts other than humans becomes infected by catching prey or eating carrion. The infection can be maintained for an indefinite period of time in small rodents through carnivorism or scavenging. It is obvious that infections in humans can be avoided by cooking all meat to at least 60°C , and preferably 70°C, to kill the zoites. This temperature also kills other parasites such as *Trichinella* (Chapter 36) and tapeworm larvae such as *Taenia* (Chapter 24).

Raw meat of almost any sort (beef, pork, lamb, horse meat) should be considered to be infected and handled accordingly. In fact, *T. gondii* has been isolated from the following:

Species	*Percentage Infected*	*Remarks*
Sheep	4–67	Many in 30% range
Goat	30–40	Fragmentary data
Ox	0–24	Mostly negative
Swine	0–43	Many in 10 to 20% range
Horse	Present	Fragmentary data

Raw meat should be handled with care. Hands,

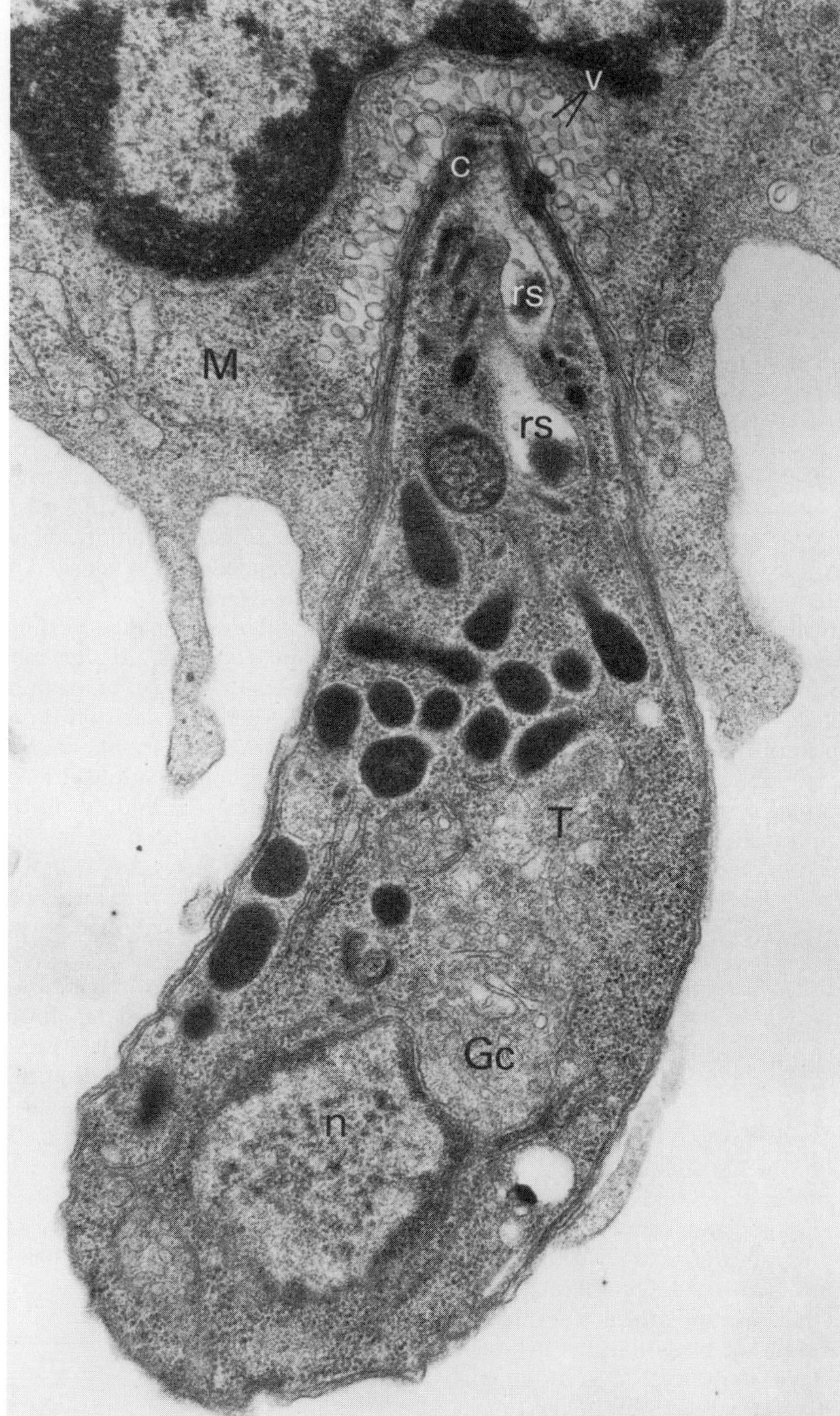

FIGURE 13.10. Penetration of a macrophage by a sporozoite of *Toxoplasma gondii*. The conoid makes contact with the plasma membrane of the cell and the rhoptries begin to empty facilitating entry. Abbreviations: c, conoid; Gc, Golgi complex; M, macrophage; n, nucleus; rs, rhoptry contents; T, *Toxoplasma* zoite; v, vesicle. [From Nichols, et al., 1983.]

utensils, and cutting boards should all be washed with soap and water to prevent transferring a possible infection to the mouth. Only well-cooked meat should be fed to cats.

There are some reports in the literature of *T. gondii* being transmitted through the milk of the mother to the newborn offspring. While this has been confirmed experimentally, milk transmission does not appear to be an important mode of transmission in human infections nor in those of other animals. Milk from dairies is highly unlikely to be a source of infection.

Treatment of individuals infected with *T. gondii* is far from satisfactory. Two drugs are commonly used: (1) a sulfonamide potentiated with pyrimethamine and (2) spiramycin. Certain other drugs such as clindamycin are used as well. It is important to note that chemotherapy has some effect in reducing the clinical aspects of toxoplasmosis but does not seem to eliminate the infection. Some of the drugs have undesirable side effects, and none, at this point, is completely effective. Better drugs are urgently needed.

TOXOPLASMOSIS IN DOMESTIC ANIMALS

Sheep

Toxoplasmosis is a widespread disease of sheep in which the major economic losses are abortion, death of the fetus, and neonatal death. *T. gondii* was first suspected as a cause of abortion in 1951 in New Zealand. Since then antibodies to *T. gondii* have been found in sheep in at least 34 countries on every continent. Outbreaks of toxoplasmic abortion have since been described in Australia/New Zealand, Asia, the United Kingdom and Europe, and North America. It is likely that the infection extends throughout the areas of the world where sheep are raised.

Specific monetary losses are difficult to calculate, but certain data allow the extent of the problem to be seen. In New Zealand, where toxoplasmic abortion was first described, almost 72% of abortions in sheep were due to *T. gondii*. Over the five year period of 1975–1980, 70,000 ewes were aborted in one sheep-raising area. In the United Kingdom, about 100,000 lambs are lost each year to toxoplasmic abortion. Several outbreaks have been described in the United States, and it appears that *T. gondii* was the major cause of abortion in these flocks.

The mode of transmission of *T. gondii* in sheep is through the ingestion of oocysts excreted by cats. Sheep are susceptible to infection at any age, even a week after being born, and usually the maximal rate of infection is seen by the time sheep are four years old.

Breeding problems arise when ewes are infected any time during pregnancy. In experimental infections, abortion takes place between 7 and 14 days after oral administration of infective oocysts. There may be mild signs of infection in the ewes, but the major effect is on the developing lamb in which infection is seen in many tissues including the placenta and the brain.

Abortions are more likely to take place in sheep that are kept close to the farmhouse, where there may be domestic cats, than in sheep on range. Also, infections are more likely to occur in fall and winter than in summer. This fact no doubt relates to survival of the oocysts, which live longer when the weather is cool rather than hot. Sheep are usually bred in fall and carry their lambs through the winter to be born in spring; thus the breeding cycle and the likelihood of there being viable oocysts in the area are coordinated. Some outbreaks of abortion have been reported when sheep have been fed a commercial feed that had been contaminated with feces of cats.

Control of toxoplasmic abortion in sheep revolves around immunity. Once a ewe has been infected, she becomes immune to challenge and probably retains that immunity for life. Vaccination has been attempted using a variety of antigens, and some success has been experienced in preventing abortion. Monensin, an antibiotic which is active against intestinal coccidia, was fed to ewes during pregnancy and reduced abortion more than 35% compared to the unmedicated group.

Goats

Many of the same problems that have been seen in sheep due to *T. gondii* have also been reported in goats. Abortion and other breeding problems have been the source of the majority of losses.

Cattle

Although the ox can be infected with *T. gondii* and the organism recovered from tissues after experimental inoculation, cattle seem to be relatively refractory to infection nor are they associated with toxoplasmosis in humans to any significant extent. Studies on seroprevalence are unreliable because of an unknown factor in the blood of the ox that interferes with the tests. Clinical case reports of toxoplasmosis in cattle have generally been criticized for lack of conclusive evidence on the presence of the causative agent. It is likely that some sporadic illness and infections occur naturally in cattle, but toxoplasmosis probably is not an enzootic problem. How the presence of *Neospora cani-*

num (see the following) has distorted our vision of toxoplasmosis in cattle is not known.

Swine

Toxoplasmosis in domestic pigs has become recognized in recent years as an economic problem. Infections have been seen in both newborn pigs and in growing swine. Natural outbreaks have been reported in many countries, but interestingly, Japan seems to be especially hard hit by toxoplasmosis. In growing swine, heart, lungs, brain and lymph nodes are the organs most often severely affected. Experimental infections have shown that *T. gondii* can be transmitted from the sow to the piglet during gestation.

The sources of infection of swine have not been clearly defined except in a few outbreaks. Oocysts have been shown to contaminate soil and feed in some instances, but there is a good deal of conjecture as to where most infections come from. Scavenging on carrion is probably a source, and it has been suggested that tail-biting among pigs is another means of becoming infected.

Control of toxoplasmosis in swine revolves around the following:

1. Controlling cats and cat feces
2. Eliminating carcasses of dead pigs and other animals from pens

Cats on farms are often shadowy apparitions that live their lives close to humans, but without much direct contact. They live, love and give birth in barns and buildings; they hunt mice and birds, and they may eat livestock feed as it is accessible to them. They defecate where it is convenient: in buildings, out in the open, or in feed containers. All of this sets the stage for gross contamination of the environment where swine are raised.

Where swine are raised on concrete, slabs are cleaned daily or nearly daily and contamination with a variety of infectious agents is kept to a minimum. This also helps to eliminate oocysts of *T. gondii*. But where pigs are in muddy pens, it is more difficult to control infectious agents in general. Any feed given to pigs must be kept in containers that prevent cats from getting in them. Also, the area should be patrolled daily to make sure that any carcasses of pigs or rodents are removed and disposed of either by burying or burning.

RELATED ORGANISMS

Among the seven species of *Toxoplasma* established by Levine (1977) are *T. hammondi*, which was originally described as *Hammondia hammondi*, discussed early in this chapter, and *T. bahaiensis*. *T. hammondi* has a cat–rodent cycle in which the intermediate host is an obligate one. Meronts in the muscles are relatively large (100 to 340 μm in length) and similar to *Sarcocystis* when examined at the EM level. A number or rodents as well as the dog, pig, and a marmoset are known to be intermediate hosts. *T. hammondi* is not pathogenic in the cat, but causes disease and sometimes death in experimental mice.

The definitive hosts of *T. bahaiensis* are canids, the mink, and the guinea pig. Intermediate hosts are various ruminants, the dog, and the guinea pig. There is probably an obligate two-host cycle. Little or no pathogenesis has been described.

SARCOCYSTIS AND SARCOCYSTOSIS

A number of genera of tissue coccidia have isosporoid oocysts and two-host life cycles: *Sarcocystis*, *Besnoitia*, and *Frenkelia*, for example (Table 13.1). The sarcocysts of *Sarcocystis* have been known for well over 100 years since they were first described by Miescher in the muscle of mice in 1843. One hundred and thirty years were to pass before the life cycles of these organisms were fully described.

Among the many species in this general category are some that are of medical or economic importance, but their impacts on human and animal health are only now being clarified. For example, in 1961 an outbreak of disease in a dairy herd near Dalmeny, Ontario, resulted in the deaths of 17 in a herd of 36 animals; 8 other affected animals survived. The only significant infectious agent found was an organism that looked like *Toxoplasma gondii* but could not be confirmed serologically. The relationship to *Sarcocystis* was clarified by an investigation of another outbreak in New York State, similar to the Dalmeny disease, in which eight yearling heifers died. Typical *Sarcocystis* sporocysts were found in the feces of a dog on the farm. During the years between the description of Dalmeny disease and the conclusion that it was caused by *Sarcocystis*, information had developed on life cycles and the potential pathogenesis of a number of species. It is now clear that *Sarcocystis* is a ubiquitous organism, that a number of species cause disease in their hosts, and that there are losses at slaughter in a variety of food animals.

In early studies on those *Sarcocystis* spp. infecting ruminants, the alternate host was found to be a carnivore or, in two instances, humans. The pattern then became clear for *Sarcocystis* in general that the intermediate host was a herbivore and the definitive host was a carnivore, or at least a meat eater, since humans are not classified as carnivores. In all instances, the two-host cycle is obligatory, unlike *T. gondii,* in which it is optional. The general pattern of herbivore—carnivore or prey—predator transmission has been demonstrated in a number of other cycles as well. For example, *Frenkelia buteonis* (syn. *Isospora buteonis)* of hawks has a vole (*Microtus agrestis)* as its intermediate host. *Sarcocystis idahoensis* has a cycle that alternates between deer mice (*Peromyscus maniculatus*) and the gopher snake (*Pituophis melanoleucus). Sarcocystis rileyi,* known to be widespread in the somatic muscles of ducks, has been found to have skunks as its definitive host.

Because knowledge of life cycles has developed so rapidly and because oocysts and sarcocysts have been associated in unexpected combinations, nomenclature in the group is difficult to deal with. The problem lies in (1) the separate descriptions of muscle stages and fecal stages, sometimes when methods and descriptions were only rudimentary, (2) subdivision of species, as it has been determined that similar oocysts comprise more than one species, (3) the problem of determining in each instance which of the original names has priority according to the rules of zoological nomenclature, and (4) differences of opinion among investigators as to what constitute valid generic and specific characters We will look here at a single species as a representative of the group.

Name of Organism and Disease Caused

Sarcocystis cruzi (syns. *S. bovicanis, S. fusiformis, Isospora bigemina,* and *I. hominis*) causes sarcocytosis, sarcosporidiosis, and Dalmeny disease.

Hosts and Host Range

Definitive hosts are canids in which the intestine is parasitized by the sexual stages of the life cycle. The intermediate host is the domestic ox, in which the parasites are located principally in the somatic muscles.

Distribution and Importance

Cosmopolitan. The prevalence of infection seems to approach 100% in cattle, and cattle are infected by at least two other species of *Sarcocystis, T. gondii,* and *Neospora caninum,* so we know that they nearly always harbor the zoites of some species of tissue coccidium. A number of outbreaks of disease have been described and additional outbreaks continue to be reported. Losses to the livestock industry are still unknown. Cattle are condemned at slaughter for eosinophilic myositis, a condition in which the muscles of the animals have a grossly seen greenish discoloration. It has been well documented that eosinophilic myositis is the result of *Sarcocystis* spp. infection.

Morphology

Sporocysts in the feces of the definitive host are 10.8 by 16.3 μm. Other closely related species such as *S. fusiformis, S. tenella,* and *S. miescheriana* have sporocysts that are almost the same size (Fig. 13.1).

The sarcocysts in the tissues of the intermediate host (Fig. 13.2) lie in a parasitophorous vacuole (PV) and are too small to be seen with the naked eye. The sarcocysts are thin-walled and may or may not have a hairy (hirsute) appearance (Table 13.1)

Life Cycle

The definitive host becomes infected with the ingestion of infected tissues of an ox or bison by a dog or other canid (Fig. 13.11). The merozoites (bradyzoites) are released in the small intestine and invade enterocytes. The zoites round up and form gamonts; they differentiate into micro- and macrogamonts and fertilization takes place.

Unlike most other coccidia, sporulation of oocysts of *Sarcocystis* takes place within the cells of the host. Sporocysts, and an occasional oocyst (Fig. 13.1), first appear in the feces in 7 to 14 days after infection.

The intermediate host becomes infected by ingestion of sporocysts, which contaminate its food or water. The bradyzoites are digested out of the sarcocyst in the small intestine and they move from the intestine to the circulatory system. The first generation of merogony takes place in small arteries in several organ systems of the body. Each meront produces a hundred or more merozoites starting 7 days after infection and continuing until about day 26.

The second generation of merogony takes place in capillaries of a number of organ systems starting 19 days after infection and continuing until day 46. The meronts are small and produce only from 4 to 37 merozoites.

The second generation merozoites move through the circulatory system to striated muscles where they develop within the myocytes. Early in the infection of muscle cells, multiplication is in so-called *metrocytes* (mother cells) (Fig. 13.3), which are rapidly multiplying forms. The metrocytes lose many of the specific structures such as the conoid, rhoptries, and micronemes and increase the number of certain organelles, such as ribosomes, indicating a high level of metabolic activity.

As multiplicaton reaches its end, the metrocytes are

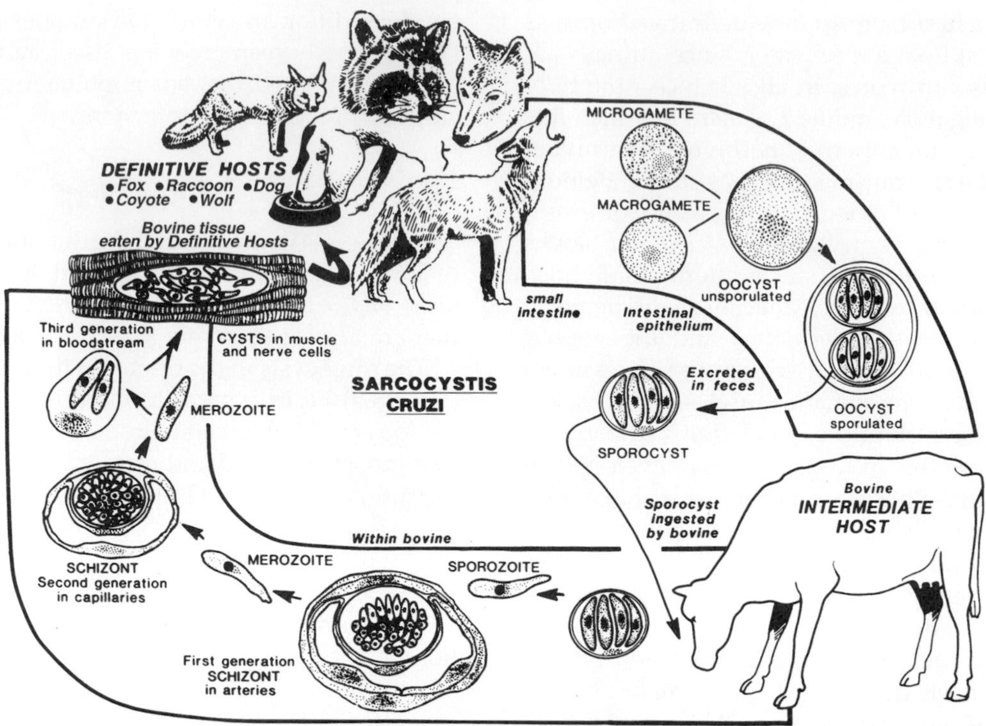

FIGURE 13.11. Life cycle of *Sarcocystis cruzi* of the ox and dog. Completion of the *Sarcocystis* life cycle requires two hosts—an intermediate host (ox) and a definitive host in which gamogony takes place (dog or other canid). [Courtesy of Dr. J. P. Dubey, Agricultural Research Service, Beltsville, Maryland.]

replaced by bradyzoites which regain all of the organelles of a typical apicomplexan (Fig. 10.1 and 13.3B). The bradyzoite is the infective stage and the infection cannot be transmitted until bradyzoites are present in the muscles.

The developmental period in the intermediate host is quite long. About 86 days are required before bradyzoites are seen in the myocytes. Thus, more than three months are required for the completion of the life cycle from oocyst to oocyst.

Diagnosis

In the definitive host, diagnosis is determined by finding sporocysts in the feces. Flotation techniques using a medium of high specific gravity are normally employed to concentrate the sporocysts so that they can be found under a compound microscope.

In the intermediate host, the presence of infection is determined by the following:

1. Finding sarcocysts in striated muscles (somatic, cardiac, esophagus)
2. Performing serology to find antibodies to *Sarcocystis*
3. Observing clinical signs of infection
4. Completing the life cycle by feeding tissues to the proper definitive host

Sarcocysts are normally found at postmortem examination by digesting tissues in pepsin-HCl or preparing tissues for histologic examination. The digestion procedure is relatively easy and inexpensive and has been used extensively in epidemiologic surveys. Digestion is highly reliable and more than 90% of cattle are found to be infected by this method.

Histology takes time and is costly to perform. It is sometimes necessary to examine the sarcocyst structure at the EM level to make a presumptive species identification. Two serologic tests are in use: Indirect Hemagglutination Test (IHA) and an Enzyme-Linked Immunoabsorption Assay (ELISA). The ELISA is widely used and is reliable. The information gained can be used in surveys for prevalence of infection or to determine if sarcocystosis is the cause of an outbreak of disease.

In certain types of investigations it may be necessary to complete the life cycle and look for sporocysts in the feces of the definitive host. Tissues, usually striated muscles, are fed to potential definitive hosts, and sporocysts are looked for in the feces until they are either found or the time of development is long past. The host range of *Sarcocystis* in the definitive host is narrow, and usually only one or a few species produce sporocysts upon inoculation. New species of *Sarcocystis* are continually being found and named, and there is every reason to believe that new species will continue to turn up even in common hosts such as domestic animals.

Host–Parasite Interactions

As we have seen with the intestinal coccidia such as *Eimeria* spp., *Sarcocystis* is genetically programmed to move through a series of stages to reach an endpoint in both the definitive and intermediate hosts. When the bradyzoite stage is reached in the intermediate host, development stops; in some species slow division and growth of the sarcocyst may continue for as many as four years. Unlike *Toxoplasma gondii*, development cannot be reactivated in an immunosuppressed host. The bradyzoite continues development only when it is ingested by the proper definitive host. The only development that takes place in the definitive host is gamogony and production of oocysts, which then undergo sporogony within the host.

S. cruzi is probably the most pathogenic species that we know of. Little damage is seen in the definitive host, but the intermediate host may suffer from a variety of signs of infection.

In the susceptible ox, a wide range of clinical signs have been described. Pathogenesis revolves around the following:

1. Cellular destruction
2. Inflammation
3. Immunopathology
4. Edema
5. Fever
6. Anemia
7. Abortion
8. Eosinophilic myositis
9. Toxin production

Meronts growing within cells cause death of the cell when merozoites are formed and released from it. This is especially true during the early merogonies in the vascular system and other organs such as the liver, depending on the species of *Sarcocystis*. A good deal of cellular debris is released at times when cells are ruptured.

A number of kinds of pathogenesis are interrelated: inflammation, immunopathology, and eosinophilic myositis. The inflammatory process itself is sometimes damaging and various aspects of the immune response lead to further damage to the host through release of lymphokines and cytokines. Tumor necrosis factor (TNF or cachectin) gives rise to wasting, for example. Delayed hypersensitivity is probably involved in the pathogenesis of eosinophilic myositis.

Anemia is a result of both hemorrhage and hemolysis. In the early stages of experimental infections, blood is released into the tissue spaces and is readily seen in organs such as the intestine and lymph nodes. Although the cause of most of the anemia is not known, red cell production begins again when the clinical phase abates.

The mechanism of abortion has not been described. In some instances, the fetus is infected, in others parasites have not been found. Be that as it may, abortion is common when animals are infected during pregnancy.

Eosinophilic myositis (EM) is often seen in cattle and some other domestic animals at slaughter. The cut surface of the muscle shows a greenish cast in reflected light. Animals showing EM are condemned for human consumption and instead go for pet food. It has been theorized that EM is a manifestation of delayed hypersensitivity.

Toxin production has been claimed off and on for many years, but unequivocal evidence for toxin(s) has not been forthcoming.

Epidemiology and Control

The levels of infection with sarcocysts in various domestic animals approaches 100%; this is true in cattle, sheep, and swine. Even animals on short-grass range where the carrying capacity may be one cow and calf per 30 acres (12.1 hectares) or more, virtually all cattle are infected. Obviously it takes only a low level of contamination with oocysts to infect nearly all cattle grazing on the area.

Oocysts survive many weeks or months under good conditions: 75% or greater humidity, temperature from about 5 to 12°C, and oxygen (anaerobic conditions are detrimental). As is true with most other coccidia, the oocyst/sporocyst stage is highly resistant to environmental insult.

In broad terms, control of sarcocystosis involves blocking the interface between the intermediate and definitive hosts. Outbreaks of sarcocystosis in dairy animals have involved contamination of corrals and loafing sheds with feces of cats or dogs. Companion animals become infected by feeding on carcasses or offal from home-slaughtered animals. This kind of contact must be eliminated (see also hydatid disease in Chapter 24).

Human infections with *S. suihominis* or *S. hominis* result from eating inadequately cooked pork and beef, respectively. Although neither infection is life threatening, serious diarrhea results. Individuals can protect themselves by eating only meat that has been heated to at least 60°C.

On range, as in western North America or the steppe of Eurasia, removing the carcasses of dead animals removes the probability of wild canids (coyote, fox, wolf) from feeding on the carcasses and becoming infected with *S. cruzi*.

There is no chemotherapy for sarcocystosis, and while immunity can be induced in livestock, there is no vaccine. Thus, we are left with management as a means of preventing sarcocystosis.

Related Organisms

Table 13.1 lists a number of common species of *Sarcocystis* as well as three other genera, *Frenkelia*, *Besnoiti*, and *Neospora*, all of which have two-host cycles and isosporoid oocysts. It should be borne in mind that this is only a sampling of species. Nearly any herbivorous or omnivorous and many carnivorous animals have sarcocysts in the extraintestinal tissues. If domestic animals are a measure, each species of host probably has two or more species of *Sarcocystis*.

Humans serve as the definitive host for two species, *S. hominis* and *S. suihominis*, but what of humans as intermediate hosts? In all of the medical literature there are 46 confirmed infections of humans with sarcocysts. There are probably seven types of sarcocysts that were identifiable, so several species probably are present. Most of the cases come from the Asian tropics and only two from the United States. Humans seem to be incidental hosts and some investigators think that primates other than humans are the normal hosts. In any event, little pathology has been described, and the number of cases on record indicates that sarcocystosis is not important in human health.

Sarcocystis riley has been known for many years as a parasite of ducks. Hunters especially are acquainted with this parasite, and when they take a duck that is heavily infected, they discard it. The breast muscle can be seen to be heavily infected when it is laid bare; one sees rice-grain-like sarcocysts just under the fascia of the muscle. The economic losses are difficult to determine, but a significant proportion of ducks in the flyways of North America are infected. The life cycle was completed in the middle 1980s and the definitive host was found to be the striped skunk, *Mephitis mephitis*. Control programs are not feasible under the circumstances of transmission in the wild, but hunters most certainly perpetuate the infection by discarding the carcasses of infected ducks.

Besnoitia is a widespread parasite that is economically important in Africa, the Middle East, and Kazakhstan. *B. besnoiti* is common in ruminants and other

TABLE 13.1 Some Common Species of Tissue Coccidia and Their Hosts

Genus and species	Definitive hosts	Intermediate hosts	Sarcocyst wall
Sarcocystis cruzi	Dog, coyote, red fox, raccoon, wolf	Ox, bison	Thin, smooth to hairy
S. hirsuta	Cat	Ox	Thick, striated
S. hominis	Human, rhesus monkey, chimpanzee (?)	Ox	Thick, striated
S. tenella	Dog, coyote, red fox	Sheep	Thick, striated
S. gigantea	Dog	Sheep	Thin
S. medusiformis	Cat	Sheep	Thin
S. capricanis	Dog, coyote, red fox, crab-eating fox	Goat	Thick, striated
S. hircicanis	Dog	Goat	Thin, smooth to hairy
S. miescheriana	Dog	Swine	Thick, striated
S. suihominis	Human and nonhuman primates	Swine	Thick, stiated
S. odocoileocanis	Dog, red fox, gray fox, wolf (?)	White-tailed deer	Thick, striated to inverted *T*
S. hemionilatrantis	Dog, coyote	Mule deer	Thin, smooth
S. rileyi	Striped skunk	Ducks	Thin to thick
S. dispersa	Barn owl, long-eared owl	House mouse	Thin to thick
S. cuniculi	Cat	European rabbit	Thick, striated
Frenkelia microti	Buzzard	Rodents (16 spp.) European rabbit	Thin, lobulated, in CNS only
Besnoitia besnoiti	Cats	Ox, zebu, goat, wildebeest, kudu, impala	Thick, nonseptate, in many organs
Neospora caninum	Dog	Dog, ox, sheep, goat	Thick, undulating in nerve cells

herbivores where it causes disease of the skin and internal organs. The definitive hosts are felids of a number of species and transmission to the intermediate host is by ingestion of oocysts. There is a vaccine which is fairly effective. Control is attempted largely through use of the vaccine. The large number of species of wild ruminants that serves as the intermediate host prevents a management control program from being effective.

NEOSPORA AND NEOSPOROSIS

Name of Organism and Disease Associations

Neospora caninum, the cause of neosporosis and abortion.

Hosts and Host Range

This organism has been found in a number of domestic animals such as the dog, ox, sheep, goat, and horse. In addition, *N. caninum* has been transmitted experimentally to the cat, mouse, rat, and gerbil.

Geographic Distribution and Importance

Cosmopolitan. Found in North America, Scandinavia, and other parts of western Europe, Australia and New Zealand, South Africa, and Japan.

The importance of *Neospora* is still unfolding. It was found first in dogs as an infection that was similar to toxoplasmosis, but the organism was different structurally and antigenically. The infection manifested itself most seriously as a neuromuscular disease and a central nervous system disease. As knowledge has developed, *N. caninum* has been found to be a cause of abortion and stillbirths in cattle and is now considered to be the single most important cause of bovine abortion in the United States. Specific economic losses have not yet been determined.

Morphology

The oocyst is an isosporoid type with two sporocysts each of which has four sporozoites. The oocysts are spherical to subspherical 10–11 μm. Merozoites—tachyzoites and bradyzoites—(Fig. 13.12 and 13.14) are the only other stages known and these are from cysts in the tissues of the various hosts listed earlier. Tachyzoites are 3 to 7 by 1 to 5 μm and range from being globular to crescent-shaped (Fig. 13.13). Bradyzoites are 6 to 8 by 1 to 1.8 μm. Tachyzoites are similar to those of *T. gondii* and other coccidia except that they have 8 to 18 rhoptries, which may extend posterior to the nucleus. Bradyzoites are similar to tachyzoites except that they have fewer rhoptries.

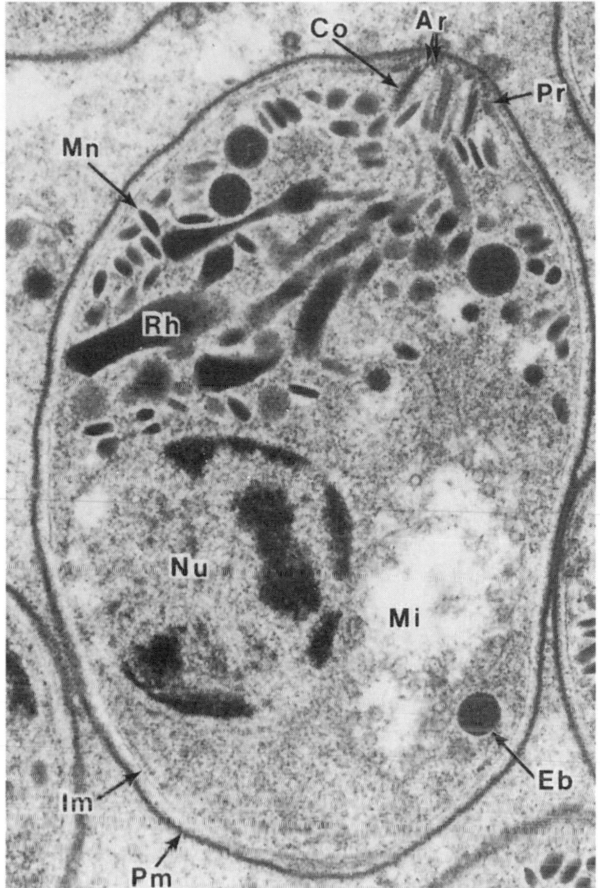

FIGURE 13.12. A tachyzoite of *Neospora caninum* from the skin of a naturally infected dog. There are a large number of rhoptries (Rh), and the micronemes tend to line up at the pellicle oriented at 90°s to it. [From Speer and Dubey, 1989.]

The tissue cysts that contain bradyzoites are found only in neural tissue and may be as long as 107 μm (Fig. 13.15). The wall of the tissue cyst is 1 to 4 μm (that of *T. gondii* is less than 1 μm).

Life Cycle

The definitive host is the dog which becomes infected by the ingestion of infected tissues of intermediate hosts. In experimental infections, oocysts were found in the feces of dogs at 8 or 13 days after infection and continued to be shed for as long as 19 days although a patent period of 10 days was more common. Oocysts were shed in an unsporulated state, and sporulated in three days.

Multiplication of the tachyzoites is by endodygeny only (Fig. 13.13).

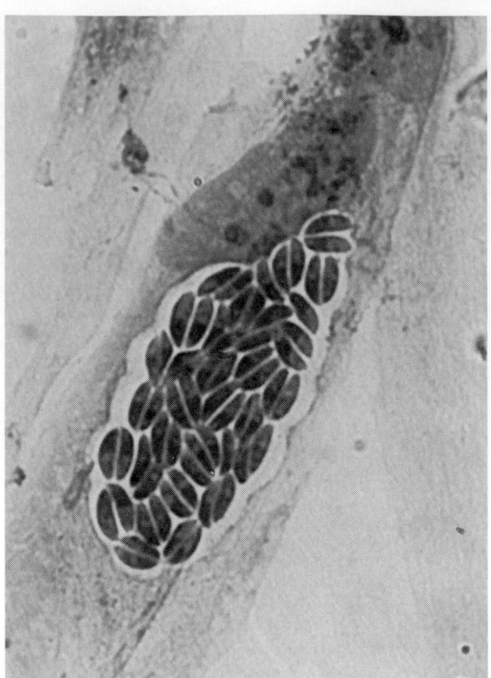

FIGURE 13.13. A group of tachyzoites of *Neospora caninum* in a fibroblast cell in culture. Note that nearly all of the zoites are paired up having undergone endodyogeny. [From Dubey and Lindsay, 1993.]

Diagnosis

Since neosporosis is a relatively newly recognized disease, it is important keep it in mind and to distinguish it from toxoplasmosis. The two diseases are similar clinically, and it is necessary to study tissue sections both at the light and EM level and to take serum for serology.

The zoites of *Toxoplasma* and *Neospora* are so similar at the LM level that a specific diagnosis is not possible; however, at the EM level, the structure of the zoites can be seen and a diagnosis made (Fig. 13.14)

An indirect fluorescent antibody (IFA) test has been developed that is generally specific at the higher titers. However, there is cross-reactivity with *Toxoplasma gondii* and *Babesia gibsoni* (Chapter 15) at lower titers. An immunohistochemical test is also accurate in diagnosing *N. caninum* infection.

Host–Parasite Interactions

N. caninum damages its host by destroying the cells in which it develops. Early in an infection, tachyzoites are found in many types of cells including macrophages, fibroblasts, endothelial (lining) cells of blood vessels, muscles cells (myocytes), and neural cells. Later in the infection, when bradyzoites are found,

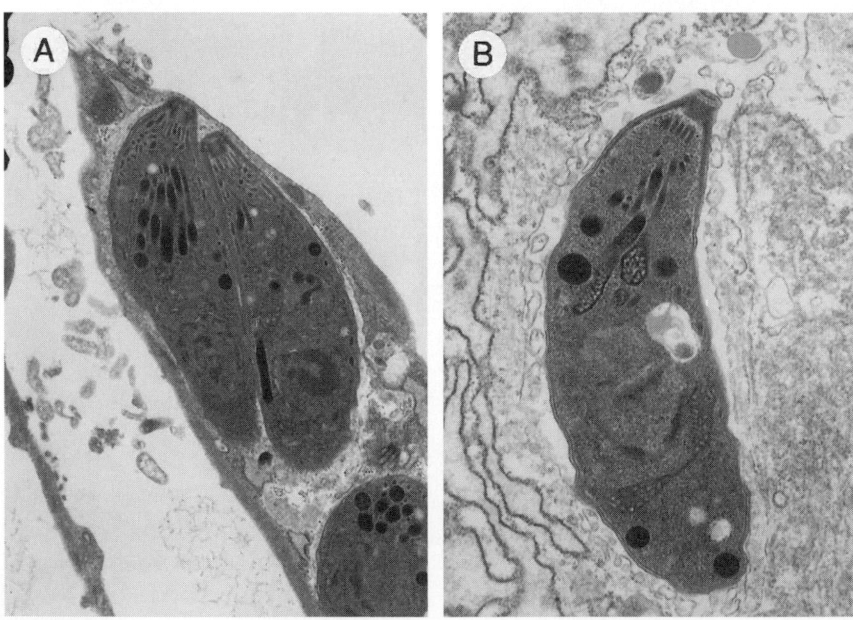

FIGURE 13.14. Comparison of bradyzoites of *Neospora caninum* (A) and *Toxoplasma gondii* (B) in TEM preparations. Note the large number of rhoptries (R) in *Neospora* and only two or three in *Toxoplasma*. The rhoptries of *Toxoplasma* also have less dense areas at their posterior ends. [From Dubey and Lindsay, 1993.]

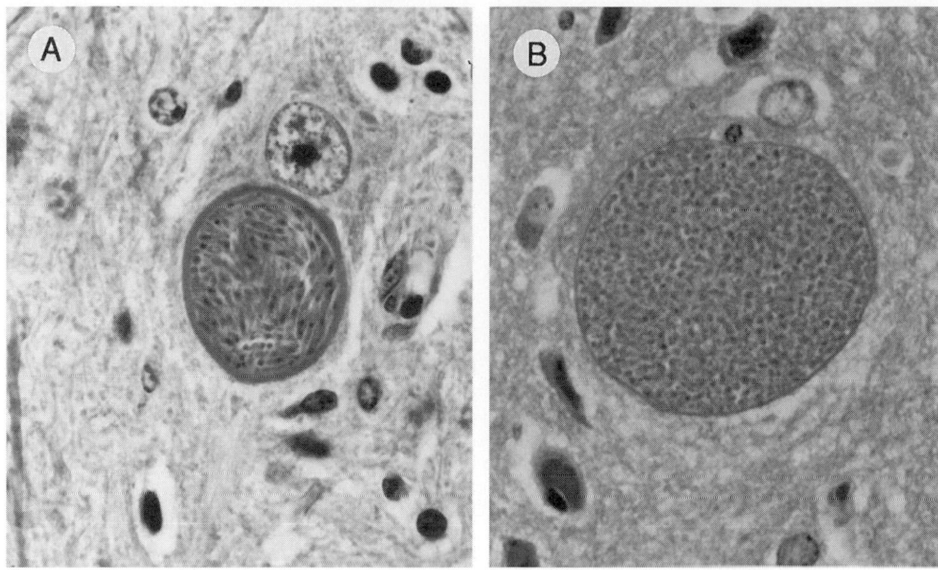

FIGURE 13.15 Tissue cysts of *Neospora* (A) and *Toxoplasma* (B) as seen in LM. Cysts of *Neospora* have relatively thick walls, but those of *Toxoplasma* are less than 1 μm in thickness.

the infection is restricted to neural cells. The result of infection of neural cells is paralysis, muscular weakness, and incoordination.

The infection is also transmitted from the pregnant dog or cow to the developing fetus. The result may be abortion, stillbirth, or an affected newborn that may die.

In addition to antibodies that can be used in diagnosis, there is some effective immunity that develops upon infection. There is some variability among host species, but in some instances, a dam that was infected during one pregnancy does not transmit the infection to her offspring during the next pregnancy.

Epidemiology and Control

Little is known about the transmission of *Neospora* under natural conditions. In addition to transmission by the oocyst, it can be transmitted by inoculation subcutaneously, intraperitoneally, intramuscularly, or by mouth. It is also transmitted from the pregnant dam to the offspring. *Neospora* elicits the production of antibody and some immunity results, as well.

Treatment with various sulfonamides and antibiotics have been only partially successful. Some reduction in clinical signs has been seen, but the host is not cleared of the infection. Better chemotherapy is clearly needed.

At this point, there is no effective control strategy.

Readings

Dubey, J. P. (1987). Toxoplasmosis. *Vet. Clin. North Am. Small Anim. Practice Parasitic Infect.* **17**(6), 1389–1404.

Dubey, J. P., and Beattie, C. P. (1988). *Toxoplasmosis of Animals and Man.* CRC Press, Boca Raton, FL.

Dubey, J. P., and Lindsay, D. S. (1993). Neosporosis. *Parasitol. Today* **9,** 452–458.

Dubey, J. P., and Towle, A. (1986). *Toxoplasmosis in Sheep: A Review and Annotated Bibliography.* Commonwealth Institute of Parasitology.

Dubey, J. P., Carpenter, J. L., Speer, C. A., Topper, M. J., and Uggla, A. (1988). Newly recognized fatal protozoan disease of dogs. *J. Am. Vet. Med. Assoc.* **192,** 1269–1285.

Dubey, J. P., Lindsay, D. S., and Speer, C. A. (1998). Structures of *Toxoplasma gondii* tachyzoites, bradyzoites, and sporozoites and biology and development of tissue cysts. *Clin. Microbiol. Rev.* **11,** 267–299.

Joiner, K. A., Fuhrman, S. A., Miettinen, H. M., Kasper, L. H., and Mellman, I. (1990). *Toxoplasma gondii:* Fusion competence of parasitophorous vacuoles in Fc receptor-transfected fibroblasts. *Science* **249,** 6411–6416.

Levine, N. D. (1977). Taxonomy of *Toxoplasma. J. Protozool.* **24,** 36–41.

Nichols, B. A., Chiappino, M. L., and O'Connor, G. R. (1983). Secretion from the rhoptries of *Toxoplasma gondii* during host–cell invasion. *J. Ultrastruct. Res.* **83,** 85–98.

Pfefferkorn, E. R. (1990). Cell biology of *Toxoplasma gondii.* In *Modern Parasite Biology* (D. J. Wyler, Ed.). Freeman, New York.

Roberts, T., Murrell, K. D., and Marks, S. (1994). Economic losses caused by foodborne parasitic diseases. *Parasitol. Today* **10,** 419–423.

Sharma, S. S. (1990). Immunology of *Toxoplasma.* In *Modern Parasite Biology* (D. J. Wyler, Ed.). Freeman, New York.

CHAPTER

14

Malaria in Humans and Related Organisms

Malaria is considered by many to be the most important infectious disease of humans on a worldwide scale. It is most common in tropical and subtropical regions of the world but is established in some temperate climates as well. During the late 1930s and early 1940s about 300 million persons were infected at any one time in the world. With the development of second generation insecticides, especially DDT, as well as good antimalarial drugs, the probability that malaria could be controlled became obvious. DDT was the perfect insecticide, it was highly effective against a broad spectrum of insects, it was (seemingly) non-toxic to humans as well as to domestic and other animals, it had a long residual action, and it was inexpensive. Thus, the campaign was launched at first to reduce the ravages of malaria, and then in the early 1960s to eradicate it from the face of the earth. In truth, a great portion of the areas where malaria was endemic were made safe and in some instances eradication succeeded. But all did not fall into place as neatly as was forecast. The fundamental story of this chapter is to present what is a highly complex disease, how the factors interact, and why malaria is now resurging in many tropical countries.

SPECIES OF *PLASMODIUM*

Name of Organism and Disease Associations

The four species of *Plasmodium* that normally infect humans are shown in Table 14.1.

Hosts and Host Range

For practical purposes, the species in the Table 14.1 are found only in humans. Some other primates have been found to be infected with organisms indistinguishable from these, but the importance of these hosts as reservoirs of infection is still an open question. A number of primates other than humans have been infected experimentally with human malaria organisms, and humans have also served as an experimental or accidental host for malarias derived from other primates. Control programs are designed on the premise that the human is the only host.

Geographic Distribution and Importance

Malaria is a cosmopolitan disease in tropical and subtropical areas of the world (Fig. 14.1); as indicated in the previous section, certain species are more common in some areas than in others. The importance of malaria can hardly be overstated. Prior to extensive control programs following World War II, at least 300 million persons were infected worldwide at any one time. About 1% of those persons died from the infection; that means between 2 and 3 million persons died each year from malaria. In addition, it greatly increased susceptibility to other diseases.

During the time of the Roman Empire, the low-lying lands near Rome were a source of anopheline mosquitoes, which maintained a constant transmission of the organism, and the so-called bad air associated with swamps gave malaria its name. Some evidence has been presented that as the Roman Empire went into decline, mosquito breeding areas increased, leading to

TABLE 14.1 The Species of *Plasmodium* Infecting Humans

Name	Disease	Distribution
Plasmodium vivax (Grassi and Felletti, 1890) Labbé, 1899	Benign tertian malaria; vivax malaria	Cosmopolitan in tropical areas except in parts of tropical Africa; most common species in subtropical and temperate areas
P. falciparum (Welch, 1897) Schaudinn, 1902	Malignant tertian malaria; falciparum malaria, blackwater fever; aestivoautumnal malaria	Tropical and subtropical areas of Africa and Asia; prior eradication in United States and Mediterranean
P. malariae (Laveran, 1881) Grassi and Felletti, 1890	Quartan or malariae malaria	Principally in southeast Asia; also in African and Indian subcontinent; rare in Western Hemisphere
P. ovale Stephens, 1922	Ovale or tertian malaria	Tropical Africa on the west coast and in Ethiopia

greater transmission of malaria, which hastened the further decline of the empire.

During World War II, nearly 500,000 military personnel had malaria. In the conflict in Korea (1950–1953) 6119 cases were reported in military personnel in Korea, but more than 20,000 cases were reported after the personnel had returned to the United States. The war in Viet Nam gave much the same picture, with 16,105 cases encountered in military personnel in the United States after they returned from southeast Asia. Many times more lost man-days in Viet Nam were due to malaria than to combat casualties as such. Many other military campaigns have had equal or greater casualties from malaria, and the outcomes of wars have been influenced more by this disease than by combat wounds.

With the development of control methods starting in the early part of this century and gaining momentum in the late 1930s, malaria was significantly controlled in many localized areas throughout the world. With the development of dichlorodiphenytrichloroethane (DDT), large-scale control of malaria vectors was achieved during the 1950s and early 1960s. In 1955 there were 200 million to 225 million malaria cases worldwide, and more than 2 million deaths annually. Malaria has been eradicated in some areas and nearly eradicated in others; however, there has been a resurgence in many of the developing countries of the

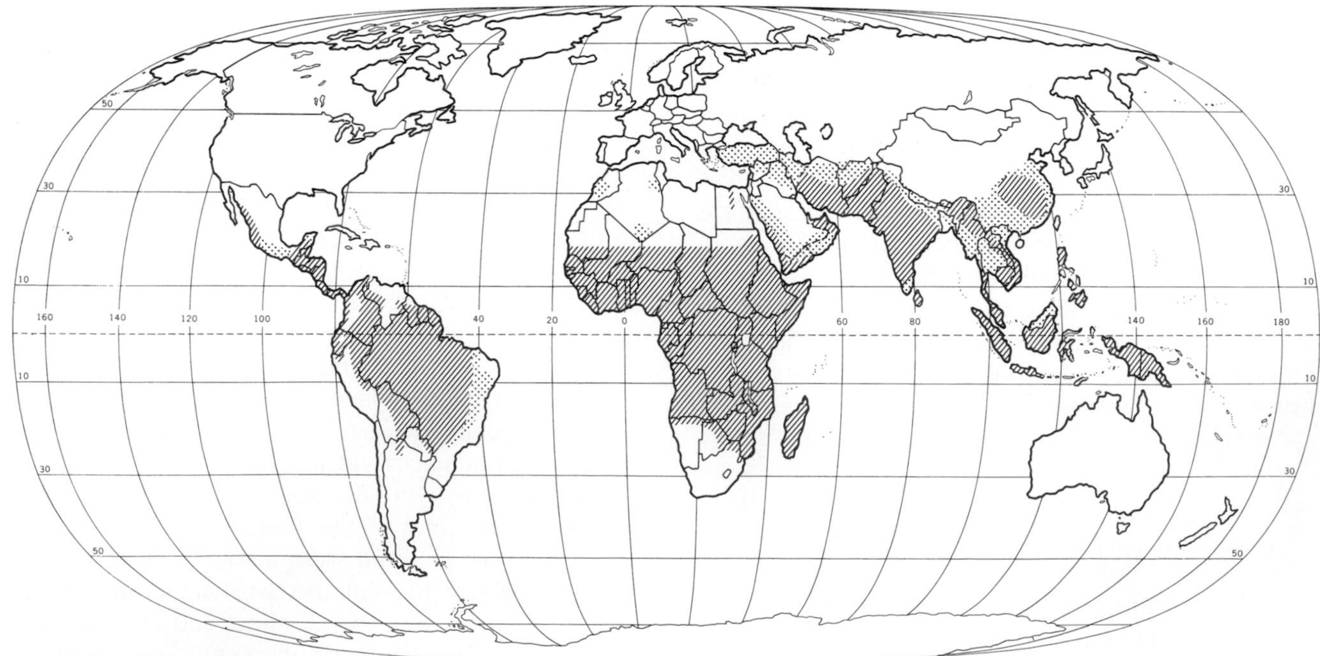

FIGURE 14.1 Map of the world showing malarious areas. Diagonal lines represent areas of frequent transmission and stippled areas represent areas of infrequent transmission.

world. India, for example, had only 40,000 cases in 1966, but the number had risen to 5.8 million by 1976.

With the resurgence of malaria in certain endemic areas, investigators have been recalculating the number of cases and deaths so as to give a current perspective on the importance of the disease. Some data estimate the annual cases of malaria at more than 400 million worldwide. Of these, about half are caused by *Plasmodium falciparum*, the most pathogenic of the four species infecting humans. The annual deaths from malaria are then estimated at 2 million to 3 million persons annually at the present time.

Life Cycle

The pattern of development in members of the genus *Plasmodium* follows the generalized life cycle for an apicomplexan set forth at the beginning of Chapter 10. In *Plasmodium* as opposed to *Eimeria*, a mosquito vector is required for completion of the cycle. Maturation of the gamonts, fertilization, and sporogony take place in the mosquito, the definitive host. Merogony and gamogony take place in the vertebrate host, the intermediate host (Fig. 14.2).

The life cycle of *Plasmodium vivax*, the cause of benign tertian malaria, is used as being representative of all four species. There are some important differences between *P. vivax* and the other three human species, which will be discussed later.

When a mosquito takes a blood meal, the long proboscis probes in the skin of the host, searching for a capillary; at the same time, salivary fluid originating in glands in the thorax is injected to keep the blood from clotting. During the injection of salivary fluid, sporozoites (Fig. 14.3A) are carried from the salivary glands into the skin or directly into the bloodstream. The sporozoites remain in the circulating blood for only about 30 minutes.

The sporozoites enter liver cells and begin their exoerythrocytic (EE) development (Fig. 14.3B, Tab. 14.2). The sporozoites transform into meronts (cryptozoites) and multiply by schizogony. At least one more asexual generation occurs in liver cells, and these generations are called *metacryptozoites*. In *P. vivax*, the number of asexual generations that takes place in the liver is probably limited, and once the merozoites leave the liver, other generations of merozoites do not return to the liver cells for development.

At eight days after sporozoite infection, merozoites derived from the EE cycle begin to appear in the circulating red blood cells (Tab. 14.2). This is the end of the prepatent period. Further development occurs in the erythrocytes.

When *P. vivax* is first seen in the circulating red cells, there are asexual stages only, and all phases of merogony may be seen at any one time. As the infection progresses during the next week or so, the asexual stages tend to become synchronized, so that a blood film taken at any one time shows a preponderance of organisms in the same stage of merogony. Also, as the infection continues, a small number of merozoites develop into sexual stages (gamonts, or gametocytes) in the circulating red cells.

Merogony (schizogony) has a 48-hour cycle in *P. vivax*, that is, 48 hours from the time a merozoite enters a red cell until the daughter cells are produced. Merozoites are perhaps 2 μm long when they attach to the surface of the host red cell. They penetrate by using the components of the apical complex and specific receptors on the red cell. Once inside, the merozoite rounds up to form the early meront, a so-called ring stage. The blue ring, 2 to 4 μm in diameter, has what appears to be a clear vacuole in the center and a single round nucleus, which stains red in Romanowsky stains (methylene blue and eosin) (Fig. 14.4).

As the ring begins to grow, it becomes more irregular in shape, the vacuole becomes less definite and pink stippling (Schüffner's dots) form in the cytoplasm of the red cell. The meront (trophozoite) ingests hemoglobin by pinocytosis and by pinching off small bits. The hemoglobin is digested and the undigested portion remains as tiny black granules that sometimes appear greenish because of their refractile quality. The hemoglobin residue is hemozoin and is characteristic of infections with *Plasmodium* and its close relatives.

Nuclear replication takes place through an amitotic splitting of the nuclear material. This is the stage usually called a *presegmenter*, in which nuclear replication occurs, but no cytoplasmic division. In *P. vivax* a so-called mature presegmenter has 12 to 18 (maximum of 24) nuclei (Tab. 14.3).

Merozoite formation takes place in such a way that each nucleus is encased in an envelope of cytoplasm and plasma membrane. The segmenter stage is reached when the merozoites form.

Forty-eight hours after a merozoite enters a red cell, 12 to 18 merozoites have formed, the red cell breaks down, and the merozoites are released to seek new host red cells. During the breakdown of the red cell, hemozoin, red cell membranes, and metabolic byproducts are released into the bloodstream of the host. Since there is synchrony in development, a large number of red cells break down at nearly the same time; the chills and fever characteristic of clinical malaria are brought about by this massive release of toxic materials. The reproductive potential of *P. vivax* can be appreciated by calculating the possible increase over an eight-day period. If we assume that one merozoite pro-

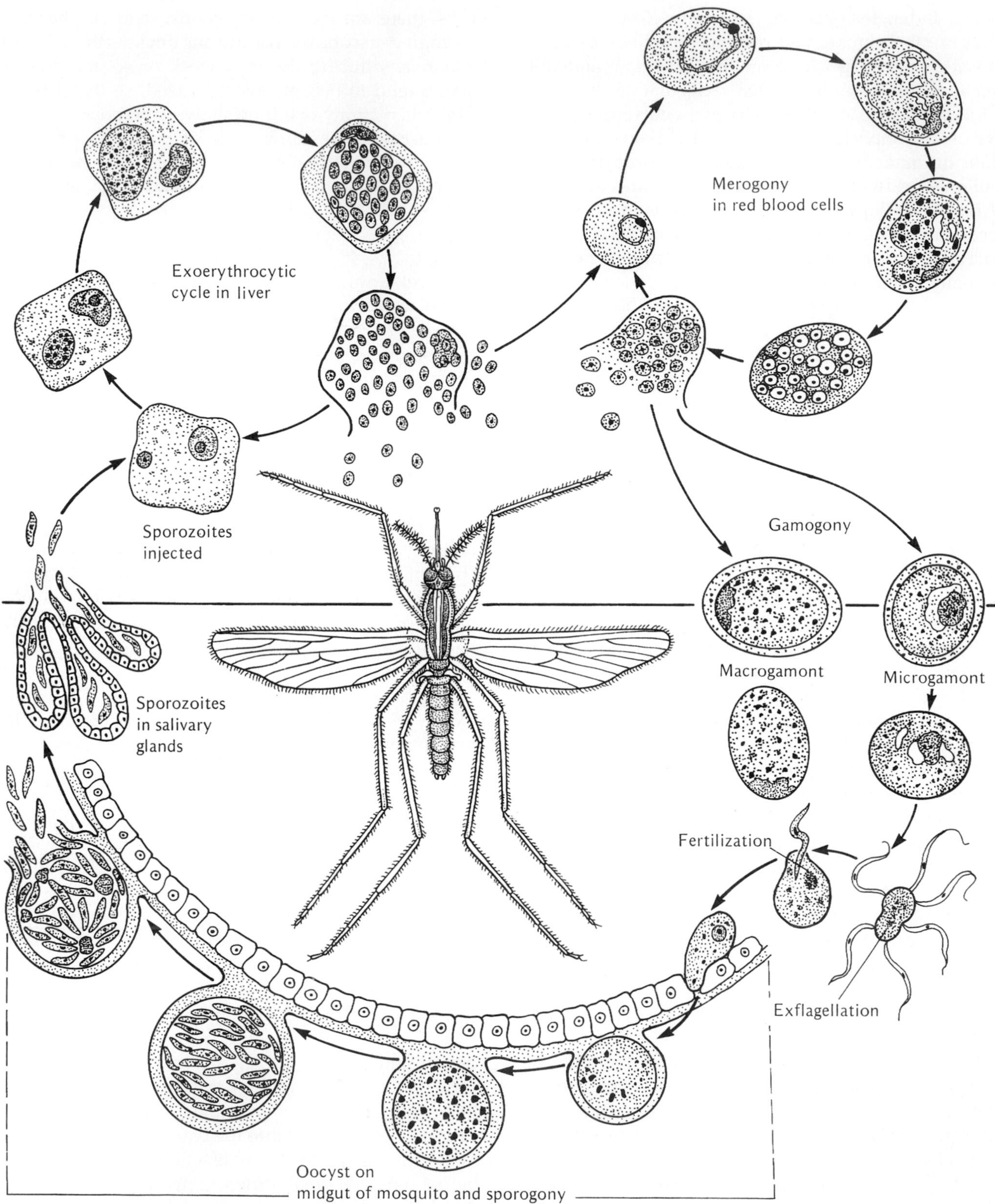

FIGURE 14.2 Life cycle of *Plasmodium vivax* in humans.

duces 18 daughter cells in 48 hours and that all of the daughter cells invade and reproduce at the same level, one merozoite will have increased to more than 10,000 during eight days.

Gamonts begin to appear in circulating red cells three to five days after the infection has become patent. It is not until this time that the infection can be transferred successfully to a mosquito vector.

Gamonts have a relatively short life in the bloodstream; if they are not picked up by a mosquito within about 48 hours of their formation, they die. They do not undergo any further development as long as they remain in the bloodstream of the vertebrate host.

When an uninfected mosquito takes a blood meal from a person, both sexual and asexual stages are ingested. The meronts die and do not participate in the transfer of the infection to a new host. The gamonts undergo change quite soon after ingestion by a mosquito. Although the organisms are haploid, nuclear activity takes place in both macrogamonts and microgamonts. As a result of reduced temperature and a change in the blood pH, nuclear division begins in the microgamonts within minutes after the blood has reached the midgut of the mosquito. Within 15 minutes, exflagellation has been completed with the formation of six to eight motile, threadlike microgametes, each about 10 μm long and with a single nucleus in the center. The microgametes swim off in search of a macrogamete.

The changes in the macrogametocytes or macrogamonts are not as striking as in the microgamonts. The nucleus moves to the periphery of the gamont and protrudes slightly at the surface to form a cone. The microgamete enters the macrogamete at the point where the nucleus protrudes. Fertilization has taken place, a zygote has been formed, and the organism is now diploid.

The zygote is called an *ookinete* (Fig. 14.3C), and it moves from the lumen of the mosquito gut to the periphery and squeezes between gut cells. During the next ten days to three weeks, sporogony occurs. Within a day or so the ookinete has laid down a membrane and nuclear division has begun; this is the oocyst stage (Fig. 14.3D). Meiosis takes place 2 to 3 days after the oocyst has formed. Sporogony is a schizogonic process in which more than 10,000 sporozoites may be formed in each oocyst.

The uninucleated sporozoites (Fig. 14.3A) are about 15 μm in length when they escape from the oocyst. They spread throughout the hemocoel of the mosquito, and those that enter the salivary glands are in a position to be injected into a new host when the mosquito takes a blood meal.

The life cycle described here is that of *P. vivax*, but there are some differences among species that are important because of the effect on the host or how they affect transmission.

EXOERYTHROCYTIC (EE) CYCLE

All species of *Plasmodium* affecting humans have stages in the liver, and none are able to reenter liver cells once they have entered red cells (Tab. 14.2).

Of particular interest is the fact that *P. falciparum* has only a single EE generation and does not retain a liver infection after the erythrocytic phase has begun. The residual liver infection serves as a source of parasites for relapses that may occur some years following infection with *P. vivax* and *P. ovale* (see Relapse and Recrudescence).

The prepatent periods given are the minima for each species, and there may be considerable variation in the time after infection when parasites are first seen or when the clinical attack may occur. In *P. vivax*, the initial attack may not occur until three or four months after infection with some geographic isolates. Treatment with antimalarials may also extend the prepatent period.

There are both morphological differences (see Morphology and Diagnosis) and differences in time of replication among the species during the blood phase of the cycle (Tab. 14.3).

RELAPSE AND RECRUDESCENCE

It has been known for a long time that persons who have suffered from an attack of malaria may later suffer another attack without having been reinfected. This recurrence of malaria may be either a relapse or a recrudescence. These two phenomena and are defined as follows:

Relapse: The reappearance of parasitemia in a sporozoite-induced infection following adequate blood schizonticidal (meronticidal) therapy.

Recrudescence: Reactivation after a period of relative inactivity.

The principal difference to be noted is that in relapse, the parasites have unequivocally been eliminated from the circulating blood cells, whereas in recrudescence the parasites probably remain in the circulating blood cells. The implication is that the infection is retained somewhere other than the erythrocytes if relapse occurs.

Among the species of *Plasmodium* infecting humans,

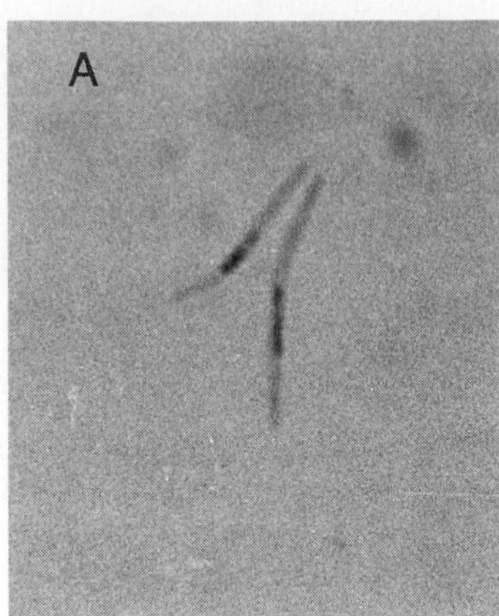

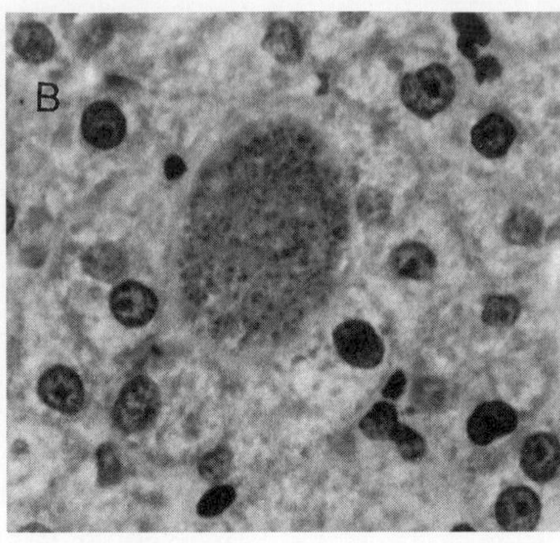

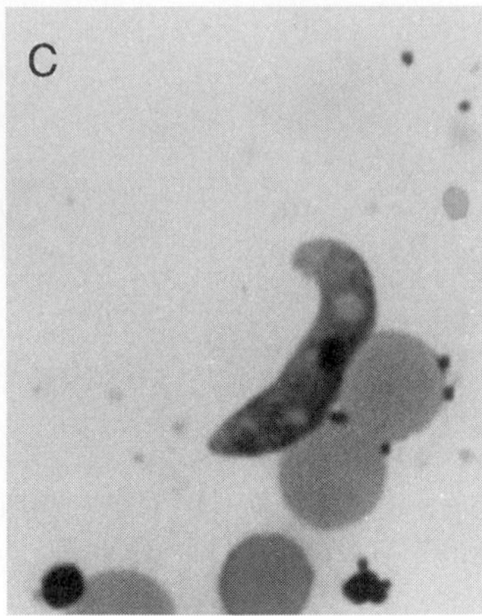

FIGURE 14.3 Life cycle stages of *Plasmodium*. (A) Sporozoite; (B) Exoerythrocytic meront (schizont) in the liver of a vertebrate; (C) Ookinete formed in the midgut of a mosquito and migrating to the wall of the midgut where it will form an oocyst, five red blood cells in the photo are still intact; (D) Oocysts on midgut of mosquito; (E) Human brain showing a capillary clogged by red blood cells infected with *Plasmodium falciparum*; each tiny dot in the Y-shaped capillary represents one malarial parasite.

P. vivax and *P. ovale* have true relapse. *P. malariae* has only recrudescence and *P. falciparum* has neither.

In *P. malariae* infections, malaria can recur after long periods of time, sometimes years, but if there has been adequate treatment of the blood stages, the patient will be cleared of infection.

Literally decades of investigation were required to find out what stage was retained and where they are located in *P. vivax* and *P. ovale*. (*Note:* most of the work has been done with *P. vivax* since *P. ovale* is rare.) Over time, the following was found:

1. As a result of massive blood transfusions, the parasites do not remain in the peripheral blood.
2. Treatment of experimental animals with drugs such as the 8-aminoquinolines, which kill sporozoites, eliminates relapse.
3. Blood transfusion during the prepatent period fails to produce infections in the recipients, but the donors may later suffer relapse.

The evidence supports the hypothesis that a stage called a *hypnozoite*, (sleeping zoite), which is a somewhat modified sporozoite, is the dormant stage in the liver of the host. The hypnozoites have been found histologically in the liver and there is little doubt that the liver infection is the source of organisms that may later cause relapse. What allows it to remain in an undifferentiated state for years? What stimulus causes it to begin development? If waning immunity is not the major factor in relapse, what is?

Morphology and Diagnosis

The blood stages of *Plasmodium* (Fig. 14.4 and Tab. 14.3) are looked for and examined in making a positive diagnosis of malaria. Diagnosis of malaria is based on the following:

1. Finding malarial parasites in stained blood films
2. Clinical signs and symptoms
3. Serological tests for the presence of antibody to *Plasmodium*
4. Finding the DNA of *Plasmodium* in the blood.
5. The patient's recent presence in a malarious area

Of these, finding the organisms is the only certain means of determining that a person is suffering from malaria. The other four are important factors in leading a diagnostician to suspect malaria.

Host–Parasite Interactions

Damage to the Host

During the early phase of the infection of humans with *Plasmodium* spp., there is no discernible damage. After the organisms begin to leave the liver and appear in the circulating blood, mild symptoms are experienced. Within about a week after patency, the parasites increase in number and their replication in the red cells becomes synchronized. It is at this point that the malarial paroxysm is seen—the typical chills and fever of a malarial attack. *Plasmodium vivax*, *P. ovale*, and *P. falciparum* have much the same generation time: 48 hours. On the other hand, *P. malariae* has a 72-hour generation time, and the paroxysms occur every three days (Fig. 14.5).

As the clinical phase of malaria progresses, more and more red blood cells are destroyed, and anemia becomes evident. While this hemolytic anemia is an

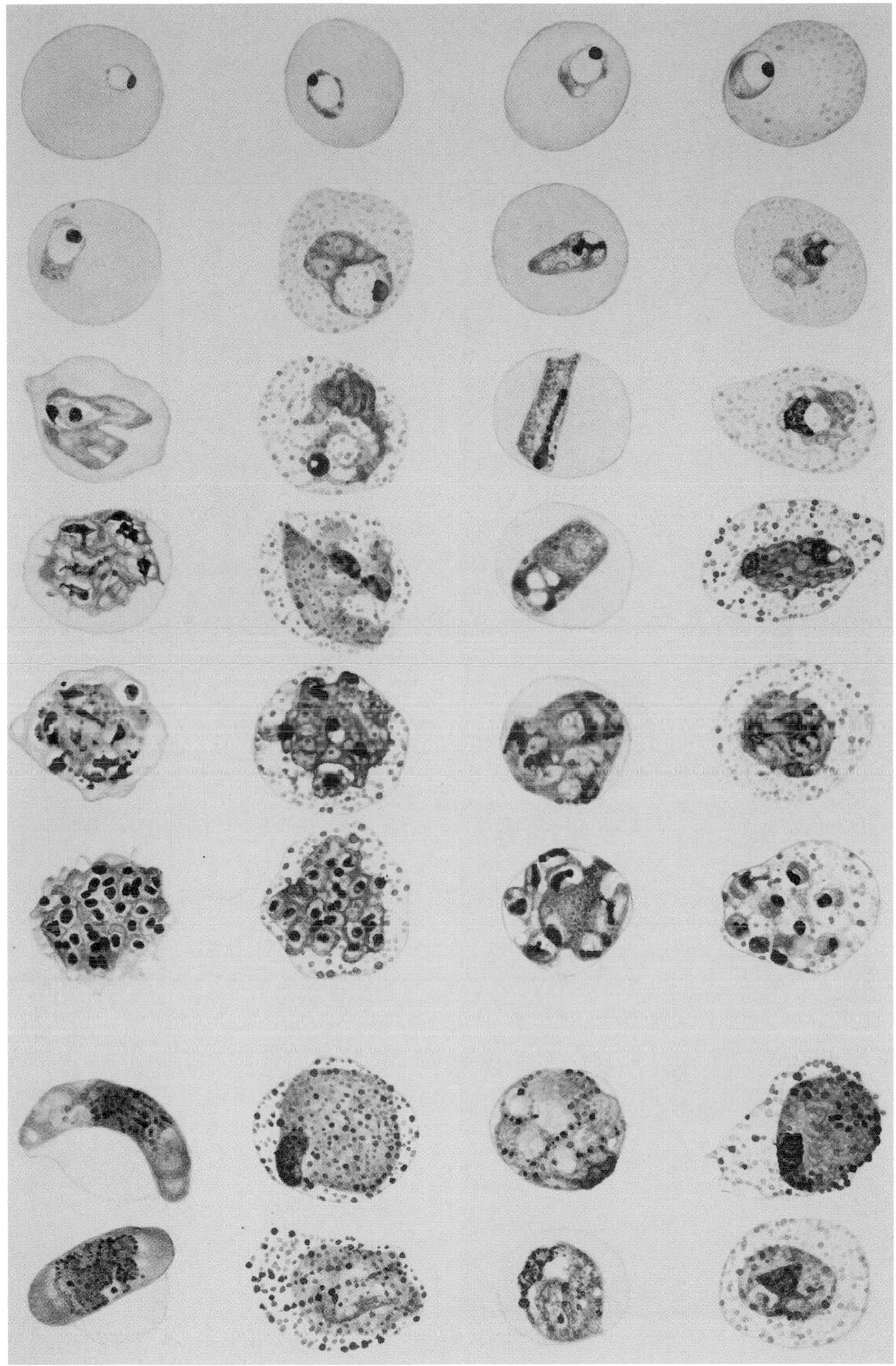

FIGURE 14.4, Part 1 Human malarial parasites as they appear in blood films. The ring stages are at the top and the various stages of merogony in the next five rows. The bottom two rows show the macro- and microgametocytes, respectively. [Reproduced by permission from L. W. Diggs, D. Sturm, and A. Bell, 1972, *The Morphology of Human Blood Cells*, 4th ed. Abbott Laboratories, North Chicago, IL.]

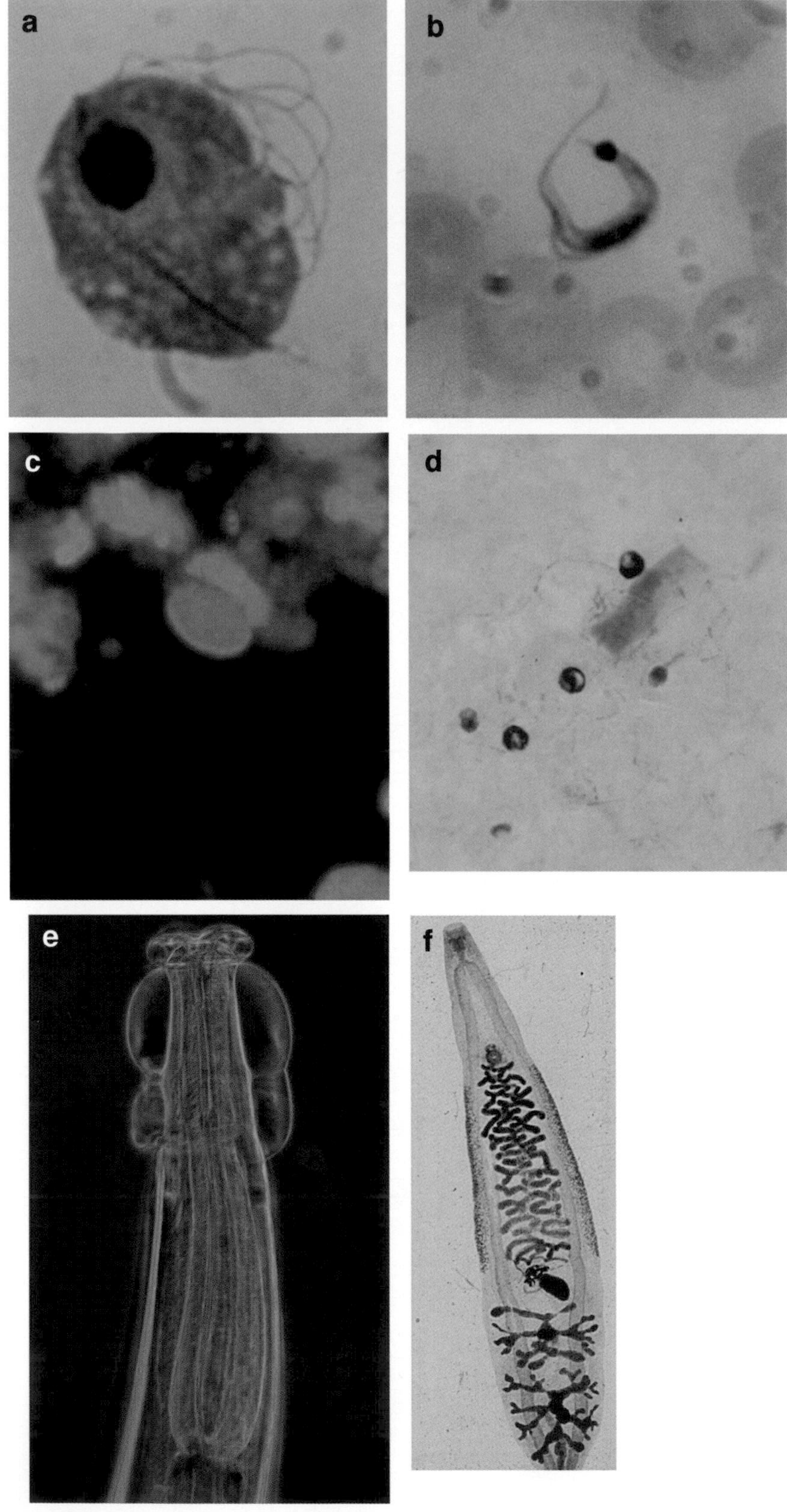

FIGURE 14.4, Part 2 (a) *Trichomonas vaginalis,* Giemsa stain; (b) *Trypanosoma cruzi,* trypoomastigote, Giemsa stain; (c) *Giardia duodenalis* cyst (lime green) in water sample — indirect flourescent antibody; (d) *Cryptosporidium parvum* occysts (red) in cal fecal smear — acid fast stain; (e) *Oesophagostomum radiatum* head and esophagus — darkfield; (f) *Clonorchis sinensis* — carmine stain.

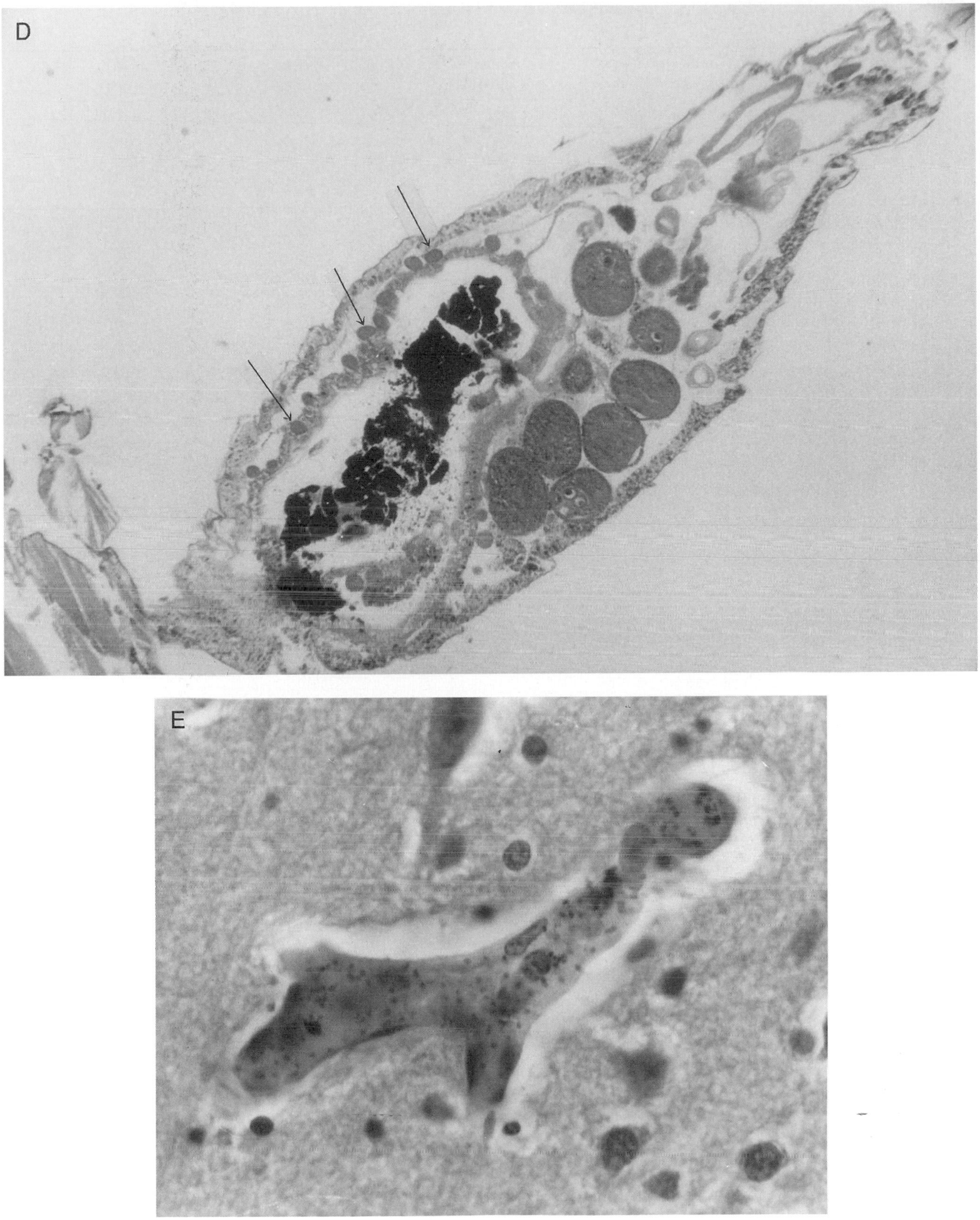

D

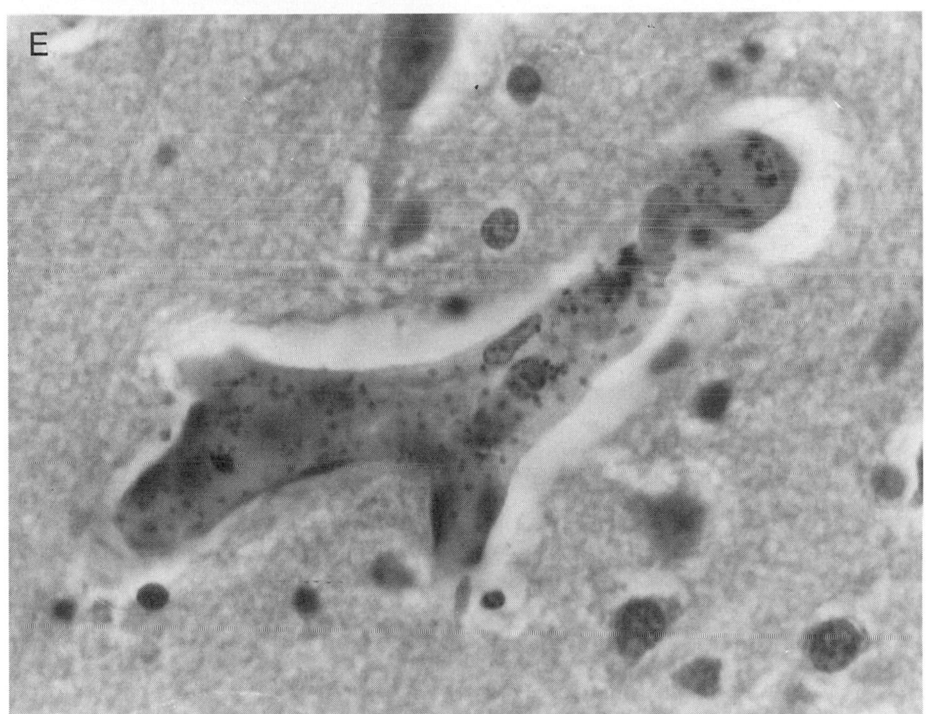

FIGURE 14.3 (*Continued*)

TABLE 14.2 Reproductive Potential, Prepatent Periods, and Liver Infections in the Species of *Plasmodium* Infecting Humans

Species of plasmodium	Number of EE generations	Merozoites/ Sporozoite	Prepatent period (minimum in days)	Liver infection retained
vivax	2[b]	1,000	8	Yes
falciparum	1	40,000	5.5–6	No
malarie[a]	2[b]	2,000	11–12	No
ovale	2	15,000	9	Yes

[a]Some information on *P. malariae* is not available and data have been taken from *P. inui*, a closely related species that infects higher primates.
[b]There are at least two EE generations; there may be more, but the exact number is not known.

obvious result of malaria, other pathologic effects are also seen as the disease continues. It has been shown that the observed anemia is more profound than mere destruction of red blood cells would indicate; it is likely that there is some effect on the hemopoeitic centers in the bone marrow. The liver and spleen both become enlarged and the liver is damaged. The kidneys are also subject to damage and glomerulonephritis is commonly seen.

Immunity and Vaccination

Immunity to infections with *Plasmodium* has beneficial effects but also some adverse effects on the host.

The beneficial effects of immunity to malaria are the following:

1. Prevention of infection, reinfection, or superinfection with the same species or strain
2. Reduction of multiplication of the parasite
3. Destruction of parasites
4. Aid in the repair of tissue

Immunity appears to act in reducing the number of parasites in the blood during a series of paroxysms. Over a period of about two weeks in a *P. vivax* clinical infection, the numbers of parasites are reduced and the paroxysms become less severe, ultimately disappearing. Thus, immunity developed during the initial stages of the infection reduces the effect on the host and controls the infection.

Premunition is a condition in which a host must retain an infection with an infectious agent in order to maintain resistance to reinfection. Malaria seems to be a good example of premunition. If an individual is cleared of infection by treatment with drugs or through development of a sterile immunity naturally, the immunity wanes in a few months and the person becomes completely susceptible to reinfection. In areas where there is likely to be year-round exposure to sporozoites of *Plasmodium*, malarial attacks are seldom seen in adults; children suffer from attacks, but as they become older, immunity and continual reinfection hold the clinical symptoms in check.

Development of a vaccine against malaria has been the objective of a number of research groups for a good many years, but a good vaccine for human use has not yet appeared on the market. The problems lie in the following:

1. The short time after a person has been cleared of infection when effective immunity is retained
2. The lack of cross-protection between species of *Plasmodium*
3. The lack of cross-protection between strains of the same species
4. The role of the HLA proteins in the efficacy of a vaccine

The proteins of *Plasmodium* spp. infecting humans are poor antigens and they do not raise the level of immunity sufficiently to produce an adequate response after the infection has waned. In many of the common bacterial or viral diseases such as measles, smallpox, or diphtheria, clinical disease is followed by sterile immunity, which is retained usually for the life of the person. Such is not the case with *Plasmodium*, and the lack of good, natural immunity has hampered the development of an artificial vaccine.

The rather poor antigenicity of *Plasmodium* spp. not only hampers development of both natural and artificial immunity but may also have detrimental effects on the host. Many eukaryotic parasites that have long developmental times are poorly antigenic. The hypothesis that has been set forth is that parasites that take more than ten days or two weeks to reach the stage when they can be transmitted to a new host must be poorly antigenic or they would be removed by the host defenses.

In an evolutionary context, parasites that are poorly antigenic would be favored for survival, and antigens that the host can readily recognize would drop out over a period of time. One possible result would be

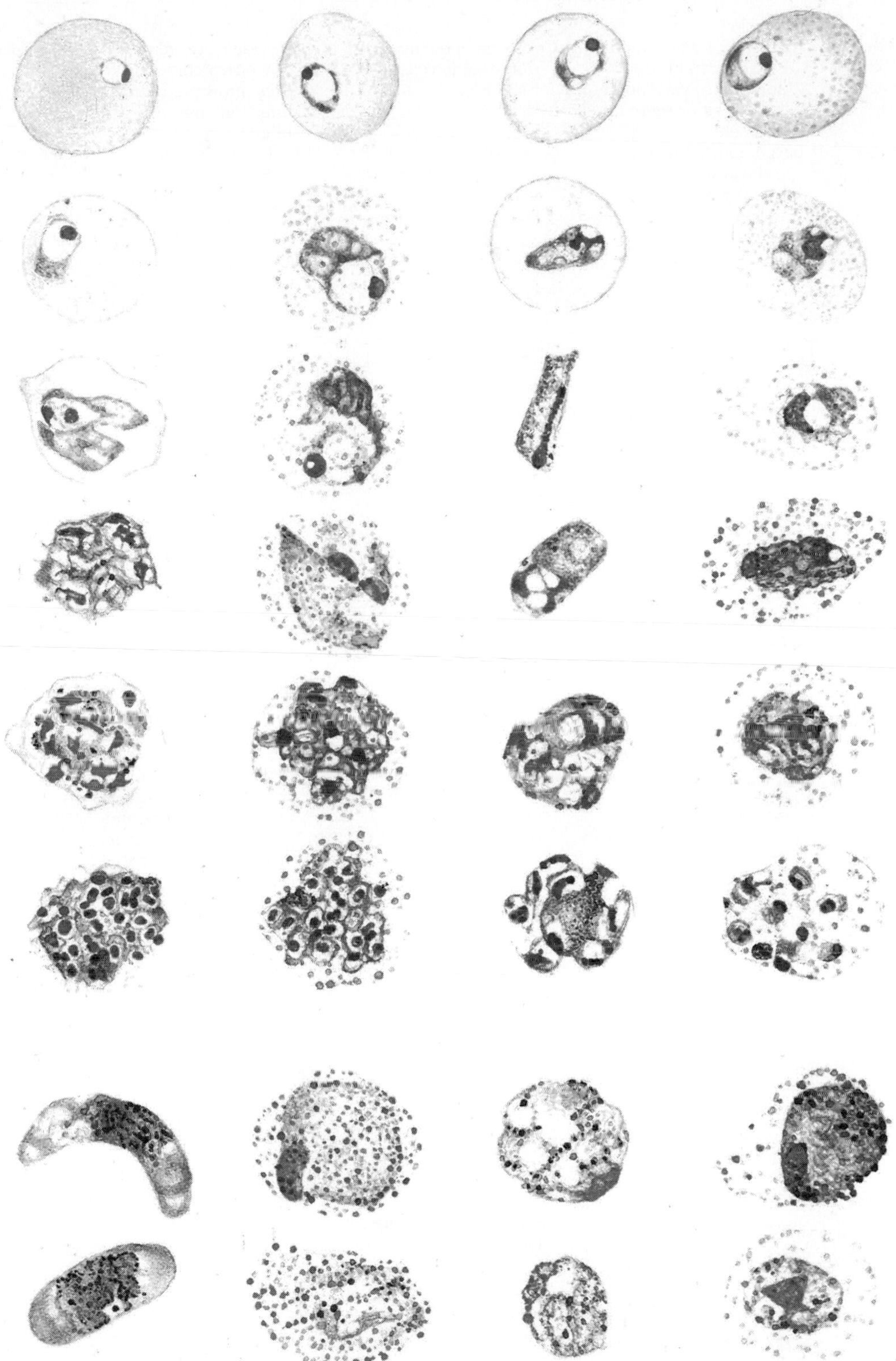

FIGURE 14.4 Human malarial parasites as they appear in blood films. The ring stages are at the top and the various stages of merogony in the next five rows. The bottom two rows show the macro- and microgametocytes, respectively. [Reproduced by permission from L. W. Diggs, D. Sturm, and A. Bell, 1972, *The Morphology of Human Blood Cells*, 4th ed. Abbott Laboratories, North Chicago, IL.] See also color plate.

TABLE 14.3 Characteristics of the Species of Malaria Infecting Humans

State or period	Plasmodium vivax	Plasmodium malariae	Plasmodium falciparum	Plasmodium ovale
In Man				
Early trophozoite or ring	Relatively large; usually one chromatin dot, sometimes two; often two rings or more in one cell	Compact; one chromatin dot; double cell infections rare	Small, delicate; sometimes two chromatin dots; multiple red cell infection common; appliqué forms frequent	Compact; one chromatin dot; double infection uncommon
Large trophozoite	Large, markedly ameboid; prominent vacuole; pigment in fine rodlets	Small; often band-shaped; not ameboid; vacuole inconspicuous; pigment coarse	Medium size; usually compact, rarely ameboid; vacuole inconspicuous; rare in peripheral blood	Small; compact, not ameboid, vacuole inconspicuous; pigment coarse
Young schizont or presegmenter	Large; somewhat ameboid; chromatin masses numerous; pigment in fine rodlets	Small; compact; chromatin masses few; pigment coarse	Medium size; compact; chromatin masses numerous; pigment granular; rare in peripheral blood	Medium size; compact; chromatin masses few; pigment coarse
Mature schizont or segmenter	Larger than normal red cells; may have double rosette	Smaller than normal red cells; single rosette	Smaller than normal red cells; single rosette	Larger than *P. malariae*; irregular rosette
Number of merozoites	8–24, usually 12–18	6–12, usually 8	8–26, usually 8–18	6–16, usually 8
Microgametocytes (usually smaller and less numerous than macrogametocytes)	Spherical; compact; no vacuole; single large nucleus; diffuse coarse pigment; cytoplasm stains light blue	Similar to *P. vivax* but smaller and less numerous	Crescents usually sausage-shaped; chromatin diffuse; pigment scattered, large grains; nucleus rather large; cytoplasm stains darker blue	Similar to *P. vivax* but somewhat smaller; never abundant
Macrogametocytes	Spherical; compact; larger than microgametocyte; smaller nucleus; pigment same; cytoplasm stains darker blue	Similar to *P. vivax* but smaller and less numerous	Crescents often longer and more slender; chromatin central; pigment more compact; nucleus compact; cytoplasm stains darker blue	Similar to *P. vivax* but somewhat smaller; never abundant
Pigment	Short, rather delicate rodlets irregularly scattered; not much tendency to coalesce	Seen in very young rings; granules rather than rods; tendency toward peripheral scatter	Pigment granular; early tendency to coalesce; typical single solid mass in mature trophozoite; coarse scattered "rice grains" in crescents	Similar to but somewhat coarser than *P. vivax*
Alterations in the infected red cell	Enlarged and decolorized; Schüffner's dots usually seen	Cell may seem smaller; fine stippling occasionally seen	Normal size but may have "brassy" appearance; Maurer's dots (or clefts) may be seen; host cell of crescent barely seen	Enlarged and decolorized; Schüffner's dots (or James's stippling) early and prominent at all stages; numerous oval-shaped red cells; or crenated margins
Length of asexual phase	48 hours or a little less	72 hours	36–48 hours	48 hours or a little longer
Prepatent period:	Usually 13–17 days	Usually 28–37 days	Usually 8–12 days	Usually 14–16 days
Minimum	8 days	14 days	5 days	8 days
Usual incubation period	8–31 days, average 14	28–37 days, average 30		11–16 days, average 14
Interval between parasite patency and gametocyte appearance	3–5 days	7–14 days; appearance irregular and numbers few	7–12 days	12–14 days; appearance irregular and numbers few
In the Mosquito				
Developmental period in mosquito	16–17 days at 20°C (68°F); 10 days at 25°C (77°F); 8 days at 28–30°C (82.4–86°F)	30–35 days at 20°C; 25–28 days at 22–24°C (75.2°F)	22–23 days at 20°C; 10–12 days at 26.7°C (80°F)	16 days at 25°C
Young oocyst (pigment)	Fusiform pigment, often in chain	Rounded or angular masses; golden brown	Square or rectangular blocks; black	Coccobacillary in form, with 15–30 grains
Sporozoites (considerable size variations in different mosquitoes)	About 8 μm	Relatively large; about 12 μm; chromatin diffuse	About 9 μm	Larger than *P. malariae*

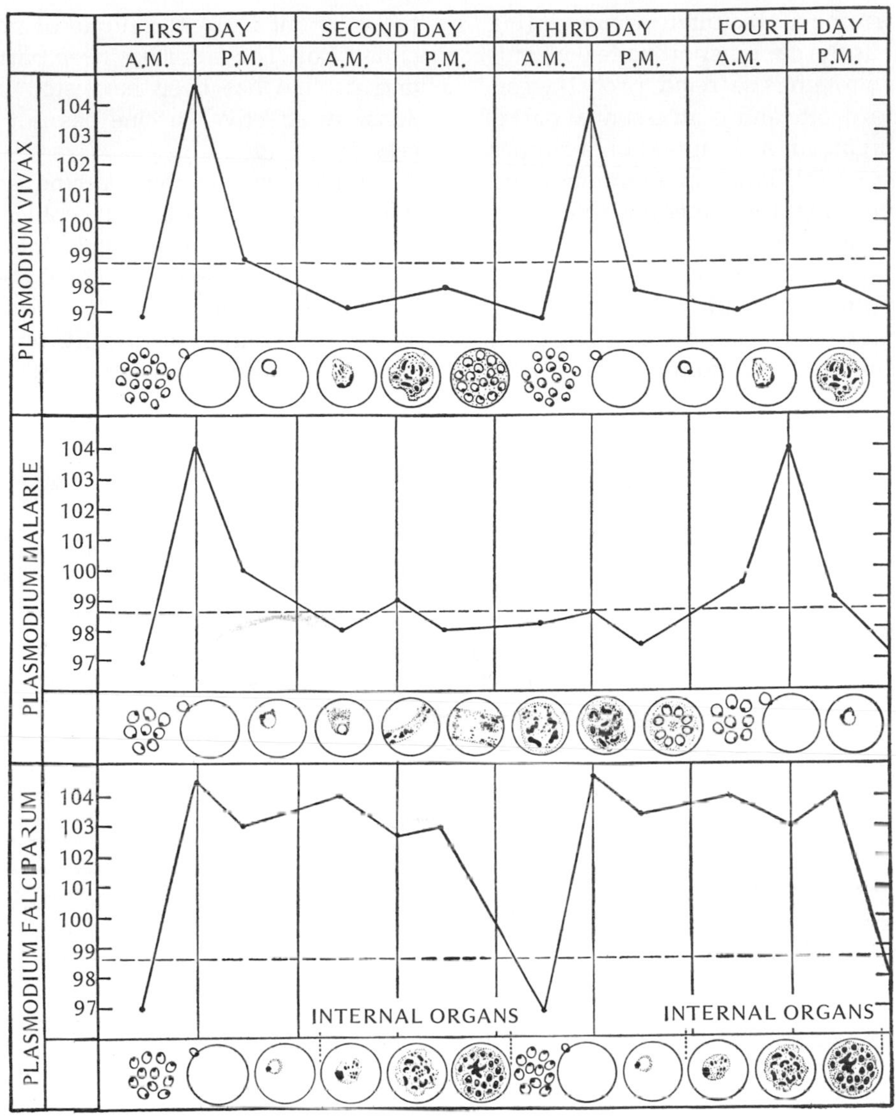

FIGURE 14.5 Body temperature and the developmental stages of malaria in the bloodstream. [Redrawn from Belding, 1965.]

that not only would the parasite be poorly antigenic, but it might mimic the host proteins as a means of "hiding" from the immune response. *Plasmodium* spp. are clearly poorly antigenic, and it has been found that some species have proteins similar to those of their hosts. The disease called *blackwater fever* is a manifestation principally of *P. falciparum* infections in which there is lysis of red cells that may be sufficiently severe to cause the death of the host. It is theorized that the host becomes hypersensitive (allergic) to its own red cells because of their similarity to the proteins of the parasite. The reaction is thereby turned against the host to its detriment.

Blackwater fever occurs in areas where there is a high prevalence of *P. falciparum* infection and is manifested, in part, by black urine. The dark color represents hemoglobin from lysed red cells. Most often it is seen in persons who reside in highly endemic areas and have long-term, continuous exposure to *P. falciparum*. A person who has an attack of blackwater fever has about a 25% chance of dying if untreated, and once an individual has had an attack, additional attacks are likely.

Attempts to make vaccines have targeted the proteins of the sporozoites, merozoite, and the gametocytes. Attacking each stage in the blood cycle has its advantages, but the sporozoite has been the object of most vaccination programs.

For more than 50 years it has been known that immune serum from a patient with malaria reacts against the sporozoite by forming a precipitate around it (Fig. 14.6). This is known as the circumsporozoite (CS) antigen or protein. This protein is secreted, probably continuously, by the sporozoite and is an essential part of the motility of the organism as it moves on a surface. Sporozoites are stopped and killed by immune serum, and it has been thought that this protein would be the logical choice for inclusion in a vaccine.

A number of means have been used over the years to make a large amount of CS protein including (1) irradiating sporozoites to weaken but not kill them, (2) growing sporozoites in cell culture, and (3) the recombinant DNA technique of producing it in vaccinia virus. The latter has been particularly successful and protein has been harvested in useful amounts. Alas, an effective vaccine has not been entirely successful.

Should an effective vaccine against malaria be developed, there are still problems to be faced. If the objective is to completely interrupt transmission of malaria in an area, 99.9% of the population must be made immune. Consider that in a disease such as measles, which is directly transmitted from one person to another, only about 80% of the population

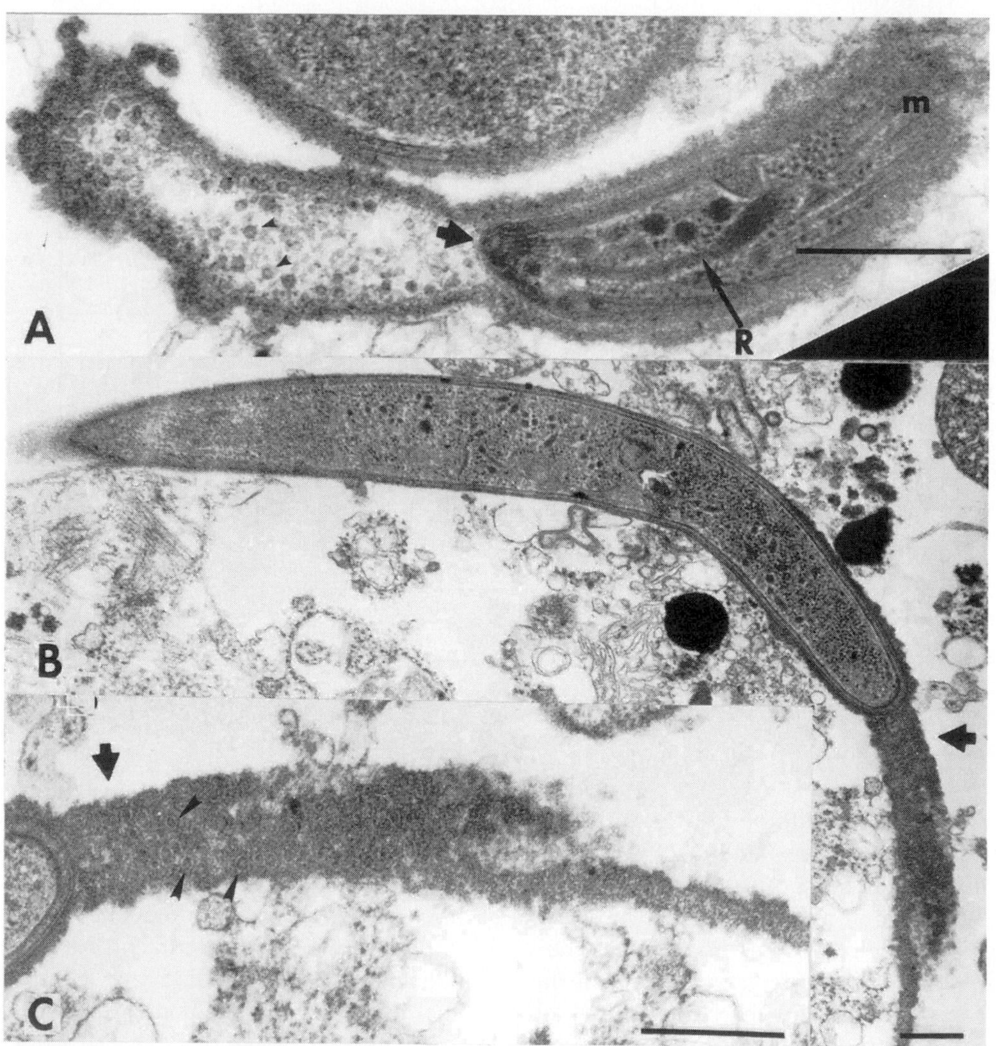

FIGURE 14.6 Circumsporozoite protein or antigen (CS) being shed from the surface of a sporozoite of *Plasmodium berghei* of rodents. The protein is produced at the anterior end (A) of the organism (thick arrow), and there are small particles in the secretion (small arrow heads). The CS protein is shed from the posterior end of the sporozoite (B) (thick arrow) and reacts with antibody to form the CSP (circumsporozoite precipitate) (C) (thick arrow). The CS protein is important in immunity developed by the host as well as in the motility of the organism Abbreviation: R—rhoptry. [From Stewart and Vanderberg, 1991.]

must be immunized to block transmission. Now, malaria occurs in areas that have little public health infrastructure, are economically poor, and reaching all of the people is difficult, especially at certain times of the year. Obtaining nearly complete immunity in the population becomes at least difficult and perhaps impossible.

Stable and Unstable Malaria

Another aspect of immunity relates to stable and unstable malaria. Stable malaria describes the situation where there is continuous transmission on a year-round basis. Nearly everyone in the community is continually exposed and reexposed to the bites of infected mosquitoes. Some individuals may fall ill for short periods of time but are generally not incapacitated after immunity is established during childhood.

In unstable malaria, transmission occurs seasonally, usually in summer. This was the situation in the southern United States until the mid-1940s when eradication was complete. Many, but not all, persons in a community would come down with malaria and eventually recover as immunity developed. By the next summer, they would have lost their immunity and become susceptible again. The stage was set for another outbreak as mosquito populations increased with the warm weather.

Consider that a vaccine might move a community from stable to unstable malaria unless a high level of immunity could be maintained both in individuals and in the population. The difficulties in economic terms, delivery of the vaccine at an appropriate time, and keeping track of individuals who may move about point up the fact that immunity may be less than protective. If a medical or public health person returns, say, to a village where stable malaria had turned to unstable malaria, it is likely that little cooperation would be forthcoming.

EVOLUTION IN THE ELEMENTS OF MALARIA

The interactions of human, *Plasmodium*, and mosquito represent a fascinating aspect of evolution in action. Each of the participants has developed mechanisms for coping with attempts to harm it or remove it completely from the population. Let us look at each separately:

Humans

Three genetic changes are seen in humans, which confer greater or lesser degrees of resistance to malaria.

Sickle Cell

The sickle cell name comes from the observation that a person with the trait has some distorted, elongate red cells. Sickle cell trait is a single-locus mutation that is generally lethal in the homozygous condition but confers some resistance to falciparum malaria in the heterozygous condition. The sickle trait results in a change in the protein portion of the hemoglobin molecule such that glutamic acid is replaced by valine.

The current view on the mechanisms of action of the sickle cell trait is as follows:

1. Homozygous red blood cells are changed to the sickle shape as a result of the formation of needle-like crystals of hemoglobin when exposed to the low oxygen tension present in tissues. The malarial parasites are mechanically disrupted by the hemoglobin needles and thus are destroyed. Usually the homozygous sickle cell individual dies from anemia, not from malaria.
2. Individuals heterozygous for sickle cell anemia have small knobs on red blood cell surfaces. These knobs are induced by the malarial parasites, and they cause infected red blood cells to stick to narrow peripheral capillary walls. These infected cells, stuck as they are, remain in low oxygen tension longer than uninfected cells. This lowered oxygen tension causes sickling of the red blood cell along with leakage of potassium from the cell. It is thought that a lowered potassium level kills the malarial organisms. Uninfected red blood cells have no knobs on their membranes and thus continue to move throughout the circulatory system. The infected cells are selectively removed, thus providing an individual heterozygous for sickle cell anemia with an effective means of coping with malaria. Unfortunately, progeny from heterozygotes face the prospect of perhaps dying from either malaria or sickle cell anemia, depending on whether they are homozygous against or for sickle cell anemia. Only the heterozygous children will survive in an endemic malarious area. Sickle cell trait is obviously not a "good solution" for genetic resistance to malaria, but it does exemplify the evolutionary pressure exerted in hyperendemic areas where falciparum malaria may cause severe sickness or death may occur in 10% of infants. In central Africa as many as 20%

of persons in some populations have the sickle trait, and in some places in the Middle East, as many as 30% have the trait; it is not true that only black Africans have the sickle trait.

Glucose-6-Phosphate Dehydrogenase Deficiency in Red Cells

Not a great deal is known about this deficiency, but children with it have lower parasitemias than normal children.

Duffy Blood Group

This factor is a single-locus mutation and persons having the Duffy blood group *negative* phenotype are completely resistant to *vivax* malaria. The genotype is present in about 90% of west African natives and in about 70% of African Americans. It has been known for generations that many blacks are resistant to malaria, and the Duffy blood group appears to be the explanation. The mechanism appears to reside in receptors on the red cell surface to which the *P. vivax* attaches; in Duffy-negative cells, the receptors are lacking and the parasite cannot attach and therefore cannot enter the red cell. There is no evidence that a person who is Duffy negative has any ill health related to it so it is a much better solution than the sickle cell trait.

Parasites

The only known change that has been found in the causative agent is drug resistance. In many parts of the world where drugs have been administered to a large proportion of the human population for a long period of time, strains of *Plasmodium falciparum* resistant to chloroquine have been found. As time has passed, additional drug resistances have been found including resistance to quinine. Drug resistance in *P. falciparum* has spread to all parts of the world where this species is found.

Mosquito

Since World War II, mosquitoes have been subjected to a great deal of evolutionary pressure from insecticides. With any rapidly reproducing organism with a short life span, one might expect that it could evolve rapidly enough to develop survival techniques. Within a few years after the wholesale use of DDT was begun, resistant populations began to emerge. Since then, populations resistant to all of the other major insecticides have been found, and in some cases the mosquitoes are resistant to more than one compound. This is a physiological resistance in which the insects are either able to metabolize the insecticide rapidly or are unaffected by the usual concentrations used. The other means of resistance is behavioral resistance. Much of malaria control depends on spraying dwellings with insecticides, such as DDT, which have a long residual action. Most of the mosquitoes that are good vectors of malaria enter dwellings, take a blood meal, and then rest on the nearest surface to digest the meal; the DDT on the surface will kill them. Because there is a range of behaviors in the population, some mosquitoes fly out of the house and thereby do not contact the treated surfaces. It is clear that these mosquitoes will be favored for survival, and populations have in fact been selected for flying out of dwellings to find resting surfaces. They survive to return later and transmit *Plasmodium*.

Each of the members of the *Plasmodium*-human-mosquito triangle has been subjected to pressures by the other members and responded with means of surviving and passing their DNA to the next generation. Before the technologies of synthetic drugs and insecticides were developed, humans appeared to be the only member that developed resistant mutations. It is only during the past 50 years that intense pressure has been placed on the vector and the causative agent.

Epidemiology and Control

The elements in the transmission of malaria are the causative agent, the vector, humans, and the environment. The characteristics of each and the ways in which they interact determine whether malaria will occur in a particular area and what the pattern of transmission will be. The distribution of malaria in the world is determined to a great extent by the distribution of the mosquito vectors. Only the Anophelinae (Chapter 47) serve as vectors of human *Plasmodium*.

Control of Malaria

Control of malaria in, its simplest terms, directs efforts at the following:

1. Personal protection
2. The vector
3. The parasite

By far the technologically simplest of these efforts is personal protection, which involves the following:

1. Screening of houses or sleeping under mosquito netting
2. Use of insect repellents
3. Avoiding mosquitoes by either not going where they are abundant or staying indoors

when they are most likely to bite (i.e., at dusk and dawn for many species)

In the tropics, many houses are not built for easy installation of screens; screens may also be prohibitively expensive, and some persons will not install them because they reduce the amount of air moving through the house.

For practical purposes, repellents are most useful in the short term, if one is going into an area where mosquitoes are abundant or must be out at night when mosquitoes are biting An interesting method of repelling insects was developed by the U.S. military by impregnating a mesh jacket with repellent; the jacket can be worn to repel flying insects or placed on the ground to repel crawling arthropods such as ticks.

Bed nets (mosquito nets, mosquito bars) can be highly effective in preventing malaria and other diseases transmitted by flying insects. Like the mesh jacket, the current practice is to impregnate the net with a synthetic pyrethrin, which will both repel and kill mosquitoes. Nets must be reimpregnated periodically.

Insecticide-impregnated bed nets were tested in The Gambia, West Africa. Child mortality was reduced by 40% in villages where they were used, except for one location where mortality was not reduced. The overall reduction in mortality was 18% when the area of failure was included in the data.

The cost of nets and impregnation remains a problem. Exclusive of the nets, the cost of impregnation is $2.41 (US), but villagers were willing to pay only $1.00 for the impregnation. When there was no cost for impregnation, the use of the nets rose to 77%. It is estimated that it would cost $120,000 to impregnate all bed nets in The Gambia, but these costs are beyond the financial capability of the government.

Although members of the Anophelinae are widely distributed, some even being found in cold northern climates, they are principally found in warm and hot climates. Of something less than 400 species and subspecies of *Anopheles*, about 65 are known to be vectors of *Plasmodium* spp. of humans. In the Western Hemisphere, there are two vectors extending from all of North America south through most of Mexico. For Central America, a much smaller area, there are five proven vectors. In Europe there are four vectors in the northern part, but seven in the Mediterranean area. Thus, in the warmer areas more species can transmit the parasite; more species means that more different ecological niches will be inhabited, thereby increasing the probability that a potential vector will be found in any one locality.

Mosquitoes are holometabolic insects. All of the larval stages and the pupae are aquatic. The time from egg to adult varies from perhaps three or four days to several weeks, depending on the species and rearing conditions of temperature and food. Adults may live a month or more, but only a minority do so. In order to complete transmission, a female mosquito must take at least two blood meals. Blood is required for the maturation of significant numbers of eggs, and a female takes a blood meal, oviposits within a few days, takes another blood meal, and oviposits a second brood. A long-lived female may lay five or more batches of eggs.

The potential for explosive epidemics in areas where unstable malaria exists is exemplified by both accidental and purposeful transmission. In one experiment, a single mosquito infected 40 persons. In a case report, late in the Korean War a marine suffered a malarious attack while camping near a girls' camp in the Sierra mountains of California. He was in the vicinity for only a single night during the paroxysm, but 35 girls later came down with malaria. In Syria, a man suffered a relapse with *P. vivax* and there were 52 known cases acquired from this single individual.

Non-mosquito-borne malaria has been a problem at various times. It first came to light in the late 1930s in New York City when an outbreak of malaria occurred; investigation revealed that the infection was transmitted among individuals who were heroin users and had passed the infection through shared needles. There have been about 200 cases in New York, and a few other outbreaks have been reported. From 1958 to 1977 there were 56 needle-borne cases of malaria in the United States, 47 of which occurred in 1971, during the Viet Nam War.

Malaria transferred by blood transfusions has not been a serious problem, but there are a few sporadic instances on record. Over the 20 years from 1958 to 1977 there was an average of 2.5 cases of transfusion malaria in the United States. It is suggested that persons who have had falciparum malaria may safely donate blood one year after an attack and those who have had vivax malaria may donate blood after three years. Those who have had *P. malariae* should not be donors. Most blood banks will not accept blood from a person who has had malaria, and in our opinion that is the proper decision to make unless the need for blood overrides the risk.

Prenatal transmission of malaria can occur, but is not common. It is seemingly a rare occurrence for either sporozoites or meronts to pass from the maternal circulation to the fetus through the placenta.

Treatment

In the history of medicine, the treatment of malarial paroxysms with quinine may well be the first instance in which a substance had a specific curative effect against an infectious agent. The myth is often repeated that the Countess of Chinchon was afflicted with malaria in Peru in about 1640. She was given the bark of a local tree by her physician and experienced a miraculous cure. She was so enthusiastic over the results of this treatment that she carried some of the tree bark back to Spain and was instrumental in establishing it as a cure for malaria.

In reviewing the history of malaria, Russell et al. (1963) relate that while the Countess was in Peru with her husband she was in remarkably good health, never suffered from malaria, but died during the return trip before reaching Spain. The traditional story is a myth whose source is unknown. The real story is more interesting, if somewhat less romantic than the myth.

The Amerinds in South America probably used the bark of cinchona and other trees to reduce fever. Since malaria did not exist in the Western Hemisphere until European colonization, the Amerinds did not use it originally against malaria. The first documented use of the bark of *Cinchona ledgeriana* against malaria was in 1600 when a Jesuit missionary, Juan Lopez, was cured of a malarious attack. The first cinchona bark reached Europe in 1632, probably taken there by Jesuits, and was widely used in treating fevers.

During the early years of colonization and exploration of the New World, plants were transported back and forth between the Old World and New World in great profusion. Likewise, there was considerable trade in potential medicinals. One of the tree barks was that of *Myroxylon peruiferum*, the extract of which was used to reduce fever, and a brisk trade grew up by the mid-1600s. Demand outstripped supply, and traders began to substitute the bark of *Cinchona ledgeriana*, which looked much like *M. peruiferum*. Physicians thought that they were using a single medicinal, but results were inconsistent and therefore confusing. Ultimately, it was determined that the fake had specific activity against intermittent fevers, and *C. ledgeriana* was established as the source of the active ingredient for treating malaria.

Carolus Linnaeus, the Swedish botanist who established binomial nomenclature for naming plants and animals, named *Cinchona ledgeriana*. He erred twice, first in perpetuating the myth of the countess's involvement in discovering a cure, and then in misspelling her name.

Extracts of cinchona bark contain more than 20 alkaloids, but only 4 of them have a significant effect on *Plasmodium*. The one with the highest level of activity is quinine, a quinoline derivative. Quinine was used for 300 years as the only drug for malaria until a concerted search was made for alternatives in the 1920s. Only in recent years has it been well documented that *Plasmodium* has shown resistance to quinine.

Quinine has a good effect against all species of *Plasmodium*, but it has some serious side effects such as ringing in the ears, deafness, dizziness, and various effects on vision. The side effects can be serious in some individuals, but the real stimulus toward finding substitutes was the interruption of the German supply of quinine in World War I.

The first useful synthetic antimalarial was an acridine, quinacrine (Atabrine, Mepacrine), used extensively in World War II as a suppressant and a chemotherapeutic. Although it is a highly effective drug, quinacrine has side effects such as discoloration of the skin and gastrointestinal disturbances.

Quinacrine was replaced by the quinolines when they were developed in the late 1940s. The quinolines have structures similar to quinine, and there are two groups of substituted quinolines, the 8-aminoquinolines and the 4-aminoquinolines. The 4-aminoquinolines are represented by chloroquine and amodiaquine. The 8-aminoquinolines are represented by pamaquine, pentaquine, and primaquine.

Since the development of these compounds, other groups of chemicals have also been found to have efficiency: pyrimidines (pyrimethamine, sulfadiazine), sufones (dapsone), and biguanides (proguanil). Broad spectrum antibiotics such as tetracycline have some curative effect.

The most recent antimalarial to gain acceptance is artemisinine or Quinghaos, which came out of traditional Chinese medicine. The plant *Artemesia annua* had been used traditionally in China to treat a variety of illnesses. In the 1980s it was found to have curative effects against malaria. Artemisinine is a sesquiterpene lactone and acts by inhibiting protein synthesis.

Chloroquine rarely causes side effects, but since about 1960, more and more isolates of *P. falciparum* have been found to be resistant to it. The major malarious areas of the world all have chloroquine-resistant falciparum malaria. Dapsone was originally used against Hansen's disease (leprosy), and has been found to be effective against drug-resistant *P. falciparum*, but regrettably it appears to be carcinogenic. None of the drugs currently cleared for use has a significant effect against sporozoites, that is, none is sporonticidal.

Antimalarials are used as

1. Therapeutics
2. Prophylactics
3. Suppressives

Therapeutic drugs are administered during a malarial paroxysm so that the parasites can be cleared from the blood quickly and the patient can begin to recover clinically. Prophylactic or suppressive administration of drugs is done on a long-term basis with a low dosage of the compound. The purpose is to prevent the appearance of clinical symptoms (suppression) or to kill the parasites in an early stage of development (prophylaxis). Chloroquine can be given both to treat an attack and to suppress the development of malaria.

Current malaria chemotherapy recommends using chloroquine to destroy blood merozoites plus primaquine to destroy liver stages. Mefloquine is used to treat chloroquine-resistant falciparum malaria. It is effective in a single dose but must be used with care because of side effects. It has also been used to treat resistant vivax malaria, but must be used with a merontic idal (antischizontal) drug such as primaquine to prevent relapses.

This discussion has taken only a general approach to chemotherapy of malaria. Although recommendations for the drugs to use under different circumstances have not changed radically, they do vary somewhat from year to year. For those living in or planning to visit a malarious area, a physician or local health department should be consulted for current recommendations.

The problem of drug resistance is becoming greater as large numbers of persons receive suppressive as well as therapeutic quantities of drugs. Quinine has been used for more than 300 years and is just now developing resistance. Quinine is exceptional among drugs, however; in nearly all instances where drugs have been used against nearly any kind of parasitic agent, microbial, protistan, helminthic, or arthropodal, resistance has been seen within a few years of introduction. The agents causing malaria are merely examples of the general principle. *Plasmodium* quite readily developed resistance to proguanil and pyrimethamine; resistance was first seen in them in the late 1940s and early 1950s, respectively. By 1977 chloroquine-resistant *P. falciparum* had been found in 8 countries of South America and 11 Asian countries; resistant forms were found in East Africa in 1979. In about 1995, reports began to surface indicating that *P. vivax* had developed drug resistance. It is now clear that resistance has developed in patchy areas of southeast Asia, the southwest Pacific, Burma (Myanmar), and the island of New Guinea (which contains the political entities of Irian Jaya and Papua New Guinea); resistance is suspected in India and Indonesia.

Mosquito Control

Efforts directed against the vector mosquito may be aimed at the larva or the adult. Different methods are required for each.

Much of the early effort to reduce the incidence of malaria was directed at the larval stages. In the early 1900s there were no effective insecticides for use against adult mosquitoes. Currently measures to reduce populations of preadult mosquitoes may be categorized as follows:

1. Chemical
2. Environmental management
3. Biological control

Control of adult mosquitoes is based on use of insecticides. Details of mosquito control are discussed in Chapter 47.

ERADICATION OF MALARIA

Eradication of a disease agent means that the organism is completely eliminated from a geographic or political area. Eradication is not to be attempted lightly, and success has been achieved with only a few infectious agents and in only limited areas. One of the few successes is that of smallpox, which was eradicated finally in 1977.

By the late 1940s, knowledge and techniques had developed to the point where eradication was being discussed. The factors that allowed consideration of an eradication program were the following:

1. The limited host range of *Plasmodium* spp. Those in humans infect only humans.
2. The anopheline vectors were almost always species that rested in dwellings after feeding.
3. DDT had been developed in the late 1930s and tested during World War II, so its characteristics were known. Its high toxicity for insects and its long residual action made it ideal for mosquito control.
4. Good chemotherapeutic and chemoprophylactic agents had been developed and tested during and after WWII. There was, therefore, a good armamentarium of drugs that could be used as part of the overall effort.

In 1955 the World Health Organization (WHO) launched a program whose objective was to eradicate malaria on a global scale (Fig. 14.7). The phases of program were as follows:

1. Preparation
2. Attack
3. Consolidation
4. Surveillance

The principles involved in these four phases of malaria eradication are the logical progression of actions

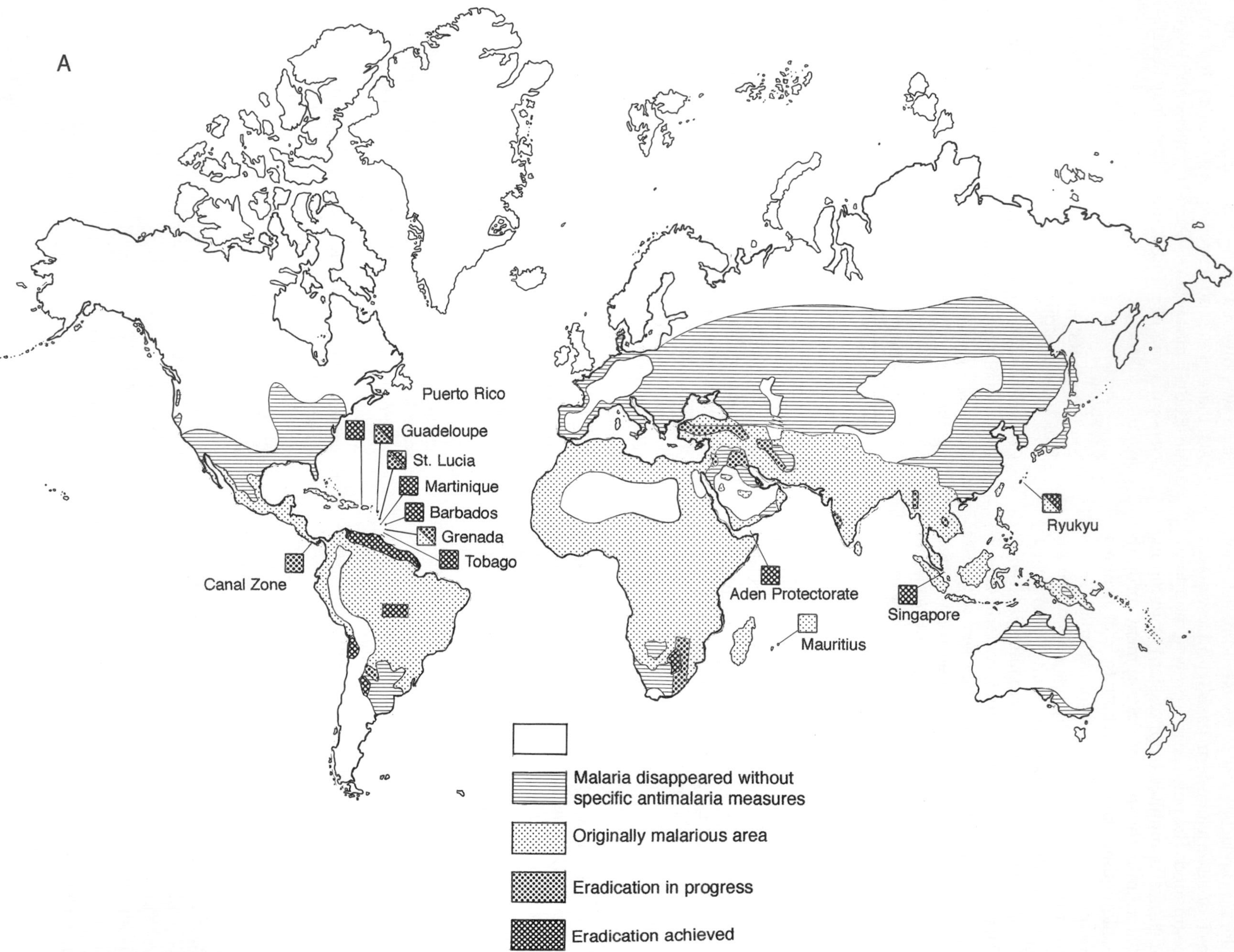

FIGURE 14.7 Global eradication of malaria. (A) Areas of the world where eradication has been achieved. Compare to Figure 14.1. (B) Phases in the eradication of malaria.

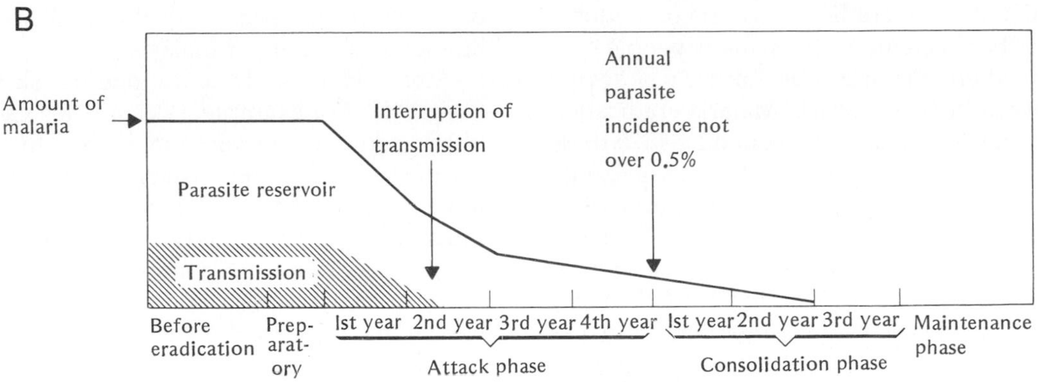

FIGURE 14.7 *(Continued)*

to take in setting up a control or eradication program for any transmissible disease.

1. *Preparation. Time: 18 months.* This is the phase for gathering information, personnel, and facilities. The extent and severity of malaria in the human population must be determined by blood film, splenic index, and public health records. The principal vector(s) of malaria must be determined and their biologies worked out. The general plan is developed, budgets are constructed, personnel are engaged, and facilities of all sorts are found, purchased, or built.

2. *Attack. Time: 4 years.* The principal thrust in the attack phase is against the anopheline vector through spraying of houses with insecticide. As large a segment as possible of the population is given prophylactic drugs such as chloroquine, and all clinical cases are treated therapeutically. Interruption of transmission should take place during the second year of the attack—that is, there should be no new cases of malaria after this time.

3. *Consolidation. Time: 3 years.* With transmission interrupted in the major part of the area, pockets of infection can then be located and eliminated. Residual spraying of some dwellings is continued. Seven years from the beginning of the attack phase, the residual or latent infections in the human population should have been almost completely eliminated. Mosquito control should keep the population of vectors, at least those associated with humans, at a low level. Even if a few persons in the population suffer from relapse or recrudescence, their number should be so small that the probability of transmission is insignificant.

4. *Surveillance. Time: 2 years or indefinitely.* Assuming that a good public health organization is in place, there should be adequate personnel to monitor and treat the occasional case or small outbreak that may occur as a result of importation of malaria.

Eradication of malaria was begun in the late 1950s by WHO. Eradication has been accomplished in the United States, some islands in the Caribbean Sea, Western Europe, Australia, and a few other countries. Note that where eradication has been successful, the countries are either affluent, on the margins of the endemic areas, or geographically isolated. Success was not experienced in the tropical areas of the Americas, Africa, Asia, and the Pacific islands. This is not to say that the impact of malaria has not been lessened, but the original objective has not been reached.

Why has eradication not been achieved when the finest minds in malariology, public health, and entomology reasoned that it could be done? The answer seems to be partly biological, but to a greater extent it is politicoeconomic. It has been pointed out that the following are requisites for malaria eradication in an area:

1. There is a single vector that seeks resting sites within houses.
2. There is a relatively high economic level in the country, and a relatively well-educated population.
3. There is a sufficient supply of trained personnel (physicians, entomologists, laboratory technicians, etc.).
4. The government is stable.
5. The government is determined to eradicate malaria and has the power to do so.

Although the absolute importance of some of these points may be debated, they have generally been found to be relevant to eradication programs. Where formerly endophilic mosquitoes were selected for exophilism through spraying of houses, control programs have become more difficult. Where public health officials have been poorly trained, malaria broke out again. Where governments shifted funds during the surveillance phase to what appeared to be more pressing problems, malaria resurged.

Despite the failure to eradicate malaria on a global scale, progress has been made; thus, many people who live in areas where malaria was formerly a severe threat are now at little or no risk. Malaria eradication was begun in the Americas in 1958, and by 1970 there were only 8346 cases of malaria in all countries, only 9% of which were contracted locally (autochthonous). In South America, 55% of the population by 1970 was living in areas where malaria was either in the consolidation or surveillance phases. In the United States, eradication was achieved in the early 1950s, but imported cases have recurred almost every year in small numbers. More recently, a few autochthonous are reported each year; usually the source of infections are immigrants from regions where malaria is endemic.

The situation in Africa is not as good as in the Americas. Of the 250 million inhabitants of Africa, 230 million originally lived in malarious areas. As of 1974, only 4.43 million were living in areas where malaria had been eradicated and 19.7 million were protected by some measures. About 90% of the population lacked the protection of an organized public health program.

There are a number of examples of eradication programs that almost succeeded. Sri Lanka had about 2.5 million cases of malaria annually prior to eradication programs. By 1963 the number was down to 16; but efforts were reduced, and in 1975 there were more than half a million cases. India's malaria cases were reduced from 75 million to 125,000 by 1965, but in 1975 the number was back up to 4 million. With deforestation in the Amazon Basin continuing apace, malaria has been imported by workers and settlers and anopheline habitat has improved so that they are flourishing.

EPIDEMIOLOGIC MODELS

Since malaria is so widespread and the costs of control are so high, it is important to determine how best to use available resources. Malaria seems to be the first disease in which concerted efforts were made to use quantitative methods for predicting the results of control (Bailey, 1982). As early as 1909, only 11 years after he described the development of *Plasmodium* in the mosquito, Sir Ronald Ross made the first attempt to write a mathematical expression for malaria transmission. He concluded that it was not necessary to eradicate the vector, but only to reduce its numbers below a certain threshold to break the cycle of transmission. Ross further refined his original equation, but nearly 40 years passed before a number of investigators in different institutions, attacking the problem simultaneously, began to refine both the mathematics and the biological elements of malaria.

Any model should allow one to ask the question, "What if?" For example, "What if we vaccinated 90% of the population against malaria?" In one model at least (May, 1983), the answer is, "not enough," since more than 99% need to be vaccinated in order to stop transmission. And that is precisely the kind of information, if it is accurate, that a public health administrator needs in order to use resources as efficiently as possible. Going back to the early part of this section, a number of possible points in the cycle of transmission of malaria can be attacked. For ultimate success to be achieved in control, the method used and the intensity of its application must be determined.

Notable Features

Working with human malaria has many difficulties, not the least of which had been the necessity of working with the organism in its normal host. However, if the organism could be cultivated outside the host, developmental, therapeutic, physiological, and biochemical studies could be done. As early at 1912, attempts were made to maintain the malaria organisms outside of its host. Survival and perhaps a few generations of merogony was the best that could be obtained for many years. Although progress was made in cultivation, and biochemical studies were done on surviving blood stages, knowledge accumulated slowly, while studies were done on bird and rodent malarias. Finally, in 1976, Trager and Jensen developed methods whereby *Plasmodium facliparum* could be maintained in continuous in vitro culture. Their methods are widely used in drug development and molecular studies on human malaria organisms.

OTHER HAEMOSPORINA

Although our greatest concern here is malaria of humans, related infections occur in other primates, rodents, birds, and reptiles. The bird malarias have been especially important in the development of knowledge on malaria and in searching for potential antimalarial drugs. The mosquito transmission of *Plasmodium* was accomplished by Sir Ronald Ross in 1898, working with *Plasmodium relictum* in sparrows. The exoerythrocytic (EE) cycle of *Plasmodium* was first worked out with bird malaria, and it became clear that such a cycle was probably also present in human malaria. During World War II, bird malaria species (especially *P. gallinaceum*, *P. cathemerium*, and *P. relictum*) were used in screening potential antimalarials.

The bird malarial parasites were good models for laboratory study, but it was felt that a species that infected mammals would be a better model because it would probably be more like the species in humans. A search was begun shortly after World War II and *Plasmodium berghei* was described from an African rodent by Vincke and Lips in 1948. The organism was adapted to laboratory mice and has since become the subject of thousands of studies on all aspects of the infection.

Haemoproteus and *Leucocytozoon*

Haemoproteus and *Leucocytozoon* are parasites of birds whose life cycles are similar to that of *Plasmodium* except that asexual stages do not appear in the circulating blood cells; the asexual stages remain in internal organs such as the muscles, spleen, and lung (Tab. 14.4). The gamonts (gametocytes) of *Haemoproteus* occur in erythrocytes, whereas those of *Leucocytozoon* are in leukocytes or erythrocytes, depending on the species (Bennett et al., 1975). These cells cannot be recognized with certainty as either white blood cells or red blood cells, because they are significantly altered by the time the infected cells reach the circulating blood.

In any locality, a sample of birds will show perhaps a 10% prevalence of infection with parasites in the genera *Plasmodium*, *Haemoproteus*, and *Leucocytozoon*, and they are generally nonpathogenic, so far as is known. Many are known only from their blood cell stages (Fig. 14.8) and have not been studied experimentally. A few species are pathogenic and cause losses in both domesticated and wild birds.

In most instances, members of these two genera have been described from wild birds, but in some domestic birds losses have been observed. For example, *Leucocytozoon smithi* is a parasite of turkeys, and poults are especially susceptible to infection. *Leucocytozoon simondi* is found in ducks and is highly pathogenic to ducklings, which die quite suddenly after showing initial signs of infection.

Haemoproteus has generally been considered to be nonpathogenic, but studies of *H. meleagridis* in the turkey have shown that birds are severely weakened by the infection and may die (Atkinson, 1991).

Control of pathogenic infections of *Haemoproteus* and *Leucocytozoon* in domestic birds is at least difficult and sometimes impossible. Most of the vectors are biting midges and black flies (Chapter 47). Both kinds of flies can generally migrate at least a kilometer from breeding sites, and it is necessary to find and treat the source. If it is possible to raise birds in tightly screened houses, they can be protected from the flies. Treatments have been developed for only a few species of the parasites.

Hepatozoon, Klossiella, and Other Adeleins

The order Adeleida contains organisms of seemingly heterogenous heritage and character. Some are

TABLE 14.4 Some Haemosporina of Birds. (*P. = Plasmodium, H. = Haemoproteus, L. = Leucocyotzoon, RBC = Red blood cell, WBC = White blood cell*)

Name	Hosts		Pathogenic	Meronts	Gamonts
	Vertebrate	Vector			
P. cathemerium	House sparrow and other passerine birds	Mosquito	Highly	RBC	RBC
P. circumflexum	Passerine and other birds	Mosquito	No	RBC	RBC
P. gallinaceum	Jungle fowl, chicken, and other galliforms	Mosquito	Highly	RBC	RBC
P. hermani	Bobwhite quail	Mosquito	Moderately	RBC	RBC
P. juxtanucleare	Galliform, passerine and anserine birds	Mosquito	Highly	RBC	RBC
P. natutinum	Many birds	Mosquito	Variable	RBC	RBC
P. relictum	Passerine columbiform anserine and other birds	Mosquito	Moderately to highly	RBC	RBC
H. columbae	Columbiforms	Hippoboscids	Slightly	Endothelial cells of blood vessels	RBC
H. meleagridis	Turkey	Biting midge	Moderately	Muscle spleen	RBC
H, sacharovi	Columbiforms	Hippoboscids	Slight	Spleen	RBC
L. simondi	Anserines	Black fly	Highly	Many organs	WBC, RBC
L. marchouxi	Columbiforms	Black fly	Moderately	Many organs	WBC, RBC
L. smithi	Turkey	Black fly	Highly	Spleen, liver gut	WBC, RBC

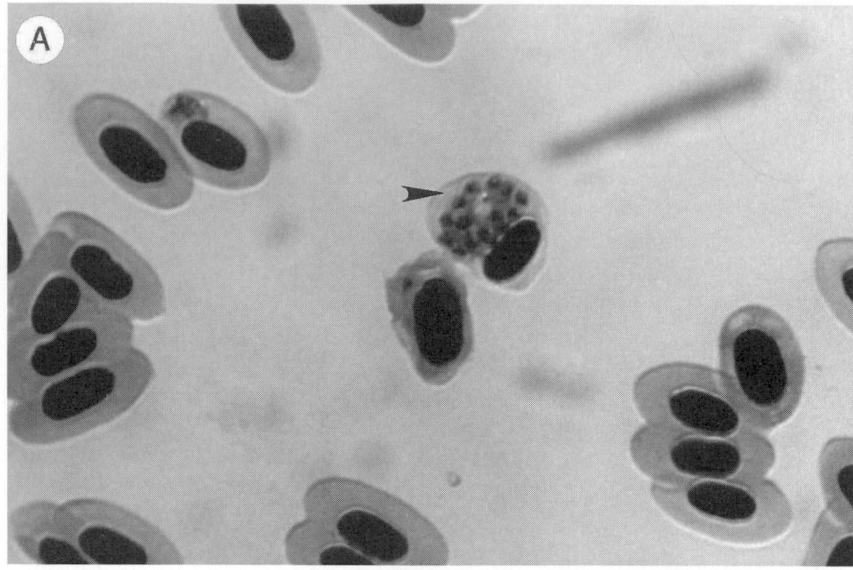

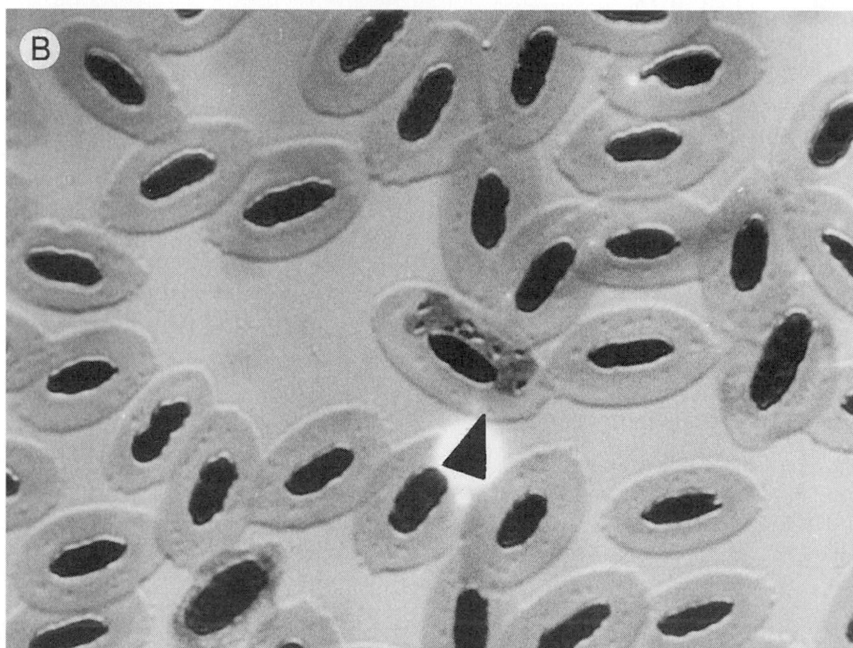

FIGURE 14.8 Some species of *Plasmodium* (A), *Haemoproteus* (B) , and *Leucocytozoon* (C) in the peripheral blood of birds as seen in LM. Erythrocytes of birds are elliptical and nucleated. The apicomplexan parasites lie in the cytoplasm of the red cell.

transmitted directly, as are the intestinal coccidia (Chapter 12), others are vector borne, but the vectors are eaten (sporozoites are not injected into the skin). The suborder is defined by the fact that the gamonts develop in syzygy, (i.e., similar to the gregarines, Chapter 11) and usually six or fewer nonmotile microgametes are formed. A few members are intestinal parasites, but most adeleins reproduce in extraintestinal sites, and gamonts are often in circulating blood cells.

Klossiella equi is a cosmopolitan parasite of the horse, zebra, and ass. Infection takes place by ingestion of sporocysts. and sporozoites infect many organs of the body. There are probably several merogonous generations, but eventually the merozoites find their way to the kidney and undergo sexual reproduction with the formation of sporocysts that are passed with the urine. Developmental stages are found usually incidentally at postmortem examination of horses, and they are considered to be incidental findings since *K. equi* appears to be nonpathogenic.

Hepatozoon canis is a cosmopolitan parasite of dogs,

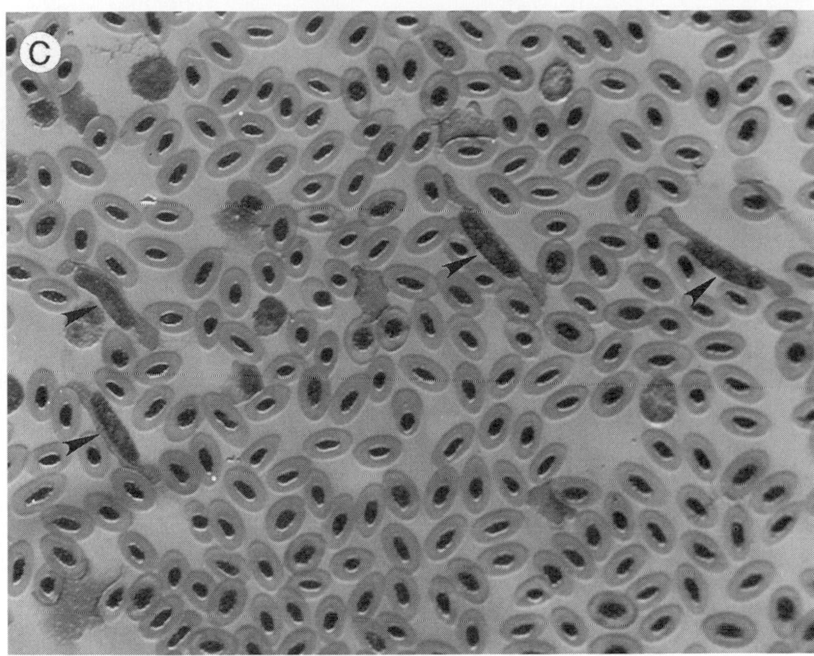

FIGURE 14.8 (*Continued*)

but it has also been reported from a number of other carnivores such as the cat, jackal, hyena, and palm civet; whether the same species occurs in all of these hosts is problematic. Merogony takes place in the spleen, bone marrow and liver; gamonts form in polymorphonuclear leucocytes. (Fig. 14.9). The vector is the brown dog tick, *Rhipicephalus sanguineus* (Chapter 51). *H. canis* is moderately pathogenic causing fever, anemia, enlarged spleen, and sometimes paralysis. Control involves eliminating ticks from areas where dogs may

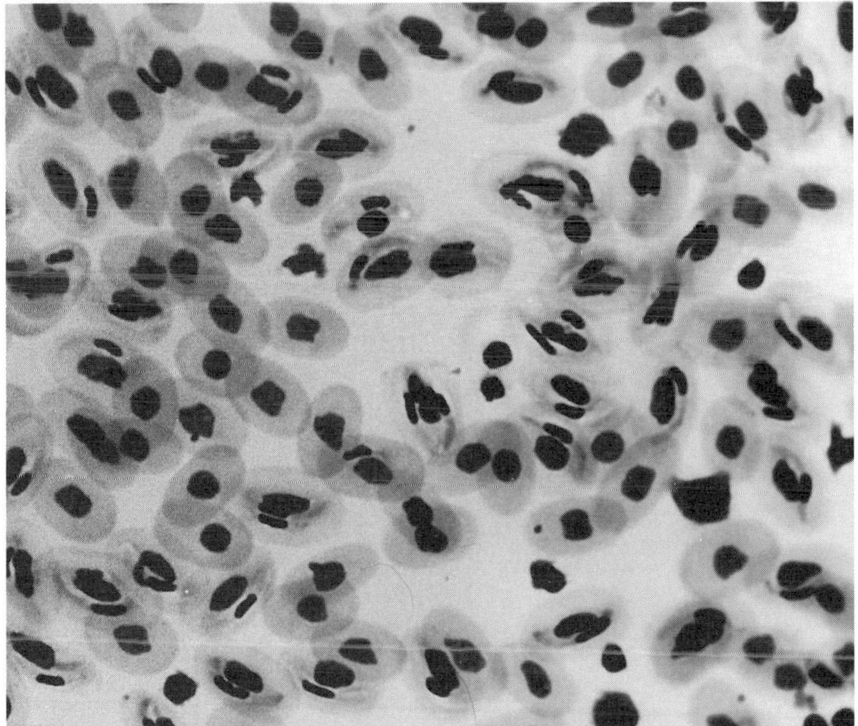

FIGURE 14.9 The blood cell parasite *Hepatozoon,* in the red blood cells of the cottonmouth snake, *Agkistrodon piscivorus leucostoma.* Erythrocysts of snakes are elliptical and nucleated; the haemogregarines are elongate, nucleated organisms that lie in the cytoplasm of the red cell.

pick them up. A number of other species of *Hepatozoon* have been reported from rodents.

Haemogregarina and *Karyolysus* are parasites of herptiles where the gamonts and, in some species, meronts are found in the red blood cells (Fig. 14. 9). *H. stepanowi* is a parasite of turtles and is transmitted by leeches; both meronts and gamonts are found in the red cells.

A number of species of *Karyolysis* have been described, and in those life cycles that are known, transmission takes place by mosquitoes or acarines that are eaten by the reptile. There are often two poikiothermic vertebrates in the life cycle; the first host is a lizard or frog and the second a snake. These organisms are probably nonpathogenic, but data are sparse. Clarification of the systematics of the bloodstream adeleins has been done by Smith (1996).

Readings

Aikawa, M. (1988). Fine structure of malaria parasites in the various stages of development. In *Malaria* (W. M. Wernsdorfer and I. McGregor, Eds.), Vol. 1, pp. 97–129.

Atkinson, C. T. (1991). Vectors, epizootiology, and pathogenicity of avian species of *Haemoproteus* (Haemosporina: Haemoproteidae). *Bull. Soc. Vector Ecol.* **16,** 109–126.

Bailey, N. T. J. (1982). *The Biomathematics of Malaria.* Macmillan, New York.

Belding, D. L. (1965). *Textbook of Clinical Parasitology*, 2nd ed. Appleton–Century–Crofts, New York.

Bennett, G. F., Laird, M., Khan, R. A., and Herman, C. M. (1975). Remarks on the status of the genus *Leucocytozoon* Sambon, 1908. *J. Protozool.* **22,** 24–30.

Breuer, W. V. (1985). How the malarial parasites invade the host cell, the erythrocyte. *Int. Rev. Cytol.* **96,** 191–238.

Bruce-Chwatt, L. J. (1973). Global problems of imported disease. *Adv. Parasitol.* **11,** 75–114.

Coatney, G. R. (1971). The simian malarias: Zoonoses, anthroponoses, or both? *Am. J. Trop. Med. Hyg.* **20,** 795–803.

Coatney, G. R. (1976). Relapse in malaria—An enigma. *J. Parasitol.* **62,** 3–9.

Cowman, A. F., and Foote, S. J. (1990). Chemotherapy and drug resistance in malaria. *Int. J. Parasitol.* **20,** 503–513.

Diggs, L. W., Sturm, D., and Bell, A. (1972). *The Morphology of Human Blood Cells*, 4th ed. Abbott Laboratories, North Chicago, IL.

Fallis, A. M., Desser, S. S., and Khan, R. A. (1974). On species of *Leucocytozoon. Adv. Parasitol.* **12,** 4–67.

Friedman, M. J., and Trager, W. (1981). The biochemistry of resistance to malaria. *Sci. Am* **268,** 154–164.

Garnham, P. C. C. (1966). *Malaria Parasites and Other Haemosporidia.* Blackwell, Oxford.

Gibbs, W. W. (1993). Back to basics. Mapping malaria's genome may help to produce a vaccine. *Sci. Am.* **268,** 134–136.

Gilles, H. M., and Wartell, D. A. (Eds.) (1993). *Bruce-Chwatt's Essential Malariology*, 3rd ed. Arnold, London.

Harrison, G. (1978). *Mosquitoes, Malaria and Man: A History of the Hostilities since 1880.* Dutton, New York.

Knell, A. J. (1989). *Malaria.* Oxford Univ. Press, Oxford.

Krier, J. P. (Ed.). (1980). *Malaria*, 3 Vols. Academic Press, New York.

May, R. M. (1983). Parasitic infections as regulators of animal populations. *Am. Sci.* **71,** 36–43.

Oaks, S. C., Jr., Mitchell, V. S., Pearson, G. W., and Carpenter, C. C. J. (Eds.) (1991). *Malaria. Obstacles and Opportunities.* Natl. Acad. Press, Washington, DC.

Rosenthal, P. J. (1998). Proteases of malarial parasites: New targets for chemotherapy. *Emerging Infect. Dis.* **4,** 49–57.

Russell, P. F., West, L. S., and Manwell, R. D. (1963). *Practical Malariology*, 2nd Ed. Oxford Univ. Press, London.

Smith, T. G. (1996). The genus *Hepatozoon* (Apicomplexa: Adeleina). *J. Parasitol.* **82,** 565–585.

Stewart and Vanderberg (1991). Malaria sporozoites release circumsporozoite protein from their apical end and translocate it along the surface. *J. Protozool.* **38,** 411–421.

Trager, W., and Jensen, J. B. (1976). Human malarial parasites in continuous culture. *Science* **193,** 673–675.

Walliker, D. (1983). The genetic basis of diversity in malaria parasites. *Adv. Parasitol.* **22,** 217–259.

Wernsdorfer, W. H., and McGregor, I. (Eds.) (1988). *Malaria, Principles and Practice of Malariology*, 2 vols. Churchill-Livingston, London.

CHAPTER

15

Piroplasmea and Piroplasmosis

Members of the class Piroplasmea are principally parasites of vertebrate blood cells and are transmitted by ticks. They are tiny organisms, seldom more than 3 or 4 μm long and are most often seen as parasites of circulating erythrocytes. Most of the species are found in mammals, but they are known also from reptiles and birds.

The importance of the piroplasms on a worldwide basis is difficult to overstate. Significant losses from piroplasms in cattle, sheep, and goats are continually experienced in nearly all parts of the world. All of the major land masses are enzootic areas for piroplasmoses, and livestock losses continue to be severe despite control programs. Infections with members of the genera *Babesia* and *Theileria* present formidable problems in the tropical and subtropical areas of South America, Africa, Asia, the Middle East, and Europe. It is the dryer areas of the world that can best be used by grazing animals where ticks are abundant and where piroplasmoses are also enzootic.

In this chapter we will look at a few of the piroplasms of herbivores, dogs, and humans as accidental hosts. However, it should be kept in mind that piroplasms are widely spread among vertebrates and ticks.

The class Piroplasmea contains organisms that are parasites of various kinds of cells of the blood system and are transmitted by ticks (Chapter 51). They are small, even for apicomplexans, and the apical complex is reduced usually to a polar ring and rhoptrics and a small conoid (Fig. 15.1). Those piroplasms that parasitize red cells do not form hemozoin, as do most members of the genus *Plasmodium* and other Haemosporina; hemozoin is the black, refractile pigment often seen in infected red cells (Fig. 14.4). Transmission by ticks has some implications of interest. In all of the cases we know of, ticks are the vectors of piroplasms. In a number of species, such as *Babesia bigemina*, the piroplasm is transmitted from one generation of ticks to the next by infection of the ova (transovarially or TOT) in the female tick. Some piroplasms have been found to be transmitted serially through many generations of ticks without ever passing through a vertebrate host. It has been suggested that the piroplasms are, in fact, parasites of ticks and the vertebrates are merely accidental hosts.

BABESIOSIS OF DOMESTIC ANIMALS

Name and Disease Caused

Babesia bigemina causes Texas cattle fever, red water fever, splenetic fever, piroplasmosis, and babesiosis.

Hosts and Location

The normal vertebrate host of *B. bigemina* is the ox (*Bos taurus*), but some other animals can be infected either transiently or at low levels of parasitemia. In the vertebrate, the piroplasms inhabit erythrocytes only. Ticks of the family Ixodidae (hard ticks) are vectors of *B. bigemina* (Chapter 51). In North America the one-host tick, *Boophilus annulatus*, is the vector.

Morphology

In the ox, the parasites are seen in red blood cells as piriform or teardrop-shaped organisms about 3 μm

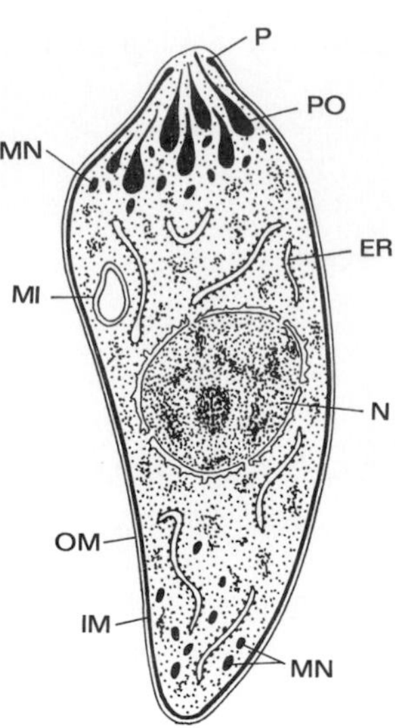

FIGURE 15.1 A diagram of a zoite of *Babesis* sp. showing the conoid, rhoptries, and micronemes.

long (Fig. 15.2). The nucleus stains red, and the cytoplasm blue with Romanowsky stains. They appear not unlike a ring stage of *Plasmodium*, with the cytoplasm being a wisp of blue surrounding what seems to be a vacant area. In the tick, the parasites vary from forms that are about 1 μm up to the vermicules, which are 11 μm long.

Life Cycle

Babesia bigemina, like the other piroplasms, is transmitted from one vertebrate host to the next by means of ticks that serve as biological vectors. In the ox, the parasite develops in erythrocytes and the single trophozoites multiply by binary fission. In a blood film, one most often sees two pear-shaped organisms with their tails near one another (Fig. 15.2). Some time after division, the red cell breaks down and the trophozoites enter uninfected cells.

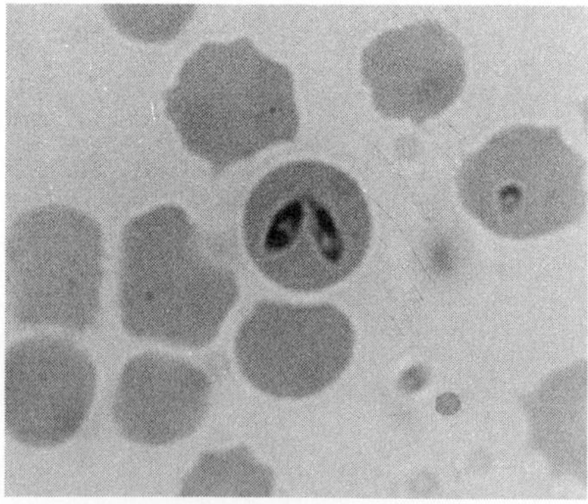

FIGURE 15.2 *Babesia bigemina* in the blood of an ox as seen in a Giemsa-stained preparation in LM.

Development in the tick is considerably more complicated than that which takes place in the mammal. Two important points should be recognized about the development of *B. bigemina* in the tick:

1. Transovarial transmission (TOT) occurs in the tick; that is, a female tick infected as an adult transmits the infection to her offspring and the second generation of ticks then transmits the infection to an uninfected ox.
2. TEM studies have revealed that sexual reproduction occurs in *Theileria* and *Babesia.* In the tick, the gamonts differentiates into male and female forms, and syngamy takes place to form a zygote; this is the so-called kinete.

Differentiation into gamonts occurs in the erythrocytes and these are seen as more rounded forms (as in Fig. 15.5, #6). These ovoid stages transform into "ray bodies" within a day in the gut of the tick, and nuclear division takes place with 4-nucleated organisms resulting. Apparently the two types of ray bodies fuse to form the zygote or kinete (Figs. 15.5, #9; 15.7) and further multiplication takes place by a budding process. The organisms now invade many tissues of the tick including the salivary glands and the ovaries. In the case of *Babesia bigemina,* infection of the ovaries is crucial in ensuring transmission.

Those kinetts that enter the cells of the salivary glands undergo further multiplication and produce sporozoites, the infective stage. In ticks which transmit babesias by the stage-to-stage mode can transmit the infection when they feed following the molt. In TOT transmission, the ovaries are infected and the parasites enter ova where they remain quiescent. In general, one-host ticks, which are vectors of babesias, transmit the parasites by TOT and two- or three-host ticks transmit babesias by the stage-to-stage mode.

During embryonation of the egg, further replication of the piroplasm occurs. In this case, multiplication is by schizogony in the intestinal cells of developing and larval ticks.

It is only after the larval tick has fed and molted to the nymphal stage that transmission of the piroplasm is likely to take place. When the nymphal stage has been reached, the parasite then moves to the salivary glands of the host and continues to replicate. Thus, 8 to 10 days after the larva attaches, an ox may be infected, but not before. Having reached an uninfected ox, *B. bigemina* enters erythrocytes and multiplies.

Diagnosis

During the acute phase of the infection, parasites are readily found in a stained film of peripheral blood.

If the animal has gone through the clinical phase and become immune, parasites are seldom seen in blood films. In such a case, serological tests such as a complement fixation test can be used to determine whether the animal has been infected.

Animals infected with *B. bigemina* become listless, fail to eat properly, and are anemic. If the breakdown of red cells has been massive, hemoglobin passes through the kidneys and the urine is red. Since the signs of infection may be similar to those of a number of other diseases, the search for parasites in the blood cells should be continued.

Host–Parasite Interactions

B. bigemina lives and reproduces only in the red blood cells of the host. As it develops and divides, it consumes some of the content of the erythrocyte and the red cell breaks down, releasing the parasites, which then invade other erythrocytes. Much of the damage to the host revolves around the breakdown of erythrocytes and the consequent anemia; however, effects are seen in other organs as well, such as the spleen, which becomes enlarged, and the liver, which becomes enlarged and yellowish.

There is considerable difference between reactions of young and mature animals to infection with *B. bigemina*. In most diseases, young animals are more severely affected than older ones, but the reverse is true in babesiosis. Young animals usually show mild clinical signs of infection but recover within a week or so. They are then resistant to further infection and remain free of clinical signs for life. The immunity that develops is not a sterile immunity, however; a low level infection is retained and a state of premunition is achieved. In premunition, the host retains immunity by virtue of residual infection.

Mature animals suffer severe clinical effects when they are infected as adults. Mortality from babesiosis may exceed 75% in some populations.

Epidemiology and Control

Control of tick-borne piroplasmoses is based on the following:

1. Tick control through acaricidal treatment of hosts
2. Chemotherapy of infected hosts
3. Avoiding areas where, or times when, ticks are present
4. Test and slaughter of infected animals
5. Quarantine of infected animals or of areas where infected animals are present
6. Inspection and certification that animals are tick-free before allowing their movement

The control and ultimate eradication of Texas cattle fever from the United States is a saga that began in the 19th century when James Law established veterinary medicine as a curriculum at Cornell University. It was here that the early leaders in animal diseases in the United States were trained. Men such as Daniel E. Salmon, John R. Mohler, and Cooper Curtice (Fig. 15.3) became the core of the group that was to attack the problem.

Texas cattle fever was a severe problem in the southeastern states and Texas during the middle 1800s. Losses by cattle raisers were considered by some to be intolerable, but there were also losses outside the enzootic area. This was the era when the American cowboy myths were spawned and when cattle were driven long distances to pastures or to market.

When cattle were trailed north to markets, there were losses in animals pastured along the trails where the disease was not ordinarily seen. The owners of such animals were understandably angry because their animals died from a disease contracted from the cattle trailed through the area. Their protests stimulated a study of the cause of the disease.

Some early work was undertaken by members of the Bureau of Animal Industry (USDA) and Salmon suggested that Texas cattle fever was infectious and transmitted by ticks. The decision was made to attack the problem, and in 1891 Dr. Theobald Smith and Dr. Frederick L. Kilbourne were sent to study the mechanism of transmission and the causative agent.

Smith and Kilbourne not only described the causative agent of splenetic fever but also proved that the tick *Boophilus annulatus* (syn. *Margaropus annulatus*) transmitted the agent.

Further work by Cooper Curtice showed transovarial transmission of *B. bigemina* and set the stage for an avalanche of studies by both USDA investigators and personnel at state experiment stations throughout the Southeast. By the turn of the century, sufficient information was at hand to attack the problem, and in 1903 the secretary of agriculture quarantined all cattle south of a line where *B. annulatus* was known to overwinter (Fig. 15.4). Cattle could not be moved north of this area unless they had been treated with an acaricide and found to be free of ticks.

In 1906 a program of eradication of *Boophilus annulatus* from the United States was established. It was concluded that there was sufficient information on the tick to make eradication possible. Once the ticks were eradicated it was reasoned that the *B. bigemina* infection would die out of its own accord.

The decision was clearly a good one, but not without its difficulties. For example, in 1933 (Fig. 15.4), after nearly 30 years of work, there were sizable areas of

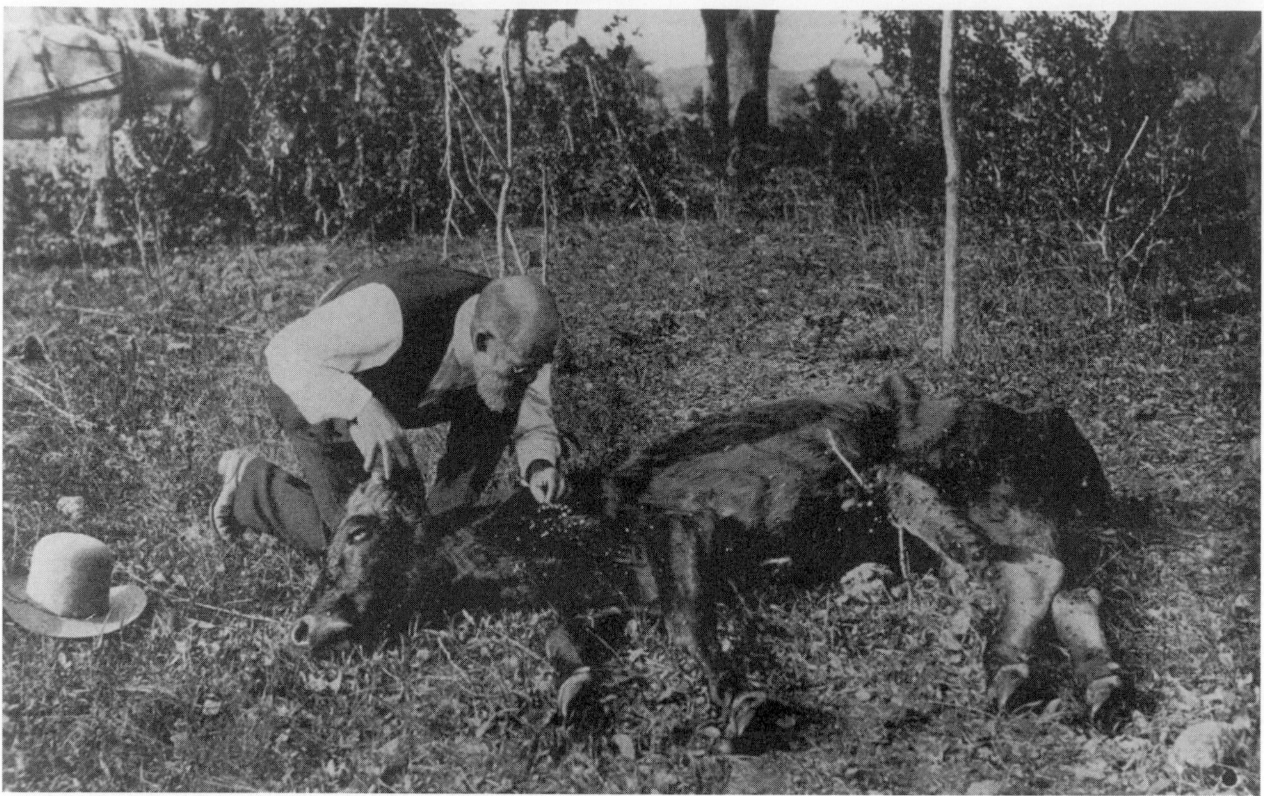

FIGURE 15.3 Cooper Curtice, a USDA veterinarian, examining an animal that had died of Texas cattle fever (date about 1892).

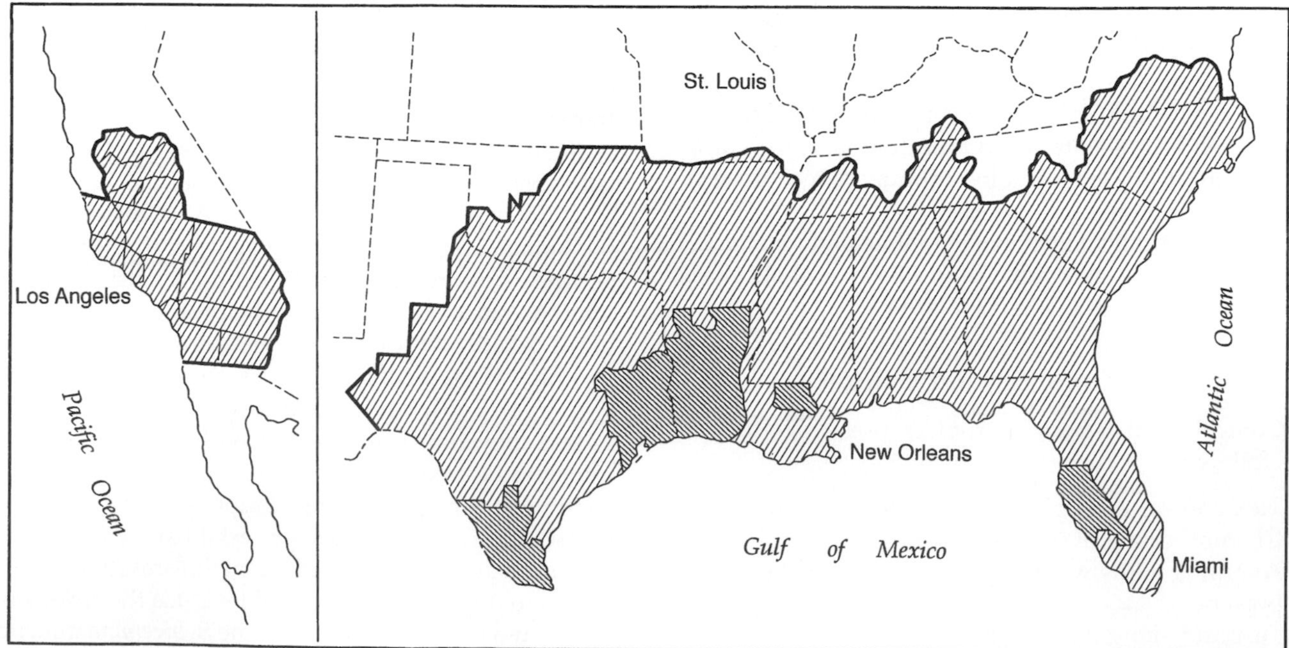

FIGURE 15.4 Map of the 1933 cattle tick quarantine area in the United States. (Lighter areas represent the limits of the distribution of Texas cattle fever and the darker areas in the south represent the distribution in 1933 after about 30 years of eradication efforts.) Only parts of Texas, Louisiana, and Florida remained infected at that time, and these were to be declared disease-free by 1939.

Texas and Florida that still had ticks. Also, not all livestock raisers were in favor of the stringent federal regulations of quarantine, dipping, and inspection.

The papers of Fred C. Bishopp at Colorado State University contain documents originating from the Bureau of Animal Industry and from cattlemen's newspapers of the time. In a USDA news release of 1916 the following is stated:

> As a result of ten years' experience in tick eradication, the Federal officials in charge of the campaign are convinced that the hearty cooperation of the people themselves is absolutely essential to success. The Department of Agriculture's representatives in the field, therefore, have been warned of the danger of beginning systematic work in any county before public opinion is ready to lend vigorous support to the enterprise. It frequently happens that a few of the more progressive farmers are earnest advocates of tick eradication, while the rest of the community may be either indifferent or actually hostile. In a number of instances in the past when tick eradication has been begun under these circumstances it has been found necessary, after two or three years, for the Federal government to withdraw its men because the results of their work were, to a great extent, nullified by popular indifference. To make a success of eradication, all cattle in the county must be dipped regularly. In practice, this is only possible when the great majority of the people are so strongly in favor of the work that they will insist upon the enforcement of the necessary regulations.

The term "actually hostile" is used with good reason. In the summer of 1915 three dipping vats in one county of Alabama were dynamited, apparently by a few dissidents who were not in agreement with the vote of 9 to 1 in favor of cooperating in the eradication program. In some other instances, federal inspectors were shot at. However, the program was skillfully managed by the Bureau of Animal Industry by putting the major responsibility for joining the program on the states and counties and then providing the expertise needed to implement eradication.

The program had two crucial parts:

1. Quarantine to prevent movement of animals
2. The lure of increased income if redwater fever were eradicated

There was a continuous stream of hard data from the state experiment station workers and persuasive articles in various farm periodicals advocating eradication. In a bulletin of the Arkansas Agricultural Experiment Station of 1908, W. Lenton discussed tick eradication during the previous year and attempted to persuade livestock raisers as follows: "If every farmer understood this question and was willing to spend a few cents and a few minutes' time each week between now and the first of next November, every tick in Arkansas could be killed by that date." Except during winter, cattle could be sent to market only for slaughter, not for fattening in northern feedlots. Lenton went on to state that "there is practically only one outlet for such cattle: they must go as 'canners.'" Other papers comparing untreated and treated cattle said that for an expenditure of about $3 an owner could realize $10.

Eradication of Texas cattle fever was possible because certain factors came together:

1. The distribution of the sole vector in North America was limited. The original habitat of *B. annulatus* was Florida, and the tick had been spread by movement of domesticated animals. Therefore, it was distributed mostly at the margin of its possible range in areas where there was frost in the winter. Some of the methods used in control, such as leaving animals off contaminated pastures for a period of time, as well as the residue of populations in Texas and Florida (Fig. 15.4) in the early 1930s, support this view. At its northern limits, *B. annulatus* died out on pasture during the winter but migrated northward during the spring and summer with the movement of cattle.
2. There was relative resistance among young animals. Immunity and premunition could be induced in young animals by transfusing them with blood from older infected animals. Such purposeful infection allowed the introduction of stock into enzootic areas, but it presented no risk of transmission to other animals once the tick population had been eradicated.
3. Effective technology to control ticks was developed. Although some of the early topical treatments for ticks such as petroleum were somewhat effective, they also could be toxic. The development of effective dips containing arsenic trioxide was crucial. The other side of the coin was that there was no effective treatment for use against *Babesia*. Thus, there were no alternatives to tick control.
4. There is only one host for *B. bigemina*. If an infectious agent has a broad host range, the probability of eradication being successful approaches zero.

During the eradication phase, all cattle in counties cooperating in the program were required to be dipped in an approved acaricide every two weeks during the tick season. They could not be moved unless they had been dipped and inspected. When a county was declared tick-free, cattle could then be moved at will. Livestock raisers joined the eradication program so that they could send their cattle to feedlots and obtain more money than if they were sent directly to slaughter. Eradication of Texas cattle fever from cattle in the continental United States was considered to be complete by 1939.

At present, the United States is still free of *B. bigemina* infection in cattle, but Mexico has the disease. Therefore, all cattle entering the United States from

Mexico must be dipped in an approved acaricide and inspected before they are allowed to cross the border. Such programs are carried out by personnel of the Animal and Plant Health Inspection Service (APHIS) of the USDA.

A number of compounds or classes of compounds have been developed for use against babesias. All drugs are administered by injection and have various undesirable side effects.

Trypan blue was first used early in the 20th century; it must be given IV and stains tissues blue-green. The effect lasts for several months. Oddly enough, species larger than 3 μm are susceptible to trypan blue, but those smaller than 3 μm are not.

Acriflavine and acaprin have been in use for more than 40 years. With these drugs parasites are reduced in number but not eliminated. The host, therefore, becomes premunized and resistant to reinfection. Among the most effective drugs are various aromatic diamidines (stilbamidine, pentamidine, berenil), which have a relatively low risk of serious side effects.

Tick control has evolved from the use of dips containing some fairly hazardous materials in the early part of the 20th century to technologically sophisticated methods of applying systemic acaricides (Chapter 51). The livestock dip most used during the Texas cattle fever eradication program was based on arsenic trioxide. During the middle 1930s rotenone was used extensively, but it was not until the 1940s, when the organochlorine insecticides (DDT, lindane) were developed, that highly efficacious and low-risk compounds were available. Instead of completely immersing animals in a dipping vat, it was then possible to treat them by spraying, if care was taken to wet the animals thoroughly.

The development of the systemic organophosphate compounds (coumaphos, ruelene, fenthion) allowed wholly new approaches to getting the acaricide to the tick. Animals can be sprayed with an organophosphate compound, but it is not necessary to reach the tick directly because the acaricide is absorbed through the skin and reaches the tick through the bloodstream. A more recent approach uses the application of a concentrated solution or suspension of acaricide to only a limited area of the animal's body. Plastic ear tags impregnated with an organophosphate insecticide may also be attached to the ears of cattle to control ticks for as long as three months.

RELATED ORGANISMS

A number of other species of *Babesia* are also parasites of ruminants. In cattle, *B. bovis, B. divergens,* and *B. major* are found in various parts of the Eastern Hemisphere and in South America.

Four species of *Babesia* have been reported from sheep in various parts of the world: *B. crassa, B. foliata, B. motasi,* and *B. ovis.*

BABESIOSIS IN HORSES

Name of Organism and Disease Caused

Babesia caballi causes equine piroplasmosis.

Hosts and Host Range

This parasite infects not only horses but other equids as well.

Distribution and Importance

B. caballi is distributed in areas with warm climates; It is found in both the Eastern and Western Hemispheres.

Morphology

The erythrocytic forms are 2 to 5 μm long, generally piriform.

Life Cycle

In the horse, the parasites are found in the red blood cells, where they multiply by binary fission. Only one or two trophozoites are found in each red cell. In the tick, the life cycle is similar to that of *B. bigemina. B. caballi* can undergo either transtadial (stage-to-stage) or transovarial transmission; on a global basis, many species of ticks serve as vectors of *B. caballi.* In the two- and three-host ticks there is transtadial transmission, and transovarial transmission in the one-host ticks.

Diagnosis

The only certain means of diagnosis is by finding the parasites in the blood of an infected animal. A number of serological tests have been developed that allow an investigator to determine whether an animal has been infected and with what species; however, the best evidence is finding the parasite.

Host–Parasite Interactions

Unlike *B. bigemina* infection, with which mortality exceeds 75%, mortality due to infection with *B. caballi* is less then 50% overall. Also, different isolates have different levels of pathogenesis.

Epidemiology and Control

On a global basis, there are about 10 species of ticks that serve as vectors of *B. caballi*. In the United States, Central America, islands of the Caribbean, and South America, *Dermacentor nitens* is the vector.

B. caballi was introduced into the United States around 1960, most likely from Cuba, but it was not diagnosed in horses until 1961. It spread quickly through southern Florida, with up to 200 cases found annually in the United States in the 1960s and early 1970s. Infections have also been found in other states, but these are considered either to have been imported or become infected in Florida and been shipped to other areas.

The establishment of *B. caballi* in the United States illustrates the principle of ready transmission of an agent when imported into an area where a good vector already exists.

When *B. caballi* was found in a racehorse, a program of quarantine, testing, and tick control was instituted by APHIS. The outbreak was contained, but not without considerable cost. It is unlikely that *B. caballi* would establish in parts of the United States other than southern Florida and Texas. The question might legitimately be asked whether the effort at control is economically justifiable. The answer is affirmative because of the continual movement of horses, especially racehorses and show horses. Even though *D. nitens* would not establish permanently in cooler areas of the country, it could spread the infection during the summer months. The economic losses might then be far greater than the costs of control.

A number of drugs administered by injection are effective against both acute and chronic infections.

Name of Organism and Disease Caused

Babesia canis causes canine babesiosis or piroplasmosis and malignant jaundice.

Hosts and Host Range

Several species of canids, both domestic and wild, are natural hosts; it also infects a number of other carnivores. Ixodid ticks are the vectors, and seven species have been implicated. In North America and many other areas of the world *Rhipicephalus sanguineus*, the brown dog tick, is the principal vector (Chapter 51).

Distribution and Importance

B. canis is a cosmopolitan parasite, principally in warm climates. It has been reported from the United States mostly in southern states but, less frequently, as far north as New Jersey. In many tropical and subtropical areas of the world the prevalence in dogs is high. *B. canis* is a highly pathogenic parasite of dogs.

B. gibsoni is found in Asia and has been reported from North America. It is also pathogenic in dogs.

Morphology

Among piroplasms, *B. canis* is quite large; when piriform, they are as large as 5μm and the round ones are about 3 μm in diameter. The shape is variable.

Life Cycle

The development in the red cells of the vertebrate host is by binary fission. In the tick, development is similar to that of *B. bigemina*, with transmission by *R. sanguineus* being both transtadial and transovarial (Fig. 15.5).

Diagnosis

As with other babesioses, finding the parasite in the erythrocytes is the definitive evidence. Clinical signs of infection with *B. canis* are quite variable. Red cell destruction gives rise to anemia and sometimes hemoglobin in the urine; animals are weak and lethargic; fever is usually present. Beyond these rather obvious signs, there may be gastrointestinal ulceration, central nervous system involvement, and bleeding from the ears or muzzle. Both young and mature animals may be infected, but younger animals show less severe clinical effects than older ones on initial infection.

Host–Parasite Interactions

The damage to the dog varies with the strain of parasite and the age of the dog. The breakdown of the red cells (hemolysis) is the most obvious sign, and it has widespread effects. Anemia, splenic enlargement, kidney damage, and impaired circulation in some organs all result from the hemolysis. If an animal survives the infection, it becomes immune and remains refractory to reinfection through premunition.

A number of drugs have been used against *B. canis*, but acaprin and phenamidine appear to be the most effective.

Epidemiology and Control

Rhipicephalus sanguineus, a three-host tick, is the most important vector of *B. canis*. It is found in most parts of the world, although it is probably native to

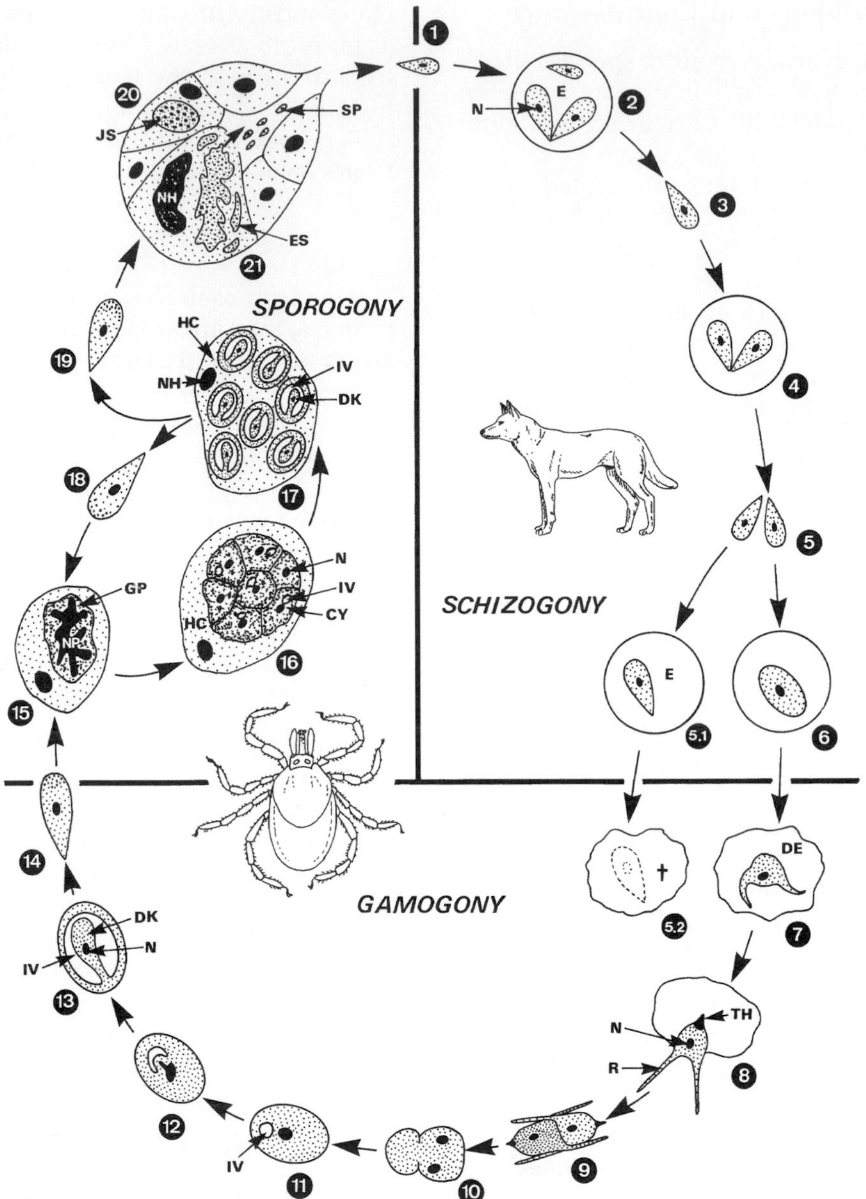

FIGURE 15.5 Diagram of the life cycle of *Babesia canis*. An infectious tick introduces sporozoites (1) into the blood of its host and the sporozoites undergo binary fission in the erythrocytes (2–4); the merozoites differentiate into gamonts also within RBCs (5, 6). When infectious blood is ingested by a tick, gamogony and fertilization occur in the gut of the tick (7–13), and then the kinete (14) enters cells of the salivary gland where sporogony takes place (15–20). Abbreviations: CY, cytomere; DE, digested erythrocyte; DK, developing kinete; E, erythrocyte; ES, enlarged sporont forming sporozoites; GP, growing parasite or polymorphic stage; HC, host cell; IV, inner vacuole; N, nucleus; NH, nucleus of host cell; R, raylike protrusion; SP, sporozoite; Th, thornlike apical structure; YS, young meront. [From Mehlhorn, H., and Schein, E., 1993.]

Africa. Although it is a warm-climate tick, it is extremely hardy. The ticks will not establish in colder climates, but they may colonize houses. Thus, in the Rocky Mountain area of the United States, *R. sanguineus* is sometimes found in houses, where it completes its life cycle quite well.

The host range of *R. sanguineus* also aids in its broad distribution. Although it prefers dogs, it has been found on 11 species of large herbivores, three carnivores other than the dog, rodents, lagomorphs, bats, 12 kinds of birds, reptiles, and two primates including humans. It is, however, an uncommon parasite of humans.

Throughout much of its range, there appears to be no concerted effort to control *B. canis* infections in dogs. Individual animals may be treated, and the obligation for control ultimately falls on the individual owner. If animals are confined to a fairly small area such as a city house lot, the best approach to preventing infection with *B. canis* is to control ticks by the following measures:

1. Treating animals with an acaricide
2. Using a flea and tick collar on the animal
3. Applying an acaricide to the premises

If an animal is taken into an enzootic area, it should be watched carefully for signs of infection and then treated if found to be infected. The dog should then develop immunity and be resistant to reinfection.

BABESIA INFECTIONS IN HUMANS

Name of Organisms

Four species of *Babesia* have been found as parasites of humans:

Name	*Normal host*
B. bovis	Ox
B. divergens	Ox
B. equi	Horse
B. microti Microtus	(rodent)

Cases of infection in humans have been reported from Yugoslavia, Scotland, Ireland, France, and the United States. More than 28 cases of human babesiosis have been reported from the United States, Britain, Yugoslavia, and France.

The first three instances of infection with *Babesia* in humans were all in persons who had had their spleens removed. The spleen is a major line of defense against piroplasmosis in domestic animals and also appears to serve the same function in humans. These infections were therefore looked on as oddities in persons who were not able to respond immunologically to the infection. Then, in 1969 a woman on Nantucket Island, Massachusetts, was found to be infected with what ultimately was determined to be *B. microti;* she was clinically ill, but had not had a splenectomy.

An investigation of how the woman became infected brought about a significant change in our viewpoint of babesiosis in humans. Nantucket is a small island a few miles off of Cape Cod. It has a year-round population of a few hundred persons and a large tourist influx during the summer. As of 1976 seven persons had been found on Nantucket to be infected with *B. microti.* Not all had clinical symptoms, but those who did were typical: chills, fever, headache, lethargy, muscle pain.

Of six species of rodents and lagomorphs examined on Nantucket for the presence of piroplasms, only two, the vole (*Microtus pennsylvanicus*) and the white footed mouse (*Peromyscus leucopus*), were found to be infected with *B. microti.* The prevalence in the rodents was high—5 of 5 voles and 31 of 39 mice. *Ixodes scapularis* (syn. *Ixodes dammini*) is the vector on Nantucket, where about 5% of ticks have been found to have piroplasms in their salivary glands.

The importance of piroplasmosis in humans is still undetermined. The first individuals found to be infected with *Babesia* died because they could not respond immunologically in a normal manner. None of the persons on Nantucket died as a result of the infection, but some felt ill for months and were incapacitated by the disease. Also, they had no association with livestock. The association rather was with rodents, but it was peripheral. The known distribution of *B. microti* infections in humans is being extended; in addition to Nantucket Island, infections have been found on Cape Cod, and on Long Island, New York. A case of transfusion-induced babesiosis has been reported from Washington state in the United States.

Piroplasms are common in various animal groups. A study done in Maryland, for example, showed that 29 of 30 raccoons were infected with *B. procyoni* and all of 13 skunks were infected with an organism morphologically similar to *B. caballi.* Other studies on rodents have confirmed that *Babesia* is common.

Diagnosis

Diagnosis of *Babesia* infection in humans presents some problems. The organisms are small and sometimes present in only a small percentage of red cells. They may be mistaken for ring stages of *Plasmodium,* particularly *P. falciparum.* Except in individuals who are immunologically incompetent, such as those who have been splenectomized or may be taking corticosteroids, the parasitemia may be at a low level. Thus, if a physician requests a differential white blood cell count for a person showing rather vague symptoms, the laboratory technician may well miss the infection. Alternatively, in an area where malaria is endemic, a misdiagnosis of malaria may be made. It is possible to differentiate infections serologically, but there are few laboratories in the world with the antigens to carry out the tests; the Center for Disease Control in Atlanta, Georgia, is the principal one in North America.

Treatment for babesiosis in humans is not satisfactory. Chloroquine has been used with some apparent success clinically, but is not considered to have much effect on the parasites. Pentamidine has been used with some success. Diminiazene aceturate, used in live stock, was administered to a man suffering from babesiosis, he was cured, but suffered neurologic sequelae that may have been caused by the drug (Teutsch *et al.*, 1980).

THEILERIOSES AND EAST COAST FEVER

Name of Organism and Disease Associations

Theileria parva causes East Coast fever, corridor disease, and bovine theileriosis.

Hosts and Host Range

Domestic cattle and both domestic and wild buffalo are hosts. In the mammalian host the organisms replicate in lymphocytes and also parasitize red cells, but they do not multiply there.

Geographic Distribution and Importance

The original distribution of East Coast fever was from South Africa northward to Kenya in the area of Africa where drainage is toward the Indian Ocean. Control programs have limited the range, particularly in the southern portion of the enzootic area.

T. parva has a reservoir in the African buffalo (*Syrlcerus caffer*), and these animals are a constant source of infection for domestic cattle, both the ox and the zebu.

East Coast fever has been a serious threat to livestock in East Africa for many years; mortality in domestic cattle may exceed 90%.

Morphology

The forms that occur in the lymphocytes multiply, and are referred to as Koch's bodies or Koch's blue bodies. They average 8 μm, are roundish, and are multinucleate.

The forms found in the red cells are nonmultiplying and probably are gamonts. They are tiny organisms, no more than 1 by 2 μm, and with shapes varying from rods to broad ovals. The nucleus is a red dot and the cytoplasm a little wisp of blue in Romanowsky stains; multiple infections of red cells are common.

Life Cycle

T. parva and other theilerias are so small that studies of development have been difficult to do; therefore, there are aspects of development that are still in doubt (Fig. 15.6). The following is a brief discussion of the major aspects of development in the ox and the tick.

Upon entry into the mammal, when an infected tick takes a blood meal, the sporozoites are filtered out in lymph nodes, usually in the neck region (e.g., prescapular nodes). The organisms undergo schizogony in the lymphocytes and cause nuclear and cytoplasmic division of the lymphocytes. Some of the merozoites enter red cells, but replication does not occur here. However, it is the erythrocytic parasites that can be transferred successfully back to a tick.

When a clean tick feeds on an infected animal, the parasites in the red cells escape and undergo transformation. As with *Babesia* spp., *Theileria* also undergoes sexual development in the tick. A gamont and zygote have been described (Fig. 15.7).

Ultimately, the parasites enter the cells of the salivary glands of the tick and are ready to be injected into a clean host.

In *Theileria* spp. there is only stage-to-stage transmission in the tick. Usually the tick is infected as a larva.

Diagnosis

Determining whether an animal is infected is based on the following:

1. Clinical signs
2. Finding the organism in a peripheral blood film
3. Finding the organism in a smear made from a lymph node biopsy
4. Serological tests

In the face of suspicious signs of infection such as fever, swollen lymph nodes, and emaciation, it is best to make both a blood film and a lymph node puncture from the animal. A Romanowsky stain will reveal the typical form in the erythrocytes. The forms in the lymphocytes are typically multinucleated schizonts.

The serological tests indicate whether the animal is infected but cannot differentiate among species of piroplasms.

Host–Parasite Interactions

Much of the damage to the mammalian host in *T. parva* infections involves the lymph system: lymph nodes and spleen. However, other organ systems such as the kidney, lungs, and liver are also affected.

A wide range of virulence occurs in different isolates of *T. parva,* and there are some differences in the ways in which the host is affected. As with *Babesia* infections, older animals are more severely affected than younger ones.

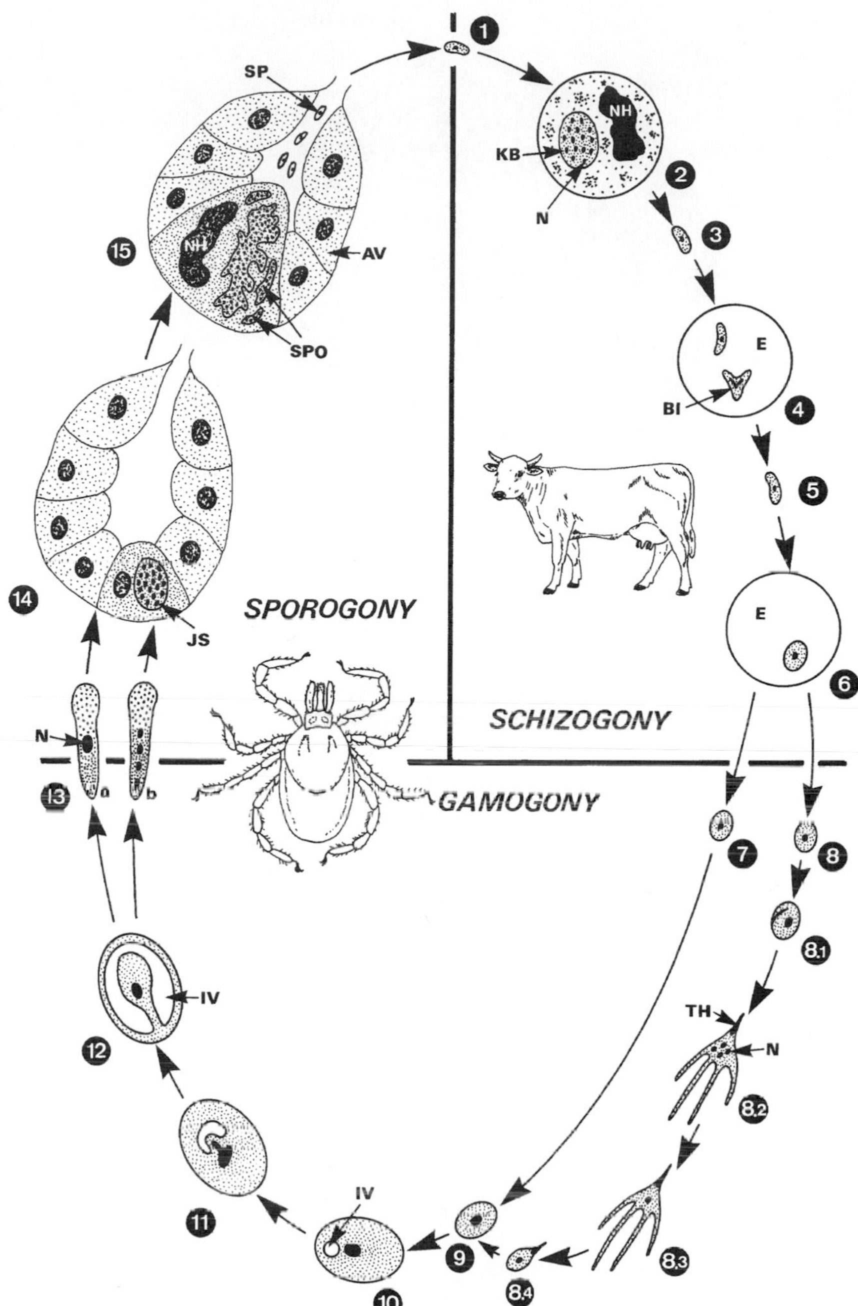

FIGURE 15.6 Diagram of the life cycle of *Theileria parva*. The life cycle takes place in both erythrocytes and leucocytes of the mammalian host. When an infectious tick feeds, the sporozoites (1) are introduced into the body and infect leucocytes (2) where they multiply The early gamonts then infect RBCs (3–6). After ingestion by a tick, gamogony and fertilization occur in the gut (7–13); multiplication then occurs in the cells of the salivary glands (4, 15). Abbreviations: AV, alveolar cell of the salivary gland; BI—binary fission; E—erythrocyte; IV, inner vacuole; KB, Koch's body or meront; N, nucleus; NH—nucleus of the host cell; SP, sporozoite; SPO, sporont; Th, thornlike apex; YS, young sporont. [From Mehlhorn, H., and Schein, E., 1993.]

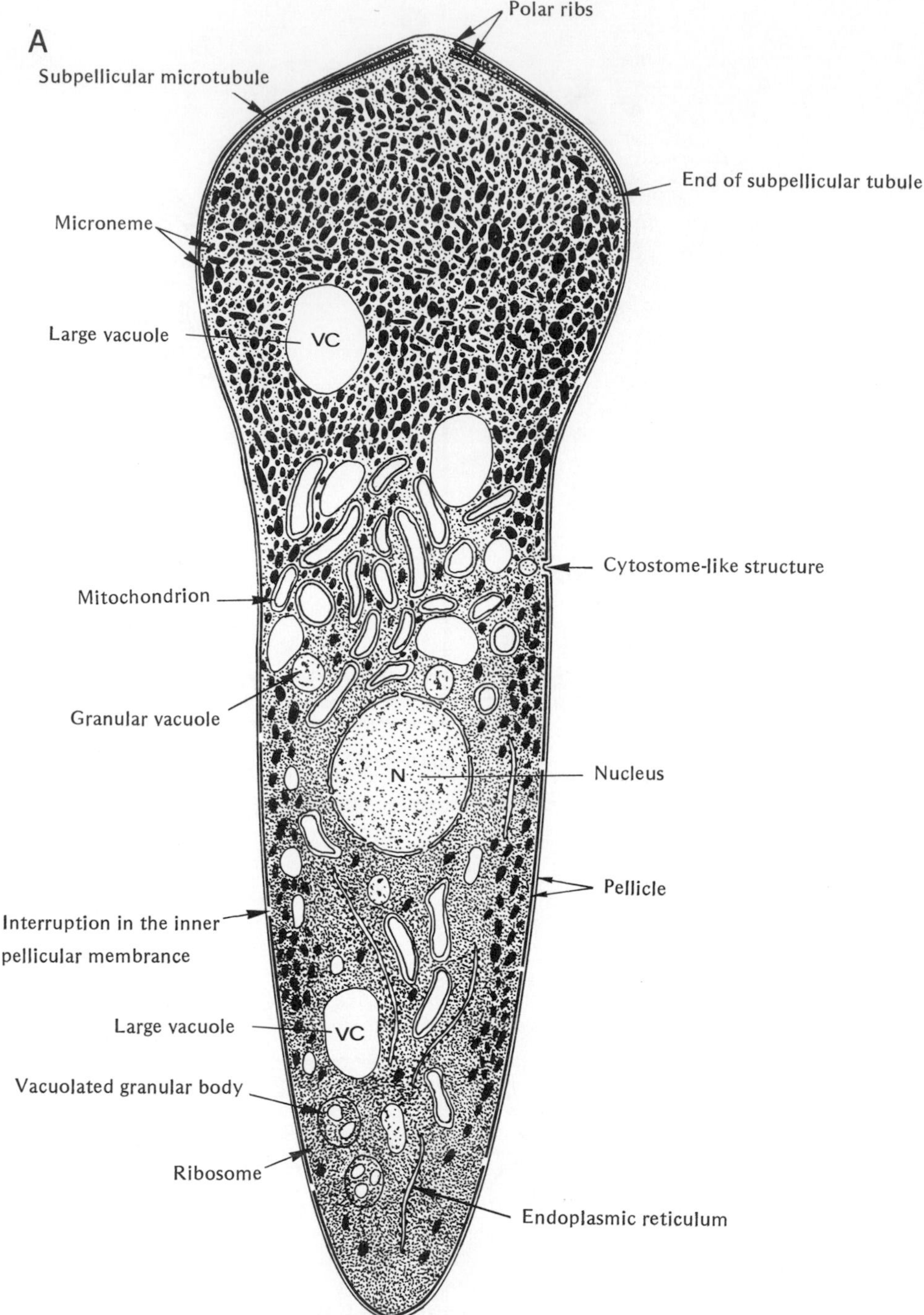

FIGURE 15.7 Stages of *Theileria parva* in the tick. (A) a zygote or kinete, and (B) a microgamont, as seen in TEM. [From Mehlhorn, et al., 1975.]

Immunity develops in animals that survive the infection, and it appears to be a sterile immunity. In some of the other species of *Theileria*, there is premunition, that is, some organisms are retained. Immunization with a mild strain has been attempted, but it does not usually provide adequate protection. Unlike in most infections, the tick vector usually remains infected for a relatively short period of time.

There is no satisfactory treatment for *Theileria parva* infections. A variety of drugs have been tried for all the species of bovine *Theileria*, and though some, such as tetracyclines, seem to prevent rapid multiplication

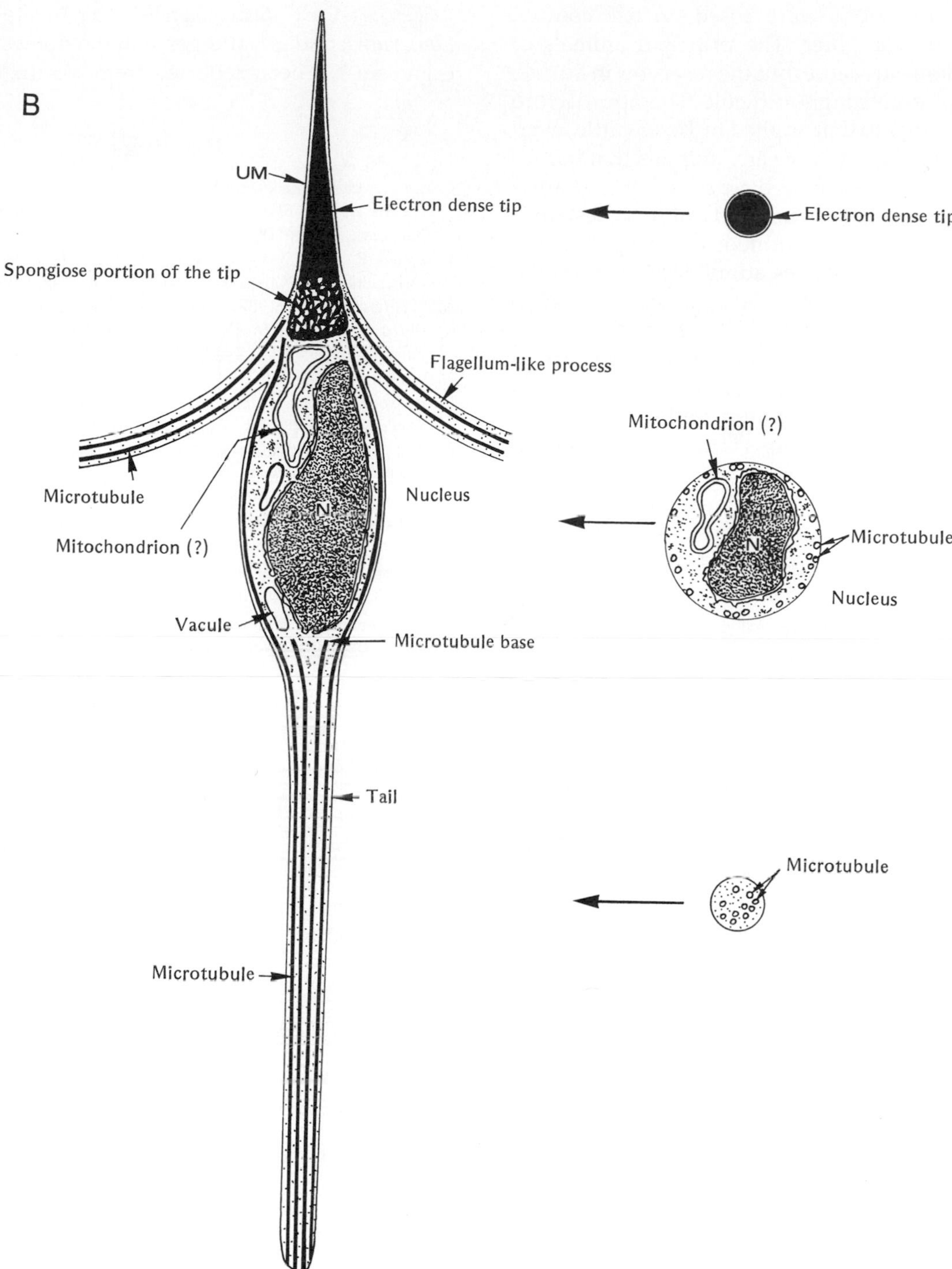

FIGURE 15.7 *(Continued)*

of the parasites, there is no good treatment for clinically affected animals.

Epidemiology and Control

There are three aspects to treatment that need to be considered:

1. Treating the ox to eliminate the infection with the parasite
2. Treating the ox to eliminate infestation with ticks
3. Treating the area to reduce populations of ticks while off of the host

The control programs for East Coast fever begun

in the 1920s and 1930s were based on tick control, quarantine, and slaughter. The principal animals of concern are domestic cattle, but the reservoir in buffalo makes control exceedingly difficult. The approach to control was similar to that applied in Texas cattle fever: to control ticks and not move any animals that harbor ticks. As the control began to have an effect, and areas were found to be free of infected cattle, a test-and-slaughter program was instituted. It is a drastic step to take and one that requires administrators with the courage of their convictions. Cattle owners are reimbursed for any animals that are killed, and adequate indemnity is essential for the success of a program. It should be emphasized also that even now there is neither satisfactory artificial immunization against nor treatment for *T. parva* infections. The armamentarium of control measures is therefore limited. The second-generation insecticides (DDT and lindane, etc.) allowed tick control to be done much more easily and effectively.

Related Organisms

Theileria infections in cattle are caused by at least three species in addition to *T. parva*. *T. annulata* is distributed in North Africa, parts of southern Europe, and southern Asia. Its vectors are species of *Hyalomma*. It is probably second to *T. parva* in importance and causes death rates up to 90% of those animals that are infected, although it is usually much lower. *T. mutans* is cosmopolitan, but rare in North America, and is only mildly pathogenic. *T. velifera* is an African species.

Other ruminants, both domestic and wild, have been found to harbor theilerias, also. *T. ovis* and *T. lestoquardi* are in the sheep and goat. *T. tarandi* is found in the reindeer. *T. equi*, of the horse was formerly called *Babesia equi*, but its life cycle has been shown to be that of the genus *Theilieria*.

T. felis (syn. *Cytauxzoon felis*) is a parasite of the lynx, *Lynx rufus*, and is pathogenic in the domestic cat. This organism has been reported from North America.

Readings

Commonwealth Bureau of Animal Health (1973). *Bovine Theileriosis. An Annotated Bibliography*. Commonwealth Agricultural Bureau, Farnham Royal, UK.

Healy, G. R., and Gleason, N. (1976). Human babesiosis: Reservoir of infection on Nantucket Island. *Science* **192,** 479–480.

MacWilliams, P. S. (1987). Erythrocytic rickettsia and protozoa of the dog and cat. In *Vet. Clin. North Am. Small Anim. Practice Parasitic Infect*. **17**(6), 1443–1461.

Mehlhorn, H., Weber, G., Schein, E., and Buscher, G. (1975). Elektronmicroskopische Untersuchung an Entwicklungs stadien von *Theileria annulata* (Dshunknowsky and Luhs, 1904) im Darm und in der Hämolymphe von *Hyalomma anatolicum excavatum* (Koch, 1844) *Z. Parasitenk.* **48,** 137–150.

Mehlhorn, H. (1982). The life cycles of piroplasms and related groups. In *Parasites—Their World and Ours* (D. F. Mettrick and S. S. Desser, Eds.). Elsevier Biomedical, New York.

Mehlhorn, H., and Schein, E. (1984). The piroplasms: Life cycle and sexual stages. *Adv. Parasitol.* **23,** 37–103.

Mehlhorn, H., and Schein, E. (1993). The piroplasms: "A long story in short" or "Robert Koch has seen it." *Eur. J. Protistol.* **29,** 279–293.

Mehlhorn, H., and Schein, E. (1998). Redescription of *Babesia equi* Laveran, 1901 as *Theileria equi* Mehlhorn, Schein 1998. *Parasitol. Res.* **84,** 467–475.

Piesman, J., and Spielman, A. (1980). Human babesiosis on Nantucket Island: Prevalence of *Babesia microti* in ticks. *Am. J. Trop. Med. Hyg.* **29,** 742–746.

Purnell, R. E. (1977). East Coast fever: Some recent research in Africa. *Adv. Parasitol.* **15,** 83–132.

Ristic, M. (1979). *Babesiosis.* Academic Press, London.

Shortt, H. E. (1973). *Babesia canis:* The life cycle and laboratory maintenance in its arthropod and mammalian hosts. *Int. J. Parasitol.* **54,** 1095–1098.

Teutsch, S. M., *et al.* (1980). Babesiosis in post-splenectomy hosts. *Am. J. Trop. Med. Hyg.* **29,** 738–741.

World Health Organization (1987). Parasitic diseases: Human babesoisis. *Weekly Epidemiol. Rec.* **62,** 226–227.

Young, A. S., and Morzaria, T. P. (1986). Biology of *Babesia. Parasitol. Today* **2,** 211–219.

CHAPTER

16

Myxozoa and Microspora

The two phyla discussed in this chapter have superficial similarities in their resistant spores, but beyond that, they are quite distinct in their structures, development, life cycles, and the hosts that they parasitize (Tab. 16.1). Some years ago they were placed in a single taxon, the Cnidospora, named because of the coiled filaments that the spores of both groups possess (Fig. 16.1). As knowledge and microscopy advanced, particularly with the development of the electron microscope and recent molecular techniques, it became clear that the Microspora had only asexual development and a spore derived from a single cell.

The Myxozoa, on the other hand, have an elementary kind of sexual development, and the spores are multicellular in origin. The polar capsules resemble the nematocysts of the Cnidaria or jellyfish. and it is now clear that the Myxozoa have affinities to that phylum. Evidence comes from studies at both the LM and TEM levels and from molecular data on the nucleic acid sequence of the 18s ribosomal DNA gene. The data show that the three genera of myxozoans that were tested lie close to a parasitic cnidarian, *Polypodium.* Although myxozoans are highly evolved, they still can be readily placed in the phylum Cnidaria (Fig. 1.21).

Since these two phyla of parasites are still thought of together, and because of their traditional classification, we discuss them in the same chapter although the Myxozoa can no longer be thought of as protists of any ilk.

MYXOZOA

All of the Myxozoa are parasitic, and their hosts are nearly always fish, although a few species of amphibia and reptiles and a scattering of invertebrates are also infected. In addition to being parasitic, the Myxozoa are characterized by having a resistant spore with one to six coiled polar filaments; two to six plates or valves form the outer covering of the spore (Figs. 16.2 and 16.3). Development within the host is both asexual and sexual, large schizonts or trophozoites reproduce by schizogony or by budding. Spores are multicellular in origin and arise within the schizonts or plasmodia. Myxozoa are both coelozoic and cytozoic, but in some instances it is not possible to tell whether they are actually within cells.

Myxozoa are economically important because they infect fish harvested for food. There are production losses and deaths, and some fish must be discarded because they are unsightly and not considered to be fit for human consumption. No myxozoan species is known to infect humans or otherwise to be a hazard to human health.

The known life cycles of the Myxozoa have been described as being direct. That is, the spores are released into the environment, usually with the death of the host, and the spores are then ingested by another susceptible host. This concept was badly shaken, as were parasitologists, with the discovery that not only does *Myxobolus cerebralis* (discussed later) have two hosts in its life cycle, but in the alternate host, a small aquatic annelid, it has a completely independent life cycle and the forms myxozoan spores of a different taxon.

More than 1000 species of Myxozoa have been described. Most of them are in teleost (bony) fish but the importance of most of them is not known. In this chapter, we consider some examples of myxozoans of economic importance and discuss the group generally.

TABLE 16.1 Comparison of the Phyla Microspora and Myxozoa

	Microspora	Myxozoa
Trophic Stage		
Level of organization before sporogenesis	Simple plasmodium; all nuclei are equipotential and all become nuclei of sporoplams	Complex plasmodium: part of the nuclei differentiate with surrounding cytoplasm into generative cells, which later undergo sporogenesis; the rest of the nuclei and plasma provide "food and shelter" until sporogenesis is completed, then they degenerate
Presence of cytoplasmic organelles	Only ergastoplasmic lamellae and smooth-membraned vesicles; no pinocytosis observed	Mitochondria, typical Golgi, ergastoplasm, fibrils, microtubules, large variety of vesicles and granules; no centriole; pinocytosis observed
Spore		
Degree of complexity	Sporoplasm produces protective shell and organelles for extrusion	Sporoplasm protected by differentiated sister cells, which produce shell and polar capsules
Extrusible apparatus	Tubule + polaroplast + polar cap + posterior vacuole; 1 set to each spore	Filament within a polar capsule produced by a capsulogenic cell; one to six in each spore
Function of filament	Injection of sporoplasm into host cell	Anchorage of spore to the gut epithelium
Mechanism of extrusion	Osmotic event; no universal agent for experimental triggering	Prebuilt pressure; triggered by urea
Composition of shell	Chitinous	Proteinaceous

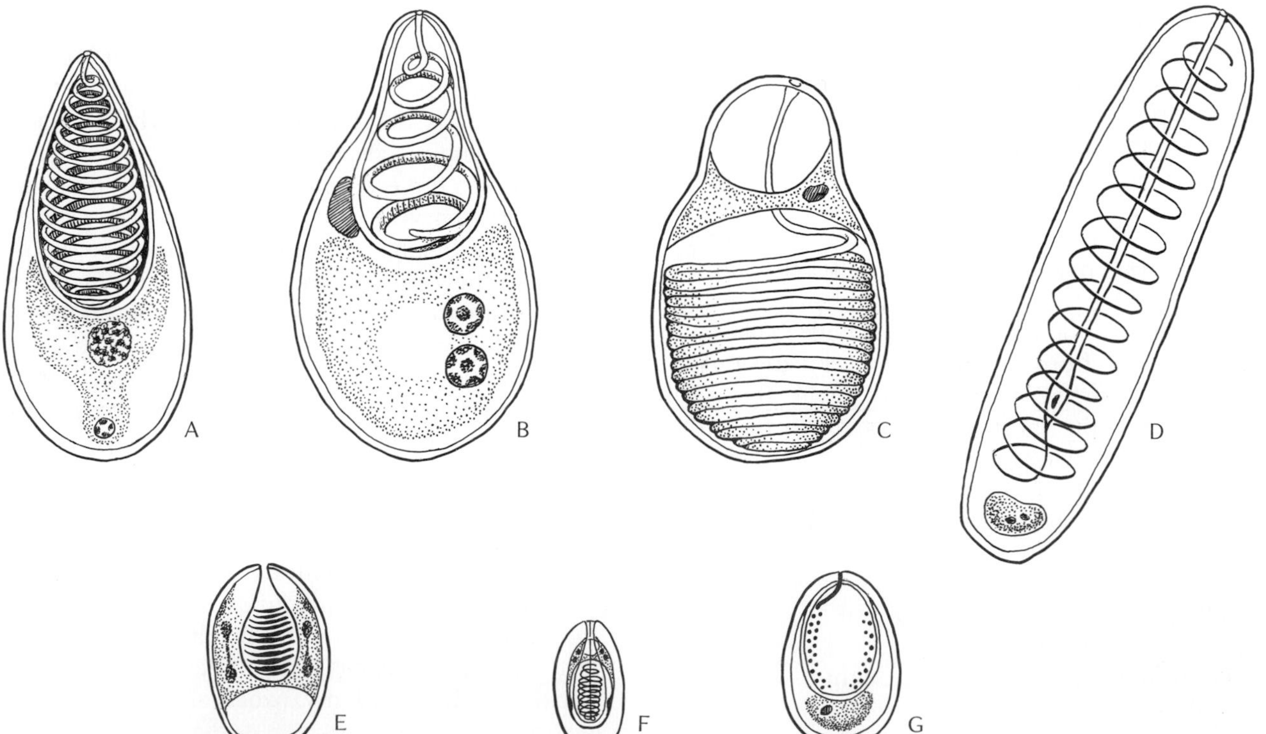

FIGURE 16.1 A selection of spores of (A to D) Myxozoa and (E, F, G) Microspora. (A) *Stempellia magna* from the mosquito, *Culex;* (B) *Myxobolus toyamai* from the carp, *Cyprinus carpio;* (C) *Plistophora longifilis* from the fish, *Barbus;* (D) *Mrazakia argoisi* from the amphipod, *Asellus;* (E) *Thelohania giardi* from the crustacean, *Crangon;* (F) *Nosema bombycis* from the silkworm, *Bombyx mori;* (G) *Nosema apis* from the honeybee, *Apis mellifera.* [Redrawn with modifications from Kudo, 1924.]

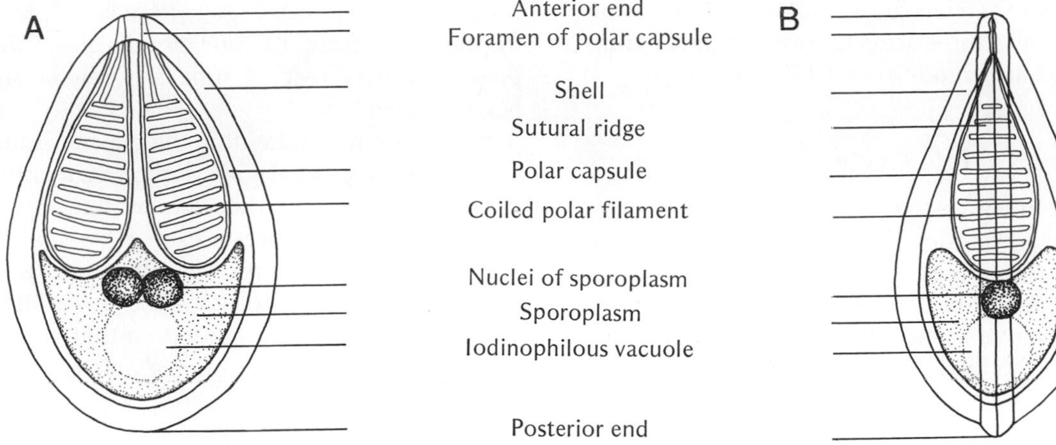

FIGURE 16.2 Diagram of a myxozoan spore viewed from the front (A) and side (B). The spore envelope is comprised of two valves each of which is formed by a cell. The two polar capsules containing filaments are also each formed by a cell. There are typically two nuclei in the sporoplasm, the infective portion of the spore. [Redrawn from Kudo, 1924.]

Identification of Myxozoa is based principally on the structure of the spore (Figs. 16.1 and 16.2)

Name of Organism and Disease Caused

Myxobolus cerebralis (syn. *Myxosoma cerebralis, Triactinomyxon gyrosalmo*) causes whirling disease, twist disease, and black disease in salmonid fish.

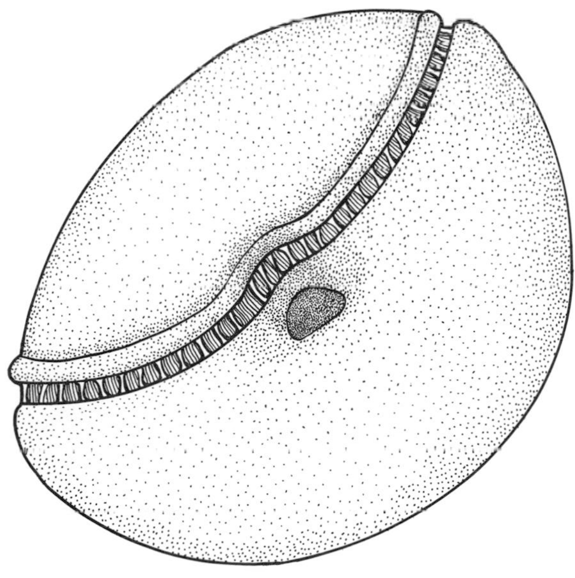

FIGURE 16.3 A spore of *Myxobolus cerebralis* based on SEM.

Hosts and Host Range

Salmonid fish (trout, salmon, steelhead, etc.) of many species are the hosts, and the organism develops in the cartilage of the head and axial skeleton. The alternate host is an annelid of the family Tubificidae such as *Tubifex tubifex*.

Distribution and Importance

Worldwide. The original location of this parasite was in western Europe, but the infection has spread to North America, South America, Britain, and New Zealand. The infection is not generally pathogenic to fish in its original European host, the brown trout, *Salmo trutta*, but infections in many other species of trout are pathogenic and have caused extensive losses especially in hatcheries.

Morphology

Spores produced in fish are 6 to 10 μm in diameter, oval, and have two valves and two polar capsules (Fig. 16.3); the polar capsules contain a coiled filament, which is extruded upon entry into a host. The spores have a mucous envelope; in SEM the opening for the extrusion of the polar filament can be seen.

Spores produced in the annelid host, the so-called triactinomyxon form, are about 36 μm long by 10.5 μm and have three polar capsules each of which has a coiled filament; this spore contains 30 to 50 spherical sporozoites. The epispore is an extension of the three valves of the spore and it is drawn out into an extension of about 90 μm and three arms like an anchor or grappling hook that are an additional 170 μm longer.

Life Cycle

When spores are ingested by a salmonid fish, factors in the gut cause extrusion of the polar filaments; the filaments slow down the passage of the spore through the intestine (Fig. 16.4). The sporozoites escape from the spore and move by ameboid movement through the gut wall to the final site of development. *M. cerebralis* develops in cartilage, where large plasmodia (or trophozoites) form. By four months after infection, the plasmodia may reach 1 mm in diameter, and spores begin to develop.

Spores are formed within the plasmodium and they are multinuclear in origin. They presumably reach the outside when the fish dies. Experimental evidence has shown that when spores are eaten by tubificid worms (Annelida: Oligochaeta) they reproduce and become infective for fish. The early work on the life cycle has been confirmed and extended so that it is now clear that the two hosts are obligate and morphologically

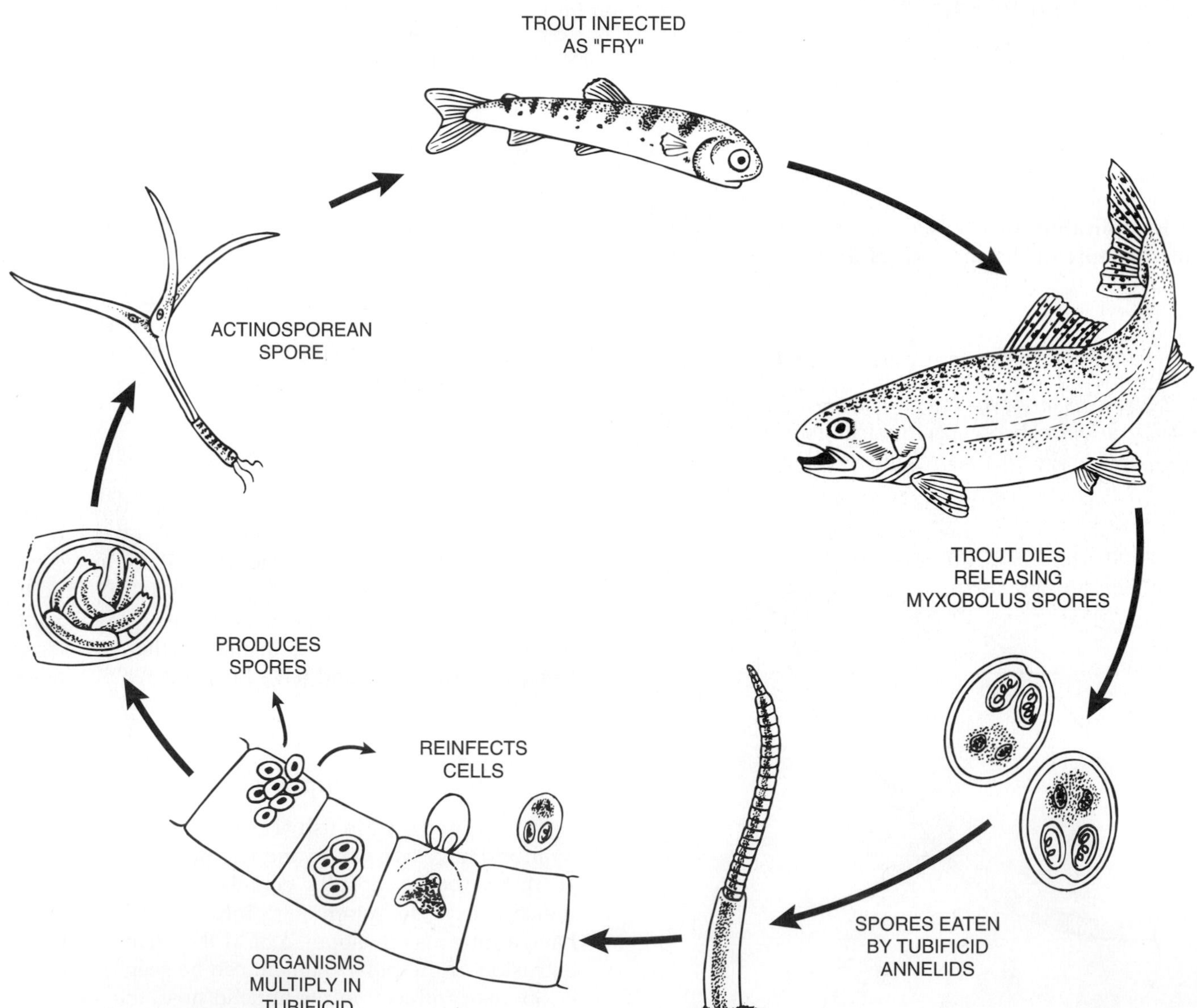

FIGURE 16.4 Life cycle of *Myxobolus cerebralis* Trout are infected as "fry," or newly hatched fish, with the actinosporean type of spore. When the fish dies as a result of the infection, it releases *Myxobolus* spores which have developed in its cartilaginous tissues. This type of spore is eaten by annelids in the genus *Tubifex* in which further multiplication takes place. The actinosporean spores are infectious for trout.

entirely different spores are produced in each host. The spores float in the water so that they can readily be eaten by susceptible fish.

In the formation of the spore, a sexual process called autogamy occurs. Two nuclei form in the sporoplasm of the spore and they fuse shortly after release from the spore.

Diagnosis

Finding the typical spores in cysts in cartilage is the surest method of determining whether *M. cerebralis* is the cause of a disease. Digestion methods are used to free the spores, or tissue sections can be examined under a compound microscope to identify the organism.

Research is ongoing with respect to developing a rapid diagnostic method. Use of polymerase chain reaction (PCR) and DNA identification represent the major thrust of these studies. Skeletal distortions and the typical swimming in circles are cause for suspicion that whirling disease is present.

Host–Parasite Interactions

In the normal host, *Salmo trutta*, the brown trout of central Europe, the pathogenesis is minor; however in the rainbow trout, *Salmo gairdneri*, and other North American trout, pathogenesis can be severe. The parasite develops in cartilage, and the location of the infection determines the effect on the host. The lesions result principally from the breakdown of cartilage and the consequent pressure on nervous tissue or sense organs. For example, when the cartilage surrounding the inner ear is weakened, the balance of the fish is disturbed and typical whirling is observed. If the caudal portion of the vertebral column is affected, there may be pressure on the nerves and the posterior portion of the fish turns dark because control of the nerves serving the chromatophores is lost. Fish lose coordination, various parts of the skeleton become distorted, and they sink exhausted to the bottom. Predation or death soon occurs.

Upon entry into a host, the polar filaments are extruded, but the stimuli for extrusion are poorly understood. In *Myxosoma cartilaginous* of bluegill (Centrarchidae), the filament can be extruded by 1% or stronger KOH, by 0.26% or stronger NaOCl (bleach), or by the quarternary ammonium disinfectant Roccal. Such stimuli are unrelated to conditions that the spores encounter in the gut or gills of a fish. Urea often triggers the extrusion of the polar filament, but this is not a physiological trigger either in freshwater fish.

After being triggered, the sporoplasm leaves the spore capsules and migrates to the tissue, where development occurs. If it is gut, presumably the sporoplasm simply enters nearby tissue. On the other hand, there is little information on how the sporoplasms reach cartilage, muscle, kidney, liver, or other organs.

Once in the tissues, development follows, but even then, information is fragmentary and sometimes conflicting. Kudo's *Protozoology* (1966) illustrated two quite different life cycles of *Sphaeromyxa sabrazesi*, a parasite of the gallbladder of the seahorse and other fish. Much of the difficulty with precise descriptions of the life cycles lies in the inability to produce infections artificially.

Epidemiology and Control

Control of whirling disease is based on the following:

1. Preventing infected fish from being transported into areas where the disease is not found
2. Constructing concrete raceways in fish hatcheries
3. Cleaning a raceway after a generation of fish has been released from it
4. Raising young fish (fry and fingerlings) in spore-free water as long as possible

Infection of rainbow trout with *M. cerebralis* is a good example of what may happen when animals or their products are moved around the world. Infection of salmonid fish with this parasite has been known since early in the 20th century, but it was not discovered in North America until about 1952 in fish in the eastern United States. By the middle 1960s whirling disease was found all across the United States, especially in hatchery fish.

It is likely that *M. cerebralis* was transferred to North America with brown trout imported from Europe. In addition, rainbow trout are good disseminators of the organism because they become heavily infected; following World War II, a market developed in Europe for rainbow trout and they were shipped widely for table use.

The hardiness of the spores is important in spreading infection. Spores are known to survive freezing, so even frozen fish may be a source of infection for fish in a new locality if scraps of fish reach free-flowing waters. Frozen fish were probably the vehicle for spreading the disease from Europe to the Western Hemisphere. The spores also pass through the intestinal tracts of other fish and of birds and remain viable; this mechanism probably spreads the infection locally.

The triactinomyxon spores are also hardy as are the tubificid hosts. The annelids can be dried or frozen and remain alive. Thus, the infection can be transported in mud containing the worms. It is not surprising that the organism causing whirling disease has been transported around the world; rather it is surprising that it did not take place until 45 years ago.

Preventing the introduction of fish infected with *M. cerebralis* requires careful diagnostic methods and monitoring. Eggs can be shipped to a hatchery if they are in an early stage of development. Sentinel fish can be placed in cages in a raceway to determine whether the spores are present there.

Building concrete raceways in a hatchery is expensive, but they can be cleaned readily. Silt accumulates on the bottom of raceways and tubificids colonize the area since it has the silty conditions and organic matter that they prefer. But all of that material can be removed between batches of fish.

Young fish are most susceptible to infection, but after they are about 6 cm long, the skeleton calcifies and they are less likely to suffer the damaging effects of whirling disease.

Notable Features

Whirling disease presents a number of instructive features in biology, biopolitics, and economics. During the explorations of the world in the 16th to 18th centuries, plants and animals were transported willy-nilly from one area to another. This was especially true between North America and Western Europe where plants were sent in both directions to determine whether they would thrive and provide new sources of food.

In the case of fish, they have been moved not only between continents, but also within continents to habitats where they had not originally been found. Trout have been moved into mountainous areas to which they could not migrate by themselves. Mountain lakes that could not otherwise be reached are stocked by helicopter with exotic trout. Water control systems then changed stream flows so that certain river courses now have water year-round instead of becoming nearly dry from mid-summer to early winter.

In the Western United States, trout fishing is not only a sport, it is also a big business. People travel from all over the world to fish in pristine mountain lakes and streams. For example, the value of trout fishing in Montana is estimated to be $270 million annually.

The introduction of whirling disease threw those who fish as well as the sport fishing industry into a conflict with state departments of wildlife and the federal Fish and Wildlife Service. Each group blames another for ruining fisheries. State and federal authorities have tried to determine who the culprit(s) is in introducing the disease. Fishing groups have railed against the scientists and bureaucrats for all sorts of real and imagined sins. Conservation activists point to greed as the motivation of nearly everyone in spreading the disease through planting fish indiscriminately both by those responsible for managing sport fisheries as well as fishermen themselves who thought that they could make improvements in fishing.

The finding that the whirling disease organism has two completely separate cycles, in the fish and in the tubificid worm, has created taxonomic problems that remain unsolved. Myxozoa are classified based on spore structure, and the group that has two valves and two polar capsules (e.g., *Myxobolus*) is far separated from the group that has three valves and three polar capsules (e.g., *Triactinomyxon*). We now find that they are, or at least some of them, in the same taxonomic group. A new name, *Triactinomyxon gyrosalmo,* was proposed in 1984 for the cause of whirling disease when the tubificid host was clearly shown to be a part of the cycle. However, *Myxobolus cerebralis* has priority since it was described in 1905.

There are at least five species of *Myxobolus* in trout affecting various organ systems. There are seventeen or more species of myxozoans that infect the cartilage of fish other than salmonids. Transmission studies have been completed with only a few of these species. Likewise, there are only relatively few species of Actinosporea (of which *Triactinomyxon* is a member), and almost none of them has been studied intensively. Questions abound as to which actinosporeans relate to which myxosporeans since we know little about life cycles, host range, or distributions. Several lifetimes of research await persons willing to enter a difficult and arcane field.

Other Myxozoa

As indicated earlier, of more than 1000 species of Myxozoa that have been described, the pathogenesis of only a few is known. Among freshwater fish, especially those in hatcheries or relatively small lakes, the effect on populations has been documented in a few instances; however, such information on marine fish is even more sketchy.

Some of the same manifestations are seen in myxozoan and microsporan infections. The bodies of the hosts are distorted, there may be tumorlike growths, or the muscle may become unsightly. The names of some of the infections indicate the signs of infection: "wormy" halibut, which occurs along the Pacific coast of North America, is caused by *Unicapsula muscularis;* "boil disease" is caused by *Myxobolus pfeifferi* in barbel; "tapioca disease" of salmon is caused by *Kudoa thyristes.*

Additional species of *Myxobolus* are being reported

to have two host life cycles. For example, *M. cotti* of the bullhead, *Cottus gobio*, also has tubificids as an alternate host and produces actinomyxon spores, which are different from those of *M. cerebralis*. *M. articus* of Pacific salmon is transmitted by *Stylodrilus herighianus*, an oligochaete in the family Lumbriculidae.

MICROSPORA

The phylum Microspora contains a number of obscure, but nonetheless important, parasites of a wide array of hosts. All Microspora are parasitic principally in insects and fish but occasionally in mammals, including humans. They are transmitted from one host to the next as a tiny spore, from which the group obtains its name.

The spores are typically quite small (Fig. 16.1). Most of them are ovoid or ellipsoid and range in size from about 4 to 8 mm long to 3 to 5 μm wide. A few, such as *Stempelia magna*, have spores that are 14 by 4.5 μm, and some, such as *Perezia lankesteriae*, a hyperparasite of the gregarine, *Lankesteria ascidiae*, have spores as small as 2.5 μm.

The spore has a smooth outer wall, and unlike the Myxozoa there are no valves or sutures. The sporoplasm has a single nucleus and a hollow filament coiled inside the spore (Fig. 16.5). This coiled tubule is everted when the spore enters the body of a potential host and actually injects the sporoplasm into a cell. The tubule, when everted, may be from 25 to 500 μm long, depending on the species, but most are 100 μm or less long; the diameter is about 0.1 μm.

Spores are usually ingested by a host, but sometimes the sporoplasm is injected through the integument (in small aquatic invertebrates). Whatever the mode of entry, when the filament is triggered, the sporoplasm escapes from the spore by moving down the length of the tube. What triggers extrusion of the tubule is not well known. Under experimental conditions, a change in osmotic pressure, drying, and mechanical pressure have all been used. The precise conditions in a host have not been determined.

Once inside a host cell, the sporoplasm undergoes merogony (Fig. 16.6). There are one or more merogonous generations, and then sporogony takes place. Depending on the species, a lesser or greater number of spores may be formed. Note that the spores are formed within the parasite, not by the formation of a wall surrounding the whole parasite. The spores reach the outside most often with feces or urine, but they may also do so through the integument or when the host dies and breaks down through natural processes.

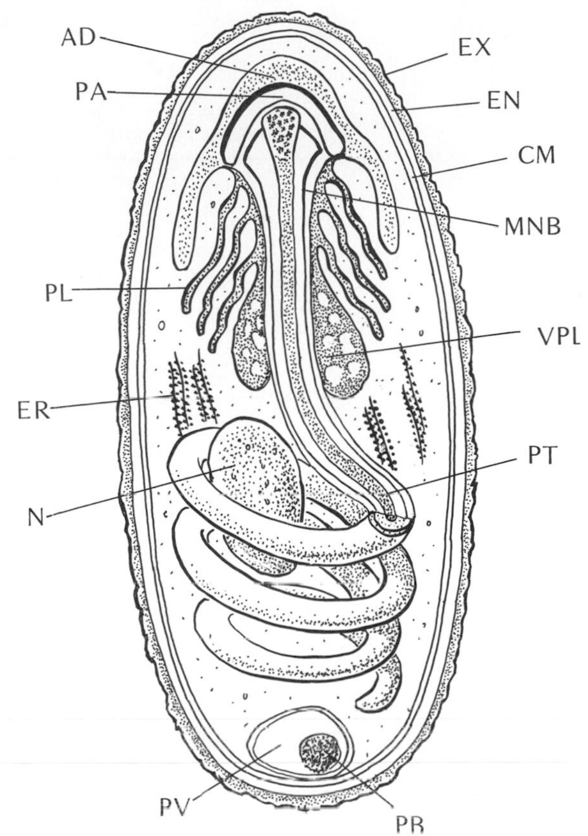

FIGURE 16.5 A diagram of a microsporan spore as revealed by electron microscopy. AD, anchoring disk of the polar tubule; EN, endospore; EX, exospore; MNB, manubrioid part of the filament; N, nucleus; PA, polar aperture; PB, posterior body; PT, polar tube; PL, lamellae of the lamellar polaroplast; PV, posterior vacuole; ER, endplasmic reticulum densely populated with ribosomes; VPL, vesicular part of the polaroplast.

There are between 500 and 600 described species of Microspora, and perhaps 200 additional species are known but not adequately described. New ones are being added continually and it is clear that only a small percentage of species has been described.

Although economically important Microspora have been known for more than a hundred years, only recently has their pervasive importance been recognized. We know now that they have a great deal of potential for controlling populations of economically important insect pests and that they are common in fish and mammals among whom they cause disease. Microspora are also important to human health, especially among those persons whose immune systems have been compromised through a genetic defect, a disease that affects the immune system such as AIDS, or drug treatment.

Microspora have an important place in the history of biology and in the development of knowledge of infectious agents. During the early 1860s a disease

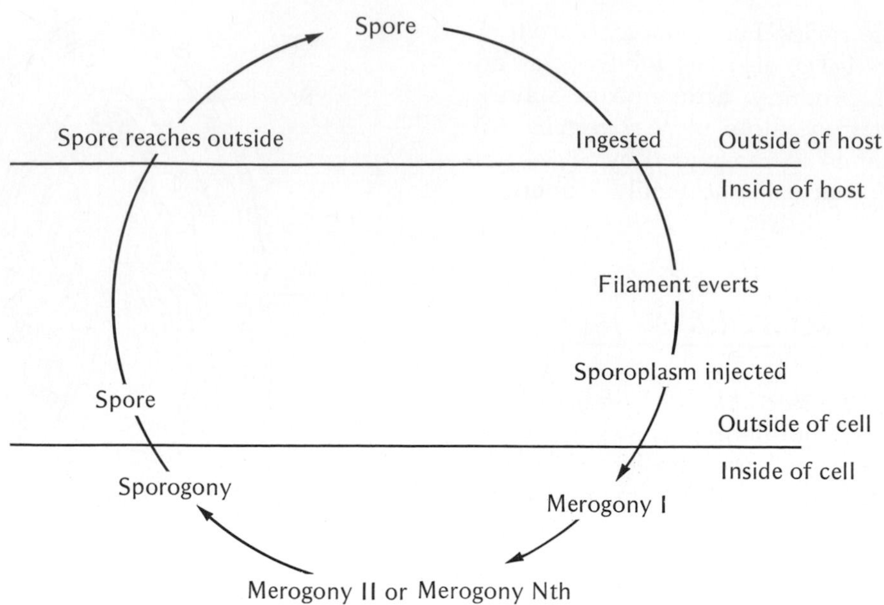

FIGURE 16.6 Generalized life cycle of a microsporan.

called pébrine swept through the silkworm-raising industry of Europe and nearly eliminated it. In France there was concern that the silk industry might disappear, and Louis Pasteur was asked to look at the problem. For a period of about five years, from 1865 to 1870, Pasteur studied the transmission of *Nosema bombycis,* the cause of pébrine. Through the experiments and observations of Pasteur and his students, methods were developed to diagnose the infection in silkworms and to rear them free of infection. Pasteur had previously worked in chemistry and on fermentation of wine, but after his studies on pébrine, he entered the world of infectious diseases and his great discoveries in bacterial and viral diseases followed.

In this chapter we deal only with a few species of Microspora that are important to humans for either their harm or potential benefit.

Name of Organism and Disease Associations

Nosema bombycis causes silkworm disease, pébrine, and Flechenkrankheit.

Hosts and Host Range

The normal host is *Bombyx mori,* the silkworm, but infections can be established in other insect species as well.

Morphology

The spores are oval and measure 3 to 4 by 1.5 to 2 μm (Fig. 16.1).

Geographic Distribution and Importance

Cosmopolitan. *N. bombycis* is a highly pathogenic parasite that has decimated the silkworm industry at various times and places.

Life Cycle

The spores are ingested by larvae and the polar filament injects the sporont into the cells of the gut. The sporoplasm transforms into a trophozoite and under goes merogony. There is more than one merogonous generation, and then the merozoites reinvade cells to form sporonts. Each sporont gives rise to only a single spore. Spores may be formed as early as 48 hours after infection.

Host–Parasite Interactions

All tissues of the larvae are infected and there may be a range of effects. In heavy infections the larvae die, or they may not be able to spin a cocoon. In lighter infections the life cycle of the insect may be completed, but the organism can be transmitted from mother to offspring through the egg, causing the newly hatched larva to die.

Diagnosis

The larvae have a speckled surface, as though covered with flakes of pepper (pébre). This sign is good evidence of pébrine, but other conditions such as bacterial infections cause similar changes in the larvae. The most certain method of diagnosis is by finding the characteristic spores in the tissues of the larva or of the adult. The animal is teased apart and the spores are looked for under the higher powers of a compound microscope.

Epidemiology and Control

Pébrine is spread by contamination of an area with spores that are ingested by silkworms. As a general rule, spores are released to the outside when a host dies and disintegrates. Since the host produces a huge numbers of spores, the environment becomes heavily contaminated and the disease spreads rapidly. Because of carryover from one generation to another through transovarial transmission, control and eradication pose difficult problems.

Pasteur's work developed principles that are still valid today: good diagnosis and use of only clean replacement stock. Pasteur and his students studied the transmission of the disease and determined that the so-called seed or eggs of the silkworm were a principal source of infection. It was reasoned that if it were possible to obtain eggs free of infection, they could be used the year following an outbreak to establish a healthy colony. Thus, Pasteur's recommendations were to use eggs only from adults known to be free of infection. He did this by keeping each batch of eggs identified with a particular adult female. If we were dealing with large farm animals, we would call this a "quarantine, test and slaughter program." Although the terms may be different, the principles are the same. Fortunately, the spores of *N. bombycis* do not remain alive from one season to the next outside a host. If the area is cleaned and allowed to remain vacant until the next spring, one can begin anew.

Name of Organism and Disease Associations

Nosema apis causes Nosema disease, dwindling diseases, nosematosis, and winter losses.

Hosts and Host Range

The principal host is the honey bee, *Apis mellifera*, but it may infect 13 or more species of insects.

Morphology

Spores are ellipsoidal, measure 4 to 6 by 2 to 4 μm, and have a long polar filament with up to 44 coils (Fig. 16.1G).

Life Cycle

The sporoplasm infects cells of the midgut of the bee. There are two merogonous generations. The meronts are long chainlike organisms, and the second generation has four double nuclei. Spores are produced about seven days after infection.

Distribution and Importance

Cosmopolitan. This organism causes serious disease in honey bees and causes losses in various times and places.

Diagnosis

A number of diseases of bees caused by bacteria, fungi, and viruses may have effects similar to those of Nosema disease. It is essential to distinguish which disease is the cause of losses because the methods of treatment and control will vary. Often it is necessary to submit bees to a laboratory that specializes in diagnosis of their diseases.

Nosematosis is a disease of adult bees and is usually seen by the beekeeper as a dwindling in the population of adult bees in the hive. Weak, dying, and dead bees are seen around the hive. The only certain method of diagnosis is to find the typical spores in the tissues of affected bees, although if the midgut of the bee is swollen and pale, the disease would be suspected.

Host–Parasite Interactions

N. apis principally affects the intestinal tract of the insect, but it also affects the Malpighian tubules. The normal gut function is disrupted and the bees become weak and cannot fly as strongly as they normally would. Since there is always some turnover in a hive of bees, the losses are not usually recognized until the disease is well established. Thus, the number of bees in an affected hive dwindles.

Epidemiology and Control

Because the infection with *N. apis* is spread from one bee to the next through fecal contamination, four measures are essential for minimizing losses from Nosema disease:

1. Purchasing only clean bees
2. Early diagnosis
3. Treatment
4. Cleaning the hives after an outbreak

The bee industry in the United States is regulated

so that in each state there is a system of inspection and certification of the health of a newly purchased colony. There is also periodic inspection of hives to ensure continued freedom from infectious diseases. Such strict regulation may seem excessive until one considers that the bee industry in the United States in 1973 was estimated to have a value of $2.1 billion. Of this total, $2 billion was for use of bees as pollinators of various crops such as fruit trees and alfalfa. Honey accounted for $106 million and the rest was beeswax. The importance of bees has brought the assurance that bees purchased from reliable raisers are free of Nosema disease as well as other diseases.

If nosematosis or other disease is suspected, prompt diagnosis is essential. Help in diagnosis may be obtained from the state college of agriculture or the state apiarist, sometimes located in the same place. Once a positive diagnosis has been obtained, fumagillin helps to control the disease.

Wintertime is especially difficult for bees because they must survive on stored honey for several months. If the colony has been weakened through nosematosis or other infectious disease, winter losses may be excessive. The question of keeping infected bees over the winter must therefore be addressed. Fumagillin usually gives good control of nosematosis, but the hive and surroundings remain contaminated for a considerable period of time. To ensure minimal risk, the hive should either be destroyed or thoroughly fumigated in fall, and then clean bees should be purchased in spring.

Name of Organism and Disease Associations

Encephalitozoon cuniculi (syn. *Nosema cuniculi, E. negri*) causes encephalitozoonosis.

Hosts and Host Range

This organism was originally described from the European rabbit, *Oryctolagus cuniculi,* but it infects, either naturally or experimentally, laboratory mice and rats, guinea pigs, the domestic dog, and perhaps humans. Experimentally the organism did not develop in three rhesus monkeys, and an apparent *Encephalitozoon* in a squirrel monkey was morphologically different from *E. cuniculi.* At this point, lack of data on the host range and differing structures in different species of hosts leaves in question how many species actually infect various mammals.

Infections are widely disseminated in the host. Most often the central nervous system and kidney are infected, but in heavy infections all tissues may have organisms in them.

Distribution and Importance

E. cuniculi infections are common in laboratory animals, especially rabbits; up to 84% of 51 rabbits were found to be infected in one study.

The effect on individuals and populations of animals is difficult to determine; however, outbreaks of encephalitozoonosis have been reported in both rabbits and dogs.

The high prevalence in laboratory experimental animals is disturbing, because it is essential that no extraneous factors invalidate data when experimental animals are used. It is known that hosts that are not immunologically competent may be affected by *E. cuniculi,* and there are some instances in which tumors have been invaded by microsporans and their size has been reduced (an unexplained observation). *E. cuniculi* is not normally looked for, and what role it may play in affecting the outcome of experiments is unknown.

Morphology

The oval spores average 2.5 by 1.5 μm, and have a relatively thick outer wall and a short polar filament of 20 to 25 μm.

The merogonous stages are quite small, ranging from about 1 μm up to 2.5 by 4 μm (Fig. 16.7).

Life Cycle

Transmission of the agent takes place by mouth and the polar filament probably everts in the intestine of the host. How the infection spreads to various other organ systems is not known. The number of merogonous generations is not clear; it appears that there might be continuous merogony if the infection is widespread in a host. Each sporont gives rise to two uninucleated spores. It has been demonstrated that spores may pass with the urine if there is infection of the kidney; experimental animals have been infected through urine containing spores. Whether spores may reach the outside through other routes is not known. Prenatal transmission seems to take place since rabbits taken by cesarean section and raised under gnotobiotic conditions have been found to be infected.

Diagnosis

Infections with *E. cuniculi* are almost always found through histologic examination of tissues. Since the organisms are so small and their distinguishing features are so difficult to see, a person experienced in identifying members of the group should be consulted. There are staining characteristics that can be used to differentiate the organism from other intracellular organisms.

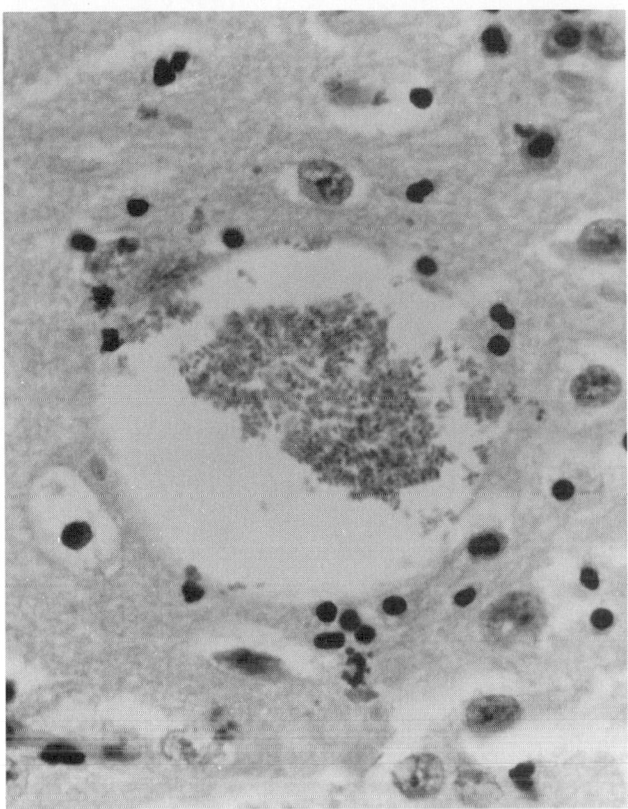

FIGURE 16.7 Meront of *Encephalitozoon cuniculi* in the brain of a rabbit. Note the large parasitophorous vacuole in which the meront lies and that there is a slight cellular response around the meront.

Host–Parasite Interactions

In most instances, *E. cuniculi* infection is inapparent. Sometimes it becomes a fulminating, fatal infection, however. Deaths are mostly in young animals.

The effects of infection are predominantly in the central nervous system and secondarily in the kidney; other tissues may also be affected. The signs of infection are related principally to damage to the brain: incoordination, weakness, convulsions, and abnormal behavior. None of these is diagnostic for encephalitozoonosis.

Epidemiology and Control

No treatment is known. The only known means of transmission are through urine containing spores and prenatal transfer. Even laboratory animals derived from supposedly uninfected mothers have been found to be infected. Prevalence of infection varies widely in laboratory animals, and the prevalence in uncaged animals is not known. At this point there are no recommendations for controlling the infection.

MICROSPORAN INFECTIONS IN HUMANS

Until recent times microsporan infections in humans were so rare that they were they were not discussed in parasitology textbooks. Some infections were known from mammals other than humans, such as *Encephalitozoon cuniculi* infections in laboratory rabbits (Fig. 16.7). Similar to cryptosporidiosis, sporadic microsporan infections had been recognized in persons lacking fully competent immune systems, but the advent of the HIV pandemic brought the infections to the attention of parasitologists and clinicians.

Name of Organisms and Disease Associations

Eight species of Microspora have been associated with human infections:

Name of organism	Organ system infected
Encephalitozoon cuniculi	Liver, peritoneum, various blood cells and vascular endothelium
E. hellum	Eye, several organs including kidney, and other parts of the urinary system, and respiratory system
Enterocytozoon bienusi	Gastrointestinal, and its adjuncts, respiratory system
Nosema conori	Disseminated infection
N. corneum	Eye
N. ocularum	Eye
Septata intestinalis	Intestine
Pleistophora sp.	Somatic muscle

In some clinical reports, the organisms were identified only to the generic level, and in others the organisms were determined to be Microspora, but they were not identified further.

Hosts and Host Range

Data are lacking on the normal hosts of the microsporans infecting humans. It is not known whether some or all of the organisms have humans or other species as their normal hosts. *E. cuniculi* has been known from the rabbit, rodents, and primates including humans for some time; it has also been identified in birds. However, the infections described in clinical cases prior to the description of *E. hellum* may not, in fact, be *E. cuniculi.*

Microspora are widely distributed throughout the animal kingdom, especially in insects. It is possible that human infections result from exposure to spores from invertebrates, and insects would be the prime suspects since they are so ubiquitous.

The use of microsporans for biological control has a good deal of potential, but the requirement that humans and livestock should not be susceptible to infection is a difficult hurdle to clear in the commercial development of such agents. Even though microsporans of insects may possibly infect humans, there are no data to support the suspicion. Likewise, when an attempt is made to obtain clearance of a microsporan for use in controlling an economically important insect, proving that it does *not* infect humans or other mammals is exceedingly difficult, if not impossible.

Geographic Distribution and Importance

Cosmopolitan. Sporadic infections in humans have been reported, but the overall importance to human health is not known. Except for a few instances, infections in humans have been reported only from persons whose immune systems are somehow compromised.

Diagnosis

The means of determining whether an individual is infected with a microsporan are as follows:

1. Finding the spores in bodily secretions and excretions
2. Finding the developmental stages in biopsied tissue or at postmortem examination
3. Finding antibodies in the serum of patients
4. Allowing stages to develop in cell culture

None of these means is satisfactory at this point. Unlike other protistan cysts and helminth eggs, the spores of microsporans do not float in media of high specific gravity, nor are they readily concentrated by sedimentation. Feces, sputum, or tracheal washings can be spread in slides and the material stained with various dyes, which can differentiate the spores, to an extent. These slides should be scanned under an oil immersion lens or at least under a high dry objective of a compound microscope. Those spores of species that have been found in humans are typically 1 to 2 μm in length, barely bigger than most bacteria. If only a few are present on a slide, it requires a good deal of skill to separate the extraneous material from the spores when examining it.

Most diagnoses are probably made from tissues obtained either ante- or postmortem. The stages can be seen at the LM level, but EM gives details that are not readily seen at the LM level. Since so little is known of these organisms, examining the endogenous stages and spores at the EM level is an important part of diagnosis. Even so, a specialist in the group should be consulted.

A variety of serologic tests has been developed, but they are of limited use. It is possible to differentiate between *E. cuniculi* and *E. hellum*, but it is uncertain what information is provided to the investigator about other species. Serosurveys have shown that as many as 42% of persons may have been exposed to *E. cuniculi*, but it is not known what cross reactions there may be.

Only *Encephalitozoon hellum, Nosema corneum,* and *Septata intestinalis* have been grown in cells. If something does come up in culture it then should be studied at the EM level to determine what species may be present. If nothing grows, the investigator knows only that the cultures were negative.

Because of the obscurity of the Microspora, they do not readily come to the mind of the clinician unless he or she is accustomed to treating persons with compromised immune systems. Even then, the signs and symptoms are similar to many other infections. Finding the spores or developmental stages is the crucial bit of information needed to make a positive diagnosis.

Host–Parasite Interactions

In nearly all of the cases of microsporan infections described in humans, the person has not been immunocompetent. It is likely that many immunologically normal individuals are infected with microsporans, but the infection never reaches a clinical phase, or the disease remains mild and is resolved quickly.

In three instances, individuals infected with Microspora were found to be immunologically normal. In one there was a self-limiting diarrhea caused by *Enterocytozoon bienusi.* In the other two there was keratitis (inflammation of the cornea of the eye) caused by *Nosema corneum* or *N. ocularum.* In this superficial location, in a tissue with limited vascularity, it is not surprising to find an opportunistic infection.

In all other instances, where the immune status was determined, the immune response was not normal. In some cases there was congenital impairment of the immune system, in others, the person was taking an immunosuppressive drug. Most often, microsporan infections have been seen in HIV-positive persons.

Persons who are HIV positive often have disseminated infections that lead to severe disease and death. More than 20 cases of microsporan infections have been described in HIV patients. The circumstance is similar to other opportunistic infections in AIDS patients; they show infections with *Pneumocystis carinii, Cryptosporidium,* and *Toxoplasma,* among others, and microsporans represent another group of agents that would not normally be important to human health, so far as we know.

Epidemiology and Control

Treatment remains at an elementary trial-and-error level of knowledge. Albendazole, a benzimidazole used to treat nematode infections, has been observed to be effective against *Septata intestinalis*, but the data are only anecdotal. Some fungicides such as fumagillin may have effect, but, again, the data are poor. For example, patients with keratoconjunctivitis treated with fumagillin showed improvement. It is not known what the result would have been if no treatment was given.

Since it is not known what the normal hosts are of the organisms infecting humans, it is not known how infections are obtained, or from what hosts. In some respiratory infections, the number of organisms was greatest in the upper part of the respiratory tree and decreased the farther toward the alveoli; it was concluded that the organisms entered the upper part of the respiratory system and moved posteriorly as the infection developed. It could be concluded that infection takes place by ingesting or inhaling the spores. But from what source?

Because so little is known about epidemiology, control is therefore not possible to formulate. There seems not to have been any infections acquired from HIV patients by their caregivers. This may mean only that a healthy immune system prevents the infection from reaching the clinical stage.

Clinical infections in humans with microsporans have been known for only about 30 years. As with cryptosporidiosis, Hanta virus infections, toxoplasmosis in certain domestic animals, among others, we may be seeing another emerging disease. What may unfold as time passes remains to be seen.

MICROSPORA AS BIOLOGICAL CONTROL AGENTS

Around 1920, a number of Microspora were found that were pathogenic for harmful insects. As an example, among many Microspora described by Richard R. Kudo was *Nosema anophelis*, which attacked the fat bodies of larval mosquitoes. It reduced stored fat in the larvae so that they were unable to complete development. It appeared that the system might be manipulated to control mosquito populations. (Insecticides such as DDT were still 20 years in the future.) Newspapers, ever alert to a story, declared that the scourge of mosquitoes and the diseases they carry would soon be a thing of the past. It is clear that such a desirable state has not yet arrived despite the passage of 70 years.

Probably three principal factors delayed development of this kind of biological control:

1. Unwillingness of administrators to commit public funds to development of such agents
2. Relatively primitive technology in biology
3. Development of fairly good insecticides in the 1930s and then the development of organochlorine insecticides (DDT, lindane, dieldrin) in the 1940s

The course of research and development is inevitably influenced by social, political, and economic forces. So it is with biological control in general. The commitment of funds to such a program was probably inconceivable when technology for mass-producing insects and their parasites was still not developed to a high level. Likewise, systems for the delivery and broadcasting of the parasites were still to be developed. In the years before World War II, economic conditions militated against such programs. During and immediately following the war, development of second-generation insecticides was explosive; it appeared that our insect problems could be taken care of through more and better chemicals. In fact, the control achieved was truly miraculous.

Then, as the 1960s unfolded, it became clear that pesticides were hazardous to many more than their target organisms. As tighter regulations were imposed and the technological climate changed, biological control became an attractive adjunct and alternative.

Some organisms have been approved for use and others are in the stage of field testing for efficacy and safety. *Nosema locustae* has been approved for control of grasshoppers and is offered to them in a grain bait containing the spores. A number of species have been used with some success in controlling insect pests of coniferous trees; in these cases, the spores are sprayed onto the foliage in liquid.

Nosema algerae was field tested for the control of anopheline mosquito vectors of malaria. Regrettably, the spores sink rapidly in water and are out of the feeding territory of the mosquitoes it is meant to infect; attempts are being made to keep the spores at the surface of the water.

Problems continue in the development of Microspora as biological control agents. Clearance for use requires proof of both efficacy and safety. Efficacy is the easier to demonstrate; this can be done in both laboratory and field tests. Safety is difficult to prove since it is necessary to determine the host range of the potential product and to show that there are no harmful acute or chronic effects on any animals important to humans, including humans. In most instances, the expense of obtaining clearance for such a product can be borne only by a large commercial company, and the company must be able to see an adequate return on its investment. The question that managers inevitably ask is, can we predict that there will be a long-term market for a product that continues to multiply in the pests it aims to control? If we sell one batch of spores, is there any need to sell more the next season? The answer is a qualified yes. When a pest is recognized as a potential problem in a certain area, the rapid amplification of the infectious agent can be accomplished most readily by introducing large numbers into the environment.

MICROSPORA OF FISH

The two principal animal groups that serve as hosts of Microspora are insects and fish. A large number of species of Microspora have been described from fish, and the prevalence of infection is high. The genera most often seen in fish are *Glugea, Pleistophora,* and *Nosema.*

The effects on individual hosts vary from inapparent to severe interference with normal functions and death. For example, *Nosema branchiale* has been reported from a number of species of cod (Gadidae), but even though there were 60 cysts on a single gill arch in heavily parasitized fish, there did not seem to be any detrimental effect. *Pleistophora ovariae* infects the ovaries of golden shiner and causes low-grade losses when these minnows are raised as fish bait. On the other hand, *Glugea anomala* contributed to a mass die-off of stickleback in Russia.

Microspora may infect nearly any organ system of fish including the gut, reproductive system, muscles, gills, brain, and eye. *Glugea stephani* is a common parasite of flounder in temperate waters, and it causes extensive damage to the intestine of the host. The effect is to cause almost complete replacement of the normal tissue of the gut with huge numbers of cysts containing the spores. *Glugea hertwigi* parasitizes not only the gut but also the gonad; fish are then unable to reproduce. A number of species, such as *Pleistophora macrozoarcidis,* cause tumorlike deformities or xenomas (tumors formed of tissue other than that of the animal) on the surface of fish.

The losses from microsporan infections in fish arise from the following:

1. Failure to grow properly
2. Death losses, or weakening so that the animals are readily removed by predation
3. Failure to reproduce
4. Discarding fish for aesthetic reasons

As we have seen with quite a number of diseases, determining the extent of losses, or placing an economic value on them, is difficult. However, there are a number of instances, quite well documented, in which there have been losses. In flounder off Cape Cod, Massachusetts, the young of the year were heavily infected, but the second-year fish had little infection; it was concluded that the young fish died in their first year. A massive die-off of smelt (*Osmerus*) was observed in Quebec in which 85% of the fish were affected. Sindermann (1970) has concluded that the "effects [of the Microspora] on the host are among the most severe of any parasite group" on marine and estuarine fish.

Readings

Cali, A. (1970). Morphogenesis in the genus *Nosema.* Proc. 4th Int. Colloq. Invert. Pathol., pp. 431–438.

Cox, J. C., Hamilton, R. C., and Attwood, H. D. (1979). An investigation of the route and progression of *Encephalitozoon cuniculi* infection in adult rabbits. *J. Protozool.* **26,** 260–265.

Desportes-Livage, I. (1996). Human microsporidioses and AIDS: Recent advances. *Parasite* **3,** 107–113.

Gray, F. H., Cali, A., and Briggs, J. D. (1969). Intracellular stages in the life cycle of the microsporidian *Nosema apis. J. Invertebr. Pathol.* **14,** 391–394.

Hoffman, G. L. (1970). Intercontinental and transcontinental dissemination and transfaunation of fish parasites with emphasis on whirling disease (*Myxosoma cerebralis*). In *A Symposium on Diseases of Fishes and Shellfishes* (S. F. Snieszko, Ed.), pp. 69–81. American Fisheries Society, Washington, DC.

Hoffman, G. L., Putz, R. E., and Dunbar, C. E. (1965). Studies on *Myxosoma cartilaginis* n. sp. (Protozoa: Myxosporidia) of centrarchid fish and a synopsis of the *Myxosoma* of North American freshwater fishes. *J. Protozool.* **12,** 319–332.

Kent, M. L., Margolis, L., and Corliss, J. O. (1994). The demise of a class of protists: Taxonomic and nomenclatural revisions proposed for the protist phylum Myxozoa Grassé, 1970. *Can. J. Zool.* **72,** 932–937.

Kudo, R. R. (1920). Studies on Myxosporidia. A synopsis of genera and species of Myxosporidia. *Illinois Biol. Mongr.* **5,** 239–503.

Kudo, R. R. (1924). A biologic and taxonomic study of the Microsporidia. *Illinois Biol. Monogr.* **9,** 83–344.

Kudo, R. R. (1966). *Protozoology,* 5th Ed. Charles C. Thomas Publisher, Springfield, Illinois.

Lom, J. (1970a). *Protozoa Causing Diseases in Marine Fishes,* Spec. Publ. No. S, pp. 142–160. American Fisheries Society, Washington, DC.

Lom, J. (1970b). Protozoa causing diseases in marine fishes. In *A Symposium on Diseases of Fishes and Shellfishes* (S. F. Snieszko, Ed.), pp. 101–123. American Fisheries Society, Washington, DC.

Lom, J. (1990). Phylum Myxozoa. In *Handbook of Protoctista* (L. Margulis, J. O. Corliss, M. Melkonian, and D. J. Chapman, Eds.), pp. 36–52. Jones & Bartlett, Boston.

Markiw, M. E., and Wolf, K. (1983). *Myxosoma cerebralis* (Myxozoa: Myxosporea) etiologic agent of salmonid whirling disease requires tubificid worm (Annelida: Oligochaeta) in its life cycle. *J. Protozool.* **30,** 561–565.

Pakes, S. P. (1974). Protozoal diseases. In *The Biology of the Laboratory Rabbit* (S. H. Weisbroth, R. E. Flatt, and A. L. Kraus, Eds.), pp. 264–286. Academic Press, New York.

Siddall, M. E., Martin, D. S., Bridge, D., Desser, S. S., and Cone, D. K. (1995). The demise of a phylum of protists: Phylogeny of Myxozoa and other parasitic Cnidaria. *J. Parasitol.* **81,** 961–967.

Sindermann, C. J. (1970). *Principal Diseases of Marine Fish and Shellfish.* Academic Press, New York.

Sprague, V. (1977). Classification and phylogeny of the Microsporidia. In *Comparative Pathobiology* (L. A. Bulla, Jr., and T. C. Cheng, Eds.), Vol. 2, pp. 1–30. Plenum, New York.

Sprague, V., and Vavra, J. (1977). *Systematics of the Microsporidia.* Plenum, New York.

Sprague, V., and Vernick, S. H. (1971). The ultrastructure of *Encephalitozoon cuniculi* (Microsporida, Nosematidae) and its taxonomic significance. *J. Protozool.* **18,** 560–569.

Strano, A. J., Cali, A., and Neafie, R. C. (1976). Microsporidiosis. In *Pathology of Tropical and Extraordinary Diseases*, pp. 336–339. AFIP Press, Washington, DC.

Vavra, J., and Sprague, V. (Eds.) (1976). *Biology of the Microsporidia.* Plenum, New York.

Weber, R., Bryan, R. T., Schwartz, D. A., and Owen, R. L. (1994). Human microsporidial infections. *Clin. Microbiol. Rev.* **7,** 426–461.

PART

2

PLATYHELMINTHES

CHAPTER

17

Introduction to the Flatworms and Aspidobothrea

The phylum Platyhelminthes includes a variety of free-living and parasitic flatworms of relatively primitive structure. Within the limitation of being aquatic or living at least in moist environments, they have successfully invaded a variety of ecological niches. The mostly free-living members, the Turbellaria, seem to be the stem forms for the parasitic classes, the flukes and the tapeworms (Fig. 17.1).

Flatworms have certain characteristics that are important for classification and identification. The platyhelminthes are members of the group referred to as acoelomate bilateria. Bilateral symmetry is found in nearly all of the parasitic metazoa, but the fact that they lack a body cavity (acoelomate) allows one to identify them readily in whole mounts or in tissue sections. The organ systems are embedded in a connective tissue network (parenchyma) which, together with the tegument or outer covering, allows their identification as members of the phylum.

The excretory system is based on the *flame cell* or *protonephridium* (Figs. 17.2 and 17.3). It is primarily osmoregulatory and functions adequately in small animals. The pattern of distribution of flame cells within an individual is sometimes used for classification and identification.

The nervous system is not usually seen in standard preparations of flatworms; it is composed of ganglia at the anterior end and two longitudinal nerve cords, with cross-commissures, running the length of the body (Fig. 17.4). Cephalization occurred first (phylogenetically) in the flatworms. In the Turbellaria, there is development of a head and associated sense organs such as eyes and tactile cilia (Fig. 17.5). In an evolutionary context, this is the first time that animals met the environment head on. Cephalization is somewhat less important in the parasitic flatworms than in the free-living ones, but a dominance of the head is still shown and movement is made with that portion anterior.

The digestive system in most platyhelminthes is incomplete. The mouth enters a blind sac, so that the residue of any food ingested must be excreted through the mouth.

The greatest number of platyhelminthes are hermaphroditic or monoecious. The sexes are separate in a few instances, such as the blood flukes and a small number of tapeworms. The reproductive systems are used almost more than any other structures for identification and classification of parasitic flatworms.

Classification, especially at higher levels, is currently experiencing increased scrutiny due to the use of computer-based cladistic analyses of morphological characteristics and data from molecular biology. We have chosen a conservative taxonomic approach until more complete analyses are available.

All of the major groups of parasitic platyhelminthes belong to the superclass Neodermata, which includes those platyhelminthes that cast off ciliated epidermis at the end of the free-swimming larval phase of the life cycle. That ciliated epidermis is replaced by an external *syncytial tegument*. These organisms are then divided into two classes, the Trematoda and the Cercomeromorphae. The latter has a hooked posterior end of the larvae, the *cercomer*, while the Trematoda does not have this posterior hooked structure on its larvae.

The class Trematoda includes a diverse group of

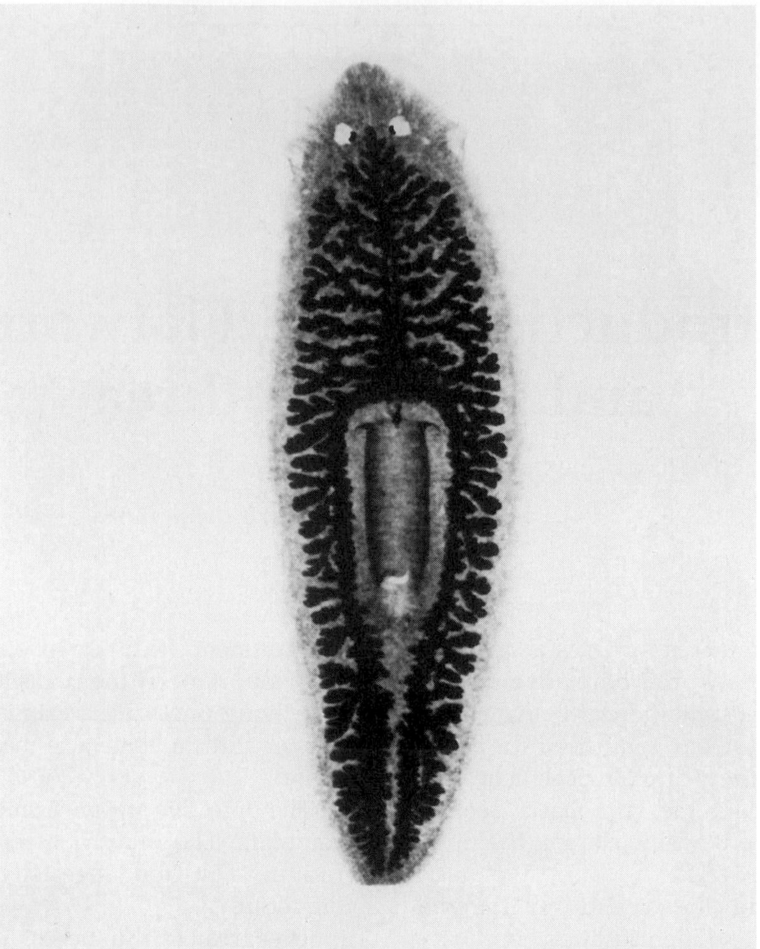

FIGURE 17.1 A free-living turbellarian. Note the pair of eyespots in the anterior region and that much of the body cavity is filled with the branching, incomplete intestinal tract.

flatworms that are all parasitic. They are small to medium-sized with most being from 2 to 30 mm long. Some adults are less than 1 mm in length, and at the other extreme a few flukes exceed 10 cm and one has been reported to be over 12 m long. They are generally flat and rather leaf-shaped. All but one or two flukes have incomplete digestive tracts and, with few exceptions (e.g., Schistosomatidae), are hermaphroditic.

Within the class Trematoda, there are two subclasses, Aspidobothrea, and Digenea. They are differentiated on the basis of the structure of both adults and larvae and on life cycle patterns.

The subclass Aspidobothrea is a rather obscure group found primarily in freshwater clams (Unionidae) but occasionally in both freshwater and marine snails and fish and in freshwater turtles. They are endoparasites mostly of the vascular, digestive, or excretory systems of their hosts. They are frequently found by students in preserved clams used for dissection of nonvertebrate animals. The members of the group can be recognized readily by the large ventral adhesive organ, which is compartmentalized. Most of them fall within a size range from 1 to 3 mm in length; some are twice as long as wide and others are nearly as broad as long. Their life cycles are not well known; however, both direct and indirect cycles have been described.

The subclass Digenea is the largest group and the most important medically and economically. The habitats in which its members are found have the greatest range both for hosts and habitats outside of the hosts. With few exceptions, the definitive hosts are vertebrates and the first intermediate hosts are mollusks. Recognition of adult members of the subclass is relatively simple, because they are all endoparasites and both the Monogenea and Aspidobothrea have distinctive holdfasts. For example, a leaflike worm found in

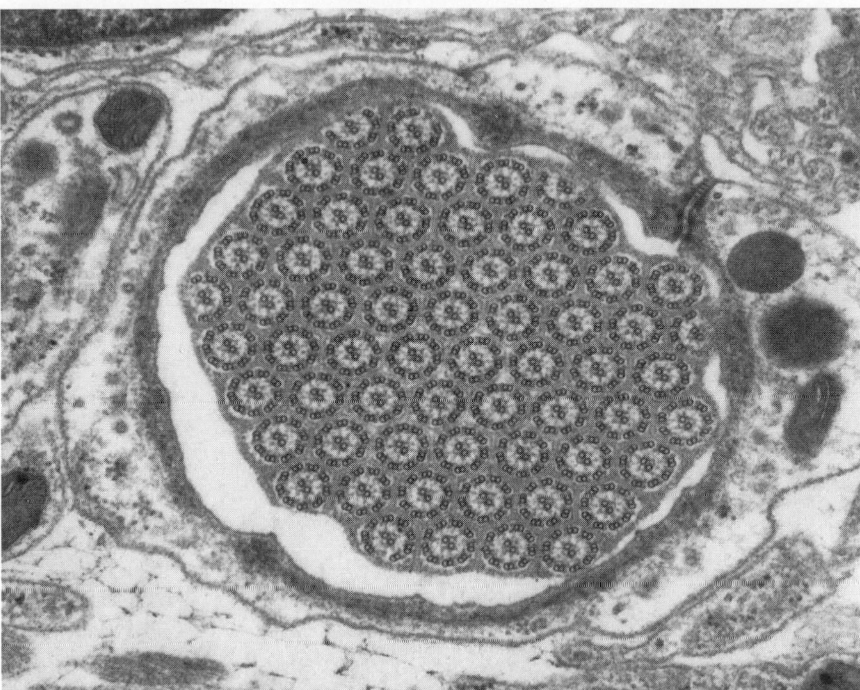

FIGURE 17.2 A cross-section of a flame cell as seen in TEM. The bundle of cilia is surrounded by a tubule made up of a single layer of cells.

the digestive system of a higher vertebrate will nearly always be a digenetic fluke.

CLASS TREMATODA, SUBCLASS ASPIDOBOTHREA

The subclass Aspidobothrea, also called Aspidogastrea and Aspidocotylea, contains a small number of species that have features of digeneans and monogeneans, but the digenean affinities are strongest. Aspidobothreans are primarily endo- and ectoparasites of mollusks, but also are parasites of elasmobranchs, teleosts, and turtles. No aspidobothreans are known to be of medical or economic importance.

Morphology

Adult aspidobothreans have a characteristic ventral disk with one to four rows of alveoli (Fig. 17.6) or a single row of suckers. Hooks are not present. The ventral disk is isolated from the dorsal body by a longitudinal septum, another characteristic structure composed of muscle and connective tissue. Reproductive organs are similar to those of the Digenea, with one exception: the oviduct is divided into compartments by numerous septa; this feature is apparently unique to the aspidobothreans.

Life Cycle

The life cycles of the aspidobothreans are probably direct; one life cycle has been completed in the laboratory. Adults (Fig. 17.7) produce eggs; some have opercula and others do not. Eggs may be ingested or hatch, releasing a characteristic larva, the *cotylocidium*, which has a posterior sucker (Fig. 17.8), and they may be ciliated or not. The cotylocidium develops directly into the adult by growth of the posterior sucker into the adult ventral disk. Most aspidobothreans parasitize mollusks. Those in vertebrates may have been ingested while still inside the mollusks; however, *Lobatostoma ringens* remains immature in mollusks and becomes gravid only in the teleost host, and *Cotylogaster occidentalis* produces more viable eggs in fish than in mussels. Thus, the tendency toward a two-host life cycle may be developing in some aspidogastreans.

Aspidobothreans have similarities to monogeneans, including direct life cycles without alternation of generations, and with digeneans, including morphologic similarities and having both mollusk and vertebrate hosts. Distinct aspidobothrean characteristics include the ventral disk, the longitudinal septum, the septate oviduct, and direct development in mollusks. The Aspidobothrea have many archaic features that merit separate taxonomic status, but they have enough features in common with the Digenea to imply that they are closely related and probably diverged from primi-

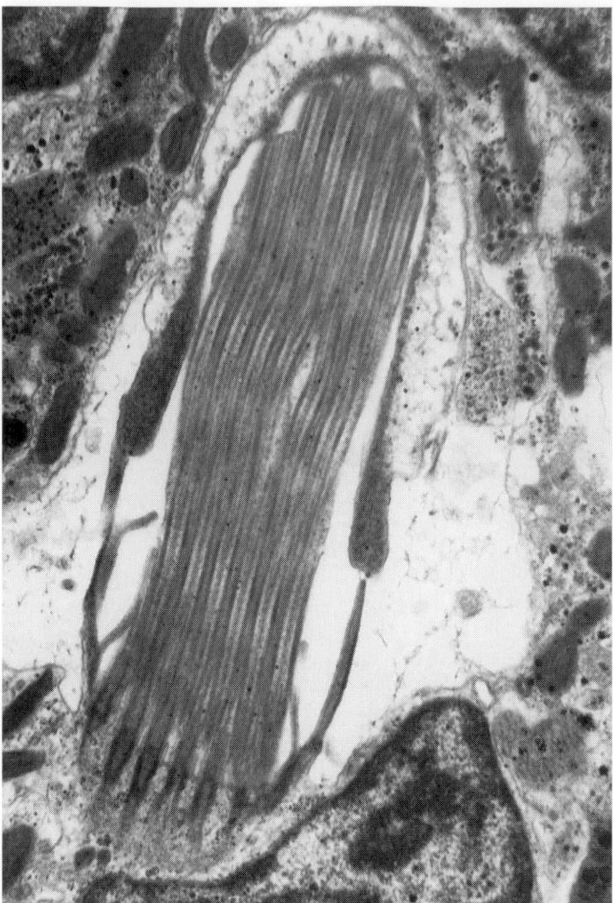

FIGURE 17.3 A longitudinal section of a flame cell as seen in TEM. The cilia are rooted at the lower left of the frame and extend down the tubule.

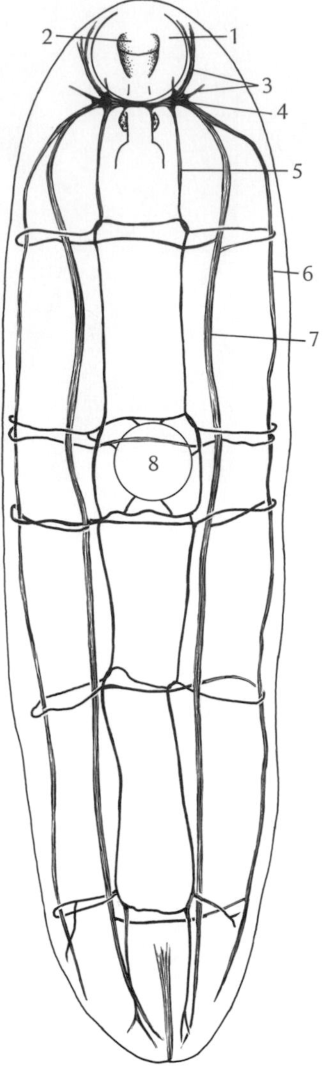

FIGURE 17.4 A diagram of the nervous system of a digenetic, distome fluke. (1) oral sucker, (2) mouth, (3) anterior nerves, (4) anterior ganglion or "brain", (5) ventral nerve chord, (6) lateral chord, (7) dorsal chord, (8) acetabulum. Note the relatively greater innervation of the oral and ventral suckers. [Redrawn from Hyman, 1951.]

tive Digenea. Further, the aspidobothreans are inferred as primitive parasites because they can survive for a long time in simple media outside a host, they have low host and site specificity, they have a complex nervous system, and there are only a few species. All of these characteristics are different in the successful parasitic groups such as the Digenea.

GENERAL FEATURES OF DIGENETIC FLUKES

The subclass Digenea includes the flukes that are of greatest importance to humans because of either the medical or economic losses they cause. Included in the group are the blood flukes or schistosomes, which are generally considered to be among the most serious helminth human parasites on a worldwide basis. In the case of livestock, the common liver fluke causes economic losses in sheep- and cattle-raising areas of the world. Also, a number of flukes (echinostomes, heterophyids) normally found in other animals may occur in humans and sometimes cause severe illnesses.

Evolution and Life Cycle

There is so much diversity in the structures of adults and life cycles of Digenea that students often cannot see the forest for the trees. The major recognition features of the adults do not always relate to taxonomic affinities (Fig. 17.9), and the life cycles include perhaps six larval stages, some of which reproduce asexually and most of which are found in snails.

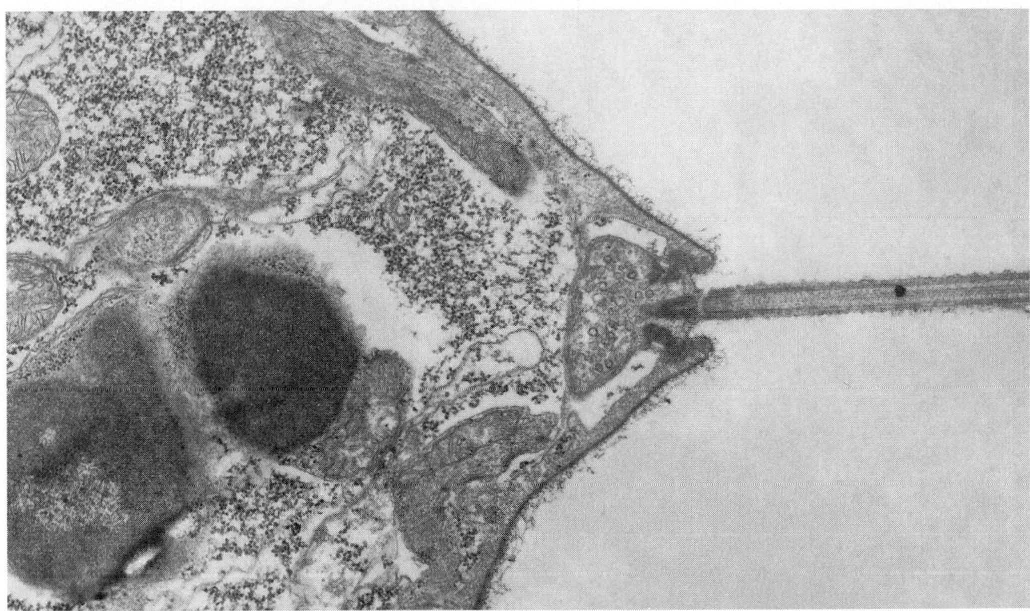

FIGURE 17.5 A sensory cilium on the tegument of a digenetic fluke as seen in TEM.

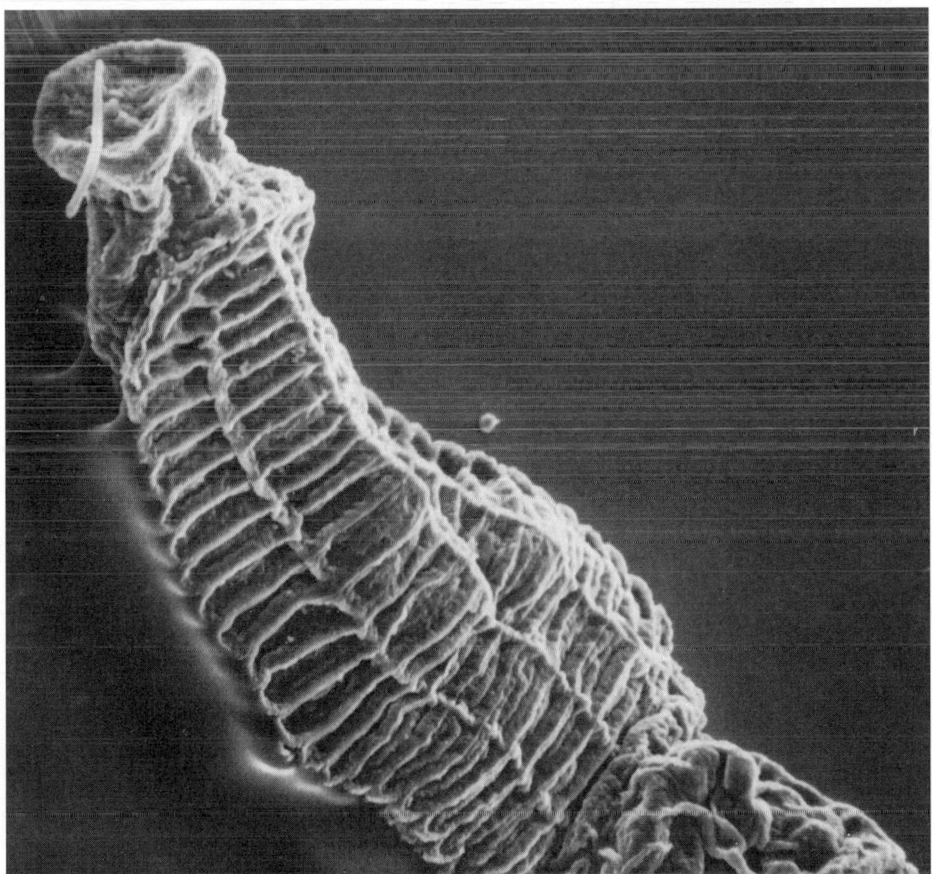

FIGURE 17.6 View of the ventral surface of the aspidobothrian fluke, *Aspidogaster conchicola,* as seen in SEM. The mouth is at the upper left and almost the whole ventral surface is covered by the holdfast organ. [Courtesy of Dr. Tyler A. Woolley.]

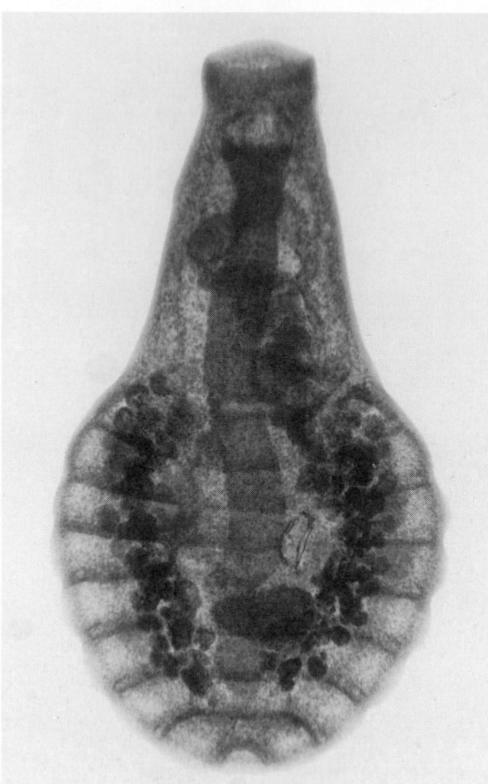

FIGURE 17.7 A whole mount of an adult aspidobothrian fluke, *Coltylaspis insignis.* as seen in LM.

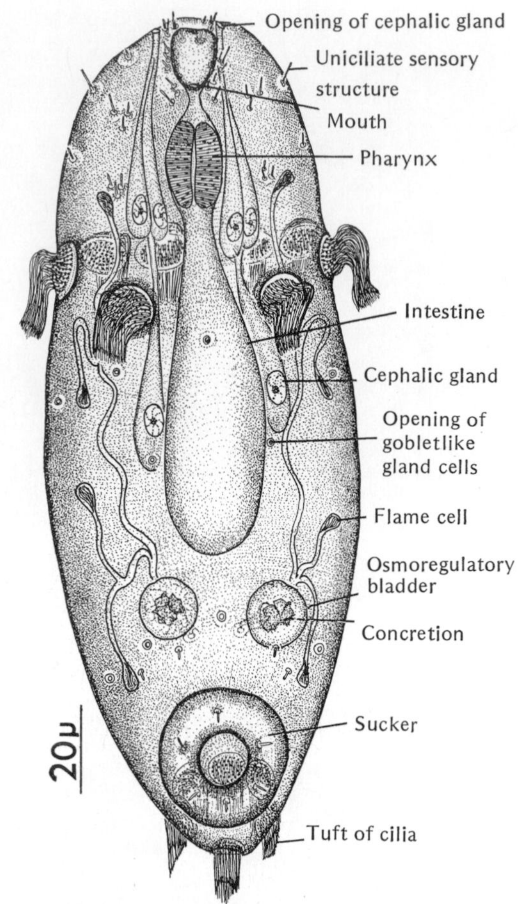

FIGURE 17.8 Diagram of the cotylocidium of *Cotylogaster occidentalis*, an immature stage of a aspidobothrean. [Redrawn from Fredricksen, 1978.]

The crucial step of making sense out of the group lies in the conclusion that gastropod mollusks (snails) were the original hosts of those flatworms that later became the Digenea. Among the many hundreds of life cycles of digenetic flukes that are known, only a small percentage use animals other than snails as their first intermediate hosts. In a few cases, bivalve mollusks, mostly freshwater clams of the family Sphaeriidae, rarely a scaphapod, and in one case a marine annelid, are first intermediate hosts.

The precursors of the Digenea were most likely free-living flatworms of the class Turbellaria. Although some members of the Turbellaria, such as the Temnocephala, are parasitic, most are free living and feed on decaying organic matter, both plant and animal. As detritus feeders, they feed on dead snails. It is not much of a step for such an animal to crawl into the mantle cavity or the pulmonary chamber of the snail and to find conditions where predators are few and food is adequate. Once having established a symbiotic relationship, the partnership would have evolved so as to damage the snail minimally or even to benefit it.

A possible scenario for the evolution of the life cycles of digenetic trematodes is briefly as follows. The forms from which the Digenea arose were most likely free-living rhabdocoel Turbellaria. These animals were ectocommensals in the mantle cavity of aquatic snails. The earliest parasites penetrated the integument and entered the viscera of their snail hosts.

The presence of the tailed, juvenile stage, the *cercaria*, in nearly all of the life cycles of the Digenea implies that the adult or preadult forms of these protoparasites escaped from the snail and moved away. Those cercariae of present-day trematodes that lack tails have lost them secondarily. The free-living adults produced eggs that hatched to motile juveniles and these, in turn, sought out snails to serve as hosts (Fig. 17.10).

Thus, the juvenile entered the viscera of snails, became sexually mature, and then escaped to lay its eggs. There is ample precedent among parasites, especially arthropods, but also in some parasitic Turbellaria, for direct life cycles in which the preadults are parasitic and the adults are free living.

The reasoning entailed in the addition of larval stages (*sporocyst, redia*) is somewhat more tenuous than

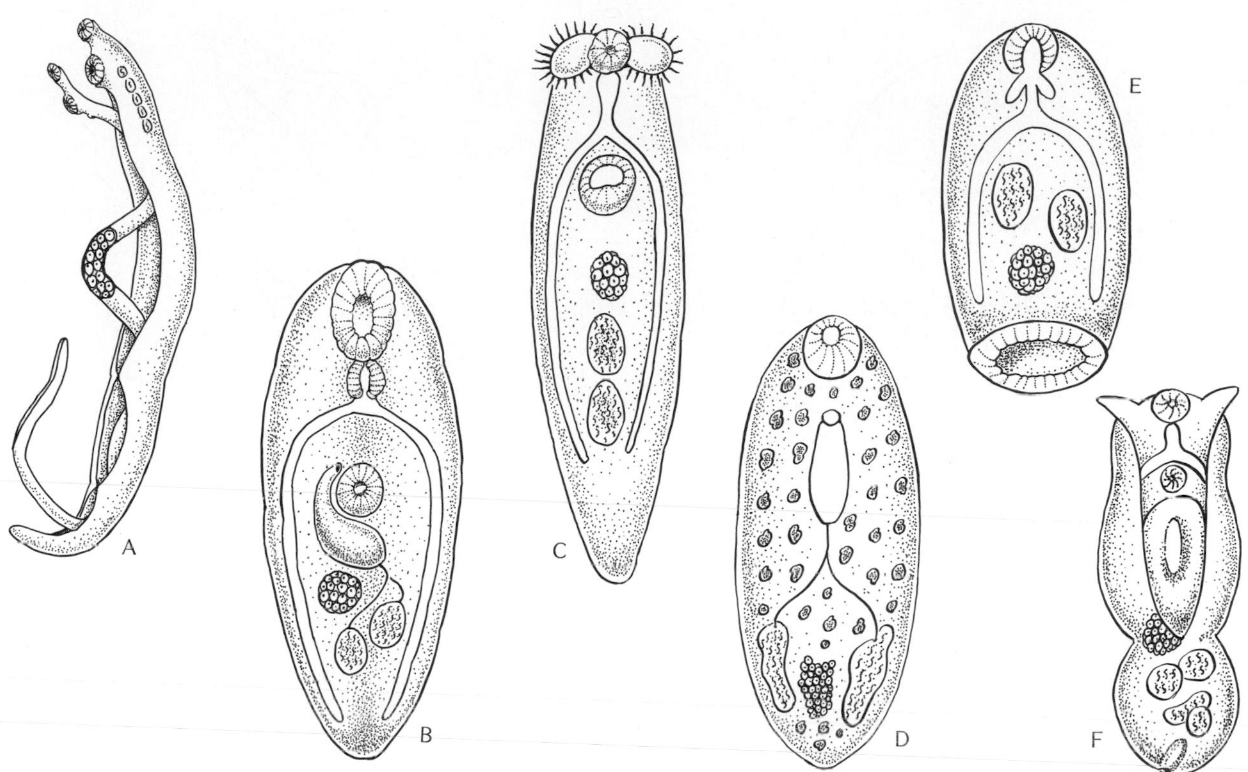

FIGURE 17.9 Diagram of the basic body types of adult digeneans. (A) schistosome; (B) distome; (C) echinostome; (D) monostome; (E) amphistome; (F) holostome.

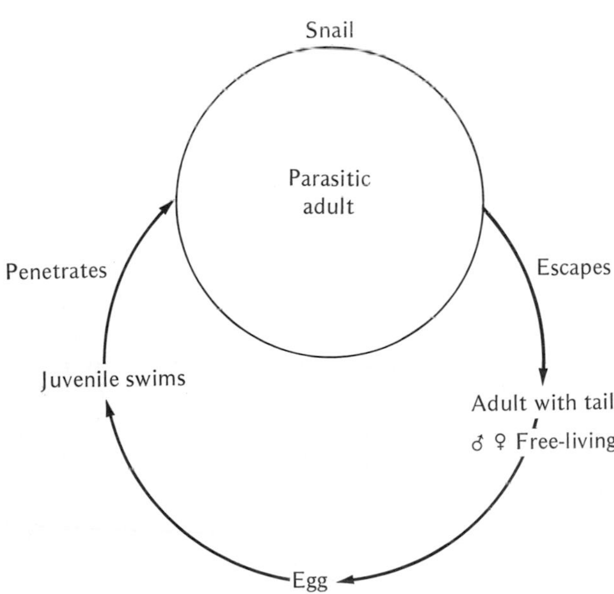

FIGURE 17.10 Hypothetical one-host life cycle of a protodigenean fluke.

the acquisition of a parasitic relationship with snails in the first place. Basically, there developed two generations of adults in a snail: the first parasitic and viviparous and the second free-living and oviparous. The life cycle, then, had established alternate generations: viviparous and oviparous. The viviparous generation subsequently lost the male system and its female system dedifferentiated into a fragmented ovary, now represented by scattered germ cells (Fig. 17.11). The gut was lost when feeding through the body surface became more efficient. The life cycle stage, which is the end product of the viviparous parasitic generation, is the sporocyst (Fig. 17.12). The means by which further larval generations (daughter sporocyst, redia) were added is highly conjectural and will not be considered here.

The redia is more complex than the sporocyst in that it has a gut, albeit simple, and usually some small tegumentary projections, the *ambulatory buds* (Fig. 17.13). Although the redial stage obtains nutrient through the body surface, it also ingests host tissues. As the life cycle progresses through its series of larvae, each succeeding stage becomes structurally and functionally more like the adult.

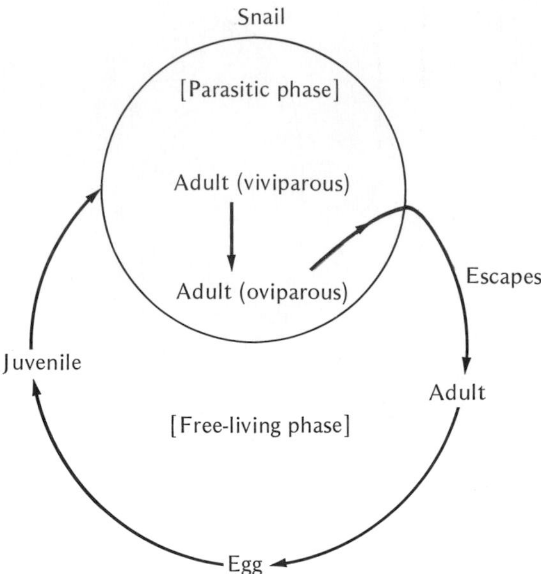

FIGURE 17.11 Hypothetical origin of the generations of the life cycle of a digenean fluke.

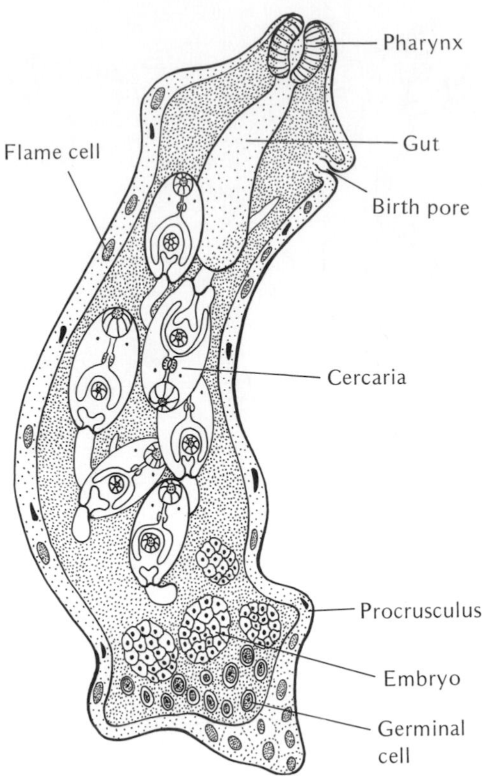

FIGURE 17.13 Diagram of a daughter redia of a digenetic fluke. This would be typical of a fluke such as *Clonorchis*, which produces cercariae from a redia.

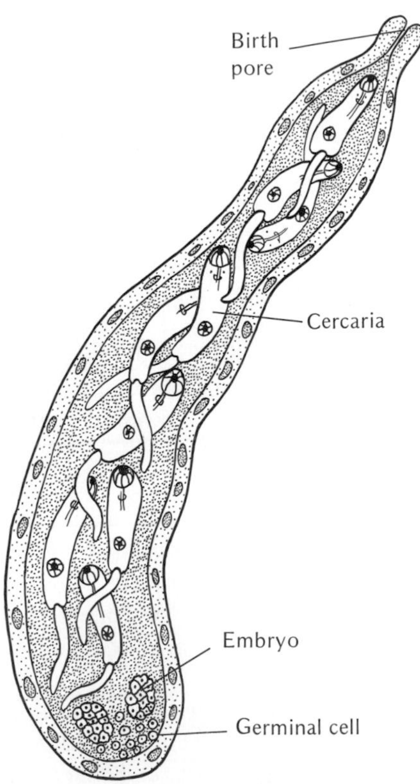

FIGURE 17.12 Diagram of a sporocyst of a digenetic fluke. This would be typical of a schistosome fluke in which the sporocyst produces cercariae.

Having established a life cycle with alternation of generations, one parasitic and the other free living, the next problem is to introduce the second host. It is most likely that the first chordate hosts were bottom-feeding fish such as the cyclostomes (jawless, primitive fish). The near-ubiquity of tails on cercariae indicates that the free-living generation escaped from the snail to be eaten by the second host rather than while still in the snail. The swimming or creeping adults were preadapted to parasitism and found the intestinal tract of their cyclostome hosts to be similar to their free-living niche: low in oxygen, rich in organic matter, and dark. Those individuals capable of surviving and continuing to lay eggs in the gut of such hosts would have an adaptive advantage in having their eggs distributed over a wide area and would be protected from predation by other animals. By now, the ability to absorb food through the tegument may have been well established. Obligatory parasitism was just a step away. Then came all the trappings of membership in the fraternity of parasites: holdfast structures, close ecological and physiological dependence on a host, and evolution with the host.

With such an evolutionary perspective, the present day digenetic trematode life cycle gains a degree of

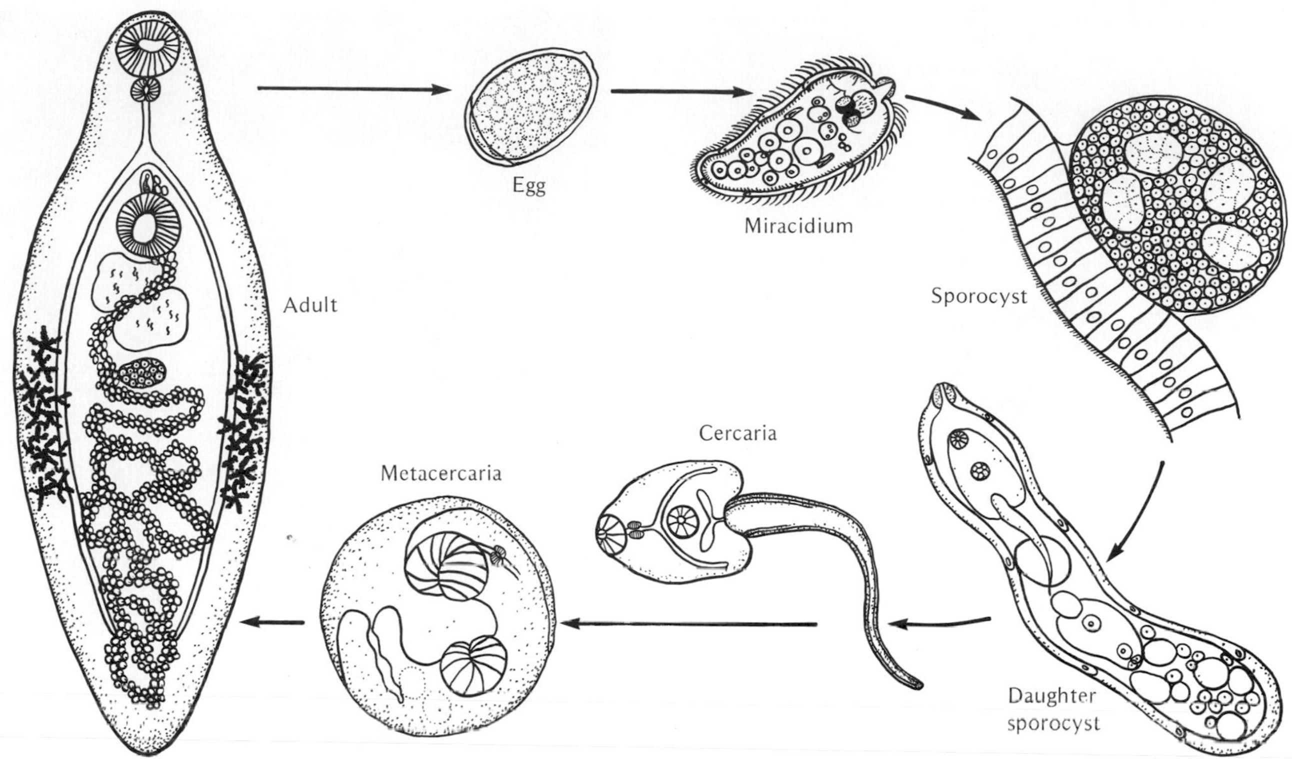

FIGURE 17.14 Diagram of the life cycle of a digenetic fluke.

rationality. The basic stages are egg, miracidium, sporocyst, redia, cercaria, usually metacercaria, and adult (Fig. 17.14). Egg, miracidium, cercaria, and adult occur in all life cycles, but there is considerable variation in the sporocyst and redial and metacercarial generations. For example, sporocysts can give rise to daughter sporocysts or rediae or cercariae. In some instances, the sporocyst generation has dropped out and the first stage in the snail is a redia, which may give rise to daughter rediae and then to cercariae. The principal points to remember are that both sporocysts and rediae are reproductive and the reproduction is asexual. For any one miracidium entering a snail, a few hundred to several thousand cercariae are produced. Additional hosts may be added in the form of second and third intermediate hosts, but reproduction takes place only in the snail and in the final or definitive host. If additional intermediate hosts are added to the cycles, they fit into a food chain, and they either concentrate preadults or move them up to a trophic level where there is a high probability that they will be eaten by the proper definitive host.

Adult Structure

Adult flukes are nearly all monoecious, that is, they have both male and female reproductive systems in the same individual. Most are macroscopic, but a few are so small that a dissecting microscope is needed to find them, or at least to see them well enough to distinguish them from extraneous material. In life they are usually flattened, although some, such as the amphistomes (Fig. 17.9), are rotund. Some structures can be seen when the animals are alive, but fixed and stained preparations are essential for accurate identification.

In a stained, sexually mature digenetic trematode, the features that are most striking are the intestine, ventral sucker or acetabulum, and the reproductive systems (Fig. 17.15). The gut is usually incomplete (no anus); the mouth is most often located at the anterior end and is surrounded by an oral sucker. There may or may not be a muscular pharynx followed by an esophagus. The intestinal ceca are most often thin-walled structures extending through the greater length of the body. In some flukes the ceca are branched (*Fasciola*, Fig. 19.2) or unite near the posterior to form a loop (Cyclocoelidae); in a very few instances (Campulidae) there is an anus.

The ventral sucker or acetabulum is an organ of attachment and does not serve in feeding. Whether or not it is present, its size and location are important in the identification of any trematode.

The male reproductive system is relatively simple.

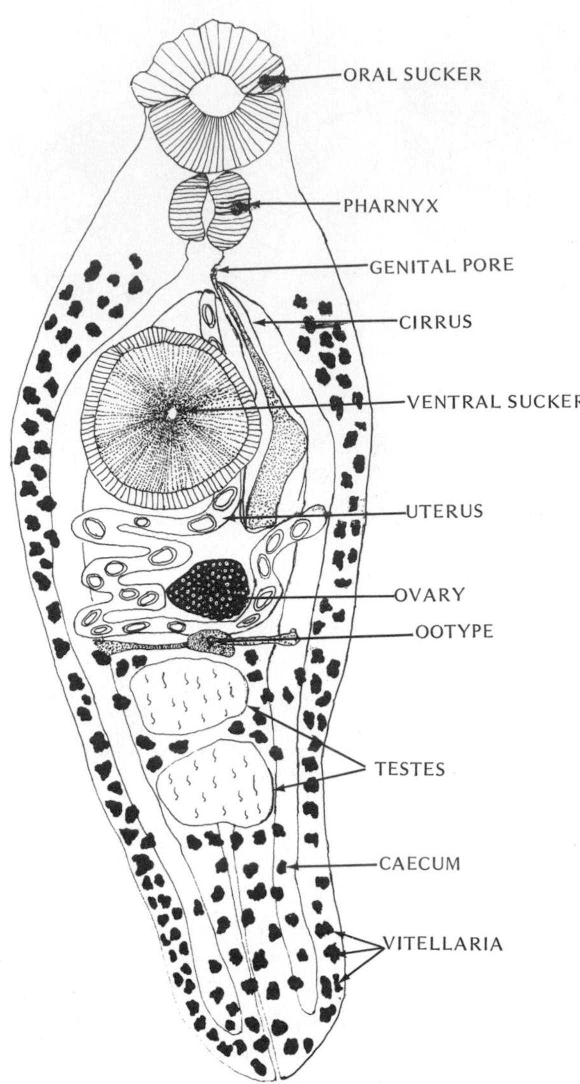

FIGURE 17.15 Diagram of an adult digenetic trematode.

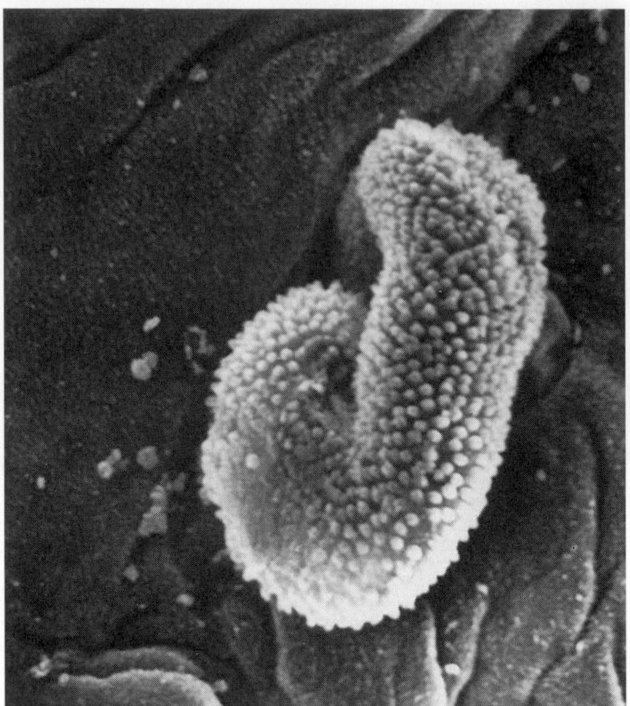

FIGURE 17.16 Self-fertilization in a digenetic fluke as seen in SEM. The cirrus protrudes from and then reenters the genital pore.

It usually consists of two testes, each with a vas efferens that may join to form the vas deferens as they extend anteriorly. The male system terminates at the cirrus, the intromittent organ. Sperm coming from the vas deferens are stored in the seminal vesicle and transferred through the protrusible *cirrus* to the genital pore of the female system. Variations in the male system used in classification and identification are the number, size, shape, and location of the testes and the presence or absence of the cirrus sac, as well as whether the seminal vesicle is external or internal (Fig. 17.16).

The female system has a number of components in which there is considerable variation from group to group. The crux of the whole system is the *ootype* into which the products of the ovary, vitelline glands, and Mehlis' gland are introduced and where fertilization takes place (Fig. 17.15). Sperm are stored in a seminal receptacle until needed. The ovary is usually single and the ova move from it to the ootype, where they are fertilized.

The vitellaria are located at the lateral margins of the body and their cells produce yolk, which serves as energy storage for the eggs, and a proteinaceous material, which will become one of the egg capsules. The products of the vitelline glands are carried by ducts that join the lateral vitelline ducts at about the level of the ovary. The lateral vitelline ducts either enter the ootype directly or enter a vitelline reservoir where the material is stored. For purposes of identification, the location of the vitelline glands and how they are clustered are both important.

Mehlis' gland is a rather diffuse group of secretory cells surrounding the ootype and with openings into the ootype.

Following fertilization, the egg shell or capsules are laid down around the zygote. Vitelline cells cluster around the fertilized egg; these vesicles contain a proteolytic enzyme, which activates a phenol oxidase. The phenol oxidase in association with an alkaline secretion from Mehlis' gland cause the tanning of the egg capsule. The size and shape of the egg are determined at this time by the shape of the ootype. Fertilization, clustering of vitelline cells, and the beginning of tanning of the egg capsule all take place in less than four seconds in a fluke such as *Fasciola hepatica*; this is a remarkable mass-production factory, which may operate 24 hours a day for a decade or longer in some digenea. As the egg moves into the uterus, further changes take place in the eggshell, most likely by quinone tanning of the protein layer.

The uterus is most often a long, winding, looping structure that contains hundreds or sometimes thousands of eggs. Eggs move from the ootype into the uterus and move forward until they are released from the genital pore in the region of the cirrus. Sperm from the male system of the same individual (Fig. 17.16) or from another individual enter the genital pore and pass the full length of the uterus to be stored in the seminal receptacle.

Features used in identification are the location of the uterus and the extent of its development. In some species such as *Nanophyetus* (Fig. 20.6), the uterus has only a few loops and fewer than a half dozen eggs, whereas in others such as *Clonorchis* (Fig. 19.8) there are many loops and more than a hundred eggs.

In *Dicrocoelium* (Fig. 19.6) the uterus loops posteriorly (descending loop) before it turns anteriorly (ascending loop), also a constant characteristic. The presence or absence of a muscular structure, the metraterm, near the opening of the uterus is also a constant and identifying characteristic.

About the only portion of the excretory system that can be seen in stained, adult flukes is the excretory bladder near the posterior end. The bladder is usually seen as a vacant or poorly stained area surrounded by parenchyma; its size and shape are used in identification.

Body shape, spination, and the oral and ventral suckers are all important in identification of adult flukes but do not necessarily relate to the taxonomic position of any one individual. Early systems of classification were based on whether there was an oral sucker only (monostomes) or also a ventral sucker (distomes). The location of the oral and ventral suckers determined whether the animal was a gasterostome (mouth in the middle) or an amphistome (suckers at either end). This terminology is not only entrenched but also useful because one can refer to an echinostome and immediately produce a mental picture of a fluke with spines surrounding the mouth (Fig. 20.3). The echinostomes represent the extreme of spination in the digenea; identifying characteristics are the presence or absence of spines on the body and their location. Sometimes it is necessary to examine the margins of an animal carefully under a compound microscope in order to see the spines.

Cercariae

Cercariae are easy to collect either by crushing snails or allowing them to shed cercariae naturally. Because cercariae have many morphological characteristics similar to those of adult flukes, the cercarial "types" often provide valuable information about the trematode fauna in a certain locality. Representative cercarial types are illustrated in Figure 17.17.

CLASSIFICATION OF THE PHYLUM PLATYHELMINTHES

Phylum Platyhelminthes

Dorsoventrally flattened Bilateria, without coelom, circulatory, respiratory, or skeletal systems; with flame cell or protonephridia, parenchyma filling all spaces between organ systems.

Superclass Neodermata

Ciliated epidermis cast off at end of free-swimming larval phase and replaced by nonciliated, syncytial tegument.

Class Trematoda

Tegument syncytial without rhabdoids, body undivided, one or more suckers, digestive tract with intestine commonly branched, all parasitic, mainly in digestive tract of vertebrates.

Subclass Digenea

All endoparasitic, two or more hosts in life cycle, the first host usually a snail, larval polyembryony, most with two suckers including an oral sucker, no hooks.

Order Strigeata

Cercariae usually fork-tailed, cercariae encyst in second intermediate host, excretory pores in tips of tail furcae. *Schistosoma*

Order Echinostomata

Cercariae with single tail, cercariae encyst in the open, primary excretory pore in anterior half of tail. *Echinostoma, Fasciola*

Order Plagiorchiata

Cercariae without caudal excretory vessels, stylet present or absent. *Dicrocoelium, Nanophyetus, Paragonimus*

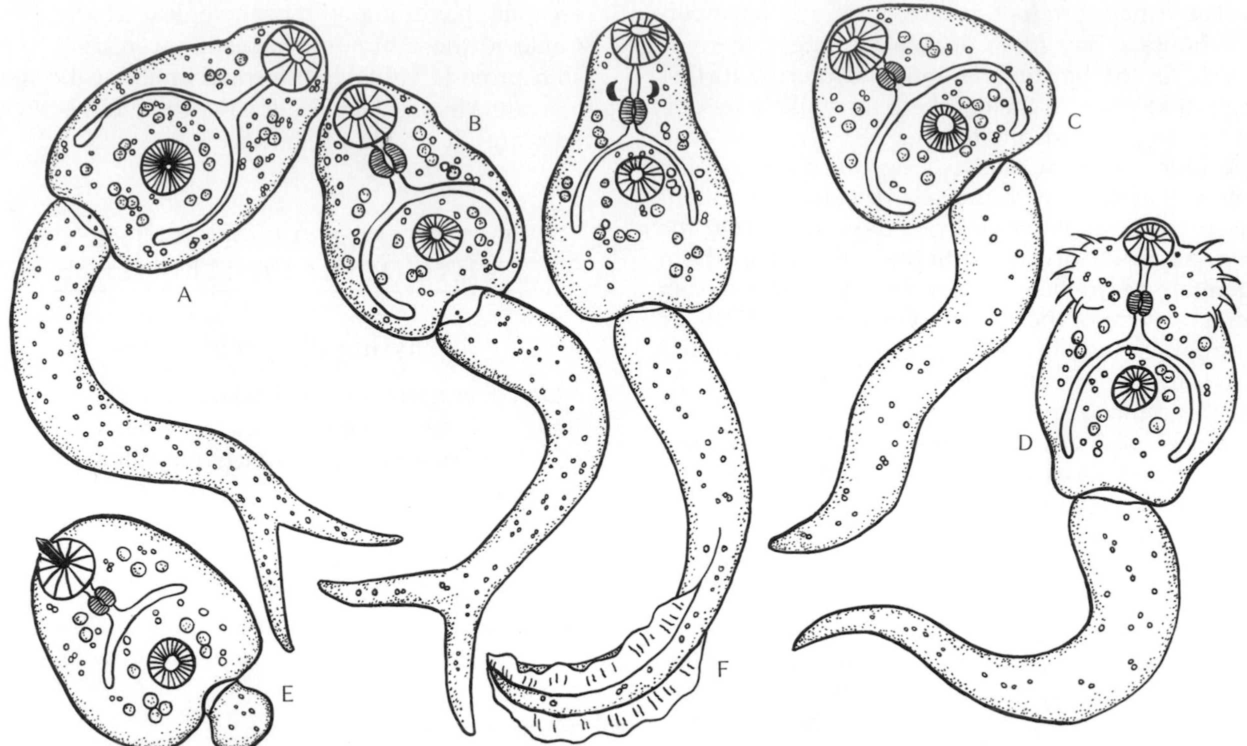

FIGURE 17.17 Diagrammatic representation of some of the types of cercariae of digenetic flukes. (A) apharyngeate furcocystis, (B) pharyngeate furcocystis, (C) gymnocephalus, (D) echinostome, (E) xiphidiomicrocercous, (F) ophthalmopleurocercous.

Order Opisthorchiata

Cercariae with caudal excretory vessels during development, stylet absent. *Clonorchis, Opisthorchis*

Subclass Aspidobothrea

Oral sucker absent, anterior end without paired adhesive structures, with a large ventral sucker divided by septa or one row of suckers, no hooks, ecto- and endoparasites most with direct life cycles, without metamorphosis, parasites of mollusks, fishes, and turtles. *Cotylogaster, Aspidogaster*

Class Cercomeromorphae

Posterior end of larva, the cercomer, armed with hooks.

Subclass Monogenea

Oral sucker absent or weak, anterior end usually with a pair of adhesive structures, posterior end with an adhesive disk usually provided with hooks or clamps, gut usually simple, all parasitic on aquatic vertebrates, especially fishes, or rarely on aquatic invertebrates, life cycles direct.

Order Monopisthocotylea

Opisthaptor single but may be subdivided by septa and usually developed directly from larval haptor, one to three pairs of large anchors plus marginal hooklets, oral sucker absent, genitointestinal canal absent, eyes often present. *Gyrodactylus, Entobdella, Dactylogyrus*

Order Polyopisthocotylea

Opisthaptor with multiple suckers, clamps, or anchor complexes, larval haptor reduced or absent, mouth usually surrounded by suckers, genitointestinal canal present, eyes usually absent. *Octomacrum*

Subclass Cestoda

Endoparasites without rhabdoids, body usually segmented, adhesive structures usually limited to anterior end, no mouth or digestive tract, embryo with hooks, life cycle usually has two or more hosts, most definitive hosts are vertebrates.

Cohort Gyrocotyliidea

Cercomer with ten equal-sized hooks (Fig. 22.18). Thick, monozoic worms with a single set of reproductive organs and a single, anterior, cuplike, muscular holdfast (Fig. 22.19). They are found in large intestines of chimeroid fishes in both the Atlantic and Pacific Oceans. *Gyrocotyle*

Cohort Cestoidea

Six large hooks on cercomer, cercomer invaginates during development. Male genital pore and vagina proximate.

Subcohort Amphilinidea

Worms with flattened, monozoic bodies without an anterior holdfast. Cercomer with six large hooks and four small hooks. The anterior end has a boring mechanism, which enables penetration of host body cavities. Worms are found in body cavities of Acepenseridae (sturgeons) in Europe and North America, siluroid fishes in India, and a tortoise in Australia. *Amphilina*

Subcohort Eucestoda

Monozoic and polyzoic. Single or multiple sets of reproductive organs. Six-hooked larva. True scolex present. Parasites of fishes, amphibians, reptiles, birds, and mammals; one genus matures in the coelom of freshwater oligochaetes. *Diphyllobothrium, Taenia, Echinococcus*

Readings

Trematoda

Brooks, D. R. (1989). The phylogeny of the Cercomeria (Platyhelminthes, Rhabdocoela) and general evolutionary principles. *J. Parasitol.* **75,** 606–616.

Brooks, D. R., and McLennan, D. A. (1993). *Parascript. Parasites and the Language of Evolution.* Smithsonian Inst. Press, Washington, DC.

Brooks, D. R., Bandoni, S. M., Macdonald, C. A., and O'Grady, R. T. (1989). Aspects of the phylogeny of the Trematoda Rudolphi, 1808 (Platyhelminthes: Cercomeria). *Can. J. Zool.* **67,** 2609–2624.

Dawes, D. (1956). *The Trematoda.* Cambridge Univ. Press, New York.

Ehlers, U. (1985). Phylogenetic relationships within the Platyhelminthes. In *The Origin and Relationships of Lower Invertebrates* (S. C. Morris, D. G. George, R. Gibson, and H. M. Platt, Eds.), pp. 144–158. Oxford Univ. Press, Oxford.

Ehlers, U. (1986). Comments on a phylogenetic system of the Platyhelminthes. *Hydrobiologia* **132,** 1–12.

Erasmus, D. A. (1972). *The Biology of Trematodes.* Crane, Russak, New York.

Gibson, D. I. (1987). Questions in digenean systematics and evolution. *Parasitology* **95,** 429–460.

Pearson, J. C. (1972). A phylogeny of life-cycle patterns of the Digenea. *Adv. Parasitol.* **10,** 153–189.

Rohde, K. (1990). Phylogeny of Platyhelminthes, with special reference to parasitic groups. *Int. J. Parasitol.* **20,** 979–1007.

Rohde, K., Hefford, C., Ellis, J. T., Baverstock, P. R., Johnson, A. M., Watson, N. A., and Dittmann, S. (1993). Contributions to the phylogeny of Platyhelminthes based on partial sequencing of 18s ribosomal DNA. *Int. J. Parasitol.* **23,** 705–724.

Schell, S. C. (1985). *Handbook of Trematodes of North America North of Mexico.* Univ. Idaho Press, Moscow.

Smyth, J. D., and Halton, D. W. (1983). *The Physiology of Trematodes,* 2nd ed. Cambridge Univ. Press, Cambridge, UK.

Yamaguti, S. (1958). *Systema Helminthum. Vol. 1. Digenetic Trematodes of Vertebrates, Parts 1 & 2.* Interscience, New York.

Yamaguti, S. (1971). *Synopsis of Digenetic Trematodes of Vertebrates,* Vols. 1 and 2. Keigaku, Tokyo.

Aspidobothrea

Blair, D. (1993). The phylogenetic position of the Aspidobothrea within the parasitic flatworms inferred from ribosomal RNA sequence data. *Int. J. Parasitol.* **23,** 169–178.

Fredericksen, D. W. (1972). Morphology and taxonomy of *Cotylogaster occidentalis* (Trematoda: Aspidogastridae). *J. Parasitol.* **58,** 1110–1116.

Fredericksen, D. W. (1978). The fine structure and phylogenetic position of the cotylocidium larva of *Cotylogaster occidentalis* Nickerson 1902 (Trematoda: Aspidogastridae). *J. Parasitol.* **64,** 961–976.

Hyman, L. (1951). The invertebrates: Platyhelminthes and Rhynchocoela, the acoelomate bilateria. Vol II. McGraw-Hill, New York.

Rohde, K. (1972). The Aspidogastrea, especially *Multicotyle purvisi* Dawes, 1941. *Adv. Parasitol.* **10,** 78–151.

CHAPTER

18

The Blood Flukes or Schistosomes

The schistosomes are different from most other members of the Digenea in that the sexes are separate. The term schistosome or *Schistosoma* means split body and refers to the fact that the males have a ventral groove called a gynecophoric canal. Adults of the family Schistosomatidae are found in the blood vessels of vertebrates, both birds and mammals. A related family, the Spirorchiidae, has turtles as definitive hosts and is also dioecious.

The blood flukes are important to humans primarily as the cause of human disease in many tropical and subtropical areas of the world, but also as economically important parasites of cattle and other large domesticated animals.

As parasites of humans or other animals, the blood flukes lie in venules, usually in the lower abdomen, where they copulate, and the females lay eggs which reach the outside in either feces or urine. There is only a single intermediate host, a snail, and the fork-tailed cercariae reach the definitive host by actively penetrating the unbroken skin.

Current estimates are that 200 million persons are infected with members of the genus *Schistosoma*, the blood flukes. This number has remained fairly constant for some years. There have been local successes in controlling the infections, but at the same time, the prevalence of infection has increased in other areas.

It should always be kept in mind that infection and disease are not the same. There is probably no infectious disease in which infection invariably progresses to severe disease. There is instead a spectrum of responses that ranges from inapparent infection through mild clinical signs and symptoms to death. Schistosomosis fits this general pattern, and in addition, the infections in humans are frequently present for the greater part of a person's life. The effect on a person is directly related to the number of worms harbored, but the effect may be modified by the species and strain of the worm and the person's age, nutritional status, and previous exposure to the parasites. In most cases, there is repeated exposure over a period of years and long-term, chronic disease results. Therein lies the problem of assessing the importance of schistosomosis in human populations. There may be periods in an individual's life when there is incapacitation from an acute phase of the disease, but by and large the infections result in long-term damage to internal organs: large intestine, bladder, and liver. The person probably will continue to work, although productivity may be reduced, and the days lost from work will be greater than for a comparable uninfected individual. Death may not be a direct result of blood fluke infection but rather of other infectious agents attacking a body already debilitated.

SCHISTOSOMA MANSONI, S. JAPONICUM, AND *S. HAEMATOBIUM*

Name of Organism and Disease Association

Schistosoma mansoni, S. japonicum and *S. haematobium* are the most important human blood flukes causing the disease schistosomosis, schistosomiasis, or bilharziasis. Of lesser importance are *S. mekongi, S. malayensis,* and *S. intercalatum,* which also cause human schistosomosis.

Hosts and Host Range

Schistosoma mansoni is found in Africa, the Middle East, South America, and a number of Caribbean islands (Fig. 18.1). The first intermediate hosts are planorbid snails *Biomphalaria* spp. and *Tropicorbis* sp. Humans are the principal definitive hosts, but reservoir hosts include rodents, opossum, monkeys, and baboons.

Schistosoma haematobium is found in Africa and the Middle East (Fig. 18.1). The intermediate hosts are *Bulinus* spp., *Physopsis* spp., and *Planorbarius* sp. Humans are the only significant definitive hosts.

Schistosoma japonicum is found in Japan, China, Taiwan, the Philippines, and Indonesia (Fig. 18.1). Snail hosts are various species of the genus *Oncomelania*. Unlike *S. mansoni* and *S. haematobium*, *S. japonicum* has an extremely wide range of definitive hosts. Seven orders of mammals are naturally infected, including humans, cattle, sheep, goats, horses, dogs, cats, rats, pigs, and others.

Geographic Distribution and Importance

The human schistosomes are distributed through some of the countries of the world at the lower end of the economic scale (Fig. 18.1), or at least the parasites are found in relatively poor rural people. Many countries of tropical and subtropical Africa that already have severe economic problems are further handicapped by widespread infection among their farmers. In parts of South America, 12% of the deaths in hospitals were due to the consequences of schistosomiasis. In Tanzania, 20% of persons in some areas have serious damage to the urinary system and can be expected to live only a few years. In Tanzania, Zanzibar, Nigeria, and Egypt the pathological changes in children are likely to have their most serious effects in adolescence and early adulthood, just when these young people are likely to have completed schooling and are ready to become productive members of society.

At current estimates of world population, 1 person in 20 is infected with blood flukes. But in determining the impact on a people, it is necessary to investigate a specific area in detail, to determine not only the prevalence of infection but debility and death losses as well.

Morphology

The important members of the genus *Schistosoma* found in humans are *S. haematobium, S. mansoni*, and

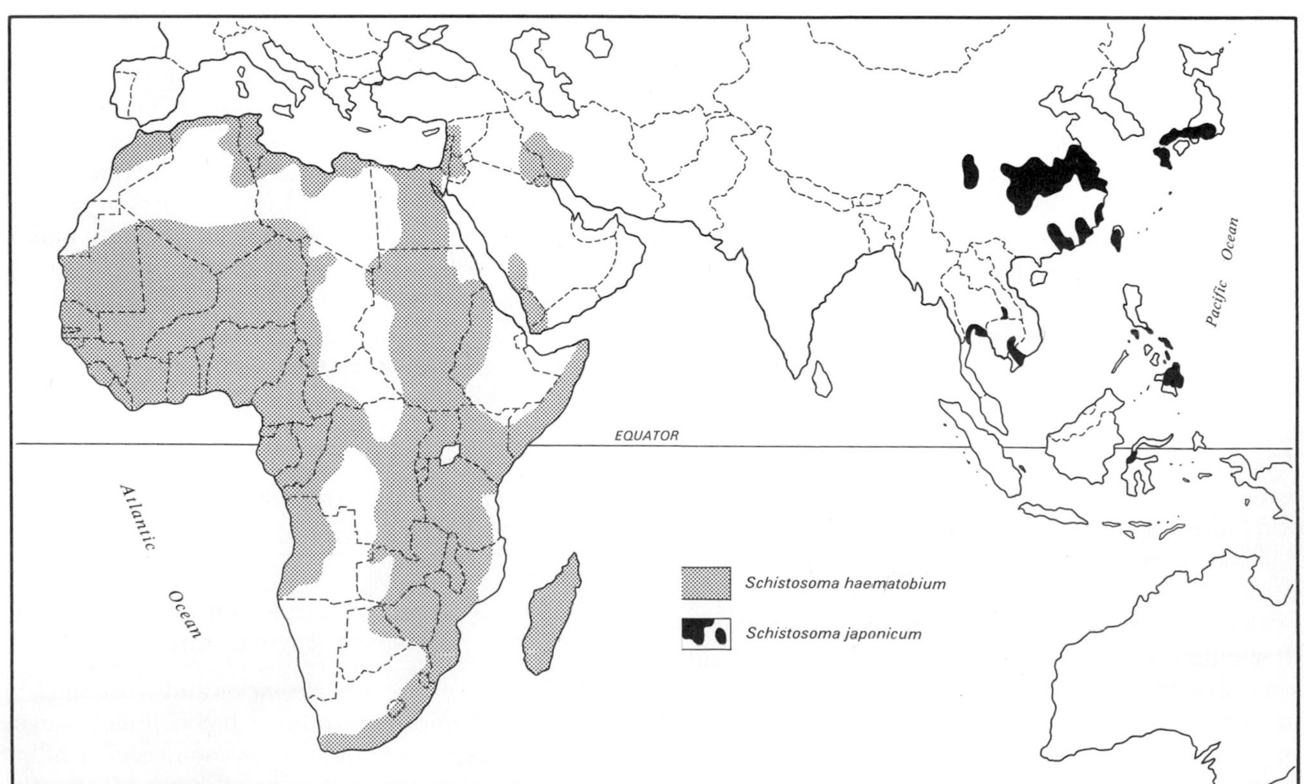

FIGURE 18.1 Geographic distribution of human schistosomosis. [Redrawn with modifications from Ansari, 1973.]

S. japonicum. They are slender worms about 16 mm long (Tab. 18.1), which can be identified by both male and female characteristics (Fig. 18.2). The females are slender, round in cross section, and 15 to 30% longer than the males. The males have lateral extensions of the body posterior to the ventral sucker, which form a gynecophoric canal in which the female worms lie (Fig. 18.3).

The eggs can be distinguished from one another on the basis of both size and other characteristics (Tab. 18.1). The most distinctive feature used for identification is the spine (Fig. 18.4). In *S. haematobium* the spine is terminal, in *S. mansoni* it is subterminal, and in *S. japonicum* it is a small, subterminal knob that may be lacking entirely in some populations.

Although there are differences among the species, the cercariae cannot easily be distinguished from one another. Cercariae have a body about 180 mm long and a forked tail (Fig. 18.5). There are oral and ventral suckers, a genital primordium in the posterior portion of the body, and a protonephridial system consisting of four or five pairs of flame cells. The intestinal system consists of the mouth, esophagus, and rudimentary intestinal ceca. Three kinds of glands have been noted in the cercariae: escape glands located in the anterior portion of the body, preacetabular glands, and postacetabular glands. The escape glands allow the cercariae to penetrate the epithelium of the snail host in order to reach the outside. The latter two sets of glands secrete substances that aid in the penetration of the definitive host and are discussed in somewhat more detail in the section on life cycle.

Not all furcocercous or forked-tail cercariae are members of the genus *Schistosoma*. Those in the family Schistosomatidae have both oral and ventral suckers and lack both eyespots and a pharynx, while most other furcocercous cercariae have a pharynx (e.g., Strigeidae and Diplostomidae).

Life Cycle

The development of the schistosomes of humans follows a pattern that is similar for all three species (Fig. 18.6). The male and female adults in the definitive host move against the blood flow into small mesenteric venules until they can move no farther. Egg laying begins and may continue for a decade or more. The eggs move toward the lumen of the organ, probably by a combination of muscular action of the organ and release of enzymes through pores in the eggshells (Fig.

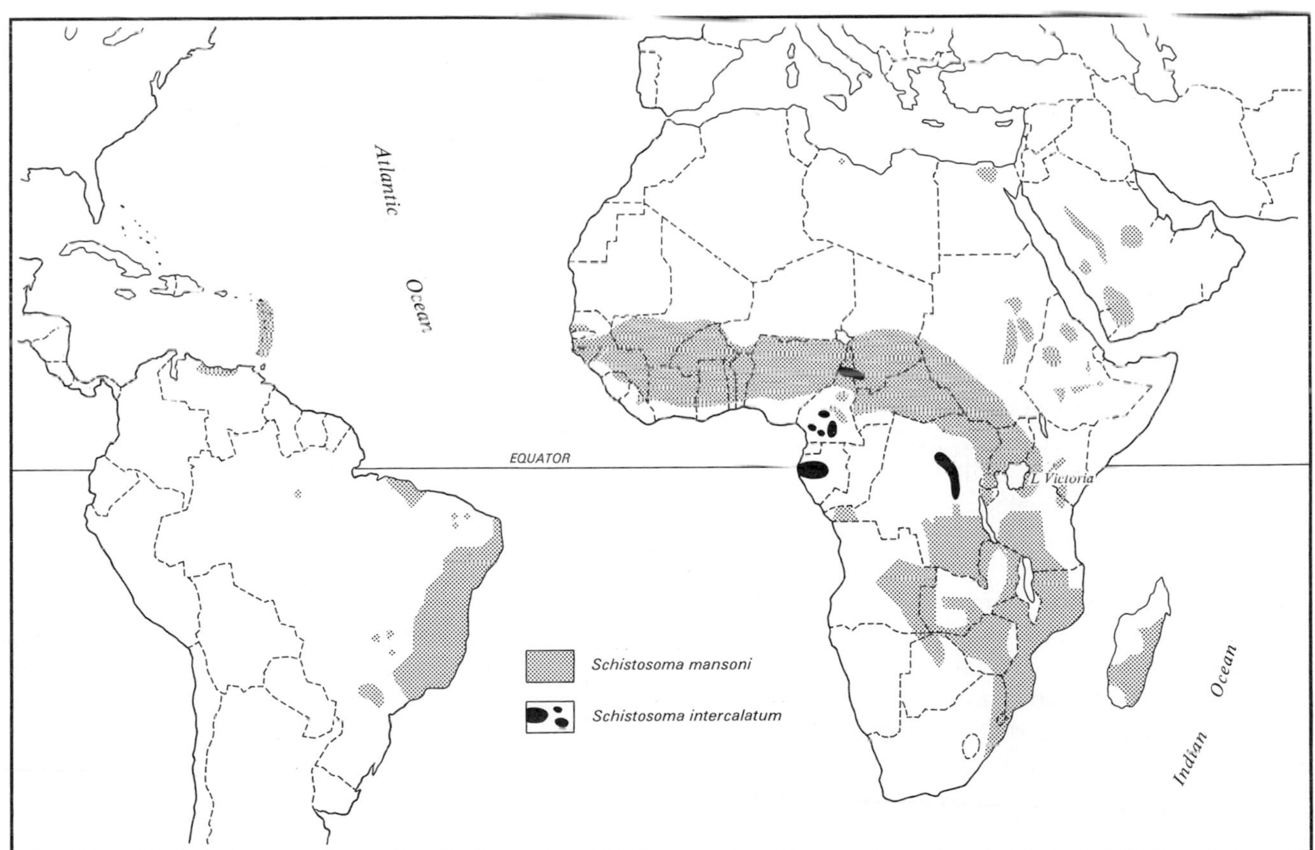

FIGURE 18.1 *(Continued)*

TABLE 18.1 Characteristics of *Schistosoma* spp. of Humans

	haematobium	*japonicum*	*mansoni*	*intercalatum*
Adults				
Male				
Length (mm)	10–14	12–20	6–12	11–14
Number of testes	4	7	6–9	2–7
Posterior union of intestinal ceca	Midbody	Posterior to midbody	Anterior to midbody	
Tegument	Scattered tubercules and blunt, short spines	Minute spines	Numerous tubercules and large, sharp spines	Short, blunt spines
Female				
Length (mm)	16–20	16–28	7–17	13–24
Ovary	Posterior to midbody	Midbody	Anterior to midbody	Midbody
Number of eggs in uterus	20–100	50 or more	1 usually	10–100+
Eggs produced/female/day	?	1400–3500	100–500	?
Location in host				
Primary	Bladder and pelvic plexuses	Both superior and interior mesenteric veins	Veins of small and large intestine near ileocecal junction	Portal and mesenteric veins
Secondary	Portal and mesenteric veins	Portal vein	Hemorrhoidal and hepatic veins	?
Prepatent period in weeks	10–12	5–7	7–8	?
Eggs				
Length (μm)	112–170	70–100	114–175	140–240
Width	40–70	50–65	45–68	50–85
Color	Golden brown	Golden brown	Golden brown	
Spine	Terminal	Subterminal knob or none	Subterminal	Terminal
Passed in	Urine	Feces	Feces	Feces

18.7). They are laid undeveloped, but have fully formed miracidia within several days. They reach the lumen of the organ, either gut or bladder, and pass to the outside with feces or urine.

The eggs are ready to hatch immediately on reaching the outside and do so mostly under the influence of lowered osmotic pressure; eggs hatch at 0.1% NaCl, but are almost completely inhibited from hatching at 0.6% NaCl. Eggs hatch well at 28°C, but are inhibited from hatching at 4°C and 37°C. Light also is a stimulus for hatching.

The miracidia escape from the egg capsules and swim in the water and actively seek snails to penetrate. Upon finding a suitable snail, the miracidia penetrate the soft tissues of the foot; in the case of the blood flukes, unlike some other digenea, the whole miracidium enters the body of the snail (Fig. 18.8). After penetration, the ciliated cells disappear, and transformation into the first generation or mother sporocyst takes place.

The first-generation sporocysts generally remain in the foot of the snail near the point of penetration; they are nonmotile, convoluted sacs less than 1 mm long.

Within two to six weeks, daughter, or second-generation, sporocysts form in the central cavities of the mother sporocyst. The daughter sporocysts are somewhat larger than the mother sporocysts, and are motile. In *S. mansoni*, 200 to 400 daughter sporocysts form in each mother sporocyst. At this time, the mother sporocyst degenerates, releasing the daughter sporocysts, which migrate into the digestive gland or ovotestis of the snail (Fig. 18.9).

Cercariae form in the central cavity of the daughter sporocyst and leave through a pore at the posterior end. Cercariae may be produced as early as 20 days following infection, but usually take four to seven weeks, and they can continue to be produced for more than a year, although the life span of an infected snail is often only one to two months. Production of cercariae depends on the size of the snails; the larger the snail, the greater the production of cercariae. Table 18.2 shows reproduction in the snail and also the differ-

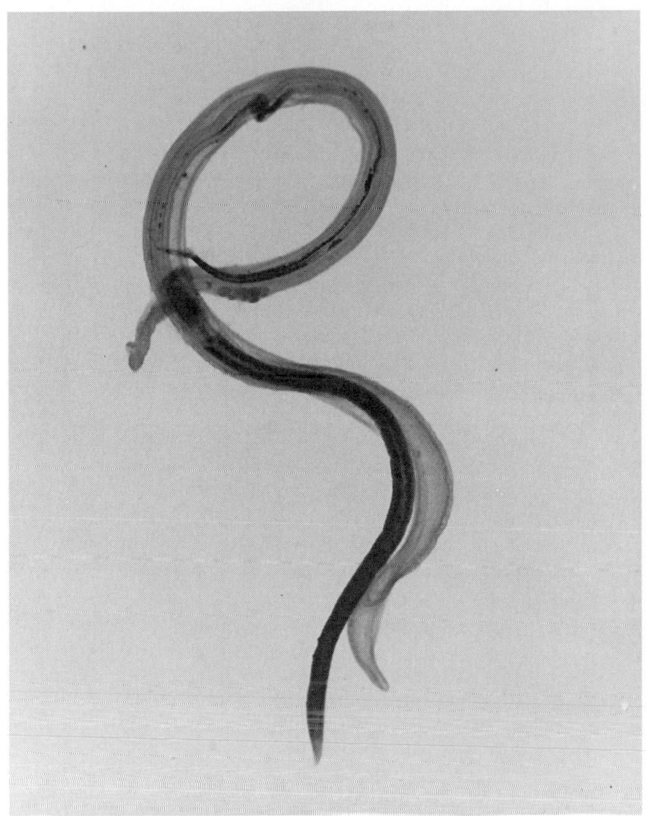

FIGURE 18.2 A male and female of *Schistosoma mansoni* in copula.

ences in cercarial production depending on species and location.

To give some idea of the contamination of water with cercaria, let us take the example of *S. mansoni* and assume that there are 100,000 snails in the vicinity of a community. Then we can see what the contamination of the area might be. A number of surveys on the prevalence of infection in snails indicate that 10% prevalence may be expected in some places. This means that 10,000 snails in the area are infected. If we take 1000 cercaria per day as the low end of production of cercariae, there are 10 million cercariae in the water at any one time. At the high end, 30 million cercariae are ready to infect persons entering the water. Considering the numbers, tipping the balance in favor of the parasite even slightly is likely to bring about an overall increase in the worm burdens of members of the community. We will look at this problem in some detail in the section on epidemiology and control.

The cercariae tend to accumulate in the area of the mantle collar of the snail, that is, close to the head of the snail in the region where escape to the outside is simple. The cercariae break out of the epithelium and reach the water. Unicellular escape glands located in the anterior portion of the body are seen only in the unemerged cercariae and presumably are instrumental in the organism's breaking out of the snail tissue. As is true for many trematodes, the cercariae of the blood

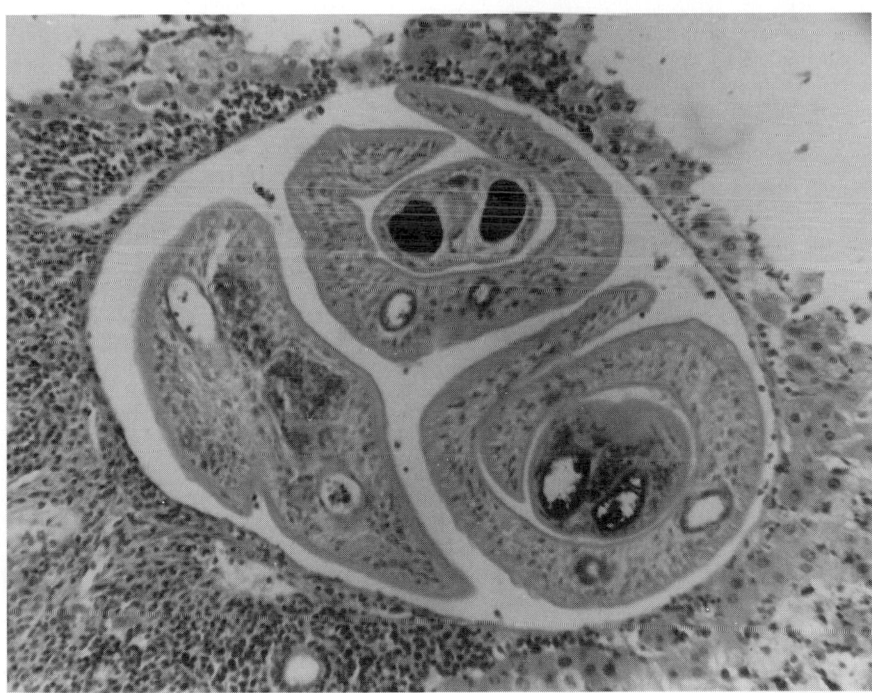

FIGURE 18.3 A histologic section showing cross sections of two male flukes holding females in the gynecophoral canal (right) and a single male (left). The adults lie in a venule, which has a relatively thin wall.

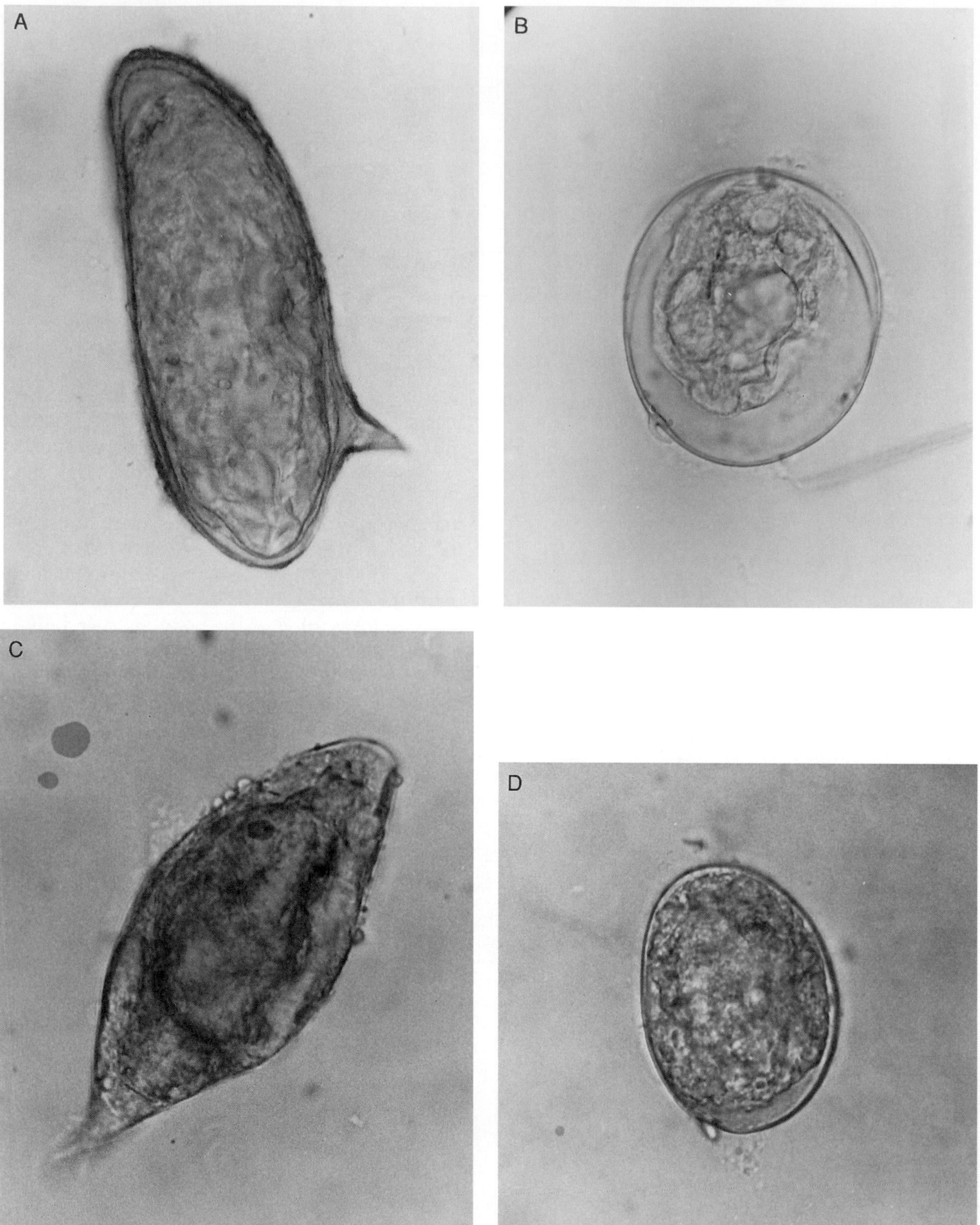

FIGURE 18.4 Eggs of (A) *Schistosoma mansoni,* (B) *S. japonicum,* (C) *S. haematobium,* and (D) *S. mekongi.*

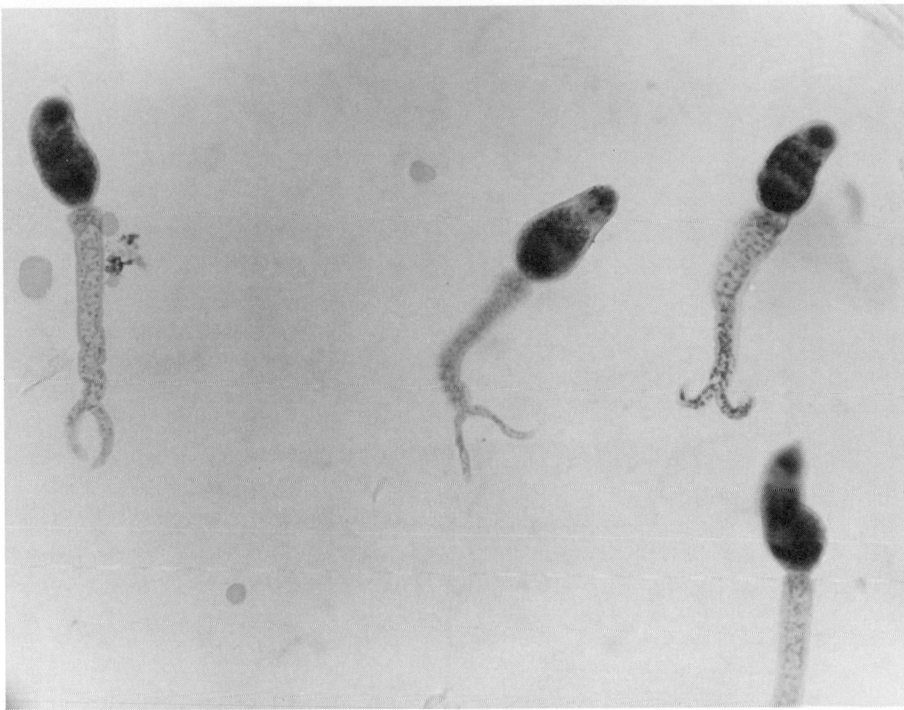

FIGURE 18.5 Furcocercous cercariae of *S. mansoni.*

flukes tend to leave the snail at certain times of the day: *S. mansoni* and *S. haematobium* between 9:30 a.m. and 2:00 p.m. and *S. japonicum* between 10:30 p.m. and 2:00 a.m.

The function of the cercaria is to move from the intermediate host through a hazardous environment to the definitive host. The cercariae swim in the water by means of their tails and actively seek a host to penetrate. They can survive about a day, but infectivity declines in a few hours if they fail to find a host. When they contact human skin, cercariae are stimulated to penetrate by warmth, skin surface lipids, and perhaps light. They shed their tails and begin the process.

Penetration takes place using the secretions of the pre- and postacetabular glands. The postacetabular glands secrete a substance that is probably a mucopolysaccharide. This material spreads out from the oral sucker, allows the attachment of the organism to the skin, and may prevent the diffusion away of enzymes. The cercariae often enter the unbroken skin through hair follicles or sebaceous glands. The cercariae penetrate the skin at least partly through the muscular action of the oral sucker. Once the organism is in the skin, the preacetabular glands secrete a substance that causes a softening of the skin's keratin layer.

The time required to begin penetration of the skin is remarkably short. As little as 3-minute exposure in water containing cercaria followed by drying of the skin permits large numbers of cercariae to penetrate the skin of mice. They reach the subepithelial layers within 30 minutes.

Once the organisms penetrate the skin, lose their tails, and secrete the substances from the various glands, they are considered to be *schistosomules*. Schistosomules are clearly different from cercariae in their ability to tolerate high osmotic pressure, their ability to survive in serum, and their appearance, which is wormlike. The schistosomules are carried by the circulatory system to the lungs about a day after penetration. They then migrate to the liver. Development takes place in the liver and as the worms approach sexual maturity, they begin to migrate down the hepatic portal vein into the smaller vessels, draining the lower intestine or bladder. Sexual maturity may be reached as early as seven weeks following infection, depending on the species (Tab. 18.1).

Studies on egg production in schistosomes have been done in both human and animal infections. The data from human infections are limited in many ways, but they are consistent with animal studies. Egg production per female worm per day ranges from 22 to 3500. The highest figure was found in *S. japonicum* infections in hamsters. An *S. mansoni* female produces perhaps 500 eggs per day, whereas *S. haematobium* probably produces fewer than 100.

There are some problems that the maturing worms

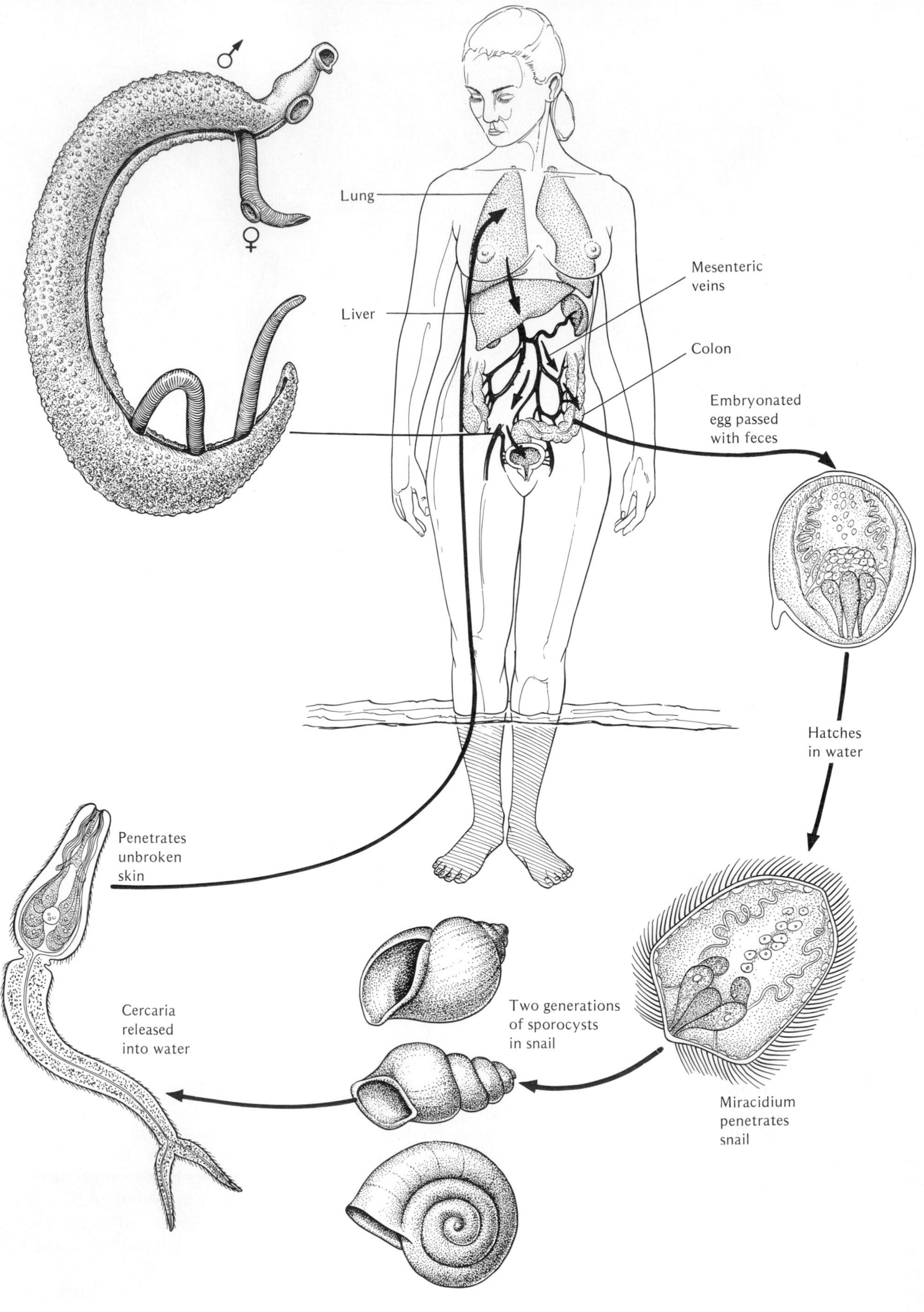

♂
♀
Lung
Liver
Mesenteric veins
Colon
Embryonated egg passed with feces
Hatches in water
Miracidium penetrates snail
Two generations of sporocysts in snail
Cercaria released into water
Penetrates unbroken skin

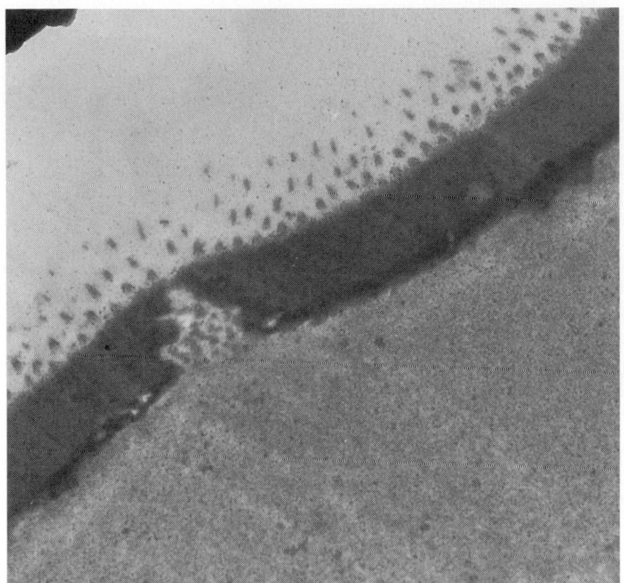

FIGURE 18.7 The egg shell of *Schistosoma mansoni* (black strip) as seen in TEM. A pore breaches the egg shell allowing antigens to leak from the interior of the egg into the tissues of the human host causing a foreign body response.

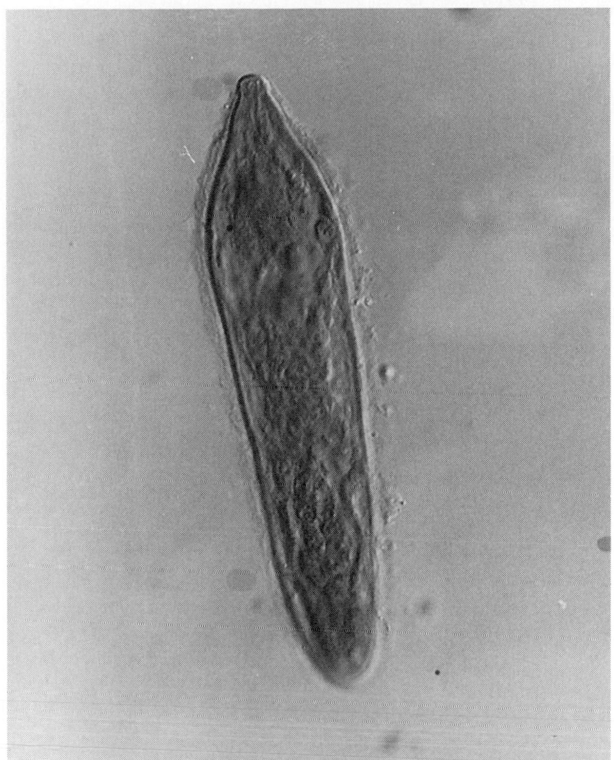

FIGURE 18.8 Miracidium of *Schistosoma mansoni* as seen in LM. The organ used for penetrating snail tissue is at the top of the picture.

need to solve. First, the sexes are separate in the schistosomes. Sex is genetically rather than environmentally determined. Therefore, a worm needs to find one of the opposite sex. The worms also tend to locate in specific abdominal organs, but there is little information on stimuli that cause them to migrate to one place or another.

A second problem facing the worms as they mature is how to survive for a long period. Since they have relatively long prepatent periods in the vertebrate host, they must be able to avoid its immune response. The solution they have evolved is an ingenious one: They adsorb host antigens from the host's serum onto their surfaces or produce antigens almost identical to that of their host. The worm antigens are almost completely covered or masked by this subterfuge and the worms are not recognized as nonself. Shedding of the outer portion of the double tegument membrane may also eliminate antigen-antibody complexes. The effectiveness of these techniques is attested to by the fact that worms may live for more than 10 years in a human host. This unique adaptation is called concomitant immunity.

Diagnosis

Diagnosis of infection with members of the genus *Schistosoma* is based on the following:

1. Clinical signs and symptoms
2. A history of living in an endemic area
3. Serological tests to look for antibodies
4. Finding the characteristic eggs

Signs and symptoms of schistosomosis are similar to those of a number of other diseases. Persons suffering from schistosomosis usually are anemic and have diarrhea and an enlarged spleen and liver. In *S. haematobium* infections, most of the damage is to the urinary system; there is painful urination, sometimes with the passage of blood.

Serological tests are useful during the prepatent period and in chronic cases in which eggs cannot be found. The most common and conclusive means of diagnosing schistosomiasis is finding the characteristic eggs. Although three species are considered to be the

FIGURE 18.6 The life cycle of a blood fluke. [Redrawn with modification from the Ciba-Geigy pamphlet, *The Life Cycle, Clinical Picture and Treatment of Schistosomiasis.* With permission.]

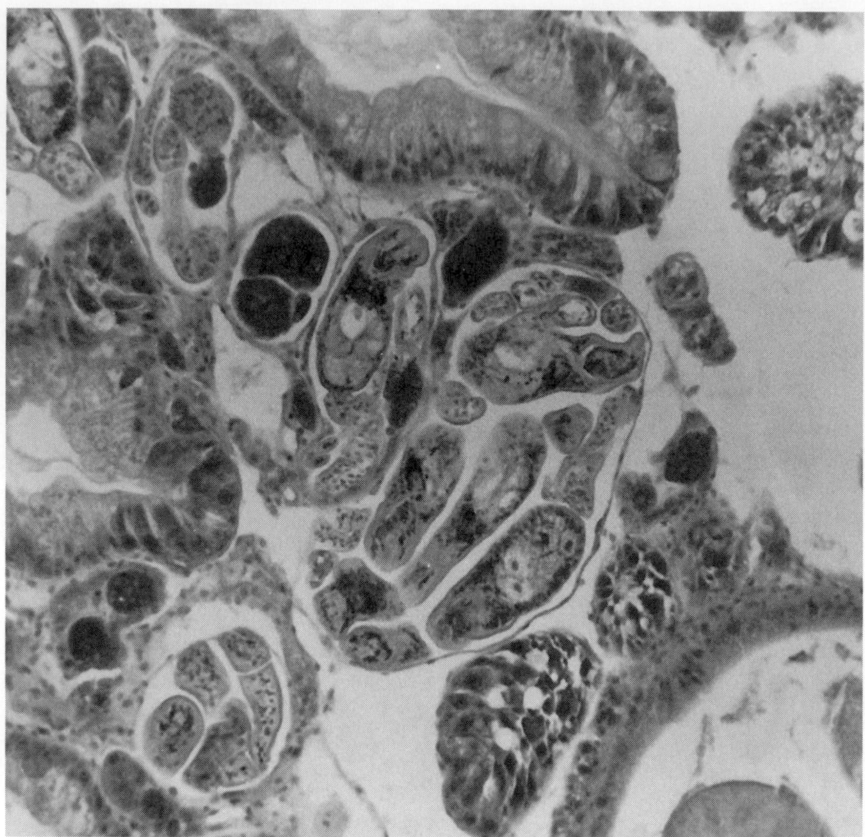

FIGURE 18.9 A histologic section of the digestive gland of a snail showing daughter sporocysts of *S. mansoni*. The sporocysts contain developing cercariae.

major human parasites, *S. intercalatum* and *S. mekongi* are also found in humans, and species normally found in domestic animals sometimes parasitize humans (Tab. 18.1). The eggs of these latter worms can usually be distinguished from the usual human parasites.

Methods of finding eggs depend on the species and the stage of the infection. If *S. haematobium* is expected, a urine sample should be taken, centrifuged, and the sediment examined microscopically for the characteristic terminally spined eggs. The sample should be taken during early afternoon, a time when the greatest number of eggs per unit volume of urine is passed. For *S. japonicum* and *S. mansoni*, fecal samples are examined by sedimentation methods designed to remove the greater portion of the fecal debris by screening or decanting. In long-standing infections, eggs may not be seen in the feces; the method then used is rectal biopsy. One or two snips of rectal mucosa are taken (the procedure is painless if properly done) and the tissue is examined microscopically while pressed between two slides.

Testing viability of eggs is important in determining the stage of infection. In some long-standing infections, dead eggs may be found in feces, urine, or biopsies. Viability may be determined by direct examination of the eggs to look for flame cell action in the miracidia, or eggs may be induced to hatch. As indicated earlier, eggs are passed with fully formed miracidia, and the

TABLE 18.2 Cercarial Production by Schistosomes in Various Species of Snails

Snail	Parasite	Location	Daily	Total
Biomphalaria glabrata	*S. mansoni*	Brazil	1000–3000	30,000–180,000
B. globosus	*S. haematobium*	W. Africa	400	12,000–24,000
Oncomelania	*S. japonicum*	Japan	15–150	450–9000

eggs hatch when exposed to low osmotic pressure. A standard method involves mixing the feces with physiological salt solution to break it up, then diluting with 10 volumes of water and placing the material in a darkened 1-liter Florence flask that has a short side arm near the top (Fig. 18.10). The flask is left for two to three hours and then a light is shown on the side arm; the miracidia will collect in the side arm. Diagnosis not only refers to determining whether an individual is infected, but also to the prevalence of infection in a community. A variety of approaches has been used to determine the prevalence and the incidence of infection in a population. Fecal and urine examinations, autopsy records, serological testing, and skin testing are the major means of screening.

Host–Parasite Interactions

Damage to the definitive host is organized according to the following time sequence:

1. Prepatent period
2. Egg deposition and extrusions
3. Tissue proliferation, repair, and degenerative effects

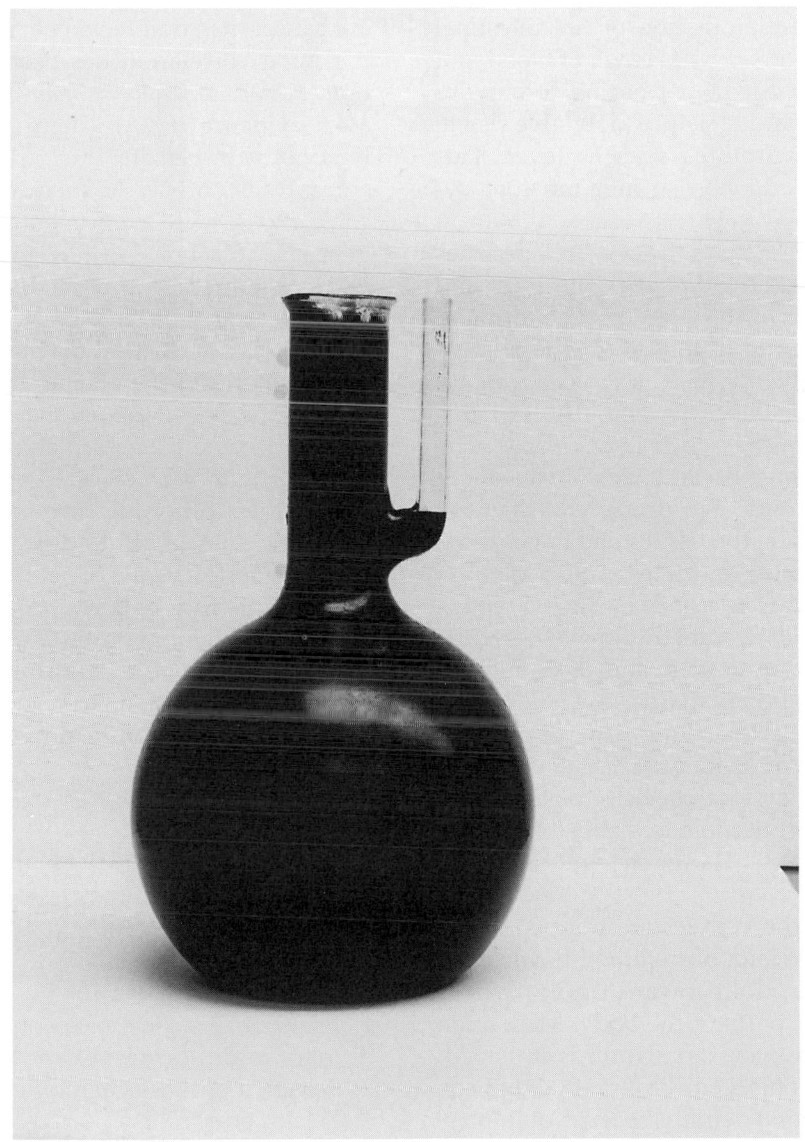

FIGURE 18.10 A side-arm flask used to collect schistosome miracidia from feces or urine. The flask is covered so that the interior is dark; when the miracidia hatch from the egg, they swim to the light at the side arm where they can be collected by pipet.

In the prepatent period, two complexes of signs and symptoms can be seen: invasion of the skin by cercariae and migration of the maturing worms from the liver to the venules in the lower abdomen. Penetration of the skin by cercariae is usually without visible effect unless there is massive invasion or the person is immune. In the nonimmune person, there may be small hemorrhages (petechiae), mild itching, and rash at the site of penetration. In the immune person, there is a local reaction by leukocytes, principally eosinophils, indicative of an allergic reaction that develops within 24 hours of infection. Unless the individual has been infected by a large number of cercariae, the symptoms are mild until the worms begin to migrate into the venules. At this time, diarrhea and fever develop. Diarrhea, symptomatic of inflammation of the intestinal tissues, may be accompanied by passage of blood and mucus with feces when egg laying begins. Strong immune reactions to first laid eggs probably give rise to acute schistosomosis symptoms such as fever. This may be due to overproduction of inflammatory cytokines.

Egg laying and entrapment of the eggs in the tissues cause the greatest long-term damage. The eggs and especially their products are antigenic; white blood cells surround the eggs and fibroblasts lay down connective tissue around them. This is a typical granulomatous reaction. In the liver, the end result of this response is termed *Symmer's clay pipe stem fibrosis.* The adult worms live in a nutritionally rich environment and the females are prolific egg producers. Many of the eggs are trapped inside the tissues and never reach outside the body, but 250 eggs/ml in urine is common in children infected with *S. haematobium* and 800 eggs/ml has been reported. So, despite the small size of the eggs, many remain in the tissues, and their effect is cumulative. Adult worms may live as long as 25 years. A major long-term effect is the laying down of progressively greater amounts of connective tissue in the infected organs so that they lose elasticity or the blood vessels are occluded and become less able to function normally as time passes. These changes are irreversible.

Not all eggs laid in the venules are trapped in the tissues where they were laid. Since blood flows away from the location of the adults toward the heart, eggs may be carried to other parts of the body. Most often eggs are carried to the liver, circulation is impeded, and the liver becomes enlarged. Progressive damage to the liver leads to general debility because of impairment to the many metabolic and detoxifying functions the liver normally performs. Other sites where eggs may lodge are the spleen, lungs, reproductive system, and central nervous system, including both the brain and spinal cord. In all instances, there is a granulomatous response around the eggs.

In *S. haematobium* infections, there may be destruction of the kidney following the fibrosis of the bladder and ureters. Lack of the normal peristaltic action of the ureter allows back pressure of urine to reach the kidney and may cause its destruction. In *S. japonicum* or *S. mansoni* infections in which there is extensive liver damage, an extra load is placed on the heart because of altered blood pressure. The heart may become enlarged and ultimately fail as a result of the excessive demands on it.

The evidence that schistosomes cause cancer is circumstantial. It has been noted that persons infected with *S. haematobium* have a higher prevalence of bladder cancer than uninfected persons from the same area. A similar correlation has been made for colon carcinoma in areas where *S. mansoni* is endemic. There is also evidence for a high prevalence of splenic lymphoma in persons infected with *S. mansoni*. There currently is no way of substantiating these statistical correlations with experimental studies, but the evidence is at least moderately good and should be taken into consideration in assessing the overall effects of schistosomosis.

The cellular reaction by the definitive host is both detrimental and beneficial. The reaction is directed against the eggs, and in the long-term, the infected organs become progressively less functional. The response ought to be directed against the adult worms to wall them off or kill them so that their eggs would not cause damage. But adult female worms continue to lay eggs for years. Thus, the correlation between parasite intensity (egg count) and morbidity may not be valid. Population-based chemotherapy has changed the disease dynamics. Large numbers of eggs may indicate recent reinfection but may not necessarily indicate clinical disease. Portable ultrasonography is helping to solve this problem.

Epidemiology and Control

A list of general methods used in attempting to control schistosomosis now endorsed by the World Health Organization (WHO) includes the following:

1. Provision for diagnosis and treatment at the primary health care level
2. Selective or mass chemotherapy
3. Health education
4. Control of intermediate hosts
5. Supply of sanitary drinking water and adequate health care facilities
6. Environmental modification

The basic pattern of life cycles in the blood flukes was worked out in the first decade of the 20th century; with that information came the keys to control. It was obvious that sanitary disposal of human excreta and reducing populations of snails were the steps to take. As knowledge increased, additional techniques were developed, so that more options were at hand. Each method is directed toward the same end: to break the life cycle or interrupt the chain of infection. If all snails could be removed from an endemic area, the probability of infection would approach zero. If all definitive hosts were treated and maintained free of infection for a year, the cycle would be broken.

Attempts have been made to apply statistical and computer models to predict the success of certain control programs. From a theoretical standpoint, it has been shown that the probability of infection is vanishingly small when the prevalence of infected hosts is reduced to a certain level. However, a careful critique of the present state of the art of mathematical epidemiology leads to the conclusion that we are still in the early stages of development of predictive models for schistosomosis. Computer models suggest that the most efficacious approach is a combination of treating the definitive hosts and reducing the number of snails or contact with contaminated water.

Snail control can be achieved using chemical, biological or ecological methods. Chemical control consists of introducing chemicals such as $CuSO_4$, sodium pentachlorophenate, or niclosamide into the water. These chemicals have proven to be successful for isolated, slowly flowing bodies of water. Only niclosamide is in wide use today.

Biological control, in theory, utilizes diseases and predators of snails such as sciomyzid larvae (Insecta: Diptera), or birds that may eat snails, or pathogenic bacteria. In practice, this has not worked very well.

Ecological control or environmental modification entails making the habitat unsuitable for reproduction or survival of the mollusks. In China, modification of *Oncomelania* habitat has worked well, while introduction of nonvector snails that compete with vector snails has been successful in Puerto Rico. Since the vectors of schistosomosis are aquatic and prefer to attach to plants in water where velocity is fairly slow, removal of aquatic plants and altering streambed and canal contours to increase water velocity reduces suitable snail habitat. As a rule, ecological manipulations require continual effort and monitoring and may therefore bring about only temporary reductions in populations.

Intertrematode antagonism has been investigated as a means of control of infections in snails. Schistosomes only form sporocysts inside snails, while echinostomes (Chapter 20.) produce both sporocysts and rediae in the same snails. A sporocyst is little more than a germinal sac, but a redia has a mouth, pharynx, gut, and locomotor appendages. Rediae actively attack sporocysts and eat them. In addition to direct predation, snail immunity or toxic products may also aid in biological control in the infected snails. Much remains to be learned about this unique aspect to biological control.

At present, snail control is best accomplished by chemical means (China is the exception). Despite the disadvantages of environmental contamination, the effects on nontarget species, and the possibility of reducing organisms that serve as natural control of snail populations, chemicals are often the most effective.

Control of schistosomosis is not the only motivating factor for sanitary disposal of human feces and urine. Not only are there aesthetic reasons, but there are microbial and other parasitic diseases that are transmitted by improper disposal and treatment of human wastes. Whether proper disposal of feces and urine can be effective in reducing transmission of schistosomes depends on a variety of factors. One key factor is the number of suitable hosts for a species of schistosome. In *S. haematobium*, hosts other than humans are probably not important, and therefore complete sanitary disposal would have an effect on transmission. Since *S. japonicum* and *S. mansoni* normally infect animals such as cattle and rodents, sanitation campaigns may have little effect.

Drugs such as Praziquantel, Oxamniquine, and Metrifonate are currently available to treat infected persons.

Dealing with reservoir hosts has been a vexing problem. Some reservoirs are valuable domestic animals such as cattle, sheep, and dogs. Elimination of these hosts would cause significant social and economic impacts. Rodent control has also often been difficult to accomplish due to a variety of reasons. If naturally infected reservoir hosts remain, the transmission of schistosomes will likely continue.

Preventing penetration by cercariae can be accomplished by applying topical anticercarials such as niclosamide to the skin. This acts as an impenetrable barrier; boots and rubber gloves can be used to prevent water contact.

Today there is significant understanding of immune responses against schistosomes and intense efforts have been made to develop vaccines against schistosomes, but there is still is no vaccine marketed for producing artificial immunity.

CERCARIAL DERMATITIS OR SWIMMER'S ITCH

Cercarial dermatitis has been reported from all parts of the world in tropical, temperate, and arctic climates.

RESISTANCE TO PRAZIQUANTEL

THE DISCOVERY OF PRAZIQUANTEL (PZQ) in the early 1980s and its subsequent development as an anthelmintic was a significant advance in the treatment of helminthic infections. For example, the treatment of schistosomosis has always been fraught with difficulties. The antimonial drugs developed early in the 20th century required administration by multiple injections and they were toxic in one way or another. Patients were often reluctant to complete a course of treatment, and even if they did, the infection might not be completely eliminated.

The objective, and hope, was to find a drug that could be administered by mouth, required only a single treatment, was nontoxic to humans, and was inexpensive. The first effective drug which could be administered by mouth was niridizole; it gave a cure rate of 75 to 95%. Unfortunately, a small percentage of patients exhibited neuropsychiatric changes that sometimes lasted for weeks. Oxnamiquine was developed in the early 1970s and it showed an efficacy of 85 to 95% when patients were given a single oral dose. Its side effects are generally mild (dizziness or drowsiness). Its greatest efficacy is against *S. mansoni*, but it is of lesser value against the other species.

PZQ has come about as close to the ideal as one could hope. It is efficacious against all three species of *Schistosoma* as a single oral dose, and episodes of intoxication are few and usually mild. That PZQ removes nearly all of the adult worms is the rub. PZQ is effective against adults, but is less so against the juvenile worms. If it leaves a few adults, the concern is that they may be resistant to the drug. In any one population of worms, there is a spectrum of susceptibility so that a few survive drug treatment, and one might assume that these few worms represent those which have a natural resistance to the drug. Their progeny, then, would be somewhat resistant upon further exposure to a drug.

Data are accumulating that schistosomes can become resistant to PZQ. One study showed that a resistant strain can be developed by treating mice with suboptimal dozes of PZQ. Another study found isolates of *S. haematobium* that were not eliminated from humans even after three doses of PZQ. Clinicians, parasitologists, and pharmaceutical companies will follow these unfolding events with interest and apprehension.

(Fallon and Doenhoff. 1994. *Am. J. Trop. Med. Hyg. 51:83*–88; Ismail, et al. 1996. *Am. J. Trop. Med. Hyg.* 55:214–218.)

It occurs in persons who have been swimming, wading, or working in littoral areas of both marine and freshwater environments and represents infection by schistosome cercariae of birds. In temperate climates, cases are seen most frequently in the middle and late summer, when the larval stages of trematodes have had time to develop and shedding of cercariae has reached a high level. Swimmer's itch should be suspected in persons who have an itching, papular eruption and who have been in water.

Schistosome cercariae penetrating the skin of a person or animal cause some irritation and a mild prickling sensation. In a host that has not been previously exposed to cercariae, the skin reaction is usually mild. However, in a host that has previously been exposed and sensitized, the reaction is more severe and results in raised, reddened, itching papules that may persist for three days to a week. This reaction is a hypersensitive or allergic response and may be seen in both normal and foreign hosts (Fig. 18.11).

The term *swimmer's itch* is usually reserved for cases of exposure of humans to the cercariae of schistosomes of water-associated birds and nonhuman mammals (Tab. 18.3). Infections acquired in marine environments are sometimes called *clam digger's itch.* As indicated, the first infection elicits a mild reaction, but subsequent exposures bring on more severe reactions. In foreign hosts, cercariae are trapped in the skin where the inflammatory reaction occurs, but there is some evidence that a few cercariae reach the bloodstream in some hosts and undergo a portion of their normal migration.

In some localities, swimmer's itch has been sufficiently severe that beaches have been closed or swimmers have been warned not to enter the water. Losses in these instances are primarily economic for the operations of businesses catering to vacationers. The afflicted

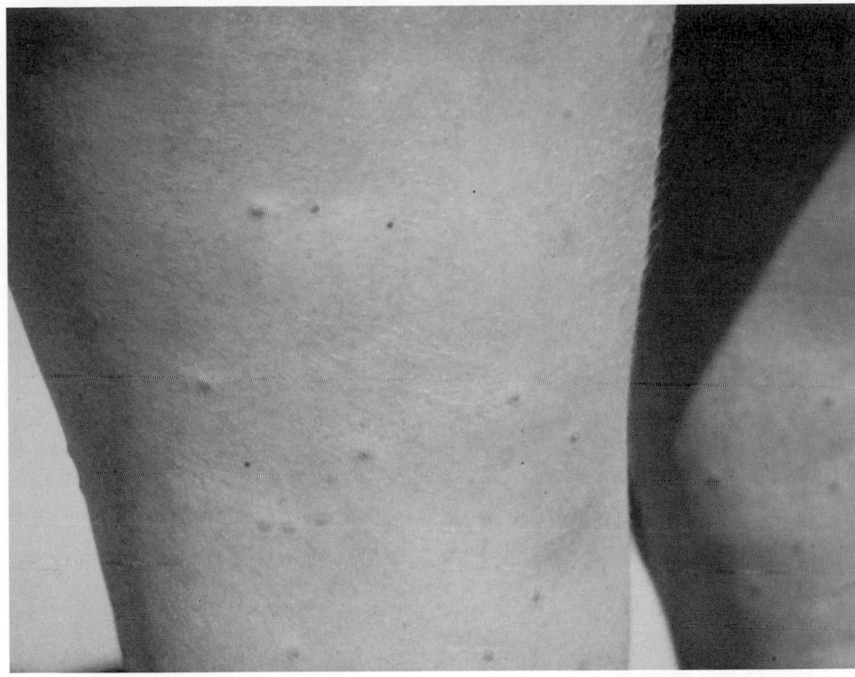

FIGURE 18.11 Human cercarial dermatitis or swimmer's itch caused by the penetration of the cercariae of a bird schistosome. At the site of penetration of a cercaria, there is a raised papule and an area of inflammation surrounding it.

individuals may suffer intensely for several days, but the effects are not lasting. Afflicted persons may be treated with topical lotions designed to reduce itching and inflammation.

Preventing swimmer's itch has two aspects: personal and community. There is some evidence that that a brisk toweling upon leaving the water may help prevent penetration of cercariae; as a general rule, cercariae find penetration easier if the skin dries slowly or repeatedly. Penetration may be prevented by applying an oily substance to the skin. At the community level, snail control programs can be effective, but they seem to have been successful only in freshwater areas, not in marine areas.

TABLE 18.3 Some Schistosomes Known to Cause Cercarial Dermatitis

Trematode	Normal definitive host	Intermediate host
Schistosomatium douthitti	Small rodents	*Lymnea* spp., *Stagnicola* spp., *Physa* sp.
Gigantobilharzia huronensis	Cardinal and goldfinch	*Physa* sp.
Trichobilharzia ocellata	Water birds	*Lymnea stagnalis*
T. stagnicolae	Water birds	*Lymnea stagnalis*
Australobilharzia variglandis	Terns, ducks	*Nassarius obsoletus*
Heterobilharzia americana	Dog, nutria, raccoon	*Lymnea cubensis*
Schistosoma spindale	Cattle	*Planorbis* sp., *Lymnea* sp., *Bulineus* sp.

A control program for cercarial dermatitis should include a determination of the parasite(s) involved and what the definitive and intermediate hosts are. A week spent in careful epidemiologic investigation may provide the key to control that would not be achieved by hasty application of a molluscicide to a wide area.

SCHISTOSOMES OF DOMESTIC ANIMALS

The schistosomes of domesticated mammals (Tab. 18.4) are basically the same in terms of life cycles and host damage as the schistosomes of humans. *S. japonicum* is found in both humans and other animals. Some of the others, such as *S. mattheei, S. intercalatum*, and *S. bovis*, have been occasionally found in humans and have been public health problems in a few instances.

Their location in the hosts are generally the abdominal veins, and heavy infections cause damage to the intestinal tract and liver. Loss of condition, reduced

TABLE 18.4 Schistosomes of Domesticated Mammals

Parasite	Principal definitive hosts	Geographic distribution
Schistosoma japonicum	Cattle, swine, dogs, humans, sheep, goats	Japan, China, Southeast Asia, Philippines
S. suis, (= *S. incognitum*)	Swine	Orient, India
S. nasalis	Cattle, sheep, goats, horses	India (one report in United States)
S. bovis	Cattle, sheep, goats, humans	Africa, Mediterranean
S. spindale	Cattle, sheep, goats, buffalo	India, Sumatra
S. indicum	Cattle, sheep, goats, equines, camel	India
S. mattheei	Cattle, sheep, equines, baboon, antelope, humans	Africa
S. intercalatum	Sheep, goats, humans, rat (*Hybomys*)	West Africa
Ornithobilharzia bomfordi	Zebu	India
O. turkestanicum	Cattle, buffalo	USSR, China, Iraq, France

milk production, and diarrhea are typical signs of infection. Diagnosis is made by finding eggs in the feces.

In *S. nasalis* of cattle, the adult worms are found in the veins of the nasal passages. In heavy infections, there is a ulceration of the nasal epithelium and a copious discharge from the nose. Partial occlusion of the nasal passages gives rise to the term *snoring disease*.

Control of schistosomes of domesticated animals is basically the same as for those of humans. Similar drugs are also often used to treat infections.

Readings

Ansari (1973). *Epidemiology and control of schistosomiasis.* Univ. Park Press, Baltimore, Maryland.

Bruce, J. L., and Sorman, S. (Eds.) (1980). The Mekong schistosome. *Malacol. Rev.* Whitmore Lake, Michigan.

Butterworth, A. E., and Hagan, P. (1987). Immunity in human schistosomiasis. *Parasitol. Today* **3,** 11–16.

Cioli, C., Pica-Mattoccia, L., and Archer, S. (1993). Drug resistance in schistosomes. *Parasitol. Today* **9,** 162–166.

Fallon, P. G., and Doenhoff, M. J. (1994). Drug-resistant schistosomiasis: resistance to praziquantel and oxamniquine induced in *Schistosoma mansoni* in mice is drug specific. *Am. J. Trop. Med. Hyg.* **51,** 83–88.

Hoeffler, D. F. (1982). Cercarial dermatitis. In *CRC Handbook in Zoonoses* (J. H. Steele, Ed.), Vol. 3, pp. 7–15. CRC Press, Boca Raton, FL.

Ismail, M., *et al.* (1996). Characterization of isolates of *Schistosoma mansoni* from Egyptian villagers that tolerate high doses of praziquantel. *Am. J. Trop. Med. Hyg.* **55,** 214–218.

Jordan, P., Webbe, G., and Sturrock, R. F. (Eds.) (1993). *Human Schistosomiasis.* CAB International, Wallingford, UK.

Loker, E. (1983). A comparative study of the life-histories of mammalian schistosomes. *Parasitology* **87,** 343–369.

Perrett, S., and Whitfield, P. J. (1996). Currently available molluscicides. *Parasitol. Today* **12,** 156–159.

Stirewalt, M. A. (1974). *Schistosoma mansoni*: Cercaria to schistosomule. *Adv. Parasitol.* **11,** 307–394.

Warren, K. S., and Hoffman, D. D., Jr. (1976). *Schistosomiasis. lll. Abstracts of the Complete Literature*, 2 Vols., pp. 1663–1974. Hemisphere, Washington, DC.

Wiest, P. M. (1996). The epidemiology of morbidity of schistosomiasis. *Parasitol. Today* **12,** 215–220.

Woolhouse, M. E., and Chandiwana, S. K. (1990). The epidemiology of schistosome infections in snails: Taking the theory into the field. *Parasitol. Today* **6,** 65–70.

CHAPTER

19

Liver Flukes

Included in this chapter are some digenetic trematodes of economic and occasional medical importance. They are grouped together principally because of the contrasts that can be seen in epidemiology and control methods. Some occur in the same geographic areas and may be found in the same hosts.

Probably the most important of these flukes, *Fasciola hepatica*, was the first digenetic fluke to have its life cycle uncovered. A. P. Thomas in Britain described the life cycle of *F. hepatica* in 1883.

FAMILY FASCIOLIDAE

Name of Organism and Diseases Associations

Fasciola hepatica, the common liver fluke, causes fasciolosis, fascioliasis, or liver rot. It may lead to secondary bacterial infections such as black disease in sheep or bacillary icterohemoglobinuria (red water) in cattle. These diseases are caused by members of the genus *Clostridium*, anaerobic spore-forming bacteria.

Hosts and Host Range

Definitive hosts include sheep, cattle, and many other ruminants; equids, swine, rabbits, hares, and marsupials are reservoirs; humans are occasionally infected. Intermediate hosts include gastropod mollusks of the family Lymnaeidae such as *Lymnaea*, *Fossaria*, and *Pseudosuccinea*.

Geographic Distribution and Importance

This fluke's worldwide distribution occurs in areas where sheep, cattle, and goats are raised and there is a niche for lymnaeid snails. In the United States, organisms are found in the Gulf Coast, the Northwest, Rocky Mountains, Florida, and occasionally elsewhere (Fig. 19.1). They are also found in Great Britain, Ireland, Continental Europe, the Middle East, the Far East, Africa, Australia, and the Caribbean area.

It is generally agreed that *F. hepatica* causes heavy economic losses in livestock worldwide, but putting a value on the global losses has not been possible. Losses are direct and indirect. Direct losses in domestic animals result from chronic and acute fluke infection. Chronic losses are mostly in the form of reduced production of meat, milk, and fiber. Direct losses include condemnation of livers at slaughter; buyers of livestock for packing plants pay less for animals from areas where flukes are endemic. Such flukey livers are used in commercial fish food, but little money is received for them.

Black disease of sheep and red water of cattle result in indirect death losses from toxins produced by the anaerobic, spore-forming bacilli *Clostridium novyi* (*Cl. oedamatiens*) and *Cl. hemolyticum*, respectively, growing in fluke-damaged livers.

In the United States, losses are estimated to be \$5.5 million per year from morbidity and mortality, and losses at slaughter are estimated at \$2.5 million per year, representing 56 million pounds of liver. In Puerto Rico 32% of cattle were found to be infected at slaughter and there was a \$1 million annual loss from condemned livers.

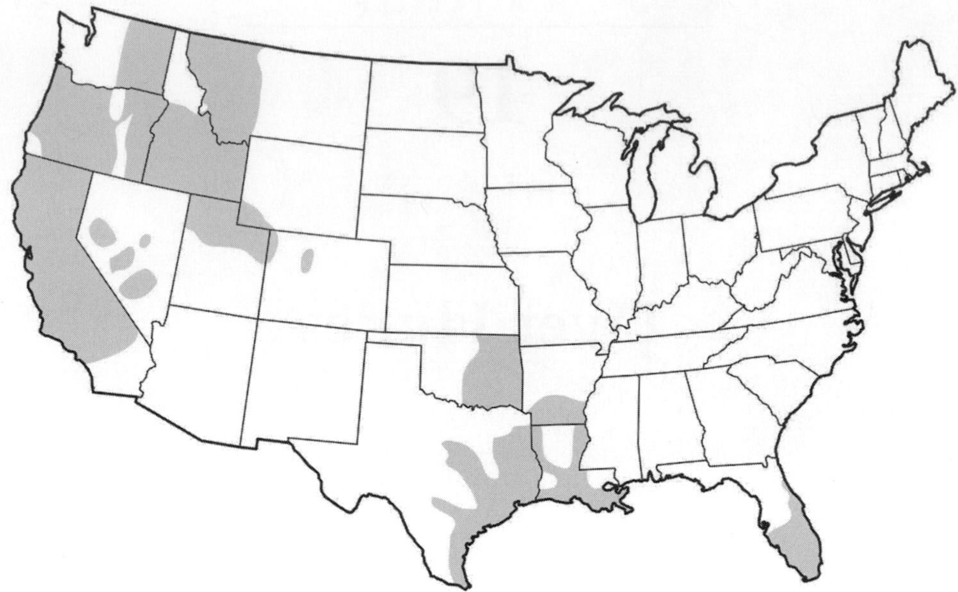

FIGURE 19.1 Distribution of *Fasciola hepatica* in the United States. [Redrawn from Malone, 1986.]

Humans are occasional hosts for *F. hepatica*, and infections are most often obtained through eating watercress (*Nasturtium officinale*) in salads. There are several hundred reports in the literature of human infections, but reports of these infections to public health agencies are not required, so their importance cannot be adequately assessed. A large outbreak in recent times occurred near Lyon, France, where there were about 500 cases. Signs and symptoms of infection in humans are relatively severe, and diagnosis is made difficult because eggs do not always appear in the feces, and eggs of echinostome flukes are similar to *F. hepatica* (Chapter 20).

Morphology

Adult flukes reach a size of 30 by 13 mm, but many are smaller. They are brown and flattened, with prominent shoulders and oral cone (Fig. 19.2). The intestine is dendritic and the ventral sucker is located in the anterior one-fifth. Most internal organs are obscured by the intestine and vitellaria even in well-stained whole mounts. *F. hepatica* can be distinguished grossly from other liver flukes on the basis of size and shape (Fig. 19.3).

Life Cycle

Eggs (Fig. 19.4) reach the outside by passing down the common bile duct and being voided with the feces. They are undeveloped when passed and require a minimum of 10 days to reach the miracidial stage. The temperatures at which development occurs are 10 to 29°C; below 10°C there is only marginal development of eggs and larval stages, and no emergence of cercariae. Miracidia (Fig. 19.5) hatch in water and penetrate the pulmonary cavity of small lymnaeid snails. One sporocyst and two redial generations give rise to gymnocephalous ("naked head") cercariae about six weeks later. The cercariae, which are set free in the water, encyst almost immediately on plants, where they form metacercariae.

Metacercariae, which are eaten with the forage, excyst in the small intestine and migrate through the gut wall to the abdominal cavity. They reach the liver about five days after infection and penetrate its capsule. Juvenile flukes migrate in the liver parenchyma, reaching bile ducts and producing eggs 8 to 12 weeks postinfection (PI). Adult flukes may live longer than 10 years in sheep, but they generally live less than a year in cattle.

Diagnosis

Finding typical eggs in feces is the method of diagnosis (Fig. 19.4); they are barrel-shaped, operculate eggs 130 to 150 by 63 to 90 μm. Operculate eggs do not reliably appear in flotation methods, and it is best to use a sedimentation technique. Eggs of *Fasciolopsis* and *Cotylophoron* are indistinguishable from *F. hepatica*, and some others are similar to them.

At postmortem examination, adult flukes are found in the gallbladder and in larger bile ducts of the liver.

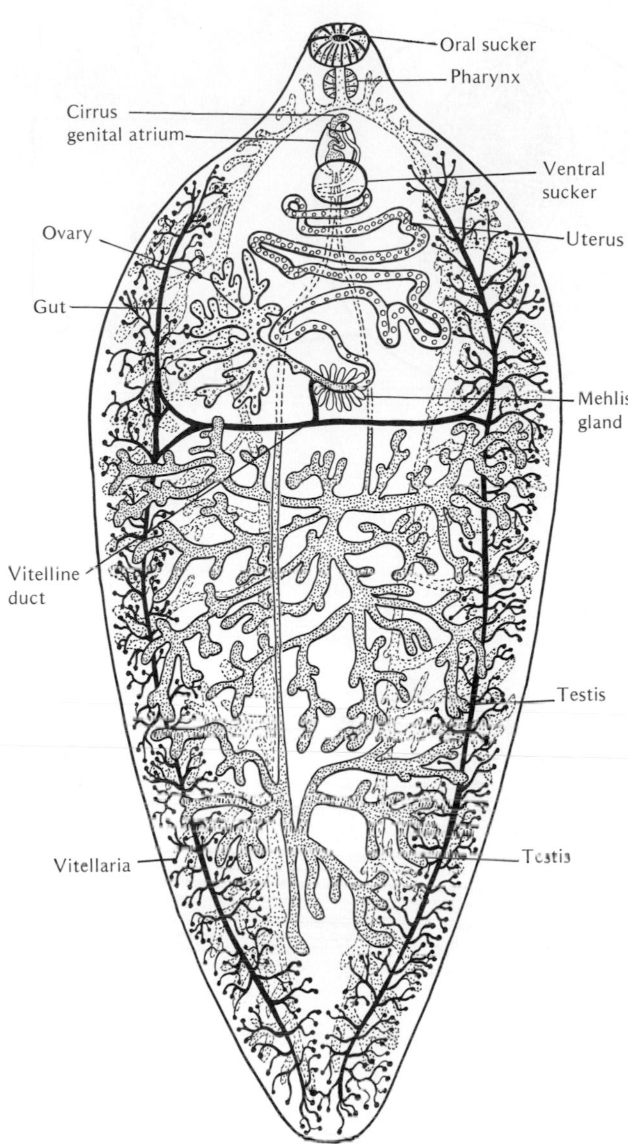

FIGURE 19.2 *Fasciola hepatica* adult.

In deaths from acute fluke infections, tracks where flukes have migrated may be seen, and it is sometimes possible to find juvenile flukes in the parenchyma of the liver.

In endemic areas, diagnosis may often be made on the basis of clinical signs such as loss of condition, anemia, and failure to gain weight. Knowing the cycle of transmission of *F. hepatica* in a particular area gives a guide to the times of year and conditions under which infection is likely to occur.

Host–Parasite Interactions

Pathogenesis as a direct result of the flukes' activities may be either chronic or acute. Acute fasciolosis occurs

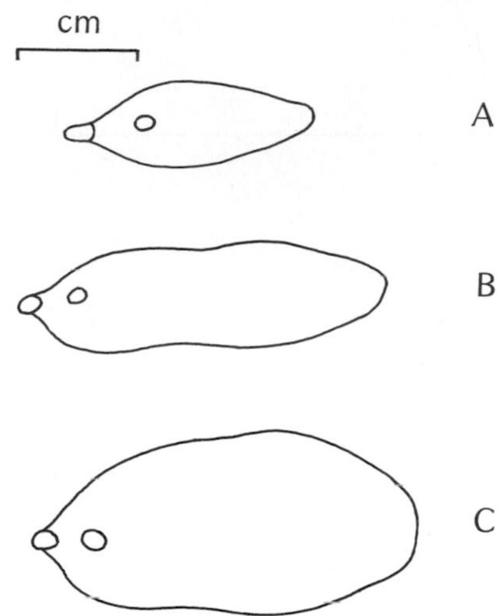

FIGURE 19.3 Outline drawings of liver flukes of large ruminants. (A) *Fasciola hepatica;* (B) *Fasciola gigantea;* (C) *Fascioloides magna.* [Redrawn from Pantelouris, 1965.]

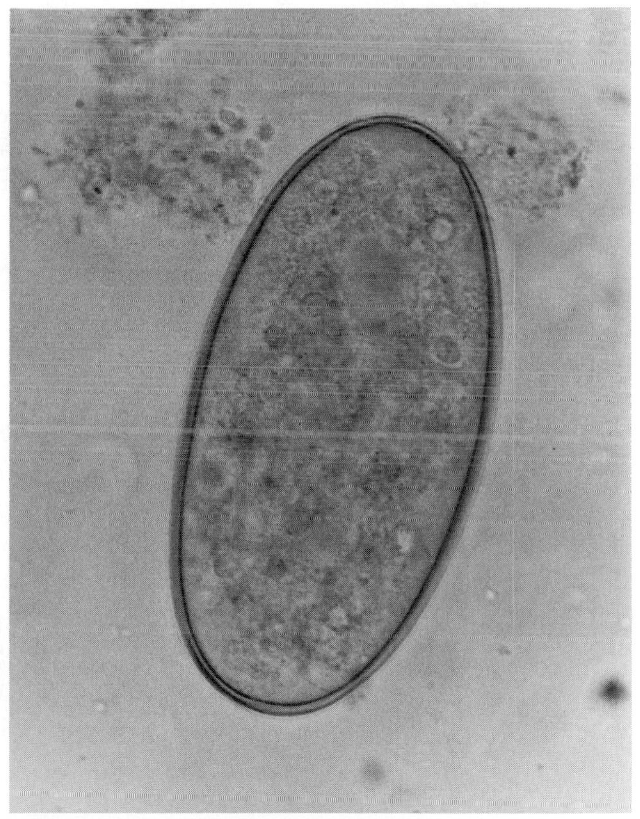

FIGURE 19.4 Egg of *Fasciola hepatica.* Eggs are passed from the host in an early stage of development and embryonate in the water or moist areas. The miracidium escapes from the egg through the operculum seen in this photograph at the upper end of the egg where the outer capsule shows two slight breaks.

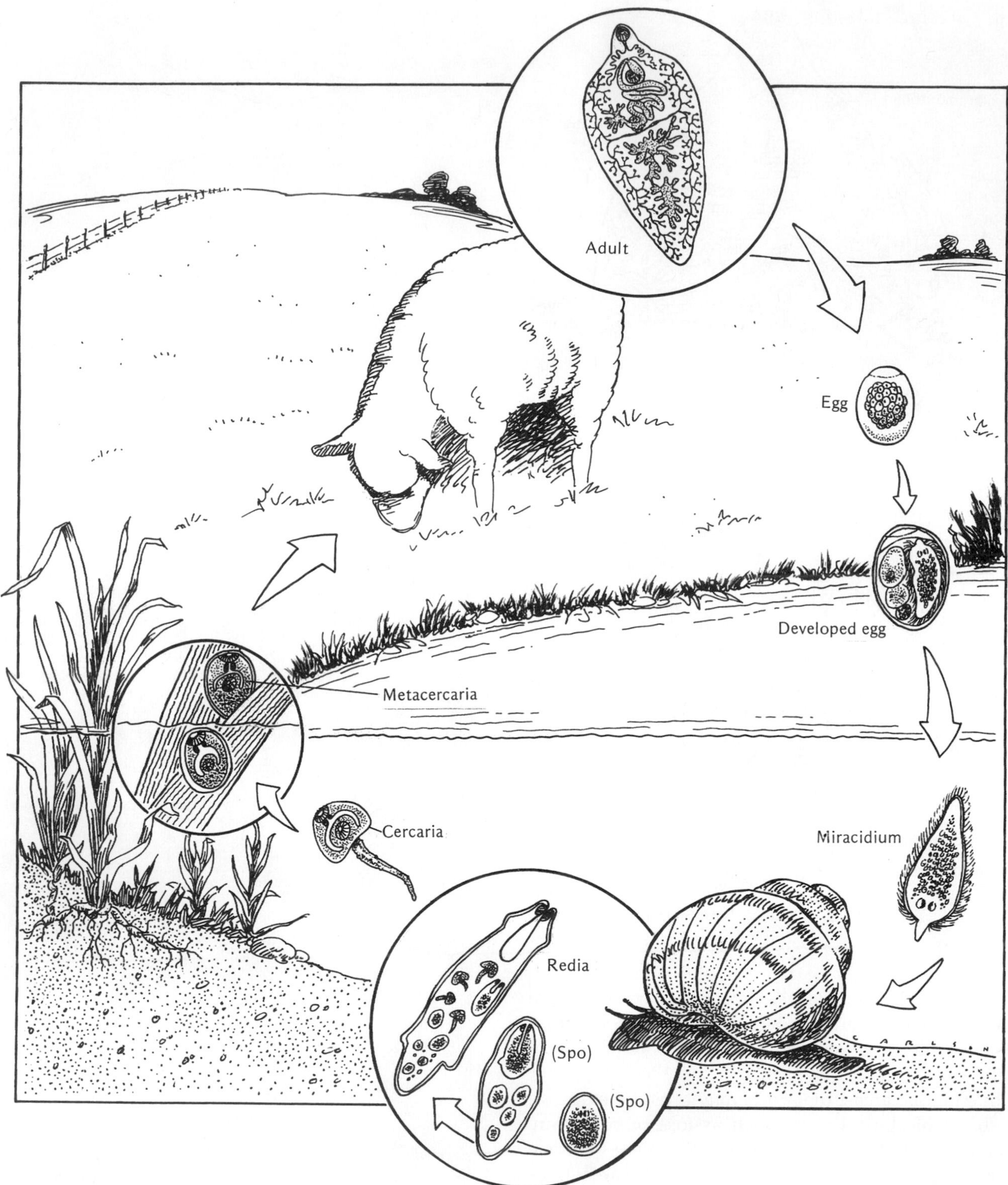

FIGURE 19.5 Life cycle of *Fasciola hepatica*.

during the preadult migration of the flukes in the parenchyma of the liver, and sometimes other organs, for about eight weeks. The time of death and severity of the damage are related to the number of metacercariae ingested; deaths occur earlier and the damage is more severe with greater numbers of flukes. In sheep, 1000 or more metacercariae ingested within a short period may cause death. Cattle are more resistant than sheep to the effects of flukes; 10,000 to 20,000 metacercariae were found to cause death.

The most striking changes in acute fasciolosis are seen in the liver, where there are hemorrhagic tracts representing the paths of the migrating juvenile flukes. The liver becomes swollen and, in some instances, may become so swollen that the capsule ruptures.

Chronic fasciolosis occurs beyond 12 weeks PI, when the flukes have reached the bile ducts and are maturing sexually. Although production losses are the usual results of chronic infections, deaths also occur. In chronic fasciolosis, the damage is primarily to the liver, but unlike the acute phase of the disease, the damage is from fibrosis (scar tissue), blockage of the bile ducts, and inflammation of the bile ducts.

The liver performs a vast array of essential functions in vertebrates, and it is axiomatic that liver damage will have severe effects. The adult flukes also cause anemia as a result of blood sucking or from hemorrhages where they graze on the mucosa of the bile ducts. The evidence is equivocal, but seems to favor a hemorrhagic anemia as opposed to a suppression in production of new red cells. The result of liver damage is failure to gain weight in young animals, weight losses in older animals, reduced milk production in cattle, and lowered fleece weights in sheep. Continuous loss of blood puts an extra burden on the bone marrow for production of red blood cells; animals on an otherwise adequate diet are likely to become progressively more anemic with the passage of time. Since more than just red cells are lost, animals become hypoproteinemic, so that the osmotic pressure of the blood is lowered and fluid is retained in the tissue spaces (edema).

Immunity to *F. hepatica* has been demonstrated, and antibodies can be found in the blood of infected animals. Observations in the field indicate that older animals become resistant to infection. Development of vaccines has been attempted, but has not yet been successful. Further efforts to develop practical immunizing agents are continuing.

Epidemiology and Control

Control of liver flukes is effected in three major ways:

1. Treatment of infected vertebrates
2. Snail control
3. Herd management through predicting outbreaks of disease

In recent years, nitroxynil and clioxanide have been found to be effective against both juvenile and adult flukes. In all drugs, higher doses must be used against juvenile flukes than against the adults in the bile ducts. The drug of choice for use in humans is bithionol.

Strategic treatment should be part of an overall control program; animals are treated after they have become infected but before the flukes have matured. To minimize the losses from black disease or red water, animals should be vaccinated against these bacterial diseases several months prior to any likelihood of being infected by flukes.

There is usually a single major snail vector in a geographic area. For example, in Britain and on the European continent, it is *Lymnaea truncatula*. In Australia, *L. tumentosa* is the most important vector, and in North America there are three important vectors, *Fossaria modicella*, *Stagnicola bulimoides*, and *Pseudosuccinea columella*, depending on the area. Before starting a control program, the vector should be determined and information developed on its reproduction and habitat preferences. For example, lymnaeid snails are air breathers (pulmonates) and are semiaquatic; they require water for breeding, die when dried out, but are likely to be found in habitats where there is only a film of water such as mudflats near a stream or pond. They are not typically found in fast-moving streams. *L. truncatula* is even found in low-lying pastures where the hoofprint of an animal can provide sufficient water for survival. This type of snail is an opportunist; reproduction is hermaphroditic and takes place all through the growing season. Therefore, populations tend to increase explosively when moisture is abundant and to crash when there is a dry period. The crucial factors in completing the life cycle are adequate moisture for the vector and temperatures above 10°C for development of the larval stages in the vector.

Chemical control of snails is most often attempted by using copper sulfate (blue stone) or sodium pentachlorophenate in the water. A simple means is to immerse a cloth bag containing $CuSO_4$ in a running stream. The problem with this method clearly is that the snails may not be in the stream or ditch but rather well out of the flow on a mudflat. The solution in Britain has been to broadcast finely granular $CuSO_4$ on pastures where snails are abundant. In Australia, high-pressure spraying of pastures with sodium pentachlorophenate has been found to be effective in irrigated areas. No molluscicide is approved for use in the United States.

The semiaquatic nature of lymnaeid snails can be exploited to bring about ecological control of snail populations. In the Rocky Mountain West, liver fluke infections are associated with irrigation, and extensive irrigation systems distribute water from mountain runoff. Irrigation ditches are constructed so that water flow is slow but constant. As systems age, they tend to erode, so that the sides slope and plants take root in or at the edges of the water. The habitat thereby becomes suitable for lymnaeid snails.

A study done during the 1930s under the auspices of the Works Progress Administration (WPA) described methods of making the ditch banks vertical and of removing vegetation to reduce the snail habitat. The methods worked and reduced snail numbers. But the study also pointed out that what works in one time and place may be entirely inappropriate in others. Consider that the WPA was instituted when the United States suffered from the worst depression in its history. Some 14 million persons were out of work, with WPA wages of about $60 per month; men were willing to shape ditch banks with shovels and to grub out weeds. During the intervening 40 years the agricultural labor force migrated to urban centers so that a ready supply of labor has gone, and agriculture has become heavily dependent on machinery for work requiring almost any earth moving. One could hardly gather the workforce, let alone pay the people living wages for their labors. Machinery, if it can be gotten into the proper areas at all, is expensive and may not be able to do the job required. Thus, this method of control can be used only in areas of the world with low wages and an excess of unskilled labor as illustrated in China for *S. japonicum* control by pick and shovel brigades.

Some aspects of habitat alteration are feasible in a developed country. Snails typically bloom in relatively restricted areas such as mudflats or boggy areas. It is usually possible to fill, drain, or fence boggy areas of a pasture at a modest cost. An owner who could cut death losses by three head of cattle by this means would have perhaps $300 more beef to market in the first year alone.

Snail control programs are difficult to put into operation under the best of circumstances. Populations bloom when there is even a slight alteration in the ecosystem favoring their survival and reproduction. Chemicals used in control have side effects on other animals in the water such as fish, and may even be toxic for livestock; our concern for environmental contamination limits the use of many toxic substances. Lymnaeid and other snails are readily carried by streams, so that recolonization takes place even if all snails have been killed. Since lymnaeids are self-fertilizing, a single snail left in an area is sufficient to repopulate it within a short time. A control program instituted by a single owner on his own premises is likely to bring little reward for the money and effort spent. The solution, then, is to obtain cooperation of all of the owners in a particular drainage so that an area-wide program can have significant effect.

The basic approach is to utilize possibly contaminated pastures before the cercariae emerge from the snails and generally to treat livestock after they have been infected but before the onset of clinical signs.

Host range, longevity, and egg production of liver flukes in definitive hosts have implications for control. In sheep, they cause relatively little host reaction (encapsulation), and the flukes may live for many years, all the while producing large numbers of eggs. Estimates are that one fluke produces about 20,000 eggs per day. Cattle, on the other hand, are relatively poor hosts in that the infection usually is retained only for months. Egg production by *F. hepatica* is also poorer in cattle than in sheep. While sheep may contaminate pastures with 2 million eggs per day per animal, cattle shed only 50,000 to 100,000 eggs per day per animal. Pasture contamination by cattle therefore increases more slowly and ends sooner than with sheep.

The difference in pasture contamination by sheep and cattle can be calculated; stocking rates for sheep on pasture are about eight times higher than for cattle. Taking the figures in the previous paragraph for egg production and assuming equal pasture utilization (one ox or eight sheep) over a two-month period, the sheep would provide 960 million eggs on the pasture, whereas one ox would deposit 4.5 million, a difference of over 200-fold. In an enzootic area, the livestock raiser must watch husbandry practices more carefully with sheep than with cattle.

As indicated in the early part of this chapter, the host range of *F. hepatica* is broad and extends to rabbits, which are common wherever livestock are raised. Although the evidence is somewhat fragmentary, it appears that rabbits cannot by themselves perpetuate fluke infections. Therefore, if a rigorous control program is instituted, it can be directed at domestic animals, only, without seriously affecting the outcome.

Other Members of the Fasciolidae

There are three additional species whose members are found in the livers or intestines of herbivores or humans. Some are found infrequently or are of little medical or economic importance. The following flukes are briefly considered, because of the losses they may cause.

Fasciola gigantica (Fig. 19.3) can be as its name implies—gigantic—up to 7.4 cm in length. It is found in

Asia and Africa and has been introduced into Hawaii where it has become the predominant species in cattle. A few human infections have been reported. The life cycle is similar to that of *Fasciola hepatica*.

Fascioloides magna is found in North America, where it is a parasite of both wild and domesticated ruminants; the normal hosts are deer. Its life cycle is basically the same as that of *F. hepatica*. In hosts other than deer, the flukes may mature, but eggs do not reach the outside; for example, in cattle and moose there is a strong encapsulating reaction by the host, which walls off the parasite. In sheep, the flukes continue to migrate through the parenchyma of the liver rather than remain in bile ducts. *F. magna* is highly pathogenic for sheep, and pathogenesis seems to result from this continual migration and damage to the animal's liver.

F. magna provides an example of interactions that may take place between wild and domestic herbivores. Deer are reservoirs of infection for domestic animals in which the parasites do not mature. The pathogenic effect in sheep is so severe that some workers recommend not raising sheep in areas where *F. magna* is enzootic in deer. *F. magna* and *F. hepatica* may be found in the same geographic area, but mature *F. magna* can be readily distinguished from *F. hepatica* by their large size (as long as 10 cm) and somewhat different shape (Fig. 19.3).

Fasciolopsis buski is a parasite of humans and swine; it is found in the small intestine. Estimates are that there are 10 million human infections in the Orient. The fluke is large, 20 to 75 mm by 8 to 20 mm, and it has a fasciolid life cycle; the snail vectors are members of the Planorbidae. Humans become infected by eating certain aquatic vegetables, or most often by peeling them with the teeth before eating them. Pathogenesis in humans is severe, resulting not only from local damage to the intestine but also from general intoxication. Control methods involve personal protection, snail control, and sanitation. Vegetables should not be peeled with the teeth or they should be immersed for 10 seconds in boiling water. Transmission is maintained by fecal contamination of fields where aquatic vegetables are cultivated. Since human excreta, or night soil, are essential to agriculture in some areas, stopping its use may not be feasible. An alternative is to hold the material for a month in a tight tank before spreading it on the fields. Obviously, snail control in agricultural fields through the use of toxic chemicals should be avoided and other means of reducing snail populations should be attempted (see *Schistosoma* control methods). Changing individuals' food preparation methods may be moderately difficult, and changing agricultural practices is even more difficult. Thus, the broader public health measures such as sanitary disposal of human excreta are clearly the greater challenge in reducing the infection rate from *F. buski*.

FAMILY DICROCOELIDAE

Name of Organism and Disease Association

Dicrocoelium dendriticum (syn. *D. lanceolatum*), lancet fluke or little liver fluke, causes dicrocoeliosis, dicrocoeliasis.

Hosts and Host Range

Definitive hosts are the sheep, goats, cattle, many wild and domesticated animals, and humans. Intermediate hosts include land snails of the genus *Cionella* (North America) and others such as *Limax*, *Helicella*, and some aquatic forms such as *Planorbis*; the parasite first inhabits the digestive gland and later the respiratory chamber. Thirty-eight species of land snails in nine families are known to be vectors. Second intermediate hosts are ants of the genus *Formica*; metacercariae are found mostly in the hemocoel but also in the nervous system. Twelve species are known to be vectors in various areas of the world.

Geographic Distribution and Importance

Distribution is cosmopolitan. Europe, Asia, Africa (Egypt), the Middle East, Australia, South America, and Caribbean islands are included, and, in North America, New York State, Pennsylvania, eastern Alberta, and Quebec in Canada.

The prevalence in Poland is 80%, and in northern France 37.5% in sheep and 46% in cattle. In the Alma-Ata region of Kazakhstan, mature, coarse-wooled sheep, merino sheep, and goats averaged 1123, 462, and 738 flukes, respectively. The prevalence of infection in goats and mountain goats was 80% and 70%, respectively.

The damage to the host is directly proportional to the number of flukes in the liver and the length of time of the infection. Black disease (see *F. hepatica* for description and etiology) sometimes occurs in infected animals. Livers are condemned at slaughter. Losses are seen in the form of reduced production of meat, milk, and fiber.

Although there are documented infections in humans, they are sporadic and probably of no real public health importance.

Morphology

Adults are 1.5 to 2.5 mm wide by 10 mm long and pointed toward the anterior, giving the common name of *lancet fluke*; the testes are anterior to the ovary; the uterus has both descending and ascending loops; vitellaria are restricted to the middle quarter of the body (Fig. 19.6).

Life Cycle

This fluke life cycle is atypical because it is terrestrial, and there are special adaptations for this terrestrial existence. Adults lie in the bile ducts or gallbladder; embryonated eggs containing miracidia reach the outside by passing down the common bile duct and are deposited with the feces (Fig. 19.7). Eggs hatch when eaten by a snail. Two generations of sporocysts give rise to cercariae about three months after infection. Cercariae are expelled from the branchial chamber of the host in a mucoid envelope called a *slime ball,* which is about 1.5 mm in diameter. Cercariae are eaten with the slime ball by ants and develop into metacercariae. Infected ants are eaten by the definitive host and the juvenile flukes reach the liver through either the common bile duct or the circulation. The prepatent period is about 70 days.

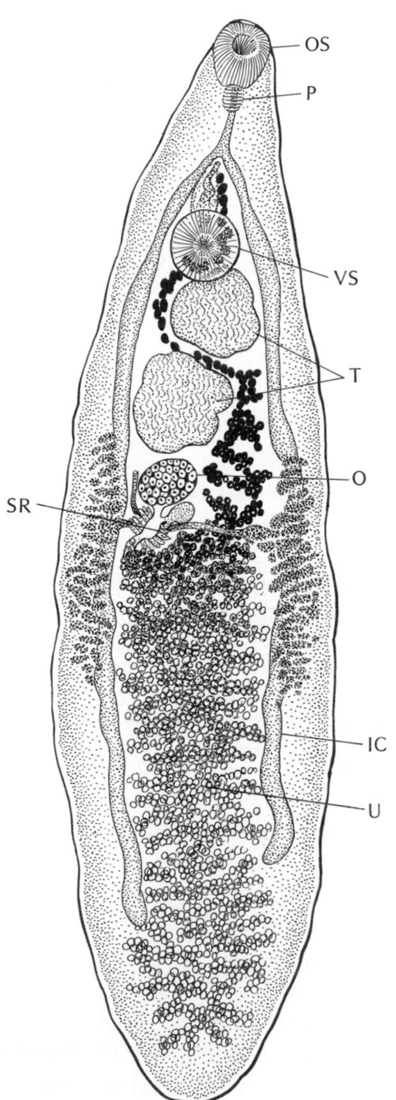

FIGURE 19.6 Diagram of an adult *Dicrocoelium dendriticum.* Abbreviations: IC, intestinal cecum; O, ovary; OS, oral sucker; P, pharynx; SR, seminal receptacle; T, testis; U, uterus; VS, ventral sucker or acetabulum.

Diagnosis

Finding eggs in the feces, embryonated, operculated, and about 26 by 41 mm is the method of diagnosis. In an enzootic area, clinical signs and symptoms may be sufficient for an experienced person to make a diagnosis.

Humans can serve as a host, but it is wise to be cautious if *Dicrocoelium* eggs are found in feces because erroneous diagnoses have been made where persons have eaten infected liver and passed eggs for a day or two.

Host–Parasite Interactions

Damage is primarily to the liver, and the changes are directly proportional to the number of flukes inhabiting the bile ducts as well as the length of time the animal has been infected. As many as 7000 adult flukes have been found in the gallbladder of a sheep, but several hundred seems to be more common. There is inflammation of the bile ducts; progressive development of connective tissue in the parenchyma of the liver leads to cirrhosis. The flukes live at least six years in sheep.

In the first intermediate host, the snail, infections are primarily in the digestive gland, but in heavy infections sporocysts are also in the lymph spaces. More than 300 sporocysts have been found in naturally infected snails; about three months are required for production of cercariae in New York and four months in Britain. Cercariae migrate to the pulmonary chamber of the snail and are incorporated into slime balls produced by the snail. Migration of the cercariae and production of slime balls seem to be caused by lowered temperatures or rain.

Successful transfer of infection from the snail through the ant to the definitive host comes about through a combination of food preferences, high infection rates in ants, and behavioral changes of infected ants. Slime balls contain 100 to 400 cercariae and are

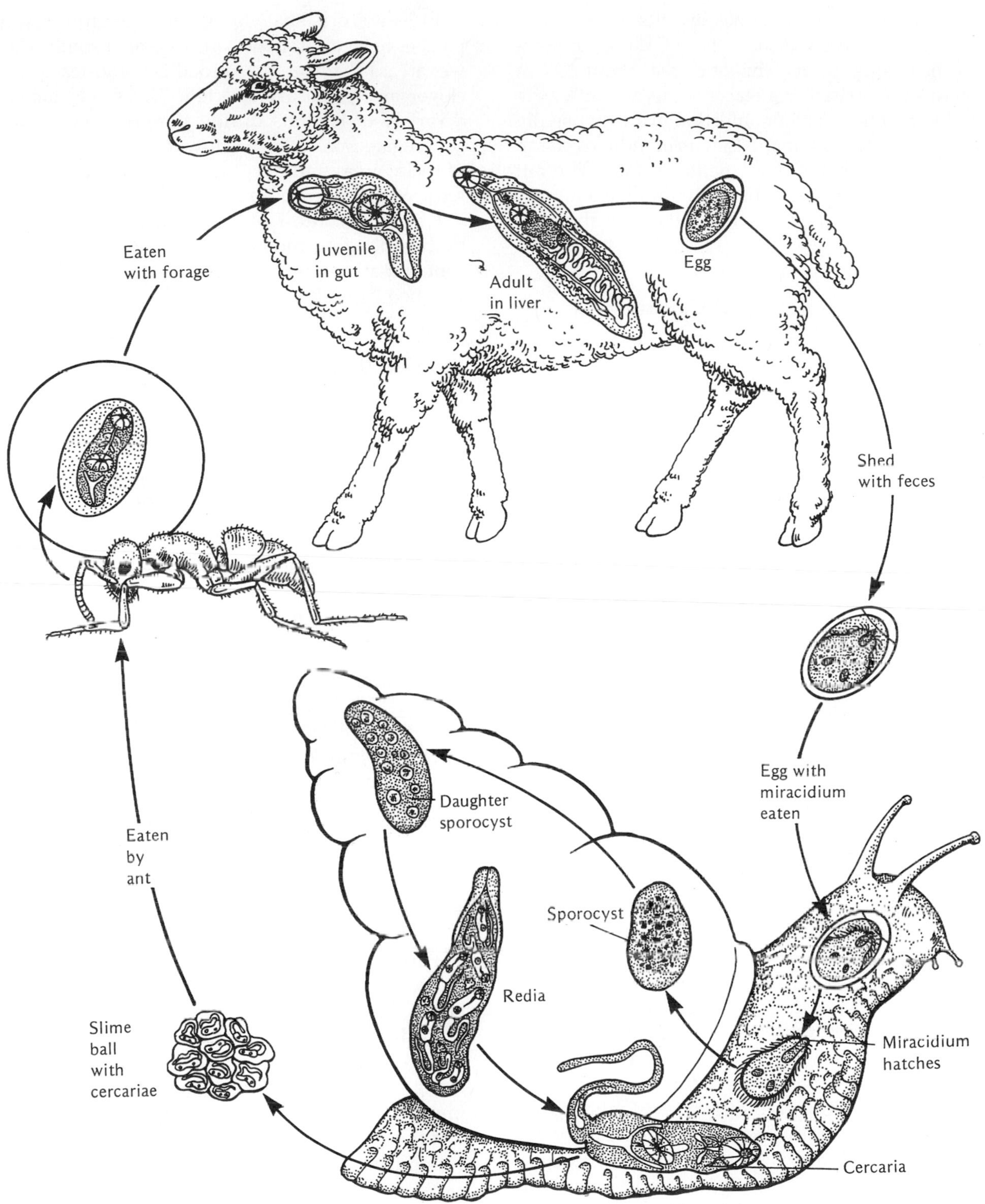

FIGURE 19.7 Life cycle of *Dicrocoelium dendriticum.*

looked on as gastronomic prizes by ants, which carry them back to the nest and share them with other members of the colony. In one enzootic area, about 30% of ants were found to harbor metacercariae, and 48% were infected in another. Further, infection in an ant usually affects the nervous system, so that its mandibles clamp into vegetation when the temperature falls. The ant remains attached to a blade of grass until the temperature rises again, thereby increasing the probability of its being eaten.

Epidemiology and Control

Control of the lancet fluke is based on the following:

1. Treatment of infected livestock
2. Snail control
3. Environmental modification

Hexachlorethane-bentonite has been the recommended treatment for many years. Hetolin removed 90% of worms in most tests. Thiabendazole is reported to remove more than 90% of adult flukes. Human infections are currently treated with praziquantel.

The lancet fluke is placed in the same chapter as the fasciolids because of the contrast it provides in solving problems of control. Both are liver flukes but they do not generally respond to the same chemotherapeutic agents. Different approaches are also required to break the cycle. The fasciolid life cycles require water at certain stages. The cycle of *D. dentriticum* is entirely terrestrial and requires only damp conditions. Control of the lancet fluke is potentially easier for a single livestock owner than control of the common liver fluke because terrestrial snails migrate more slowly than aquatic snails, which are readily carried by water.

The broad host range of both kinds of flukes presents some difficult problems, but it seems to be of greater significance in the lancet fluke than in the common liver fluke. Rodents and rabbits are not major sources of infection for domestic animals with the common liver fluke. However, the wide range of herbivorous animals that serve as normal hosts of the lancet fluke present a different situation. It is usually neither feasible nor desirable to eradicate rodents, rabbits, and large ungulates to eliminate a reservoir of infection for domestic animals. It may be possible to fence out large animals, but rodents and rabbits are almost uncontrollable.

The best approach is a combination of treatment of animals on a herd basis and pasture renovation. Oddly enough, there is little information on control of lancet flukes. In New York, plowing and reseeding of pastures reduced snail populations to about 15% of their original levels.

In New York, snails occur most often in raspberry patches or areas of shrubs; they are not usually found in wet areas. Their preferred food is broad-leafed plants; clover and grass are rejected. The snails move into a variety of habitats during the growing season but congregate in rocky areas toward the fall. Elimination of rocky areas and keeping pastures in grasses might reduce snail populations.

Chemical control of snails on pastures is feasible by broadcasting molluscicides, but toxic effects and contamination of the environment should be weighed carefully.

CLONORCHOSIS AND *OPISTHORCHOSIS*

Several flukes of the family Opisthorchiidae are important agents of human disease. These include the oriental liver fluke of humans, *Clonorchis sinensis*, and two cat liver flukes, *Opisthorchis felineus* and *O. viverrini*. Humans are occasionally infected with another opisthorchid, *Metorchis conjunctus*.

Name of Organism and Disease Associations

An important member of the family Opisthorchiidae with respect to human disease is *Clonorchis sinensis* (syn. *Opisthorchis sinensis*). The disease is called *clonorchosis*, *opisthorchosis* or *oriental liver fluke disease*.

The generic name *Clonorchis* has been and still is the subject of discussion. *Opisthorchis* was described in 1875 and *Clonorchis* in 1907; the major basis for separating them was the shape of the testes—highly branched in *Clonorchis* and lobed or only slightly branched in *Opisthorchis*. Additional species of *Opisthorchis* have been described where testes range from oval to highly branched, thereby seeming to invalidate the newer *Clonorchis* genus. There are reasons for retaining *Clonorchis*. *Clonorchis* has been commonly used in medical literature for about 70 years, and it refers to a specific disease caused by a specific parasite. Even though adult morphologies are similar, larval stages (metacercarial and cercarial flame cell patterns and body sizes) are different in each, thus giving additional support for the retention of both genera.

Hosts and Host Range

Humans are the most suitable definitive host for *Clonorchis sinensis*. Most fish-eating mammals and a few fish-eating birds can be infected, but dogs and cats are probably the most important reservoir hosts. Adults are in the liver.

Geographic Distribution and Importance

Clonorchis sinensis is found in nine countries in Asia and the former Soviet Union. It is common in Japan, Korea, China, Hong Kong, and Indochina. This distribution coincides with the distribution of the snail first intermediate host, *Parafossarulus manchouricus*, and closely related hydrorbid snails. It is estimated that there are 7 million human infections and 290 million people are at risk. Nearly 100% of people in certain villages in China are infected.

Morphology

Adult flukes are 10 to 25 mm long and 3 to 5 mm wide (Fig. 19.8). The tegument is quite transparent, which makes them ideal for studying internal structures in parasitology classes. The acetabulum is slightly smaller than the oral sucker and is located near the end of the anterior third of the body. The middle third of the body contains the vitellaria and uterus. Two highly branched testes occupy most of the posterior third of the body. A three-lobed ovary and a large seminal receptacle are just anterior to the testes.

Eggs are oval and yellow-brown (Fig. 19.9). Mature eggs are 26 to 30 mm by 15 to 17 mm and have an etched surface; an operculum fits into a shoulderlike thickening of the shell. There is commonly a small knob on the shell opposite the operculum.

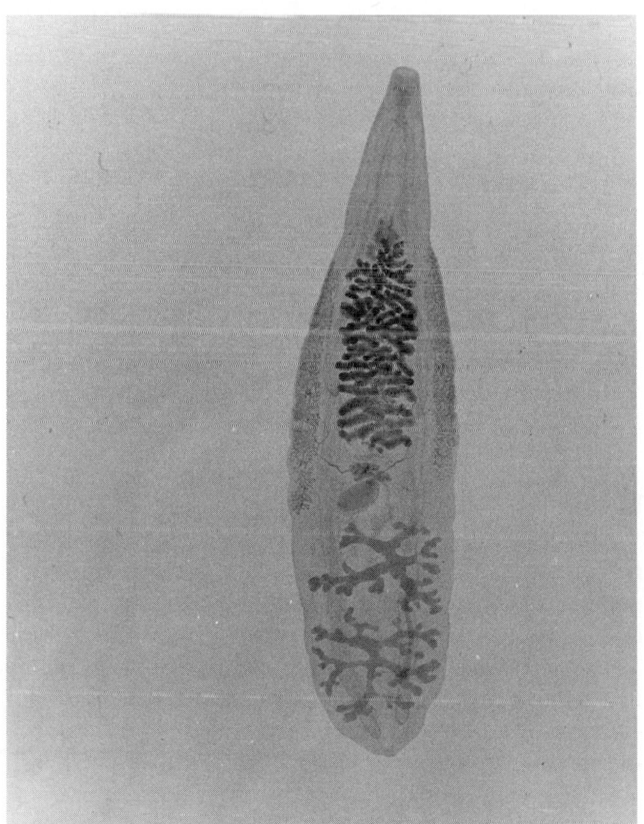

FIGURE 19.8 An adult *Clonorchis sinensis.*

Life Cycle

Fully embryonated eggs are passed in stools of infected individuals (Fig. 19.10). Eggs are ingested by the first intermediate host, *Parafossarulus manchouricus*, and closely related hydrorbid snails. When eggs hatch in the alimentary canal of the snail, miracidia penetrate the intestine and develop into sporocysts. Rediae are produced in sporocysts, leave them, and develop in the digestive gland of the snail. Oculate (one pair of eyes), lophocercous (with tail fins) cercariae mature in the digestive gland after leaving the rediae, penetrate the surface of fishes, and develop into metacercariae. Metacercariae infect 80 species of freshwater fishes, but only a dozen of them are responsible for most human infections. In addition to fishes, three species of freshwater shrimp harbor infective metacercariae and have been implicated in transmission in China. Metacercariae encyst in subcutaneous connective tissue and muscle and become infective in a month.

Definitive hosts ingest uncooked fish containing metacercariae. Metacercarial cyst walls dissolve in the duodenum or intestine and juvenile flukes migrate up the common bile duct into the small bile ducts of the liver. Egg laying begins three to four weeks after infection.

Diagnosis

A definitive diagnosis depends on recovery of eggs from feces or duodenal aspirates. Zinc sulfate flotation is recommended. There is no widely accepted serodiagnostic technique.

Clinical symptoms, along with a history of ingesting raw fish, help to confirm a diagnosis. Symptoms are classified as mild, moderate, or severe, depending on

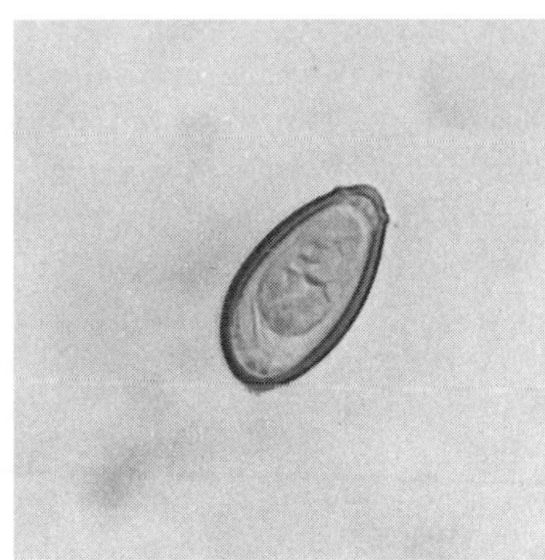

FIGURE 19.9 Egg of *Clonorchis sinensis.*

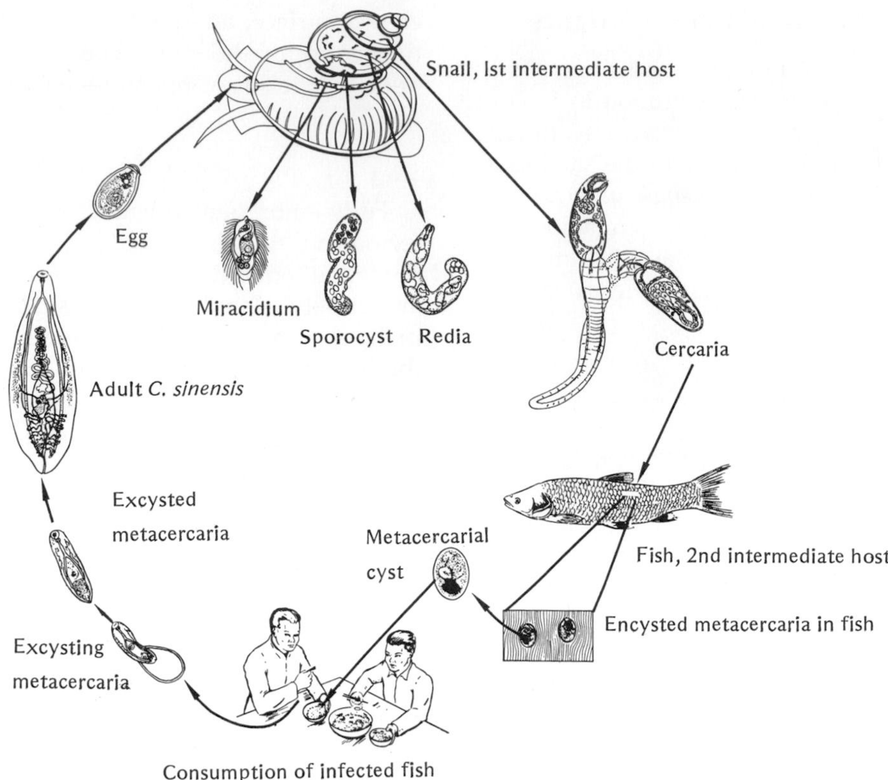

FIGURE 19.10 Diagram of the life cycle of *Clonorchis sinensis.* [From Yoshimura, 1965.]

the worm burden, length of infection, and health of the host. Light infections may be asymptomatic. Heavy infections are characterized by chills and fever, followed by liver enlargement and tenderness, sometimes with splenomegaly. Chronic heavy infections cause cholecystitis (inflammation of the gallbladder) and hepatitis (inflammation of the liver). Persons with moderate infections of 100 to 1000 flukes show appetite irregularity, diarrhea, edema, and some hepatomegaly (liver enlargement).

Host–Parasite Interactions

C. sinensis adults and ova are usually found in bile ducts; the ova apparently evoke no immune response. Occasionally an ovum can evoke a nonspecific granulomatous response in the wall of a gallbladder. More typical is hyperplasia of the bile duct epithelium and subsequent desquamation (shedding). Fibrosis (connective tissue formation) is common in infected bile ducts. Flukes occasionally invade the pancreas and may cause atrophy of the islets of Langerhans in severe infections.

C. sinensis has been implicated in bile duct cancer (cholangiocarcinoma). Patients with intrahepatic bile duct cancer in Hong Kong sometimes have chronic *C. sinensis* infections. Severe infections exert a mild but essential carcinogenic effect.

Epidemiology and Control

Control of *C. sinensis* infection in humans involves the following:

1. Treatment of individuals
2. Changing food habits
3. Snail control
4. Control or preventing infection of those reservoir hosts that have close contact with humans

Praziquantel is the drug of choice for treatment of humans.

Humans must ingest infective metacercariae in raw fish or crayfish to become infected. Raw and pickled fish are delicacies in many parts of the Orient, so millions of people are potential hosts for *C. sinensis* infections. Infection rates correlate with a community's predilection for raw fish. For example, northern Chinese do not eat raw fish, but southern Chinese do; the prevalence of infection increases from north to south even though animal reservoirs are infected throughout China. Reservoir hosts include dogs, cats, pigs, and rats.

Clonorchosis can be spread over a wide area because

of the longevity of the parasites in the definitive host. For example, a patient acquired the disease in China and lived in Panama for 40 years with no travel to an endemic area. This is the longest known duration for a *C. sinensis* infection; it indicates the need to question patients about travel.

The obvious means of control of clonorchosis is not to eat raw fish or shellfish. Unfortunately, cultural practices are difficult and sometimes impossible to change; this appears to be the case with clonorchosis. Travelers to the Orient sometimes sample indigenous foods without recognizing the hazards, and persons eating raw fish dishes stand a significant chance of becoming infected. It has been calculated that 10 g of fish contain an average of 2.6 metacercariae and that a single meal at which infected raw fish was eaten might result in the person later having 20 adult flukes.

Molluscicides to control the snail first intermediate host are generally not used because they are often harmful to important freshwater fish. Animal and human feces are important fertilizers for fish ponds in the Orient. Feces must be composted first, and the process must be rigidly controlled to prevent viable eggs from entering water. A successful composting program is operating now in China. In addition, snail populations have been significantly reduced by removal of water plants when snails lay their eggs (April to September), thereby permitting fish more easily to feed on larval snails. Thus, even though food habits are difficult to change, progress is being made by breaking the parasite life cycle at the egg and intramolluscan stages.

OTHER OPISTHORCHIIDAE

Opisthorchosis is also caused by two flukes, *Opisthorchis felineus* and *O. viverrini* (Fig. 19.11). Both are

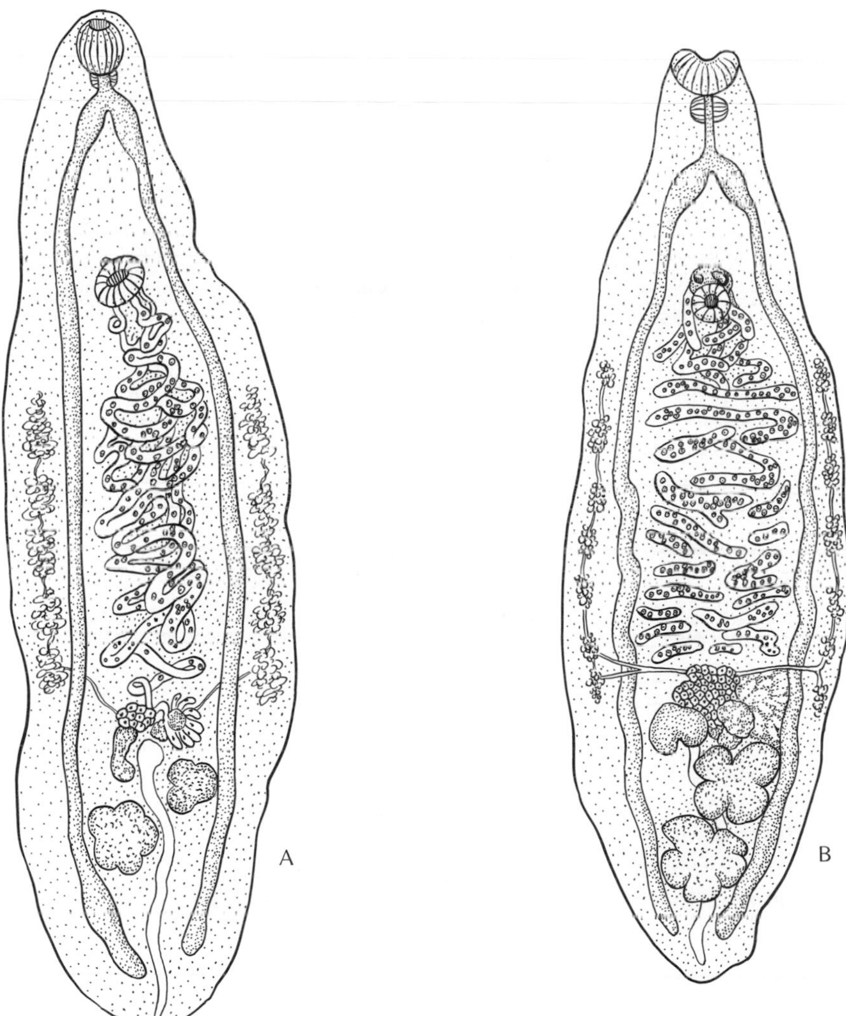

FIGURE 19.11 Diagram of the adults of (A) *Opisthorchis felineus* and (B) *O. viverrini.*

cat liver flukes that infect other mammals and humans. There are at least 8.7 million human infections of *O. viverrini* in Thailand and Laos, but it is difficult to make an accurate estimate of the number of human infections throughout the remainder of Southeast Asia. It is estimated that there are more than 3 million human infections of *O. felineus* in Europe, Russia, North Korea, and probably in Japan, India, and the Philippines.

The life cycles of *Opisthorchis* spp. are similar to that of *C. sinensis*. Bithyneid hydrorbid snails are first intermediate hosts and numerous freshwater fishes are second intermediate hosts. Definitive hosts (including humans) are infected by ingesting metacercariae in raw or undercooked fish.

Wykoff et al. (1965) compared *O. viverrini* and *O. felineus* and concluded that these species could not be distinguished on the basis of the characteristics of adults or eggs, but that they are valid species because of differences in flame cell patterns in larvae. *Opisthorchis* eggs can be distinguished from *Clonorchis sinensis* eggs because they have a smaller diameter (11 mm versus 16 mm) and a less pronounced shoulder at the operculum.

Diagnosis, clinical symptoms, and pathology of opisthorchosis are similar to those of clonorchosis. Like *Clonorchis sinensis* infections, cancer of the liver has also been linked to *Opisthorchis* infections.

Control measures are similar to those for *C. sinensis*. Praziquantel is the drug of choice to treat opisthorchosis. Because fish are a basic food in endemic areas and because of cultural preferences, raw fish is often eaten. Control must therefore be focused at other stages in the parasite life cycle. Dogs and cats are important reservoirs, so proper sanitation of human feces is not enough. Snail control appears to be the only realistic means of controlling opisthorchosis. Molluscicides cannot be used because they harm the fish used for human consumption. Therefore biological control of snails ought to be studied for reduction in the number of infections.

Amphimerus pseudofelineus (syn. *Opisthorchis guayaquilensis*) has been reported in humans and dogs in Ecuador. There is potential for a great number of human infections, because it is found in fish-eating mammals in South, Central, and North America.

Metorchis conjunctus is a North American member of the family Opisthorchiidae that occasionally infects humans. It is in the bile ducts of dog, cat, fox, mink, raccoon, and humans. The snail *Amnicola limosa porata* is the first intermediate host and the common sucker, *Catostomus commersoni*, the second intermediate host, harbors metacercariae. Fortunately, few people eat suckers, either raw or cooked; therefore, this parasite should not become a serious human health problem.

Readings

Boray, J. C. (1969). Experimental fascioliasis in Australia. *Adv. Parasitol.* **7,** 95–210.

Calero, C. M. (1967). Clonorchiasis in Chinese residents of Panama. *J. Parasitol.* **53,** 1150.

Colhoun, L. M., Fairweather, I., and Brennan, G. P. (1998). Observations on the mechanism of egg shell formation in the liver fluke, *Fasciola hepatica. Parasitology* **116,** 555–567.

Dawes, B., and Hughes, D. L. (1964). Fascioliasis: The invasive stages of *Fasciola hepatica* in mammalian hosts. *Adv. Parasitol.* **2,** 97–168.

Foreyt, W. J., and Todd, A. C. (1976). Development of the large American liver fluke, *Fascioloides magna*, in white-tailed deer, cattle and sheep. *J. Parasitol.* **62,** 26–32.

Haswell-Elkins, M. R., Sithihaworn, P., and Elkins, D. (1992). *Opisthorchis viverrini* and cholangiocarcinoma in northeast Thailand. *Parasitol. Today* **8,** 86–89.

Healy, G. R. (1970). Trematodes transmitted to man by fish, frogs, and crustacea. *J. Wildlife Dis.* **6,** 255–261.

Jensen, P. C., Mapes, C. R., and Whitlock, J. H. (1955). Pasture management and control of the lancet fluke, *Dicrocoelium dendriticum* (Rudolphi, 1819) Looss, 1899. *Cornell Vet.* **45,** 526–538.

Kendall, S. B. (1970). Relationships between species of *Fasciola* and their molluscan hosts. *Adv. Parasitol.* **8,** 251–258.

Komiya, Y. (1966). *Clonorchis* and clonorchiasis. *Adv. Parasitol.* **4,** 53–106.

Malek, E. A. (1980a). Clonorchiasis. In *Snail-Transmitted Parasitic Diseases* (E. A. Malek, Ed.), Vol. 2, pp. 67–89. CRC Press, Boca Raton, FL.

Malek, E. A. (1980b). Opisthorchiasis. In *Snail-Transmitted Parasitic Diseases* (E. A. Malek, Ed.), Vol. 2, pp. 91–105. CRC Press, Boca Raton, FL.

Malone, J. B. (1986). Fascioliasis and cestodiasis in cattle. *Vet. Clin. North Am. Food Anim. Practice* **2,** 261–275.

Ollerenshaw, C. B., and Smith, L. P. (1969). Meteorological factors and forecasts of helminthic diseases. *Adv. Parasitol.* **7,** 283–323.

Pantelouris, E. M. (1965). *The Common Liver Fluke*. Pergamon, New York.

Reinhard, E. G. (1957). Landmarks in parasitology. I. The discovery of the life cycle of the liver fluke. *Exp. Parasitol.* **6,** 208–232.

Rim, H.-J., Farag, H. F., Sornmani, S., and Cross, J. H. (1994). Foodborne trematodes: Ignored or emerging? *Parasitol. Today* **10,** 207–209.

Stoll, N. R. (1947). This wormy world. *J. Parasitol.* **33,** 1–18.

Tarry, D. W. (1969). *Dicrocoelium dendriticum*: The life cycle in Britain. *J. Helminthol.* **43,** 403–416.

Wykoff, D. E., Harinasuta, C., Juttijudata, P., and Winn, M. M. (1965). *Opisthorchis viverrini* in Thailand—The life cycle and comparison with *O. felineus*. *J. Parasitol.* **51,** 207–214.

Yoshimura, H. (1965). The life cycle of *Clonorchis sinensis*: A comment on the presentation in the seventh edition of Craig and Faust's *Clinical Parasitology*. *J. Parasitol.* **51,** *961–966.*

CHAPTER

20

The Intestinal Flukes

On a worldwide basis, between 20 and 30 million humans have intestinal infections with digenetic flukes. Most are small flukes that cause little or no pathology. It is only massive or ectopic infections that result in clinical problems. We will consider three major families in this chapter.

ECHINOSTOMATIDAE

Name of Organism and Disease Associations

Echinostomatosis is caused by flukes in the family Echinostomatidae. Possibly 8 genera and 15 species from this family infect humans (Tab. 20.1), and the potential for additional human infections is great because some adult flukes typically have low host specificity. A good example of low host specificity is the North American parasite, *Echinostoma trivolvis;* the adult parasitizes at least 26 species of birds and 13 mammals, including humans. Miracidia infect *Helisoma trivolvis*, and metacercariae are found in many snail species, fingernail clams, tadpoles, and possibly fish.

Hosts and Host Range

Some echinostomes are incidental intestinal parasites of humans. Natural definitive hosts include many birds and small mammals.

Geographic Distribution and Importance

The largest number of human echinostome infections are in the Far East (Tab. 20.1). Except for an occasional massive human infection, most cause little or no pathology. Some echinostomes in poultry and small mammals cause economic losses.

Morphology

Echinostomes are medium sized distome flukes (4–12 mm by 1–3 mm) (Fig. 20.1). The most prominent structural feature is the collar of large spines surrounding the oral sucker, from which the name, *echinostome* is derived. The number, size, and position of spines are of taxonomic value. Collar spines are present in most cercariae (Fig. 20.2), metacercariae, and adult worms (Fig. 20.3). The acetabulum is usually larger than the oral sucker; the genital pore is median, and the cirrus pouch is well developed. The uterus is entirely anterior to the ovary and vitelline follicles are abundant; a seminal receptacle is lacking.

Life Cycle

Unembryonated operculate eggs are shed in feces; miracidia hatch in about 14 days and penetrate snails. A sporocyst generation is followed by two or more generations of rediae. Many echinostome rediae possess lateral body protrusions called *lappets* or *procrusculi* (Fig. 20.4), locomotor appendages that enable rediae to crawl. Echinostome cercariae leave daughter rediae through birth pores located near the anterior end of rediae. Most echinostome cercariae have spines in patterns similar to those of the adults.

Cercariae can encyst (1) in the same snail in which they developed, (2) in other snail species, (3) on snail shells, or (4) on the surfaces of fish, bivalves, and tad-

TABLE 20.1 Major Echinostome Parasites of Humans

Organism	Source of human infection	Geographic distribution	
		Organism	Human infection
Echinostoma trivolvis	Bivalves	North America	North America
Echinostoma malayanum	Snail	Far East	Malaysia, Singapore, India, Thailand, Sumatra
Echinostoma echinatum (=*lindoense*)	Clam	Far East	Far East
Echinostoma hortense	Fish	Far East	Japan
Euparyphium ilocanum	Snail	Far East	Java, Philippines

poles. Spines can be seen on the juvenile inside the bilayered metacercarial cyst. Definitive hosts become infected by ingesting metacercariae. They pass to the intestines, excyst, and develop to adults.

Diagnosis

Initial diagnosis of echinostomatiasis is often difficult. The adult worms cause few lesions and hence few clinical symptoms. In addition, the large operculate eggs (85 mm and larger) are easily confused with the large operculate eggs of *Fasciolopsis* and *Fasciola*. A definitive diagnosis is made when adult worms are recovered after anthelmintic treatment is given.

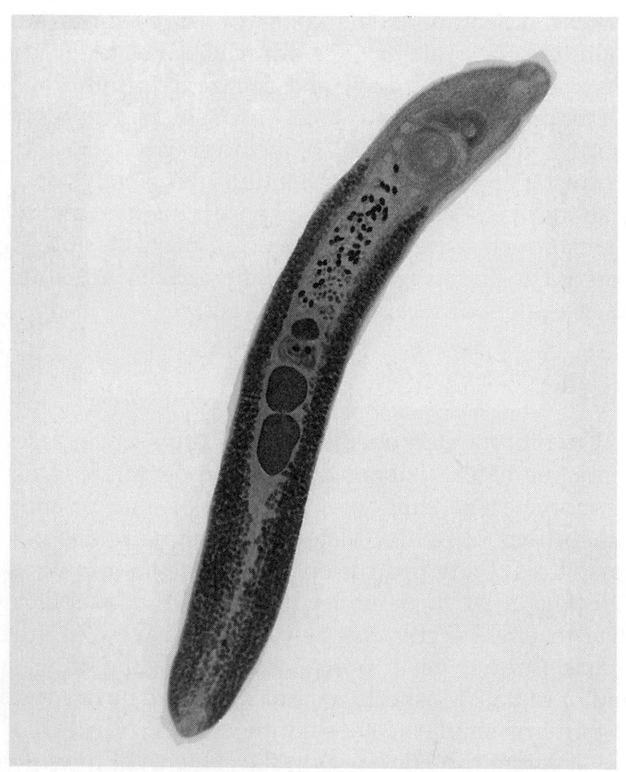

FIGURE 20.1 A photomicrograph of an adult *Echinostomum trivolvis.*

Cultivation

Attempts to culture echinostomes have been partially successful. Metacercariae of several trematode species, including *Echinostoma caproni*, have developed to maturity on chick allantoic membranes.

Host–Parasite Interactions

Most infections with adult echinostomes produce little or no clinical disease, but heavy infections cause diarrhea and abdominal pain.

Epidemiology and Control

Control of echinostomatosis is based on the following:

1. Treatment of infected persons
2. Changing food habits

Almost any vermifuge eliminates echinostomes; praziquantel is the drug of choice.

The lack of host specificity, especially in the metacercarial stage, plus the cosmopolitan distribution of echinostome species suggests that humans are at risk throughout the world. Ingesting uncooked snails, clams, tadpoles, and fish can lead to echinostomatosis. Fortunately, most second intermediate hosts harboring metacercariae are not eaten raw in most parts of the world, and so the number of human infections is far smaller than the potential risk.

A remarkable story in successful control is illustrated for an echinostome species. As recently as 1965, *Echinostoma echinatum* (=*lindoense*) infected over half of the people living around Lake Lindu in Central Sulawesi (Celebes), Indonesia (Fig. 20.5). Mollusks, especially clams (*Corbicula* spp.), were a major source of

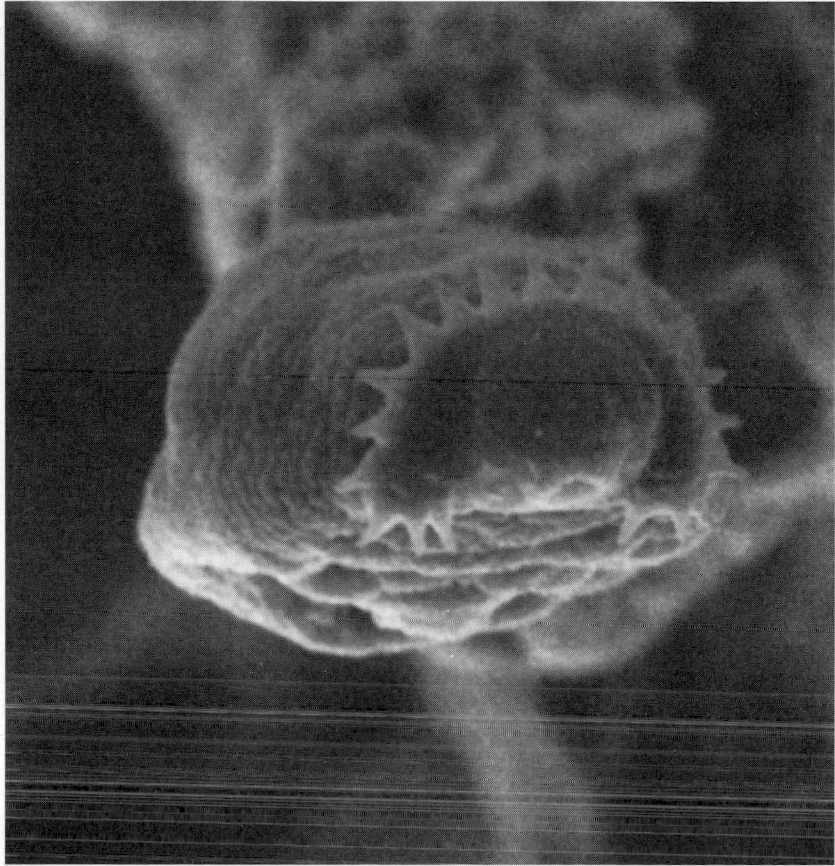

FIGURE 20.2 A "head-on" view of the cercaria of an echinostome fluke as seen in SEM. Note the collar of spines around the oral sucker.

animal protein for the people. The mujair fish *Tilapia mossambica* was introduced into the lake and rapidly became abundant. The people changed their diet from clams to fish. This fish is now a daily item in the Lindu diet and is cooked before it is eaten. Consequently, a survey in 1972 of more than 1400 people revealed no *E. echinatum* infections. Thus, infections with this human parasite were eliminated with just a change in diet. Unfortunately, the more serious parasitic disease caused by *Schistosoma japonicum* (Chapter 18) is still prevalent in the Lake Lindu population and control efforts have had limited success.

Humans are the only known definitive host for *E. echinatum*, but there must be animal reservoirs because the parasite was found in *Biomphalaria* snails in Brazil. Since people there do not eat snails at all, there must be a reservoir host maintaining the life cycle, and risk for humans is present.

Echinostome rediae have been studied extensively as potential predators of other trematode species that do not produce rediae, such as schistosomes (Chapter 18). Echinostome rediae move throughout snails and actively ingest sporocysts. Echinostomes can be used as biological control agents for other trematode species at the local level if high echinostome infection percentages in snails can be achieved in local susceptible snails. This trematode antagonism combined with other means including sanitary, clinical, and biological control might be used to control some human parasites (see also Chapter 18).

Notable Features

The organism with 37 collar spines, formerly known as *Echinostoma revolutum*, was assumed to have little host specificity and have cosmopolitan distribution. It is no longer considered so. Detailed life cycle studies on organisms recovered from the original description location revealed that the first intermediate host is only a lymneaeid snail, and the definitive hosts are birds not mammals. As a consequence of several detailed investigations, we now believe that *E. revolutum* occurs only in Europe and Southeast Asia. The organism found in North America should properly be called

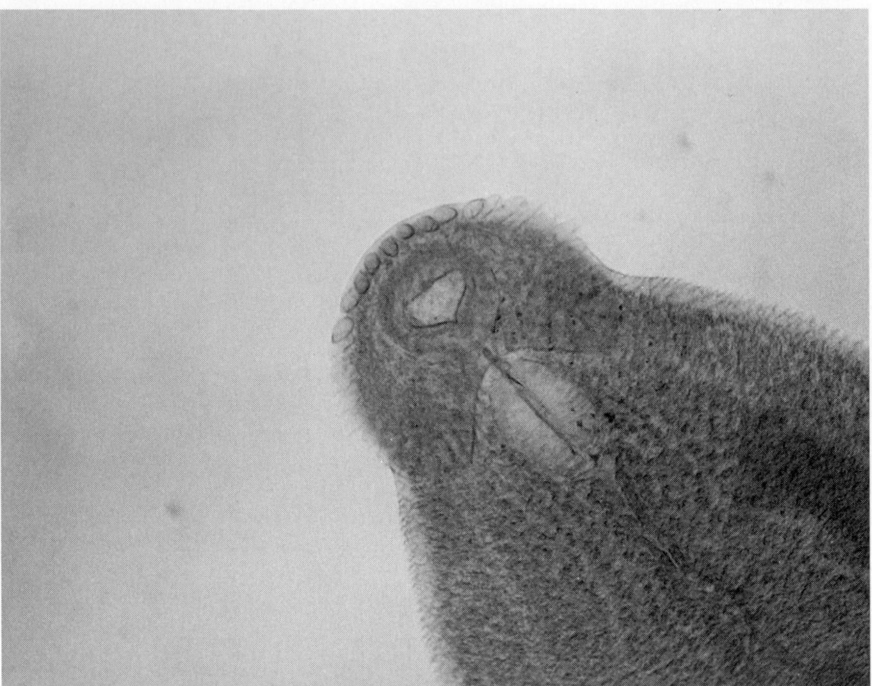

FIGURE 20.3 Anterior portion of an adult echinostome showing the collar of spines around the oral sucker and the heavy spination on the body.

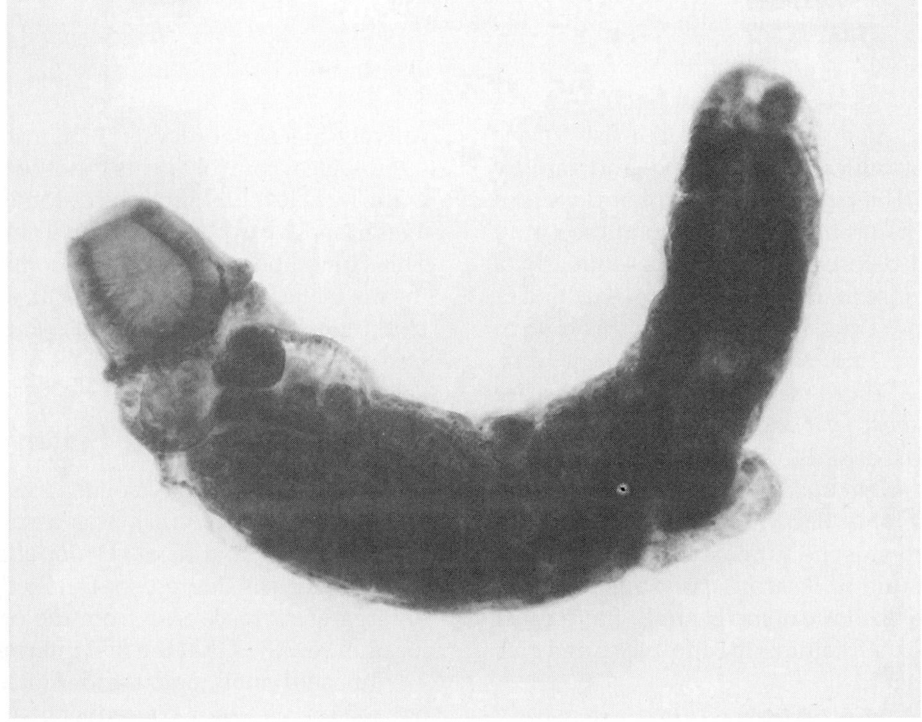

FIGURE 20.4 Redia of an echinostome fluke as seen in LM. Note the prominent pharynx at the left side and one visible procrusculus at the posterior end.

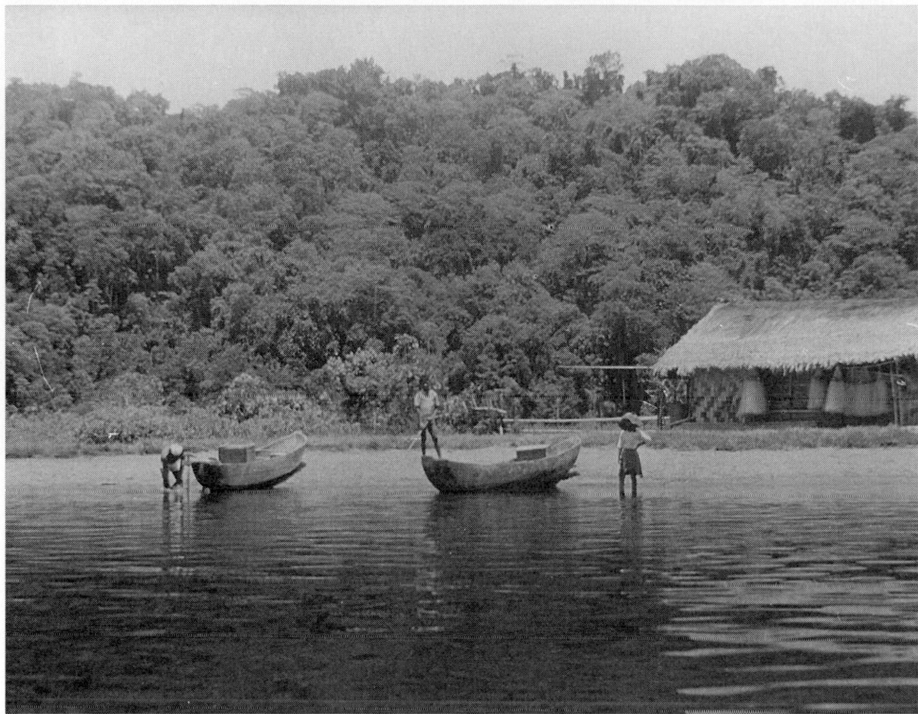

FIGURE 20.5 Lake Lindu in central Sulawesi where human infections with *Echinostoma echinatum* have been eliminated by a change of diet. [Courtesy of Dr. David Kistner.]

Echinostoma trivolvis. The confusion arose when organisms with similar morphology, but differing biology, were called the same name. Parasitology marches ever onward, if only in small, but significant steps, repairing past false notions.

NANOPHYETUS SALMINCOLA AND "SALMON POISONING DISEASE"

Name of Organism and Disease Associations

Nanophyetus salmincola is a small trematode that is the vector for a rickettsia, *Neorickettsia helminthoeca*. The infection is usually fatal to dogs, foxes, and coyotes that ingest fishes infected with flukes containing rickettsia. The resultant disease is called *salmon poisoning disease* (*SPD*), although salmon are neither poisoned nor do they cause the disease.

Hosts and Host Range

The raccoon (*Procyon lotor*) and spotted skunk (*Spilogale putorius*) are the probable principal definitive hosts. Millemann and Knapp (1970) listed 32 natural and experimental host species for the adult fluke. Occasional human infections have been reported from North America. The adult flukes lie in the paramucosal lumen of the small intestine.

Geographic Distribution and Importance

Distribution of the fluke is apparently limited by the range of the single first intermediate host to streams in Washington, Oregon, and northern California. Infections in dogs are sporadic but do cause significant losses each year.

Morphology

Nanophyetus salmincola is 0.8 to 2.5 mm long, with a cirrus sac dorsal to the acetabulum but no cirrus. Vitelline follicles are prominent and uteri typically contain 5 to 16 eggs (Fig. 20.6).

Life Cycle

Eggs are passed unembryonated and require 87 to 200 days to mature and hatch (Fig. 20.6). How miracidia infect snails is unknown. Microcercous xiphidiocercariae develop from rediae and leave the snail with exhalant water currents. Cercariae penetrate the skin of salmonid and other fish and encyst in almost all

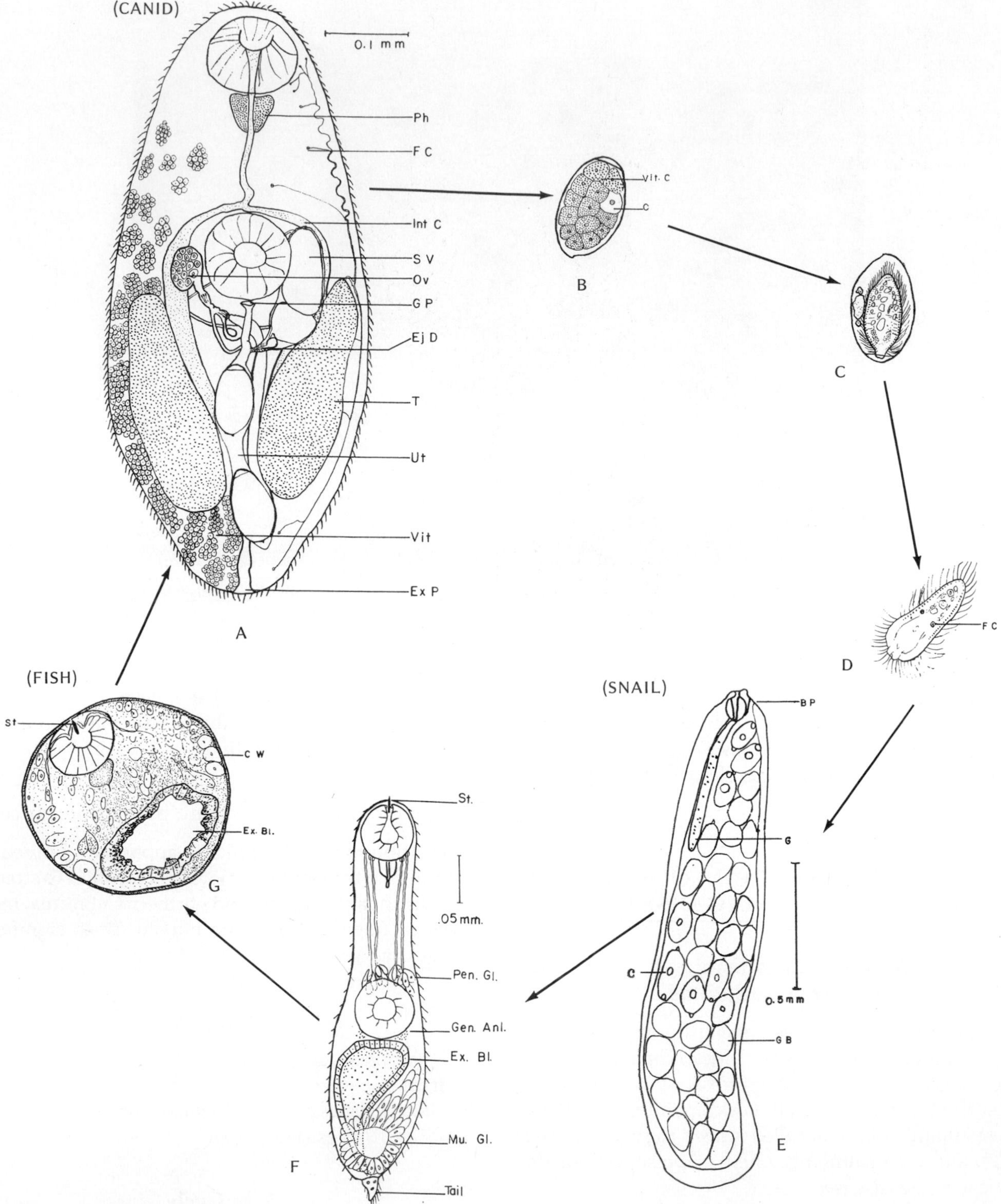

FIGURE 20.6 Life cycle and structure of the adult *Nanophyetus salmincola.* (A) adult; (B) partially embryonated egg; (C) miracidium within egg capsules; (D) free-swimming miracidium; (E) redia in snail; (F) free-swimming cercaria; (G) metacercaria in fish. Abbreviations: B P, birth pore; C, cercaria; C W, cyst wall; Ej D, ejaculatory duct; Ex B, excretory bladder; F C, flame cell; G, gut; Gen Anl, genital primordium; G P, genital pore; Int C, intestinal cecum; Mu Gl, mucus gland; Ov, ovary; Pen Gl, penetration gland; Ph, muscular pharynx. St, stylet; S V, seminal vesicle; T, testis; Ut, uterus; Vt, vitelline gland. [Redrawn from Bennington and Pratt, 1960.]

internal organs, subcutaneous tissue, and fins. Definitive hosts are infected by eating raw or poorly cooked fish containing metacercariae.

Second intermediate hosts are primarily salmonid fishes, but other fish, lamprey, and the giant pacific salamander are also infected. Taxonomy of the snail host currently is uncertain; it has been called *Oxytrema silicula*, *Goniobasis plicifera* var. *silicula*, and *Juga silicula shastaensis*.

Diagnosis

Infection with *N. salmincola* is diagnosed by examining feces for eggs. Infection of dogs with *Neorickettsia helminthoeca* is diagnosed by the appearance of clinical signs along with a history of eating raw fish. Prominent signs are fever, lassitude, and diarrhea.

Host–Parasite Interactions

By far the greatest effects of SPD are in dogs, foxes, and coyotes. Apparently only canids are seriously affected by SPD. Dogs show sudden onset of fever five to seven days after infection, fever fluctuates for a week. Dehydration and anorexia are common. Lymph nodes enlarge as the disease progresses. About 90% of naturally infected canids die within ten days to two weeks after onset of clinical signs, whereas other mammals such as the raccoon and bear may have only transient fever as an indication of low-grade infection.

The reaction to *Nanophyetus* infections in fish ranges from slight to severe lesions depending on the parasite burden. In heavy infections, almost every organ of the fish is affected, especially muscle, gills, and kidneys. Swimming ability is also affected, at least until the metacercariae encyst.

Epidemiology and Control

Control of infection with *Nanophyetus* and SPD is quite limited:

1. Treatment of infected dogs
2. Preventing dogs from eating raw salmon or their entrails

Antibiotics, including chloramphenicol and oxytetracycline, as well as sulfonamides are used to treat SPD. Canids that recover from SPD are immune to the rickettsia, but not to *Nanophyetus salmincola*.

SPD is unique because its vector is a trematode; other rickettsiae such as *Rickettsia* and *Ehrlichia* are transmitted by ticks and lice. Rickettsiae have been reported in all stages of *N. salmincola*, and there is transovarial transmission. It appears that salmon become infected while still in fresh water; they maintain both the metacercarial and rickettsial infections for three to seven years while in the ocean. The infections are then transmitted to the definitive host when the salmon return to fresh water to spawn.

The only realistic control for SPD is to keep dogs away from streams during salmon migration and not to feed dogs salmon entrails. The swiftly flowing streams make snail control using molluscicides virtually impossible. Treatment of dogs when signs of infection have appeared will help the individual dog, but will not have much effect on the general problem.

Other Subspecies

A Siberian subspecies, *Nanophyetus salmincola schikholbalowi*, has a similar life cycle; salmonids and other fishes serve as second intermediate hosts. Some human populations in Siberian villages are reported to have infection percentages of 95 to 98%. These infections result in various gastrointestinal disturbances including diarrhea and gastric pain. More than 500 parasites have been reported from one human host. No SPD organism has been found in the Siberian subspecies of fluke.

HETEROPHYIDAE

Name of Organism and Disease Associations

Some members of the family Heterophyidae cause heterophyidosis or heterophyosis. These small flukes parasitize the intestines of fish-eating birds and mammals, including humans. Most important, from a medical standpoint, are *Heterophyes heterophyes* and *Metagonimus yokogawai*.

Hosts and Host Range

Heterophyes heterophyes infects four genera of snails, *Tympanotomus, Melania, Cleopatra,* and *Pirenella* spp. The second intermediate hosts are at least 11 genera of fishes and shrimp. Definitive hosts are fish eaters including cats, foxes, wolves, weasels, birds, and occasionally humans.

Geographic Distribution and Importance

Human infections with heterophyiids are cosmopolitan. Most infections occur in Southeast Asia and are limited to areas where raw or semi-cooked fish and shrimp are eaten.

Morphology

Heterophyes heterophyes is a small (1.0 to 1.7 mm by 0.3 to 0.4 mm) fluke. The adults are densely covered with spines. The acetabulum is medial or submedial and is associated with a *gonotyl* or genital sucker, which has 60 to 90 spines on its margin (Fig. 20.7). No cirrus pouch or cirrus are present. Eggs are oval and measure 28 to 30 by 15 to 17 mm.

Life Cycle

Adults are parasitic in the intestines of cats, dogs, foxes, wolves, weasels, fish-eating birds, and humans. Eggs are passed containing fully developed miracidia. Snails (*Tympanotomus microptera, Melania tuberculata, Cleopatra bulimoides,* and *Pirenella conica*) ingest the eggs. Following sporocyst and two generations of rediae, opthalmolophocercous cercariae are released. Metacercariae encyst in muscles of fish including *Mugil* sp. and *Tilapia* sp. Definitive hosts ingest metacercariae in uncooked or undercooked fish.

Diagnosis

Finding heterophyid eggs in feces is not definitive because these eggs cannot reliably be distinguished from those of *Metagonimus yokogawai* and closely resemble those of *Clonorchis sinensis* and *Opisthorchis* spp. Therefore, the only definitive diagnosis is made by finding adult worms after administration of an anthelmintic.

Host–Parasite Interactions

Human infections usually produce mild intestinal disturbances. Extra-intestinal infections by ova and adults may cause significant clinical problems, depending on location such as heart, brain, liver, spleen, or lungs.

Infections in dogs produce mild intestinal disturbances to persistent diarrhea.

Epidemiology and Control

The drug of choice is praziquantel. Snail hosts are estuarine and brackish-water dwellers. Poor sanitation in these areas maintains infections. Multiple reservoir hosts also maintain sizable populations, rendering control efforts difficult. Realistic human prevention is achieved through education about proper cooking of fish.

Other Heterophyids

The other heterophyid most responsible for human disease is *Metagonimus yokogawai*. The snail host, *Semi-*

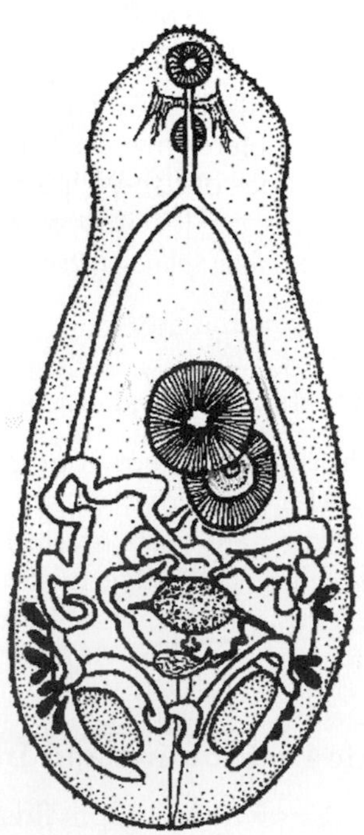

FIGURE 20.7 Adult of *Heterophyes heterophyes*. Note the gonotyl, a spiny structure surrounding the genital pore, which lies to the right of and partly covered by the acetabulum.

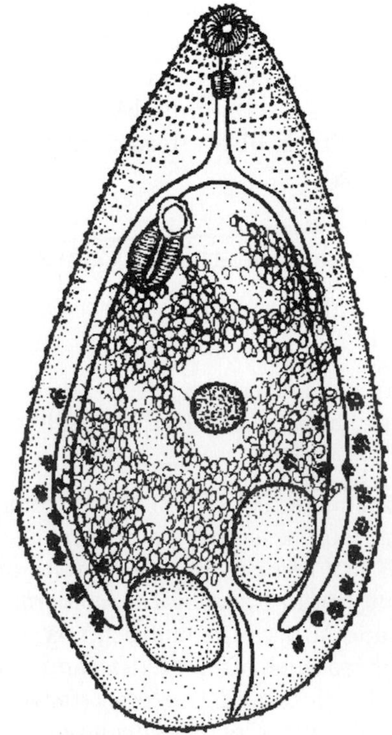

FIGURE 20.8 Adult of *Metagonimus yokogawi*.

SURVEYS

THE PARASITOLOGIC LITERATURE IS full of surveys of hosts enumerating the parasite fauna in certain animals or humans. In the literature prior to about 1960, a good deal of survey work was done, but even today, some journals publish surveys. These studies usually concentrate on either a particular locale or host, usually both. Such studies are often called "classical parasitology," a term that is somewhat derogatory.

Host examinations are often carried out by an investigator over a period of from two to ten years or more. The protists or helminths are removed from the host, prepared for microscopic examination, and identified. Lists and tables are prepared with the numbers and seasons at which all of the parasites were found as well as the organ systems where they were located.

It is certainly relevant to ask why anyone would want to do such a thing as rummaging through the carcasses of scores of dead animals—and worse, looking for worms, of all things. The answer has a number of parts.

Parasitology as a distinct science is only about a hundred years old; prior to that time, physicians, veterinarians, and zoologists investigated parasites as a part other interests. Then, as specialization became necessary, parasitology became a separate science. A good deal of intellectual curiosity was behind many of the surveys that were done in the late 19th and early 20th centuries. Many people just wanted to see what was there; it was clear that the more they looked, the more parasites they found. All scientific disciplines begin by collecting and cataloging; as knowledge accumulates, patterns begin to form and theories are set forth. The principal journal for the publication of parasitologic papers in North America, *The Journal of Parasitology*, was founded by Dr. Henry B. Ward only in 1914, and many of its early papers described new parasites and the parasitic fauna of many vertebrate hosts. It was all new and exciting.

In human and animal medicine, it is often necessary to define the problem. Let's say that there is a tropical island in the Pacific Ocean where the inhabitants have poor health and often die at an early age. A team of scientists, physicians, and technicians would come in and, through serology, clinical signs and symptoms, fecal examinations, autopsies, and statistical compilations, determine what the major illnesses are. Then, having defined the problem, solutions can be sought. The survey, of whatever sort, is essential before any other applied studies can be fruitful.

There are baseline studies that often need to be done. If a major project such as a dam, an open pit mine, or a toxic chemical storage facility is to be built, one needs to know what organisms are there at the beginning so that changes can be predicted or described later. When the high dam at Aswan in Egypt was proposed, baseline studies had already been done on the prevalence and importance of schistosomosis. Scientists were therefore able to predict that schistosomosis would become worse in the Nile River drainage, and their predictions were borne out.

Evolution is the glue that holds biology together. It is an agreed-upon principle that biologists use to elucidate relationships among organisms and to pick apart the mechanisms by which evolution proceeds. Collections are made of all kinds of animals and plants to develop further our concepts in evolution. Parasites are sometimes good material to use in these studies, and since there are more species of parasites than free-living animals, it seems right to include them in any investigation.

Perhaps, only perhaps, we have gone beyond the need to catalog parasites in various localities, but there are larger issues that may require such collections now and in the future.

sculospira libertina, is found in Formosa, Japan, Korea, East Indies, Philippines, China, and Ukraine. Similar fish-eating definitive hosts maintain the life cycle. Human infections have been reported from the Balkans, Spain, Israel, the former Soviet Union, and Indonesia. The gonotyl of this species is off-center and is fused with the acetabulum (Fig. 20.8). Other aspects of biology and control are identical with *Heterophyes heterophyes*.

Readings

Basch, P. F., and Di Conza, J. J. (1975). Predation by echinostome rediae upon schistosome sporocysts in vitro. *J. Parasitol.* **61,** 1044–1047.

Bennington, E., and Pratt, I. (1960). The life history of the salmon-poisoning fluke, *Nanophyetus salmincola* (Chapin). *J. Parasitol.* **46,** 91–100.

Chien, W. Y., and Fried, B. (1992). Cultivation of encysted metacercariae of *Echinostoma caproni* to ovigerous adults in the allantois of the chick embryo. *J. Parasitol.* **78,** 1019–1023.

Clarke, M. D., Carney, W. P., Cross, J. H., Hadidjaja, P., Oemijati, S., and Joesoef, A. (1974). Schistosomiasis and other human parasitoses of Lake Lindu in Central Sulawesi (Celebes), Indonesia. *Am. J. Trop. Med. Hyg.* **23,** 385–392.

Dawes, B. (1968). *The Trematoda.* Cambridge Univ. Press, Cambridge, UK.

Eastburn, R. L., Fritsche, T. R., and Terhune, C. A., Jr. (1987). Human intestinal infection from salmonid fishes. *Am. J. Trop. Med. Hyg.* **36,** 586–591.

Healy, G. R. (1970). Trematodes transmitted to man by fish, frogs, and crustacea. *J. Wildlife Dis.* **6,** 255–261.

Hillyer, G. V. (1981). Introduction to the trematode zoonoses. In *The Parasitic Zoonoses* (G. V. Hillyer, Ed.). CRC Press, Boca Raton, FL.

Huffman, J. E., and Fried, B. (1990). *Echinostoma* and Echinostomiasis. *Adv. Parasitol.* **29,** 215–269.

Kanev, I. (1994). Life-cycle, delimitation and redescription of *Echinostoma revolutum* (Froelich, 1802) (Trematoda: Echinostomatidae). *Syst. Parasitol.* **28,** 125–144.

Lim, H., and Heyneman, D. (1972). Intramolluscan inter trematode antagonism: A review of factors influencing the host–parasite system and its possible role in biological control. *Adv. Parasitol.* **10,** 191–268.

Malek, E. A. (1980). Echinostomiasis. In *Snail Transmitted Diseases* (E. A. Malek, Ed.), Vol. 2, pp. 245–259. CRC Press, Boca Raton, FL.

Marcial-Rojas, R. A. (1971). Rare intestinal flukes. In *Pathology of Protozoal and Helminthic Diseases* (R. A. Marcial-Rojas, Ed.), pp. 469–476. Williams & Wilkins, Baltimore.

Millemann, R. E., and Knapp, S. E. (1970). Biology of *Nanophyetus salmincola* and "salmon poisoning" disease. *Adv. Parasitol.* **8,** 1–41.

Phillip, C. B. (1955). There's always something new under the "parasitological" sun (the unique story of the helminth-borne salmon poisoning disease). *J. Parasitol.* **41,** 125–148.

Taylor, D. W. (1981). Freshwater mollusks of California: A distributional checklist. *California Fish Game* **67,** 140–163.

Ulmer, M. J. (1975). Other trematode infections. In *Diseases Transmitted from Animals to Man* (W. T. Hubbert, W. F. McCollough, and P. R. Schnurrenberger, Eds.), 6th ed., pp. 646–677. Charles C Thomas, Springfield, IL.

Velasquez, C. C. (1982). Heterophyidiasis. In *The Handbook Series in Zoonoses*, Vol. 3. CRC Press, Boca Raton, FL.

CHAPTER

21

The Lung Flukes

A number of mammals, including humans, are infected by lung flukes of the genus *Paragonimus*; Yokogawa (1982) listed more than 30 species of flukes, at least seven of which are implicated in human disease.

PARAGONIMUS WESTERMANI

Name of Organism and Disease Associations

Paragonimus westermani is the most important species infecting humans; it causes paragonimosis, paragonimiasis, pulmonary distomiasis, and endemic hemoptysis (expectoration of bloody sputum).

Hosts and Host Range

Hosts are carnivores including tigers, lions, leopards, feral cats, pigs, dogs, monkeys, and humans. Adult flukes are found in lungs, but may also be found in almost any body organ or tissue; 30 to 60% of extrapulmonary paragonimoses were either cerebral or spinal cord infections.

Geographic Distribution and Importance

The organism is distributed in China, Japan, Taiwan, Korea, the former Soviet Union, Philippines, Thailand, Indonesia, India, and Sri Lanka. In Korea alone, between 1.0 and 1.5 million people are infected.

Morphology

Adult flukes are 7 to 12 mm long with a thick, spiny tegument; a small acetabulum is located just anterior to the middle of the body. Often one must remove some tegument and vitellaria to discern the reproductive organ structure. Two posterior lobed testes are present; the ovary is also branched and is located slightly posterior to the acetabulum. There is no cirrus or cirrus pouch. The genital pore is posterior to the acetabulum. Eggs are operculate, irregularly barrel-shaped, and are 80 to 120 μm by 48 to 60 μm (Fig. 21.1) in size.

Life Cycle

Eggs are shed in sputum, or coughed up, swallowed, and then shed in feces (Fig. 21.2); they hatch in two to three weeks and remain alive for several months at low temperatures. Miracidia penetrate the first intermediate host, operculate snails of the family Thiaridae; *Semisulcospira libertina* is the most important first intermediate host. Sporocysts develop in the snail and produce mother rediae, which, in turn, produce

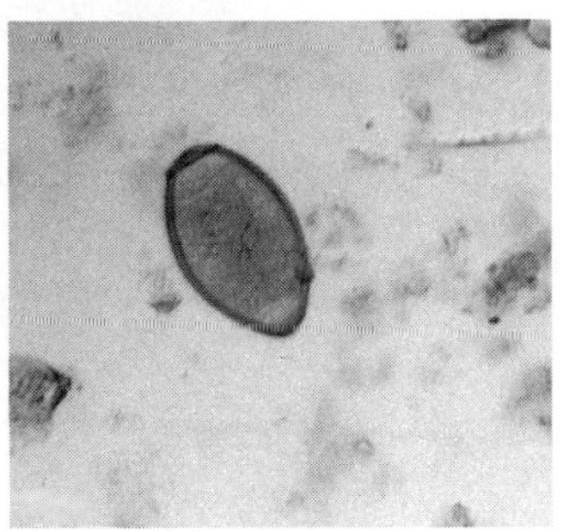

FIGURE 21.1 Egg of *Paragonimus*.

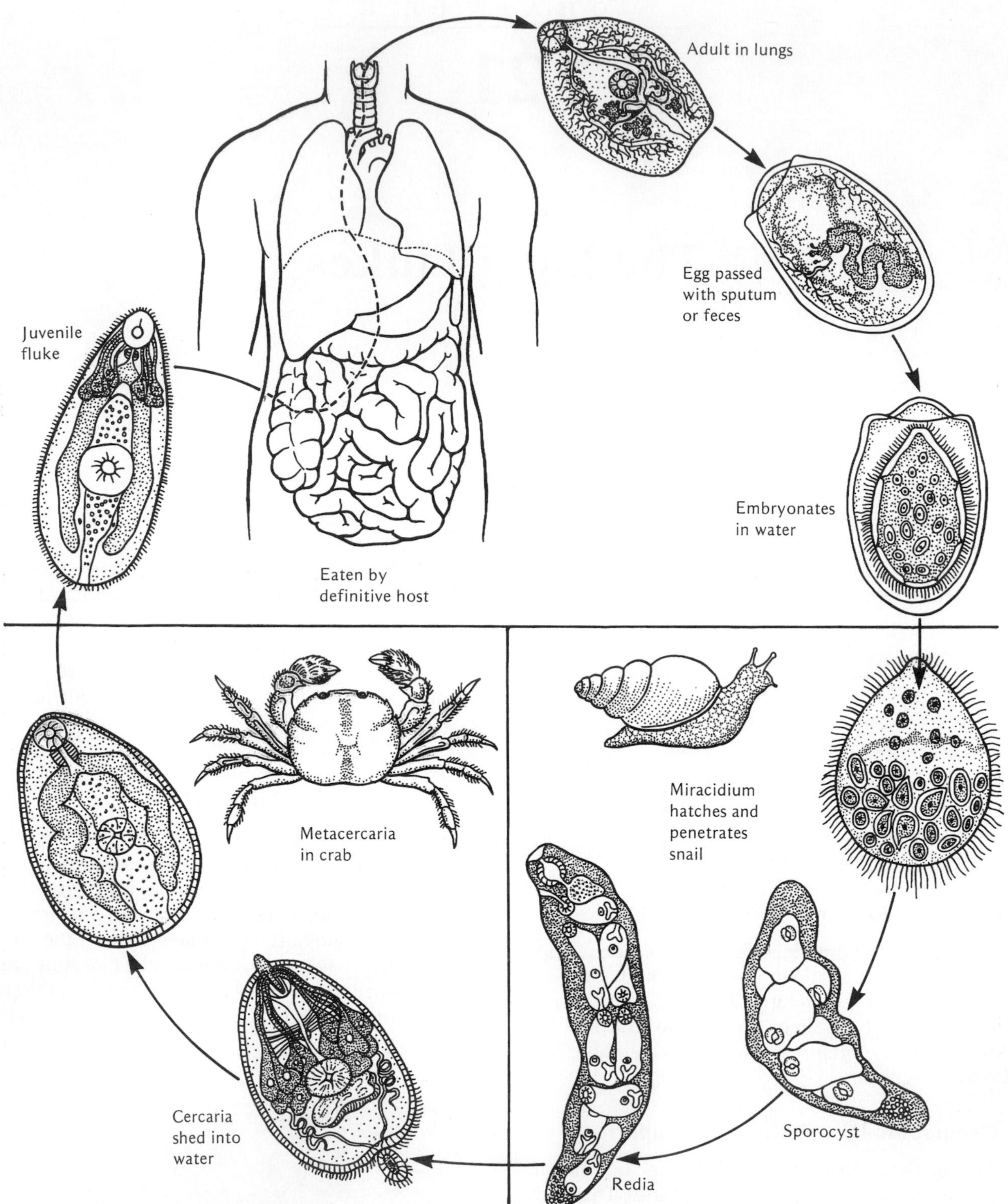

FIGURE 21.2 Life cycle and structure of *Paragonimus westermani.*

daughter rediae. Microcercous cercariae emerge from the snails approximately 13 weeks after infection.

Crayfish and freshwater crabs are second intermediate hosts for *P. westermani*. Microcercous cercariae crawl along stream beds until they are eaten or penetrate joints of the exoskeleton. If crustacea ingest infected snails, they become infected. Metacercariae encyst in the gills, legs, body muscles, and viscera.

Definitive hosts, including humans, are infected by eating raw or poorly cooked crab or crayfish containing metacercariae. When the metacercariae reach the small intestine, the juvenile flukes are activated and escape from the cyst. Juvenile flukes penetrate the intestinal walls and enter abdominal wall muscles, where they remain for 5 to 7 days and then reenter the abdominal cavity. Young flukes penetrate the diaphragm and enter the pleural cavity about 14 days after infection. Seventy days after the infection, the flukes are mature and produce eggs. Humans have also been infected by eating paratenic hosts such as wild boars, wild pigs, monkeys, and probably other small mammals.

Diagnosis

There are two methods of determining whether a patient is infected with *P. westermani:*

1. Finding eggs in sputum or feces
2. Finding antibodies to the organism in the blood

Diagnosis should include microscopic examination of sputum and feces for large operculate eggs (Fig. 21.1). Sputum should be examined following centrifugation and sedimentation in 1 to 2% NaOH. Charcot-Leyden crystals in sputum help to confirm the diagnosis; these crystals are associated with monocytes. Serodiagnostic tests have been developed to identify *Paragonimus* infections and are especially useful in diagnosing extrapulmonary paragonimiasis and in evaluating chemotherapy. Intradermal tests distinguish between paragonimiasis and tuberculosis, but not among various *Paragonimus* spp. Nor can they identify a clinical cure. The most reliable serodiagnostic tools available are complement-fixation and precipitation tests.

Host–Parasite Interactions

There are three characteristic lung lesions in paragonimosis. First are granulomata around eggs (Fig. 21.3). This host response is similar to that around schistosome eggs in liver, bladder, and intestines (Chapter 18). Granulomata typically have fibroblasts, lymphocytes, and eosinophils encircling the eggs.

The second lesions are cysts or distoma cysts in which both worms and eggs are encapsulated by fibrous granulation tissue of fibroblasts, lymphocytes, macrophages, eosinophils, and mononuclear cells. Calcification may occur in chronic paragonimosis. Apparently, two worms are necessary for formation of a cyst, but surgery usually yields cysts with only one worm. Two worms appear to be present initially, but one of the two dies during chronic infection.

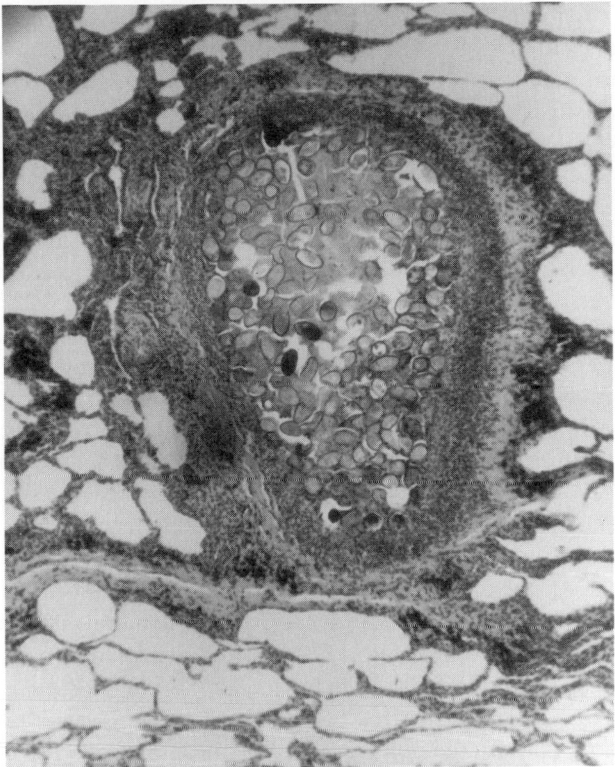

FIGURE 21.3 A histologic section of human lung showing the granulomatous response around the eggs of *Paragonimus*.

The third type of lesion is abscess cavities caused by necrosis of lung tissue and the subsequent liquefaction of this tissue and often of the worms and eggs as well.

Rarely, young worms wander in ectopic sites such as the brain, where they cause localized hemorrhage and inflammatory responses. These usually do not cause significant pathology.

Epidemiology and Control

In theory, at least, there are four methods for controlling paragomimosis:

1. Changing food habits
2. Controlling snails
3. Treating infected individuals
4. Eliminating reservoir hosts

Adequate cooking of the crustacean intermediate hosts kills metacercariae and prevents infection. Unfortunately, cultural preferences sometimes interfere with satisfactory control. In Japan crabs are usually eaten well cooked, but a common practice is to prepare vegetables using the same chopping block and cutlery immediately after preparation of the crab. Thus, metacercariae are transferred to other foods or to the mouth. In China "drunken crab" is a delicacy. Crabs are immersed in wine for about 12 hours before being eaten, resulting in infection rates approaching 100%. The raw or undercooked crab or crayfish eaten in many other parts of the world leads to paragonimosis.

In Japan 136 human cases of paragonimosis were acquired when people ate raw pork and wild boar that were paratenic hosts for *Paragonimus westermani*; metacercariae were located in the somatic muscles of these hosts.

Control of paragonimosis through eliminating the snail host has not been successful because their habitat is rapidly flowing water. Elimination of crustacean second intermediate hosts is impractical because they are both a valuable source of protein and a culinary delicacy. Adequate cooking of crabs and crayfish, cleanliness of food preparation utensils, and drug treatment for adult worms offer the most promise for control. Also, other meat from possible transport hosts must be well cooked.

The current drug of choice is praziquantel.

OTHER SPECIES OF *PARAGONIMUS*

Knowledge of the taxonomy and biology of most species of *Paragonimus* is still fragmentary. *P. miyazakii* in Japan, *P. africanus* in the Cameroon and Congo, and *P. uterobilateralis* in Nigeria are also etiological agents of pulmonary paragonimosis in humans; subcutaneous paragonimosis is caused by *P. skrjabini* in China and *P. heterotremus* in China, Thailand, and Laos.

In the Western Hemisphere human pulmonary paragonimosis was previously attributed to *P. westermani*. Only *P. peruvianus* (syn. *P. mexicanus*, *P. ecuadorensis*), found in Ecuador and Peru, is now thought to cause human paragonimiasis. The status of other Western Hemisphere *Paragonimus* species is currently uncertain.

P. kellicotti is a lung fluke widely distributed in the eastern United States and Canada. Definitive hosts include cat, dog, pig, goat, mink, muskrat, bobcat, raccoon, opossum, skunk, red fox, coyote, and weasel. *P. kellicotti* can be distinguished from *P. westermani* and other species by its ovarian shape and the thickness of the inner metacercarial wall. *P. kellicotti* occasionally infects humans.

Readings

Chung, C. H. (1971). Human paragonimiasis (pulmonary distosomiasis, endemic hemoptysis). In *Pathology of Protozoal and Helminthic Diseases* (R. A. Marcial-Rojas, Ed.), pp. 504–535. Williams & Wilkins, Baltimore.

Hillyer, G. V. (1981). Immunoserology of fascioliasis, paragonimiasis, and clonochiasis. In *Immunoserology of Parasitic Diseases* (K. Walls, Ed.). Decker, New York.

Ishii, Y. (1966). Differential morphology of *Paragonimus kellicotti* in North America. *J. Parasitol.* **52,** 920–925.

Miyazaki, I. (1982). Paragonimiasis. In *Handbook Series in Zoonoses* (J. H. Steele, Ed.), Vol. 3. CRC Press, Boca Raton, FL.

Miyazaki, I., and Habe, S. (1976). A newly recognized mode of human infection with the human lung fluke, *Paragonimus westermani* (Kerbert, 1878). *J. Parasitol.* **62,** 646–648.

Noble, G. A. (1963). Experimental infection of crabs with *Paragonimus*. *J. Parasitol.* **49,** 352.

Stromberg, P. C., and Dubey, J. P. (1978). The life cycle of *Paragonimus kellicotti*, in cats. *J. Parasitol.* **64,** 998–1002.

Yokogawa, M. (1965). *Paragonimus* and paragonimiasis. *Adv. Parasitol.* **3,** 99–158.

Yokogawa, M. (1969). *Paragonimus* and paragonimiasis. *Adv. Parasitol.* **7,** 375–387.

Yokogawa, M. (1982). Paragonimiasis. In *The Handbook Series in Zoonoses* (J. H. Steele, Ed.), Vol. 3. CRC Press, Boca Raton, FL.

CHAPTER

22

The Cercomeromorphae: The Monogeneans and the Cestodes, the Tapeworms

SUBCLASS MONOGENEA

The subclass Monogenea may be recognized by the small size of the adults, mostly from 5 mm to less than 1 mm in length, a body usually divided into two regions, the body and the opisthaptor or posterior holdfast. The oral sucker is not often well developed and internal structures are difficult to see in most stained specimens. As indicated by the name, the Monogenea have direct life cycles, that is, there are no biological vectors. The Monogenea generally are ectoparasites of aquatic, poikilothermic vertebrates, mostly fish. They are found on the gills and, less often, in the mouth, urinary bladder, and ureters. Within the limits of hosts and an aquatic environment, the Monogenea have been highly successful; thousands of species have been described from all parts of the world.

Members of the subclass Monogenea are all parasitic flatworms, most with simple one-host cycles, hence the designation "one beginning." They are typically ectoparasites of aquatic vertebrates, especially on the skin and gills of fishes. They feed on mucus, epithelial cells, and blood from wounds inflicted by their hooks. Usually they are not pathogenic, but massive infections may occur in artificial situations such as fish hatcheries and ponds, resulting in serious pathology and economic loss. *Dactylogyrus*, *Gyrodactylus*, *Microcotyle*, *Ancyrocephalus*, and *Benedenia* have caused deaths in fish by suffocation and by wounds that permitted fatal bacterial infections to develop. Whether ectoparasitic or endoparasitic, most monogeneans are both host- and site-specific.

Morphology

Adult monogeneans are oval to circular and range from 1 mm to 3 cm long. The most characteristic structure is the large, complex posterior holdfast or opisthaptor. In the subclass Monopisthocotylea, the opisthaptor is usually a single muscular disk that develops directly from the larval (oncomiracidial) haptor. Usually 1 to 3 pairs of large hooks (anchors) and 2 to 16 small hooks (hooklets) are present (Fig. 22.1). Eyes are usually present, but a genitointestinal canal is absent.

In the order Polyopisthocotylea, eyes are usually absent and a genitointestinal canal is present. The opisthaptors in this subclass are quite complex, with multiple suckers, clamps, and hooks (Fig. 22.2). The anterior holdfast, the prohaptor, is far less spectacular. It may simply have glands opening through head organs and marginal ducts, one or more muscular suckers surrounding the mouth, or head lappets.

Monogeneans are hermaphroditic and usually cross fertilize; male and female reproductive organs are similar to those of the Digenea and will not be discussed in detail here. A notable difference from the Digenea is the genitointestinal canal present in many Polyopisthocotylea. This is a tube that connects part of the intestine with the oviduct or ootype (Fig. 22.3). The function of this connecting tube remains obscure, but three suggestions have been put forth. First, many free-living Turbellaria also possess this structure, and those who work on Turbellaria regard this as evidence that eggs were once discharged via the intestine or mouth; thus, it is a primitive oviduct/uterus. Second, it may be an intestinal pouch, much like the human appendix.

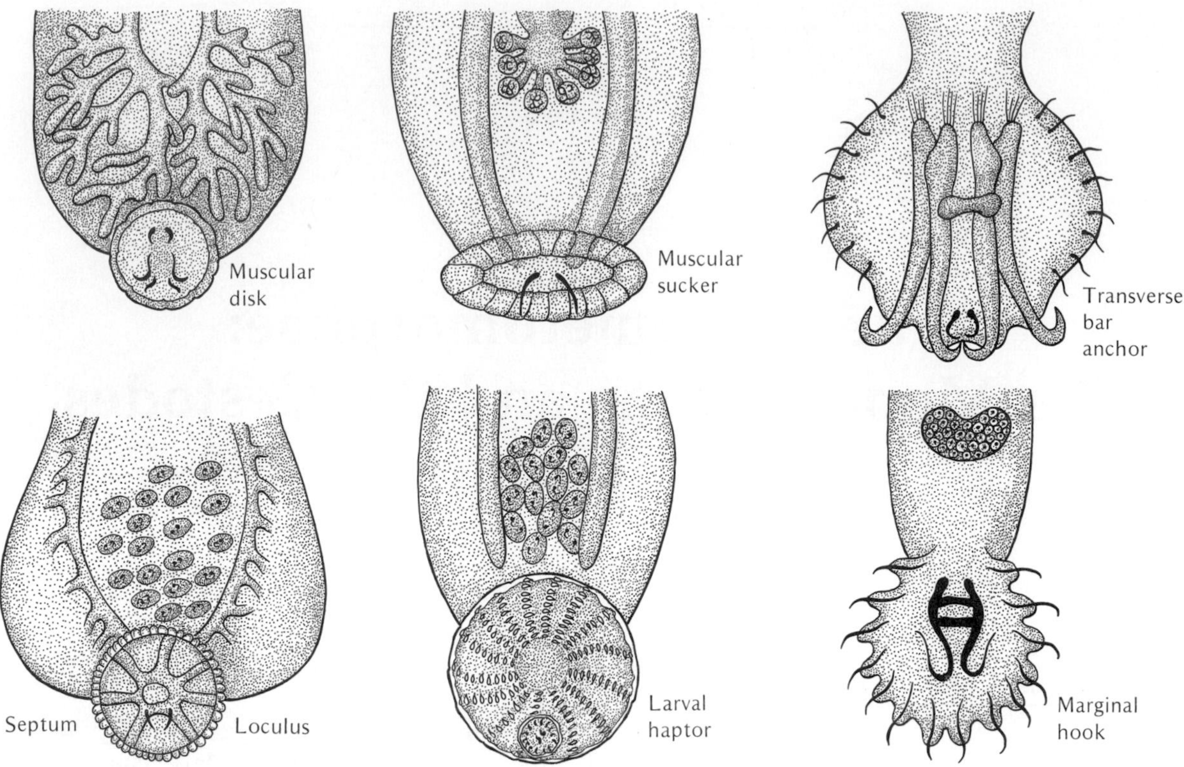

FIGURE 22.1 Opisthaptors of members of the Monopisthocotylea.

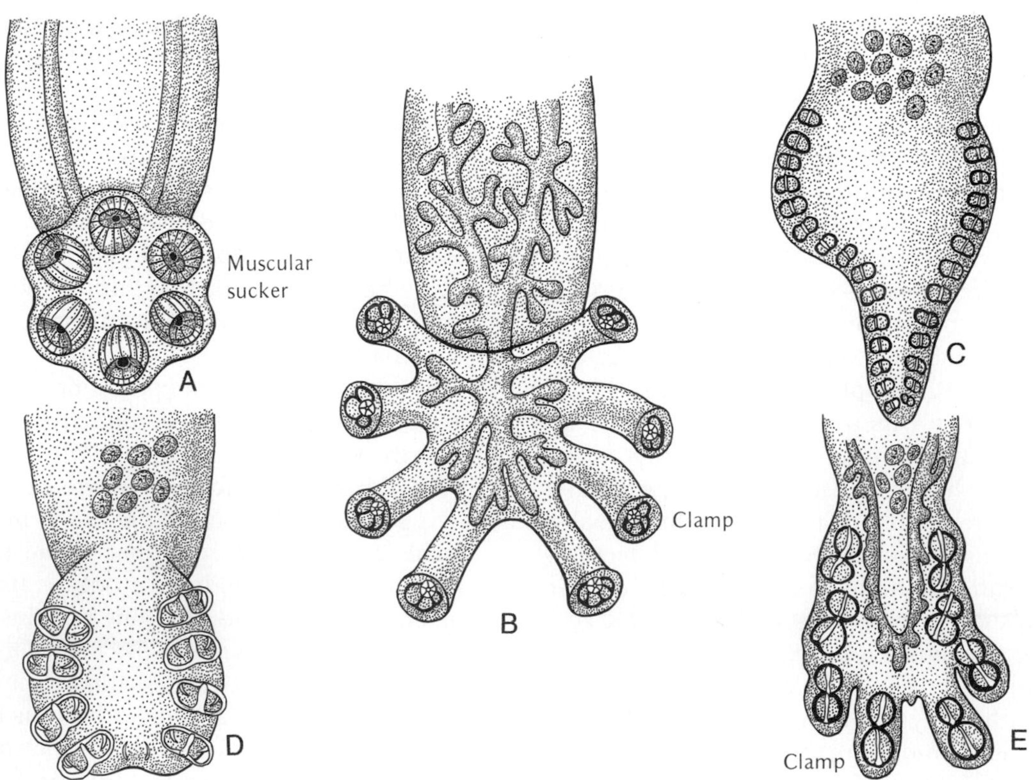

FIGURE 22.2 Opisthaptors of members of the Polyopisthocotylea.

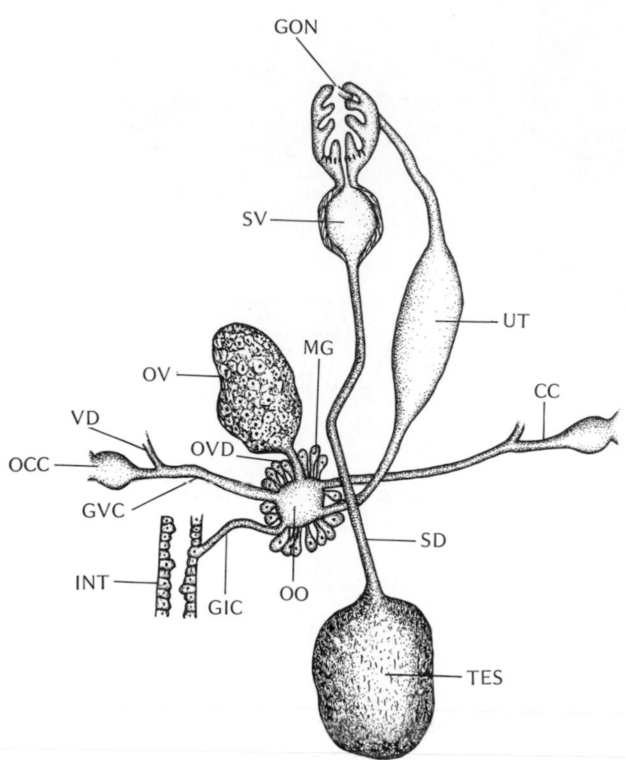

FIGURE 22.3 The monoecious reproductive system of the Monogenea. Abbreviations: CC, copulatory canal; GIC—genitointestinal canal; GON, gonopore; GVC, common genitovitelline canal; INT, intestine; MG, Mehlis' gland; OCC, opening of copulatory canal; OO, ootype; OV, ovary; OVD, oviduct; SD, sperm duct; SV, seminal vesicle; TES, testis; UT, uterus; VD, vitrelline duct [Redrawn with modifications from Cheng, T. C., 1985.]

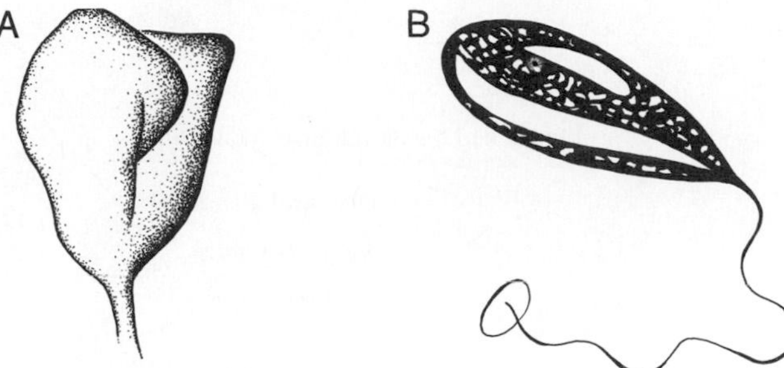

FIGURE 22.4 Eggs of Monogenea (A) *Thaumatocotyle dasybatis;* (B) *Udonella caligorum.* [Redrawn with modifications from Price, 1938.]

An intriguing third possibility was discussed by Rohde, who noted that when worms were squeezed, surplus material was discharged through the genitointestinal canal into the gut, presumably to be digested and recycled.

Life Cycle

The Monogenea have simple one-host life cycles with an egg, a ciliated larval stage, the oncomiracidium, and an adult. An exception is the family Gyrocotylidae, which has no oncomiracidium stage; members are viviparous and give birth to a subadult. Monogenean eggs are usually fusiform and have filaments at one or both ends for attachment to hosts (Fig. 22.4). The oncomiracidium hatches from the egg, swims to a new host, sheds its ciliated cells, and develops into an adult (Fig. 22.5). The oncomiracidia of *Entobodella soleae* (Fig. 22.6) can find their correct hosts in total darkness with uncanny accuracy using chemical detection of mucus on the scales of the fish. Since the fish can swim much faster than the oncomiracidia, the probability of reaching a fish would seem to be remote; however, hatching behavior in *E. soleae* is regulated to increase the odds in favor of the parasite. Most hatching occurs at dawn when the night-feeding fish (*Solea solea*) return to their daytime resting places.

Members of the family Gyrodactylidae lack the egg and oncomiracidium and instead give birth to subadults (Fig. 22.7). Inside the uterus of the subadult may be another subadult, the "grandchild"; this unusual type of reproduction is thought to be a form of sequential polyembryony.

Evolution

The Monogenea have been classified as members of the class Trematoda for many years. Most classifications included two subclasses, the Monogenea and the Digenea; however, this concept has changed in recent years. Current evolutionary schemes place weight on larval forms, emphasizing that "ontogeny recapitulates phylogeny," as promulgated by Haeckel in the 19th century. The concept that monogeneans are more closely related to cestodarian tapeworms than to digenetic trematodes is supported is supported by the following evidence:

1. The hooks of cestodes and monogeneans are stabilized by disulfide bonds and those of the digeneans are not.
2. The oncomiracidium of monogeneans and the lycophore, coracidium, and hexacanth of tapeworms are armed, whereas the digenean miracidium is not.
3. Adult digeneans typically have an infolded tegument, whereas monogeneans and cestoideans have microvilli or microtrichs on their external surfaces.
4. The monogeneans and cestodes are usually host specific for the vertebrate hosts but the digeneans are host specific for the invertebrate hosts.

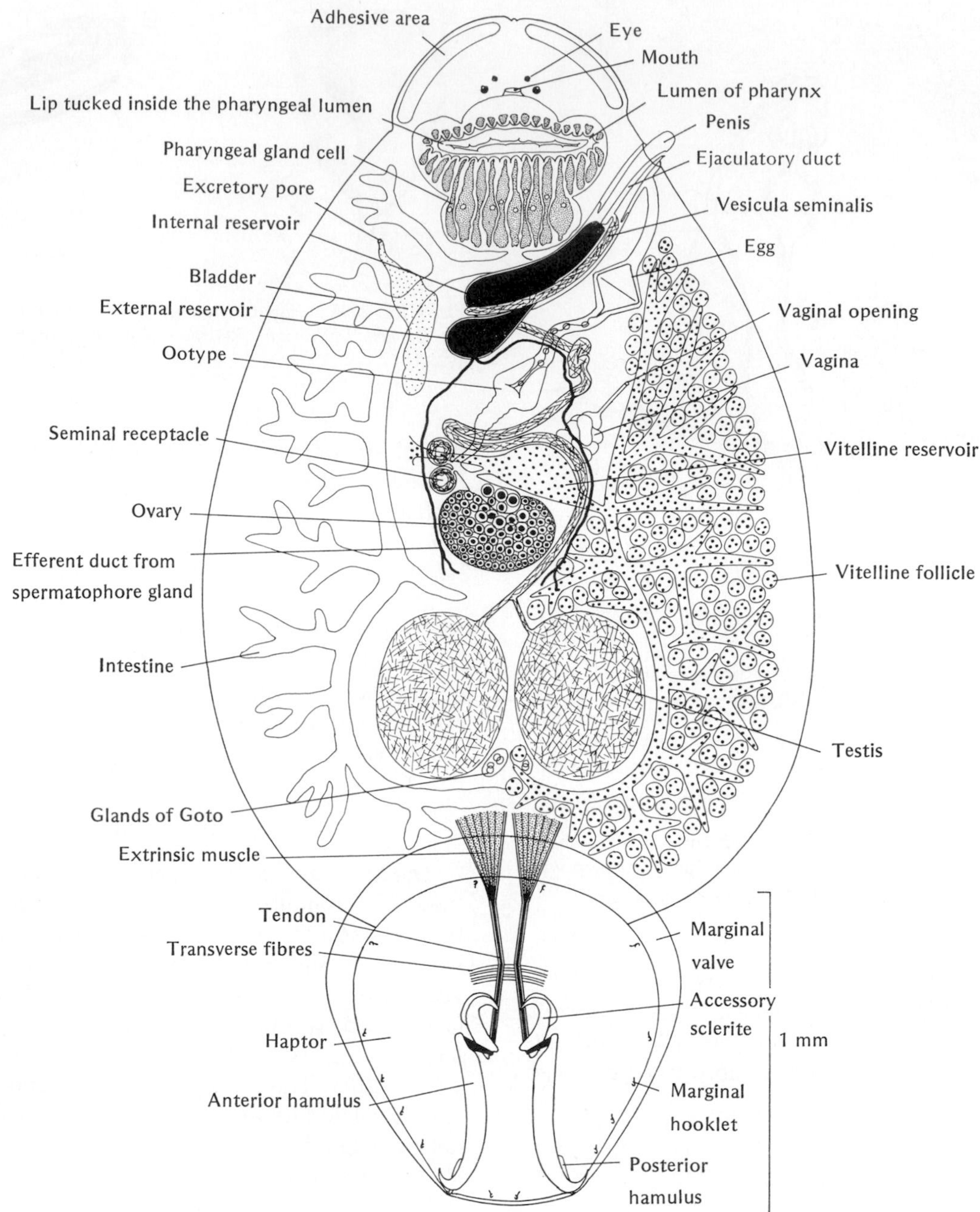

FIGURE 22.5 An adult monogenean, *Entobdella soleae,* an ectoparasite of the marine flatfish, *Solea solea.* [From Kearn, 1971, in Fallis, M.]

It is probable that the free-living rhabdocoel-like ancestors gave rise to two distinct lines: (1) the Monogenea and Cestoda and (2) the Trematoda.

REPRESENTATIVE MONOGENEANS

Gyrodactylus spp. are viviparous monogeneans that can cause serious skin and gill lesions in trout, bluegill, goldfish, and other fishes if they are crowded together in fish ponds. Newborn subadults have no cilia and closely resemble the adult; they have an opisthaptor with a pair of anchors and 16 marginal hooklets. Typically the subadults attach to the skin or gills of the same host as the parent worm. They have no cilia and thus are poor swimmers; presumably they transfer to another host when there is contact between the hosts, such as crowding in a fish pond.

Entobdella soleae (Fig. 22.5) is a more representative example of the order Monopisthocotylea than the pathogenic *Gyrodactylus* mentioned previously. *E. so-*

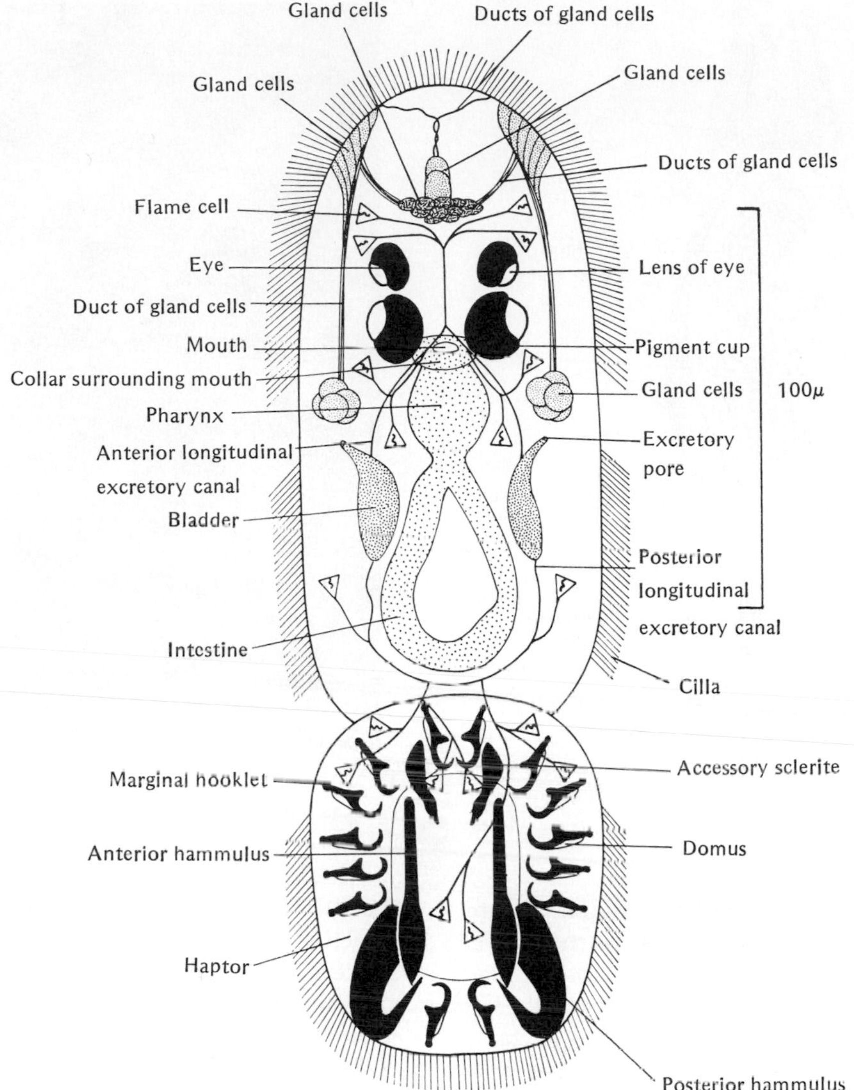

FIGURE 22.6 Oncomiracidium of *Entobdella soleae* [From Kearn, 1963.]

leae has the usual monogenean life cycle with an egg attached to sand grains, a free-swimming oncomiracidium, and an adult on the scales of the common sole, *Solea solea.* In nature, soles have 1 to 9 adult parasites per fish, but up to 200 have been counted on fish kept in aquaria. The parasite erodes only the superficial epidermis of the host; thus the danger of host secondary bacterial infection is minimal. This minimal pathogenesis is the rule for most monogeneans in nature, even those that inhabit the gills and feed on blood.

Octomacrum lanceatum (Fig. 22.8), of the order Polyopisthocotylea, has eight clamps on the opisthaptor and two small suckers on the prohaptor. It is found on the gills of suckers (genus *Catostomus*) and, although a blood feeder, it rarely causes serious damage because only a few parasites are on any fish. It has a typical monogenean life cycle with an egg, oncomiracidium, and adult.

Classification

The characteristics most often used in the subclass Monogenea are external features such as opisthaptor morphology and variations in male copulatory apparatus. This is in contrast to the class Trematoda, in which detailed examination of internal reproductive organs is required for classification.

THE CESTODES

The subclass Cestoda of the phylum Platyhelminthes contains the tapeworms. These worms have

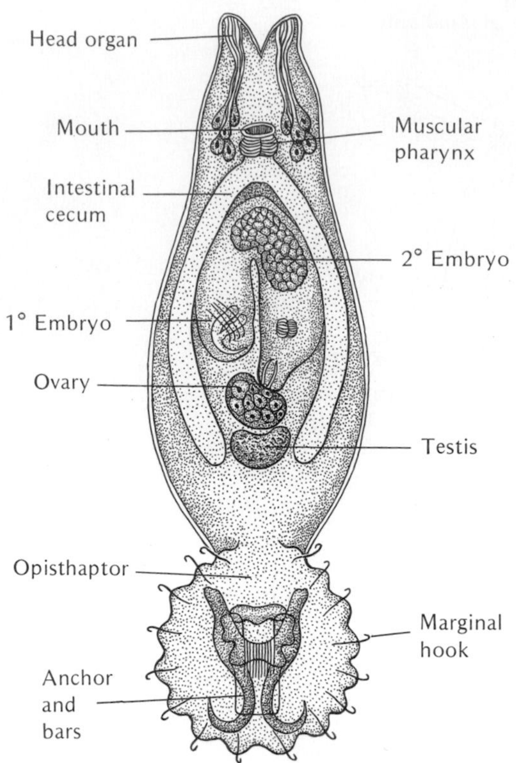

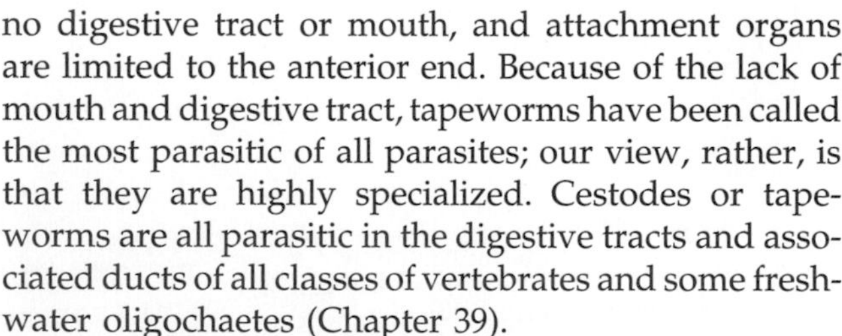

FIGURE 22.7 Diagram of an adult *Gyrodactylus rhinichthius* containing two generations of developing embryos.

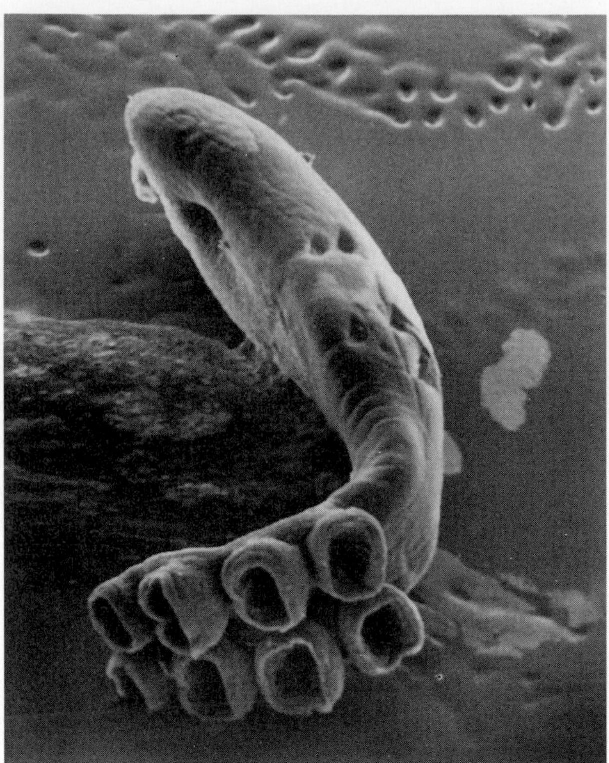

FIGURE 22.8 An adult polyopisthocotylean, *Octomacrum lanceolatum* as seen in SEM. [Courtesy of Sharon Haines.]

no digestive tract or mouth, and attachment organs are limited to the anterior end. Because of the lack of mouth and digestive tract, tapeworms have been called the most parasitic of all parasites; our view, rather, is that they are highly specialized. Cestodes or tapeworms are all parasitic in the digestive tracts and associated ducts of all classes of vertebrates and some freshwater oligochaetes (Chapter 39).

Human and animal tapeworm infections have been known since classical times. Celsus, Pliny, Aristotle, and their contemporaries recognized human intestinal flatworms (*Taenia*). Larval tapeworms were also recognized by early investigators, but they were not associated with their adult forms in humans. The Mosaic law forbids eating meat of the camel, rabbit, hare, or pig, perhaps because of bladder worms, but it was not until the 19th century that larval and adult worm relationships were described.

Morphology

The anterior end of tapeworms is called the *scolex* or *holdfast*; it has various structures for attachment including sucking depressions, hooks, and glandular areas. The sucking depressions are of three types: bothria, a pair of shallow sucking grooves typical of the Pseudophyllidea; bothridia, four leaflike, flexible structures seen in the order Tetraphyllidea; and true suckers or acetabula, four hemispherical muscular cups characteristic of several orders including the important Cyclophyllidea (Fig. 22.9). A few tapeworms lack anterior holdfast structures, but most have one of the three types mentioned. In addition, some tapeworms have an apical organ, the rostellum, which may have an additional sucker, glandular area, or hooks (those scolices with hooks are spoken of as being *armed*).

Posterior to the scolex region there are two body types. The first is a body of a single segment (monozoic) and the other is a body of many segments (polyzoic). Each segment is called a *proglottid*, and the chain of proglottids is called a *strobila*. Usually each proglottid has its own set of reproductive organs. Tapeworms have the immature proglottids closest to the scolex, then a region of sexually mature proglottids, and finally gravid proglottids that have uteri filled with eggs. This form of sequential segmentation is characteristic of the subcohort Eucestoda; however, not all tapeworms have a strobila of proglottids produced sequentially. The order Pseudophyllidea, which includes the fish tapeworm of humans, *Diphyllobothrium latum*, has proglottids that are formed "instantaneously"; Wardle

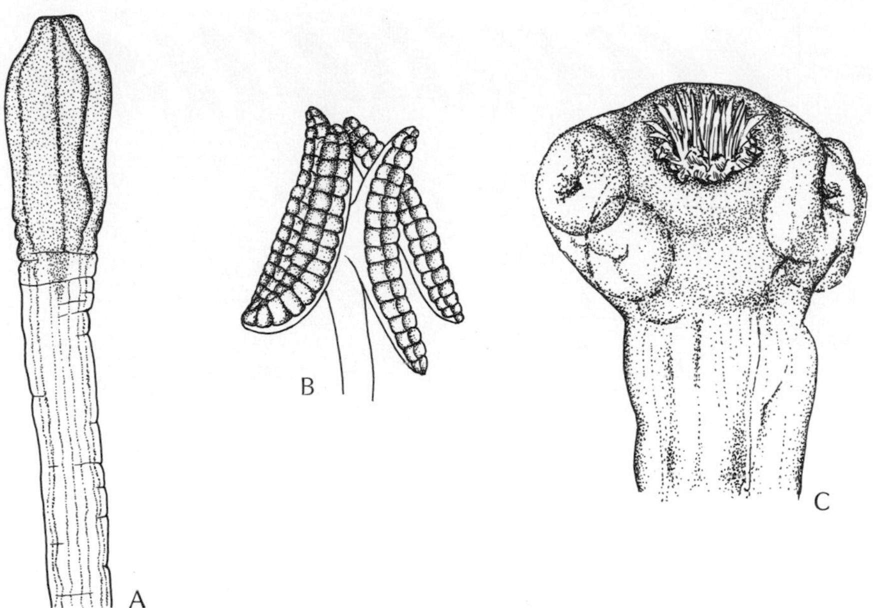

FIGURE 22.9 Tapeworm scolices or holdfasts: (A) *Diphyllobothrium latum*, a scolex with bothria; (B) *Echeneibothrium tobijei*, a scolex with bothridia; (C) *Taenia* sp., a scolex with suckers.

et al. (1974) therefore suggested that these should also be called monozoic because they were formed at one time. In addition, these proglottids lack the intervening membranous or muscular partitions characteristic of polyzoic tapeworms. In many species the proglottids overlap their immediate neighbors and are called *craspedote;* others that do not overlap are called *acraspedote.* Some tapeworms continuously shed terminal proglottids in the feces; these are called *apolytic* and those that do not are called *anapolytic.*

Since tapeworms lack both a mouth and digestive tract, all nutrients must be acquired through the external surface. This external surface is a living, multinucleate (syncytial) tegument and not an inert, secreted cuticle. The external surface is a carbohydrate glycocalyx. Beneath the glycocalyx is a limiting membrane and then an unusual type of microvillar surface projection called *microtriches* (singular, microthrix), which are visible with the electron microscope. Microtriches have characteristic dense caps that point toward the posterior of the worm and are supported by microfilaments. Beneath the microtriches is a vacuolated, syncytial cytoplasm connected to the subtegumental layer by thin protoplasmic extensions. The protoplasmic extensions pass through three muscle layers—circular, longitudinal, and oblique or transverse—before reaching the subtegumental layer. This inner layer contains tegumental cell bodies with nuclei, mitochondria, Golgi apparati, and endoplasmic reticulum cisternae (Fig. 22.10).

The function of microtriches has been the subject of considerable debate. Most workers believe that since the microtriches increase surface area 10 to 50 times, there is better nutrient absorption, similar to that of the microvilli in the cells of the vertebrate gut. The microtriches may also assist the worm in maintaining its position in the gut because of their posteriorly pointed orientation.

In cross-section the tapeworm body is seen to be filled with parenchyma. Muscle layers separate the body into an outer cortex and an inner medulla (Fig. 22.11). The reproductive organs are usually in the medulla. Pairs of dorsal and ventral excretory or osmoregulatory canals (Fig. 22.12) traverse the entire strobila from scolex to the last proglottid. The dorsal one is often smaller than the ventral, and this observation can help in orientation when studying stained specimens. Transverse canals can sometimes be seen connecting the longitudinal canals.

Most tapeworms are monoecious, although a few dioecious ones are known. In most tapeworms the male reproductive system matures first (protandry), and may prevent self-fertilization within the same proglottid. The rationale for such a system may seem obscure at first since all proglottids come from the same zygote and are thus genetically identical; however, if sperm and ova develop at different times, the opportunities for genetic change may be increased. Both self-fertilization and cross-fertilization have been demonstrated in a number of tapeworm species.

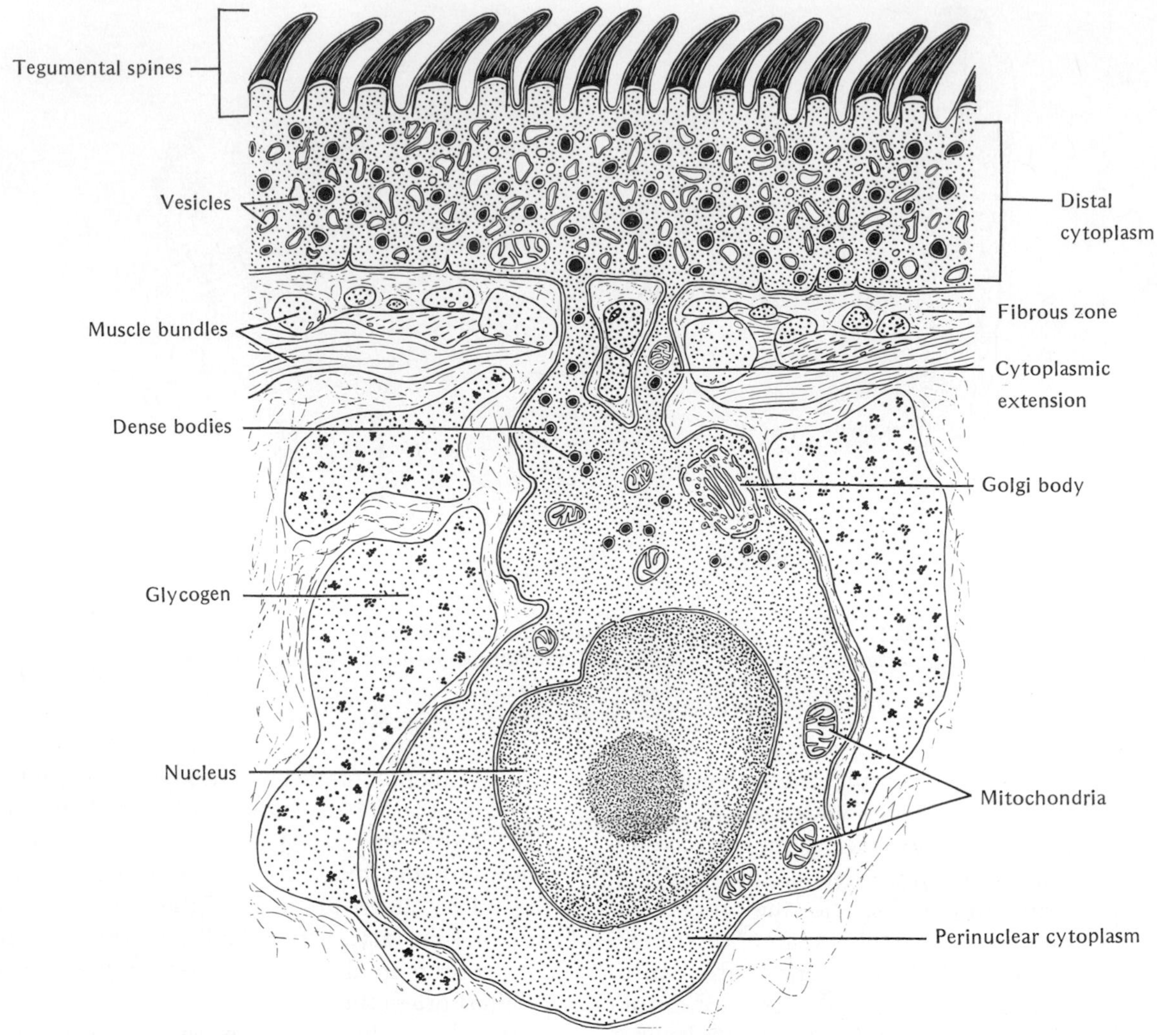

FIGURE 22.10 Diagram of the tegument of the protoscolex of *Echinococcus granulosus* [From Morseth, 1967.]

Reproductive systems in members of the Cestoda (Fig. 22.13) have the same structures as those of the Trematoda (Chapter 17) except that some tapeworms lack a uterine pore. A typical mature male system consists of numerous testes that produce sperm; vasa efferentia lead from each testis to a common vas deferens or sperm duct. Some species have a chamber for sperm storage or seminal vesicle. The male copulatory organ, the cirrus, is surrounded by the cirrus pouch. Most often the cirrus pouch and female vagina enter a common chamber, the genital atrium, and share a common opening to the outside, the genital pore.

A typical mature female tapeworm system includes a vagina leading from the genital pore to a seminal receptacle or sperm storage chamber; an ovary which produces eggs or ova; a single oviduct leading from the ovary to conduct eggs; the ootype, which is a chamber joined by the oviduct, the duct from the seminal receptacle, and is surrounded by the cells of the Mehlis' gland. The uterus leads from the ootype and may have either an opening or uteropore or end blindly. Proglottids without uteropores detach when gravid (apolysis) and break up to release their eggs. Individual differences are discussed with each particular organism.

The parenchyma of most cestodes contains structures called *calcareous corpuscles* (Fig. 22.14) because they contain calcium. In addition, inorganic components including magnesium and phosphorus and organic compounds including DNA, RNA, proteins, sugars, and enzymes have also been reported. The function of these corpuscles is unknown, but they are useful in identifying tapeworms in tissue sections. Similar structures are sometimes seen in trematodes but are contained only in the excretory canals.

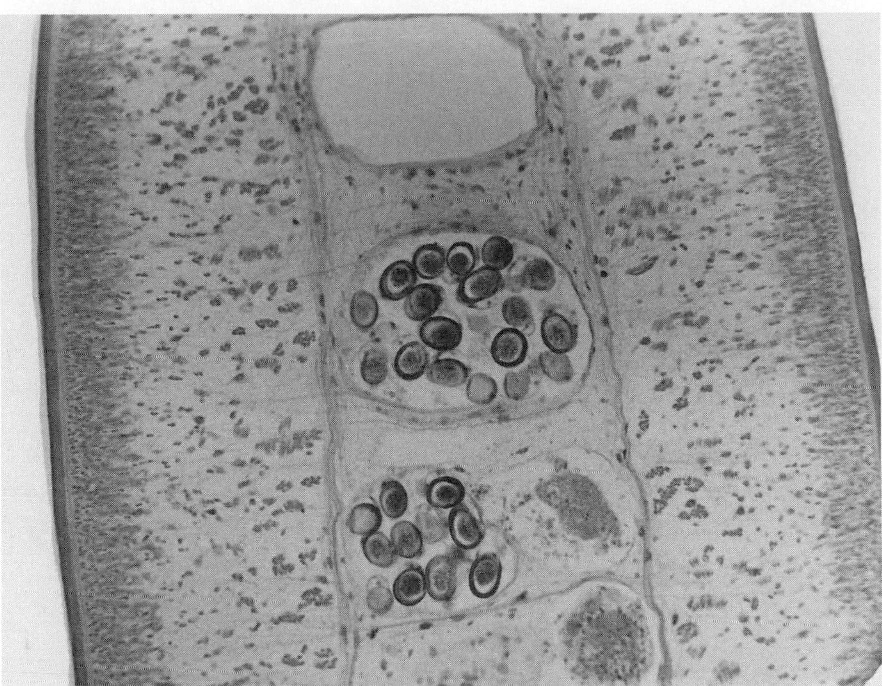

FIGURE 22.11 A histologic section of a proglottid of *Taenia taeniaformis* with eggs filling the uterus in the medullary portion of the proglottid.

The nervous system of tapeworms consists of two large nerve trunks that travel from the scolex to the end of the strobila. Lateral branches from the main nerve trunks reach all proglottids in a ladderlike fashion. The area of the genital atrium is richly supplied with nerve endings. The tapeworm "brain" is in the scolex; it consists of dorsal and ventral commissures and accessory nerves connecting with holdfast organs,

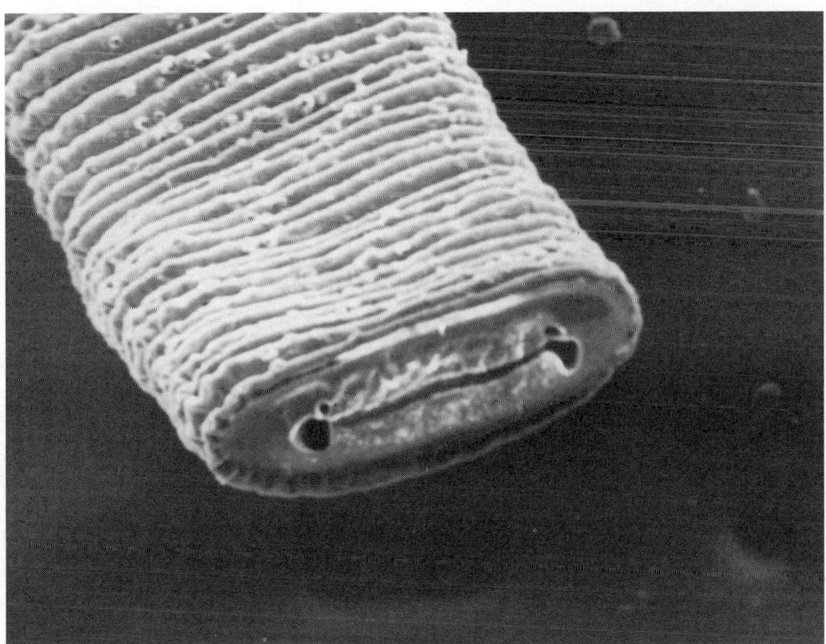

FIGURE 22.12 The cut surface of a mature proglottid of *Hymenolepis diminuta* as seen in SEM. Two small, dorsal osmoregulatory canals are located above the larger ventral osmoregulatory canals. The transverse canal joining the two ventral canals is also visible.

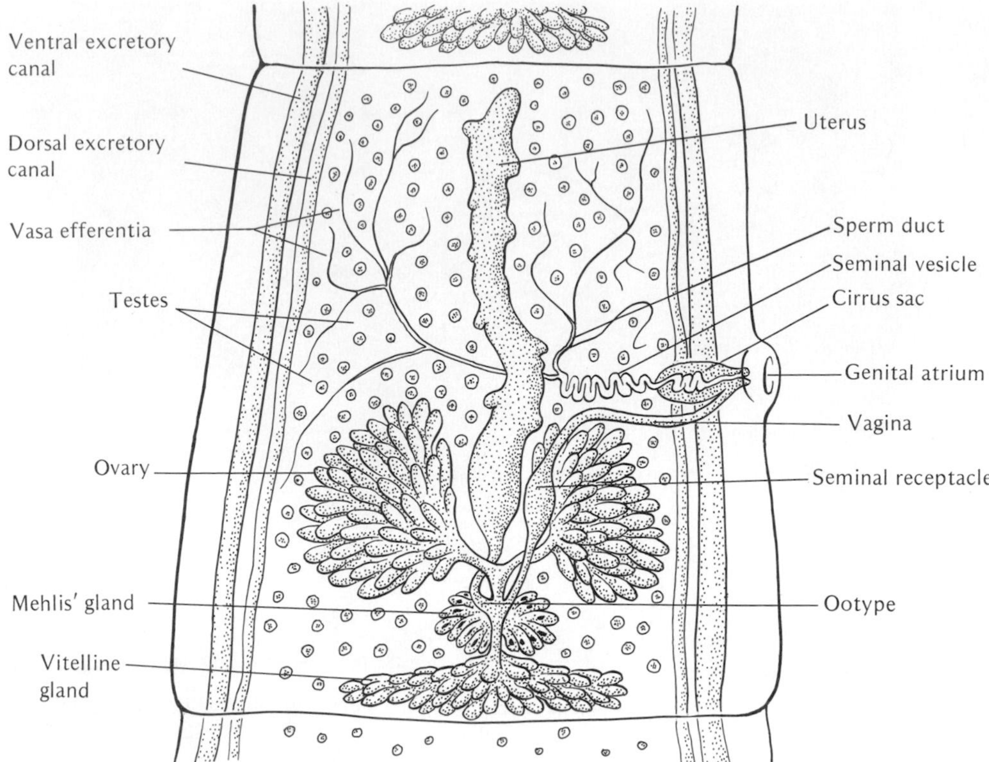

FIGURE 22.13 Diagram of a mature proglottid of *Taenia* sp.

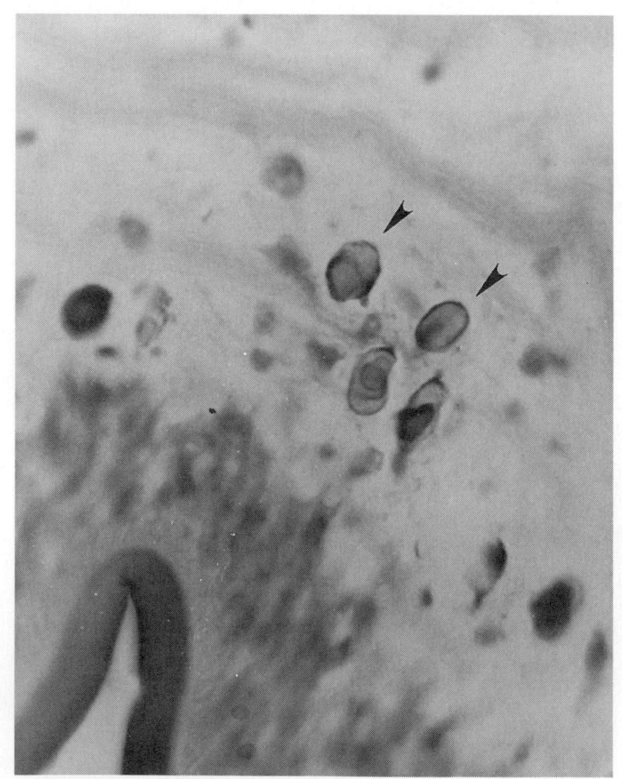

FIGURE 22.14 Oval calcareous corpuscles in the parenchyma of a proglottid of *Taenia* sp.

and so forth. Complexity varies from species to species. Externally, cestodes have a high density of uniciliate sensory cells on the scolex. The proglottids possess both uniciliate and nonciliate sensory cells (Fig. 22.15). These sensory cells are similar to those seen in other invertebrates including the trematodes (Fig. 17.5). The ciliate cells are probably tangosensory (touch) or chemosensory. The nonciliate sensory cells do not reach the tegumental surface and thus probably are not tango—or chemosensors; instead they probably monitor body deformations (stretch sensors) of the tapeworm body wall caused by worm activity, host gut peristalsis, or both.

Life Cycle

The basic life cycle patterns for tapeworms consist of a monoecious (rarely dioecious) adult, which produces an ovum. The ovum is fertilized and the resultant zygote develops into a larva called an *oncosphere;* it usually has six hooks and is also called a *hexacanth embryo.* The oncosphere usually is ingested by an invertebrate intermediate host and migrates to a parenteral location such as an insect hemocoel. The larva metamorphoses and grows as a *metacestode* (i.e., changing cestode) until signs of sexual maturity appear and a scolex with adult structure develops. Usually, a verte-

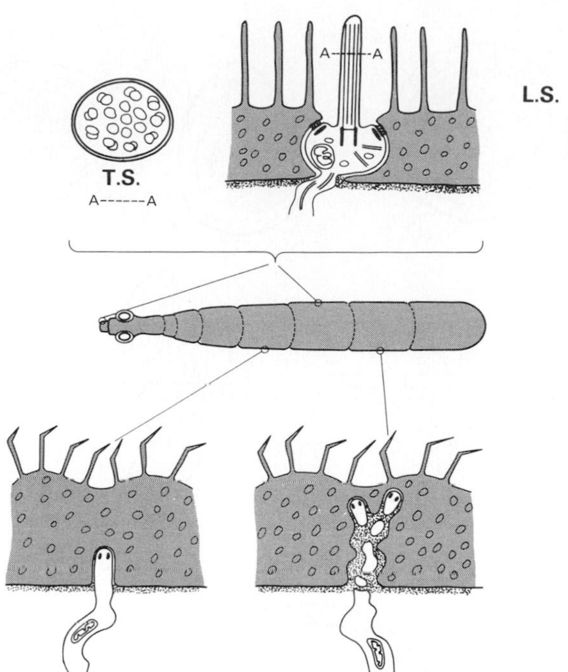

FIGURE 22.15 Tegumental sensory endings of tapeworms. Upper: tangential section (T. S.) and longitudinal section (L. S.) of a ciliated receptor. Lower: Two diagrams of nonciliated sensory receptors that are characteristic of proglottid tegument. [Redrawn with modifications from Whitfield, 1979.]

brate definitive host ingests the invertebrate containing the metacestode. Final development to a sexually reproducing adult occurs in the vertebrate digestive tract and associated ducts.

Freeman (1973) proposed terminology that is useful for organizing tapeworm metacestodes. There are two types of metacestode development, primitive and neoteric. Primitive metacestodes develop without a primary cavity or lacuna, whereas neoteric metacestodes do develop one. Primitive or solid metacestodes are subdivided into procercoids, which do not have a scolex similar to the adult, and plerocercoids, which do have a scolex similar to adult worms. Neoteric or hollow metacestodes, all in the order Cyclophyllidea, have two basic patterns of development; the cysticercoid has a lacuna filled with parenchyma and the cysticercus has a fluid-filled lacuna. There are types of metacestodes other than those just mentioned. Most notable are variations of the cysticercus, which include (1) strobilocercous, a cysticercus with some strobilization; (2) coenurus, with multiple scolices inside a nonlaminated lacuna; and (3) hydatid, with multiple scolices inside a laminated lacuna. Some oncospheres and metacestodes are illustrated here (Fig. 22.16). Variations in biology and morphology are discussed with each organism.

CESTODE NUTRITION AND SURFACE ACTIVITIES

Cestodes have been used as models for research on nutrient uptake because they have no gut. Adult cestodes acquire nutrients from the immediate external environment, the host gut, but diffusion and active transport mechanisms and probably endocytosis act as well. In addition, the tapeworm tegument must be viewed as a "digestive-absorptive interface." The outer surface of tapeworms is studded with enzymes; some are produced by the worm and are called *intrinsic digestive enzymes*. They are membrane bound and not released into the environment. Cestode surface activities are illustrated in Figure 22.17.

Diffusion is the net flow of nutrient from a region of high concentration, in this case the host intestine, to a region of lower concentration, the tapeworm interior. No energy is required for this process. Pyridoxine, a B vitamin, is acquired by simple diffusion.

Most amino acids are acquired by active transport, but diffusion may also be utilized. Active transport moves substances against concentration gradients from a region of low concentration to one of higher concentration. This process occurs only across biological membranes, requires energy, and has many features in common with enzyme-substrate interactions, including uptake kinetics and competitive inhibition. Uptake of glucose by *Hymenolepis* species is an example of active transport.

A number of parasite-produced enzymes are embedded in the tapeworm surface. One example of an intrinsic digestive enzyme is phosphohydrolase, which hydrolyzes glucose-6-phosphate to glucose; this can then be taken into the worm by active transport at specific monosaccharide sites.

An additional function of the tapeworm's surface that is beneficial for it is the ability to inactivate host digestive enzymes such as trypsin and chymotrypsin. Mammalian intestinal cells do the same thing to prevent their being digested by enzymes in the gut; presumably this is also why the tapeworms do it.

Thus the cestode tegument is a multifunctional surface that processes nutrients and takes them into the body of the worm; at the same time it protects the worm against digestive enzymes of the host.

CLASSIFICATION OF THE SUBCLASS CESTODA

Cohort Gyrocotylidea

Cercomer with ten equal-sized hooks (Fig. 22.18). Thick, monozoic worms with a single set of reproduc-

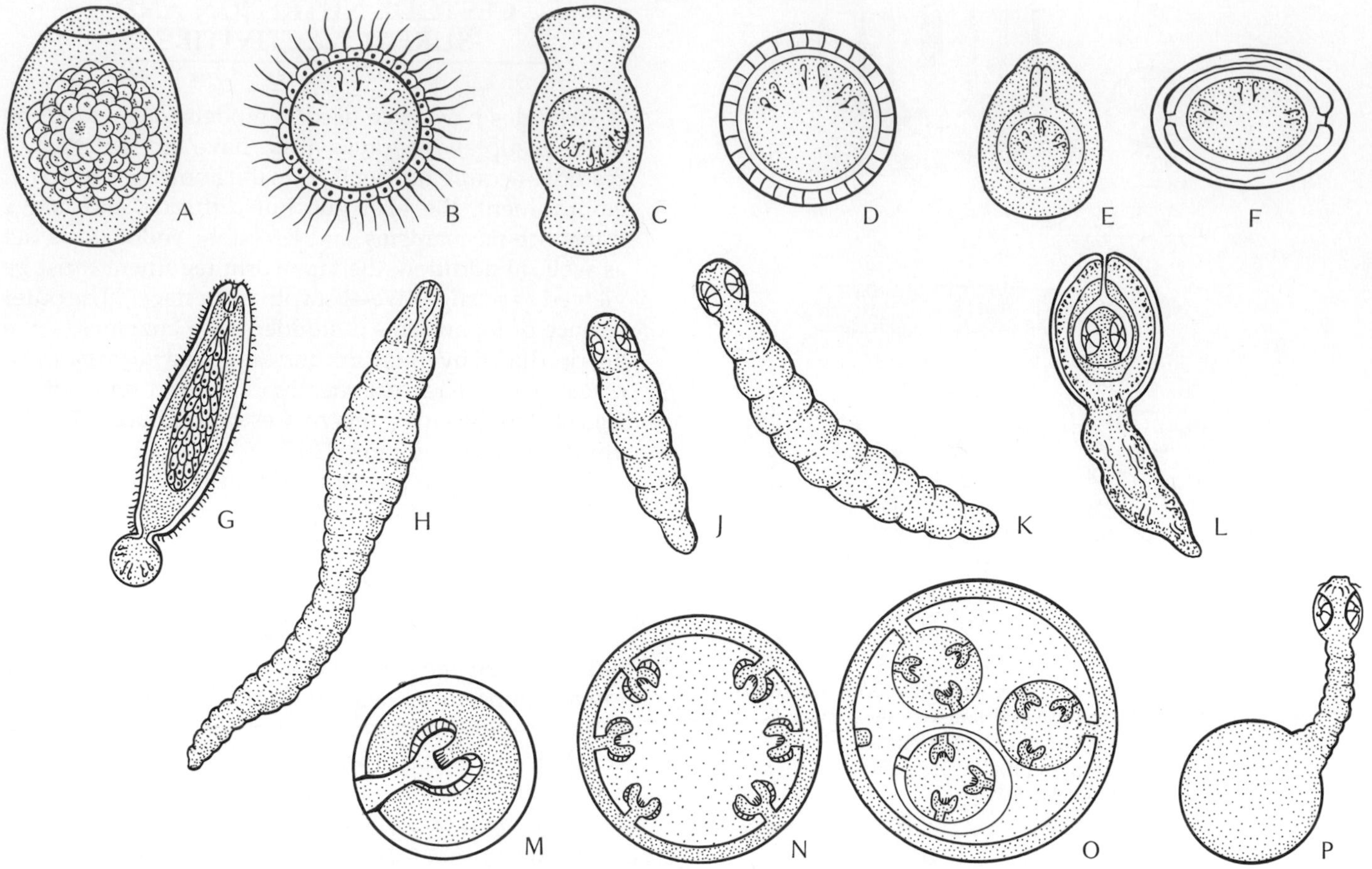

FIGURE 22.16 Diagrams of cestode oncospheres and metacestodes: (A) pseudophyllidean egg; (B) coracidium; (C) proteocephalan egg; (D) taenioid egg; (E) anoplocephalid egg; (F) hymenolepidid egg; (G) pseudophyllidean procercoid; (H) pseudophyllidean procercoid; (J) proteocephalan procercoid; (K) proteocephalan plerocercoid; (L) cysticercoid; (M) cysticercus; (N) coenurus; (O) hydatid; (P) strobilocercus.

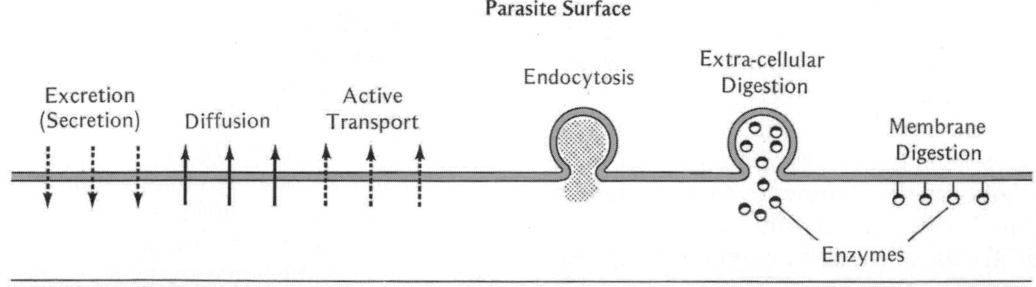

FIGURE 22.17 Activities at the cestode-host interface. A portion of interchange with the host occurs as passive diffusion such as the uptake of certain substances and excretion, but most involve active transport.

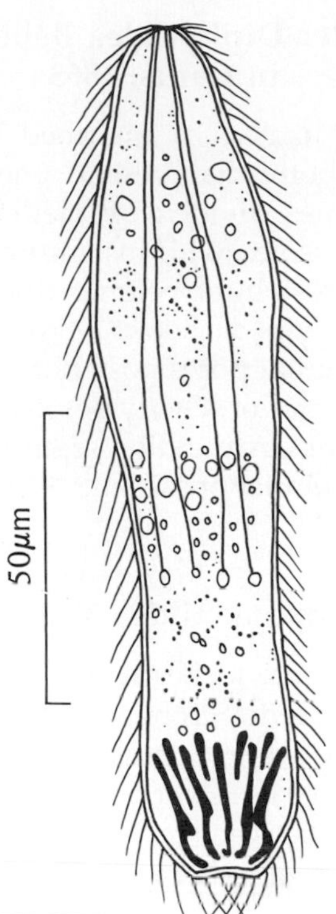

FIGURE 22.18 Diagram of a lycophore larva of *Gyrodactyle urna*. [Redrawn from Lynch, 1945.]

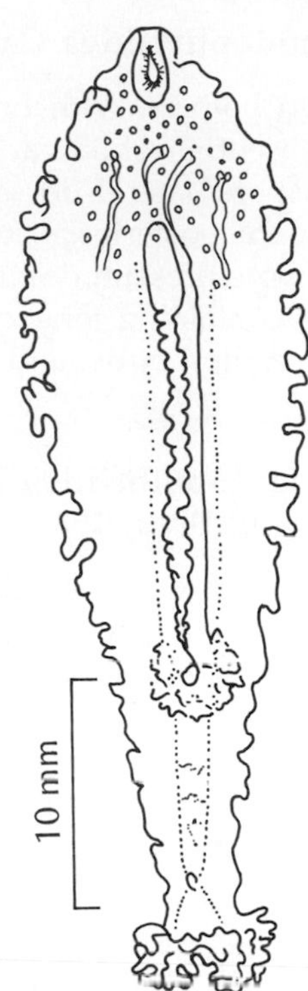

FIGURE 22.19 Diagram of an adult of *Gyrodactyle urna*. [Redrawn from Lynch, 1945.]

tive organs and a single, anterior, cuplike, muscular holdfast (Fig. 22.19). They are found in large intestines of chimaeroid fishes in both the Atlantic and Pacific Oceans.

Cohort Cestoidea

Six large hooks on cercomer, cercomer invaginates during development. Male genital pore and vagina proximate.

Subcohort Amphilinidea

Worms with flattened, monozoic bodies without an anterior holdfast. Cercomer with six large hooks and four small hooks. The anterior end has a boring mechanism, which enables penetration of host body cavities. Worms are found in body cavities of Acepenseridae (sturgeons) in Europe and North America, siluroid fishes in India, and a tortoise in Australia.

Subcohort Eucestoda

Monozoic and polyzoic. Single or multiple sets of reproductive organs. Six-hooked larva. True scolex present. Parasites of fishes, amphibians, reptiles, birds, and mammals; one genus matures in the coelom of freshwater oligochaetes.

Order Caryophyllidea Beneden in Olsson, 1893

Scolex with shallow grooves or loculi, or fimbriated, weakly developed, lacking true suckers. Strobila monozoic. Genital pores midventral. Testes numerous. Ovary posterior. Vitellaria follicular, scattered, or lateral. Uterus a coiled, median-tube opening, often together with vagina, near male pore. Parasites of teleost fishes and aquatic annelids.

Order Spathebothriidea Wardle and McLeod, 1953

Scolex feebly developed, undifferentiated, or with funnel-shaped apical organ, or with one or two hollow, cuplike organs. External segmentation absent, internal segmentation present. Genital pores ventral. Testes in two lateral bands. Ovary dendritic. Vitellaria follicular, lateral, or scattered. Uterus coiled, with ventral pore. Parasites of teleost fishes.

Order Pseudophyllidea Carus, 1863

Scolex with two bothria, with or without hooks. Neck present or absent. Strobila variable. Proglottids anapolytic. Genital pores lateral, dorsal, or ventral. Testes numerous. Ovary posterior. Vitellaria follicular, scattered. Uterine pore present, dorsal or ventral. Egg usually operculate, containing coracidium. Parasites of fish, amphibians, reptiles, birds, and mammals.

Order Haplobothriidea Joyeux and Baer, 1961

Scolex club shaped with four tentacles. Primary strobila modified at anterior to secondary stroblia and pseudescolex. Genital pore midventral. Testes numerous in two lateral fields. Ovary posterior. Vitellaria in lateral bands, joining anteriorly and posteriorly. Uterine pore usually present. Eggs operculate. Parasites of North American teleosts.

Order Trypanorhynchidea Diesing, 1863

Scolex elongate, with two or four bothridia, and four eversible (rarely atrophied) tentacles armed with hooks. Each tentacle invaginates into internal sheath provided with muscular bulb. Neck present or absent. Strobila apolytic or anapolytic. Genital pores lateral, rarely ventral. Testes numerous. Ovary posterior. Vitellaria follicular, scattered. Uterine pore present or absent. Parasites of elasmobranchs.

Order Lecanicephalidea Baylis, 1920

Scolex divided into anterior and posterior regions by horizontal groove. Anterior portion cushionlike, or with unarmed tentacles, capable of being withdrawn into posterior portion forming a large suckerlike organ. Posterior portion usually with four suckers. Neck present or absent. Testes numerous. Ovary posterior. Vitellaria follicular, lateral, or encircling proglottid. Uterine pore usually present. Parasites of elasmobranchs.

Order Tetraphyllidea Carus, 1863

Scolex with highly variable bothridia, sometimes also with hooks, spines, or suckers. Myzorhynchus present or absent. Neck present or absent. Proglottids commonly apolytic. Hermaphroditic, rarely dioecious. Genital pores lateral, rarely posterior. Testes numerous. Ovary posterior. Vitellaria follicular (condensed in *Dioecotaenia*), usually lateral. Uterine pore present or not. Parasites of elasmobranchs.

Order Diphyllidea Beneden in Carus, 1863

Scolex with armed or unarmed peduncle. Two spoon-shaped bothridia present, lined with minute spines, sometimes divided by median, longitudinal ridge. Apex of scolex with insignificant apical organ or with large rostellum bearing dorsal and ventral groups of T-shaped hooks. Strobila cylindrical, acraspedote. Genital pores posterior, midventral. Testes numerous, anterior. Ovary posterior. Vitellaria follicular, lateral, or surrounding segment. Uterine pore absent. Uterus tubular or saccular. Parasites of elasmobranchs.

Order Nippotaeniidea Yamaguti, 1939

Scolex with single sucker at apex, otherwise simple. Neck short or absent. Strobila small. Proglottids each with single set of reproductive organs. Genital pores lateral. Testes anterior. Ovary posterior. Vitelline gland compact, single, between testes and ovary. Osmoregulatory canals reticular. Parasites of teleost fishes.

Order Proteocephalidea Mola, 1928

Scolex with four suckers, occasionally with apical sucker or armed rostellum. Neck usually present. Genital pores lateral. Testes numerous. Ovary posterior. Vitellaria follicular, usually lateral. Uterine pore present or absent. Parasites of fishes, amphibians, and reptiles.

Order Tetrabothriidea Baer, 1954

Scolex with four bothridia. Genital pores lateral. Testes few to numerous. Ovary lobed, mid-proglottid. Vitelline gland compact, anterior to ovary. Uterine pore present. Parasites of marine homeotherms.

Order Cyclophyllidea Beneden in Braun, 1900

Scolex usually with four suckers, rostellum present or not, armed or not. Neck present or absent. Strobila variable, usually with distinct segmentation, hermaphroditic or, rarely, dioecious. Genital pores lateral (ventral in Mesocestoididae). Vitelline gland single, compact, usually posterior to ovary. Uterus variable. Uterine pore absent. Parasites of amphibians, reptiles, birds, and mammals.

Readings

Arai, H. P. (1980). *Biology of the Tapeworm Hymenolepis diminuta.* Academic Press, New York.

Arme, C. (1975). Tapeworm–host interactions. *Symp. Soc. Exp. Biol.* **29,** 505–532.

Arme, C., and Pappas, P. W. (1983). *The Biology of the Eucestoda,* 2 Vols. Academic Press, London.

Boeger, W. A., and Kritsky, D. C. (1993). Phylogeny and a revised classification of the Monogenea Bychowsky, 1937 (Platyhelminthes). *Syst. Parasitol.* **26,** 1–32.

Bychowsky, B. E. (1957). *Monogenetic Trematodes, Their Systematics and Phylogeny* (W. J. Hargis, Jr., Ed.). Am. Inst. Biol. Sci., Washington, DC. [Trans. from Russian]

Cheng, T. C. (1985). *General Parasitology.* Academic Press, New York.

Chitwood, M., and Lichtenfels, J. R. (1972). Identification of parasitic metazoa in tissue sections. *Exp. Parasitol.* **32,** 407–519.

Freeman, R. S. (1973). Ontogeny of cestodes and its bearing on their phylogeny and systematics. *Adv. Parasitol.* **11,** 481–557.

Hoberg, E. P., Mariaux, J., Justine, J.-L., Brooks, D. R., and Weekes, P. J. (1997). Phylogeny of the orders of the Eucestoda (Cercomeromorphae) based on comparative morphology: Historical perspectives and a new working hypothesis. *J. Parasitol.* **83,** 1128–1147.

Hoeppli, R. (1959). *Parasites and Parasitic Infections' in Early Medicine and Science.* Univ. of Malaya Press, Singapore.

Kearn, G. C. (1963). The egg, oncomiracidium and larval development of *Entobdella soleae,* a monogenean skin parasite of the common sole. *Parasitology* **53,** 435–447.

Kearn, G. C. (1971). The physiology and behavior of the monogenean skin parasite *Entobdella soleae* in relation to its host (*Solea solea*). Univ. Toronto Press, Toronto.

Khalil, L. F., and Jones, A. (Eds.) (1994). *Keys to the Cestode Parasites of Vertebrates.* CAB International, Wallingford, UK.

Llewellyn, J. (1963). Larvae and larval development of monogeneans. *Adv. Parasitol.* **1,** 287–326.

Lynch, J. E. (1945). Redescription of the species of *Gyrocotyle* from the ratfish *Hydrolagus coliei. J. Parasitol.* **31,** 418–446.

Morseth, D. J. (1967). Fine structure of the hydatid cyst and protoscolex of *Echinococcus granulosus. J. Parasitol.* **53,** 312–325.

Pappas, P. W., and Read, C. P. (1975). Membrane transport in helminth parasites: A review. *Exp. Parasitol.* **37,** 469–530.

Price, E. W. (1938). North American monogenetic trematodes. II. The families Monocotylidae, Microbothriidae, Acanthocotylidae and Udonellidae (Capsaloidea). *J. Wash. Acad. Sci.* **28,** 183–198.

Schmidt, G. D. (1986). *Handbook of Tapeworm Identification.* CRC Press, Boca Raton, FL.

Smyth, J. D., and McManus, D. P. (1989). *The Physiology of Cestodes,* 2nd ed. Cambridge Univ. Press, Cambridge, UK.

Thomas, J. N., and Turner, S. G. (1980). A reinterpretation of the evidence for contact digestion in the tapeworm *Hymenolepis diminuta. J. Physiol.* **301,** 79P–80P.

Wardle, R. A., and McLeod, J. A. (1952). *The Zoology of Tapeworms.* Univ. of Minnesota Press, Minneapolis.

Wardle, R. A., McLeod, J. A., and Radinovsky, S. (1974). *Advances in the Zoology of Tapeworms, 1950–1970.* Univ. of Minnesota Press, Minneapolis.

Whitfield, P. J. (1979). The Biology of Parasitism. Univ. Park Press, Baltimore, Maryland.

Yamaguti, S. (1963). *Systema Helminthum. Vol. IV. Monogenea and Aspidocotylea.* Interscience, New York.

C H A P T E R

23

Orders Pseudophyllidea and Proteocephala

ORDER PSEUDOPHYLLIDEA

Pseudophyllidean tapeworms are pseudopolyzoic, because they have many proglottids, but they are formed "instantaneously" (Chapter 22). The scolex has dorsal and ventral grooves called *bothria*. The proglottids are wider than they are long and usually have midventral genital openings. A separate uteropore is also present. The eggs are usually operculate and unembryonated when laid. Testes and vitellaria are scattered throughout most of the proglottid. These are among the largest tapeworms known, some reaching 30 m in length. Of particular importance are the human and animal tapeworms belonging to the genera *Diphyllobothrium* and *Spirometra*.

Name of Organism and Disease Associations

Diphyllobothrium latum (syn. *Dibothriocephalus latus*); a number of *Diphyllobothrium* spp. cause diphyllobothriosis, diphyllobothriasis, or broad fish tapeworm disease in humans; *D. latum* is the most important. Humans are the principal final host, but numerous animal reservoirs exist.

Hosts and Host Range

The principal definitive host for *D. latum* is humankind. Other species of fish-eating mammals are infected; the domestic dog may be an important reservoir. Adult worms reside in the small intestines of definitive hosts.

Geographic Distribution and Importance

D. latum is a cosmopolitan species typically present in subarctic and temperate zones. Infections decrease substantially north of the Arctic Circle and in the tropics. The original focus of infection was northern Europe, from which the worm has spread through migrations of people carrying the infections with them. Human infection reports are common from the Scandinavian countries, the Balkan countries, Europe, Asia, and especially Japan, North America, and South America (Peru and Chile). Additional cases have been reported throughout the world; most apparently result from infections acquired in the previously mentioned areas.

Current estimates of human infections worldwide are about 9 million cases, of which 5 million are in Europe, 4 million in Asia, fewer than 100,000 are in North America, and even fewer are in South America. Serious disease is uncommon, but tapeworm anemia, usually called tapeworm pernicious anemia, can result.

Morphology

D. latum is the largest tapeworm that infects humans. Adults 20 to 25 m long and 1.5 to 2.0 cm maximum width have been recorded. A large worm may have 4000 proglottids, and spent portions of the strobila are shed in feces (pseudoapolysis).

The scolex has deep dorsal and ventral bothria (Fig. 23.1), followed by a short neck, and then a strobila of broad proglottids. A mature proglottid has a separate uteropore and a male and a female genital pore, all opening on the midventral surface (Fig. 23.2). Testes

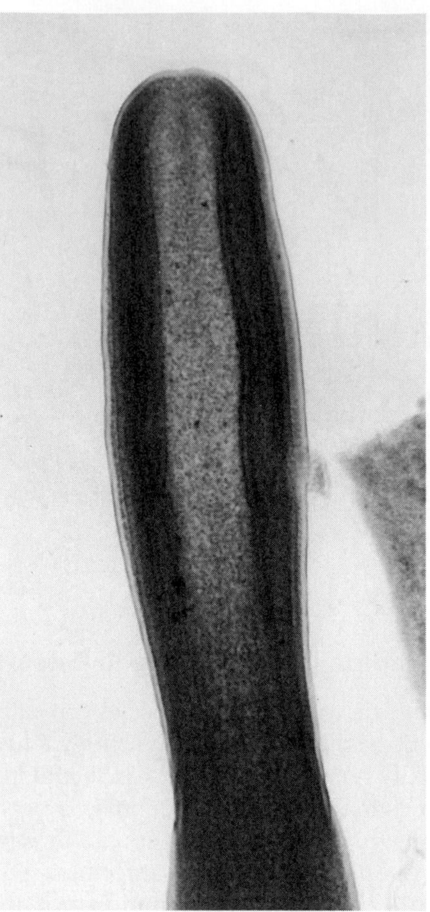

FIGURE 23.1 Scolex of *Diphyllobothrium latum* showing the bothria or grooves.

and vitellaria are scattered throughout most of the proglottid. The bilobed ovary is located in the posterior part of the proglottid; gravid proglottids appear to the naked eye to be brownish, because the anterior half is filled with uterine loops packed with eggs (Fig. 23.3). The eggs are ovoid and average 65 by 45 mm; they have an operculum at one end and a small knob at the opposite end (Fig. 23.4).

Life Cycle

Eggs are passed in the feces and take from 7 to 20 days to develop, depending on temperature and oxygen. Under anaerobic or nearly anaerobic conditions, embryonation proceeds for 5 to 6 days at 20°C, but the embryo then dies. Eggs develop better on a sandy or rocky substrate than on mud, probably because of availability of oxygen.

Hatching takes place under the influence of light after the coracidium is completely formed. Both the amount of light and its wavelength are important. Maximal hatching is seen at two wavelengths—in the yellow (500–600 nm) and in the ultraviolet (250 nm)—and only 30 to 60 seconds of light at 50 to 100 lux are required to start the process.

The spherical, ciliated coracidium is about 50 μm when it escapes from the egg capsules, but it increases in size to about 100 μm. Under good conditions, a coracidium may live five days while swimming in the water. Coracidia can tolerate salinity of 0.4% well but die quickly at 0.9%; therefore, they can live in brackish estuaries where the salinity is 0.2 to 0.4%.

First intermediate hosts are copepods, usually of the genera *Diaptomus* and *Cyclops*. About 40 species of the copepods have been infected with *D. latum*, and although there are differences in susceptibility, the host specificity is rather low. After being eaten by a copepod, the hexacanth embryo escapes from the ciliated covering and penetrates to the hemocoel, probably in the same way as the hexacanth of *T. saginatus*, by holding on with its hooks and secreting a substance to allow it to squeeze between cells. The hexacanth transforms into a procercoid, which is fully developed in about 14 days at 20°C. The procercoid is 500 to 600 μm long and about 300 μm wide, with a saclike structure at its posterior, the cercomere, which contains all that remains of the hexacanth—its hooks.

The second intermediate hosts are planktivorous fish, which eat the infected copepods. The procercoid migrates into the extraintestinal tissues of the fish and develops into the plerocercoid (Fig. 23.5), which is usually from 6 to 10 mm long. Nearly any tissue of the fish may be infected, but muscle, ovary (hard roe), and liver are especially important for transmission to humans, because these are the parts most often eaten. Different fish are important in different parts of the world (Tab. 23.1), but pike, perch, salmonids, and burbot are especially significant. The plerocercoid infection is passed from small planktivorous fish to larger predatory fish without change in the plerocercoid. It moves from the gut to the tissues of its new host and continues its existence there. A large pike or burbot can harbor 1000 plerocercoids and, in some areas, nearly 100% may be infected.

Humans or other definitive hosts become infected from eating raw or insufficiently cooked fish harboring the plerocercoid. Dogs may be important reservoir hosts in some areas, but the question remains open. The plerocercoid attaches to the intestinal wall with its primitive holdfast and grows to the adult. The worms grow at a rate of 5 cm a day and eggs are produced in from 25 to 30 days after infection. Infections may persist in humans for as long as 30 years.

Diagnosis

Finding eggs in the feces is the most certain diagnostic method. Eggs of *Paragonimus* are much like those of *D. latum* but somewhat larger.

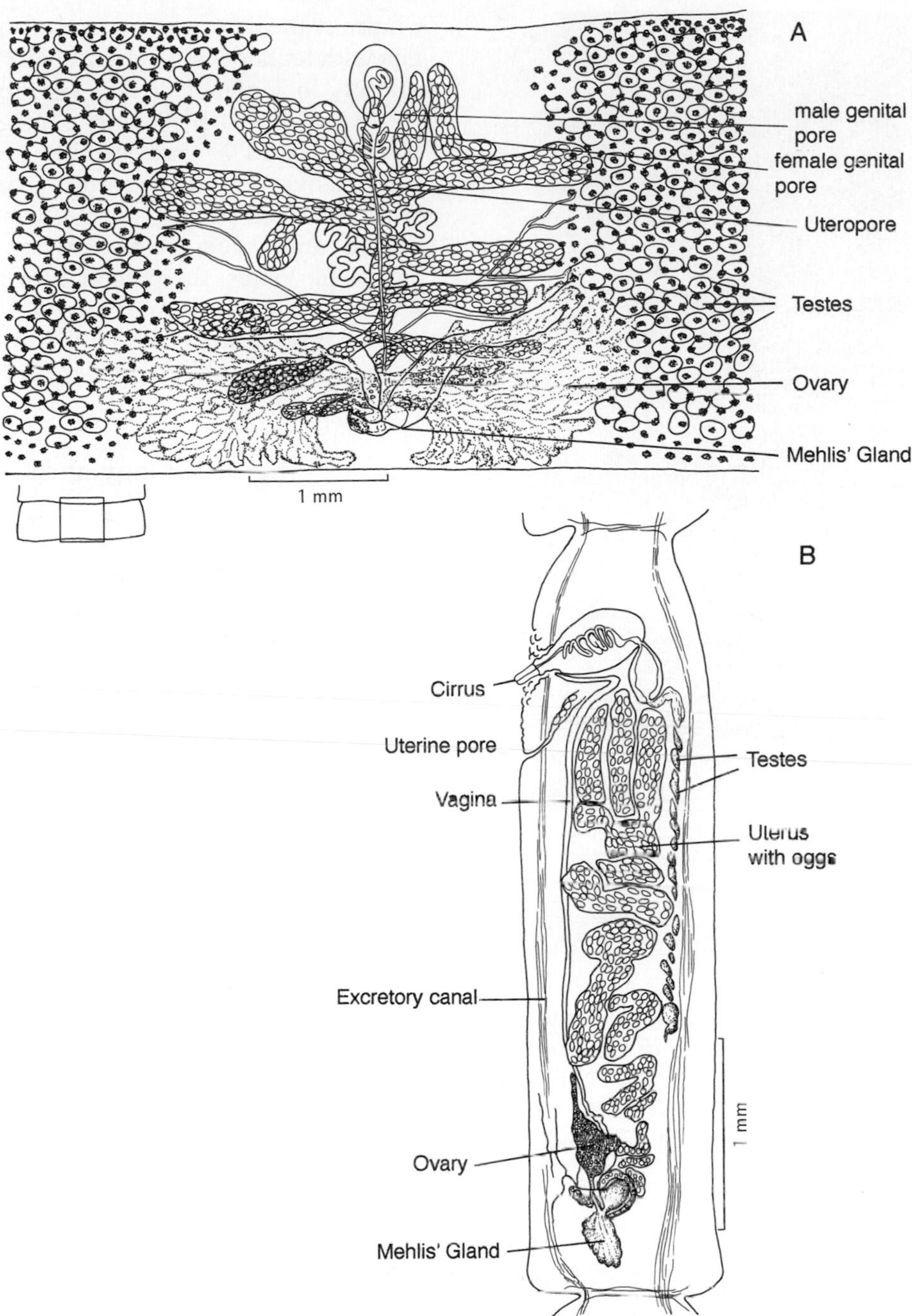

FIGURE 23.2 Diagram of gravid proglottids of *Diphyllobothrium latum:* (A) ventral view and (B) sagittal section. [Redrawn from Rausch and Hilliard, 1970.]

Host–Parasite Interactions

D. latum infections in humans usually cause little discomfort. The voracious appetite attributed to tapeworm infections is a myth, but some vague abdominal discomfort, diarrhea, and weakness may occur. *D. latum* rarely causes intestinal obstruction. There is local epithelial atrophy where the scolex is attached to the intestinal villi. When the villi are destroyed, the worm releases and moves to another site.

Tapeworm anemia, called *pernicious anemia,* is the most significant host–parasite interaction. Tapeworm anemia is rarely fatal, but von Bonsdorff (1977) recommended retaining the term *tapeworm pernicious anemia* because it is established in medical literature. He gave an interesting account of the accidental discovery of tapeworm anemia by a physician name Reyhner. The physician had a patient with "pernicious anemia" who also was passing tapeworm proglottids. When he treated the patient for the tapeworm, the anemia was

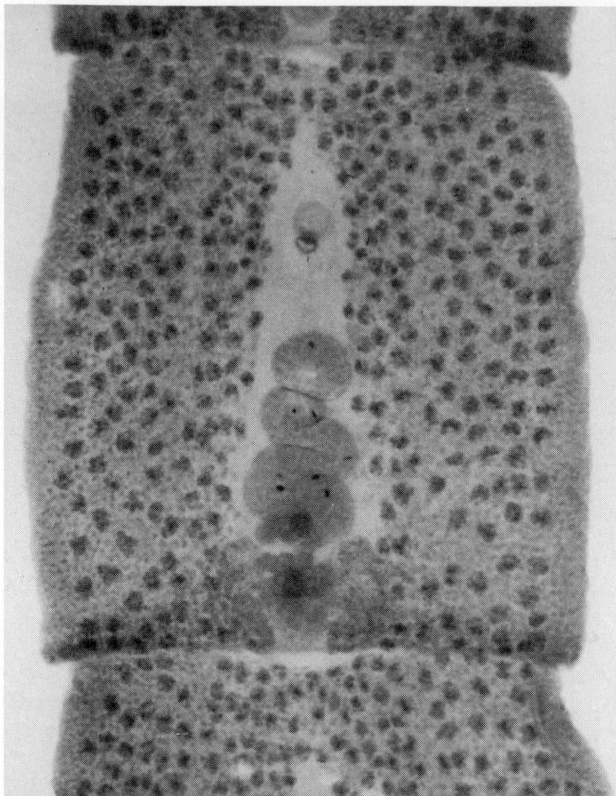

FIGURE 23.3 A stained whole mount of a gravid prolottid of *Diphyllobothrium latum* as seen in LM.

cured. His accidental bedside observation led to the discovery of a new disease.

Tapeworm anemia occurs in about 1 of 50 infected people, especially in Scandinavia; the disease results primarily from vitamin B_{12} deficiency. The worm absorbs vitamin B_{12} ingested by the host and reduces the amount of the vitamin needed for hematopoiesis.

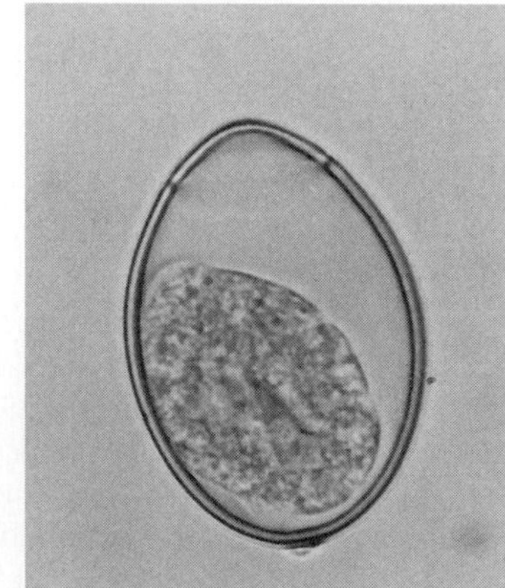

FIGURE 23.4 An egg of *Diphyllobothrium latum* with the operculum at the upper end and a small knob at the other.

Clinically the host has a macrocytic, megaloblastic anemia with leukopenia. Nyberg et al. (1961) studied 1345 subjects in Finland; of the 366 tapeworm infections (27.2%), 8 (1.9%) persons had megaloblastic anemia and another 1.1 % were borderline cases. Of the worm carriers, over 50% had a serum vitamin B_{12} concentration under 100 pg/ml; normal values are 150 to 900 pg/ml, and values below 100 are considered to be pathologic. Thus, the potential for more than the observed 2% tapeworm anemia exists. Probably the nonanemic hosts utilized stored vitamin B_{12}, and months or even years could pass before anemia developed.

Epidemiology and Control

Control of *D. latum* revolves around the following:

1. Eliminating intermediate hosts—copepods and fish
2. Treating infected persons
3. Providing proper disposal of human waste
4. Changing food habits

All but the first of these are feasible and are used in designing control programs. Although the infection is not especially hazardous to health, infected individuals should be treated in order to reduce possible contamination of the environment. As indicated, egg production of the worms is high, infections last a long time in humans, and humans are the principal definitive host. Reservoir hosts therefore will probably not be able to maintain the life cycle if human infections are eliminated. It should be noted that a few infected persons can transmit the infection to a large number of fish. At a lake in Sweden, 100% of susceptible fish were infected, but only 20 persons in the vicinity were infected (cited in von Bonsdorff and Bylund, 1982).

Modern sewage disposal, or at least efficient pit toilets, is essential for containment of any eggs that might reach the environment. Since eggs are not resistant to either freezing or drying, holding treated sludge for a period of time after treatment further reduces the probability of environmental contamination with eggs.

When campaigns to educate people about the source of infection have been instituted, changing dietary habits has been successful. For example, 34,000 infections recorded in Finland in 1959 were reduced to fewer than 2300 by 1975 following an intensive educational program. The total infection rate in Finland dropped from 20% to 1.8%. The endemic area surrounding the Great Lakes of the United States seems to have declined; infected fish have not been found. It seems likely that the habit of eating raw fish has declined. In parts of Alaska and Canada, diphyllobothriasis re-

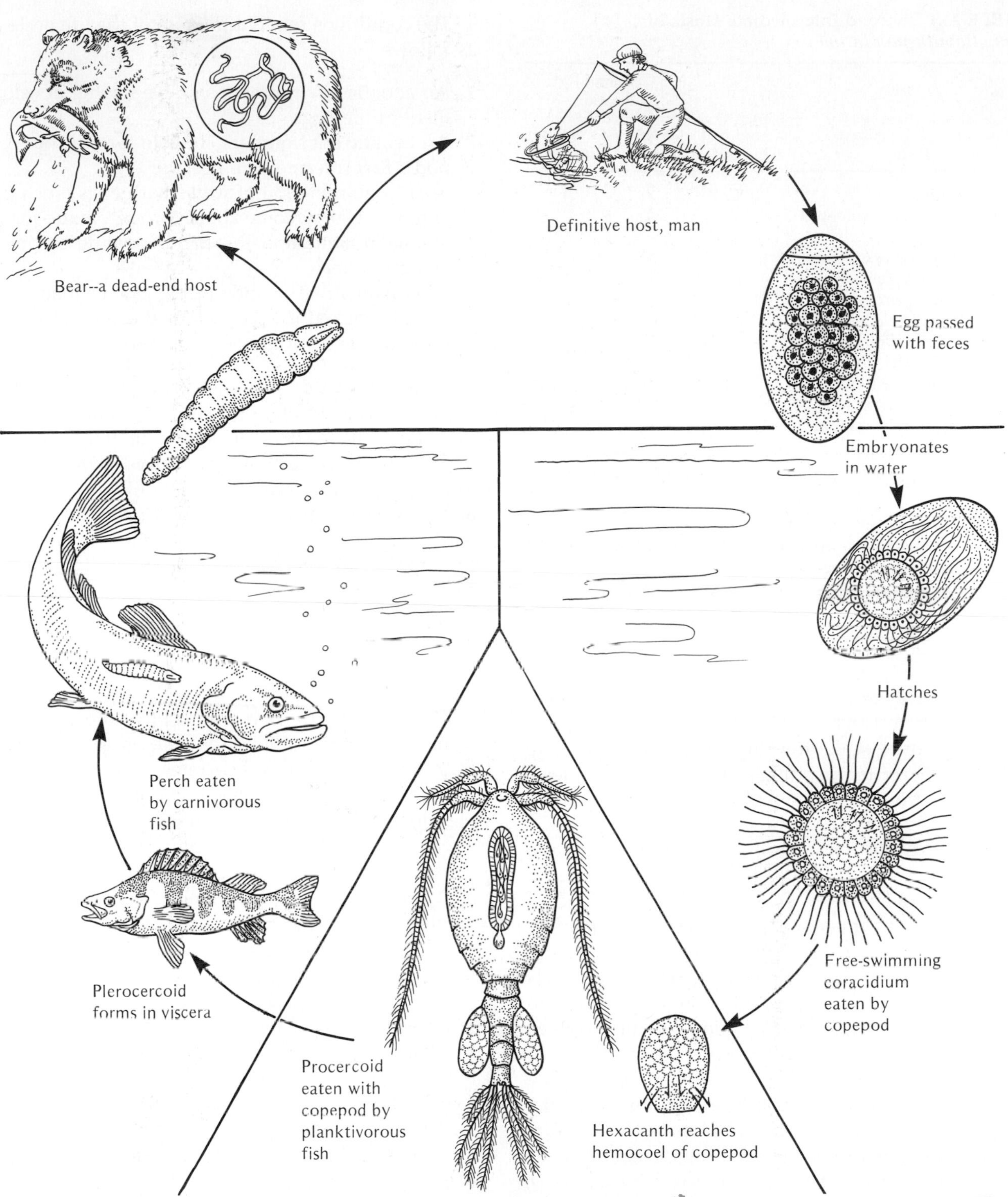

FIGURE 23.5 Life cycle and epidemiology of *Diphyllobothrium latum.*

TABLE 23.1 Second Intermediate Hosts of *Diphyllobothrium latum*

Fish	Geographical location		
	Eurasia	North America	South America
Esox lucius (pike)	X	X	
Stizostedeon vitreum (wall-eyed pike)		X	
S. canadense (sand pike)		X	
Perca fluviatilis (perch)	X		
Perca flavescens (perch)		X	
Lota lota (burbot)	X		
Lota maculosa (burbot)		X	
Onchorhynchus spp. (trout)		X	
Salmo lacustris (lake trout)			X
Salmo irideus (trout)			X
Salmo gairdneri (rainbow trout)			X

mains a problem because sewage disposal is poor and fish are still eaten raw.

Cooking fish is the most effective way of killing the plerocercoids. As with many parasites, heating to 55 to 60°C kills them; this is about the temperature at which protein coagulates and kills plerocercoids. If fish are smoked, therefore, the temperature in the smokehouse needs to reach 55 to 60°C. At the other end of the temperature scale, freezing for 24 hours or more at home freezer temperature (0°C, −18°F) kills plerocercoids. Curing fish for five days in 10% salt solution also kills plerocercoids.

Numerous folk remedies have been used to expel tapeworms; some are quite effective, but they usually have severe side effects. One example is an extract of the rhizome of a male fern, *Dryopteris felix mas*. The active ingredients are acylphloroglucinoles and a derivative; Desaspidin is in current use. The most widely used drugs are niclosamide and praziquantel. In addition to being wormed, anemic patients should be given vitamin B_{12} to replenish fully the body stores that may have been depleted.

D. latum is primarily an infection of humans, but a number of other species of mammals can also be infected. Among domestic animals, dogs, cats, and swine are readily infected, and wolves, foxes, bears, seals, and other fish-eating wild animals have been found to be infected in nature or have been infected experimentally. Epidemiological studies indicate that there is no feral cycle of *D. latum*, but rather that humans must be present for its maintenance. The role of humans seems to be to provide the right epidemiological conditions for transmission.

The conditions for continuation of the life cycle are as follows:

1. An aquatic environment suitable for the development of the eggs
2. An aquatic environment suitable for the copepod's first intermediate host
3. Fecal contamination of water with eggs (such contamination may come about through inadequate sewage treatment or through people defecating in or near water)
4. Food habits that include eating raw or inadequately cooked fish, especially those species that serve as the second intermediate host

Considering this list, one can appreciate that the conditions are not often satisfied. The aquatic system must be relatively free of organic matter so that the dissolved oxygen does not drop too low for the eggs to develop. Water temperature should be 15 to 20°C, but it can range from 4 to 25°C. Copepods are ordinarily found in waters that are still or that do not run rapidly. Infection of copepods takes place near the shoreline, so a shallow littoral area is conducive to bringing the coracidia and the copepods near one another. A threshold density of about 1000 copepods per cubic meter must be met before infection can be maintained in them.

The type of lake is important for infection of the second intermediate hosts as well as the first. Deep oligotrophic lakes have low rates of infection in fish, whereas shallow eutrophic lakes are likely to have high levels of infection even where the prevalence of infection in the human population is low.

The last element is the human, who must be considered from the standpoint of both dietary and sanitary habits. Eating raw or partially cooked fish is associated either with primitive conditions, where fuel for cooking is not available, or with areas where certain fish dishes are a traditional part of the diet. Even the preparation of fish plays a part in transmitting the infection; for example, gefilte fish is cooked before being served, but it is often tasted by the cook when it is seasoned to make sure that it is properly spiced.

Promiscuous defecation is an obvious enough problem, but even in a well-designed treatment plant, 5% of the *D. latum* eggs may be found in the effluent. Where the system is overloaded or not well run, higher numbers escape treatment. An individual infected with *D. latum* may pass from 2 million to 40 million eggs per day, and that means that a minimum of 100,000 eggs a day would survive treatment from that one person. Since we know that infections can last for 30 years, a minimum of 1 billion eggs would be disseminated into the environment even under conditions of good sewage treatment.

D. latum has been distributed from its ancestral home in northern Europe to a number of other places that have all the right conditions. The infections in Alaska were probably carried there by Russians who maintained a colony on the Alaskan coast from about 1741 to 1867, and the endemic area in the Midwestern United States was probably established by immigrants from Scandinavia.

Related Species

Human infections with pseudophyllidean tapeworms have been reported from the former Soviet Union, North and South America, Scandinavia, and Japan. In addition to *Diphyllobothrium latum*, 11 other species of *Diphyllobothrium* and 3 of *Diplogonoporus* are pseudophyllidean tapeworms that infect humans who ingest plerocercoids in fishes. The taxonomy of this group of organisms is currently unsettled, and there may be fewer species involved. *Diplogonoporus* is easily identified by its double set of reproductive organs per proglottid.

SPARGANOSIS

In addition to being a definitive host for adult pseudophyllidean tapeworms, humans can also be a transport host for plerocercoids. Unidentified plerocercoids were originally given the generic designation *Sparganum*, and the term *sparganosis* is still used for plerocercoid infections. Today most spargana are known to be plerocercoids of members of the genus *Spirometra*. Human cases of sparganosis have been reported worldwide, but most are from China, Japan, and Southeast Asia. The taxonomy of this genus is uncertain. The Far Eastern parasite is called *Spirometra mansoni* or *S. erinacei*, and the parasite found in the United States is usually called *S. mansonoides*. To add to the confusion, Mueller (1974) admitted that if the rules of zoological nomenclature were strictly followed, the generic name should be *Luehella*; but the name *Spirometra* is firmly entrenched in both parasitological and medical literature and will probably persist.

The genus *Spirometra* has a typical pseudophyllidean life cycle; the coracidium escapes from an operculate egg and is ingested by a copepod. The copepod harbors the procercoid stage. Second intermediate hosts include amphibians, reptiles, and mammals, but not fish. Definitive hosts are cats, related species, and, rarely, reptiles; they are infected by eating second intermediate hosts infected with plerocercoids.

Humans can become infected in three ways:

1. A human who drinks water containing copepods infected with procercoids will become a true second intermediate host. The procercoid will penetrate the intestinal wall and enter the subcutaneous tissue, where it will develop into a plerocercoid.
2. Humans can ingest uncooked or poorly cooked frogs, snakes, birds, or mammals containing plerocercoids. They also migrate through the intestinal wall and encyst as spargana; humans are a paratenic host in this event.
3. By pressing the flesh of an infected frog as a poultice to ulcers, wounds, or sore eyes, individuals are infected. Plerocercoids migrate from the frog to the human tissue, and once again the person becomes a paratenic host. Poulticing is a common medical practice for treatment of skin and eye diseases in Viet Nam, Thailand, and other Far Eastern countries.

Spargana are usually encapsulated by fibrous connective tissue and can appear grossly like tumors of the eye, subcutaneous tissues, or almost any visceral organ; they can cause elephantiasis-like symptoms if they locate in lymphatic ducts.

Satisfactory treatment is obtained by surgical excision of the nodule containing the parasite. Control methods include ensuring safe drinking water, cooking of frog, snake, and mammal flesh, and avoidance of poultices. All of these are difficult to accomplish with the current socioeconomic situation in the Far East. Since this disease is a zoonosis in which cats are principal definitive hosts, elimination of adult worms is impractical. Fortunately, the number of cases of sparganosis with severe lesions is small.

ORDER PROTEOCEPHALA

The order Proteocephala is composed of about 30 genera, all endoparasitic in fishes, amphibians, and reptiles as adults. The adults and the two metacestode stages, procercoids and plerocercoids, all have scolices with four suckers; in some species an additional fifth apical sucker is present as well. A distinctive morphological feature of adult proteocephalans is the lateral location of the vitellaria in mature proglottids. Most proteocephalans belong to the genus *Proteocephalus*, and one of the best known of these is *Proteocephalus ambloplitis*, a parasite of bass and perch.

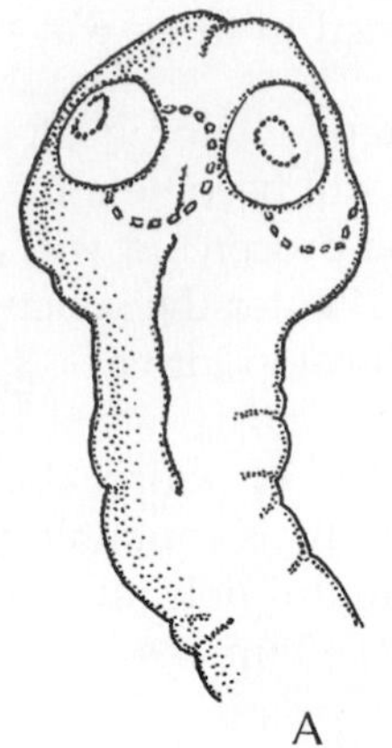

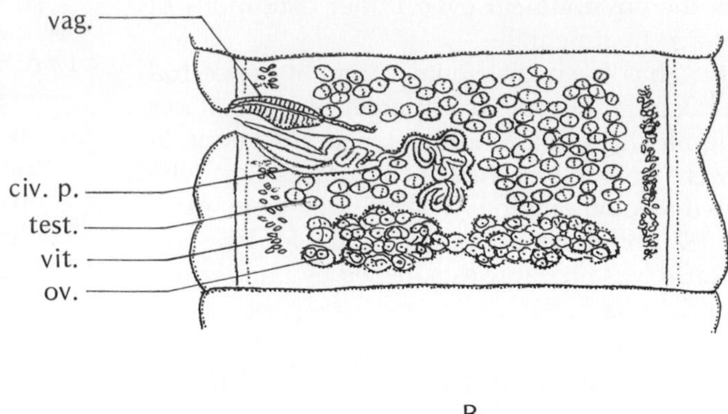

FIGURE 23.6 Morphology of *Proteocephalus* sp. (A) scolex, (B) mature proglottid. Abbreviations: civ. p, cirrus pouch; ov, ovary; test, testis; vag, vagina; vit, vitellaria [(A) Redrawn from Hoffman, G. L., 1967. (B) Redrawn from VanCleave, H. J., and Mueller, J. P., 1934.]

Name of Organism and Disease Associations

Proteocephalus ambloplitis is known as the bass tapeworm.

Hosts and Host Range

Adults are common intestinal parasites in bass, *Micropterus dolomieui* and *M. salmoides*, but are also found in the yellow perch (*Perca flavescens*), the bowfin (*Amia calva*), and other freshwater fishes.

Geographic Distribution and Importance

The bass tapeworm infects fish throughout much of North America. Wandering plerocercoids sometimes cause so much fibrosis of the gonads that bass are rendered sexually sterile (parasitic castration). Because bass are an important sport fish, this disease has received widespread attention.

Morphology

Adults have lateral genital pores and vitellaria that extend from the anterior to the posterior ends of the mature proglottids (Fig. 23.6). Adults, procercoids, and plerocercoids all bear four suckers.

Life Cycle

Usually the life cycle of *P. ambloplitis* involves three hosts. Gravid proglottids are passed in host feces; they rupture upon contact with water, releasing embryonated eggs. Eggs are ingested by crustaceans including *Cyclops* sp. and *Hyallela* sp., and procercoids develop in the hemocoel. When infected crustaceans are eaten by second intermediate hosts, centrarchid or percid fishes, plerocercoids develop in the viscera. Definitive hosts become infected by eating infected smaller fish. Often, large bass harbor numerous plerocercoids; they were once thought to be a dead end in the life cycle because it was unlikely that an even larger fish would eat them. However, Fischer and Freeman (1969) found that the usual three-host life cycle is often a two-host cycle: plerocercoids in the viscera can penetrate back into the gut of the same fish host and develop into adults.

Epidemiology and Control

The anthelminthic di-*n*-butyl tin oxide removes all gut tapeworms. The treatment must be repeated yearly in hatchery stock because visceral plerocercoids are unaffected. The best method of control is to start with clean fry for stocking purposes.

Readings

Adams, A. M., and Rausch, R. L. (1997). Diphyllobothrium. In *Pathology of Infectious Diseases* (D. H. Connor, F. W. Chandler, *et al.*, Eds.), Vol. 2. Appleton & Lange, Stamford, CT.

Andersen, K., Ching, H. L., and Vik, R. (1987). A review of the freshwater species of *Diphyllobothrium* with redescriptions and the distribution of *D. dendriticum* (Nitsch, 1824) and *D. ditremum* (Creplin, 1825) from North America. *Can. J. Zool.* **65,** 2216–2228.

Becker, C. D., and Brunson, W. D. (1968). The bass tapeworm: A problem in northwest trout management. *Prog. Fish Cult.* **30,** 76–83.

Fischer, H., and Freeman, R. S. (1969). Penetration of parenteral plerocercoids of *Proteocephalus ambloplitis* (Leidy) into the gut of smallmouth bass. *J. Parasitol.* **55,** 766–774.

Freze, V. I. (1965). *Essentials of Cestodology. Vol. V. Proteocephalata in Fish, Amphibians and Reptiles.* Izdat. Akad. Nauk., Moscow.

Meyer, M. C. (1970). Cestode zoonoses of aquatic animals. *J. Wildlife Dis.* **6,** 249–254.
Mueller, J. F. (1974). The biology of Spirometra. *J. Parasitol.* **60,** 3–14.
Nyberg, W., Gräsbeck, R., Saarni, M., and von Bonsdorff, B. (1961). Serum vitamin B_{12} levels and incidence of tapeworm anemia in a population heavily infected with *Diphyllobothrium latum. Am. J. Clin. Nutr.* **9,** 606–612.
Peters, L., Cavis, D., and Robertson, J. (1978). Is *Diphyllobothrium latum* currently present in northern Michigan? *J. Parasitol.* **64,** 947–949.
Rausch, R. L., and Hilliard, D. K. (1970). Studies on the helminth fauna of Alaska. XLIX. The occurrence of *Diphyllobothrium latum* (Linnaeus, 1758) (Cestoda:Diphyllobriidae) in Alaska, with notes on other species. *Can. J. Zool.* **48,** 1201–1219.
VanCleave, H. J., and Mueller, J. P. (1934). Parasites of Oneida Lake fishes. Part III. A biological and ecological survey of the worm parasites. *Roosevelt Wild Life Ann.* **3,** 161–334.
von Bonsdorff, B. (1977). *Diphyllobothriasis in Man*. Academic Press, New York.
von Bonsdorff, B., and Bylund, G. (1982). The ecology of *Diphyllobothrium latum. Ecol. Dis.* **1,** 21–26.
Wardle, R. A., and McLeod, J. A. (1952). *The Zoology of Tapeworms*. Univ. of Minnesota Press, Minneapolis.
Williams, H., and Jones, A. (1994). *Parasitic Worms of Fish*. Taylor & Francis, London.
Williams, H. H., and Jones, A. (1976). *Marine Helminths and Human Disease*, Misc. Publ. No. 3. Commonwealth Agricultural Bureaux, Farnham Royal, Bucks, UK.
Yamaguti, S. (1959). *Systema Helminthum. Vol. II. The Cestodes of Vertebrates.* Interscience, New York.

CHAPTER

24

Cyclophyllidea

The order Cyclophyllidea includes most of the tapeworms of medical and veterinary importance as well as most of those that infect birds and mammals. The scolex with four suckers and a compact vitelline gland are identifying features of the adults of this order. They range in size from a few millimeters long in *Echinococcus* to more than 12 m long in *Taenia saginata*. A few, such as *Echinococcus*, infect humans as larvae and in others, such as *Taenia saginata*, the beef tapeworm, humans are the definitive host. *Taenia solium* is a double threat since both larvae and adults can infect humans, occasionally simultaneously.

FAMILY TAENIIDAE

Taeniids are the most important adult tapeworms of humans, canids, and felids; in addition, humans, cattle, and swine and other hosts are infected by larval taeniids. Therefore, they are of both medical and veterinary importance.

Traditionally taeniids have been placed in several genera whose adult forms are quite similar but whose larvae are different. *Taenia* has a cysticercus (Fig. 24.1), *Multiceps* has a coenurus (Fig. 24.6), *Hydatigera* has a strobilocercus (Fig. 24.7), and *Echinococcus* has a hydatid (Fig. 24.10). An identifying feature of taeniids is the scolex with four suckers (Fig. 24.4) and a double row of hooks (Fig. 24.2). *Taenia saginata,* sometimes called *Taeniarhynchus saginata,* is identical to other members of the genus except that it lacks rostellar hooks. Wardle and McLeod (1952) retained the various genera, but with the following reservations:

> This practice opens up the question as to whether, in the absence of any practicable method of counting chromosomes, the specific and generic units of zoological classification shall be based upon readily recognizable characteristics of *adult* animal, or upon features of the life cycle and biology, a procedure while eminently desirable is rarely attainable.

Studies such as those of Verster (1967, 1969) have led to the conclusion that adult structure is more important than that of the larvae, and larval evolution may have taken place secondarily (Moore, 1981). Two genera are now accepted in the Taeniidae: *Taenia* and *Echinococcus*.

Name of Organism and Disease Associations

Taenia saginata (syn. *Taeniarhynchus saginatus, Cysticercus bovis*), causes taeniosis, taeniasis, cysticercosis, beef tapeworm, and measly beef.

Hosts and Host Range

Humans are the only definitive host. The main intermediate hosts are domesticated members of the artiodactyl family Bovidae and the reindeer, *Rangifer tarandus* (family Cervidae). Adults are in the small intestine of the definitive host; cysticerci are in the striated muscles of the intermediate host. Whether humans are infected with cysticerci, despite 12 records in the medical literature, is still an open question.

Geographic Distribution and Importance

Beef tapeworm infections in humans are cosmopolitan. It is the most common taeniid tapeworm of humans. More than 39 million infections are estimated

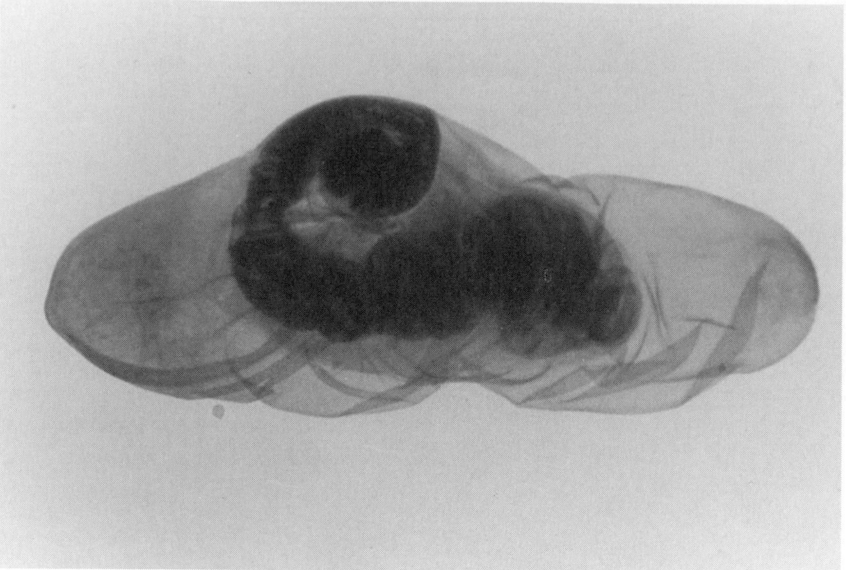

FIGURE 24.1 A whole mount of a cysticercus of *Taenia.* sp. as seen in LM.

throughout the world, and the prevalence of infection in the United States is 23 per 100,000. Infections seldom lead to serious disease; the infected persons, because they have adequate protein in the diet, usually remain in a good nutritional state

The greatest financial losses are in the beef cattle industry. An annual loss of $500,000 is estimated in the United States due to carcasses that are condemned or must be frozen to comply with meat inspection regulations. In developing countries, the loss is estimated at $25 per animal.

Morphology

Unlike other taeniids, neither the adult nor the metacestode of *Taenia saginata* has rostellar hooks, although they occur ephemerally during larval development. Adults are usually 4 to 12 m long and 12 to 14 mm wide. They have a typical taeniid reproductive system (Fig. 22.13) including a bilobed ovary; a vaginal sphincter is found in this species and *T. hydatigena* only. Gravid proglottids have 14 to 32 lateral uterine branches; the number of branches is sometimes used in identification (see Diagnosis).

The spherical eggs with their thick, striated capsules (Fig. 24.3) cannot be distinguished from other taeniid eggs with any degree of confidence.

The fully developed cysticercus is white, about 10 mm in diameter, and has a single unarmed scolex inverted in a fluid-filled bladder (Fig. 24.1). Before an association was made between the adult and metacestode of *T. saginata*, the name of the metacestode, *Cysticercus bovis*, was established. Regrettably we still have two so-called scientific names for the same organism. Both names continue to be used in the scientific literature and in meat inspection, as do the names of some other adult and larval tapeworms (Tab. 24.1).

Life Cycle

Humans become infected by eating cysticerci in raw or partially cooked beef. The scolex evaginates in the small intestine, attaches, and the proglottids begin to differentiate. About three to four months after ingesting cysticerci, gravid proglottids begin to appear in the feces. Proglottids are shed irregularly and may even crawl out of the anus; they are motile most often in the late afternoon and early evening. Cattle become infected by eating eggs while grazing; the cysticerci in the muscles reach infectivity about 60 days after being eaten.

Diagnosis

Signs and symptoms of taeniosis are rather vague and finding the eggs is the best method of determining whether a person has a taeniid infection, but an identification to species cannot be made from the eggs because they are so similar. The principal methods are as follows:

1. Perianal swabs made on three alternate days. The material is examined as a wet mount under a compound microscope.
2. Thick, stained smears of feces may be examined also.

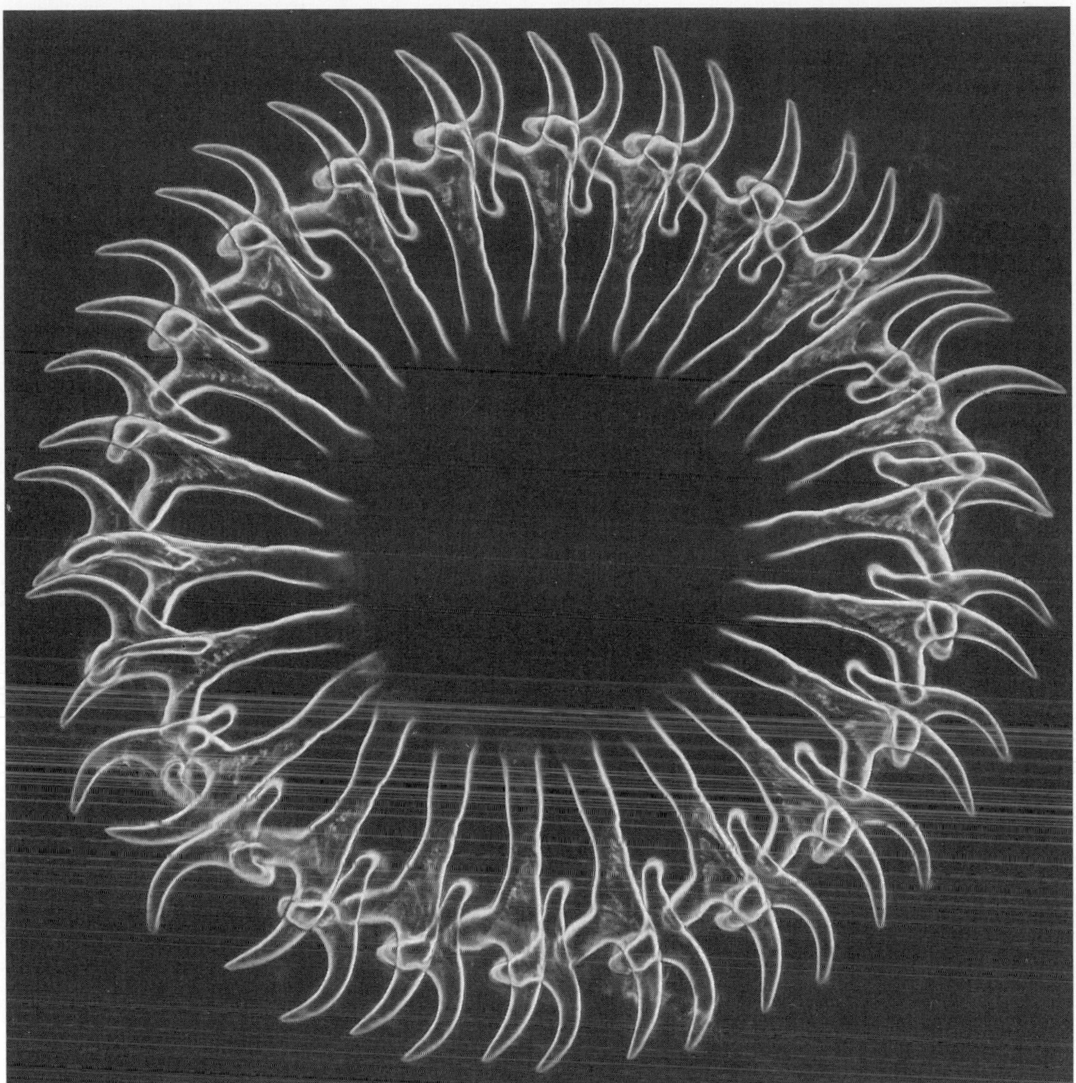

FIGURE 24.2 A whole mount of the circlet of hooks of *Taenia pisiformis* photographed in darkfield microscopy. Note the alternating large and small hooks, this is referred as a double row of hooks.

3. Eggs in feces may be concentrated by either flotation or sedimentation techniques.
4. Serological tests may be done to determine whether the person has antibodies in the blood to tapeworms. This is not a highly specific method.

The symptoms of infection with *T. saginata* do not clearly relate to a tapeworm infection. There may be abdominal discomfort, diarrhea, and frequent hunger pangs, hardly characteristics of anything specific. The most frequent sign is the discharge of proglottids, which can hardly go unnoticed. The proglottids are examined, and the characteristic bilobed ovary in the mature proglottid and the vaginal sphincter muscle in the gravid proglottid are good indications of the presence of *T. saginata*. The number of uterine branches has been used to distinguish between *T. saginata* (14–32) and *T. solium* (7–16), but it is not a reliable characteristic because of the difficulty in obtaining a good preparation and wide variation in the number of uterine branches. If a person is given an anthelmintic and worms are passed, the scolices can be examined, and if they are a taeniid type but lack hooks, the identification is almost certain.

Host–Parasite Interactions

Most *T. saginata* infections cause little damage to the host (see Diagnosis), but occasionally there is sufficient irritation to the gut to cause muscular spasms giving considerable abdominal pain. Occasionally the worms

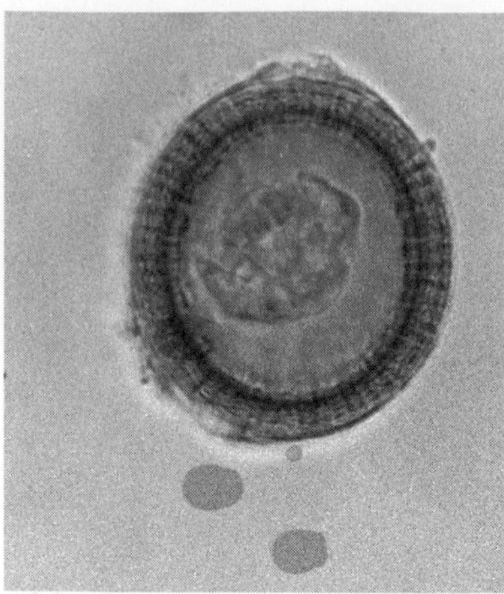

FIGURE 24.3 A taeniid egg showing the characteristic striated outer capsule. In general, taeniid eggs can not be identified to species.

migrate into the appendix, causing severe reactions leading to appendicitis.

Epidemiology and Control

In a general context, the following methods are important for controlling infections in humans:

1. A meat inspection program to find infected carcasses
2. Condemnation of heavily infected carcasses

TABLE 24.1 Tapeworm Synonyms

Name of Adult	Name of Metacestode[a]
Taenia hydatigena	*Cysticercus tenuicollis*
Taenia pisiformis	*Cysticercus pisiformis*
Taenia ovis	*Cysticercus ovis*
Taenia taeniaeformis (=*Hydatigera t.*)	*Cysticercus fasciolaris,* Strobilocercus
Taenia solium	*Cysticercus cellulosae* *C. racemosus*
Taenia krabbei	*Cysticercus tarandi*
Taenia crassiceps	*Cysticercus longicollis*
Taenia saginata (=*Taeniarhynchus saginatus*)	*Cysticercus bovis*
Taenia multiceps (=*Multiceps m.*)	*Coenurus cerebralis*
Taenia serialis (=*Multiceps s.*)	*Coenurus serialis,* *C. glomeratus*
Echinococcus granulosus	Hydatid Unilocular cyst
Echinococcus multilocularis	Alveolar hydatid Multilocular hydatid
Spirometra	*Sparganum*
Spirometra mansonoides	*Sparganum proliferum*

[a]"Scientific" names of metacestodes are in italics; the names of the metacestodes are in Roman type; names of adults are the only acceptable scientific names but the names of the metacestodes are still used.

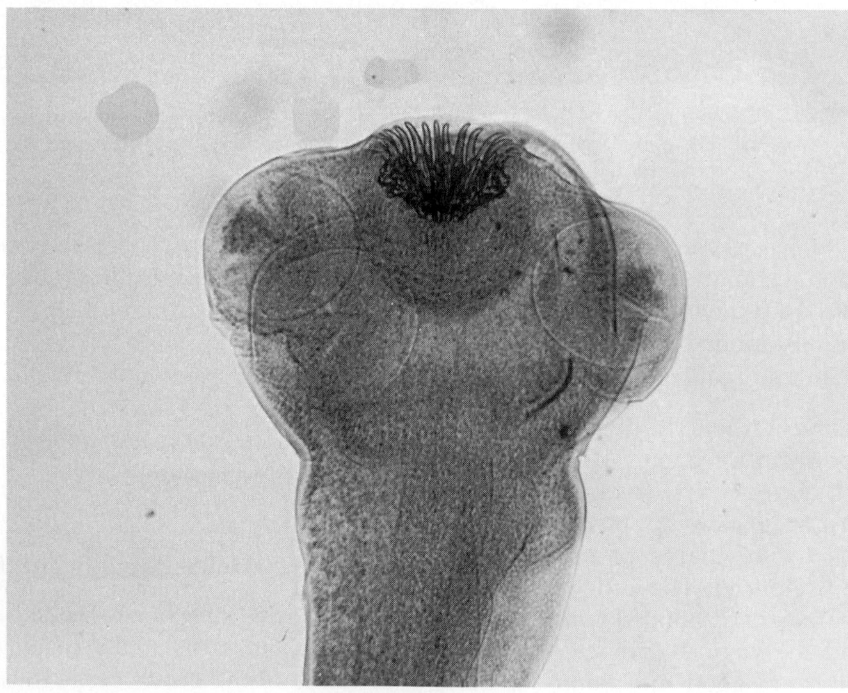

FIGURE 24.4 A whole mount of the scolex of *Taenia* as seen in LM.

3. Freezing of lightly infected carcasses
4. Awareness on the part of the consumer of the possibility of infection so that beef is eaten only when cooked sufficiently to kill the cysticerci (60°C, 140°F)

Recommendations for control of bovine cysticercosis so that infections do not reach humans include the following:

1. Treatment of any infected workers on a ranch or feedlot
2. Education of employees about the mode of transmission and personal hygiene
3. Provision of sanitary facilities that are readily accessible and will contain any infectious agent
4. Periodic examination of treated employees to ensure that they have not become reinfected
5. Preventing unauthorized persons from entering the premises

In their review of taeniid infections, Pawlowski and Schultz (1972) commented on the paradox that "infection is prevalent in developed countries because they are rich and in the developing nations because they are poor!" They were referring to the consumption of raw beef dishes such as steak tartar or rare steaks among well-to do persons and poor sanitation and lack of fuel that lead to a high prevalence of infection in both humans and cattle among poor peoples.

Many infections in cattle are acquired by indirect means. Eggs can be spread by flies or passed through the digestive tracts of birds. They can also pass sewage treatment unharmed and appear in the effluent or in sludge drying pits. In the southwestern United States, farm workers may defecate in irrigation ditches and their feces will then spread on fields when the water is turned on; if one of them carries a tapeworm infection, it can be carried some distance.

An outbreak of bovine cysticercosis in a large feedlot in California illustrates the potential losses that an owner can incur. One infected worker infected almost 5% of cattle over several months, causing a large financial loss when the cattle went to slaughter.

Although cysticerci seem not to be pathogenic for cattle, they do live for long periods, at least a year, and perhaps as long as three years so holding cattle until the cysticerci die is not feasible.

Although meat inspection detects only three-fourths of infected carcasses because of the small size of the cysticerci, the probability of infection is reduced by inspection. Beef should be cooked so that the cysticerci in its center will be killed; adequate cooking also kills other parasites such as *Toxoplasma gondii* and *Sarcocystis* (Chapter 13). In light infections, freezing the carcass is allowed to kill the cysticerci:

Time (hour)	Temperature (°C)
360	−5
216	−10
144	−15 or lower

Although the risk of infection is small where these precautions are observed, the predilection of some persons for rare beef ensures that the beef tapeworm will be with us for the foreseeable future.

The drug of choice for treatment of humans is niclosamide; it is highly effective and is usually tolerated well.

Name of Organism and Disease Associations

Taenia solium (*Cysticercus cellulosae, C. racemosis*) causes taeniosis, taeniasis, cysticercosis, and pork tapeworm.

Hosts and Host Range

Humans are the definitive host; adults live in the small intestine. Pigs are the most common intermediate hosts; dogs, monkeys, camels, deer, sheep, cats, and humans may harbor the cysticercus. Cysticerci tend to localize in striated muscle but can be found in almost any organ. Neurocysticercosis is a major human health problem in Mexico and Latin America and is the most prevalent central nervous system (CNS) parasitic disease in the United States.

Geographic Distribution and Importance

T. solium is a cosmopolitan parasite with a prevalence of infection in the human population of 2 to 3% based on a number of studies; however, in certain localities its prevalence is much higher.

It is rarely found in humans in the United States. Even though the pork tapeworm occurs less often than the beef tapeworm in humans, it is a more significant medical problem. Humans can be a host of the cysticercus as well as the adult; it is unusual, but not unknown, for the same species of vertebrate to serve as both definitive and intermediate host for a tapeworm. *Hymenolepis nana* is another example. Like the beef tapeworm, the pork tapeworm causes little intestinal damage to humans, but when the eggs are ingested, cysticerci develop in striated muscles, liver, or the CNS, often with serious or even fatal consequences. In addition, an infected person who may not have fastidious personal habits can be a source of infection for other members of a household.

About 2 to 5% of pigs are infected with *T. solium* cysticerci worldwide. Figures for economic losses to "measly pork" are difficult to obtain for most parts of the world, but they must be in the millions of dollars annually.

Morphology

Adults are 2 to 8 m long and have a typical taeniid rostellum with a double row of hooks (Fig. 24.2). The ovary in the mature proglottid has three lobes (Fig. 24.5) and the gravid uterus has 7 to 16 lateral branches. Eggs are indistinguishable from other taeniid eggs. The mature cysticerci are about 5 by 9 mm and are white; they have an invaginated scolex with hooks and a fluid-filled bladder.

Life Cycle

The life cycle of *T. solium* is the same in many respects as that of *T. saginata*; humans, the definitive host, are infected by ingesting raw or poorly cooked pork containing cysticerci. The scolex evaginates in the small intestine and attaches to the wall of the gut, where it strobilates. Gravid proglottids develop about five weeks after infection. Gravid proglottids are shed only during a bowel movement since the proglottids are only weakly motile (unlike *T. saginata*). The eggs are resistant to environmental hazards and remain alive for months. After ingestion by the intermediate host, eggs hatch in the small intestine, penetrate the intestinal mucosa, and enter small mesenteric veins. Having reached the circulatory system, the hexacanth embryos are carried throughout the body and lodge especially in the striated muscles, liver, and brain. The cysticerci reach infectivity in about two months.

When a human is the intermediate host, the person becomes infected by ingesting eggs in contaminated food or water (heteroinfection) or by carrying them on contaminated fingers to the mouth (autoinfection).

Diagnosis

See *T. saginata* when humans are suspected of being the definitive host. Cysticercosis is diagnosed by serological tests, X rays, and biopsies. In swine

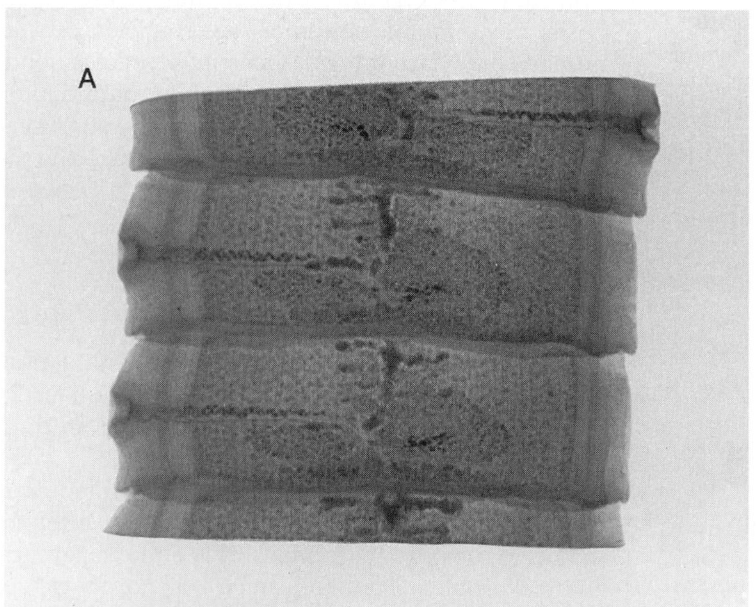

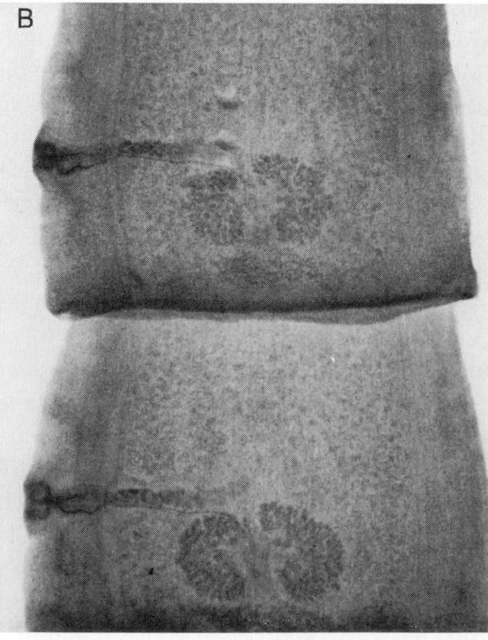

FIGURE 24.5 Stained whole mounts of proglottids of *Taenia* spp. as seen in LM. (A) *T. solium* proglottids are barely maturing. The tri-lobed ovary is characteristic of this species. (B) *T. pisiformis*. A number of diagnostic structures can be seen including the ovary, Mehlis' gland, vagina, genital atrium, seminal vesicle, and the lateral excretory canals. In both specimens the testes are seen as small rather granular structures scattered in the parenchyma from the mid-line to the excretory canals.

going to slaughter, the cysticerci are looked for in the muscles.

Host–Parasite Interactions

Intestinal infections with *T. solium* have the same clinical manifestations as those of *T. saginata*. Usually only one adult worm is present, hence, the name *solium*; but two or more are occasionally found and some persons harbor other species of tapeworms as well.

Serious effects may result from cysticercosis in humans. Although they may be found in almost any organ, cysticerci are commonly located in striated muscles, liver, the eye, and the CNS, where they most often are in the meninges and the ventricles of the brain. About 30% of human infections are in the brain; these cysticerci are usually less than 20 mm in diameter with a volume of only a few milliliters, but in one case report, a cysticercus had a diameter of 50 mm and a volume of 60 ml. In an aberrant form of *T. solium*, apparently found only in the CNS, a cysticercus has daughter cysticerci budding from the bladder wall and forming an invasive, proliferating parasite. This type of metacestode is referred to as a *racemose cysticercus* and is sometimes given the quasi-scientific name of *Cysticercus racemosis*. No viable scolices have been found in racemose cysticerci.

Living cysticerci usually elicit little inflammatory response. They damage the host by forming space-occupying lesions; that is, their growth puts pressure on the adjacent tissue and interferes with its function or causes necrosis due to reduced circulation. In the ventricles of the brain, the organisms often cause hydrocephalus because the cerebrospinal fluid cannot be properly drained. When cysticerci die, they often evoke severe inflammatory responses and persons so affected are those most often seen by physicians.

Epidemiology and Control

The following are the principal means of controlling *T. solium*:

1. Adequate cooking of pork
2. Freezing pork after slaughter and before it is marketed
3. Sanitary disposal of human waste
4. Meat inspection to find and eliminate infected carcasses
5. Prompt treatment of persons found to be infected
6. An educational program aimed at changing habits of personal hygiene so that persons do not reinfect themselves or others with whom they have contact

Intestinal infections in humans are acquired by eating inadequately cooked pork. Pigs are infected by eating the gravid proglottids passed with human feces. Since a single proglottid may have hundreds of eggs, a pig may obtain a heavy infection throughout its body by eating only a few proglottids.

These principles are much the same as would be applied in the control of *T. saginata*, but the extra hazard of humans being an intermediate host makes prompt treatment and a program designed to change human behavior essential to prevent the devastating effects of blindness and lesions in the CNS. In many parts of the developing world, pigs are kept in rather informal conditions, that is, allowed to run wild and to eat whatever they can find. They readily eat human feces, and if allowed to do so, a high prevalence of infection can develop. In addition, fuel may be expensive or some peoples prefer their pork less than well done. Serious problems hamper breaking into this cycle and blocking it. In tropical countries, animals are slaughtered and consumed usually on the same day. Freezing of meat is seldom an option. Although there are meat inspection systems for meat that is sold in markets, much is killed for local consumption. Since the definitive host range is limited to humans, emphasis on altering human behavior could have dramatically effective results. Although hosts other than the pig can be infected, they are seldom important in maintaining the cycle. Therefore, sanitary disposal of human waste and efforts to ensure cooking of pork as well as personal cleanliness should result in a reduction in the incidence of infection. If facilities and finances allow it, persons coming to dispensaries and hospitals can be examined for tapeworm infection and treated forthwith if found to be infected.

Niclosamide is the drug of choice for intestinal infections; it is highly effective and well tolerated. Cysticercosis is best treated in humans by surgical removal of the cysts, when possible. If surgery is not feasible, or if cysts rupture during surgery, mebendazole, a benzimidazole, can be administered. Praziquantel is the drug of choice for both human and porcine cysticercosis. If chemotherapy is considered, the beneficial effects should be weighed against the foreign body reaction against dead cysticerci.

Other *Taenia* Species

Taenia pisiformis is often used in parasitology classes as a typical taeniid tapeworm. This cosmopolitan worm occurs in dogs and other canids but rarely in cats. Cysticerci are in the viscera of rabbits and hares, in which they most often can be found attached to the intestinal mesenteries; perhaps 30% of cottontail rabbits are infected. Dogs that are allowed to run loose in areas where there are rabbits frequently become heavily infected. Some intestinal distress is experienced by dogs that are infected, and treatment is justified; a number of highly effective taeniacides are available. Keeping dogs from running loose is the best method of preventing infection. *T. pisiformis* is not a parasite of humans.

Taenia multiceps (syn. *Multiceps multiceps*) and *T serialis* (syn. *M. serialis*) have a coenurus metacestode that produces many protoscolices by internal budding (Fig. 24.6). The names given to the larvae are *Coenurus cerebralis* and *C. serialis*, respectively. The metacestode resembles a cysticercus in its nonlaminated outer wall but it has multiple protoscolices like a hydatid. *T. multiceps* is a cosmopolitan parasite of canids: the dog, fox, coyote, and jackal. The metacestode occurs in herbivores such as sheep, in which it is located most often in the CNS; because of pressure put on the brain or spinal cord, it produces blindness, incoordination, or circling, which giving rise to the common names of "gid" or "staggers." In the United States, giddy sheep have been a cause of significant loss to sheep raisers, but infections have not been reported for some years. A few infections have been reported in humans, especially from sheep-raising areas; presumably human infections have been acquired through close association with infected dogs. Adults of *T. serialis* are in dogs and coyotes, and the metacestodes are in rabbits and sometimes in rodents.

Taenia taeniaeformis (syn. *Hydatigera taeniaeformis*) has a metacestode called a *strobilocercus* (Fig. 24.7). The strobilocercus is elongate, with a segmented body and a small, terminal bladder; the scolex is often everted while the metacestode is still in its intermediate host. The definitive hosts are cats and the intermediate hosts are rodents; the most common cycle is between domestic cats and mice or rats on which they prey. Interestingly, infection of rats extending over many months results in a small percentage of them developing cancer of the liver. There are a few other instances in which cancers seem to be caused by helminths, such as *Spirocerca lupi*, and they have been used effectively in laboratory studies on carcinogenesis.

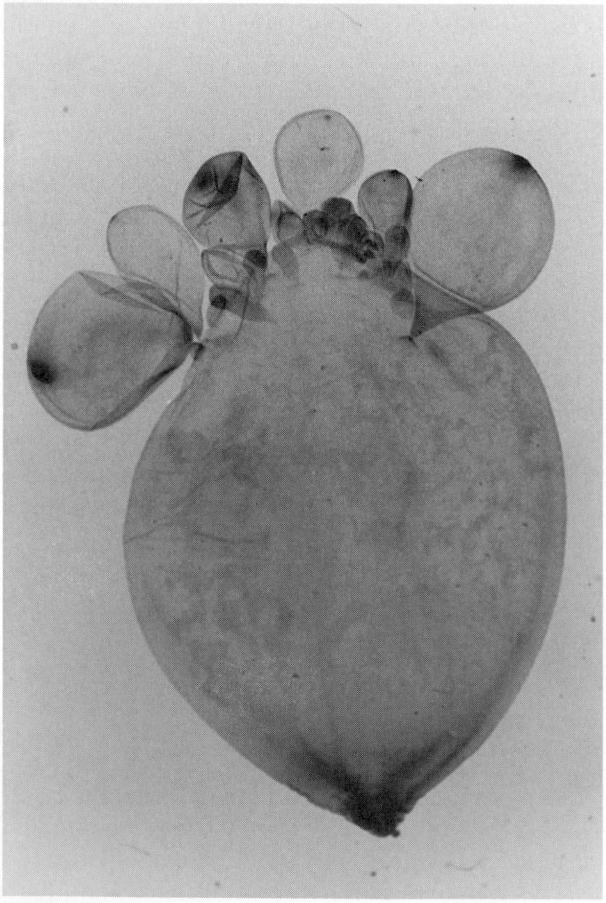

FIGURE 24.6 A whole mount of a coenurus of *Taenia multiceps* as seen in LM.

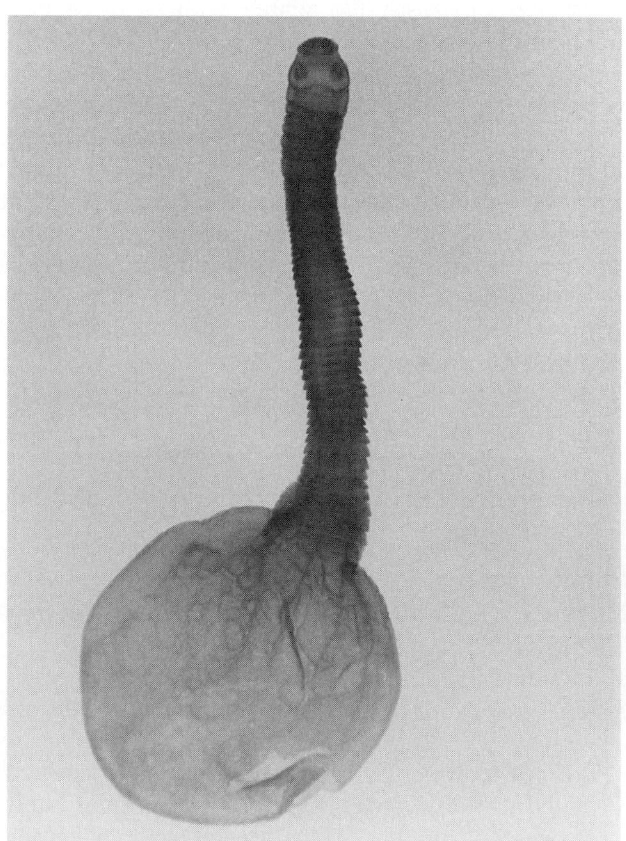

FIGURE 24.7 A whole mount of a strobilocercus of *Taenia taeniaformis* as seen in LM.

HYDATID DISEASE

Four species of *Echinococcus* ("prickly berry" for the hydatid) cause hydatid disease: *Echinococcus granulosus*, *E. multilocularis*, *E. oligarthus*, and *E vogeli*. Both *E. granulosus* and *E. multilocularis* were originally parasites of canids and their prey. *E. granulosus* originally cycled between the wolf and large ungulates such as deer, European elk, and caribou (reindeer). The northern strain maintains this association, but the European or southern strain has become adapted to domestic animals and cycles between dogs and domestic ruminants.

E. multilocularis originally cycled between foxes and microtine rodents such as *Microtus* spp., *Clethrionomys* spp., and the lemming, *Lemmus sibiricus*. Both species have been distributed beyond their original northern location, but *E. multilocularis* to only a limited extent (Fig. 24.8). Some importations such as those into Australia and parts of North America have been well documented, but much of the movement of these parasites is lost in prehistory or is unknown.

Name of Organism and Disease Associations

Echinococcus granulosus cause echinococcosis, echinococciasis, hydatid disease, hydatidosis, hydatosis, and unicystic or unilocular hydatid disease.

Hosts and Host Range

Adult worms are in the small intestines of dogs and wolves. Hydatids occur in the liver or lungs of deer and domestic ungulates; they occur in humans most frequently in lung and liver but occasionally in other organs as well.

Geographic Distribution and Importance

Two major strains of *E. granulosus* are known: the northern strain found in wolves, deer, and other wild herbivores, the cycles of which is usually referred to as the *sylvatic cycle*, and the European or cosmopolitan strain, which occurs in dogs and domestic ungulates. In the continental United States, the current major problem areas in the United States are on sheep ranches in California, Utah, New Mexico, and Arizona where humans are sometimes an incidental participant in the dog-sheep cycle. About 70% of sheepdogs surveyed in northern California were infected with adults worms, a prevalence comparable to that of the sheep-raising areas of New Zealand, Australia, China, and probably similar to that of other sheep-raising areas of the world.

Morphology

Adults are quite small, measuring 3 to 6 mm in length. The scolex has an armed rostellum, a short neck, and commonly one immature, one mature, and one gravid proglottid (Fig. 24.9). Eggs from gravid proglottids are identical to others in the family Taeniidae.

The hydatid, the metacestode stage, has a laminated outer wall that covers a thin, germinal layer (Fig. 24.10). Brood capsules bud from the germ layer into the cyst cavity—so-called endogenous budding. Protoscolices are formed in the brood capsules and remain attached to the surface from which they budded. Occasionally, daughter brood capsules form within the primary ones; these are miniature hydatids including the laminated outer wall. The term *hydatid sand* refers to hydatid contents released from a cyst; there are free-floating protoscolices and daughter brood capsules in the fluid, which give it a granular appearance. Since the protoscolices remain attached to the germinal membrane under normal circumstances, it is only in a degenerating or improperly preserved hydatid that the protoscolices are free. After surgical removal, the large and small hooks from the scolices may be measured and the metacestode identified as to species (Tab. 24.2). *E. granulosus* is the only species with a unicystic hydatid.

Life Cycle

Gravid proglottids and eggs are shed in the feces. Like other taeniid eggs, they are resistant to environmental hazards and to various disinfectants. Intermediate hosts, most often ungulates but occasionally humans, ingest eggs as contaminants of food or water or through close association with canids. Hexacanth embryos hatch in the small intestine and penetrate the intestinal mucosa to reach the circulatory system. The hexacanths are carried by the bloodstream until they lodge in small vessels, commonly in the liver or lung, where they develop into the hydatid. Cysts grow to 4 to 5 mm in about three months.

Cysts containing fully developed protoscolices must be ingested by a carnivore of the family Canidae for the adult stage to develop; bile salts of other kinds of animals are lethal to the protoscolices. The protoscolices attach to the wall of the intestine and develop to the sexually mature adults in about eight weeks.

Diagnosis

Determining whether a person is infected with a hydatid is based on the following:

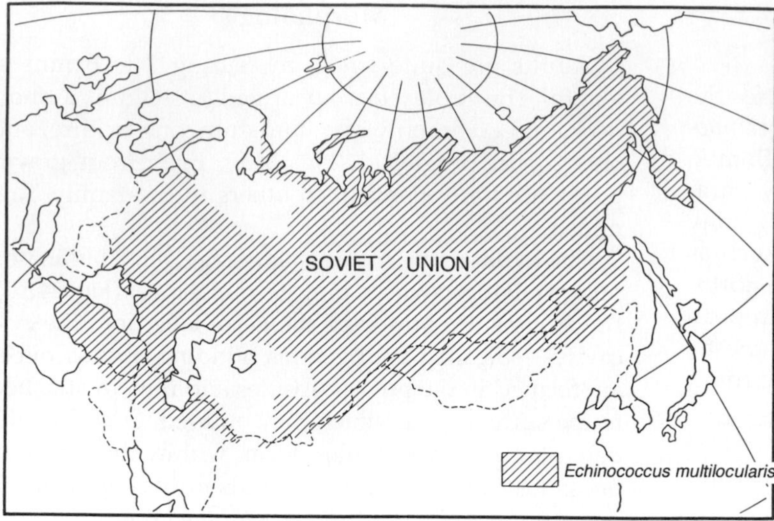

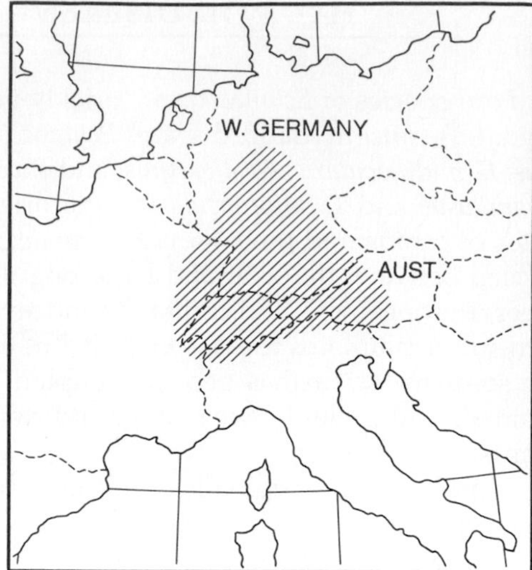

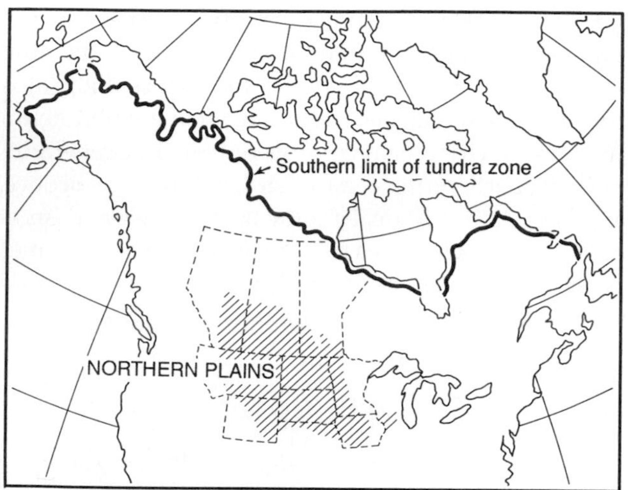

FIGURE 24.8 Distribution of *Echinococcus multilocularis.* [Redrawn with modifications from Rausch, 1967, and Wilson and Rausch, 1980.]

1. An association with dogs or wild canids
2. X-rays, ultrasound, CT scan, or NMR of the infected part of the body
3. Serology to find antibodies
4. Finding the hydatid during surgery and identifying the organism

Signs and symptoms of the infection are usually related to pressure on tissues adjacent to the growing hydatid. The effects on normal function of the organ or tissue may be similar to those of a tumor; hydatids often are mistaken for tumors. X rays show a growing mass and add information for the diagnostician. Diagnosis is made using several immunologic tests, but they are less sensitive than various imaging techniques. Because the growth of the hydatids is so slow, 10 or more years may elapse between infection and the development of clinical disease; how the infection was obtained is often obscured.

Cultivation

Early experiments in the cultivation of *E. granulosus* produced only metacestodes, not the adult worms. As work progressed, it was possible to produce adult worms from protoscolices. The worms resembled adults from natural infections, but fertile eggs were not produced.

Host–Parasite Interactions

Hexacanth embryos pass through the intestinal mucosa, reach the hepatic portal circulation, and are carried throughout the body. In the northern strain, the

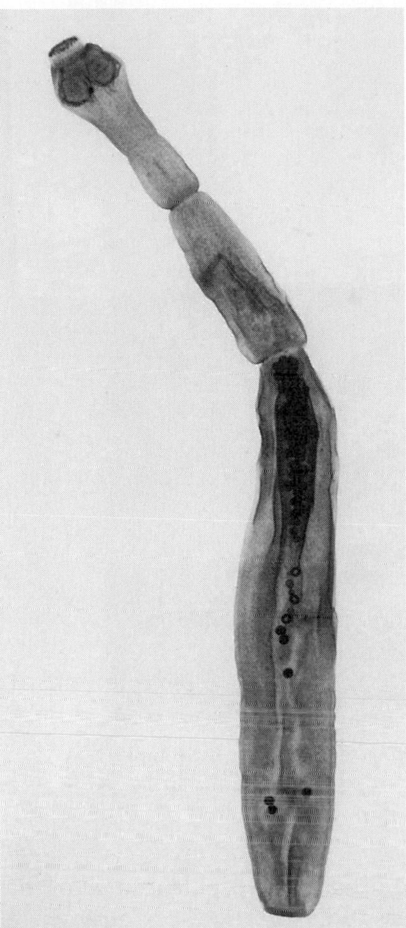

FIGURE 24.9 A stained whole mount of *Echinococcus granulosus* as seen in LM. There are usually only three proglottids: an immature, a mature, and a gravid proglottid.

cysts are found almost exclusively in the lungs of deer. In the southern strain, about 60% are trapped in the liver, 20% in the lungs, and the remainder in almost any other organ of the body including the kidney, the somatic muscle, the spleen, the cavity of long bones, and the central nervous system.

The damage to the host depends on the location and size of the hydatid. Many years may pass after initial infection before clinical signs and symptoms appear, because the cysts grow slowly. The cyst compresses adjacent tissues and reduces the blood supply, causes pain, or reduces the function of the affected part. If the cyst is untreated and occupies a crucial organ such as the brain, the space-occupying lesion may cause the death of the host.

The host responds by a foreign-body reaction and production of antibodies. The cyst becomes surrounded by connective tissue, and after considerable time it may become calcified. In addition, a host often becomes hypersensitive to the fluid that leaks from the hydatid in small amounts; this fluid contains protein and is allergenic. If a cyst is ruptured either through some normal process or during surgery, the fluid may cause anaphylaxis and immediate death.

E. granulosus is one of the few helminths for which we have an explanation of the mechanism of its host specificity. It is well known that various herbivores, swine, and humans can be intermediate but not definitive hosts. Likewise, it is known that certain carnivores (dog, fox, coyote, wolf) can only be definitive hosts. When the eggs are eaten, the outer capsules are removed by slightly alkaline conditions and the hexacanth embryos are then activated by bile, intestinal contents, or both. Activation of the embryos takes place in either human bile or intestinal juice of ruminants; they are not activated in bile or intestinal juice of dogs and cats. When the protoscolices are eaten by a potential definitive host, bile again plays a key role in their survival and establishment of infection. Bile from hare, rabbit, ox, sheep, and human cause lysis and death of protoscolices, whereas that of dog, cat, and fox has no effect on them. The key lies in the specific bile salt that predominates in the bile of a species. Thus, the conditions that the parasite meets upon entering the host are crucial in determining whether the life cycle can continue.

Epidemiology and Control

The following are the elements of a control program for hydatid disease:

1. Keeping the viscera of domestic animals from being eaten by dogs
2. Treatment of infected dogs with an effective anthelmintic
3. Education and publicity of the hazards associated with echinococcosis

The original cycle of *E. granulosus* was

Wolf ↔ Ungulate

However, with colonization of many kinds of habitat by humans and the domestication of various large ungulates, this tapeworm was carried along and a number of variations on the original natural cycle were established:

Dog ↔ Wild Ungulate
Dog ↔ Domestic Ungulate
Wild Carnivore ↔ Domestic Ungulate

In addition to the dog, some of the definitive hosts that have become integrated into the cycle are foxes in the genera *Alopex* and *Vulpes*, the hunting dog of Africa, *Lycaon pictus*, jackals in Africa and Russia, and

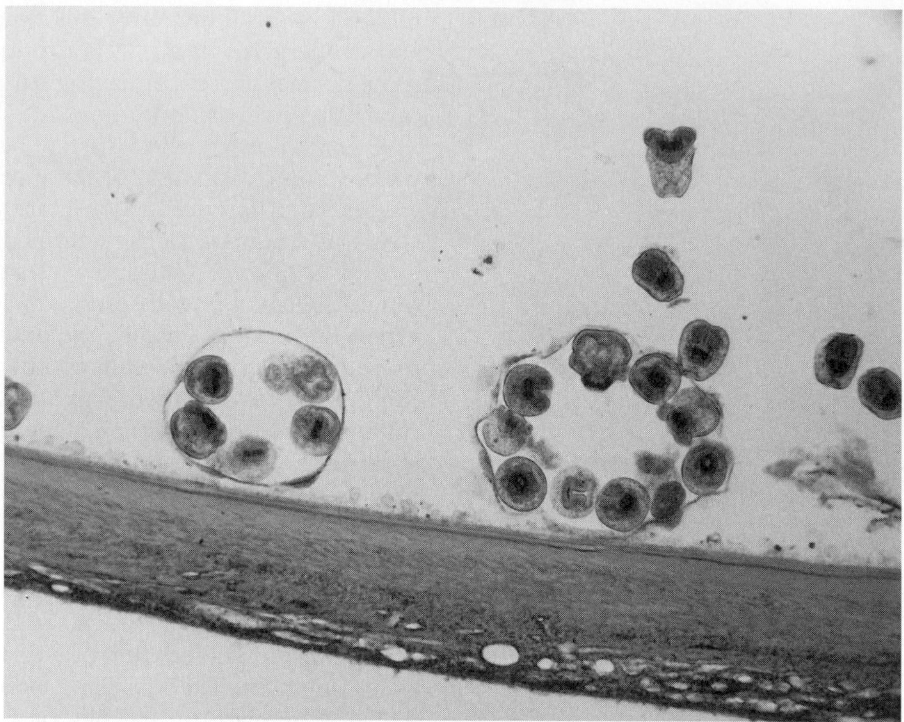

FIGURE 24.10 A portion of a unilocular cyst of *Echinococcus granulosus* showing the complex cyst wall and protoscolices floating inside it.

the coyote, *Canis latrans*. Unlike most other tapeworms, which do not have metacestode reproduction, a single hydatid may produce literally thousands of protoscolices; this increases the probability that the worm will have sufficient variability to develop in a species of host new to it. Adaptability and rapid evolution seem to be characteristics of *Echinococcus* spp.

Of the preceding cycles, the dog-domestic ungulate contains the greatest hazard to human health. Dogs may eat the entrails of animals that die or are butchered on the ranch or station. The continual shedding of eggs and the close association of humans and dog create a situation in which a person may occasionally ingest a few living hexacanths and eventually develop a damaging infection.

Hydatid disease is a problem in all of the livestock-raising areas of the world, especially where sheep are raised in large numbers. Often sheepdogs are the definitive hosts and sheep the intermediate hosts. This domestic cycle is the one most often seen and, as indicated, the one of greatest hazard to humans. Some of the major areas of infection in the United States are California, Arizona, and Utah; other areas are Australia, New Zealand, and the Middle East. It should be noted that the distribution of *E. granulosus* is essentially worldwide and with the movement of livestock it can appear nearly anywhere.

In certain areas of the world such as Iceland, Australia, and New Zealand, great strides have been made in reducing the prevalence of infection in both dogs

TABLE 24.2 *Echinococcus* **Characteristics**

Species	Distribution	Natural Hosts		Hydatid Type	Mean Protoscolex Hook Size (mm)	
		Definitive	Intermediate		Large	Small
granulosus	N. Hemisphere cosmopolitan	Canidae	Ungulates	Unicystic	22	18
multilocularis	N. Hemisphere	Canidae	Rodents	Polycystic	27	23
oligarthus	Central and South America	Felidae	Agouti	Polycystic	33	26
vogeli	Central and South America	Canidae	Paca	Polycystic	42	33

and sheep, but only Iceland has achieved eradication. Effective control requires a relatively stable, accessible population of livestock raisers and an infrastructure of parasitologists and public health personnel. If it is not possible to determine who owns what animals or if people are nomadic, various elements of the cycle will slip through the net that one wishes to erect.

In the small focus of infection in Utah, it was possible to examine and treat all dogs by sending teams of people out periodically to hold clinics. An essential part of the program was to reach both livestock and dog owners so that they would recognize the risk to human health and take action to ensure that once the dogs were treated they did not eat the entrails of any sheep that died or were butchered for home consumption. Meetings and printed materials were available to all adults. In order to make certain that the information reached all age groups, a tapeworm coloring book was produced and distributed to children in the grade schools. What parent could ignore a seven-year-old with his or her own tapeworm in hand as a trophy of the day's artistic endeavor?

Surgery is the recommended treatment for hydatid disease in human illness, but removal of a hydatid cyst must be approached with care. As indicated earlier, an individual harboring a hydatid often develops hypersensitivity to the fluid in the cyst. If the cyst is broken during surgery and the fluid leaks into the body cavity, the patient may die within minutes from anaphylactic shock, a manifestation of hypersensitivity. The other result of breaking the cyst is that the protoscolices may set up secondary sites of infection in other parts of the body (assuming that the patient survives). Following surgical excision, the area is cleansed with 3% hydrogen peroxide to kill any remaining protoscolicies.

Mebendazole has been used successfully in some individuals who have hydatids in locations that are inoperable. Adult worms in dogs are susceptible to treatment with praziquantel.

Name of Organism and Disease Associations

Echinococcus multilocularis, in the adult form, causes the same disease caused by *E. granulosus*; the metacestode causes multilocular or alveolar hydatid disease.

Hosts and Host Range

Natural definitive hosts are foxes, and the intermediate hosts are microtine rodents. Domesticated animals, especially dogs and cats, are definitive hosts and are sources of eggs that can infect humans; mice harbor metacestodes on farms and in some urban areas.

Geographic Distribution and Importance

E. multilocularis is enzootic in Alaska, Canada, central Europe, Siberia, and northern Japan and occurs widely in central North America (Fig. 24.8). Since the hydatid grows by external budding, it has often been compared to an invasive neoplasm (cancer). Similar to a cancer, if a portion becomes detached, it can be carried by the blood and establish (metastasize) in another location of the body. Untreated alveolar hydatid disease is fatal in about 75% of infections in humans; it is one of the most lethal human helminthic diseases. The primary hepatic lesions resemble cancer clinically and errors in diagnosis are common, probably resulting in a lower incidence of infection than is actually the case. Alveolar hydatid disease is a major problem in Siberia, where, for example, 22 cases per year have been reported in Kamchatka alone.

Morphology

Adults of *E. multilocularis* and *E. granulosus* are similar, but the former has fewer and smaller testes and the genital pore is slightly different. The metacestode forms in the intermediate hosts are different as well; *E. granulosus* has a unilocular cyst and *E. multilocularis* has an alveolar or multilocular cyst (Fig. 24.11). Alveolar cysts that grow in humans are not infectious since they do not form protoscolices.

Life Cycle

The life cycle pattern of *E. multilocularis* is basically the same as that of *E. granulosus* in that it is a carnivore-herbivore cycle, but the hosts and therefore the epidemiology are different. Microtine rodents such as voles (*Microtus* spp.) and lemmings (*Lemmus* spp.) are the intermediate hosts, and canids such as foxes and the coyote are the definitive hosts in feral cycles. In domiciliated cycles, dogs and cats become infected.

Diagnosis

Since the alveolar cyst grows irregularly in the tissue, usually the liver, the signs and symptoms of infection may relate to impaired liver function or to pressure and interference of the function of the liver or other organ in which it is located. Antibodies are formed and may be shown by serological methods.

Finding eggs in the feces, or adult tapeworms at

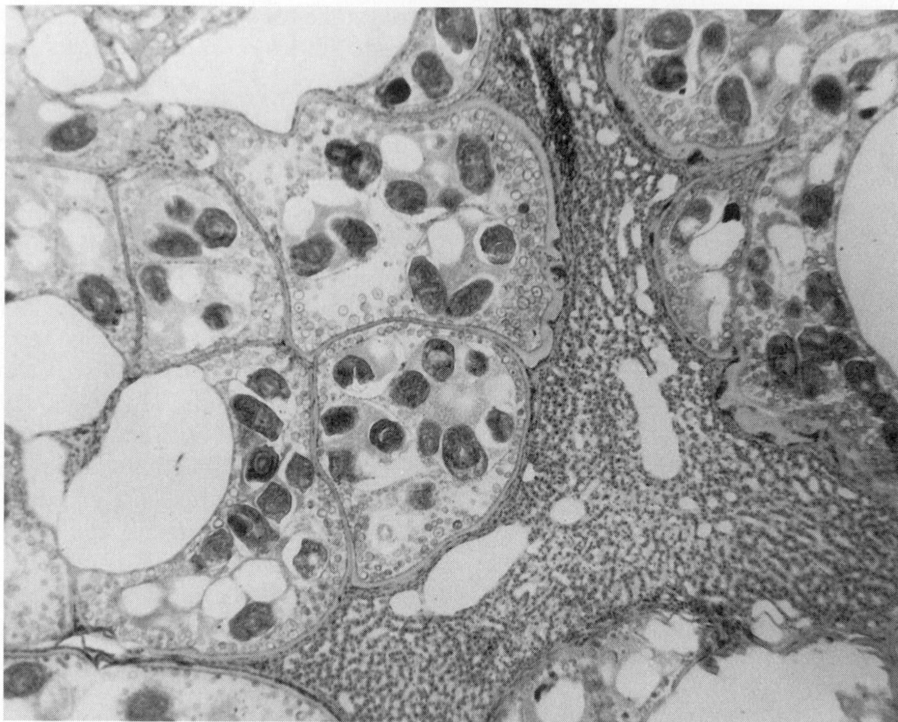

FIGURE 24.11 A histologic section of liver showing the multilocular cyst of *Echinococcus multilocularis* with some of the many loculi and protoscolices floating in them.

postmortem examination are the usual means of diagnosis in the definitive host.

Host–Parasite Interactions

The growth form of the alveolar cyst is crucial to the way in which it damages the host and to the possibility of treatment of the intermediate host. The alveolar cyst tends to grow in an irregular form through the tissue, with buds extending from the surface. The cyst is not a discrete body, as in *E. granulosus*; surgery, therefore, is often difficult, because the parasite must be dissected out of the organ. Only about one quarter of liver infections can be treated surgically. Albendazole, not yet approved by the FDA, is recommended for the treatment of inoperable hydatids. Praziquantel is the drug of choice in the definitive hosts.

Humans display three distinctly different responses to *Echinococcus multilocularis* infections. First there are those individuals who are susceptible to disease. Apparently only 10 to 30% of people exposed to *E. multilocularis* will actually develop alveolar echinococcosis. The remainder who are exposed and seroconvert are resistant to the development of the disease. Some are susceptible to infection but are resistant to disease. They develop calcified cysts that do not contain viable parasites. Others appear to be immunologically resistant to infection, even though they are seropositive. Therefore, they must have been exposed to *E. multilocularis*, but parasite development did not occur. Much remains to be learned about the details of immunology here. The laminated cyst wall apparently plays a significant role in immunogenicity.

Epidemiology and Control

The feral cycle involves wild canids such as foxes and coyote, and many of the infections with *E. multilocularis* are in fur trappers. In pelting animals, trappers may inhale the eggs thrown into the air from the pelt or get a little intestinal content on their hands. Since the eggs are quite resistant, they might remain for many weeks on a knife or equipment used to stretch hides. Some potential methods for preventing infection in humans are evident: wearing a mask to keep from inhaling eggs, washing hands, and disinfecting tools. These methods may not be practical considering that trapping of foxes in the arctic is usually done in rural, relatively primitive areas.

If a cycle occurs near human habitation, companion animals should be monitored and treated. Under some conditions, a rodent control program can be instituted near towns or ranches, but with rapidly reproducing rodents such as *Microtus*, success in reducing numbers may be elusive.

Other *Echinococcus* Species

The other species currently accepted are *E. oligarthus*, and *E. vogeli*; both have metacestodes with multiple chambers produced by external or exogenous budding. The terms *alveolar, multilocular hydatid*, and *polycystic cyst* have been used for these metacestodes.

E. vogeli produces polycystic hydatid disease in humans in Central and South America. Metacestodes differ in several respects from *E. multilocularis*: most notable is the presence of numerous protoscolices in the cysts. The normal definitive host is the bush dog, *Spethos venaticus*, and the natural intermediate host is the paco, *Cuniculus paca*.

Echinococcus oligarthus also produces polycystic hydatid disease in Central and South America, but no confirmed human infections have been reported. The adults are intestinal parasites of cats such as the jaguar (*Panthera onca*), not dogs, and the metacestodes are in rodents such as the agouti (*Dasyprocta punctata*). The habits of cats make it unlikely that humans would commonly become infected by fecal contamination with *E. oligarthus*.

FAMILY HYMENOLEPIDIDAE

Hymenolepididae comprise small tapeworms of birds and mammals throughout the world. They have long, slender strobilae, armed rostella (usually), and one to four testes per proglottid.

Name of Organism and Disease Associations

Hymenolepis (syn. *Vampirolepis*) *nana*, the dwarf tapeworm, causes hymenoleposis or hymenolepiasis.

Hosts and Host Range

This tapeworm is found in the small intestines of rats, mice, and humans.

Geographic Distribution and Importance

H. nana is cosmopolitan, and is the most common tapeworm of humans throughout the world. Relatively high infection rates in children are found in central Europe and Latin America, but range from 0.3 to 3% in the southern United States.

Morphology

This is the smallest human adult tape worm, usually 7 to 100 mm long. Adult worms have a prominent armed rostellum, a scolex with four suckers, proglottids that are wider than long, and three testes per proglottid. Eggs are 30 to 47 mm and have a thin outer shell. The oncosphere is surrounded by a membrane with two characteristic *polar knobs* and *polar filaments* (Fig. 24.12). The metacestode is a cysticercoid.

Life Cycle

Eggs of *Hymenolepis* have the hexacanth embryo formed when they pass from the host; therefore, no period of development outside the host is required. *H. nana* is unique among cyclophyllidean tapeworms in that an intermediate host is optional. Intermediate hosts are arthropods such as grain beetles or larval

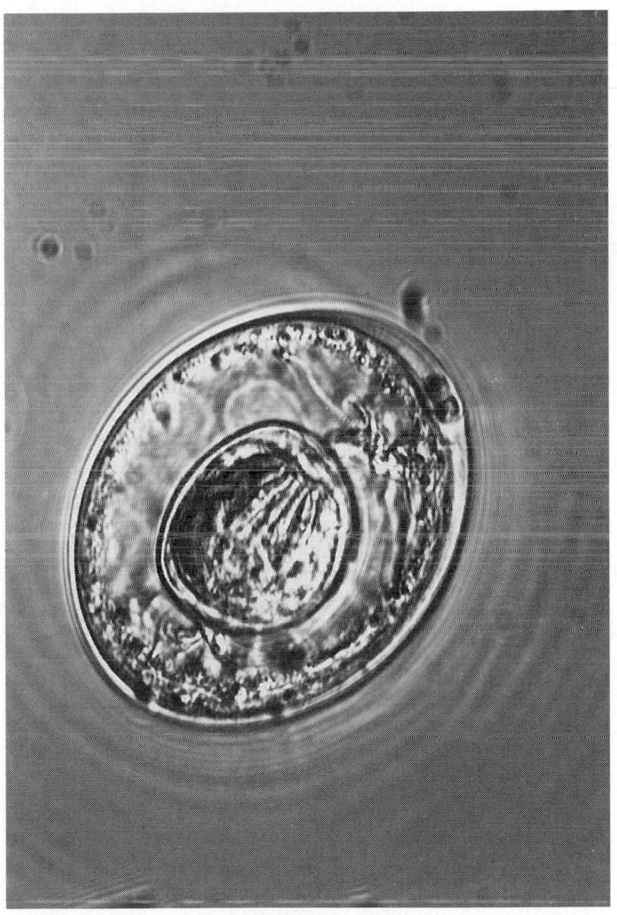

FIGURE 24.12 An egg of *Hymenolepis nana* photographed under the interference contrast microscope. The hexacanth embryo is the smaller body in the center of the egg; characteristic hooks, knobs, and filaments are present. [Courtesy of Dr. Robert Mead, University of Nevada, Reno.]

fleas; the cysticercoid develops in the hemocoels of these hosts when they ingest the oncospheres. When an infected arthropod is eaten by a person, the scolex of the cysticercoid attaches to the small intestine and develops into the adult.

The alternative method of infection of the definitive host is for a person to ingest the egg containing the oncosphere. The embryo escapes from the egg capsules in the small intestine and enters the lacteal of a villus in the small intestine. After developing for two weeks or more, the worm returns to the lumen of the intestine and forms a strobila. Eggs from gravid proglottids bring about autoinfection by hatching while still in the host and forming cysticercoids in the intestinal tissue; infections can thus become extraordinarily heavy.

Diagnosis

Both sedimentation and flotation methods concentrate eggs so that they can be found in a fecal sample. The characteristic polar knobs and filaments (Fig. 24.12) are diagnostic.

Cultivation

Hymenolepis was the first tapeworm to be cultivated in vitro, and both *H. nana* and *H. diminuta* have produced gravid proglottids from cysticercoids in culture. Also, oncospheres have produced cysticercoids in culture.

Host–Parasite Interactions

Light infections are asymptomatic, but heavy infections cause abdominal pain, diarrhea, headache and dizziness, among other vague symptoms.

The method of infection and the development of immunity are interrelated. If a cystercoid is ingested, there is little development of immunity, and through autoinfection the number of worms may become quite large. On the other hand, if eggs are ingested, immunity usually develops quickly.

Epidemiology and Control

The dwarf tapeworm is usually a household problem and control revolves around the following:

1. Determining which persons are infected
2. Treating all infected individuals
3. Cleaning the dwelling, clothing, bedclothes, bathrooms
4. Killing insects in the house and making it less attractive for them
5. Teaching measures of personal hygiene, especially to children who might not yet have developed fastidious habits

Infection with the dwarf tapeworm is not usually considered to be a public health problem but rather is a familial one and is approached in that way. The steps listed here are directed at breaking the microcosm of transmission in the household. It is important to rid all persons of their infection and to undertake preventive measures at the same time. Cleanliness and personal hygiene are the keys to ensuring that transmission is stopped. The dwarf tapeworm is often a problem in children who are institutionalized, and under this circumstance, they may not be capable of readily learning procedures of personal hygiene. In addition, publicly supported institutions often operate on minimal amounts of money and may not have the resources to maintain adequate levels of cleanliness despite the desires of their personnel.

Although both niclosamide and praziquantel are effective, the former is the drug of choice.

Related Species

Hymenolepis diminuta is a cosmopolitan parasite of rats and mice and only rarely of humans. Despite its species name, *H. diminuta* is a relatively large tapeworm, sometimes reaching a meter in length, but usually it is about 30 cm long and has an unarmed rostellum (Fig. 24.13). Intermediate hosts are insects, usually beetles, and in the laboratory, it can be propagated

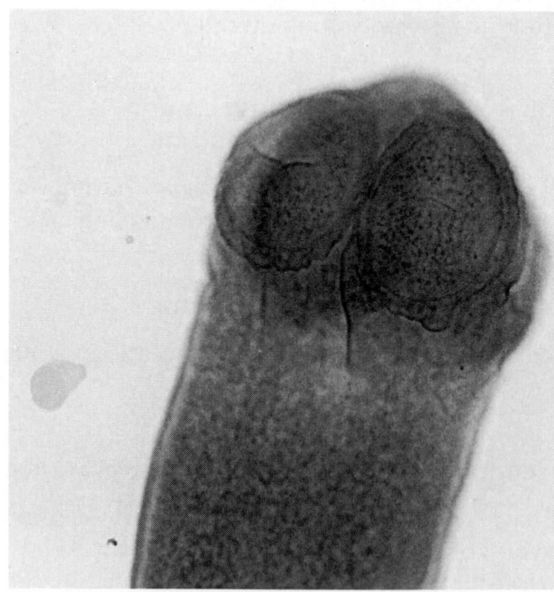

FIGURE 24.13 The scolex of *Hymenolepis diminuta* showing the unarmed rostellum.

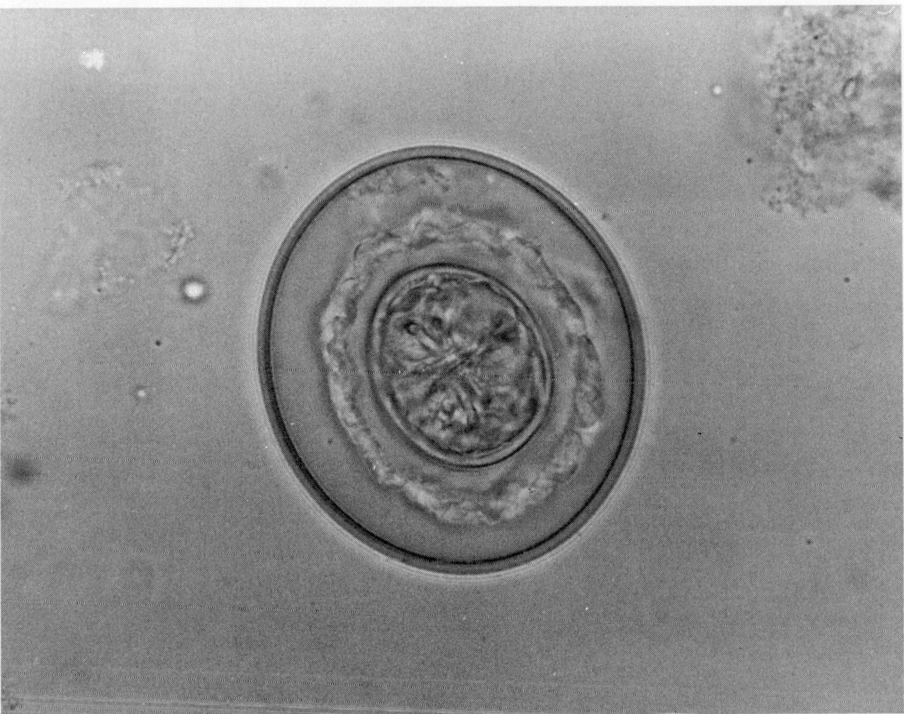

FIGURE 24.14 An egg of *Hymenolepis diminuta* showing lack of polar knobs. The hexacanth embryo is the smaller body in the center of the egg and its six hooks can be seen.

readily in the confused flour beetle, *Tribolium confusum*. Eggs resemble those of *H. nana*, but lack polar knobs and filaments (Fig. 24.14). *H. diminuta* has been used extensively in physiological, fine structural, and biochemical studies; it has been studied so much that tapeworm physiology is, in fact, *H. diminuta* physiology.

FAMILY DILEPIDIDAE

Dipylidium caninum is a cosmopolitan parasite of dogs and cats. Intermediate hosts are *Ctenocephalides canis* and *C. felis*, the common fleas of the dog and cat, which harbor cysticercoids. Adults are referred to by the common name of the *double-pored tapeworm* because they have two sets of reproductive organs (Fig. 24.15). Proglottids are passed in the feces and the egg packets (Fig. 24.16) are eaten by larval fleas. The cysticercoid develops in the hemocoel of the intermediate host. The infection is retained in the larva when it pupates and emerges as an adult flea; the definitive host is infected when it eats an infected flea. Dogs and cats are mildly affected by *D. caninum*; they usually have a rough hair coat and may have diarrhea. The proglottids are quite motile and may crawl out of the anus of the dog or cat. Since the effects are generally mild, the first sign

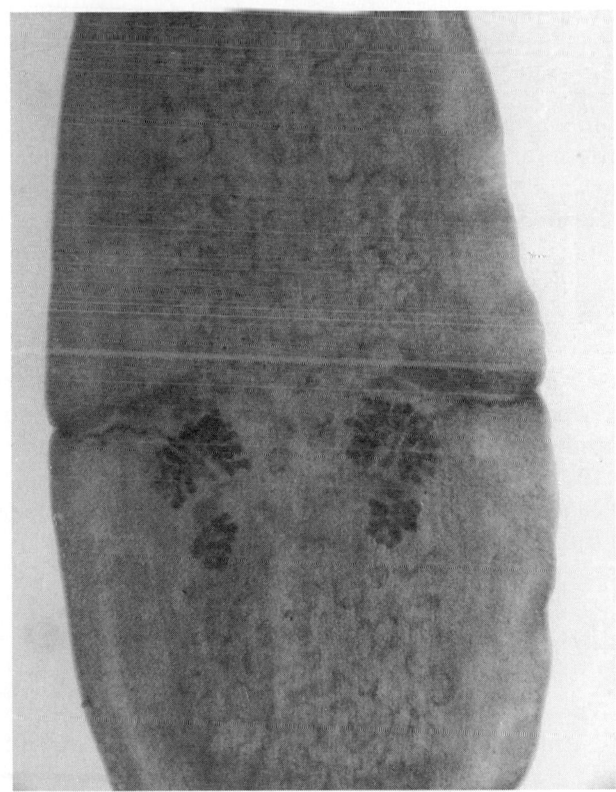

FIGURE 24.15 A stained whole mount of a mature prolgottid of *Dipylidium caninum* showing the characteristic double set of reproductive organs.

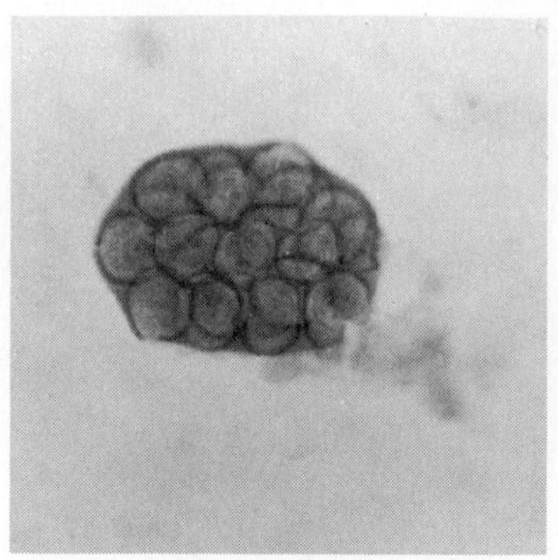

FIGURE 24.16 An egg packet of *Dipylidium caninum.*

of infection in a companion animal is likely to occur when a proglottid is found inching its way across the sofa. Diagnosis of the infection entails examining a proglottid for the typical structure of the species or finding the typical eggs in packets (Fig. 24.15).

When *D. caninum* establishes in a household, three steps should be taken:

1. All companion animals are treated. Niclosamide and praziquantel are effective.
2. Flea control is instituted by treating companion animals and by eliminating larvae from the house (see Chapter 46).
3. Companion animals are examined periodically to ensure that any reinfections are found early and treated.

In warm climates in which fleas reproduce well out of doors and they may be active year round, flea control may not be effective. Even if the inside of the house is cleaned up, the fleas outside are a massive reservoir that may be a continuing source of infection, since they live where the animals roam and defecate.

In addition to infecting companion animals, *D. caninum* occasionally infects children. There are about 100 case reports describing infections in children; moderately severe intestinal disturbances occur, such as abdominal cramps and diarrhea. Children become infected if they are closely associated with infected dogs or cats. They ingest infected fleas or parts of fleas just as the normal hosts do.

FAMILY ANOPLOCEPHALIDAE

The members of this family are mostly large organisms (more than 15 cm long) that have a scolex with large, fleshy suckers lacking hooks and one or two sets of reproductive organs with lateral genital pores. The testes are numerous and scattered in the proglottid. The eggs have a heavy hyaline outer capsule and the hexacanth embryo is encased in a *pyriform apparatus*, a distinctive structure with two fingerlike projections. Most of the life cycles use grass mites (Acarina, Oribatoidea) as intermediate hosts in which the cysticercoid develops. The definitive hosts are herbivorous animals that become infected through eating infected grass mites with the forage (Tab. 24.3).

Some of the species such as *Cittotaenia* and *Moniezia* are cosmopolitan; others such as *Thysanosoma actinoides* are limited in their distribution, in this case only the western United States.

Moniezia spp. may reach 4 m in length, but usually they are less than a meter. They may, however, occur in sheep or cattle in large numbers and are quite striking when seen at postmortem examination. When the small intestine is opened, literally handfuls of tapeworms spill out of the gut. It is tempting to lay the cause of death of the animal on something that is as striking as a huge mass of tapeworms, but that is not the case. It is axiomatic that tapeworm tissue is formed of the nutrients that would otherwise have gone to the host, but most studies point toward little weight reduction in infected animals. Some well-controlled studies indicate that young animals suffer from infections and gain less well than uninfected animals.

Thysanosoma actinoides is found in the high plains and Rocky Mountain area of the western United States as well as sporadically in other parts of the Western Hemisphere and is the cause of some economic losses in lambs. *T. actinoides* is located in the upper small intestine, and the scolex is frequently attached in the bile ducts of the liver with the strobila extending down the common bile duct into the duodenum. The intermediate hosts of the fringed tapeworm are probably bark lice (Insecta, Psocoptera), in which the cysticercoid develops. Studies on weight gains have frequently shown that uninfected animals gain a little better than infected ones, but most losses come from condemnation of livers at slaughter.

TABLE 24.3 Common Herbivorous Animals and Their Anoplocephalid Parasites

Parasite	Hosts
Cittotaenia spp.	Rabbits and hares
Moniezia benedeni	Cattle and sheep
Moniezia expansa	Sheep and cattle
Anoplocephala spp.	Equids
Thysanosoma actinoides	Deer and sheep
Monoecocestus spp.	Porcupine
Avitellina spp.	Ruminants
Stilesia spp.	Ruminants

Readings

Andersen, F. L., Chai, J.-J., and Liu, F. J. (Eds.) (1993). *Compendium on Cystic Echinococcosis with Special Reference to the Xinjiang Uygur Autonomous Region, the People's Republic of China*. Brigham Young Univ. Press, Provo, UT.

Andersen, F. L., Ouhelli, H., and Kachani, M. (Eds.) (1997). *Compendium on Cystic Echinococcosis in Africa and in the Middle Eastern Countries with Special Reference to Morocco*. Brigham Young Univ. Press, Provo, UT.

Arai, H. P. (Ed.) (1980). *Biology of the Tapeworm Hymenolepis diminuta*. Academic Press, New York.

Cook, G. C. (1988). Neurocysticercosis: Parasitology, clinical presentation, diagnosis, and recent advances in management. *Q. J. Med.* **68,** 575–583.

D'Alessandro, A., Rausch, R. L., Cuello, C., and Arestizabal, N. (1979). *Echinococcus vogeli* in man, with a review of polycystic hydatid disease in Colombia and neighboring countries. *Am. J. Trop. Med. Hyg.* **28,** 303–317.

Earnest, M. P., Reller, L. B., Filley, C. H., and Grek, A. J. (1987). Neurocysticercosis in the United States: 35 cases and a review. *Rev. Inf. Dis.* **9,** 961–979.

Eckert, J., Pawlowski, Z., Dar, F. K., Vuitton, D. A., Kern, P., and Savioli, L. (1995). Medical aspects of echinococcus. *Parasitol. Today* **11,** 273–276.

Freeman, R. S. (1973). Ontogeny of cestodes and its bearing on their phylogeny and systematics. *Adv. Parasitol.* **11,** 481–557.

Gemmel, M. A., and Johnstone, P. D. (1977). Experimental epidemiology of hydatidosis and cysticerosis. *Adv. Parasitol.* **15,** 312–369.

Gottstein, B., and Felleisen, R. (1995). Protective immune mechanisms against the metacestode of *Echinococcus multilocularis*. *Parasitol. Today* **11,** 320–326.

Greenberg, A. E., and Dean, B. H. (1958). The beef tapeworm, measly beef and sewage—A review. *Sewage Ind. Wastes* **30,** 262–269.

Laws, G. F. (1968). Physical factors influencing survival of taeniid eggs. *Exp. Parasitol.* **22,** 227–239.

Leiby, P. D., and Kritsky, D. C. (1972). *Echinococcus multilocularis*: A possible domestic life cycle in central North America and its public health implications. *J. Parasitol.* **58,** 1213–1215.

McManus, D. P., and Smyth, J. P. (1986). Hydatidosis: Changing concepts in epidemiology and speciation. *Parasitol. Today* **2,** 163–168.

Moore, J. (1981). Asexual reproduction and environmental predictability in cestodes (Cyclophyllidea: Taeniidae). *Evolution* **35,** 723–741.

Neafie, R. C., and Marty, A. M. (1993). Unusual infections in humans. *Clin. Microbiol. Rev.* **6,** 39–56.

Pawlowski, Z., and Schultz, M. G. (1972). Taeniasis and cysticercosis (*Taenia saginata*). *Adv. Parasitol.* **10,** 269–343.

Rausch, R. L. (1967). On the ecology and distribution of *Echinococcus* spp. (Cestoda: Taeniidae) and characteristics of their development in the intermediate host. *Ann. Parasitol.* **42,** 19–63.

Roberts, T., Murrell, K. D., and Marks, S. (1994). Economic losses caused by foodbourne parasitic diseases. *Parasitol. Today* **10,** 419–423.

Rybicka, K. (1966). Embryogenesis in cestodes. *Adv. Parasitol.* **4,** 107–186.

Slais, J. (1973). Functional morphology of cestode larvae. *Adv. Parasitol.* **11,** 396–480.

Smyth, J. D. (1964). The biology of the hydatid organisms. *Adv. Parasitol.* **2,** 169–219.

Smyth, J. D. (1969). The biology of the hydatid organisms. *Adv. Parasitol.* **7,** 327–347.

Smyth, J. D., and McManus, D. P. (1989). *The Physiology and Biochemistry of Cestodes*. Cambridge Univ. Press, Cambridge, UK.

Thompson, R. C. A. (1973). The post-embryonic developmental stages of cestodes. *Adv. Parasitol.* **11,** 707–730.

Thompson, R. C. A., and Lymbery, A. J. (1988). The nature, extent and significance of variation within the genus *Echinococcus*. *Adv. Parasitol.* **27,** 209–258.

Thompson, R. C. A., and Lymbery, A. J. (Eds.) (1995). *Biology of Echinococcus and Hydatid Disease*. CAB International/Univ. Arizona Press, Wallingford, UK/Tuscon, AZ.

Verster, A. (1967). Redescription of *Taenia solium* Linnaeus, 1758 and *Taenia saginata* Goeze, 1782. *Ztschr. Parasitenk.* **29,** 313–328.

Verster, A. (1969). A taxonomic revision of the genus *Taenia* Linnaeus, 1758. *Onderstepoort J. Vet. Res.* **36,** 3–58.

Voge, M. (1967). The postembryonic developmental stages of cestodes. *Adv. Parasitol.* **5,** 247–297.

Wardle, R. A., and McLeod, J. A. (1952). *The Zoology of Tapeworms*. Univ. of Minnesota Press, Minneapolis.

Wardle, R. A., McLeod, J. A., and Radinovsky, S. (1974). *Advances in the Zoology of Tapeworms, 1950–1970*. Univ. of Minnesota Press, Minneapolis.

Warren, K. S. (1974). Helminthic diseases endemic in the United States. *Am. J. Trop. Med. Hyg.* **23,** 723–730.

Wilson, J. F., and Rausch, R. L. (1980). Alveolar hydatid disease. A review of clinical features of 33 indigenous cases of *Echinococcus multilocularis* infections in Alaskan Eskimos. *Am. J. Trop. Med. Hyg.* **29,** 1340–1355.

Wilson, J. F., Diddams, A. C., and Rausch, R. L. (1968). Cystic hydatid disease in Alaska. A review of 101 autochthonous cases of *Echinococcus granulosus* infection. *Annu. Rev. Respir. Dis.* **98,** 1–15.

PART

3

NEMATODA

CHAPTER

25

Introduction to the Nematodes

Among multicellular animals, the phyla Arthropoda and Mollusca are often considered to be the most successful since they have more than a million and 80,000 species, respectively. The phylum Nematoda, or roundworms, must be considered nearly as successful as the arthropods because there are probably 500,000 species in the world, although only about 10,000 have been described. Hundreds of new species are described annually.

Success in an animal group is measured not only by the number of species it has, but also by the number of individuals. Although nematodes are both free living and parasitic, by far the greater number of species and individuals are free living. Like the English sparrow, nematodes are ubiquitous, as can be readily seen by looking at almost any environment with organic matter in it. In the soils of Utah and Idaho there are between 800 million and more than a billion nematodes per acre of soil and these include at least 35 species. Farm soils in north China contain 2 billion to 6 billion per acre. In a marine area off the Dutch coast 4.4 million nematodes were found in bottom muck; even in the lower reaches of a beach off Massachusetts there were 527 million per acre in the top three inches of sand.

Free-living nematodes have been found in almost every conceivable habitat, including aquatic and terrestrial, marine and fresh water, hot and cold water, in deep seas, and floating in the community of plants and animals in the ocean. Their only universal requirement is that there be a moderate amount of water for them to move and feed in for a part of the life cycle. Their numbers are greatest where there is a large amount of organic matter and small where the amount of organic matter is low, such as a sandy beach.

Since we are concerned here with parasites, the question might be raised of why we discuss free-living roundworms. The reason is that the basic structure and life cycle of all nematodes are remarkably homogeneous. The parasitic forms inhabit not only other animals but plants as well. The parasites of plants are of considerable economic importance in citrus fruit, pineapple, root crops such as sugar beets, and tomatoes, among others. The parasites of animals are found in nearly every animal species that has been examined and in one host or another in every organ system and structure that one might think of (excluding hair, feathers, and cornified structures).

The anatomical structure and the pattern of development of nematodes are admirably suited for invasion of many niches. Although the origins and affinities of the nematodes are not clear, it is generally agreed that the early forms were tiny aquatic animals attached to the substrate by their tails, where they trapped particulate food with bristles surrounding the mouth (Fig. 25.1).

Nematodes are elongate worms, round in cross section with a mouth at the anterior tip (Fig. 25.2) and a subterminal anus (Fig. 25.3). The body is covered with a secreted cuticle (Fig. 25.4), which is underlain by a single layer of neuromuscular cells. The nervous system consists of two ganglia dorsal and ventral to the esophagus connected by nerves that make up the circumesophageal nerve ring. Nerves run anteriorly to the sense organs and posteriorly, dorsally, ventrally, and laterally in the hypodermis. A cross section of *Ascaris* clearly shows these nerve trunks, as well as the connections of the neural portion of the neuromuscular cells with the dorsal and ventral nerve cords (Fig. 25.5).

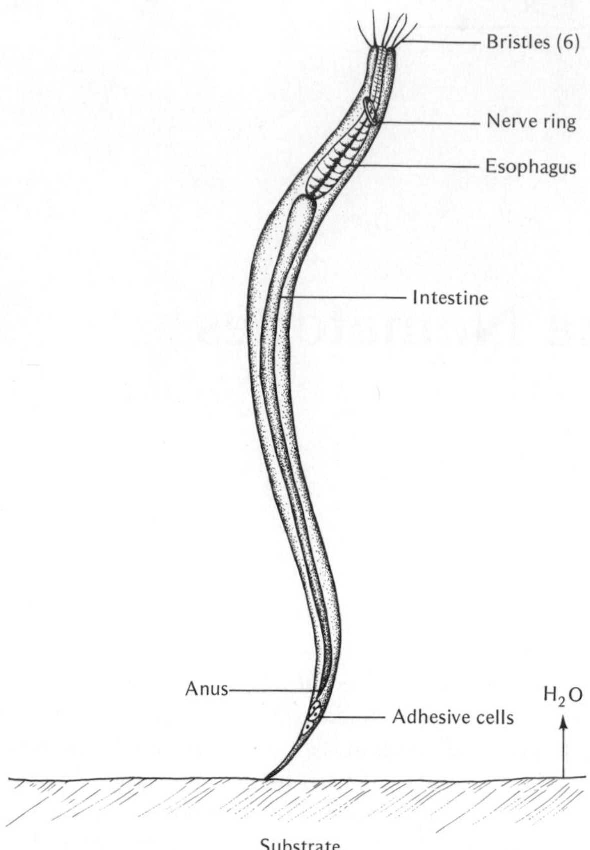

FIGURE 25.1 A hypothetical primitive nematode attached to the substrate.

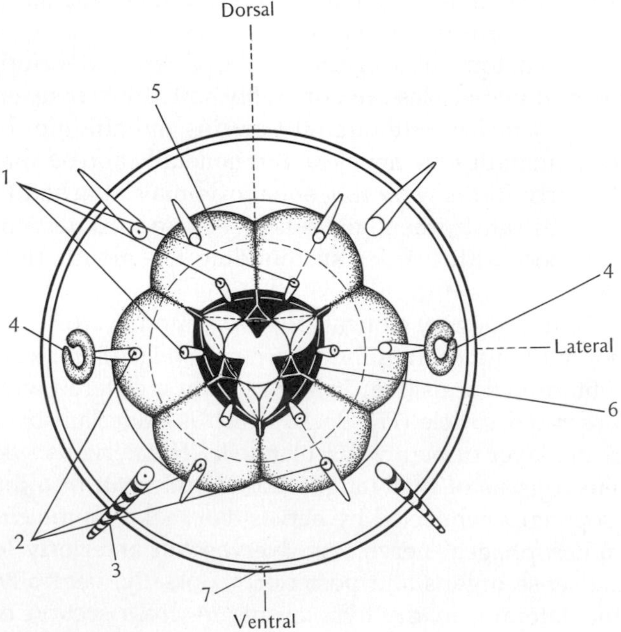

FIGURE 25.2 A primitive nematode seen *en face*: (1) Cephalic bristles; (2) inner labial bristles; (3) outer labial bristles; (4) amphids; (5) lips; (6) buccal capsule. Note tripartite pharynx.

The nerves innervate the muscles to control muscular contraction; the neuromuscular cell is unique among all animals. The amphids and lips at the anterior end and the phasmids at the posterior end of the worm are sensory structures.

The excretory system is usually composed of a gland, pulsatory vesicle, and excretory pore near the posterior end of the esophagus, but there are also longitudinal canals that run the length of the animal. Although end-products of nitrogen metabolism are excreted through this system, it serves primarily as an osmoregulatory organ.

Sexes are usually separate, although there are a few monoecious species and a few that are parthenogenetic. The female system consists of a uterus, usually with two branches, that connect to an elongate ovary (Fig. 25.3). Ova move from the ovary into the upper part of the uterus, where fertilization takes place and egg capsules are then laid down. The eggs reach the outside through the short vagina and the vulva located somewhere along the length of the body. Some species have muscular ovejectors at the vagina to expel eggs. The male system is similar to that of the female in that the testis is an elongate structure in which the spermatids are formed. They mature in the vas deferens, are stored in a seminal vesicle, are ejected by a muscular ejaculatory duct, and are passed to the female. The principal differences are that in the male system there is a common opening with the intestine at the cloaca and there are additional structures, such as copulatory spicules and the bursa, which facilitate the passing of sperm to the female. Spermatozoa lack flagella and have ameboid movement.

The basic structure of a nematode is a tube within a tube. The tubes, intestinal tract, and reproductive system lie within a cavity, the pseudocoel. The structure is closely related to a nematode's function.

In a small free-living or parasitic nematode, the esophagus constantly pumps. Small particles in the medium move into the mouth and then pass down the esophagus to the intestine. Occasionally, the muscles that keep the anus closed open the anus and allow some of the gut content to escape into the medium. In addition to feeding, the esophagus pumps fluid so as to maintain a high hydrostatic pressure in the body of the worm. This hydrostatic pressure not only maintains the round shape of the worm but is essential for its motility. A study by Harris and Croften (1957) considered the theoretical and practical importance to the nematode of maintaining a high hydrostatic pressure. The study showed that efficient motility is possible in an animal that has a simple nervous system and only a single layer of muscles because of the physical principle that a liquid is incompressible. This means that

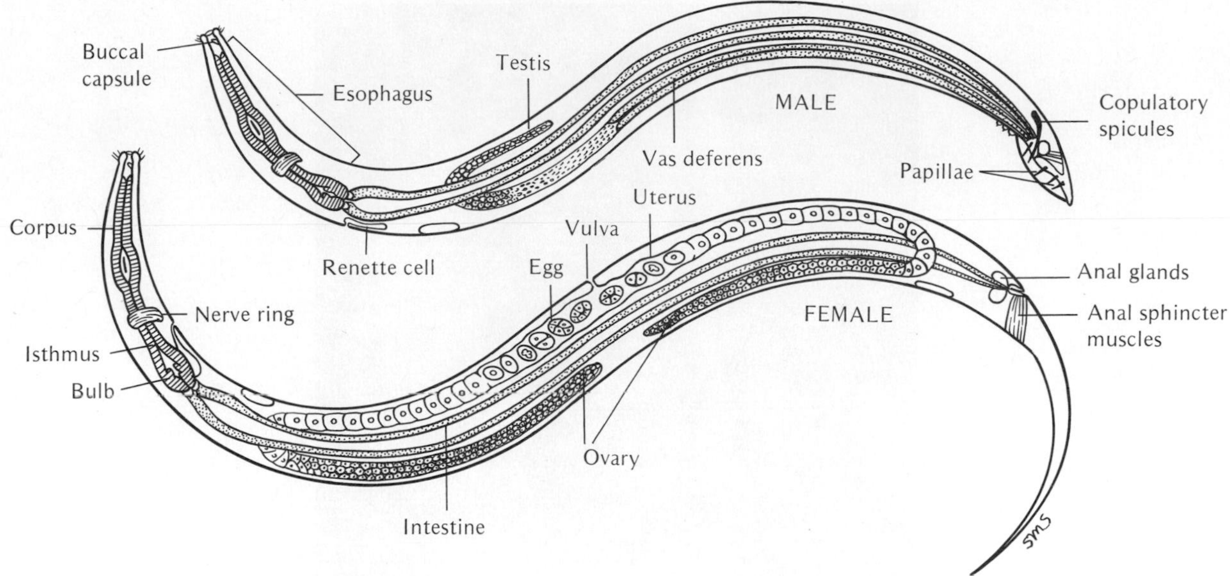

FIGURE 25.3 A diagrammatic representation of nematode anatomy, (A) female and (B) male.

any shortening or narrowing in the body's diameter will produce an immediate change in shape in another part of the body, which will either elongate or increase in diameter.

The cuticle of nematodes is important in their physiology and in relation to the host. It is secreted by the hypodermis and consists of several layers; there is some variation in the layers in various species of nematodes and in the stages of the life cycle, but a general pattern can be seen in most of them. *Ascaris suum* has been studied both at the light microscope (LM) and electron microscope (EM) levels and provides an adequate model for other nematodes (Fig. 25.4). There is a clear outer layer of cortex underlain by a matrix and then three layers of fibers. These layers are made up of cross-linked collagen. The basement membrane rests on the hypodermis.

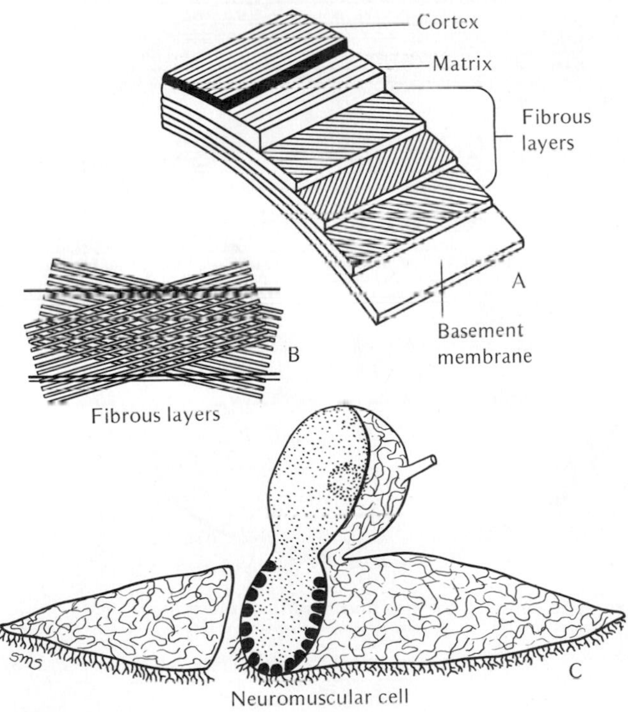

FIGURE 25.4 Structure of the nematode body wall. (A) Cuticle of *Ascaris;* (B) fiber lattice showing the oblique orientation of the fibers; (C) a neuromuscular cell as is found in *Ascaris.* [Redrawn with modifications form Crofton, M. D., 1966.]

The epicuticle is a multilayered structure exterior to the cortical layer of the cuticle; it forms the primary interface with the host. The epicuticle is important in the context of stimulating the host immune response, yet it remains poorly described from the biophysical standpoint. The fibers in the basal layer lie at an angle to one another, usually 70 to 75 degrees (Fig. 25.4B). It is this layer that controls the transfer of forces in the movement of the animal, as discussed earlier.

Cuticle and growth in nematodes are interrelated. Growth in nematodes is separated by a series of four molts. Prior to each molt, a new cuticle is formed beneath the old one. This general growth and molting pattern has been found in all nematodes that have been studied with care. After hatching from the egg, the first stage larva (L_1) feeds, grows, and then molts to the second stage larva (L_2). The process continues to the L_5, which then becomes the adult through maturation of the reproductive system (Fig. 25.6).

Molting is a complex process which is under hor-

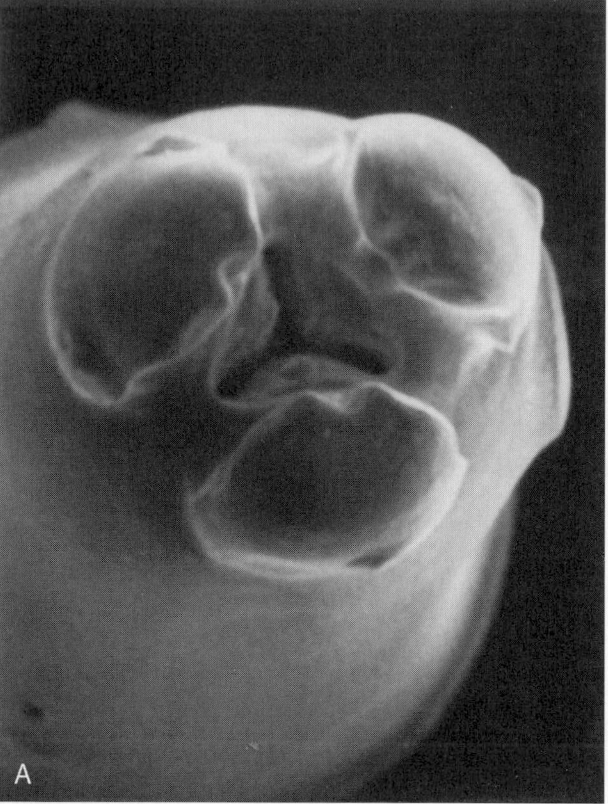

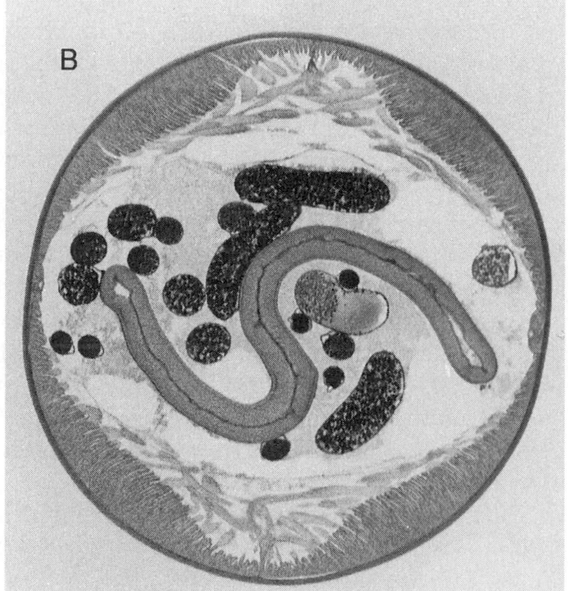

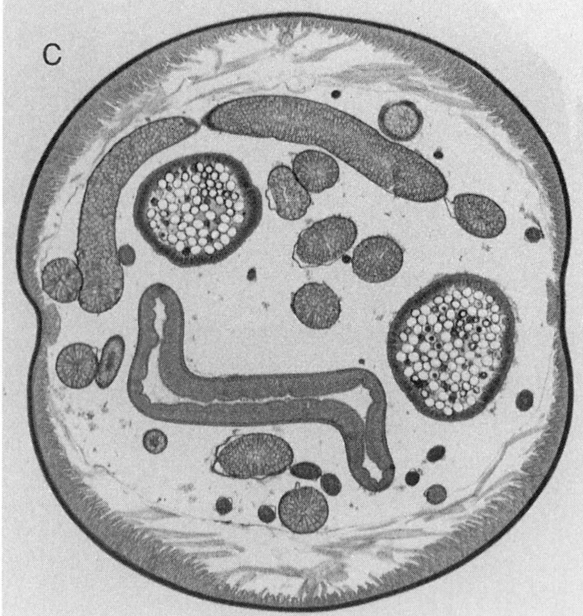

FIGURE 25.5 *Ascaris suum.* (A) Scanning electron micrograph showing the lips and triradiate pharynx; (B) cross-section of a male; (C) cross-section of a female.

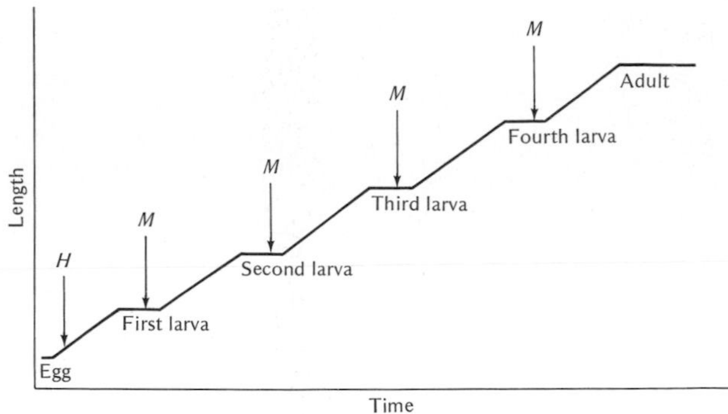

FIGURE 25.6 Growth and molting in nematodes. (H, egg hatches; M, molt occurs) [Redrawn from Lee, D. L., 1965.]

monal control, as in insects. It has been said that molting in nematodes serves the same function that it does in insects; the worm can grow only to a certain size and then must molt in order to grow larger. However, the L_5 of *Ascaris* grows from about 22 mm to 300 mm without molting, and it therefore appears that molting serves additional functions.

Regardless of the origin and function of molting in free-living nematodes, the process has been adapted to the parasitic mode of life. The typical free-living nematode moves continuously from one stage of the life cycle to the next when there is adequate food, moisture, and moderate temperature. On the other hand, the parasitic nematodes have adapted molting for control of their development and to increase the probability of completing the life cycle. As an example, the trichostrongyloid nematodes have direct life cycles in which there is a free-living phase. Eggs are shed with the feces of the host, and after they develop for a few days, the L_1 hatches. The L_1 feeds, and then molts to the L_2, which feeds and molts. The L_3 is the infective stage, which is a nonfeeding stage ensheathed in the cast cuticle of the L_2. Thus, molting has gone only halfway; the body of the L_3 has separated from the L_2 cuticle but has not crawled out of it. The L_3 remains ensheathed until it has been ingested by the proper host, at which time the sheath is shed and the L_3 invades the tissue to become a parasitic form. The same is true of vector-borne nematodes; they develop to a certain stage in the vector and continue development only when they have been transferred to the next host in the cycle. The infective stage may vary depending on the particular group of nematodes, but the same phenomenon is seen: development stops at a certain stage and continues only when the larva has received the signal that it has reached the proper environment and further development is feasible.

CLASSIFICATION OF THE PHYLUM NEMATODA

Classification and identification of nematodes are based largely on the following features:

1. Phasmids, presence or absence and structure
2. Lateral excretory canals, presence or absence (Fig 25.7)
3. Esophageal structure (Fig. 25.8)
4. Structure of the buccal capsule and lips or papillae on the anterior end (Fig. 25.9)
5. Structure of the male copulatory organs (Fig. 25.3)
6. Structure of the posterior tip of the female
7. Structure of the eggs

The phylum Nematoda has two classes, Secernentea (originally Phasmidia) and Adenophorea (originally Aphasmidia), and the division is based on the fact that the Secernentea has phasmids (structures in the caudal region of the worm, which are neuro-sensory) and lateral excretory canals and the Adenophorea lacks both. Unfortunately, the phasmids are difficult to see and the lateral excretory canals can be seen only in tissue sections. For practical purposes, in identifying nematodes one ignores both phasmids and excretory canals and uses the other five characteristics to place a specimen in the proper class, order, or lower taxon.

Class Secernentea (Phasmidea)

Phasmids usually present; lateral excretory canals; caudal glands absent; external amphids porelike, usually small; cervical papillae (deirids) usually present; caudal alae or copulatory bursa common; usually four to six pseudocoelomocytes.

Order Tylenchida

Stylet present in mouth; single excretory canal esophagus composed of corpus often with bulb, isthmus, and nonvalved glandular region.
Anguina, Heterotylenchus

Order Rhabditida

Stylet absent; excretory canals paired; esophagus usually composed of corpus, isthmus, and bulb, but the bulb is sometimes absent; transverse vagina, not heavily muscled; caudal alae, if present with papillae rather than muscular rays.
Caenorhabditis, Pelodera, Rhabiditis, Strongyloides

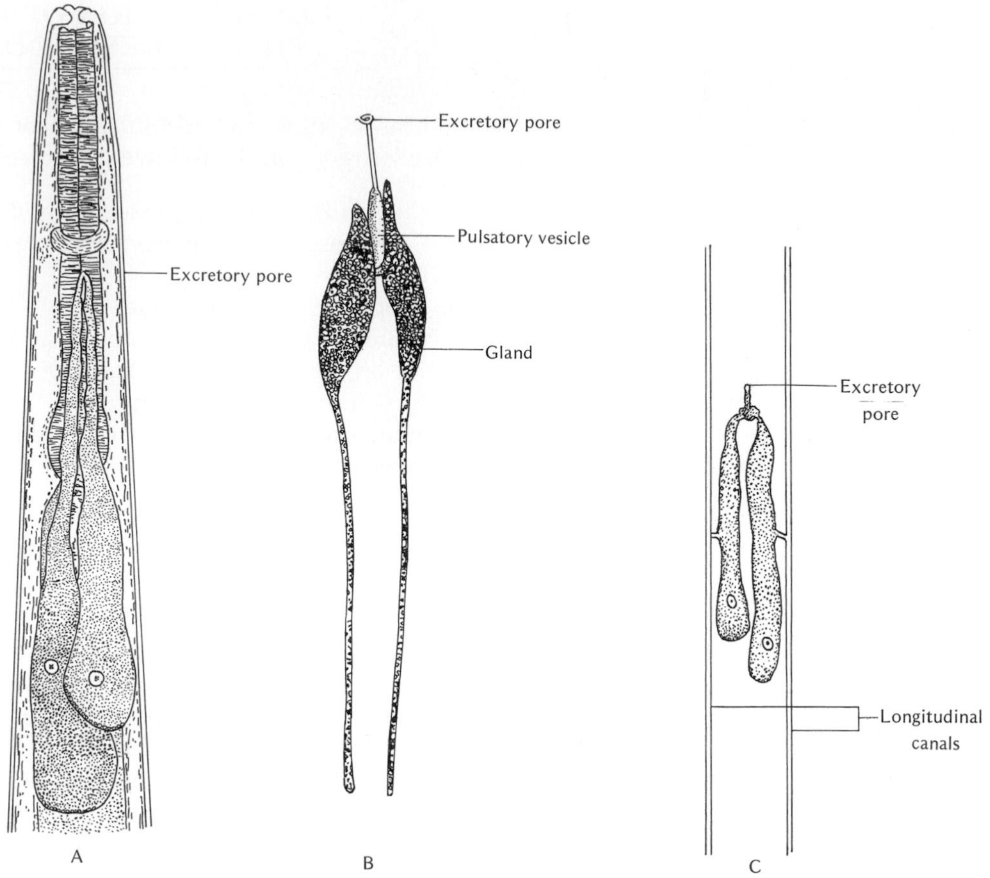

FIGURE 25.7 Nematode excretory systems. [Redrawn with modifications from Hyman, 1951.]

Order Strongylida

Corona radiata or three or six lips; buccal cavity surrounded by esophageal tissue; larval esophagus consists of pro- and metacorpus, isthmus, and bulb; adult esophagus clavate; excretory system with paired lateral canals and paired subventral glands; female with transverse or short vagina vera and single or double vagina uterina, often heavily muscled (ovejector); male with caudal alae usually containing well-developed muscular rays forming the true or strongylid copulatory bursa; two spicules, equal or subequal.

Superfamily Ancylostomatoidea

Buccal capsule subglobular, never hexagonal in transverse section; lips and corona radiata absent; oral opening unarmed or with teeth and cutting plates; bursa well developed.
Ancylostoma, Necator, Bunostomum, Uncinaria, Gaigeria, Globocephalus

Superfamily Strongyloidea

Mouth surrounded by corona radiata, sometimes six lips, oral opening sometimes hexagonal, teeth and cutting plates absent; bursa well developed.
Strongylus, Craterostomum, Chabertia, Oesophagostomum, Stephanurus, Syngamus, Triodontophorus, Oesophagodontus, Mammomonogamus

Superfamily Trichostrongyloidea

Mouth small, lips absent or surrounded by three or six small lips; often with cuticular inflation at mouth region; usually numerous longitudinal ridges; L_1 often with valved esophageal bulb and conical tail ending in a simple point; bursa well developed.
Cooperia, Cooperioides, Haemonchus, Hyostrongylus. Nematospiroides, Heligmosomoides, Nematodirus, Nippostrongylus, Ostertagia, Trichostrongylus

Superfamily Metastrongyloidea

Mouth small, sometimes even absent, surrounded by six lips or lips small; longitudinal ridges absent; L_1

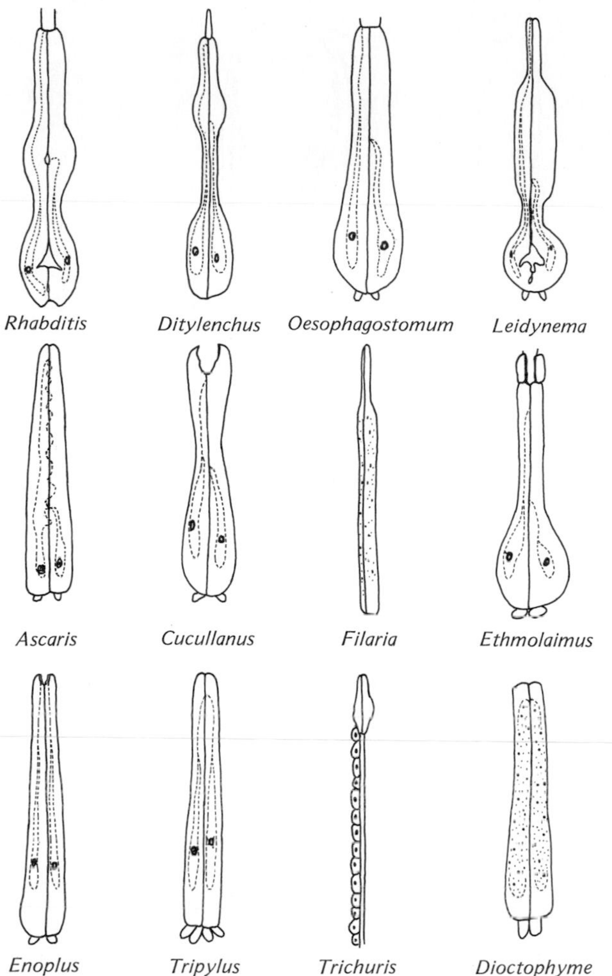

FIGURE 25.8 Esophageal structures of various nematodes. [Redrawn from Crofton, M. D., 1966.]

without esophageal bulb, tail usually asymmetrical; bursa small, rays somewhat fused; parasites of the lungs and blood vessels of vertebrates.
Angiostrongylus, Dictyocaulus, Elaphostrongylus, Metastrongylus, Muellerius, Parelaphostrongylus, Protostrongylus

Order Ascaridida

Generally heavy-bodied worms; adults with all gradations in esophageal structure from rhabditiform to cylindrical; three, two, or no lips; preanal sucker in male present or absent; caudal alae, if present, with papillae; two, one, or no spicules; generally with direct life cycles, except in Subuluroidea.
Ascaris, Ascaridia, Heterakis, Toxocara, Toxascaris, Anisakis, Contracaecum, Phocanema, Subulura

Order Oxyurida

Worms with short, stout bodies and often with elongated tails in the females giving rise to the common name of *pinworms*; males with a small number of caudal papillae and a single spicule; preanal sucker absent except in a single genus; esophagus with a large bulb; eggs often asymmetrical and embryonated while still in female; direct life cycles; parasites of the lower part of the digestive tract.
Enterobius, Oxyuris, Skrjabinema, Syphacia

Order Spirurida

Stout to threadlike worms; anterior extremity bilaterally symmetrical and lacking lateral external labial papillae; caudal papillae ventral or ventrolateral; esophagus with a short, anterior muscular portion and a long, glandular posterior portion; indirect life cycles, parasites of the anterior portion of the gut of vertebrates or of the blood and tissue spaces.

Suborder Camallanina

Larva lacking cephalic hook but with long, pointed tail and conspicuous phasmids; esophageal glands uninucleate, parasites of the gut of lower vertebrates or other organs in both lower and higher vertebrates; indirect life cycles with copepods as intermediate hosts.
Camallanus, Dracunculus, Philometra, Philometroides, Avioserpens

Suborder Filariina

Larva with cephalic hook or spine and inconspicuous porelike phasmids; esophageal glands multinucleate; parasites of the gut or extraintestinal tissues of all vertebrates; intermediate hosts are arthropods, often insects and ticks; ten superfamilies including the Filarioidea, which is most important, as it contains many parasites of humans and domestic animals. *Acuaria, Physaloptera, Stephanofilaria, Elaeophora, Wuchereria, Brugia, Thelazia, Habronema, Diplotriaena, Dipetalonema, Onchocerca, Litosomoides, Dirofilaria, Loa, Mansonella*

Class Adenophorea (Aphasmidia)

Phasmids lacking; lateral excretory canals absent; esophagus cylindrical.

Order Trichurata

Amphids pocketlike, porelike, or tuboid; excretory system poorly developed or absent; stylet present;

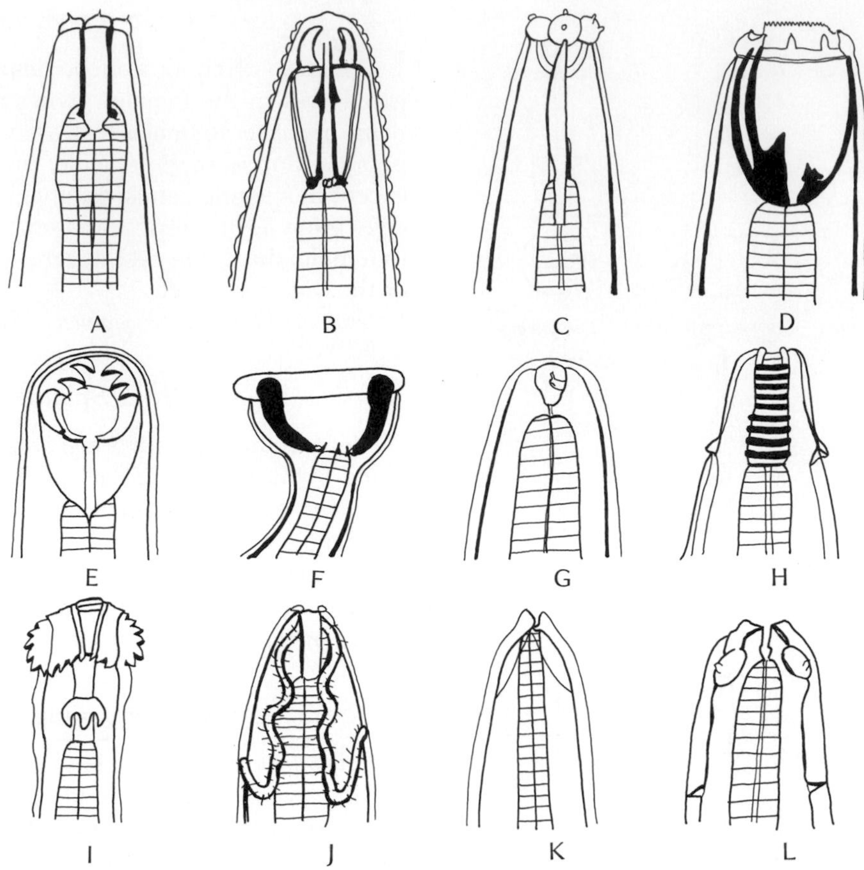

FIGURE 25.9 Head and mouth structures of various nematodes. (A) *Rhabiditis;* (B) *Rotylenchus;* (C) *Dorylaimus;* (D) *Strongylus;* (E) *Ancylostoma;* (F) *Syngamus;* (G) *Haemonchus;* (H) *Physocephalus;* (I) *Seuratia;* (J) *Acuaria;* (K) *Enterobius;* (L) *Filaria.* [Redrawn from Crofton, M. D., 1966.]

esophageal gland orifices posterior to nerve ring and uninucleate; neither caudal alae nor bursa present in male.

Superfamily Mermithoidea

Male with one or two spicules and two testes; females usually with two ovaries; larvae parasites of arthropods and adults free living.
Mermis, Romanomermis

Superfamily Trichinelloidea

Amphids porelike; esophageal glands free in body cavity forming stichostome; male with one testis and no or one spicule; female with elongate, tubular vagina and one ovary; eggs usually operculate; both adults and larvae parasitic.
Capillaria, Trichinella, Trichosomoides, Trichuris

Order Dioctophymatida

Amphids pocketlike, porelike, or tuboid; esophageal glands inside wall of cylindrical esophagus; reproductive system single in males and females; male with one spicule and caudal sucker; eggs operculate.
Dioctophyma, Eustrongylides, Hystrichis

Readings

Adamson, M. L. (1987). Phylogenetic analysis of the higher classification of the Nematoda. *Can. J. Zool.* **65,** 1478–1482.

Anderson, R. C. (1992). *Nematode Parasites of Vertebrates. Their Development and Transmission. Nos. 1–10.* CAB International, Wallingford, UK.

Anderson, R. C., Chabaud, A. G., and Wilmott, S. (Eds.) (1974). *Keys to the Nematode Parasites of Vertebrates.* Serial Publ. Commonwealth Inst., Helminthol, Commonwealth Agricultural Bureaux, Farnham Royal, UK.

Andrássy, I. (1976). *Evolution as a Basis for Systematization of Nematodes.* Pitman, San Francisco.

Behnke, J. M. (1990). *Parasites: Immunity and Pathology: The Consequences of Parasitic Infections in Mammals.* Taylor & Francis, Bristol, PA.

Bird, A. F., and Bird, J. (1991). *The Structure of Nematodes*, 2nd ed. Academic Press, New York.

Caveness, F. E. (1964). *A Glossary of Nematological Terms*. Pacific Printers, Ibadan, Nigeria.

Chitwood, B. G., and Chitwood, M. B. (1974). *Introduction to Nematology*. University Park Press, Baltimore.

Chitwood, M. B., and Lichtenfels, J. R. (1972). Identification of parasitic metazoa in tissue sections. *Exp. Parasitol.* **32,** 407–519.

Crofton, M. D. (1966). *Nematodes.* Hutchinson Univ. Library, London

Gibbons, L. M. (1986). *SEM Guide to the Morphology of Nematode Parasites of Vertebrates.* CAB International, Oxford, UK.

Harris, J. E., and Croften, D. H. (1957). Structure and function of nematodes: internal pressure and cuticular structure in *Ascaris. J. Exp. Biol.* **34,** 116–130.

Hyman, L. (1951). *The invertebrates. Vol. III Acanthocephala, aschelminthes, entoprocta.* McGraw-Hill, New York.

Inglis, W. G. (1971). Speciation in nematodes. *Adv. Parasitol.* **9,** 185–226.

Kennedy, M. W. (1990). *Parasitic Nematodes: Antigens, Membranes and Genes.* Taylor & Francis, Bristol, PA.

Lee, D. L. (1965). *The Physiology of Nematodes.* Freeman, San Francisco

Lee, D. L. (1972). The structure of helminth cuticle. *Adv. Parasitol.* **10,** 347–379.

Levine, N. D. (1980). *Nematode Parasites of Domestic Animals and Man*, 2nd ed. Burgess, Minneapolis.

McLaren, D. J. (1976). Nematode sense organs. *Adv. Parasitol.* **14,** 195–267.

Yamaguti, L. (1961). *Systema Helminthum. Vol. III. Nematodes*, Parts 1 and 2. Interscience, New York.

CHAPTER

26

Strongyloides and Other Rhabditid Nematodes

The members of the order Rhabditida are singularly unremarkable in their structure; they are small, transparent worms with little development of head or tail structures (Fig. 26.1). Their characteristics are outlined at the end of Chapter 25.

An interesting aspect of the rhabditid nematodes is their seeming transition from free-living to parasitic modes of existence. Species can be seen in this group that are completely free living but can invade hosts and develop in the skin (*Pelodera strongyloides*) or sometimes in internal organs of the host (*Rhabditis axei*). Even those that are obligate parasites (*Strongyloides* spp.) maintain a free-living sexual generation alternating with a parthenogenetic parasitic one.

Except for members of the genus *Strongyloides*, the parasitic and facultatively parasitic species in the order are of only minor medical or economic importance. We consider only one facultative parasite and *Strongyloides*.

Two species of rhabditids serve as experimental animals in fundamental biological studies. The worms are inexpensive and easy to maintain in the laboratory and they are amenable to induced mutations. *Caenorhabditis elegans* is a free-living species that has been maintained in axenic culture and is used in a myriad of genetic studies. In fact, *C. elegans* has become the fruit fly of the late 20th century in studying molecular aspects of genetics.

Because nematodes have determinate cleavage, the fate of each cell formed early in embryogenesis can be followed. The 900-odd cells in *C. elegans* have been mapped and the sources of mutations have been shown. Induced mutations have allowed the description of temperature-sensitive mutants as well as neural mutants that affect behavior, and other processes. In addition, various investigators have created transgenic *C. elegans* by introducing other nematode genes into it and having those genes expressed. This, along with the complete cosmid library now available for *C. elegans*, has permitted another dimension in genetic analysis and the potential for a more complete description of the roles of various gene products.

A second member of the genus, *C. briggsae*, has been used in nutritional studies and has been found to have about the same nutritional requirements as the parasitic species that have been studied. One might think that the parasites would have lost the synthetic abilities found in free-living species, but that seems not to be the general situation.

PELODERA STRONGYLOIDES

Name of Organism and Disease Associations

Pelodera strongyloides (syn. *Rhabditis strongyloides*); no name has been given to the infection caused, but it could be referred to as *cutaneous nematodosis*.

Hosts and Host Range

The dog, ox, sheep, and rodents are known to be hosts. The organism lives in the skin and in the orbit of the eye.

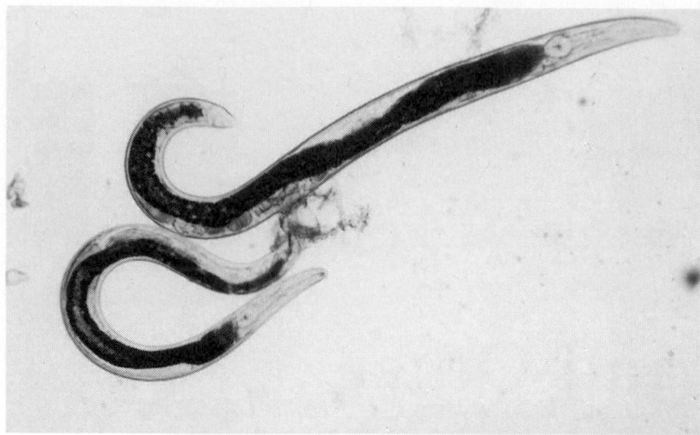

FIGURE 26.1 *Pelodera strongyloides* male and female in *copula*.

Geographic Distribution and Importance

Cosmopolitan. This species occurs infrequently in domestic animals; it causes the host some discomfort and may lead to secondary bacterial infections.

Morphology

Females are 1.3 to 1.5 mm long; males are 0.9 to 1.2 mm long (Fig. 26.1). The vulva of the female is just posterior to the midpoint of the body. The male has a pair of fused spicules 65 to 73 μm long and a rather flat, spindle-shaped gubernaculum 47 μm long. L_1s are about 180 μm long and the organism grows through a series of molts, becoming larger at each stage.

Life Cycle

At room temperature (20–22°C) the organism passes from egg to adult in about four days. Under crowded cultural conditions or drying, the L_3, and perhaps other larval stages, form *dauer* larvae, a general term for a resistant form that can survive for many months.

Diagnosis

Nematodes that enter the skin of an animal cause crusty, weeping lesions and some loss of hair. Scrapings of the area reveal the living nematodes when examined as a wet mount under a compound microscope.

Other organisms that may cause similar lesions are chewing lice such as *Bovicola bovis* or mites such as *Chorioptes*, *Psoroptes*, or *Sarcoptes*. If no nematodes are found, skin scrapings may be examined microscopically for the presence of arthropods.

Host–Parasite Interactions

In domesticated animals, the worms are limited to the skin, where they cause principally superficial damage.

Epidemiology and Control

P. strongyloides is normally a free-living organism. It becomes a parasite under conditions in which animals such as cattle or dogs are housed under unsatisfactory conditions with wet and soiled bedding. If an animal lies on wet bedding and there are bacteria growing in it, the skin becomes soft and its cornified, protective barrier breaks down. The nematodes that are normally present under such conditions move from the bedding to the skin and continue the life cycle there.

Control of *P. strongyloides* infections is directed at providing better conditions for the infected animals. When animals have clean, dry bedding, the lesions usually clear up spontaneously.

Our interest in *Pelodera* lies in its transition from a purely free-living organism to a facultative parasite. Its success as a parasite is marginal, but proper conditions allow it to invade the skin and live there for a while. The percutaneous mode of infection of *Strongyloides* spp. and the maintenance of a free-living generation illustrate the further transition perhaps from facultative to obligate parasitism.

STRONGYLOIDES INFECTIONS

Strongyloides spp. are tiny worms ranging in length from 2.2 mm for *S. stercoralis* to 9 mm for *S. westeri*; most are 3 to 6 mm long. All of the species have much the same structure and life cycle. They differ from one another in details of structure, life cycle, and pathogenesis. We use *S. papillosus* of ruminants as a typical member of the genus and then comment on other species as relevant. There are some common features of *Strongyloides* spp. that are important in dealing with them as agents of disease:

1. The small size makes them difficult to find in the intestine during postmortem examination. More than the usual care is required to look for them using a dissecting microscope in examining intestinal contents or scrapings.
2. All of the species have the potential of a homogonic cycle and a heterogonic cycle in the free-living phase (Fig. 26.2). In the homogonic cycle, the organisms develop directly to the infective L_3. In the heterogonic cycle they develop through a free-living sexual generation and then their progeny develop to the infective L_3.

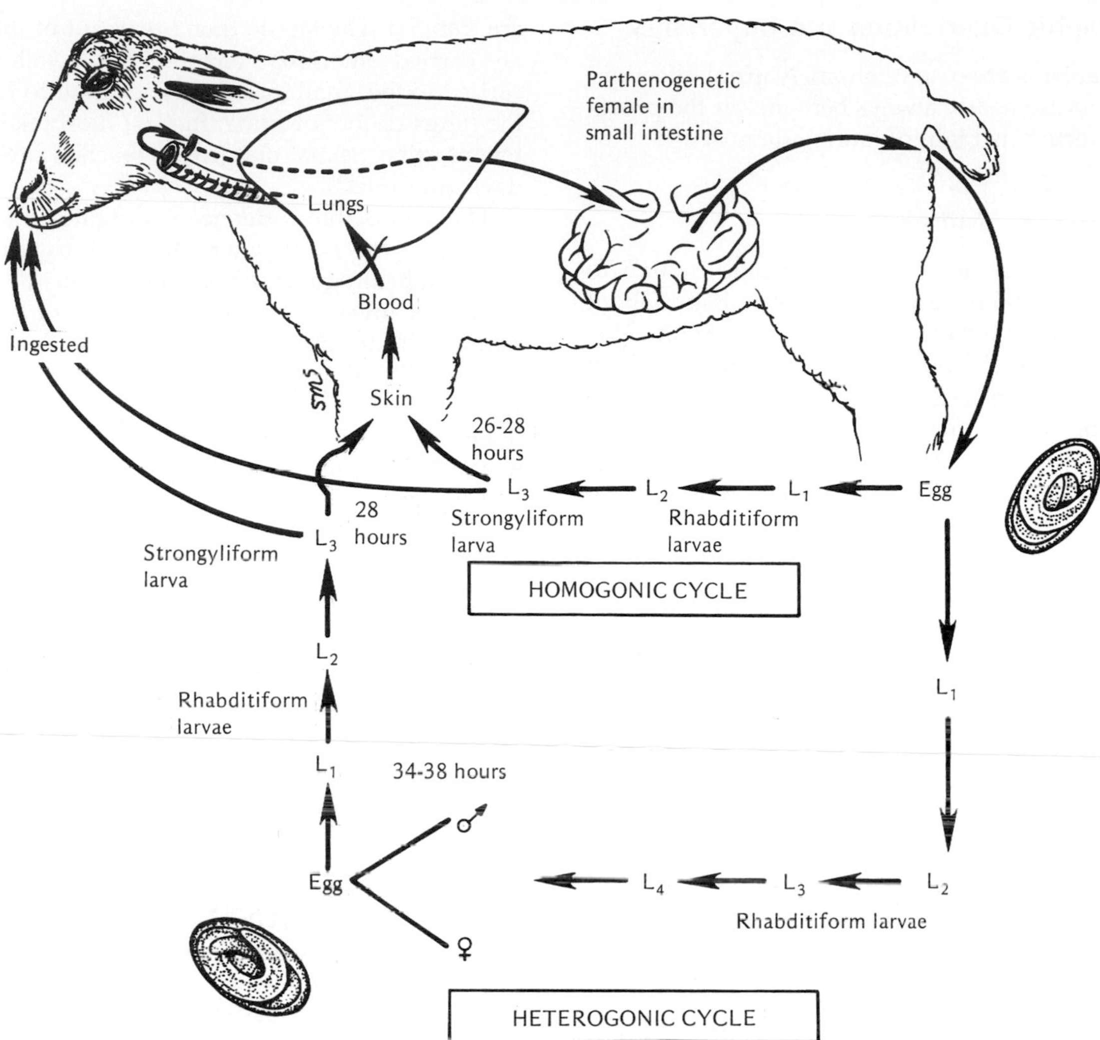

FIGURE 26.2 Diagram of the life cycle of *Strongyloides papillosus* of ruminants. The life cycles of all species of *Strongyloides* are essentially the same.

3. The parasitic phase of the cycle consists of parthenogenetic females only. A few reports of finding parasitic males have not been confirmed. Thus, there is an alternation of generations in the life cycle.

4. The free-living stages are short-lived and are detrimentally affected by adverse environmental conditions. The L_3s typically survive only a few days in the environment. *S. papillosus* L_3s were found to survive as long as 40 days at 20°C, and this can be considered to be the maximal survival time in the genus. Cold, freezing, drying, and anaerobic conditions kill the L_3s within a short time.

5. Whether the free-living stages develop directly to the L_3 through the homogonic cycle or the heterogonic cycle depends on conditions inside and outside the host. The conditions that shift the cycle through one phase or the other seem to be somewhat different for each species.

6. Any one species has only a moderate host specificity. Usually a species is found naturally in from three to six species of hosts; development may occur in experimental animals taxonomically far removed from the normal hosts.

Name of Organism and Disease Associations

Strongyloides papillosus causes strongyloidosis, strongyloidiasis, and threadworm infection.

Hosts and Host Range

Sheep, cattle, goats, other ruminants both domestic and wild, pig, and rabbits are hosts.

Geographic Distribution and Importance

The organisms are cosmopolitan. Natural infections in ruminants are nearly always benign, but the prevalence of infection is high in young animals.

Morphology

Parasitic females are 3.5 to 6 mm long by 0.05 to 0.065 mm wide and have a filariform esophagus about 0.98 mm long or about one-sixth the body length. Eggs in feces are about 55 by 35 μm and contain a fully developed L_1 when passed. The infective L_3 is 520 to 710 μm long, with a filariform esophagus 200 to 270 μm long; the L_3 is not ensheathed. All stages except the parasitic female and the L_3 have a rhabditiform esophagus, in which there is an anterior corpus, a narrow isthmus, and a distinct bulb at its posterior end.

Life Cycle

All species of *Strongyloides* have four possible phases in their life cycles (Fig. 26.2):

1. The parasitic phase in which only female worms are found in the intestine of the vertebrate host.
2. The homogonic phase is free living and the worms develop on the ground through the L_1, L_2, and then reach the infective L_3. The L_3 must then enter a host or it perishes.
3. The heterogonic phase in which there is a free-living sexual generation. Development proceeds to form males and females which copulate and lay eggs that eventually reach the infective L_3. There is only a single sexual generation.
4. In the autoinfective or retrofective phase, the homogonic worms develop to the L_3 without ever leaving the intestine of the vertebrate host. The L_3s invade the tissues of the gut and develop to parthenogenetic females.

The parasitic females lie in the paramucosal lumen of the small intestine, where they lay eggs with nearly fully developed L_1s that pass with the feces; the L_1s hatch in 6 hours at 27°C. If the organisms develop directly through the homogonic cycle, they reach the L_3 in 26 to 28 hours. If the organisms develop through the heterogonic cycle, the egg-laying adults are reached in 34 to 38 hours after leaving the host. The infective L_3s are reached about 28 hours later (Fig. 26.2).

The L_3s may be eaten with forage or may penetrate the unbroken skin. If eaten, the larvae probably remain in the gut and develop directly to parthenogenetic females. If they penetrate the skin, the L_3s enter the bloodstream and are carried to the lungs, where they are trapped. The larvae then break out of the air sacs, are carried anteriorly, coughed up, swallowed, and carried to the small intestine. They molt to L_4 either in the lungs or the intestine; the last molt takes place in the intestine. Sexual maturity is reached seven to nine days after infection.

The factors that influence the organism to develop directly to the L_3 or, alternatively, through the free-living, or heterogonic, sexual generation have been the subject of investigation by a number of workers. A number of interpretations and theories have been set forth as a result of experiments on the more common species of *Strongyloides*. Most likely in *S. papillosus* and *S. ransomi* the sex of the offspring of the parasitic females is determined by conditions in the host. The immune status of the host seems to be the most important factor in producing male and female offspring that have the potential of developing into the free-living sexual generation. Males do not appear until several weeks after the parthenogenetic females have established, and although there is a possibility that the worms produce males as they age, most of the evidence points toward immunity as the cause. Once outside the host, environmental conditions cause the female eggs to shift either to free-living adults or to the homogonic L_3s. For example, hydrogen ion concentrations below pH 5.9 or above pH 7.2 favor development directly to L_3, whereas hydrogen ion concentrations within this range favor the heterogonic cycle. As a general rule, the heterogonic cycle is favored by optimal external conditions.

Recent research on *Strongyloides* amphids has greatly advanced our understanding of these fascinating chemosensory structures in nematodes. Most recently, Schad and colleagues have described evidence that the amphids of *Strongyloides* communicate external cues that control the switching between homogonic and heterogonic development.

It was previously believed that males participated in sexual reproduction only as tokens. It was believed that sperm initiated fertilization but did not provide any genetic material This was termed obligate pseudofertilization. Newer data using *S. ratti* have shown that syngamy does, in fact, take place. In this species, at least, both parents contribute to the genome of the offspring.

Diagnosis

The most common method of diagnosis is finding the typical embryonated eggs or hatched L_1s in the feces. It is said that the L_1s fail to float in the usual flotation media used in fecal examinations, but fecal examinations on infected lambs usually show a few larvae. An alternative is to use a method such as the Baermann funnel to allow the larvae to migrate out of the feces, where they can then be collected.

Host–Parasite Interactions

Strongyloides spp. cause damage to the host at three different points:

1. At the site of penetration of the skin
2. During migration through the tissues and the lungs
3. After reaching the intestine and becoming sexually mature

In the case of *S. papillosus* specifically, little overall economic effect occurs in natural infections. However, penetration of the skin by L_1s allows the invasion of bacteria such as *Bacteroides nodosus*, one of the causative agents of foot rot in sheep. For a long time there was doubt that *S. papillosus* was pathogenic at all, but massive inocula have been found to cause considerable damage to both lambs and calves. Inocula of 10^4 or more L_3s were lethal for lambs and 2×10^4 or more were lethal for calves. Animals are not naturally exposed to that many larvae at one time.

In an epidemiological study of gastrointestinal nematodes of ruminants, eggs of *S. papillosus* are the first to appear in the feces. In lambs, for example, eggs appear within about the first six weeks or two months of life and are seen for the next five months and then disappear. Typically, they are not seen in large numbers at any time; in ewes only an occasional egg is seen.

Two factors act to limit the life of infection—immunity and age resistance. As an animal is exposed to L_3s, a skin reaction develops that traps many of the larvae in the skin. Circulating antibodies have also been found, which seem to inhibit those larvae that reach the bloodstream. Age resistance probably also acts since much larger inocula are required to produce pathogenesis as calves become older. However, it is always difficult to truly differentiate immunity from so-called age resistance.

As with many of the parasitic nematodes, study of the immunology of *Strongyloides* infection has been limited due to the inability to work with genetically identical hosts. However, adaptation of *Strongyloides stercoralis* to the mouse has been of great benefit in this regard. The ability to study this infection in mice has led investigators to a number of important findings. For example, infective larvae can be killed by protective immune responses, but they must go through a differentiation event within the host before they are susceptible to killing. That is, infective larvae that have not been adequately exposed to their host cannot be killed by the same protective immune responses that kill larvae that have had brief, but sufficient, exposure to environmental cues within the host. Also of note is the finding that these worms are killed through an effector arm of the immune response, the T helper 2 arm, which is usually only associated with deleterious immune responses such as allergy and certain other antibody responses. The complete life cycle of this parasite has also been successfully established in the Severe Combined Immunodeficiency Disease (SCID) mouse. While this particular mouse strain is devoid of an effective immune system at birth, it is possible to graft immune systems from other mammals into this mouse strain. It should be possible, therefore, to study the human immune response to the human species of *Strongyloides* within the mouse. This could prove to be very important for the design of effective vaccines, therapeutics, and diagnostic assays.

Strongyloides spp. may not complete development in hosts outside of their usual host range, but the L_3s penetrate the skin of almost any potential host. Cutaneous larva migrans has been seen in humans as a result of penetration of the larvae of *S. papillosus*, *S. stercoralis*, *S. myopotami*, and *S. procyonis*. The larvae sometimes migrate from the skin to internal organs such as the lung and cause some lung damage and eosinophilia (Loeffler's syndrome). Cutaneous larva migrans is discussed further in Chapter 27.

Epidemiology and Control

Despite experiments showing the pathogenesis of large inocula given to young animals, *S. papillosus* rarely causes damage under the conditions in which animals are usually raised. Treatment is not typically given to ruminants infected with *S. papillosus*.

The free-living stages of *Strongyloides* are most prevalent in climates that are warm and moist. The L_3s are particularly susceptible to environmental extremes. Cold, drying, and anaerobic conditions are all detrimental to the L_3s. At refrigerator temperatures of 4 to 6°C, about half (47%) of the larvae die in two days.

Name of Organism and Disease Associations

Strongyloides stercoralis causes strongyloidosis, strongyloidiasis, or threadworm infection.

Hosts and Host Range

Humans, dogs and other canids, cats, coatimundi, and both higher and lower primates are hosts. Different geographic isolates of *S. stercoralis* have different host ranges.

Geographic Distribution and Importance

Cosmopolitan, but prevalence is highest in warm, moist climates. Globally there are about 200 million infections in humans. In the United States there are about 400,000 human infections at any one time; in the rural South, up to 4% of persons may be infected. Under some conditions, infection rates can become quite high; for example, 18% of 1437 inmates in a New York mental hospital were infected; in other institutionalized persons, the prevalence ranged from 1.7% to 40% in a number of studies. In dogs in the United States, the prevalence of infection is between 1 and 2%.

Morphology

The parthenogenetic parasitic females (Fig. 26.3) are 1.7 to 2.7 by 0.03 to 0.04 mm. Eggs are 55 to 60 by 28 to 32 μm but usually hatch before leaving the host. Larvae develop through the usual stages of nematodes (Fig. 26.4).

Life Cycle

See *S. papillosus* (Fig. 26.2). The adult parthenogenetic females live in the duodenum and upper part of the jejenum of the small intestine. Even though Figure 26.2 represents the accepted view of the life cycle of *Strongyloides* spp., some qualifications must be addressed.

When the life cycles of the various species of *Strongyloides* were worked out, the pattern of migration seemed to be consistent, and it was accepted without much question for many decades. In the mid-1980s Gerhard Schad and his coworkers undertook quantitative studies on *S. stercoralis* in helminth-free dogs. When the number of larvae administered was compared to the number of larvae migrating through the respiratory tree, only a small proportion was found. The remainder of the larvae were found migrating in other organ systems: liver, nervous system, reproductive system, and so on. It has been proposed that migration is random, and that those which reach the lungs

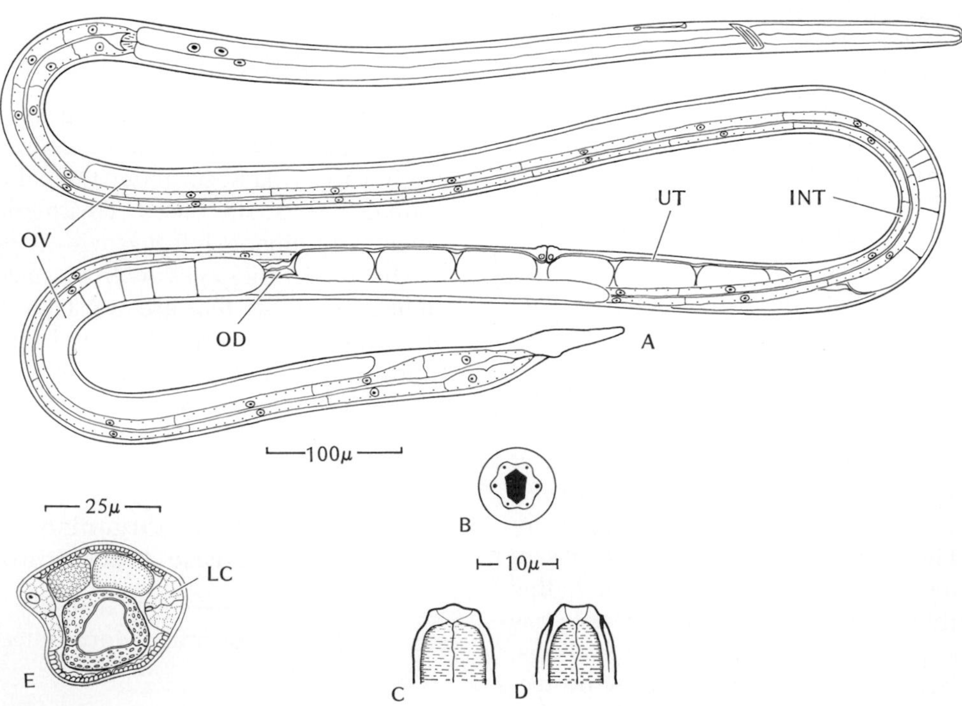

FIGURE 26.3 Parthenogenetic female of *Strongyloides stercoralis*. (A) Entire worm (INT, intestine, OV, ovary, OD, oviduct, UT, uterus containing eggs); (B) en face view; (C) lateral view of the head; (D) dorsal view of the head; (E) transverse section at the level of the ovary (LS, lateral nerve chord). [From Little, M.D., 1966a.]

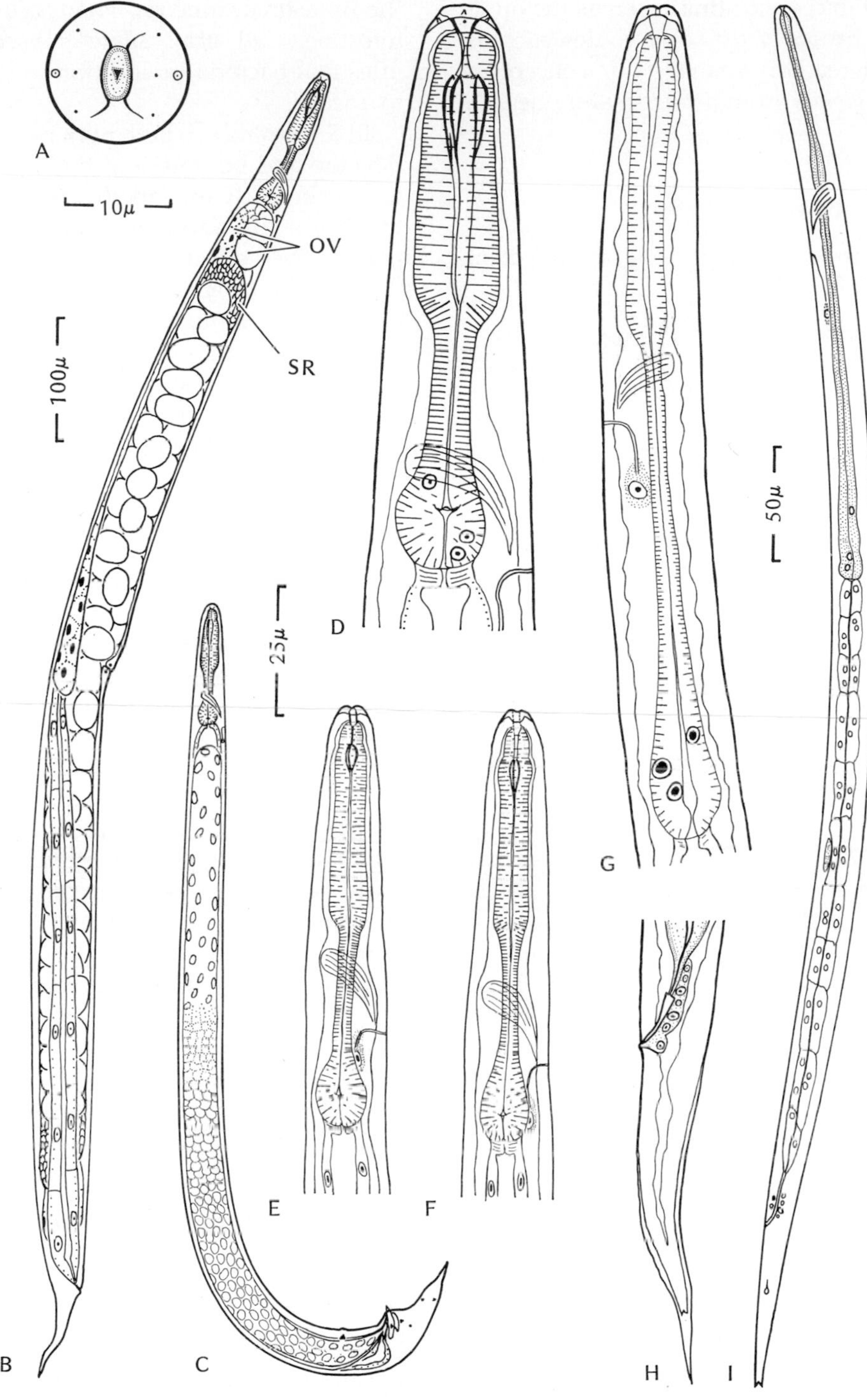

FIGURE 26.4 Free-living stages of *Strongyloides stercoralis.* (A) Free-living female, en face; (B) free-living female, lateral view; (C) free-living male; (D) anterior end of free-living female showing details of esophagus; (E) newly hatched L_1 obtained by duodenal aspiration from human; (F) L_1 from freshly passed feces; (G) L_2 in the process of developing to the L_3, the cuticle is separating at the anterior end; (H) tail of late L_2; (I) L_3 or infective or filariform larva. [From Little, 1966a.]

ultimately wind up in the intestine whereas the other reach the intestine probably by other routes such as direct migration there. This changes our concept of migration in *Strongyloides* from a purposeful one to a more random one.

Diagnosis

The common methods of diagnosing the infection in humans are the following:

1. Fecal examination by
   a. Flotation
   b. Baermann funnel apparatus
2. Duodenal aspiration
3. Sputum examination
4. Clinical signs and symptoms

The direct examination gives about 30 to 60% reliability while the Baermann increases the probability of finding a positive case to 70 to 80%. An agar plate method has been shown to be even more reliable. Duodenal aspiration is about the same as the Baermann—60 to 70%; duodenal aspiration is both uncomfortable for the patient and relatively costly. There are promising serologic tests, but they are not widely used.

Clinical signs and symptoms are so general as to be without great value except to alert the physician that an intestinal infection is underway. There is usually an enteritis that may give rise to diarrhea and abdominal discomfort. It is always useful to inquire about travel to warm countries and to keep in mind that thread-worm infections can be maintained for many years.

Infections in hosts other than humans are generally diagnosed by fecal examination only, but there may be instances in which more costly methods are justified.

Host–Parasite Interactions

The host range of *S. stercoralis* raises concerns, especially the possibility of cross-transmission between dogs and humans. No definite statement can be made about whether it is likely to occur in any one instance, because there are geographic races that vary in their host range. Experimental transmission from dog to human appears not to have been done, but there is a report of accidental transmission of *S. stercoralis* to an animal caretaker who had contact with dogs.

Although there are sometimes skin and pulmonary problems in persons infected with *S. stercoralis*, most of the damage takes place in the intestine when the worms have matured. Since the worms burrow into the intestinal mucosa, they cause damage to the intestine, and may allow subsequent invasion by intestinal bacteria in addition to the enteritis alluded to earlier.

In *S. stercoralis* in both humans and dogs, the L_3 may develop and become infective before the larvae have left the body. It appears that the worms become infective in the gut and then penetrate either in the lower part of the large intestine or in the perianal region; this type of infection is probably best referred to as *retrofection*, although the terms *hyperinfection* and *autoinfection* are used for the same process.

A number of cases have been recorded in which individuals have been overwhelmed by *S. stercoralis* infections. It has been concluded by a number of investigators that the person lacked the ability to launch a useful immune response, and that the worms then disseminated at will. However, another explanation has been proposed. It appears that the adult worms somehow regulate the size of their population to about 100 parthenogenetic females. The population turns over, but the number remains fairly constant. From a critical reading of the literature, it appears that immunosuppression by itself does not necessarily allow *S. stercoralis* to disseminate throughout the body. AIDS patients or other individuals receiving certain immunosuppressive drugs seemingly do not experience disseminated infections, but those receiving corticosteroids, or ACTH (adrenocorticotrophic hormone) do, in fact, suffer from disseminated strongyloidiasis. It was proposed that the life cycle of *S. strercoralis* is regulated by steroidal compounds, and that when the concentration of these compounds increases, the worms multiply rapidly in the host and then disseminate throughout the body. Alternatively, there may be clues available through an appreciation of the different types of immunosuppression engendered by those various means.

Epidemiology and Control

S. stercoralis is likely to be a widespread problem only in areas with warm, moist climates. Control involves the following:

1. Sanitary disposal of human waste
2. Treatment of infected persons
3. Elimination of infections in companion animals
4. Stringent measures to prevent feces of dogs from coming into contact with humans

Treatment of strongyloidosis can be challenging, particularly in case of hyperinfection. Until recently, thiabendazole was considered to be the drug of choice, but ivermectin has been shown to be superior in efficacy and does not have side effects. While ivermectin is not registered for human use, the importance of avoiding hyperinfection in AIDS patients, for example, will no doubt elicit use of the drug.

Since *S. stercoralis* is usually a significant problem in economically depressed areas, all the difficulties of implementation of control discussed in the chapters on blood flukes, ascarids, hookworms, and other intestinal parasites pertain here as well. Chemotherapy is not as distressing to the patient as in some other diseases, and it should be possible to institute treatment programs without much resistance if infections are diagnosed.

If a member of a family is diagnosed as having *S. stercoralis* infection, all of the other members of the family and companion animals in the household should be examined and treated if necessary. The reservoir of infection in hosts other than humans, especially the dog, must be addressed in the face of a familial outbreak of strongyloidosis.

Instances such as infections in institutionalized persons present a particularly difficult problem. Developmentally disabled people may not be capable of developing fastidious habits of defecation and cleanliness. The rapid development of the free living stages of *Strongyloides* makes such persons particularly prone to infection. An 18% infection rate in institutionalized persons is a case in point.

NAME OF ORGANISM AND DISEASE ASSOCIATIONS

Strongyloides ransomi causes strongyloidosis or strongyloidiasis in swine.

Hosts and Host Range.

The hosts are pigs.

Geographic Distribution and Importance

Cosmopolitan. Prevalence of infection in swine at slaughter is 10 to 14% but is undoubtedly higher in young animals; it is higher in warm, wet climates than in cool and cold climates.

Losses to *S. ransomi* are probably limited to young pigs during their first few months of life. The annual loss in swine has been estimated at $2.7 million. As more swine are raised in confined quarters, and with the use of stringent hygiene, the economic importance of *S. ransomi* should continually decrease.

Life Cycle

It is the same as that of *S. papillosus*. The principal difference from the other members of the genus is the transmission of larvae from the sow to the pigs either prenatally or in the milk.

Diagnosis

Eggs may be found in the feces by flotation methods, but in young pigs the infection is likely to be pathogenic prior to sexual maturity of the worms. In young pigs suffering from diarrhea and emaciation, it is best to examine the intestinal tissues of dead or dying animals for worms. Since a number of apicomplexan, bacterial, and viral agents cause similar signs in young pigs, those should be ruled out before concluding that *S. ransomi* is the problem.

Host–Parasite Interactions

As is true with the other members of the genus, *S. ransomi* is found in greatest numbers in younger animals. Pathogenesis occurs when large numbers of larvae are transmitted to the pigs prenatally or with milk shortly after birth. Much the same situation pertains here as with nematodes such as *Toxocara canis* and *Uncinaria lucasi*; the pregnant female accumulates larvae in her tissues, which then move to the developing offspring before birth or shortly after birth through the milk.

Damage to pigs takes place before the worms are sexually mature. There may be damage to extraintestinal tissues as the larvae migrate through them, and there is considerable damage to the intestine after the worms arrive there (Fig. 26.5).

Epidemiology and Control

In the southeastern United States, *S. ransomi* has been observed as a problem in young pigs in years when the spring was especially wet. Such conditions apparently allow large numbers of free-living stages to develop, which then accumulate in the tissues of the pregnant sow and are passed to the offspring.

The conditions under which sows are housed during pregnancy are crucial for preventing infection of their piglets. It is essential that bedding be clean and dry and that it be a material that will not hold water. Since the L_3 can be reached quickly, and skin penetration takes place readily, it is essential that contamination with feces be kept to a minimum and that it be removed within a day after deposition.

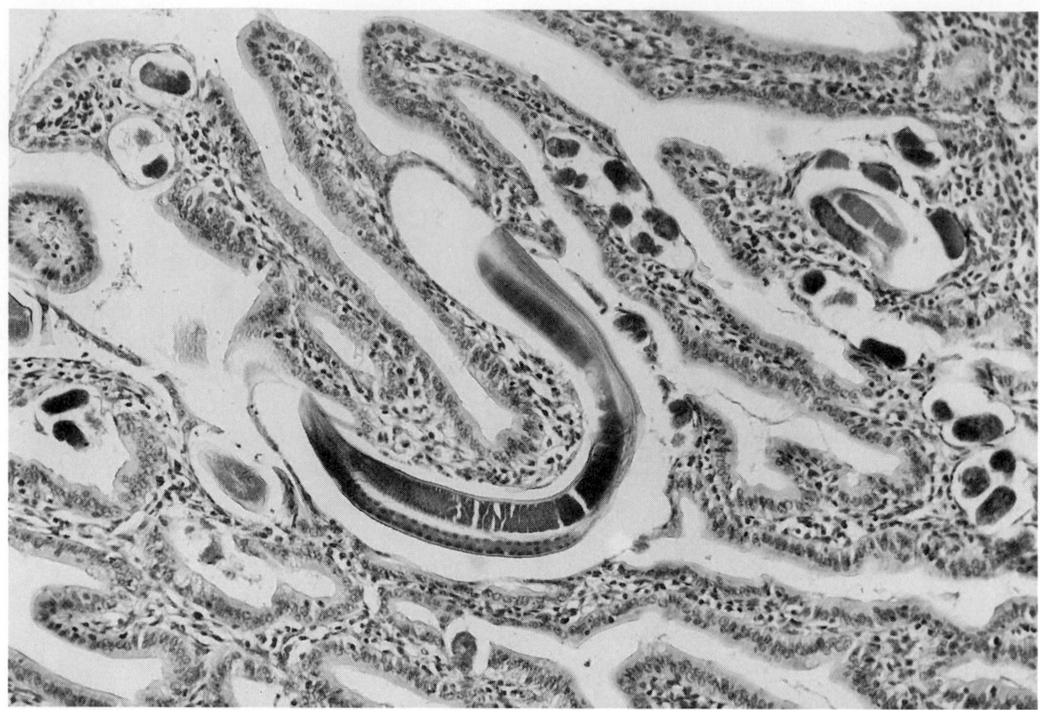

FIGURE 26.5 *Strongyloides ransomi* stages in the intestine of a young pig. [Courtesy of Dr. T. B. Stewart, School of Veterinary Medicine, L.S.U.]

Related Organisms

S. tumifaciens of the cat causes diarrhea and is associated with tumorlike changes in the large intestine. *S. westeri* of horses is a cosmopolitan parasite that probably has only a low degree of pathogenicity. *S. ratti* of rodents infects laboratory rats and has been used extensively as a laboratory model of strongyloidiasis. *S. fuelleborni* is found in higher primates and may occur occasionally in humans.

Readings

Ashton, F. T., and Schad, G. A. (1996). Amphids in *Strongyloides stercoralis* and other parasitic nematodes. *Parasitol. Today* **12,** 187–194.

Ashton, F. T., Bhopale, V. M., Smith, G., and Schad, G. A. (1998). Developmental switching in the parasitic nematode *Strongyloides stercoralis* is controlled by the ASF and ASI amphidial neurons. *J. Parasitol.* **84,** 691–695.

Basir, M. A. (1950). The morphology and development of the sheep nematode, *Strongyloides papillosus* (Wedl, 1856). *Can. J. Res. Ser. D Zool. Sci.* **28,** 173–196.

Brigandi, R. A., Rotman, H. L., Leon, O., Nolan, T. J., Schad, G. A., and Abraham, D. (1998). *Strongyloides stercoralis* host-adapted third stage larvae are the target of eosinophil-associated immune-mediated killing in mice. *J. Parasitol.* **84,** 440–445.

Datry, A., Hilsmadottiir, D. A., Mayorga-Sagastume, R., Lyagoubi, M., Gaxotte, P., Biligui, S., Chokadewitz, J., Neu, D., Danis, M., and Gentilini, M. (1994). Treatment of *Strongyloides stercoralis* infection with ivermectin compared to albendazole: Results of an open study of 60 cases. *Trans. R. Soc. Trop. Med. Hyg.* **88,** 344–345.

Genta, R. M. (1989). Global prevalence of strongyloidiasis: Critical review with epidemiologic insights in the prevention of disseminated disease. *Rev. Infect. Dis.* **2,** 755–767.

Genta, R. M. (1992). Dysregulation of strongyloidiasis: A new hypothesis. *Clin. Microbiol. Rev.* **5,** 345–355.

Georgi, J. R., and Sprinkle, C. L. (1974). A case of human strongyloidiasis apparently contracted from asymptomatic colony dogs. *Am. J. Trop. Med. Hyg.* **23,** 899–901.

Grove, D. A. (Ed.) (1989). *Strongyloidiasis, a Major Roundworm Infection of Man.* Taylor & Francis, London.

Hendrix, C. M., Blagburn, B. L., and Lindsay, D. S. (1987). Whipworms and intestinal threadworms. *Vet. Clin. North Am. Small Anim. Practice Parasitic Infect.* **17**(6), 1355–1375.

Little, M. D. (1966a). Comparative morphology of six species of *Strongyloides* (Nematoda) and redefinition of the genus. *J. Parasitol.* **52,** 69–84.

Little, M. D. (1966b). Seven new species of *Strongyloides* (Nematoda) from Louisiana. *J. Parasitol.* **52,** 85–97.

Rotman, H. L., Yutanawiboonchai, W., Brigandi, R. A., Leon, O., Nolan, T. J., Schad, G. A., and Abraham, D. (1995). *Strongyloides stercoralis*: Complete life cycle in SCID mice. *Exp. Parasitol.* **81,** 136–139.

Rotman, H. L., Schnyder-Candrian, S., Scott, P., Nolan, T. J., Schad, G. A., and Abraham, D. (1998). IL-12 eliminates the Th-2 dependent protective immune response of mice to larval *Strongyloides stercoralis. Parasite Immunol.* **19,** 29–39.

Schad, G. A., Aikens, L. M., and Smith, G. (1989). *Strongyloides stercoralis:* Is there a canonical migratory route through the host? *J. Parasitol.* **75,** 740–749.

Viney, M. E., Matthews, B. E., and Walliker, D. (1993). Mating in the nematode parasite *Strongyloides ratti*: Proof of genetic exchange. *Proc. R. Soc. London Ser. B Biol. Sci.* **254,** 213–219.

CHAPTER

27

Introduction to the Strongyles and the Hookworms

INTRODUCTION TO BURSATE NEMATODES

The unique characteristic of the members of the order Strongylida is the copulatory bursa at the posterior end of the males; it is composed of three groups of muscular rays (Fig. 27.3B, presented later): ventral, lateral, and dorsal (as shown from tbe top toward the bottom). Occasionally reference is made to a bursa in another order of nematodes, but the true copulatory bursa occurs only in the Strongylida. The bursate nematodes are generally small to medium sized, slender worms, ranging from about 2 mm to 20 mm long. Head structures range from almost none in the Trichostrongyloidea to elegant leaf crowns in the Strongyloidea and cutting plates in the Ancylostomatoidea.

The life cycles are all basically the same. With the exception of some of the Metastrongyloidea, they have direct life cycles. The eggs are passed with the feces in an early stage of embryonation (Fig. 27.5) and they develop on the ground through the L_1 and L_2 as feeding stages. When the L_2 molts to the L_3, it becomes an ensheathed, nonfeeding stage; the sheath is the cast cuticle of the L_2. Entrance into a host takes place by ingestion with contaminated food or water; the hookworms have the option of entering through the intact skin of the host. A few, such as the lungworms (s.l.), have true intermediate hosts in which development from the L_1 to the infective L_3 takes place.

THE HOOKWORMS—SUPERFAMILY ANCYLOSTOMATOIDEA

Hookworms form a fairly homogeneous group of strongyles in structure, life cycle, and epidemiology; they have large buccal capsules with cutting plates. The anterior portion of the worm is bent dorsally (Fig. 27.1) so that when one looks at the head, the dorsal teeth are at the bottom and the ventral teeth at the top (Fig. 27.2). The esophagus is strongly muscular in keeping with the food habits of pulling intestinal tissue into the buccal capsule and sucking blood. The copulatory bursa is well developed and the spicules are long and slender (Fig. 27.3). The term *hookworm* comes from the general body shape not the hooklike teeth.

The life cycles are quite similar. L_1 and L_2 are free-living, feeding stages and L_3 is the ensheathed, infective stage. Infection can take place either by mouth or by penetration of the unbroken skin. Worms penetrating the skin migrate through the bloodstream to the lungs, are coughed up, swallowed, and carried to the small intestine, where they mature. L_3s ingested with food or water usually remain in the gut and do not migrate through the body. The pattern of migration in the hookworms is similar to that of *Strongyloides* spp. (Chapter 26), and may be a more random than purposeful migration as well. The migration via the lungs does occur, but worms may reach the intestines by other routes as well.

As adults, hookworms are parasites of the small intestines of a wide range of mammals. The adults are bloodsuckers and they can remove prodigious amounts of blood from the host when worm populations are high and continuously present.

The distribution of hookworms is generally in warm, moist climates. Many of the hookworms of medical and medical veterinary medical importance are cosmopolitan in tropical and subtropical areas (Tab. 27.1); however, some have limited distribution and on occasion may be carried outside their limited range by being introduced into special niches such as mines.

There are perhaps ten hookworms of interest because of their importance in humans and domestic animals or because they demonstrate certain principles in parasitology (Tab. 27.1). Note, for example, that *An-*

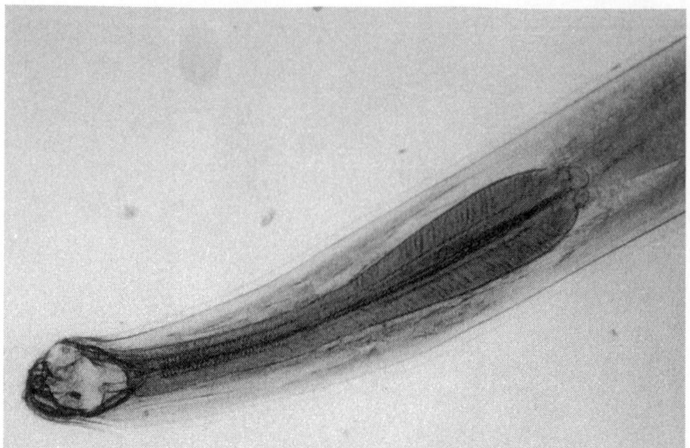

FIGURE 27.1 Anterior end of *Ancylostoma caninum* with characteristic dorsal bend of the head.

cylostoma caninum is found in warm climates, whereas *Uncinaria stenocephala* is found in colder climates. While both are parasites of dogs, the difference in distribution lies in the preferences of the free-living stages: *A. caninum* has its optimum development at about 30°C and *U. stenocephala* has its optimum at about 20°C. Therefore, *U. stenocephala* replaces *A. caninum* in the northern United States and in Canada.

U. lucasi of the northern fur seal is a pathogen of young fur seals in the Pribilof Islands of the Bering Sea just north of the Aleutian Islands of Alaska. These isolated, wind-swept islands are an inhospitable locale for a parasite we think of as being found in warm climates. Investigations of mortality showed that fur seal pups died of massive hookworm infection within the first few weeks of life. Initial research showed that contamination of the beach areas was not important for infection, but how the pups became infected was the puzzle. The landmark work of Olsen and Lyons (1965) revealed that the female seals were infected during summer and carried the larvae in their tissues for nearly a full year, passing them to their pups through the milk. Transmission in the milk also occurs in *A. caninum*, and there is some indication that human hookworms may also be passed in the milk.

In this chapter we consider only a few hookworms, but the principles apply to many other species in the group.

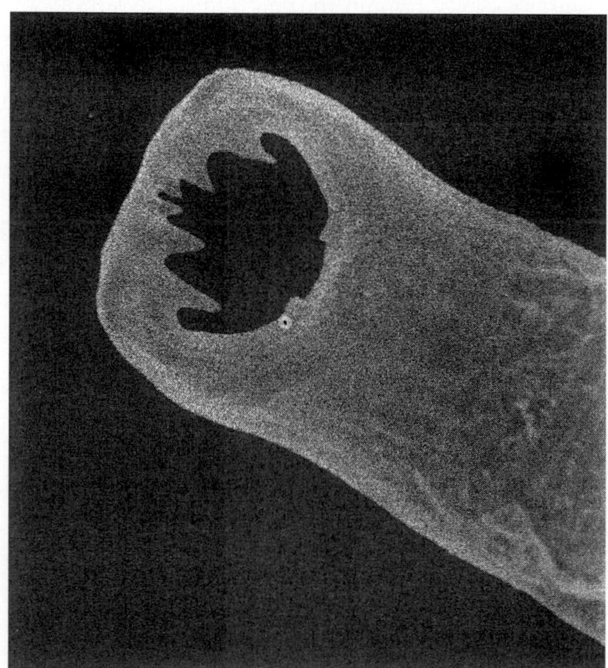

FIGURE 27.2 SEM of *Ancylostoma caninum* showing the large ventral teeth in the buccal capsule.

Name of Organism and Disease Associations

Ancylostoma caninum causes hookworm disease, ancylostomosis, ancylostomatosis, ancylostomiasis, and hookworm anemia. Additional species of hookworms are found in dogs (Tab. 27.1) but they are discussed here only incidentally.

Hosts and Host Range

A. caninum is found in a variety of canids and other carnivores; it is the more prevalent hookworm of dogs.

Geographic Distribution and Importance

Cosmopolitan in warm and temperate climates throughout the world; prevalence is high in warm climates, but infections are found in cold to temperate areas such as the northern United States and southern Canada. If we take some of the data for dogs in North America and arrange them from warm to cooler climates, we can see that the prevalence generally decreases toward the north:

Locality	Percentage Infection
Mexico	50–98
Hawaii	71
Georgia	86
Oklahoma	72
Kansas	21
New Jersey	22–27
Illinois	7
Quebec	9

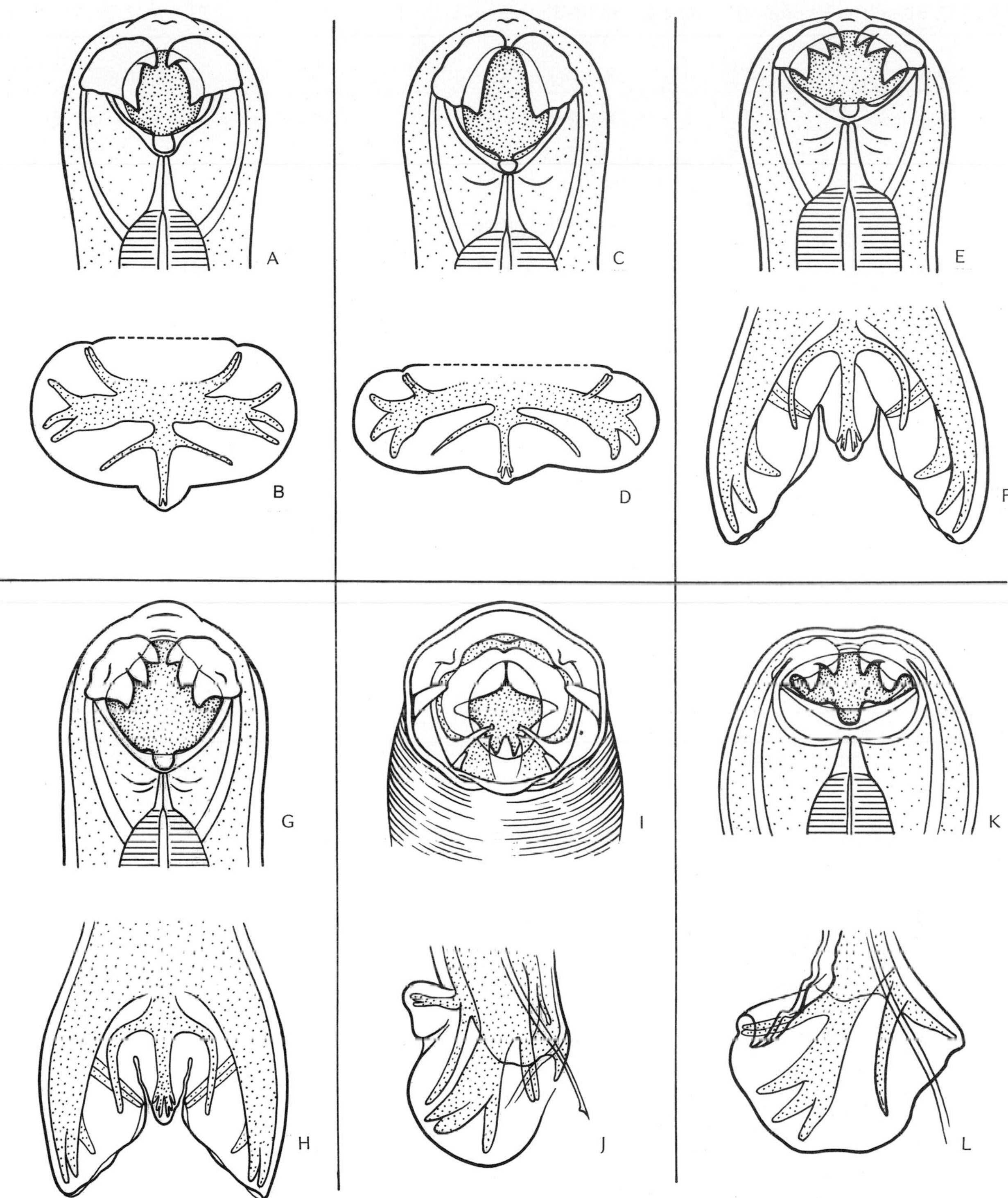

FIGURE 27.3 Hookworm male heads and bursae, respectively. (A and B) *Ancylostoma ceylanicum* (C and D) *Ancylostoma braziliense,* (E and F) *Ancylostoma caninum,* (G and H) *Ancylostoma tubaeforme,* (I. and J) *Necator americanus,* (K and L) *Ancylostoma duodenale.*

TABLE 27.1 Some Hookworms of Economic and Medical Importance

Name	Hosts	Geographic Distribution
Ancylostoma caninum	Canines and other carnivores	Cosmopolitan in warm and warm-temperate climates
A. ceylanicum	Humans, cats, dogs	Asia, South America
A. braziliense	Dogs, cats, and other carnivores	Africa, Central and South America, Gulf Coast of United States
A. duodenale	Humans and some other primates	Suptropical Europe, Asia, South America, Africa
A. tubaeforme	Cats	Cosmopolitan
Necator americanus	Humans	Tropical: United States, Central and South America, Africa, Orient, Australia
Uncinaria stenocephala	Dogs and other canines	Northern United States and Canada
U. lucasi	Fur seal	Bering Sea
Bunostomum trigonocephalum	Sheep, goats	Warm, moist climates
B. phlebotomum	Ox	Warm, moist climates
Gaigeria pachyscelis	Sheep	India, Africa

It is difficult to assess the importance of the infection of companion animals either in lost days at work or in production losses, as might be done with some other hosts such as humans or domesticated animals. However, animals become anemic and the consequences of infection can range from subclinical effects to death. There is also some hazard of skin infections in humans (see *Cutaneous Larva Migrans*).

Morphology

Male worms are 12 mm long by 0.36 mm wide and have a prominent buccal capsule and bursa. The female worms are 14 to 20 mm long by 0.5 mm wide and have a pointed tail. The buccal capsule has a pair of ventral teeth each with three points; these are usually spoken of as being three pairs of teeth (Fig. 27.3E); the dorsal teeth are within the buccal capsule. As noted in the introduction, the head of hookworms is bent dorsally and the arrangement of dorsal and ventral is reversed from what one usually expects. The large bursa is typical of the hookworms (Fig. 27.3F). A distinguishing feature is the structure of the dorsal ray; it can often be used in identifying hookworms to species. The spicules are long and slender, about 860 μm in length. The eggs average 62 x 39 μm (Fig. 27.5).

Life Cycle

Eggs are passed in the feces and reach the outside when the embryo is in an 8- or 16-cell stage. The L_1 hatches in about a day at 23°C; the L_3 is reached in four to five days at 23°C. Entrance into the host takes place by mouth or by penetration of the unbroken skin. If ingested, larvae may remain in the gut, but some migrate from gut to blood to lungs to trachea to esophagus and back to the small intestine the same pattern seen in those that enter the skin. The prepatent period is two to three weeks (Fig. 27.4).

In *A. caninum,* and some other hookworms, migrating L_3s within a pregnant bitch can traverse the placenta and infect fetuses in utero. Similarly, newborn pups can be infected as the L_3s make their way across the mammary glands and into the colostrum. It is not uncommon to see puppies suffering from acute, hookworm-induced anemia within the first few days of life as a result of transplacental and transmammary transmission of L_3s.

When adult worms are removed by, say, anthelmintic treatment, a reservoir of arrested L_3s migrate to the intestine and become mature. The exact mechanism of this populations modulation has not been described.

Diagnosis

The usual method of determining whether an animal is infected is finding typical eggs in the feces (Fig. 27.5). In areas where hookworm is a continuing problem, it should be suspected when an animal becomes listless, has a rough hair coat, and has pale mucus membranes indicating anemia.

Some of these clinical signs can be seen in other infectious diseases such as tapeworms or heavy loads of ascarids or inadequate diet. Therefore, a fecal examination is important to ensure a proper diagnosis.

Host–Parasite Interactions

Damage to the host involves the following:

1. The site of larval penetration

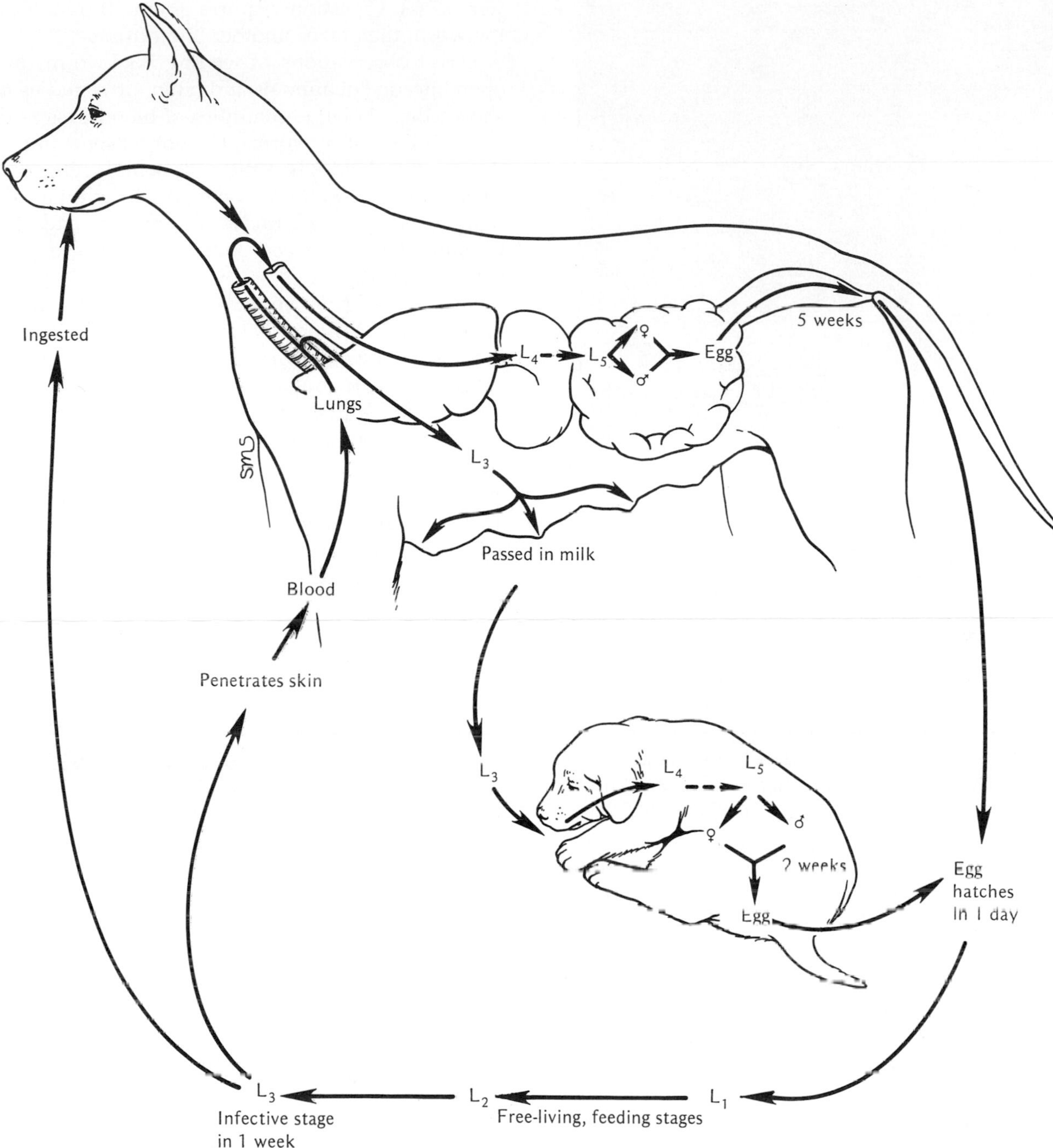

FIGURE 27.4 Life cycle of *Ancylostoma caninum* showing infection routes either by mouth or percutaneously. Newborn puppies are infected when the arrested L_3s become active and are passed in the milk.

2. Larval migration
3. The intestine
4. Extraintestinal sites

The L_3s are about 730 by 22 μm and enter the unbroken skin of the host through hair follicles, sebacous ducts, or sweat glands to reach the dermis and enter the lymphatic system. The mechanism of penetration is most likely facilitated by the secretion of a protease as has also been described for other skin-penetrating helminths. A zinc metalloprotease has been demonstrated in larvae, which were activated to move from a preparasitic to a parasitic status. Furthermore, a protein with homology to the venom allergens of hyme-

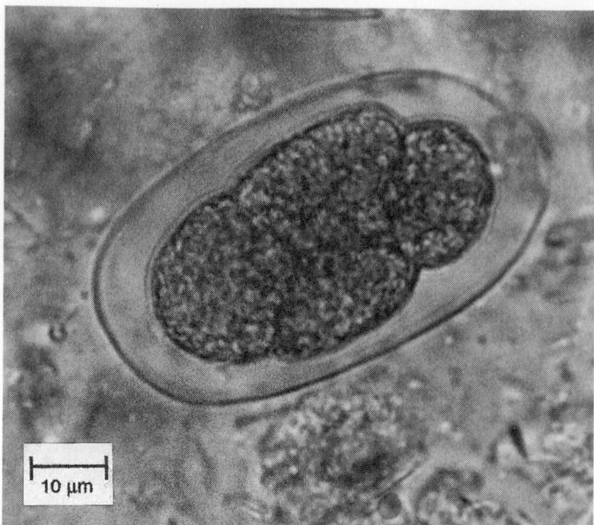

FIGURE 27.5 *Ancylostoma caninum* egg in an 8-cell stage as passed in the feces.

nopterans has been shown to be developmentally regulated and associated with the induction of the parasitic phase of the life cycle.

The larvae shed the L_2 sheath, move down the follicle or duct, and exit near the basement membrane in the dermis. In the normal host, they soon reach the circulatory system and are carried to the lungs. There is some damage to the skin where each larva enters; the greater the number of larvae, the greater the damage. Most often penetration takes place between the footpads where the skin is thin. An inflammatory response to the migrating larvae is the result. This tissue destruction is frequently exacerbated in individuals with specific immunologic hypersensitivities. In an abnormal host, such as humans, hookworm larvae may remain in the subcutaneous tissue and migrate there for some weeks (see *Cutaneous Larva Migrans*).

During migration, the principal site of damage is the lungs, where larvae break out of the capillaries into the alveoli. There may be pneumonia and coughing at this time.

In the intestine, the worms molt from L_4 to L_5 and begin to attack the intestinal mucosa. Although there is damage to the intestinal wall, diarrhea is seldom seen in hookworm infections; usually the stools are normal but may be black because of hemoglobin in them. Diarrhea can be seen when an animal is so heavily parasitized that it is near death.

Hookworms do suck blood, but strong evidence indicates that the worms feed principally on intestinal tissue. When worms feed, they pull a plug of intestinal mucosa into the buccal capsule by esophageal action (Fig. 27.6.). Digestion requires about 10 minutes and the worm then takes another bite of tissue.

Direct observations of feeding hookworms in the open intestine of animals and on in vitro studies have shown that (1) large quantities of blood pass rapidly through the gut of worms, (2) worms spew out large volumes of blood when the body wall is nipped with an instrument, (3) there is continual pumping of the esophagus of worms under observation, and (4) the intestine fails to bleed extensively where worms have detached.

Worms feed from about six different sites during a 24-hour period. Blood is lost when the capillary bed in the subepithelial layer is ruptured; blood flows out around the worm but a significant amount is ingested. The intestine quickly repairs itself and no permanent scars remain. *Ancylostoma*-specific anticoagulants have been molecularly characterized and the corresponding genes have been cloned. A factor in the blood is required for glycogenesis in the worms, so at least one substance is removed from the blood.

A high proportion of the blood that has passed through the worms is digested and recycled by the host. The important point is not how much blood leaks

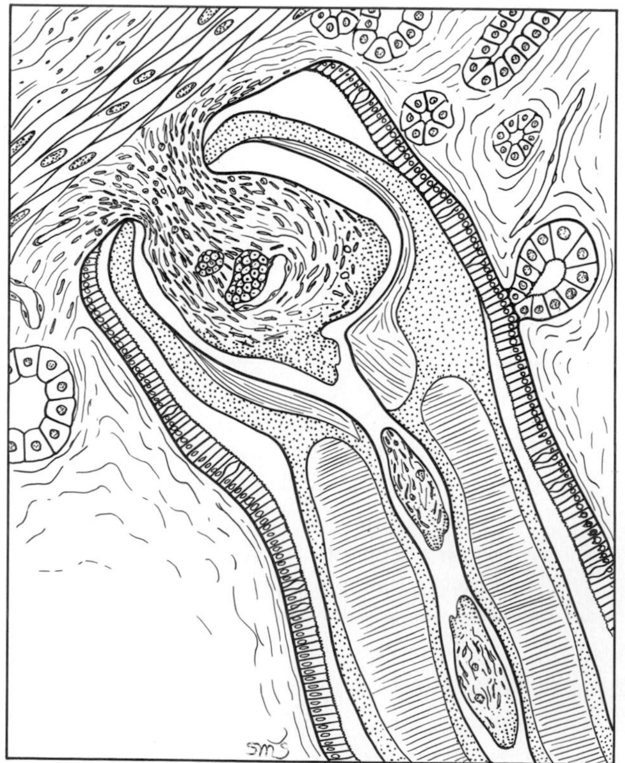

FIGURE 27.6 Sagittal section of a hookworm feeding in the intestine of the host. The worm takes in a mouthful of intestinal mucosa, pinches it off, and swallows it, all through the muscular action of the esophagus.

from the intestine into the lumen, but rather how much is ultimately lost. It can be seen (Tab. 27.2) that a huge volume of blood could be lost per year even under a moderate level of parasitism.

Obviously, the calculated blood loss is not realized, or animals could not survive even a moderate infection. The crux of blood loss lies in iron loss, as discussed later in connection with hookworm infections in humans.

Animals that have been repeatedly infected develop immunity; this observation was used to develop an irradiated larval vaccine against *A. caninum*. A series of studies growing out of the work on lungworm disease in cattle (Chapter 31) showed that vaccination against hookworms was feasible.

A hookworm vaccine was briefly marketed in the United States. Dogs were protected against clinical hookworm disease but nevertheless had adult hookworms in the intestines. The problems to be overcome for the commercial success of the vaccine were partly biological, partly economic. A number of hurdles had to be cleared before a product could be made available to veterinarians for use. For example, federal standards for biologics require near sterility, and the fecal culture method of producing L_3s led to so much contamination with bacteria that a sterile culture technique had to be developed. The more laborious procedures for sterile culture of the free-living stages had an advantage in there being less damage to the L_3s at harvest and a longer shelf life for the vaccine. Once the larvae had been irradiated, storage temperature had to be controlled at between 10 and 15°C for a maximum shelf life of 12 to 14 months. Temperatures as low as 4°C and as high as 20°C could be tolerated only briefly. Thus, special shipping containers had to be developed as well as special incubators to be placed in the veterinarian's refrigerator (normally set at 4–6°C).

After the biological problems of production, storage, and adverse vaccine reactions were overcome, the vaccine did not sell well. Part of the problem was a matter of education and part was economics. The vaccine did not produce a sterile immunity. In any event, the vaccine was withdrawn from the market in 1975 after about two years of poor sales.

TABLE 27.2 Potential Blood Loss in Hookworm Infections

Number of Worms/Lb of Body Weight	Total Number of Worms	Ml of Blood Loss/Worm/Day	Calculated Loss/Year/ 100 Worms
8–27	240–294	0.07–0.29	2.5–7.3 liters
30–64	371–972	0.01–0.09	0.36–3.31 liters

Work on the development of a useful vaccine continues. Laboratories on different continents are using techniques of antigen discovery and molecular cloning with the goal of producing a vaccine.

Epidemiology and Control

Control of hookworm disease in companion animals is based on the following:

1. Therapeutic treatment
2. Keeping animals in a clean environment
3. Surveillance by periodic fecal analysis
4. Prophylactic treatment

A number of drugs are on the market that have a high degree of efficacy, but treatment should not be given until a proper diagnosis has been made. Effective anthelmintics such as pyrantel pamoate are used both for treatment of clinical infection and as a monthly preventive in combination with other compounds such as ivermectin. These combination treatments or other single compounds such as milbemycin oxime are used once a month for the prevention of clinical levels of infection with hookworms as well as ascarids (Chapter 32) and heartworm (Chapter 34).

The development, survival, and migration of the infective stage of hookworms are crucial in the epidemiology of the infection. Adding to the complex is egg production of female worms. Hookworms produce relatively high numbers of eggs, considering their size, and they may live for more than a year. Animals may be exposed to large numbers of L_3s where there are moderate temperatures, moisture, and protection from sunlight. *A. caninum* L_3 is reached in the following time periods at various temperatures:

Temperature (°C)	Time in Days
37	2
30	2.6
23	4.5
17	9
15	22

The L_3s can live for many weeks where conditions are moist, the temperature is 20°C or lower, and there is protection from direct sunlight. Conditions detrimental to the free-living stages of *A. caninum* are temperatures below freezing and above 37°C, drying, and exposure to sunlight. The L_3s of *U. stenocephala* survive freezing better than those of *A. caninum*, and their optimal temperature of development is lower, in keeping with its location in the northern United States and Canada.

As indicated (Tab. 27.1), hookworms are more prevalent in climates that are warm and moist than in those that are cold (*U. stenocephala* excepted), dry, or both. Thus, problems are likely to be more severe in tropical and subtropical regions than in others. Untreated infections can last in a host for more than a year and contamination with L3s can build up rapidly in the summer almost anywhere.

As with the case of other strongyles, the L_3s of hookworms tend to migrate from their sites of development in the feces. This helps to place them in areas where they can more easily survive and readily reach a new host.

Companion animals allowed to roam will almost certainly become infected with hookworms in an enzootic area. Likewise, animals in kennels that lack hygienic conditions can become heavily infected.

Of these means of control, providing a clean environment is easiest with companion animals that are restricted to a fenced yard or run. Once treated and kept in clean quarters, animals do not usually build dangerously high levels of infection. They can be examined periodically and treated as needed. Animals that are allowed to roam inevitably become infected. Surveillance and regular preventive treatment are essential during summer and in warm climates.

If dogs are kept in kennels for either boarding or breeding, hookworm disease (as well as other helminthic and infectious diseases) can become severe. Kennel floors should be made of concrete or well-drained gravel; soil is unsatisfactory. Dog runs should be sloped in such a way that they will drain and be exposed to the sun for a part of the day. Cleaning by hosing with water should be done daily so that as few as possible of the free-living stages remain in the area. When control has been achieved, any animals introduced should be quarantined, examined, and treated as necessary.

Name of Organism and Disease Associations

Ancylostoma duodenale Necator americanus and *A. ceylanicum* cause hookworm disease, hookworm anemia, and ancyclostomosis.

Hosts and Host Range

A. duodenale and *N. americanus* are the principal hookworms that infect humans. Following early migration, they are found in the small intestinal lumen. Hookworms sometimes mature in abnormal hosts, and hosts other than the principal ones can be infected with human hookworms.

Geographic Distribution and Importance

Human hookworm is endemic in warm, wet climates (Tab. 27.1), but each species has some limitation on its distribution. Also, in some locations, such as in coal mines in central Europe, the distribution may either be extended or found in small pockets.

Estimates of the prevalence of infection in the human population range from 450 million to 900 million persons worldwide. In his often quoted 1947 article titled, "This Wormy World," Norman Stoll compiled data indicating that 457 million people were infected worldwide. Thus, there is an increase in the number of infected people compared to 50 years ago. Since that time, the global population has about doubled, so there is small consolation that the per capita prevalence of infection has remained about the same.

Because hookworm infection occurs in the poorest parts of the world, it interacts with other factors to impose a significant drain on the health of people. Inadequate diet and continual blood loss sap their strength and sense of well being. Other helminthic and protozoan infections are common in warm climates, so that any one person is almost certain to harbor at least one pathogenic parasite, and many have several. So-called polyparasitism makes for health problems that are difficult to sort out and alleviate.

Hookworm disease was found to be a significant cause of ill health in the southeastern United States at the early part of the 20th century. Fundamental studies on hookworms supported by the Rockefeller Foundation and the control programs that were instituted resulted in a decline of infection from 4.5 million persons in 1910 to 1.75 million in 1935. However, there are still pockets of relatively high infection in the United States where 12 to 15% of children have been found to be infected. Current data are rather scattered, but there was been a decline in the Southeast from 42% to perhaps 4% in prevalence from early in this century to mid-century.

Morphology

In general size, the two principal human hookworms are similar but can be differentiated statistically:

	A. duodenale	*N. americanus*
Male	8–11 × 0.45 mm	6–9 × 0.3 mm
Spicules	2000 μm	900–1000 μm
Female	10–18 × 0.6 μm	9–11 × 0.35 μm
Eggs	40 × 60 μm	30–40 × 60–76 μm

The two can readily be differentiated by examining the ventral teeth (Fig. 27.3 I, K), but differentiation from other closely related species may be difficult. *A. duodenale* needs to be differentiated from *A. ceylanicum*, and the similar *A. braziliense*. These two latter species have been confused for some time and reports of *A. braziliense* in humans may be erroneous in some instances.

N. americanus is the only member of this genus that has been reported from humans, but there are some similar species such as *N. suillus* from swine that are found in the same geographic areas.

Life Cycle

Similar to that of *A. caninum*.

Diagnosis

The principal means of determining whether a person is infected with hookworms is by examining the feces for characteristic eggs. The technique most often used is a flotation method, but sedimentation can also be used.

In some instances, it is important to determine the level of infection in an individual or a community, and quantitative egg counts can provide useful information. Taking a number of studies into account, "light" infections are represented by egg counts up to about 2000 eggs/g of feces. Above 2000 eggs/g infections are considered to be "heavy." There is often a direct correlation between the number of worms and the number of eggs per gram of feces; there is also a direct correlation between the number of worms and the severity of anemia. Neither correlation is necessarily linear, but the number of eggs per gram of feces can be used as a guide to possible clinical disease.

The clinical sign of anemia coupled with fatigue are suggestive of hookworm infection in an endemic area. Diarrhea is not a sign of hookworm disease in humans.

Host–Parasite Interactions

The ways in which hookworms cause damage to their human hosts may be described as follows:

1. *Primary*, in which the signs and symptoms are directly related to the worms:
   a. Skin penetration
   b. Migration through the lungs and pharyngeal regions
   c. Presence of worms in the small intestine, where they cause direct effects
   d. Inflammation of somatic muscles in which larvae may be held in a state of arrest
2. *Secondary*, in which disturbances of the physiology and/or blood of the host result from chronic infection.

Penetration of the skin causes a slight lesion at the site, which may cause no more than an itching or prickling sensation; however, upon subsequent infection there is likely to be a more severe reaction due to hypersensitivity.

As the worms break into the alveoli of the lungs and migrate anteriorly, there may be some chest pain and inflammation of the pulmonary and pharyngeal tissues.

When the worms reach the small intestine, abdominal pain occurs, among other gastrointestinal signs and symptoms.

The most significant aspect of hookworm infection is anemia as a result of long-standing infection. The severity of hookworm anemia is related most directly to the number of worms and the nutritional status of the person. In general, anemia results from depletion of iron stores and the inability of the person to maintain a normal amount of hemoglobin.

Removal of blood by human hookworm can be calculated as follows:

Species	Blood Loss	
	ml/worm/day	ml/100 worms/year
N. americanus	0.01–0.04	365–1,460
A. duodenale	0.05–0.3	1,825–10,950

One hundred worms is not generally considered to be a severe infection despite what appears to be dramatic loss of blood. At some level, this blood is recycled, as described earlier. In addition, a well nourished host is capable of compensating for blood loss through ongoing synthesis. The more anterior the site of the worms in the small intestine, the greater the recycling; if the worms lie in the lower part of the small intestine, there are greater real losses.

An inexorable loss of iron depletes iron stores so that eventually there is insufficient iron to make hemoglobin (Fig. 27.7). The normal amount of hemoglobin (15 g/100 ml of blood) is maintained until iron reserves have been depleted; then there is a decline in hemoglobin to a point where the individual stabilizes at about 50% of normal hemoglobin. A person with such anemia lacks energy and frequently demonstrates pale mucous membranes.

There are other factors contributing to hookworm disease, but they are beyond the scope of this discussion.

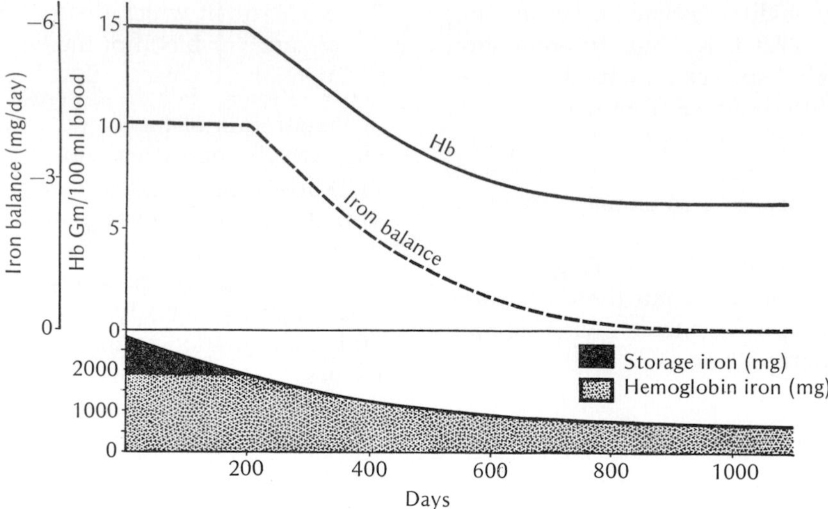

FIGURE 27.7 Iron depletion and the development of hookworm anemia in humans. When stored iron is depleted, the ability of the host to make hemoglobin is reduced to that available in the diet. [Redrawn from Roche and Layrisse, 1966.]

As discussed in the section on *A. caninum*, a high level of protective immunity can be developed in the dog; however, there is no conclusive evidence for protective immunity in humans. A considerable body of circumstantial evidence points to there being a protective immunity. The evidence suggesting a protective immunity is based on the following:

1. Epidemiologic studies
2. Observations after treatment
3. Comparison to infections in other hosts such as dogs

The epidemiologic pattern of hookworm infection in the human population is an increasing prevalence of infection up to about age 10 years and then a leveling off or decline until age 30 or 40 years; finally, there may be an increase in prevalence in elderly people. The pattern of acquisition and maintenance of worm infection is the same in dogs and people; therefore, it can be postulated that, like dogs, humans appear to develop immunity upon repeated or prolonged exposure to infective larvae. Following treatment, adults tend to have relatively low worm burdens, but children under 10 years of age reacquire high levels of infection.

Because there is good immunity, the issue of developing a vaccine should be addressed. With the constant drain on the health of as many as 900 million infected persons around the world, a hookworm vaccine would be a great benefit to those countries where the prevalence is high. Studies in dogs have laid a groundwork that perhaps can be transferred to humans.

The prepatent period in hookworm infections is generally 20 to 50 days, depending on the species, and it generally has been held that once they have entered a host, the worms develop inexorably toward sexual maturity. However, it has been shown that development may not proceed until some months later. When *A. duodenale* infects a host, sexual maturity can be delayed as long as 40 weeks after infection, nearly six times the usual period. This work was done in the region of Calcutta, India, where there is a rainy season followed by a long, hot, dry season. Persons who become infected during the wet season harbor preadult worms all through the dry season; egg production commences shortly before the rains begin. It is not known whether the long prepatent period is inherent in the worms or whether they somehow sense seasonal change from inside the host and then commence reproduction. Whatever the mechanism, the worms have been selected so that they do not jeopardize their resources until there is a high probability that the life cycle will be completed. This phenomenon of delayed or arrested development or hypobiosis has long been known in trichostrongyles of domestic ruminants (Chapter 30), but this was the first clear-cut instance of arrested development in a nematode parasite of humans.

Epidemiology and Control

A total campaign against hookworm disease requires the following:

1. Mass chemotherapy

2. Sanitary disposal of human waste
3. Wearing shoes
4. Administration of iron salts
5. Ensuring adequate dietary protein

A number of highly effective anthelmintics are available for use in humans, including piperazine and benzimidazoles. Treatments are generally well tolerated and can be used in mass treatment programs.

Transmission of hookworm in the human population and the development of disease are dependent on a combination of the following biological and climatic factors and human culture:

1. Egg production of the female worms
2. Longevity of adult worms
3. Development and survival of the free-living stages as related to weather and climate
4. Immunity of the definitive hosts
5. Nutritional level of the human population
6. Technological and economic level of the area

The potential contamination with the free-living stages of hookworms is truly great. *A. duodenale* produces 10,000 to 30,000 eggs/female/day and *N. americanus* produces 5000 to 10,000 eggs/female/day. In areas where hookworm is endemic, egg counts of 2000 eggs/g of feces are common. An adult human produces perhaps 100 g of feces in a day, so that one person might contaminate the area with 200,000 eggs every day. In rural Venezuela about 7% of the population had eggs in excess of 2000 eggs/g of feces. A few persons in a population may produce 15,000 eggs/g of feces. Since worms may live in the host for as long as a year, the potential contamination of soil is horrendous.

Moderate temperatures of about 15 to 35°C, adequate oxygen, and some moisture promote the devel opment and survival of hookworm free-living stages. Sandy or sandy-loam soils allow good survival of infective larvae.

Freezing, high temperatures (above 37°C), drying, and exposure to sunlight are all detrimental to the survival of the free-living stages. When exposed to any one of these conditions, larvae die within a few days.

Hookworm free-living stages are similar to other strongyles in their pattern of development and behavior. The L_1s and L_2s remain in feces, where they feed, grow, and molt. The L_3s tend to migrate and move out of the feces. They move toward subdued light and require a film of moisture in which to move. If there is minimal moisture, a larva may carry along the droplet of water surrounding it and be held to it by surface tension.

Dispersal of feces deposited on the ground takes place through a combination of weather and microbial and invertebrate animal activity. Invertebrates are the most important in the early dispersal of feces and in warm climates; beetles seem to be the principal agents that break up and carry feces away. In the southern United States, for example, dung beetles (family Scarabeidae) and burying beetles (family Silphidae) can remove the feces of a family of four to six persons during the warm part of the year. It is still not clear whether the beetles are detrimental or beneficial to the development and survival of hookworm free-living stages.

A concern in the disposal of fecal material lies in the use of some of the macrolide antibiotics (e.g., ivermectin) used as anthelmintics. These compounds are also used as insecticides and may have a detrimental effect on dung beetles. In warm climates, the principal biological dispersal agent might be removed from the ecosystem. This was also observed in livestock fed juvenile hormone analogs such as methoprene; their feces failed to break down except through weathering.

During the middle part of the 19th century anemia in coal miners was recognized. Investigations by Italian parasitologists, in the main, showed that people working in mines suffered from hookworm anemia. Working conditions in mines in the 19th century were unbelievably bad, and sanitation was poor. People sometimes worked only partly clothed in cramped, hot, humid, dark mines. If people defecated in the mines, someone was likely to come along later and be exposed to the infective larvae. This example, however dated, underscores the fact that special conditions lead to infections with hookworm where they would not ordinarily be expected.

Hookworm disease and the prevalence of infection are greatest in the less developed countries of the world, especially those with warm climates. Where there is little sanitary disposal of human waste, subsistence farming, and too little money for the purchase of shoes, hookworms are prevalent.

We tend to think of sanitary disposal of human waste as a panacea for control of intestinal infections, but as was shown 60 years ago, nearly complete disposal is needed before there is significant reduction in transmission of hookworms. This does not mean that the attempt should not be made, but it should be recognized that success in a control campaign may come slowly.

Oddly enough, help sometimes comes from unexpected sources. Hookworm infection in Egypt has declined because of the availability of inexpensive plastic shoes. The protection that these shoes provide seems to have reduced the prevalence of hookworm infection. Merely running an educational campaign on the importance of wearing shoes would probably have had little impact, but the availability of inexpensive, comfortable shoes has helped to reduce the prevalence of infection.

Related Organisms

A common hookworm of the cat and bobcat is *A. tubaeforme,* which has about the same geographic distribution as *A. caninum*. Mice can serve as paratenic hosts; larvae administered to mice accumulate in the lungs and remain viable for months. When an infected mouse is eaten by a cat, the worms continue their migration and mature in the small intestine.

Hookworms are common in ruminants in warm, wet climates. *Bunostomum phlebotomum* is a parasite of the ox and zebu while *B. trogonocephalum* is found in sheep and goats. *Gaigeria pachyscelsis* has been reported from a number of species of domestic and wild ruminants in Africa and India. *Globocephalus urosubulatus* is found in pigs in many parts of the world.

CUTANEOUS LARVA MIGRANS

Human skin may be invaded by a number of species of nematode larvae with the result that skin lesions develop at the site of entry. The larvae remain in the skin and cause inflammation, which may last for a few weeks. The pattern is typical for a number of helminth parasites that may invade a foreign host: the normal migration is altered.

The principal hookworms causing cutaneous larva migrans are *A. braziliense, Uncinaria stenocephala,* and *Bunostomum phlebotomum*; *A. caninum* and *A. ceylanicum* play only minor roles. The rhabditoid nematode, *Strongyloides papillosus,* also causes skin lesions in humans (Chapter 26).

In addition to the technical term *cutaneous larva migrans,* the disease is also referred to as *larva currens, plumber's itch, ground itch,* and *creeping eruption.*

The common names for the disease are descriptive not only of the conditions under which a person may become infected but also of the appearance of the skin. The larvae penetrate the skin, sometimes remaining in place, but often wandering in the skin, causing inflamed, sinuous tracks. Repeated infections may give rise to a more severe reaction at the site of entry indicating the development of hypersensitivity.

Readings

Ball, P. A. J. (1966). The relationship of host to parasite in human hookworm infection. In *The Pathology of Parasitic Diseases* (A. E. R. Taylor, Ed.), pp. 41–48. Blackwell, Oxford.

Behnke, J. M. (1987). Do hookworms elicit protective immunity? *Parasitol. Today* **3,** 200–206.

Booth, M., and Bundy, D. A. P. (1992). Comparative prevalences of *Ascaris lumbricoides, Trichuris trichiura,* and hookworm infections and the prospects for combined control. *Parasitology* **105,** 151–157.

Croll, N. A., Matthews, B. E., and Smith, J. M. (1975). Hookworm behaviour: Larval movement patterns after entering hosts. *Int. J. Parasitol.* **5,** 551–556.

Crompton, D. W. T. (1989). Hookworm disease: Current status and new directions. *Parasitol. Today* **5,** 1–2.

Gilles, H. M., and Ball, P. A. J. (1991). *Hookworm Infections.* Elsevier, New York.

Hawdon, J. M., Volk, S. W., Rose, R., Pritchard, D. I., Behnke, J. M., and Schad, G. A. (1993). Observations on the feeding behavior of parasitic third-stage hookworm larvae. *Parasitology* **106,** 163–169.

Hawdon, J. M., Jones, B. F., Hoffman, D. R., and Hotez, P. J. (1996). Cloning and characterization of *Ancylostoma*-secreted protein. *J. Biol. Chem.* **217,** 6672–6678.

Kalkofen, U. P. (1987). Hookworms of dogs and cats. *Vet. Clin. North Am. Small Anim. Practice Parasitic Infect.* **17**(6), 1341–1354.

Loukos, A., Opdebeeck, J., Croese, J., and Prociv, P. (1994). Immunologic incrimination of *Ancylostoma caninum* as a human enteric pathogen. *Am. J. Trop. Med. Hyg.* **50,** 69–77.

Miller, T. A. (1971). Vaccination against canine hookworm diseases. *Adv. Parasitol.* **9,** 153–183.

Miller, T. A. (1978). Industrial development and field use of the canine hookworm vaccine. *Adv. Parasitol.* **16,** 333–342.

Miller, T. A. (1979). Hookworm infection in man. *Adv. Parasitol.* **17,** 315–384.

Nawalinski, T. A., and Schad, G. A. (1974). Arrested development in *Ancylostoma duodenale*: Course of a self-induced infection in man. *Am. J. Trop. Med. Hyg.* **23,** 895–898.

Olsen, O. W., and Lyons, E. T. (1965). Life cycle of *Uncinaria lucasi* Stiles, 1901 (Nematoda: Ancylostomatidae) of fur seals, *Callorhinus ursinus* Linn. on the Pribilof Islands. *J. Parasitol.* **51,** 689–700.

Pritchard, D. I., McKean, P. G., and Schad, G. A. (1990). An immunological and biochemical comparison of hookworm species. *Parasitol. Today* **6,** 154–156.

Roche, M., and Layrisse, M. (1966). The nature and causes of hookworm anemia. *Am. J. Trop. Med. Hyg.* **15,** 1031–1102.

Schad, G. A. (1994). Hookworms: Pets to humans. *Ann. Intern. Med.* **120,** 434–435.

Schad, G. A., Chowdhury, A. G., Dean, C. G., Kochar, V. K., Nawalinski, T. A., Thomas, J., and Tonascia, J. A. (1973). Arrested development in human hookworm infections: An adaptation to a seasonally unfavorable external environment. *Science* **180,** 502–504.

Schad, G. A., and Warren, K. S. (Eds.) (1990). *Hookworm Disease, Current Status and New Directions.* Taylor & Francis, London.

Stanssens, P., Bergum, P. W., *et al.* (1996). Anticoagulant repertoire of the hookworm *Ancylostoma caninum. Proc. Natl. Acad. Sci. USA* **93,** 2149–2154.

CHAPTER

28

Strongyles of Horses

As with other grazing animals, horses acquire gastrointestinal nematodes on pasture starting when they begin to take some grass but are still taking milk from the dam. Under circumstances in which animals are crowded on lush pastures, the populations of worms can become high and cause both illness and death. In many geographic areas, it is a constant battle to keep worms at an acceptable level.

The control of nematodes in horses presents some interesting problems because of peculiarities of pathogenesis in different species, different times of acquisition of other species, and interactions among populations of parasites.

The worms that are of greatest concern in horses are the so-called strongyles, members of the superfamily Strongyloidea, family Strongylidae; they usually are separated into two groups, the large strongyles and the small strongyles. The large strongyles are *Strongylus vulgaris*, *S. equinus*, and *S. edentatus*, which range in size from 15 to 45 mm in length. The small strongyles, also frequently called "cyathostomes," encompass 16 genera and about twice that many species; most of them fall within a size range of 10 to 20 mm in length. Other nematodes of importance in horses are *Parascaris equorum* (syn. *Ascaris equorum*) (Chapter 32) and the pinworm, *Oxyuris equi* (Chapter 33). The larval forms of *Gasterophilus intestinalis* and *G. nasalis* (Insecta, Diptera, Gasterophilidae) (Chapter 49), usually called bots, are also intestinal parasites and are often treated at the same time as nematodes.

THE LARGE STRONGYLES

Name of Organism and Disease Associations

Strongylus vulgaris, *S. equinus*, and *S. edentatus* are large strongyles or palisade worms that cause helminthosis, strongylosis, and colic.

Hosts and Host Range

Equids in general are the hosts. Although the emphasis here is on the horse, these parasites are found in the ass, zebra, mule, and other members of the family as well. The adults are in the lumen of the cecum and colon. Preadults are in the tissues of the gut or in other locations such as the mesenteric arteries, liver, and pancreas, depending on the species (see Life Cycle).

Geographic Distribution and Importance

Large strongyles are cosmopolitan in distribution. *Strongylus* spp. cause the greatest losses from helminths in horses; *S. vulgaris* is the most important of the three. The prevalence of infection with one or more of these worms approaches 100% in foals, but the pathogenesis seen in any one host is directly related to the intensity of infection.

The dollar losses from morbidity and mortality with large and small strongyles could be estimated to exceed $10 million (U.S.) per year. However, these costs pale in view of the costs associated with anthelmintic and veterinary care, which exceed $100 million per year.

Morphology

As members of the Strongylidae, the large strongyles have a large, almost globular buccal capsule and a modification of the lips into a comblike structure called a *leaf crown* or *corona radiata*. These species have both an external leaf crown at the anterior tip of the body and an internal leaf crown just posterior to the external one and quite a bit smaller (Fig. 28.1).

S. vulgaris. Males are 0.75 to 0.95 by 11 to 16 mm.
Females are 1 to 1.4 by 20 to 25 mm.

S. equinus. Males are 1.1 to 1.3 by 26 to 35 mm.
Females are 1.8 to 2.3 by 38 to 55 mm.

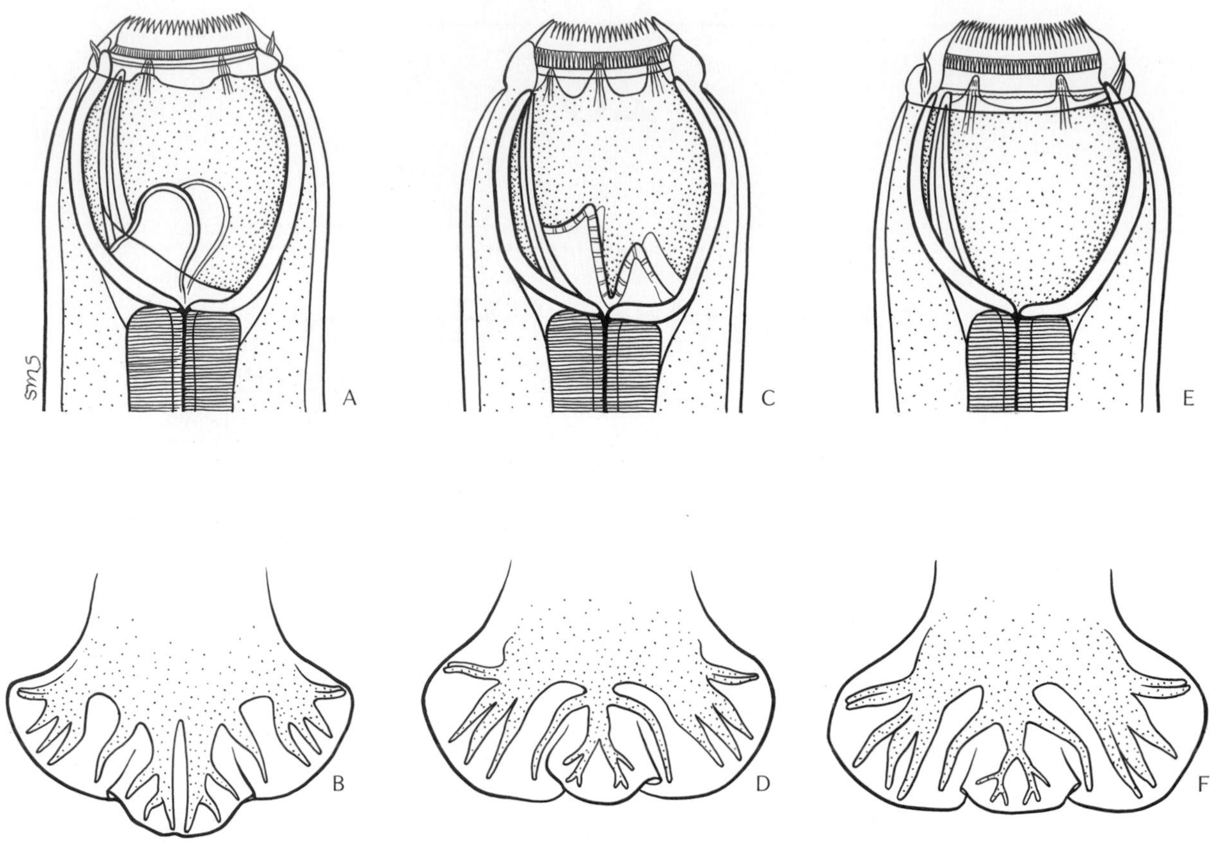

FIGURE 28.1 Heads and bursae of the large strongyles of horses. (A and B) *Strongylus vulgaris;* (C and D) *S. equinus;* (E and F) *S. edentatus.*

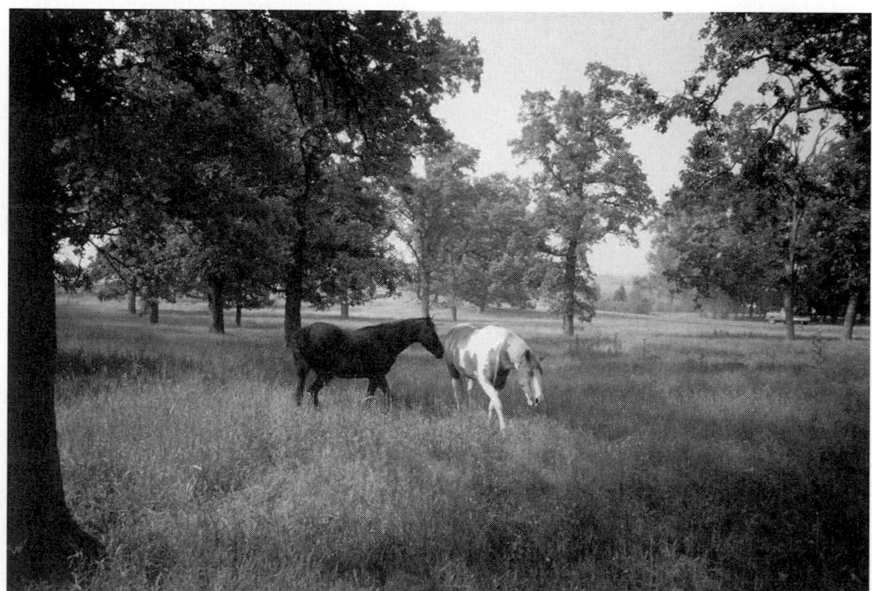

FIGURE 28.2 Horses on pasture in Wisconsin. A habitat where transmission of gastrointestinal nematodes would readily take place. The grass is lush, and the pasture is shaded; moisture is retained, and the free-living stages of nematodes are not exposed to the heat of the sun.

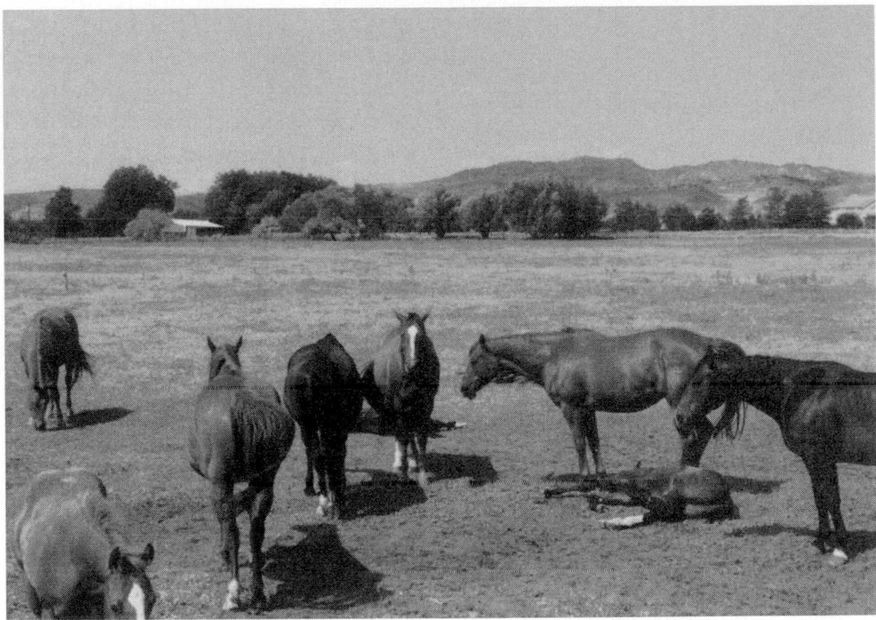

FIGURE 28.3 Horses on pasture in the semi-arid portion of the western United States. Precipitation in this area is less than 45 cm. Forage is rather sparse; sunlight reaches the ground causing drying and heating of the soil.

S. edentatus. Males are 1.3 to 1.5 by 23 to 28 mm.
Females are 1.6 to 2.2 by 33 to 44 mm.

The worms are usually differentiated from one another by the head structures, but there are differences in the male copulatory structures as well (Figs. 28.1B, D, and F).

Life Cycle

The eggs pass with the feces in about a 16-cell stage and hatch within a day or two, releasing the L_1. The ensheathed L_3 can be reached in two to three days at 35°C, but usually requires a week or two at lower temperatures. The L_3 is ingested with forage or water. After being ingested, the L_3 enters the wall of the intestine, but each of the three species of large strongyles has a different site of development in the host from this point on.

S. vulgaris. The larvae most likely migrate from the intestinal tissue to arterioles in the gut and then move upstream through the lining, or intima, of the arterioles to the mesenteric artery; they migrate in the arterial walls for two to four months and then move downstream to the colon. They enter the lumen, complete development to maturity, and begin to lay eggs. The prepatent period is about six months.

S. equinus. The larvae migrate into the wall of the gut until they lie under the serosa or outer layer, where they grow and molt. After several days they leave the nodules and migrate to the liver, then the pancreas or the peritoneal cavity. They mature to the adult stage penetrate the wall of the large intestine and, upon reentry to the gut, begin reproduction. The prepatent period of *S. equinus* is about nine months.

S. edentatus. After burrowing through the wall of the intestine, the L_3s of *S. edentatus* migrate to the liver via the portal veins. They molt, grow, and migrate to the liver where they remain for about two months. They then leave the liver, migrate to the peritoneal cavity, and eventually return to the wall of the intestine. They penetrate the wall of the intestine, mature, and begin reproduction. The prepatent period for *S. edentatus* varies from six to eleven months, no doubt due to the variable lengths of time that the immature parasites spend in migration.

Diagnosis

The following should be taken into account when determining whether an animal or group of animals should be treated for strongyle infections:

1. General physical condition
2. Clinical signs
3. Clinical history of the animal(s)
4. Unique husbandry or environmental circumstances (Figs. 28.2 and 28.3)

5. Fecal egg counts

As indicated late in the section on epidemiology and control, a program of routine, periodic treatment is usually recommended.

A veterinarian or parasitologist, or one who works with horses closely, recognizes the usual yet nonspecific signs of helminthosis which may include rough hair coat, loss of condition, failure to eat properly, pale mucous membranes indicating anemia, diarrhea, and indications of abdominal discomfort.

If these signs are seen, and if the fecal egg count is high, treatment is justified. The dilemma is determining what is a high egg count. Also, the preadults, which cause much of the problem, do not produce eggs. The preadults damage the host in their migrations, or in hypobiosis, in the case of cyathostomes. Some investigators recommend treating horses when egg counts reach 500/g of feces, others recommend it at 1000/g, but egg counts much higher than those may be seen in horses that are clinically normal.

The eggs of the three *Strongylus* spp. and of the small strongyles cannot be distinguished from one another (they all look much like hookworm eggs; see Fig. 27.5). This further clouds the interpretation of fecal egg counts. However, the eggs of *Parascaris* and *Oxyuris equi* are distinct, as are those of the tapeworms sometimes found in equids.

If it is important to determine which strongyles are present in a host, the eggs and larvae can be allowed to develop in the feces and then the L_3s can be identified based on their unique morphologies.

Only a part of diagnosis is aimed at the health of the individual; the other part is herd health and prevention of infection in young animals, which must be taken into account in determining the severity of infection and the benefits that may accrue. Overall, the most important reason to treat for strongyle-infected horses is to prevent excessive pasture contamination with infective larvae.

Host–Parasite Interactions

Although we deal with the large strongyles as a group, they affect the host in different ways and to differing degrees. As adults, all three species attach to the wall of the large intestine, where they ingest intestinal mucosa and suck blood; the host may become anemic or the lesions where intestinal mucosa has been removed may become infected. The damage to the host from the adults can be serious enough, but the damage by the preadult stages is greater and more difficult to deal with.

S. vulgaris is the most pathogenic of the three species. As the worms migrate and grow in the arteries leading to the gut, including the large mesenteric artery, they cause blood clots to form in the artery. Normally, the slick internal surface of the artery prevents the clotting cascade from starting; however if that surface is damaged somehow by the worms, a clot forms and it may continue to increase in size almost indefinitely. This clot, attached to the surface of the blood vessel, is called a *thrombus* (pl. *thrombi*). It impedes the normal flow of blood, causing either blockage or ballooning of the artery, or both. The resulting pathological condition is called an *aneurysm*. Aneurysms may also result directly from damage to the arterial wall when the worms migrate there. The more important the artery or the greater number of aneurysms formed, the more the tissue downstream lacks an adequate blood supply. Thrombi may break loose and, as emboli, travel farther down arterial vessels where more blockage may occur.

There may be tissue necrosis for lack of adequate blood supply or the gut may telescope on itself. The animal feels pain, develops a fever, fails to eat properly, and may roll on the ground. This syndrome of abdominal pain in horses is relatively common and *S. vulgaris* is frequently the source of the problem.

As is true with helminths in general, the greater the number of larvae ingested by an animal, the greater the damage. In experimental infections with from 2500 to 5000 larvae administered in a single dose or doses of 250 larvae given every four to five days to a total of 6250, the effects on foals were severe. Animals lost weight, had fever, diarrhea, and colic. At the postmortem examination there were severe lesions in the intestinal tract, and the blood vessels had damage from thrombi and embolisms.

S. edentatus ranks behind *S. vulgaris* as a cause of damage. The nodules produced by its encysted larvae may cause bleeding and interfere with the blood supply to the intestine, depending on their location. The animal may have considerable blood loss into the abdominal cavity and may show colic and persistent diarrhea because of interference with normal intestinal function.

S. equinus causes less but not negligible damage compared to the other two species by encysting under the peritoneal lining. Its major damage is to the liver and pancreas, in which the L_4s develop.

Immunity to larval *Strongylus* spp. probably develops on repeated infection.

Epidemiology and Control

The approach of most equine strongyle control programs falls into the category of preventive public health. That is, the goal is prevention of excessive pasture contamination thereby reducing the risk of exposure to infective larvae. The following program has been modified somewhat from Drudge and Lyons (1978):

1. Treat all horses on the premises.
2. Quarantine and treat any horses introduced to a farm before allowing them to be with the residents.
3. Treat horses regularly. In areas where there is a high density of horses and year-round transmission of parasites, treat mares every six to eight weeks. In colder climates, year-round treatment is not necessary.
4. Do not treat foals. Treating young animals has no effect on their acquiring infective larvae or the preadult stages, which are most damaging.
5. Use alternate drugs so that problems with anthelmintic resistance are reduced. Alternating classes of drugs, at least annually, is believed to be effective. Follow the directions on dosage and other procedures so that full efficacy and safety will be achieved.
6. Physically disperse manure, keep pastures mowed, and move stock to different pastures whenever practical.
7. Monitor the efficiency of the program by periodic fecal egg counts.
8. Modify the program depending on the environmental conditions. For example, a single animal fed in a barn is at very different risk from animals pastured together in a warm climate.
9. Retain the services of a veterinarian who is skilled in diagnosis and treatment not only of helminthoses but of other diseases as well.

A variety of drugs developed in fairly recent times have been highly effective against strongyles of horses. Among them are the benzimidazoles, but the worms have tended to become resistant to the drug. Ivermectin, a macrolide antibiotic, is one of a group of compounds called avermectins, which are fermentation products produced by *Streptomyces avermitilis.* Ivermectin and some related compounds have been found to be highly effective against both large strongyles and cyathostomes. Despite efficacy, there is some concern about development of resistance to ivermectin. Although certain anthelmintics, such as moxidectin and fenbendazole, have recently obtained product label claims for efficacy against arrested larvae, many anthelmintics work neither against hypobiotic larvae nor active, migrating larvae.

A number of problems must be overcome in developing a control program for large strongyles:

1. A relatively small number of infective larvae can have severe effects on foals.
2. The free-living stages quickly reach L_3 during the growing season.
3. The free-living stages are quite hardy, living for months and even overwintering in areas where there is only occasional frost.
4. Egg production by adult worms is strikingly high, and an adult horse with only a low-grade infection may contaminate the pasture with millions of eggs in a day. There are seasonal differences in the number of eggs in the feces of animals; it is highest in summer.

CYATHOSTOMES OR SMALL STRONGYLES

Name of Organism and Disease Associations

Small strongyles or cyathostomes include 16 genera and more than twice that number of species in equids. Some of these are *Cylicocercus, Cylicocyclus, Poteriostomum, Triodontophorus,* and *Cyathostomum.* Strongylosis and helminthosis are the diseases caused.

Geographic Distribution and Importance

Cosmopolitan, although some species have been reported only from certain localities. These worms are often not considered to be as important as the large strongyles. While that may be true on a worm-to-worm basis, the cyathosomes are increasingly appreciated for their importance in equine disease.

Morphology

Most species are 10 and 20 mm long, but some males may be as short as 5 mm, and have stout bodies. Small strongyles are members of the superfamily Strongyloidea but have relatively small buccal capsules. The variations in leaf crowns and male genitalia are the principal means of distinguishing among the genera and species (Bowman, 1995).

Life Cycle

The life cycle is direct (see *Strongylus* spp). Upon entering the host, the infective larvae do not leave the gut but enter the intestinal tissue and develop; they return later to the lumen of the large intestine as adults. The prepatent period may be as short as 6 weeks in some species or as long as 50 weeks in others. A large population of larvae may to through a hypobiotic stage or a period of arrested development.

Diagnosis

See *Strongylus* spp.

Host–Parasite Interactions

Damage to the host by the adult small strongyles is relatively small but is not to be ignored. Some horses suffer from malabsorption due to larval-associated nodules in the tissue of the colon. Horses may have over a hundred thousand of these small nodules which, collectively, pose a threat simply due to nutritional competition with the host.

The adult worms such as *Cyathostomum* spp. are said to suck blood, but other genera and species seem to graze on intestinal epithelium or to ingest gut contents.

Arrested Development in Cyathostomes of Equids

Gibson's (1953) study on arrested development in small strongyles of horses, described in the essay titled *Arrested Development,* was important in itself but led to further observations in other nematodes as well.

Epidemiology and Control

See *Strongylus* spp. The same principles of development and survival of the free-living stages that were discussed in connection with *Strongylus* spp. pertain to the small strongyles.

Control programs for large strongyles remove small strongyles at the same time. Certain anthelmintics are more effective than others in removing hypobiotic larvae.

Readings

Bowman, D. D. (1995). *Georgi's Parasitology for Veterinarians,* 6th ed. Saunders, Philadelphia.

Drudge, J. H. (1972). Metazoal diseases, endoparasitisms. In *Equine Medicine and Surgery* (E. J. Catcott and J. F. Smithcors, Eds.), 2nd ed., pp. 157–179. American Veterinary, Santa Barbara, CA.

Drudge, J. H., and Lyons, E. T. (1978). Equine parasites—Problems and control. *Practicing Vet.* **49**(3), 5–9.

Drudge, J. H., Lyons, E. T., and Szanto, J. (1966). Pathogenesis of migrating stages of helminths with special reference to *Strongylus vulgaris.* In *Biology of Parasites* (E. J. L. Soulsby, Ed.), pp. 199–214. Academic Press, New York.

Gibson, T. E. (1953). The effect of repeated anthelmintic treatment with phenothiazine on the faecal egg counts of housed horses, with some observations on the life cycle of *Trichonema* spp. in the horse. *J. Helminthol.* **27,** 29–40.

Jacobs, D. E. (1986). *Color Atlas of Equine Parasites.* Lea & Febiger, Philadelphia.

Klei, T. R., Torbert, B. J., Chapman, M. R., and Ochoa, R. (1982). Irradiated larval vaccination of ponies against *Strongylus vulgaris. J. Parasitol.* **68,** 561–569.

Levine, N. D. (1980). *Nematode Parasites of Domestic Animals and Man,* 2nd ed., pp. 100–114. Burgess, Minneapolis.

Soulsby, E. J. L. (1965). *Textbook of Veterinary Clinical Parasitology. Vol. 2. Helminths.* Davis, Philadelphia.

CHAPTER

29

Nodular Worms, Kidney Worms, and Other Strongyloidea

The worms discussed in this chapter have elegant mouth structures such as leaf crowns, as seen in the strongyles of horses, or other elaborations of the buccal apparatus (Fig. 29.5, presented later). The nodular worms have received their name from the fact that many of them produce a strong foreign body reaction in the intestinal tracts of their hosts leading to the formation of a granulatoma of a few millimeters in diameter up to 10 mm or more. Those worms found in domestic animals are the most important overall, and they usually lie in the large intestine where the larvae burrow into the mucosa. There are only a few reports of members of this group as human infections, but *Oesophagostomum bifurcum* has been found at a relatively high level of prevalence in West Africa, and it may be an overlooked infection of humans in developing countries.

NODULAR WORMS OF LARGE FARM ANIMALS

Name of Organism and Disease Associations

Oesophagostomum spp. See Table 29.1 for a list of species in sheep, goats, cattle, and swine. Nodular worm, pimply guts, knotty guts, oesophagostomosis, and oesophagostomiasis are caused by the organisms.

Hosts and Host Range

Most species have been reported in only a few closely related species of hosts, but in a few instances they are found in families of closely related hosts (Tab. 29.1).

Geographic Distribution and Importance

Cosmopolitan. Some species have been found only in restricted localities, but the species of economic importance seem to be found worldwide. Although these worms are likely to be found almost anywhere, they cause problems in areas that are relatively warm and wet. In the United States, for example, they can be a major problem in areas east of the Mississippi River where the winters are not severe. The worms are a continuing problem in Britain even as far north as Scotland.

Economic losses are due to production losses associated with morbidity and mortality.

Morphology

These worms are members of the superfamily Strongyloidea, subfamily Oesophagostominae, and as such have leaf crowns; but unlike other members of the family, they have a relatively small buccal capsule (Fig. 29.1). The vulva of the female is near the posterior end and the males have a large bursa with slender spicules.

Life Cycle

The life cycle is direct. Embryonated eggs hatch to release the L_1s; the L_1s and L_2s feed, grow, and molt. The ensheathed L_3 (Fig. 29.6, presented later) is the infective stage, which is ingested with the forage. The L_3s enter the tissues of the lower part of the small

TABLE 29.1 ***Oesophagostomum*** **Species in Farm Animals**

Species	Hosts
Oe. columbianum	Sheep, goat, alpaca, antelope
Oe. venulosum	Sheep, bighorn sheep, goat, chamois, argali, camel, alpaca, vicuna
Oe. multifoliatum	Sheep, goat
Oe. asperum	Goat
Oe. radiatum	Ox, zebu, water buffalo
Oe. dentatum	Pig, peccary
Oe. brevicaudum	Pig
Oe. georgianum	Pig
Oe. quadrispinulatum	Pig
Oe. maplestonei	Pig
Oe. rousseloti	Pig
Oe. granatensis	Pig
Oe. hsungi	Pig

intestine or, more frequently, the large intestine, where they encyst. Most species return to the lumen of the gut during the L_4 and then molt to become the L_5 and adult. In initial infections, the L_4s return to the lumen of the gut in about one week and the patent period begins at about three weeks.

In previously infected animals, the prepatent period is extended and the larvae may remain in the tissues for months.

Diagnosis

Oesophagostomosis is generally a herd problem, and determining whether it is the causative agent is based on the following:

1. Herd history
2. Fecal egg counts
3. Clinical signs
4. Postmortem examination

The history of the herd and the signs of disease are helpful. Animals crowded on moist or wet pastures in enzootic areas are likely to pick up L_3s of various strongylid nematodes including *Oesophagostomum* spp. In warm, wet climates such as the southeastern United States, nodular worms may be prevalent. Diarrhea, loss of condition, and anemia are common signs and symptoms of gastrointestinal helminthoses; *Oesophagostomum* infection is no exception.

In some species nodules form in the wall of the gut, and these can be felt just inside the rectum of an animal. Not all species cause this reaction, however, and it represents relatively long-standing infections.

Fecal egg counts give a hint as to the cause of the problem but are not a reliable diagnostic method. There are two caveats:

1. Eggs of *Oesophagostomum* cannot readily be distinguished from those of other strongyles.
2. Much of the damage may arise before egg production begins particularly when larvae are encysted in noidules.

The most reliable way of determining the cause of the disease is to perform a postmortem examination. If an investigation is made at a farm or ranch, recently dead or moribund animals may be examined. Sometimes the only alternative is to perform complete postmortem examinations on a few of the most debilitated animals.

Host–Parasite Interactions

Some generalizations can be made about the nodular worms, but their damage to the host may vary with the species in question. Much of the damage, whether nodules are formed or not, is caused when the larvae are in the tissues of the gut. This is a foreign-body tissue reaction, and the greater the number of larvae, the greater the corresponding gut malfunction.

In instances such as *Oe. columbianum* of sheep, long-term damage arises from nodule formation. In an animal previously unexposed to *Oesophagostomum*, the worms mature and begin to produce eggs about three weeks after infection. As infection continues and as additional L_3s are acquired, the larvae are retained in the tissue and a strong inflammatory response occurs. A granuloma (a swelling containing white cells, fluid, and connective tissue) forms around each larva, and this pocket often becomes infected with bacteria. The nodule may reach 5 mm or more in diameter and extends to the muscular layers of the gut; with time it becomes hard and calcified. The gut loses its ability to function normally in the vicinity of each nodule. Resorption of water and inorganic balance are disturbed; the result is diarrhea. Nodule formation is a sign of immunity. However, as is emphasized in a number of instances in this book, the immune response is not always beneficial, or the results may be mixed.

Epidemiology and Control

Control of nodular work infections is based on the following:

1. Knowing that the worm occurs in a specific region
2. Chemotherapy to reduce pasture contamination

Treatment for nodular worm is only partly success-

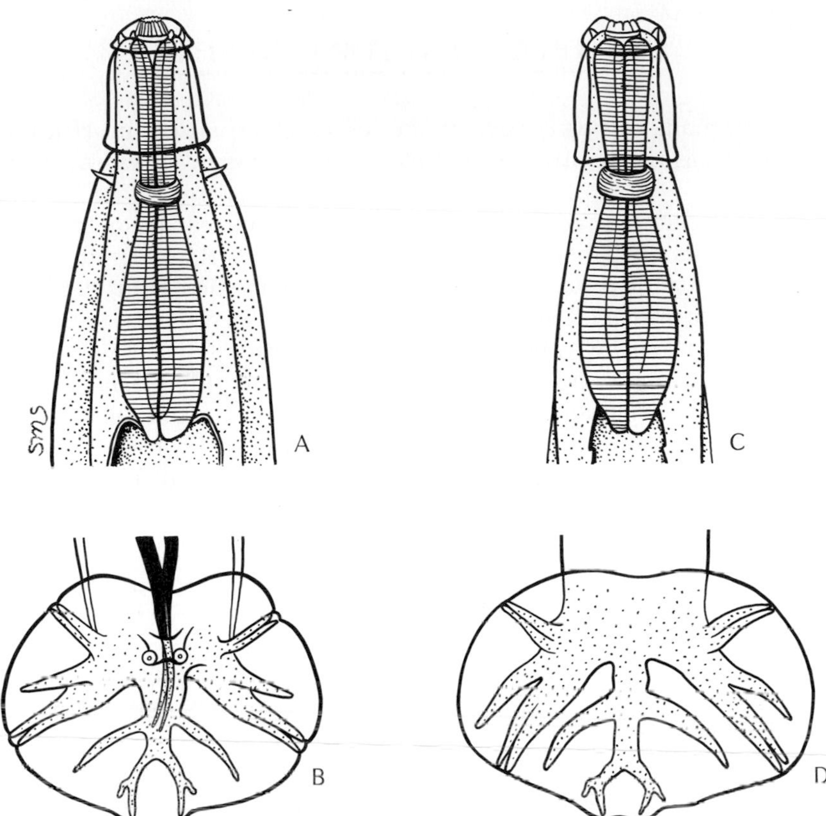

FIGURE 29.1 Heads and bursae of two nodular worms. (A and B) *Oesophagostomum columbianum* of sheep, goats, and some other ruminants. (C and D) *Oe. venulosum* of sheep and other ruminants.

ful, and as in the case of other nematodes in grazing animals, the correct use of drugs is strategically focused on the prevention of contamination of pastures with large numbers of L_3s. Most modern anthelmintics are virtually 100% effective against adults but they vary in their efficacy against preadults. Much of the damage to the host is caused by larvae, and more efficient drugs are needed.

Oesophagostomosis is a wet or moist-climate disease and usually occurs in areas where winters are relatively mild, with infrequent frost or failure of the ground to freeze hard for long periods. Patent infections can be retained for more than 100 days, so animals that go into the winter with an infection can seed pastures with eggs the following spring.

Young animals are especially susceptible to infection, and the best means of preventing infection is to treat the adults as a herd health measure. As a specific example, let us look at a herd of sheep that is at risk of infection with *Oe. columbianum*. The objective is to prevent seeding pastures so that ewes are treated before they go out on pasture in the spring. Some worms may mature during the pasture season; ewes are treated at least once during that time. Monitoring the herd by fecal egg count gives some information on the need to treat. Then, when animals come off of pasture in fall, the whole herd—ewes, lambs, and rams—is treated so that the animals can go into the winter with as little as possible draining them during pregnancy or feeding to market weight.

KIDNEY WORM OF SWINE

Name of Organism and Disease Associations

Stephanurus dentatus causes kidney worm disease although the worm is not strictly a parasite of the kidney, but typically in the perirenal area where it damages the ureter.

Hosts and Host Range

Swine are the hosts. The organism has been reported occasionally from other hosts such as the ox and ass

SELF-TREATMENT FOR PARASITES

A CHANCE OBSERVATION made during behavioral studies on chimpanzees in Africa has opened an area of investigation that has importance in the treatment of parasitic diseases and in the evolution of knowledge in medicine.

A free-ranging group of chimpanzees in the Mahale Mountains near Lake Tanganyika in Africa had been studied for several years for, among other things, food habits. It appeared that certain plant foods were taken not for their nutritional value, but rather for their medicinal properties. Then, in 1987, an adult female chimpanzee, accompanied by her male infant, was observed to be lethargic, rested frequently while foraging, showed mild diarrhea, and had dark-colored urine.

At one point she selected a plant known as "bitter leaf" because of the taste of its leaves, bark, stems, and roots. The plant is *Veronia amygdalina* (Compositae). She removed a part of the bark of some branches and sucked out the liquid. Her son picked up a few pieces of the *V. amygdalina* but discarded them immediately after tasting them. The following day the female resumed foraging with her group and behaved as if she had fully recovered from her illness.

Further studies showed that there were a number of steroid glycosides in *V. amygdalina*, and that some of these compounds have activity against certain parasites and a tumor. Ingestion of the liquid from the pith of *V. amygdalina* seemed to reduce the number of eggs of *Oesophagostomum stephanostomum* in observations on free-ranging chimpanzees.

Quite a different tactic of removing *Oe. stephanostomum* has also been documented at Mahale in which chimpanzees ingest leaves of *Aspila* spp. and some other genera. They may ingest from a few to more than 50 leaves by folding them and swallowing them whole. The leaves pass through the intestinal tract more or less unchanged. SEM studies showed that the leaves of these plants have tiny, thornlike process on them, and it has been suggested that the spines mechanically remove the strongyles. In fact, worms have been found adhering to the surface of leaves passed with the feces.

It is especially interesting to note that tribes all across Africa use decoctions of *V. amygdalina* for a variety of intestinal complaints. One could speculate that before humankind and the chimpanzee diverged from one another evolutionarily that their progenitor had discovered *V. amygdalina* for use against intestinal worm infections. If the use of the plant carried through several million years, that would mean that internal medicine (i.e., the diagnosis and treatment of disease) had its inception some millions of years before the present.

Additional information may be found in Huffman, M. A., et. al. 1996. *Int. J. Primatol.* **17,** 475–503, and Huffman, M. A., et al., 1997. *Primates* **38,** 111–125.

usually after aberrant larval migration. The principal location of the adults is in the perirenal fat and around the ureters, but it may be found in nearly any organ system of the body, especially while the preadult stages are migrating.

Geographic Distribution and Importance

The kidney worm is cosmopolitan in warm, wet climates throughout the world. Losses arise from production losses, mortality, and condemnations of carcasses at slaughter. The widespread nature of the infection in tropical and subtropical areas suggests that the production losses in the developed economies and morbidity and mortality in subsistence societies in less developed countries are both critically significant.

Morphology

Males are 1.2 by 20 to 30 mm long and females are 1.8 by 30 to 45 mm long; they have rather mottling of light and dark because the color of the internal organs shows through the cuticle. The broad, cup-shaped buccal capsule has a single leaf crown at the anterior tip and six teeth in the base of the capsule (Fig. 29.2).

Life Cycle

The kidney worm has a typical strongylid free-living phase, with the L_3 being reached about three days after the eggs pass from the host with the urine. Unlike most other strongyloids, *S. dentatus* has three options for reaching the definitive host:

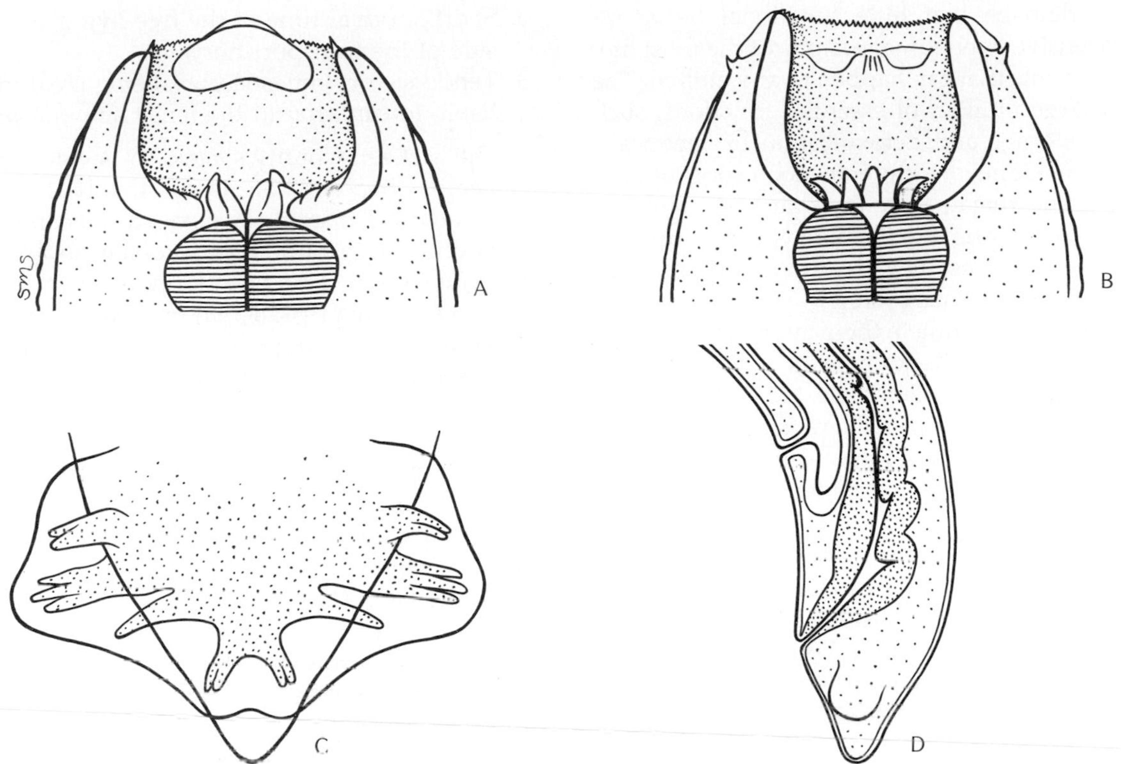

FIGURE 29.2 *Stephanurus dentatus*, the kidney worm of swine. (A) Dorsal view of head; (B) lateral view of head; (C) bursa of male worm; (D) tail of female.

1. It can be eaten with contaminated food or water
2. It can penetrate the unbroken skin of the pig
3. It can be eaten by earthworms (e.g., *Eisenia foetida*) and use them as transport hosts, which are later eaten by pigs

If the L_3 is eaten directly or with an earthworm, the larva passes from the gut to the mesenteric lymph nodes, where it remains for 10 to 32 days becoming a well-developed L_4 before it migrates to the liver via the circulatory system.

If the larva penetrates the skin, it reaches the liver through the circulatory system in 8 to 40 days. The larva migrates in the liver for a least two months, and they have been reported to remain there for as long as nine months.

The larva leaves the liver by passing through its capsule into the peritoneal cavity. Although there is some random migration, the larva that completes the life cycle reaches the region of the kidney, where it matures. The female penetrates the wall of the ureter with the posterior part of her body, and the eggs pass out with the urine. Egg laying can begin as early as four months after infection, but it usually takes more than six months.

Diagnosis

During the patent period, eggs are in the urine. Before egg production begins, one must rely on the history of the animals and the knowledge that kidney worm occurs in the vicinity. If dead or dying animals are available, a postmortem examination may be done; worms should be looked for in the liver, peritoneal cavity, larger blood vessels, and the perirenal fat.

Host–Parasite Interactions

Damage to the host revolves around three events in the life cycle:

1. Skin penetration
2. Larval migration
3. Egg laying

Skin damage by the penetrating larvae is relatively minor, but there may be some inflammation at the site.

The long period of larval migration causes the major damage. The larvae remain during much of the prepatent period in the liver and literally chew their way through it with the well-developed buccal structures of the L_4. Experimental inocula of 10,000 L_3s caused so much liver damage that little functional tissue remained. Extensive liver damage is one of the most life-threatening events that can happen to any animal. The liver has a large number of essential functions, such as glycogen storage and detoxification of chemicals, and in severe kidney worm infections, not enough functional tissue remains for the animal to survive. The larvae may migrate into the blood vessels, causing thrombi and embolisms; they are also found occasionally in the central nervous system.

When the larvae complete their migration and mature in the vicinity of the kidney, they cause lesions there. Usually a male and female are found near a ureter in a pus-filled nodule. There is damage to the ureter and sometimes the kidney during egg laying since the tissue is penetrated. The lumen of the ureter may be constricted.

Animals that do not succumb to kidney worm infection gain poorly; even under moderate experimental infections of 200 to 1000 L_3s, infected pigs gained about 1/2 lb less per day than uninfected pigs. A 65-lb difference between an infected and an uninfected animal is about $25 (U.S.) at present prices.

Epidemiology and Control

Control of swine kidney worm is based on the following:

1. Chemotherapy
2. Environmental management
3. Importing clean stock and shipping them before the patent period begins

Several anthelmintics may be used to eliminate the kidney worm. These drugs can have a variable effect on migrating larvae, but adult worms are readily killed.

The limited geographic areas where kidney worm is found tell a good deal about the hardiness of the free-living stages. The climate must be warm and moist; at 11°C and below the larvae are harmed, at 20°C only slight development occurs, and optimal development occurs at 25 to 27°C. Earthworms are transport hosts, but they also protect the larvae from drying, thereby increasing the length of time that they survive.

Two major problems must be addressed in designing control programs for kidney worm:

1. The prepatent period is about six months.
2. The adults may live for two years and shed eggs into the environment during that time

On the other hand, some characteristics of the parasite and the host, as well as the efficacy of contemporary drugs, are helpful in designing a program:

1. Narrow host range
2. Short survival time of the free-living stages (outside of the transport host)
3. Tendency of domestic pigs, being creatures of habit, to run around the fence line in a pasture

The McLean County system for swine raising, discussed in Chapter 32 on *Ascaris*, involves farrowing in clean quarters from a clean sow and keeping the animals on clean ground. The problem in applying the McLean County system to kidney worm is obtaining a clean sow. Egg production may continue for at least two years, and in pregnant sows, there is a rise in worm egg production six to seven weeks prior to farrowing, further contributing to contamination of pastures.

In the southeastern United States, a system was developed in which young, unbred sows (gilts) are purchased from areas where kidney worm does not exist. Six months after the litter is born, the sows and young pigs are shipped out and another group of clean gilts is brought in. Thus, all of the animals are removed from the farm before egg production commences. After three or four farrowings, the residual free-living stages should have died out, the farm should then be clean, and conventional hog raising can be started again. Although this system involves extra costs, it works.

In a tropical area, it is unlikely that such a system could easily be established. In the United States, the enzootic areas are the southeastern states and Hawaii. In the Southeast, gilts can be purchased from clean areas farther north and shipped in. In the tropics or less developed countries, clean stock might not be readily available. If such a program were to be instituted, it would need to be done by importing clean swine to a central facility where they could be raised and then provided to farmers as needed. Such a program assumes that feral swine are not present or that owners could fence in their animals and not allow them contact with any others.

Because much of swine production in North America is done in confinement with excellent hygiene, and modern drugs are very effective against this parasite, the economic importance of the kidney worm is more limited than in the past. This "gilt only" system, however, is still relevant in much of the world. It is also an example of how to apply ingeniously the biological knowledge of a parasite to developing control programs while at the same time not incurring significant additional expense.

STRONGYLOIDS OF THE PHARYNX AND TRACHEA

The genera *Syngamus*, *Cyathostoma*, and *Mammomonogamus* contain about 35 species of worms that are found in the pharyngeal region, nasal passages, middle ear, or trachea of birds and mammals. Some of them have been reported from humans, but these seem to be only sporadic infections.

The best known of the group is *Syngamus trachea*, a parasite of the trachea of galliform and other birds; it seems to have a low degree of host specificity. The cycle is both direct and indirect, with a wide array of invertebrates including earthworms, snails, and various insects serving as transport hosts. When large numbers of worms are located in the trachea, passage of air is impeded and the birds gasp for air—thus, the common name of *gapeworm*. *S. trachea* is a problem if chickens or other birds are raised as farm flocks; with the development of battery raising of chickens in the United States and other high-technology countries, the prevalence of gapeworm declined. The infection is easily recognized by finding the worms in the trachea at postmortem examination (Fig. 29.3). The male and female remain permanently in copula. When necessary, an anthelmintic may be administered in the feed with good effect.

RELATED ORGANISMS

Primates including humans are infected with *Ternidens deminutus*, a strongylid that is found in the large intestine of higher primates in the warmer climates of the Eastern Hemisphere. The females of this worm are 1.2 to 1.6 cm long and 0.6 to 0.7 mm wide. There is a small buccal capsule in which there are two small leaf crowns and three teeth at the entrance to the esophagus. The adults suck blood and cause anemia in heavy infections.

Oesophagostomum bifurcum (Figs. 29.4, 29.5, and 29.6) parasitizes the large intestine of monkeys. It forms nodules and causes diarrhea, and the eggs are not distinguishable from those of hookworms being 51 to 72 μm x 29 to 40 μm. In the Sahelian region of Togo and Ghana in West Africa, *Oe. bifurcum* has been found as a human infection in 17.3% of individuals of all ages. The prevalence peaked at 33.9% of women 30 to 39 years of age and 21.4% of males aged 10 to 19 years. The worms cause large granulomata in the intestinal tract or in the abdominal cavity; surgery can remove the masses.

Chabertia ovina is a parasite of the large intestine of both domestic and wild ruminants in all parts of the world. This worm has a large, globular buccal capsule the opening to which is surrounded by two leaf crowns that have a multitude of tiny projections. Most of the damage caused by *C. ovina* is during larval development when heavily infected hosts show diarrhea, often with blood, lose condition, and become

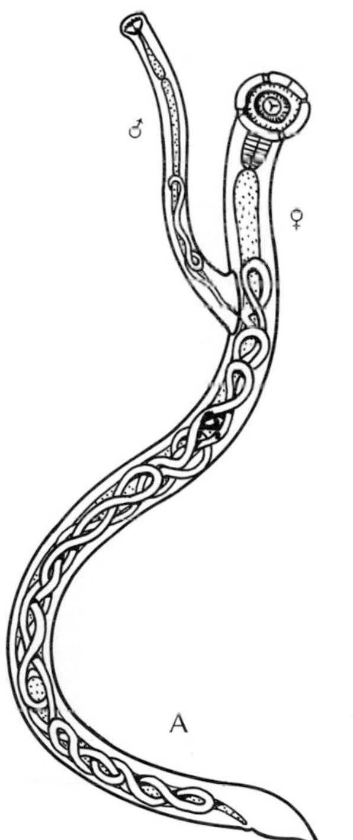

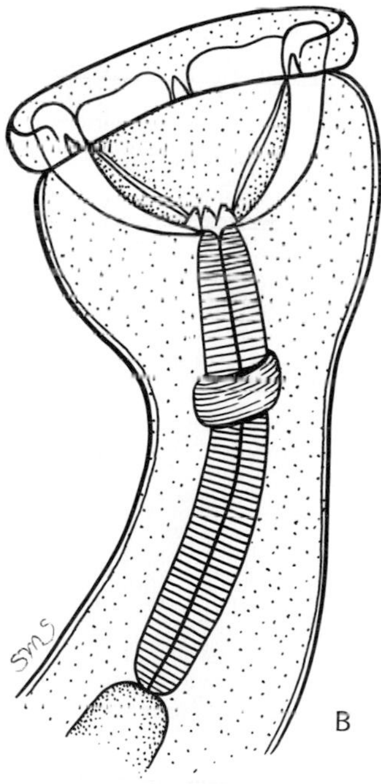

FIGURE 29.3 *Syngamus trachea*, the gapeworm of fowl. (A) Male and female in copula; (B) buccal capsule of the female.

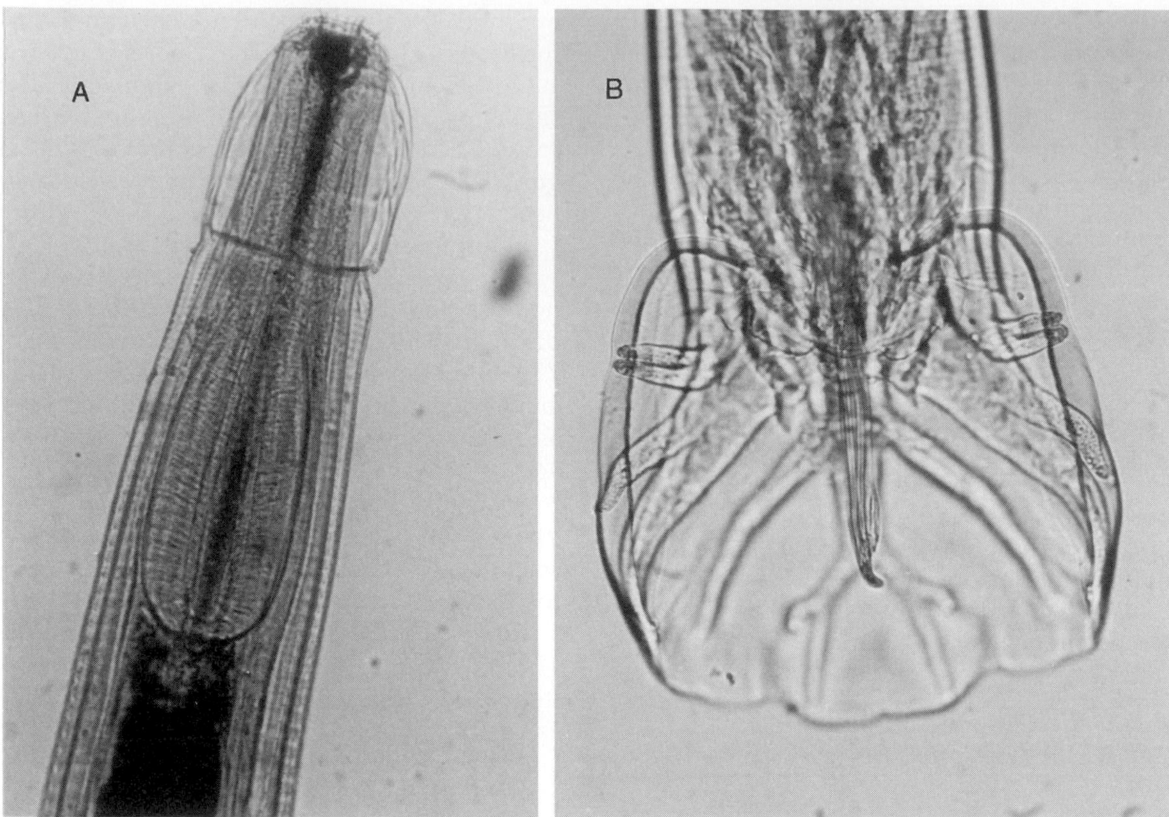

FIGURE 29.4 *Oesopohagostomum bifurcum*, a parasite of humans in West Africa, (A) Pharyngeal and esophageal structure shows a buccal capsule and a stout, muscular esophagus. (B) Copulatory bursa and spicules of the male. The bursal rays show quite well in this preparation. [Photomicrographs of *Oe. bifurcum* courtesy of Prof. Coby Blotcamp, Leiden University. From Polderman, A. M., et al., 1991.]

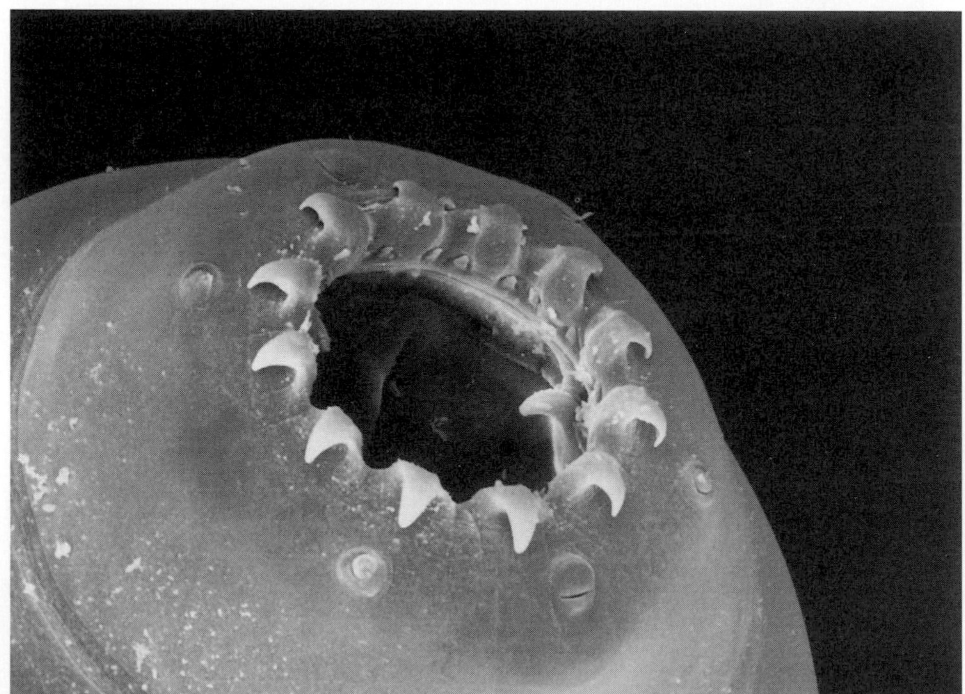

FIGURE 29.5 *Oesopohagostomum bifurcum*. SEM of the head portion of an adult worm. The leaf crown, typical of members of the superfamily Strongyloidea, shows well. [Photomicrographs of *Oe. bifurcum* courtesy of Prof. Coby Blotcamp, Leiden University. From Polderman, A. M., et al., 1991.]

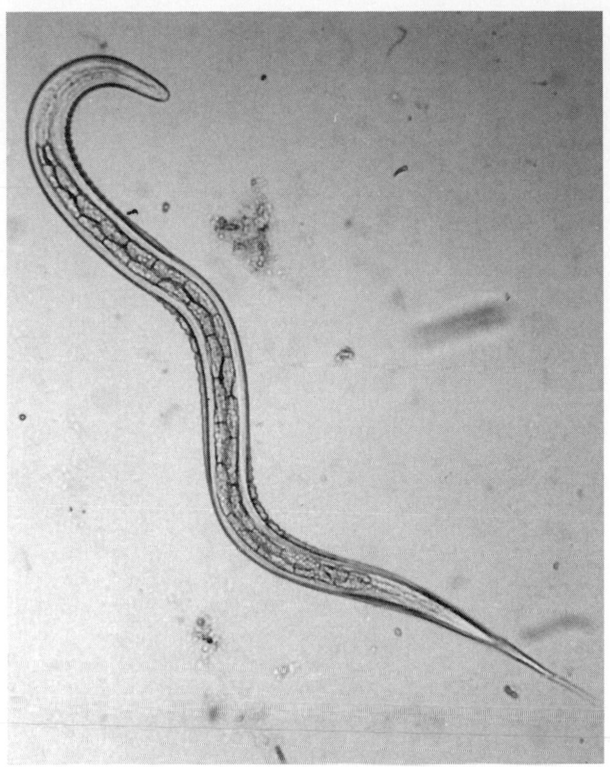

FIGURE 29.6 The third stage infective larva (L_3) of *Oesophagostomum bifurcum*. This L_3 is typical of the infective stage of other strongyles; there are minor differences among them, but all are basically the same. [Photomicrographs of *Oe. bifurcum* courtesy of Prof. Coby Blotcamp, Leiden University. From Polderman, A. M., et al., 1991.]

anemic. The adults suck blood and cause some damage to the intestinal wall but seem not to be as damaging as the larvae.

Readings

Batte, E. G., Harkema, R., and Osborne, J. C. (1960). Observations on the life cycle and pathogenicity of the swine kidney worm (*Stephanurus dentatus*). *J. Am. Vet. Med. Assoc.* **136,** 622–625.

Fernando, M. A., Stockdale, P. H. G., and Remmier, O. (1971). The route of migration, development and pathogenesis of *Syngamus trachea* (Montagu, 1811) Chapin, 1925, in pheasants. *J. Parasitol.* **57,** 107–116.

Lichtenfels, J. R., and Tromba, F. G. (1972). The morphogenesis of *Stephanurus dentatus* (Nematoda: Strongylina) in swine with observations on larval migration. *J. Parasitol.* **58,** 757–766.

Long, P. L., Current, W. L., and Noblet, G. P. (1987). Parasites of the Christmas turkey. *Parasitol. Today* **3,** 361–366.

Polderman, A. M., Krepel, H. P., Baeta, S., Blotkamp, J., and Gigase, P. (1991). Oesophagostomiasis; A common infection of man in northern Togo and Ghana. *Am. J. Trop. Med. Hyg.* **44,** 336–344.

Waddell, A. H. (1969). The parasitic life cycle of the swine kidney worm *Stephanurus dentatus* Diesing. *Aust. J. Zool.* **17,** 607–618.

CHAPTER

30

Trichostrongyles of Cattle, Sheep, Goats, and Other Ruminants

The strongyles discussed here as a group are among the most important helminth parasites of grazing animals. Although there is variation in the species composition found in a particular kind of habitat, there is usually a mixture of five or six species in any one locality. It is important to recognize at the outset that any one grazing animal may have a few hundred or a few thousand worms, but these worms often cause no discernible damage to the host. Only under certain conditions are production and death losses observed. The trichostrongyles exemplify, as well as any group, the role of weather and climate in enzootic and epizootic infections with helminths.

The trichostrongyles are members of the superfamily Trichostrongyloidea and are characterized as having a small buccal capsule and a large copulatory bursa with stout, heavily sclerotized spicules. Their life cycles are direct; L_3s are ingested with the forage.

If problems with trichostrongyles arise in grazing animals, there may also be problems with lungworms (Chapter 31), nodular worms (Chapter 29), and hookworms (Chapter 27). High host density on lush, moist pastures favors the free-living stages of all of these worms and increases the probability of large numbers of L_3s being ingested.

Name of Organism and Disease Associations

Six principal genera are found in domestic ruminants (Table 30.1); eleven additional genera are of minor importance or are localized. The diseases they cause are referred to generally as helminthosis or helminthiasis, but when one worm predominates, the generic name is often used; thus, *Haemonchus* spp. cause haemonchosis and *Trichostrongylus* spp. cause trichostrongylosis. A frequent sign of heavy infection is diarrhea, and terms such as *black scours* may be applied to infections with *Trichostrongylus* or *Nematodirus*.

Hosts and Host Range

The hosts listed in Table 30.1 are the principal domesticated ruminants, and it should be noted that most of the species infect all three hosts. There is a moderate degree of host specificity in most species since most will infect many ruminants and sometimes even nonruminants such as horses or humans in a few instances.

Geographic Distribution and Importance

Most species are cosmopolitan, but a few, such as *Nematodirus battus*, which is found in Britain and a few areas in North America, have limited distribution.

Although death losses occur from this complex of worms, the main losses are in livestock production, in reduced weight gain, and in a lowered production of fiber. Annual losses for the United States in sheep and cattle are measured in the hundreds of millions of dollars. About one-third of the loss is due to deaths and two-thirds from production losses (i.e., meat, milk, and fiber). It is difficult to obtain accurate figures for these annual losses either in the United States or globally since so much of the economic loss is associated with subtle effects or diminished production rather than overt disease or death. For example, there might be a 1kg production loss per head in a flock of 1000 lambs when the lambs are weaned. The owner fails

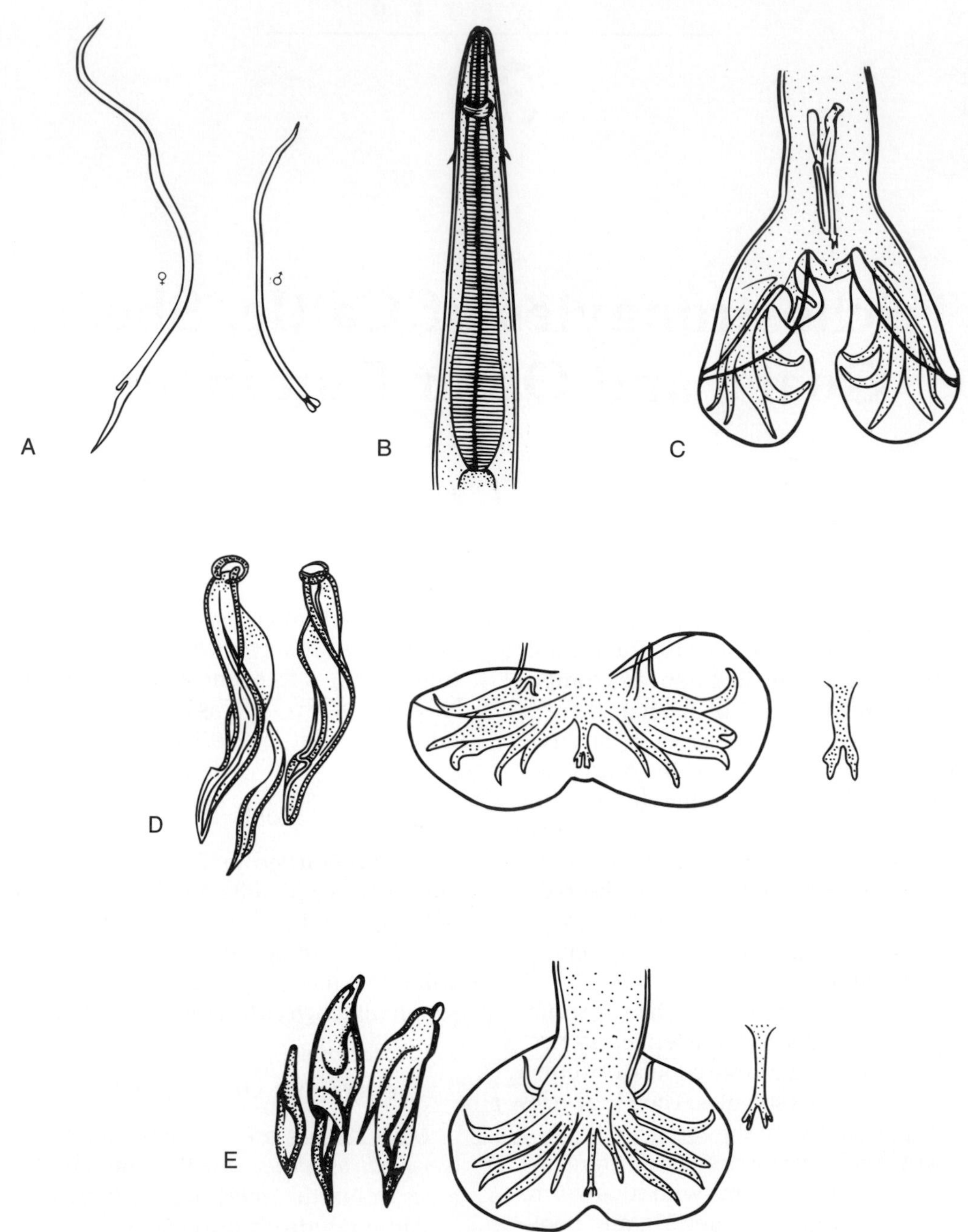

FIGURE 30.1 Identifying characters of some common trichostrongyles. *Haemonchus contortus*, (A) male and female three times normal size; (B) anterior end of adult worm showing nerve ring, cervical papillae, and esophageal structure, a tiny stylet lies in the small buccal capsule but is not shown here; (C) bursa of the male; (D) *Trichostrongylus colubriformis*. Left to right: spicules, gubernaculum, bursa, and dorsal lobe of the bursa; (E) *Trichostrongylus axei*. Left to right: gubernaculum, spicules, bursa and dorsal lobe of the bursa.

to realize the benefit of selling an additional ton of livestock weight.

Another approach to determining losses is to look at "worm production." Just as grain or meat production can be calculated, the amount of nutrient that is diverted into production of worms and worm eggs can also be determined. Boughton (1957) calculated that annual worm production in livestock in the United States amounts to 7000 tons of nematodes and 1000 tons of eggs. Further calculation showed that these

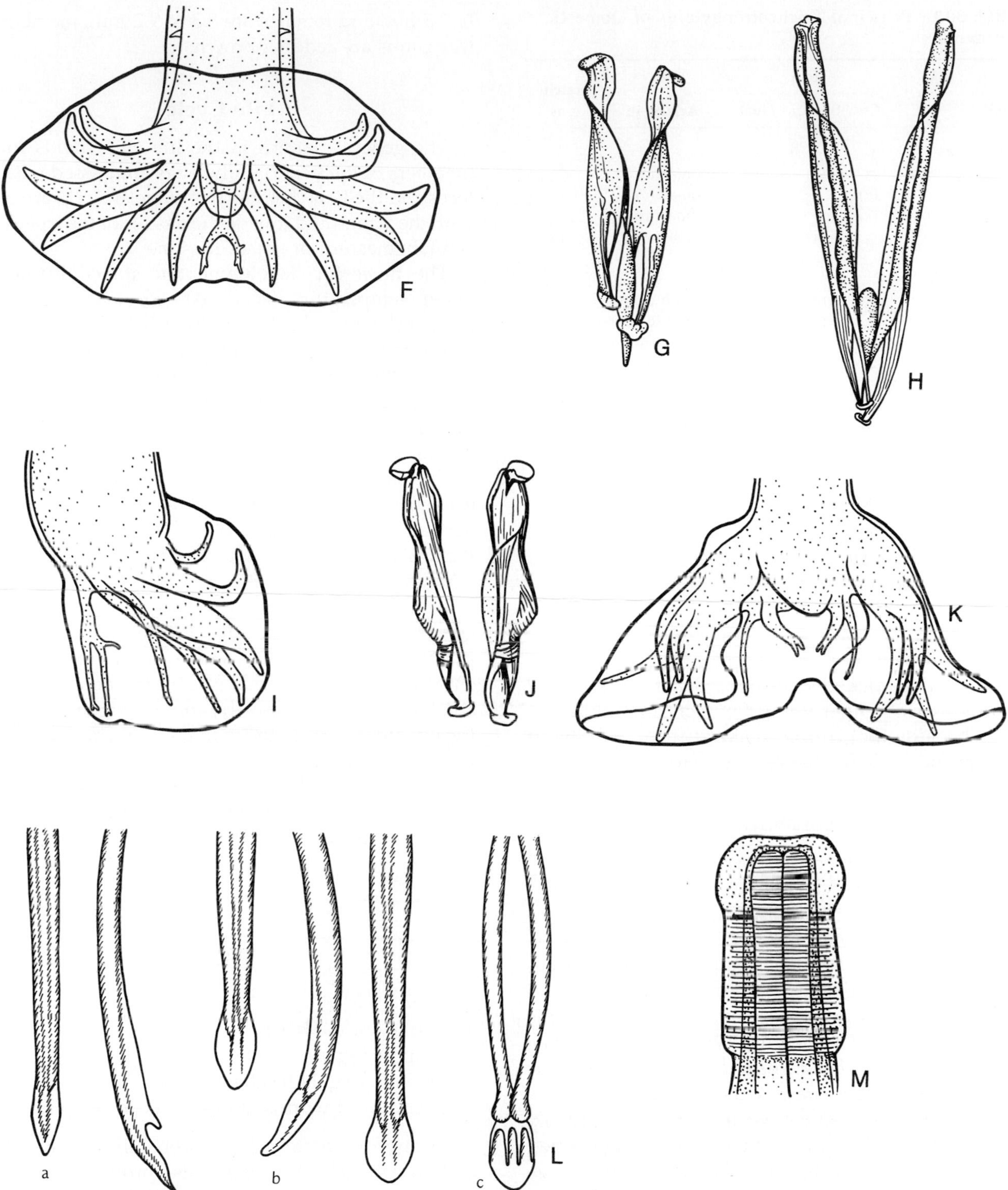

FIGURE 30.1 (*Continued*) *Ostertagia trifurcata* (F) bursa; (G) spicules; *Ostertagia circumcincta*; (H) spicules; *Cooperia*; (I) *bursa*; *Cooperia onchophora*; (J) spicules; *Nematodirus battus*; (K) *bursa*; (N) head; tips of the spicules of *Nematodirus* (a) *N. fillicollis*, (b) *N. spathiger*, (c) *N. battus*.

TABLE 30.1 Principal Trichostrongyloids of Domestic Ruminants

Parasite	Host			Adults in	Hatches as
	Ox	Sheep	Goat		
Haemonchus contortus	x	(x)	x	Abomasum	L_1
H. placei	(x)	x	x	Abomasum	L_1
Ostertagia ostertagi	(x)	x	x	Abomasum	L_1
Telodorsagia. circumcincta	x	(x)	(x)	Abomasum	L_1
Trichostrongylus colubriformis	x	(x)	x	Small intestine	L_1
T. vitrinus	x	(x)	x	Small intestine	L_1
T. longispicularis	(x)	x	x	Small intestine	L_1
T. axei	x	x	x	Abomasum	L_1
Nematodirus spathiger	x	(x)	x	Small intestine	L_3
N. filicollis	x	(x)	x	Small intestine	L_3
N. helvetianus	(x)	x	x	Small intestine	L_3
N. battus		(x)		Small intestine	L_3
Cooperia curticei		x	x	Small intestine	L_1
C. oncophora	(x)	x		Small intestine	L_1
C. punctata	(x)	x		Small intestine	L_1

(x) = Principal host.

worms and eggs had a value of $144 million (1957 dollars). Is this calculated loss merely a trivial exercise? Apparently not. Other lines of evidence point to economic benefits that can be realized when subclinical worm burdens are further reduced through treatment.

Morphology

Worms of the superfamily Trichostrongyloidea all have a small buccal capsule and a large bursa. The paired spicules are stout and heavily sclerotized; in addition to the spicules there is a dorsal sclerotization of the cloaca called a gubernaculum, which serves as a guide when the spicules are protruded. A good deal of variation occurs in the copulatory apparatus of the males (Fig. 30.1). The females within a genus often cannot be differentiated from one another; specific identification is therefore based on males.

These are long slender worms which are usually colorless, but in the case of the bloodsucking species, the blood can be seen through the body wall; *Haemonchus* is referred to as the barber-pole worm, because of the intertwined red intestine and the white ovary or testis. *Trichostrongylus axei* males are 2.3 to 6.0 mm long by 50 to 60 μm wide; females are 3.2 to 8.0 mm by 55 to 70 μm. *T. colubriformis* males are 4.3 to 7.7 mm and the females are 5.0 to 8.6 mm. *Haemonchus* males are 10 to 20 mm by 0.4 mm and females are 18 to 30 mm by 0.5 mm. *Ostertagia ostertagi* males are 6.5 to 7.5 mm and females are 8.3 to 9.2 mm; members of this genus are reddish-brown.

Life Cycle

The general pattern in the life cycle holds for all members of the superfamily: eggs are passed with the feces and the L_3 is the infective stage. The L_3s are eaten with the forage and invade the tissues of the true stomach (abomasum) or small intestine.

The times for development to infectivity at any given temperature vary. At constant conditions, *Haemonchus* may reach L_3 in three days, whereas *Nematodirus* may require ten days. Also, *Nematodirus*, unlike most of the other genera, remains within the egg capsules until it hatches as an L_3; the stages outside the host in this genus rely on stored food for development and survival.

The site of development is somewhat different for each species, and the stimuli for exsheathment differ as well. As discussed in other sections of this book, the host provides a stimulus that triggers the transition from the free-living to the parasitic phase of the cycle. The stimulus for *Haemonchus* is CO_2 under reducing conditions in balanced salt solution, whereas *Trichostrongylus* require CO_2 and acid pepsin for exsheathment; these worms inhabit the abomasum and small intestine, respectively, and the triggers represent the conditions just anterior to the site where the worm normally establishes.

The prepatent period for most of the worms is 14 to 18 days upon initial infection. With a subsequent infection, due to immunity or other undefined factors, the prepatent period may be stretched out for weeks or months.

Diagnosis

Diagnosis is based on a number of factors:

1. History of the herd
2. Clinical signs
3. Trichostrongyle fecal egg counts
4. Recovery of worms at postmortem examination

In any one area, a high probability exists that a certain complex of worms cause problems in certain ages of animals at certain times of the year (Table 30.2). Thus, if anemia occurred in animals during the middle of the pasture season, *Haemonchus* would be suspected. If only the lambs in a flock of sheep had severe diarrhea either early or late in the pasture season, *Nematodirus* would be a good bet.

If animals are dead or moribund, a postmortem examination of a few of them is the surest way of de-

TABLE 30.2 Survival of Sheep Nematode Larvae on Temperate Zone Pastures[a]

Type of weather	Survival		
	Optimum[b]	Intermediate	Minimum or None[b]
Warm, moist (summer weather with high maximum temperature and adequate rainfall)	*Cooperia* *Haemonchus* *Oesophagostomum*[c] *Trichostrongylus*	*Nematodirus* *Ostertagia*	
Warm, dry (summer weather with high maximum temperature and low rainfall or drought)		*Cooperia* *Nematodirus* *Trichostrongylus*[c]	*Haemonchus* *Oesophagostomum*[c] *Ostertagia*
Cool, moist (early spring or late fall weather with moderate temperatures and adequate rainfall)	*Nematodirus* *Ostertagia* *Trichostrongylus*	*Cooperia* *Haemonchus* *Oesophagostomum*[c]	
Cool, dry (early spring or late fall weather with moderate temperatures and low rainfall or drought)	*Nematodirus*	*Ostertagia* *Trichostrongylus*	*Cooperia* *Haemonchus* *Oesophagostomum*[c]
Over winter in regions where subfreezing temperatures occur	*Nematodirus* *Ostertagia*		*Cooperia* *Haemonchus* *Oesophagostomum*[c] *Trichostrongylus*

[a]From Levine (1963).
[b]Optimum survival = survival of many larvae for two or more months during the grazing season or over winter. Intermediate survival = survival of many larvae longer than one month but less than two months during the grazing season. Minimum or no survival = survival of few or no larvae after one month or less during the grazing season or over winter.
[c]Presumably, *Oe. columbianum*, not *Oe. venulosum*.

termining what the species and number of worms are. Weight loss, diarrhea, and anemia are typical signs of helminthosis in ruminants, but other infectious agents and some intoxications can also cause the same signs. Therefore, it is essential that other causes of disease be kept in mind when performing a postmortem examination.

Fecal egg counts have utility in epidemiologic studies and in diagnosis when the data are conservatively interpreted. The factors that must be taken into account are the following:

1. Egg counts in cattle rarely exceed 300/g of feces, whereas in sheep they are often 1000/g or higher.
2. Different species of worms produce eggs at different rates. A rough rule of thumb is as follows:

Genus	Eggs/female worm/day
Haemonchus	5000
Bunostomum	5000
Trichostrongylus	1000
Nematodirus	300

(Note: these figures were complied from various sources and are intended only as a general guideline.)

3. Helminthosis is sometimes seen prior to sexual maturity of the worms, such as in *Ostertagia* and *Oesophagostomum* infections.
4. Egg production varies from season to season. Winter time is usually associated with low egg production, and counts often rise in spring.
5. Some eggs can be differentiated from one another quite readily. However, a great deal of skill (and perhaps imagination) is required to differentiate among *Haemonchus*, *Trichostrongylus*, *Bunostomum*, *Cooperia*, and *Oesophagostomum*. *Nematodirus*, *Strongyloides*, lungworm larvae, and *Trichuris*, as well as tapeworm eggs and fluke eggs, can be readily identified.

Although we consider the trichostrongyles in this chapter, the gastrointestinal nematodes include hookworms such as *Bunostomum*, *Oesphagostomum* the nodular worm, the threadworm *Strongyloides*, *Trichuris* the whipworm, and members of the Metastrongyloidea, the lungworms. A nearly pure infection with a single species of worm may occur, but this is exceptional. In nearly all helminthoses there is a mixture of half a dozen species or more. Lungworms, especially in warm, wet climates, are often part of the parasite mix that causes economic losses. Thus, the need for worm counts becomes clearer. In sheep, 1000 to 2000 worms is not usually cause for concern, but when perhaps 5000 worms are present, helminthosis is probable. In cattle, the numbers are higher and worm counts in excess of 5000 are not uncommon in normal animals, but when the number is 10,000 or greater, the worms cause losses.

Host–Parasite Interactions

In considering damage to the host, one must take into account not only the trichostrongyles, which are the subject of this chapter, but also the nodular worms (Chapter 29), hookworms (Chapter 27), *Strongyloides* (Chapter 26), and lungworms (Chapter 31).

Because helminthosis is typically caused by a complex of species, the signs and symptoms of infection are usually diarrhea, weight loss, anemia, and dehydration. But the underlying question is, how do the worms damage the host? A part of the answer is that each species among the major pathogens causes damage in a different way. In addition, each species causes more than one type of damage. We can categorize the way that worms damage the host in the following way:

1. Stage of life cycle
   a. Larvae
   b. Adults
2. Type of damage
   a. Anemia
      (1) Blood loss: *Haemonchus, Ostertagia, Bunostomum*
      (2) Suppression of red cell formation: *Trichostrongylus*
   b. Tissue damage
      (1) Fluid loss
      (2) Inorganic ion imbalance
      (3) Reduced efficiency of feed conversion
      (4) Secondary invasion by microbial agents
   c. Immunopathology
      (1) Nodule formation: *Oesophagostomum*
      (2) Hypersensitivity *Haemonchus*

Further complicating the pathologic processes are the following factors:

1. Age of animals
2. Breed of animals
3. Quality of the feed
4. Immune status of the herd
5. Reproductive stage of the herd (pregnant, milking or not)
6. Other stressors such as harsh weather or coinfection with viruses, for example
7. Number of worms in the host(s)

Let us first look at individual species and what we know about their mechanism of damage. Among the simplest is that of anemia caused by blood loss. In *Haemonchus, Bunostomum*, and *Ostertagia* the worms suck blood and essentially exsanguinate the host when the intensity of infection is high. In *Haemonchus*, blood sucking begins during the L_4. Some of the better studies on blood loss in haemonchosis estimate a blood loss of 0.05 to 0.08 ml/day/worm. It is sometimes said that up to 500 worms in the abomasum of a sheep will not cause significant damage, but using the previous figures, that means there is a loss of from 25 to 40 ml of blood/day and from 3750 to 6000 ml during a 5-month pasture season. If this is scaled up to a clinical level where there may be from 10,000 to 50,000 *Haemonchus* in one animal, the daily blood loss could be from 500 to 4000 ml. Obviously such a loss cannot be sustained for more than a short period. In these cases of uncomplicated haemonchosis, there is a loss of not only red cells but also of serum proteins; the result is anemia, which can readily be seen in the pale mucus membranes and the accumulation of fluid in the tissue spaces. Serum proteins maintain the osmotic pressure of the blood; when proteins are lost, fluid is not returned from the tissue spaces to the blood vessels but instead accumulates. This is best seen in ruminants in a sign called *bottle jaw*, an accumulation of fluid in the submandibular region (Fig. 30.2).

Anemia is often seen in infections with species such as *Ostertagia, Trichostrongylus*, and *Cooperia*, which are known to suck little (*Ostertagia*) or no blood. The mechanism leading to anemia seems to lie in damage to the intestine, so that there is leakage of fluids from the tissue into the lumen. Although in most instances the proteins that are lost to the lumen would be digested and recycled, it appears that the diarrhea associated with helminthosis reduces the time for digestion to occur, as well as the ability of the gut to take up nutrients. The result is a heavy loss of protein through the digestive tract. Studies on naturally infected animals indicate that they have adequate stores of everything except protein for production of hemoglobin.

Damage to the intestinal tissue of the host leads not only to anemia but also to fluid loss, inorganic molecule imbalance, dehydration, and inefficiency in feed conversion. There may also be secondary invasions by bacteria if the intestinal epithelium has been damaged.

Damage to the intestinal tissue by the larval stages and the adults can readily be seen microscopically. Worms invade the glands of the mucosa, or sometimes the submucosal areas, depending on the species. The study of histologic sections reveals that there is cell death in the vicinity of the larvae. Other techniques such as electron microscopy have shown that the tight junctions between epithelial cells are broken and fluid leaks from the tissue to the lumen. The traumatized gut further loses surface by reduction of villi.

Animals treated with a good anthelmintic are

ARRESTED DEVELOPMENT IN PARASITES

When the life cycles of parasites are described you might infer that they run at a regular pace from egg to adult and then begin egg production in helminths, or from sporozoite to sporozoite in apicomplexans. It is as if a ball were set in motion and it proceeded to roll across a smooth surface without being impeded. But life is not like that.

Parasites respond to signals in the host and the environment. They have evolved to survive and prosper, and natural selection retains those that are fit. In some instances, the life cycle of a parasite is stretched out in order to prepare for the next season when hosts will be available. In other instances parasites respond to conditions within the host such as immunity or the presence of other parasites to delay their maturation.

In 1953 a seminal paper was published in the British *Journal of Helminthology*, T. E. Gibson studied nematode parasites of horses. He found that there was a population of larvae of small strongyles in the intestinal tissues that became sexually mature only when adults were removed. He treated mares with phenothiazine, a popular anthelmintic of that day, and found that adults were eliminated, egg counts dropped to zero and then began to rise as larvae matured. Repeated treatment of the mares, who were housed in a barn and not reinfected, showed the same pattern. He concluded that a population of larvae retained in the intestinal tissue was incapable of maturing as long as adults were present. It was not clear whether immunity was involved, or whether the larvae sensed that adults were present and that there was insufficient room for more adults.

At about the same time, other British workers studied the phenomenon of "spring rise" in sheep. It had been known for many years that fecal egg counts of the stomach worm, *Haemonchus contortus*, remained low during the winter in pregnant ewes. As they approached lambing time, fecal egg counts increased. A series of studies showed that *H. contortus* larvae became sexually mature as the egg counts rose. These larvae had been acquired during the previous growing season but had not matured. Thus, as lambs were born, pastures were contaminated with the free-living stages of the parasite.

In the 1960s, outbreaks of ostertagosis were seen in cattle in winter in Scotland and northern England. The culprit was *Ostertagia ostertagi*, a stomach worm of cattle. It was found that the normal two-week prepatent period of *Ostertagia* was lengthened when the cattle were infected in late summer and fall. The worms became mature and caused disease during the winter.

A series of innovative studies by Gerhard Schad and coworkers on hookworm in India showed that this parasite of humans also has arrested development. The usual prepatent period in hookworm infections in humans is about forty days. But Schad found that it was lengthened to almost six months in India. This long prepatent period seems to be tied to the dry season in the vicinity of Calcutta. If the worms matured at their usual rate, they would have produced eggs that would be exposed to extremely dry conditions, so they have been selected to wait until the wet season to become mature.

Protozoa also adapt to climate. *Plasmodium vivax*, now seemingly eradicated from Siberia, once was a serious health problem there. It was found that the usual prepatent period of *P. vivax* was stretched out to three or four months in isolates obtained from that region. The parasites remained in the liver until there was an increased probability that a mosquito would be present to transmit the organism to another host.

relieved of nearly all of their worms and recover clinically within a matter of several days. However, a common observation is that the ability of animals to grow normally, regain lost weight, and convert feed efficiently has been compromised. Some sort of long-term damage to the gut or liver seems to have taken place.

Immunity is usually beneficial to the host, but it can be detrimental also, as has been noted in connection with other eukaryotic parasites: *Schistosoma* spp. and various filarioid nematodes. The nodules that develop around *Oesophagostomum* larvae (Chapter 29) are a case in point. The parasites are successfully walled off, but the gut is left permanently damaged and not able to function normally.

Hypersensitivity, one form of immunity, is a mixed bag of benefit and damage. In the case of certain worms of ruminants, particularly *Haemonchus contortus* of

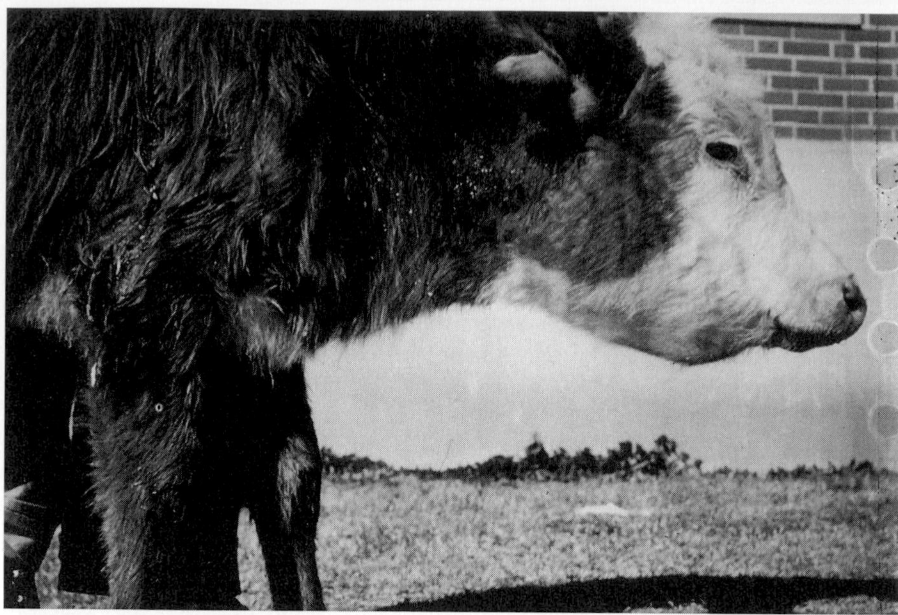

FIGURE 30.2 "Bottle jaw" in a calf. This condition is a submandibular accumulation of fluid as a result of hypoproteinemia and is frequently seen in heavy infections with *Haemonchus*.

sheep, hypersensitivity is the cause at least in part of the so-called self-cure reaction. In a certain percentage of sheep with established infections of *Haemonchus*, the whole adult population may be shed spontaneously. Most often self-cure occurs when sheep receive an inoculum of L_3s; the gut becomes highly motile and hyperemic (congested with blood) and the worms are shed two to four days later. Evidence supports the concept that the L_3s trigger a type of allergic response with release of histamine, production of mucus, and other typical reactions. Some animals are resistant, for a time, to reinfection, but others may be reinfected immediately after self-cure.

A good and useful immunity develops to gastrointestinal nematodes on repeated infection. It is not generally manifested as a sterile immunity, such as one typically sees in viral infections, but rather it serves to mitigate against clinical disease. An animal that has been infected is relatively resistant to challenge, but some of the worms in the challenge inoculum develop. Immunity is manifested in the following ways:

1. Killing some worms
2. Reduction in egg laying of adult females
3. Stunting in the growth of worms
4. Inhibition of development of preadult worms

Most of the immune response is directed against the larvae; in some studies, adults were removed (other than self-cure), but the major action is to kill or prevent development of larvae. The cuticle, or epicuticle, of nematodes is often antigenic. That is, molecules within these structures often provoke an immune response. It is not at all clear, however, that those are the immune responses associated with protective immunity. Indeed, antibody responses to microfilariae (Chapter 34) are typically damaging to the host. Other antigens that may be important to immune protection against nematodes include the excretions and secretions of larvae, including molecules associated with molting and the migration of L_3s and L_4s.

It is interesting to note that one group of thoroughly researched helminth antigens are those inside the gut of *Haemonchus contortus*. It has been demonstrated that if ruminants hosts are immunized with antigens prepared from the gut of *Haemonchus* that parasites can be seriously damaged or killed. It appears that when the parasite ingests blood that contains antibody to its own gut antigens, the resulting antibody-mediated damage destroys the parasite. This is consistent with the so-called hidden antigen approach used in developing vaccines against ticks (Chapter 51).

Inhibition of larval development is an important factor in both epidemiology and clinical disease. There is undoubtedly a strong immunologic component in this inhibition, but there are also other factors such as host physiologic state and interaction among the parasites themselves that influence inhibition and its release.

One of the first known instances of larval inhibition was observed as part of the "spring rise" phenomenon in sheep in Britain. It had been observed as early as the 1930s that toward the end of winter or in early spring, pregnant ewes not yet on pasture showed a striking increase in fecal egg counts. In the 1950s it was finally found that spring rise came about through the maturation of *Haemonchus* larvae that had lain dormant for many months, probably since the animals had been taken off of pasture in late fall. The larvae developed partially and then stopped. Toward the end of pregnancy and at the time when animals would be going out on pasture, development resumed and the worms became sexually mature. The question is whether maturation results from (1) a lowering of the level of immunity, (2) a response to hormonal levels in the ewe, (3) an inherent annual rhythm in the worms, or (4) a change in larval physiology as the weather changes at the end of the pasture season. All except the last of these are still open issues, and in other instances such as hookworm and *Ostertagia* there may be a difference in larvae, depending on the season.

A second case of inhibited development occurs in *Ostertagia* infections in cattle. Egg laying in *Ostertagia* infections begins 16 to 23 days after administration of L_3s. In single infections, clinical signs of diarrhea and weight loss closely coincide with the maturation of the worms. This uncomplicated event is referred to as Type I ostertagosis. In Type II ostertagosis, the appearance of clinical signs is delayed for weeks or months by retention of fourth-stage larvae in the tissue of the abomasum. Typically, animals have been on pasture and have come off at the end of the grazing season to be fed hay or other wintertime feed. The animals may remain normal until late winter or even early spring and then come down with clinical ostertagosis coinciding with the maturation of the inhibited L_4s. In many cases, the presence of larvae in the gastric glands destroys the function of these glands, and profound disease may result prior to the reinitiation of maturation of the L_4s.

Epidemiology and Control

The following are approaches that have been taken to control harmful populations of nematodes in ruminants:

1. Periodic treatment
2. Stock rotation, also known as *pasture rotation*
3. Grazing of pastures by nonsusceptible species
4. Killing the free-living stages on pasture
5. Maintaining a high level of nutrition
6. Immunization

Helminthosis in domestic livestock is a herd problem and is approached as such. All of the animals in a herd are treated, though some may not be in immediate need of treatment.

Several modern anthelmintics can be used to kill intestinal nematodes, typically the adult stage. The most successful anthelmintics developed in the past three decades are (1) the benzimidazoles, such as thiabendazole, and (2) the macrolide antibiotics such as ivermectin. Various drugs in these two classes have been used in different formulations, all generally intended to make administration of the drugs easier and therefore more likely to be used. Drugs have been added to animal feed or feed supplements, but making drugs that can be poured onto the backs of animals have been more practical on a herd-wide basis than those drugs administered orally.

Drugs for killing intestinal nematodes are now highly effective. Various formulations make it practical to treat large numbers of animals with minimal labor and minimal trauma to the animals. The spectrum of activity of the drugs is quite broad and they not only kill adults but may kill larvae of nematodes and some ectoparasites such as lice as well.

Despite having reach a seeming anthelmintic utopia, we have managed to create other problems. For example, using broad spectrum drugs aggressively and without switching periodically to other drugs has allowed drug resistance to develop. There is no substitute for integrating the use of anthelmintics with knowledge of the biology of the parasites in order to obtain optimal control of disease.

A considerable body of literature exists on the development and survival of the free-living stages of the trichostrongyles, especially *Haemonchus*, *Trichostrongylus colubriformis*, *T. axei*, *Ostertagia circumcincta*, *O. ostertagi*, *Nematodirus spathiger*, and *N. battus*. Other nematodes of ruminants—*Strongyloides*, *Dictyocaulus*, and *Bunostomum*—have been studied extensively (Gibson, 1966; Gordon, 1948, Levine, 1963, 1980; Michel, 1969; Ollerenshaw and Smith, 1969; Rogers and Sommerville, 1963, 1968; Thomas, 1974).

The reason for these numerous and classical studies resides in the crucial role that the free-living stages play in maintaining infection and in allowing clinical infections to develop. The basic questions asked by all of these studies were the following: Under what conditions do animals become infected, and how can the system be manipulated so that animals will not develop harmful infections? Despite many avenues of investigation, these questions are at the core of all the studies.

Data are gathered in a variety of ways on the free-living stages and on the worm burdens actually found in naturally infected animals.

Free-Living Stages

1. In the laboratory the time to reach infectivity and the length of survival of infective stages are studied under constant, controlled conditions.

2. In the field eggs and larvae are placed on pasture under the fluctuating conditions found in nature. Materials are placed out at various times and then retrieved periodically, and survival and development are determined. Often pasture clippings are examined for L_3s and calculations are made on the number of infective larvae that might be ingested in a day by an ox or a sheep.

3. Purposely contaminated pastures are grazed periodically by sentinel animals. The concept of a sentinel animal is that a susceptible animal is exposed to the infectious agent under natural conditions of transmission for a period and then examined for evidence of infection. A series of groups of, say, five animals are allowed to graze a contaminated pasture each for a week or so and then examined for the presence of infection either by fecal egg count or by postmortem examination.

Worm Populations

The kinds of worms that are likely to cause problems in ruminants vary with the geographic/climatic area. One way of finding out what worms are present is through the use of "parasite profiles," (Fig. 30.3). These data are for sheep, and one might expect somewhat different results for cattle. Note that *Haemonchus* is the principal parasite in Beltsville, Maryland, *Cooperia* in Auburn, Alabama, and *Ostertagia* in Moscow, Idaho. The situation is somewhat different in Lexington, Kentucky, and in College Station, Texas, where a number of species are more or less evenly distributed in proportion to the population of nematodes.

Parasite profiles are useful as a rough index of which worms one might expect to be important; however, development of such a profile does not constitute an epidemiologic study. A properly designed epidemiologic study focuses on carefully conducted host examinations of an adequate sample of adults and young of both sexes taken at various seasons of the year.

In the broad sense, development to infectivity of the free-living stages of nematodes depends on temperature, moisture, and oxygen. We can generalize rather loosely and state that for trichostrongyles a temperature of from 10 to 35°C (50 to 95°F) allows development. Development is too slow to be significant at temperatures below 10°C (50°F) and at temperatures above 35°C (95°F) they are harmful to the free-living stages. Moisture needs are not so consistent; some worms require water, others can get along with a saturated atmosphere, and some do well at 50% saturation. Oxygen is required by all worms; if the environment becomes anaerobic through excess water and bacterial action, development is inhibited and eventually the free-living stages are killed.

When individual requirements for development and survival are examined, a pattern emerges of what each species requires and can tolerate (Table 30.2), so that it is possible to see the factors that affect populations of various genera of gastrointestinal nematodes. For example, *Cooperia*, *Haemonchus*, *Oesophagostomum*, and *Trichostrongylus* do well where there is a warm, moist summer, but they survive poorly, or not at all, where winters are hard. *Nematodirus* and *Ostertagia*, on the other hand, do well in climates that are more difficult (i.e., cold and dry).

Various approaches have been taken to refine the climatic and meteorologic conditions that affect transmission. In Australia, heavy dependence on the sheep industry made control of infectious diseases a national priority, and the pioneering work of Clunies Ross and H. Mc.L. Gordon laid the groundwork used by parasitologists and livestock raisers around the world. Gordon (1948) used bioclimatographs to describe and predict when transmission would occur. A bioclimatograph (Fig. 30.4) plots mean monthly temperature in a weather shelter against mean monthly precipitation. If we look at the plot for Urbana, Illinois, we see that a dot is placed at the junction of the temperature and precipitation for each month and the months are then connected sequentially with a line. June, July, August, and September have temperatures between 20 and 25°C and 75 to 100 mm precipitation. As the fall progresses, the temperature declines to about 0°C and precipitation to about 50 mm. One can then use a bioclimatograph together with laboratory data on a species of worm to predict when transmission will take place. As noted in the figure legend, *Haemonchus* is transmitted when the precipitation is 50 mm or higher and the temperature is above 15°C.

Bioclimatographs are useful, but they also have some serious drawbacks. Weather shelter data are easy to obtain since records are readily available in nearly any locality. The principal problem is that the temperature is taken 1.5 m above the ground. The real activity is in the plants and at the soil surface; as someone said, "very few sheep have become infected in a weather shelter."

A number of factors are important in the grass and at the soil surface where grazing animals actually become infected. Temperature is stable: seasonal and daily fluctuations are not as great as in the air. Moisture is

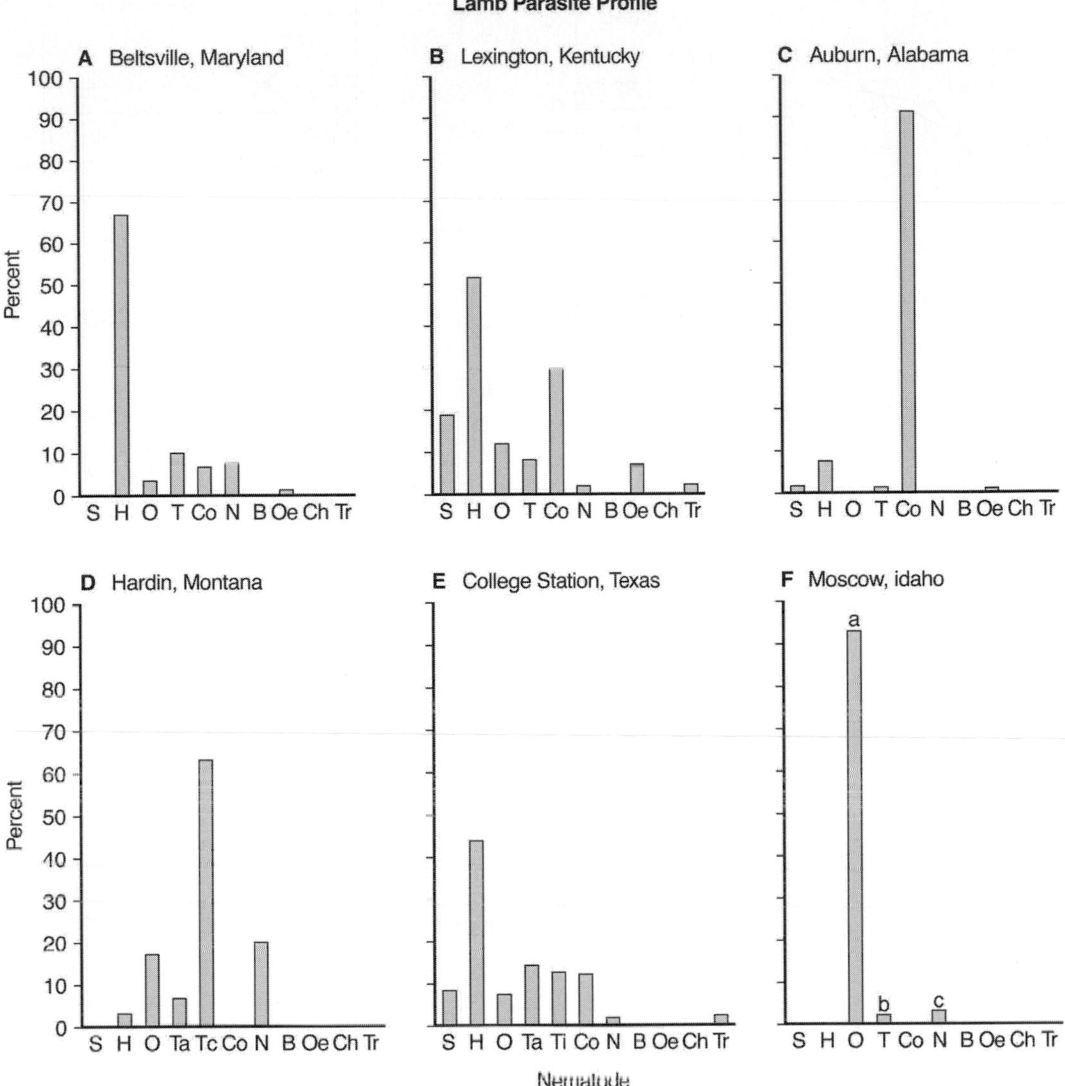

FIGURE 30.3 Parasite profiles of sheep from different region of the United States. (A) Beltsville, Maryland; (B) Lexington, Kentucky; (C) Auburn, Alabama; (D) Hardin, Montana; (E) College Station, Texas; (F). Moscow, Idaho. (a, 90% *Ostertagia circumcincta*; b, usually less than 1%, c, usually less than 3% in adult sheep). Abbreviations: B, *Bunostomum;* Ch, *Chabertia;* Co, *Cooperia;* H, *Haemonchus,* N, *Nematodirus;* O, *Ostertagia;* Oe, *Oesophagostomum;* S, *Strongyloides;* T, *Trichostrongylus;* Ta, *Trichostrongylus axei;* Tc, *Trichostrongylus colubriformis;* Ti, intestinal species of *Trichostrongylus;* Tr, *Trichuris.* [A, B, C, E, and F from Levine, N. D., 1980; D from W. C. Marquardt, unpublished data.]

relatively constant and may be present when there has been no rain for a long period; even nightly dew can provide water for a portion of the day. Plants provide protection from the harmful effects of ultraviolet irradiation and heat from the sun. To deal with these factors, Levine (1963) (Fig. 30.5) looked at available moisture in various climates of North America. In a temperate climate of, say, the Midwestern United States, the soil becomes dry toward the end of the growing season; then, with cooler weather it begins to recharge with moisture. By the beginning of the growing season, the soil is saturated in a locality such as Urbana, Illinois. In some areas such as Lubbock in west Texas, the soil does not saturate; there is enough moisture for growth of grass and other plants tolerant of arid conditions, but the soil is dry most of the time. Moisture in the soil continually moves out by transpiration from plants and evaporation from soil. If there is water in the soil, there will be moisture near the lower portions of the plants and at the soil surface where the worms are.

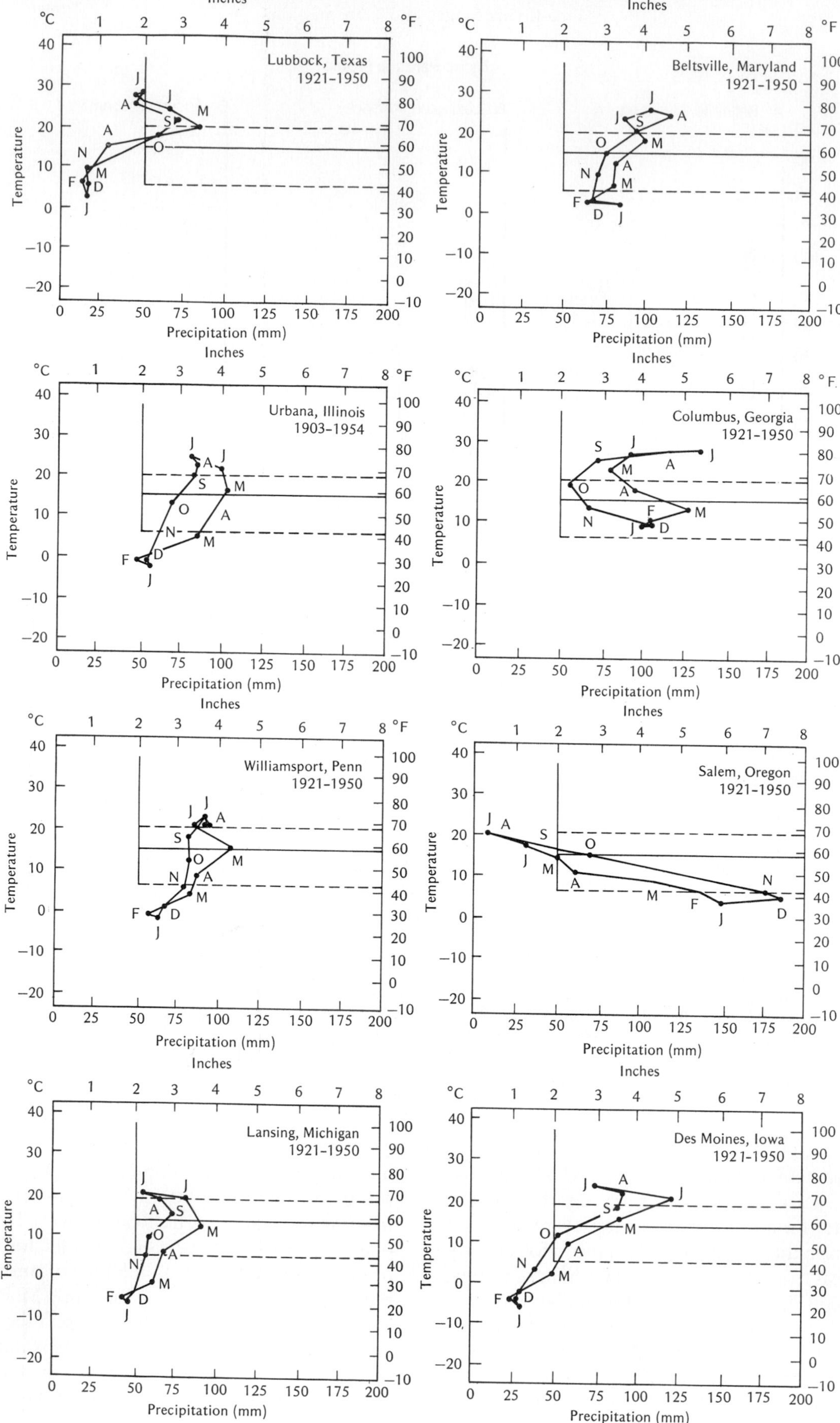

Lubbock, Texas 1921–1950
Beltsville, Maryland 1921–1950
Urbana, Illinois 1903–1954
Columbus, Georgia 1921–1950
Williamsport, Penn 1921–1950
Salem, Oregon 1921–1950
Lansing, Michigan 1921–1950
Des Moines, Iowa 1921–1950
Inches
°C
°F
Temperature
Precipitation (mm)

The data on moisture availability and on temperature were carried one step further (Fig. 30.6) to allow prediction of the conditions under which transmission of *Haemonchus* and *Trichostrongylus* might occur in various climates.

On a global basis, *Haemonchus contortus* and *H. placei* probably cause more losses than any other species of nematodes in ruminants. *Haemonchus* is a heavy egg producer; estimates as high as 5000 eggs/day/female worm give an idea of the amount of pasture contamination that it can cause when an animal has 1000 to 10,000 female worms in its abomasum. *Haemonchus* is also relatively long lived in the host; an individual may live for months, and the spring rise phenomenon further contributes to heavy pasture contamination of L_3s when young, susceptible, immunologically naive animals begin to graze.

Despite the fact that *Haemonchus* prefers warm, moist conditions, it is often found in climates where its presence would be unexpected. For example, *Haemonchus* is a problem in the Red River Valley of North Dakota near Fargo. The bitter winters of this area in great part kill the free-living stages, but the infection can be maintained in ewes over the winter. An outbreak of haemonchosis occurred in Montana on irrigated pasture and in animals kept on a low island in a stream. In areas where animals water from troughs, spilled water may allow a lush growth of grass in a small area; animals like this grass and it may have large numbers of infective larvae. Since worms are always present in ruminants, the potential for a rapid increase in the population is also great.

With *Haemonchus* the adult animals maintain a moderate population of worms and pass the infection to younger animals during the pasture season. The situation with *Nematodirus* exemplifies a different epidemiologic picture. *Nematodirus* is found in significant numbers only in lambs. If host examinations are done on ewes, few or none are found; this prevalence mainly in younger animals is one reason for carefully designing an epidemiologic study.

During the mid-1950s it was found that outbreaks of diarrheal disease in lambs in Great Britain were caused by *Nematodirus battus*. Few worms were found in ewes, but lambs were subject to overwhelming infections. The question was, how did the lambs acquire such massive infections? The answer revolves around the slow development of the free-living stages and of their remarkable resistance to environmental insult. *Nematodirus* does not hatch until the L_3 has been reached, so it is somewhat different from most of the other trichostrongyles that have free-living, feeding L_1s and L_2s. Even under optimal conditions, *Nematodirus* L_3s do not hatch for two weeks, whereas *Haemonchus* can reach L_3 in as few as four days. Careful studies by British workers showed that eggs deposited on pasture during late summer and fall do not reach infectivity until late winter or early spring, at which time they appear in massive numbers. Sheep husbandry calls for lambs to be born just about the time that ewes and lambs go on pasture in the spring. Thus the most susceptible members of the population were being exposed to massive numbers of infective larvae. The concept developed from these investigations was that there is a lamb-to-lamb transfer in *Nematodirus battus*; the ewes are not important. The infection in last year's lamb crop is the source of infection for this year's lamb crop.

With *Haemonchus*, other trichostrongyles, and *Nematodirus*, clinical disease comes about through the exposure of susceptible animals to large numbers of infective larvae over a short period of time. In *Haemonchus*, *Trichostrongylus*, and *Ostertagia*, the infection comes from the ewes (Fig. 30.7); on the other hand, in nematodirosis, the infection comes from the long development and simultaneous hatching of the L_3s as the lambs begin to take solid food (Fig. 30.8). In both cases there is a steep rise in the number of L_3s on the herbage. Much has been said about the buildup on pasture of free-living stages through successive generations of worms; calculations have been made showing how such an increase occurs. The problem is that it does not happen that way at all in climates with definite seasonal changes. What the graphs show is the sudden appearance of L_3s at a particular time of year. Depending on the species, the time of year varies, but the general principal is that the preinfective stages accumulate on pasture during hard times and develop slowly toward L_3. Then, when moisture or temperature

FIGURE 30.4 Bioclimatographs from various localities in the United States. Temperature is plotted against precipitation for each month of the year sequentially. Temperatures are given in both Celsius and Fahrenheit and precipitation in both English and metric units. *Haemonchus* can be transmitted during the times when precipitation and temperature both fall between the dotted horizontal lines. Compare the two top graphs for Lubbock, Texas, and Beltsville, Maryland. At Lubbock precipitation allows transmission of *Haemonchus* in perhaps two or three months of the year while at Beltsville, *Hasemonchus* can be transmitted during at least five months. [Redrawn from Levine, 1963.]

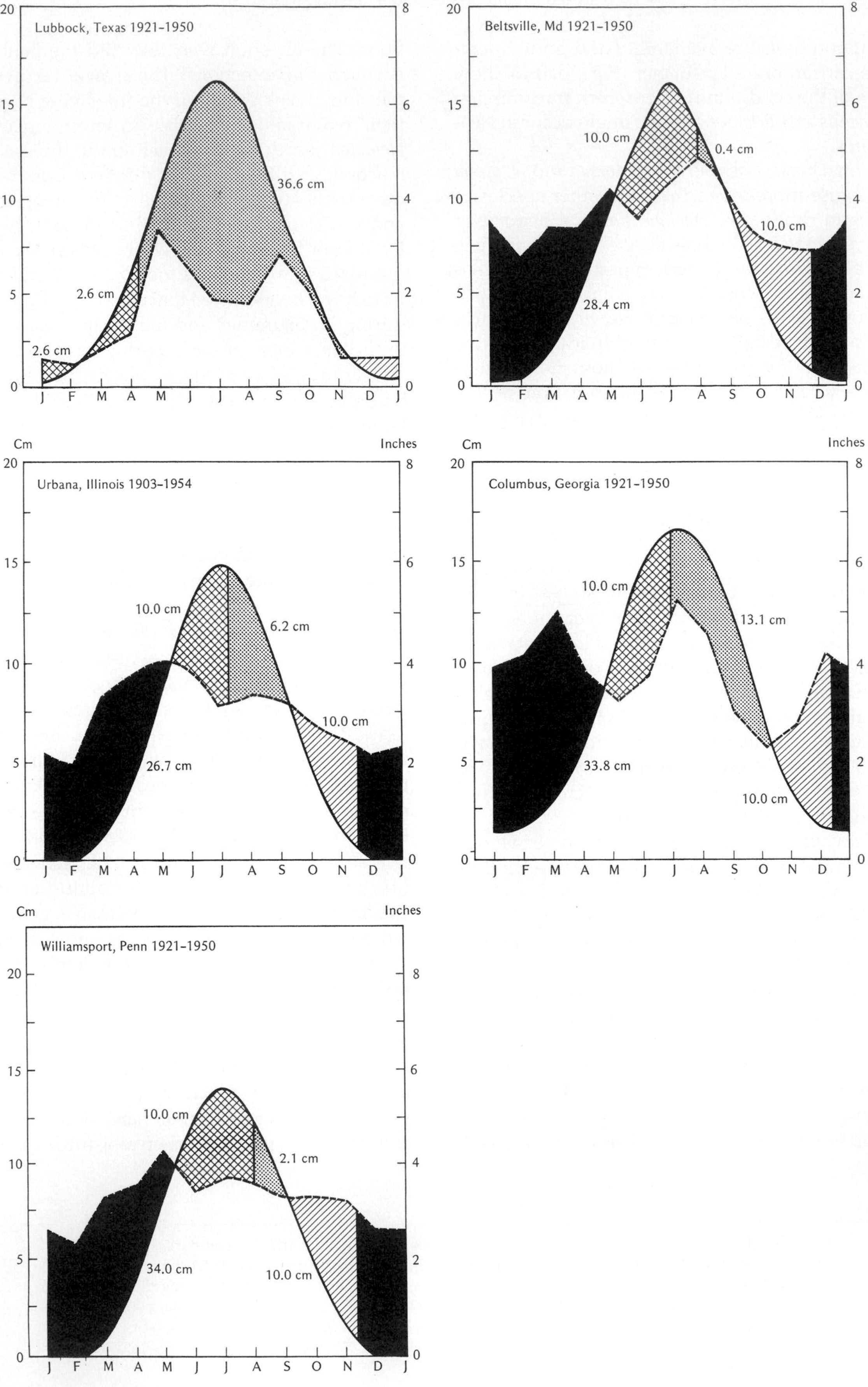

Cm
Inches
Lubbock, Texas 1921–1950
36.6 cm
2.6 cm
2.6 cm
Beltsville, Md 1921–1950
10.0 cm
0.4 cm
10.0 cm
28.4 cm
Urbana, Illinois 1903–1954
10.0 cm
6.2 cm
10.0 cm
26.7 cm
Columbus, Georgia 1921–1950
10.0 cm
13.1 cm
33.8 cm
10.0 cm
Williamsport, Penn 1921–1950
10.0 cm
2.1 cm
34.0 cm
10.0 cm
J F M A M J J A S O N D J

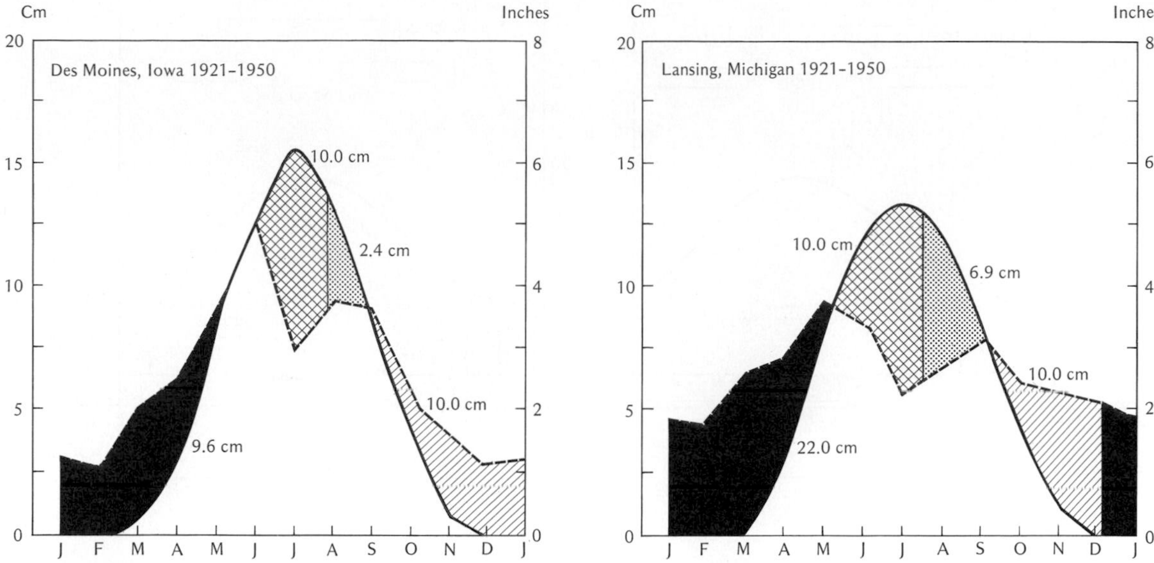

FIGURE 30.5 Potential evapotranspiration and available moisture for various localities in the United States. Compare Lubbock Texas with Beltsville, Maryland, and note that the soil is saturated from December to May at Beltsville while it never saturates at Lubbock. The soil is dry at Lubbock for seven months of the year while at Beltsville it is dry only for a short time toward the end of the growing season. [Redrawn from Levine, 1963.]

reaches the proper level, the development continues to infectivity like a thunderclap.

Species of worms differ in development and survival, as do the nutrition, immunity of the hosts, and turnover or inhibition of populations in the hosts. The objective of a control program is to prevent financial loss; eradication of worms of grazing animals is not a feasible goal. Therefore, a livestock owner lives with the problem, recognizes that there is a continual threat of loss, and tries to minimize it.

Among the methods that have been used, stock rotation (pasture rotation, hurdling, pasture spelling) allows animals to graze for a period less than that required for development to the L_3 and then animals are moved to clean pasture. Animals are moved through a series of pastures and then returned to the first one, presumably when the free-living stages have died out. The principal problem is that animals cannot be left off of pasture long enough during the growing season for the free-living stages to die. In fact, if animals are returned to the original pasture a month later, the population of L_3s is likely to be at its peak. Stock rotation alone, at the end of a number of careful investigations, does not control nematodes but does allow good utilization of pasture forage.

The best approach to minimizing losses is to know what worms are likely to cause problems and when it is likely to happen (Ollerenshaw and Smith, 1969). An epidemiologic investigation is done to determine what worms are present and then to monitor both the health of the animals and worm populations. Animals are then treated before there are significant losses. Theoretically, the animals will have developed immunity through subclinical infections and if they are watched for signs of helminthosis, the nutritional level can be maintained so as to minimize the effects of the worms.

A key to control is the development of immunity. In haemonchosis and nematodirus disease, lambs are subjected to large numbers of infective larvae before they can develop effective immunity. The goal of many research groups has been to facilitate the development of immunity so that animals can withstand infection. There has been some recent success with experimental vaccines for haemonchosis. These successes remain far from a commercial product, and it remains unclear whether a vaccine against a single species of worm would have a practical role. Whatever product is eventually developed, it will most likely aid the acquisition of immunity that occurs through natural exposure and will be coupled with strategic anthelmintic treatment.

The proposal has sometimes been made that rather than have animals graze on pasture, it would be better to bring the pasture to them. The so-called zero grazing or feeding green chop consists of cutting forage and bringing it to animals kept in corrals or buildings where the possibility of their becoming infected with worms is exceedingly low. Additional benefits are that

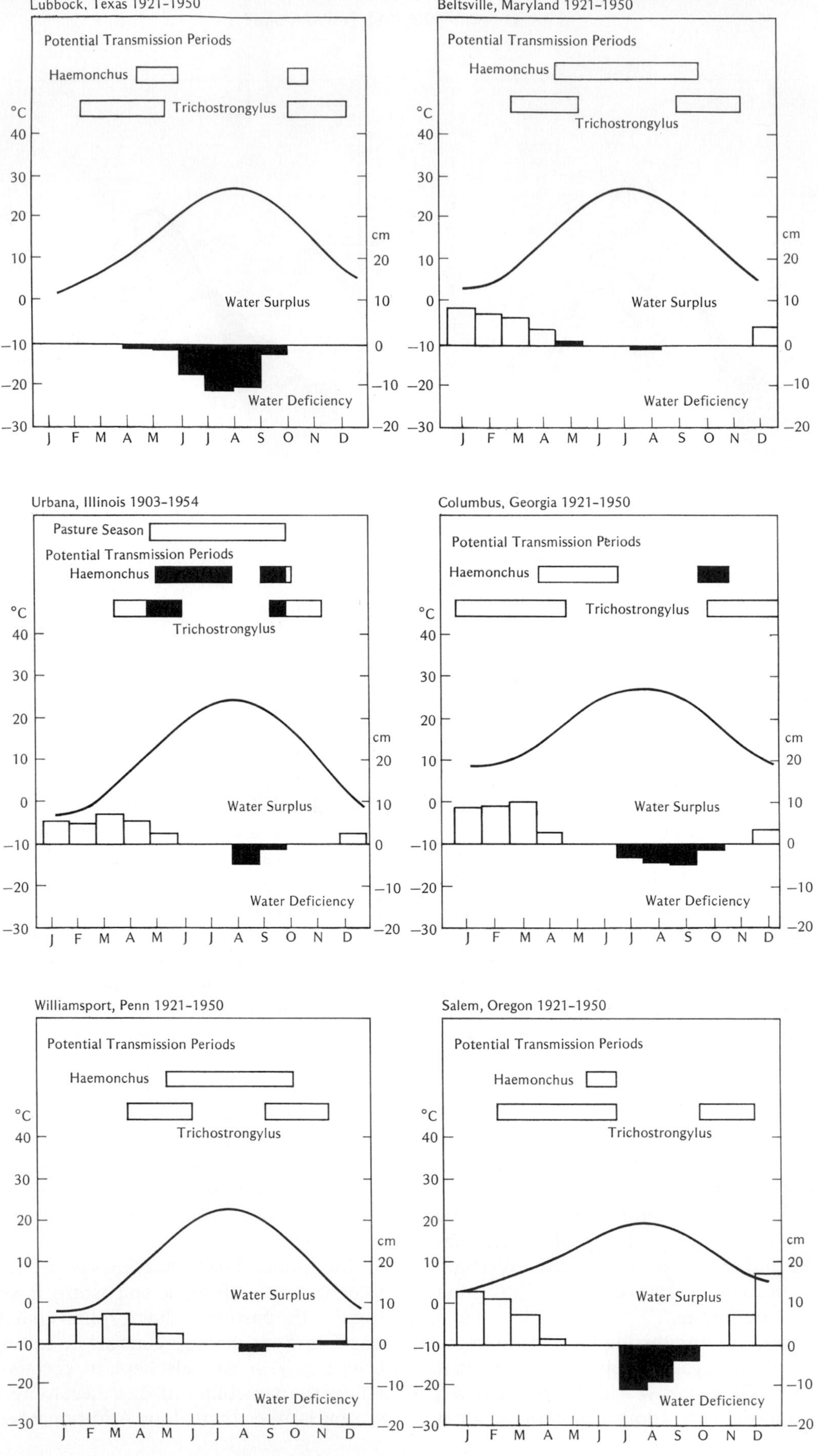
Lubbock, Texas 1921–1950
Potential Transmission Periods
Haemonchus
Trichostrongylus
°C
cm
Water Surplus
Water Deficiency
J F M A M J J A S O N D
Beltsville, Maryland 1921–1950
Potential Transmission Periods
Haemonchus
Trichostrongylus
Water Surplus
Water Deficiency
Urbana, Illinois 1903–1954
Pasture Season
Potential Transmission Periods
Haemonchus
Trichostrongylus
Water Surplus
Water Deficiency
Columbus, Georgia 1921–1950
Potential Transmission Periods
Haemonchus
Trichostrongylus
Water Surplus
Water Deficiency
Williamsport, Penn 1921–1950
Potential Transmission Periods
Haemonchus
Trichostrongylus
Water Surplus
Water Deficiency
Salem, Oregon 1921–1950
Potential Transmission Periods
Haemonchus
Trichostrongylus
Water Surplus
Water Deficiency

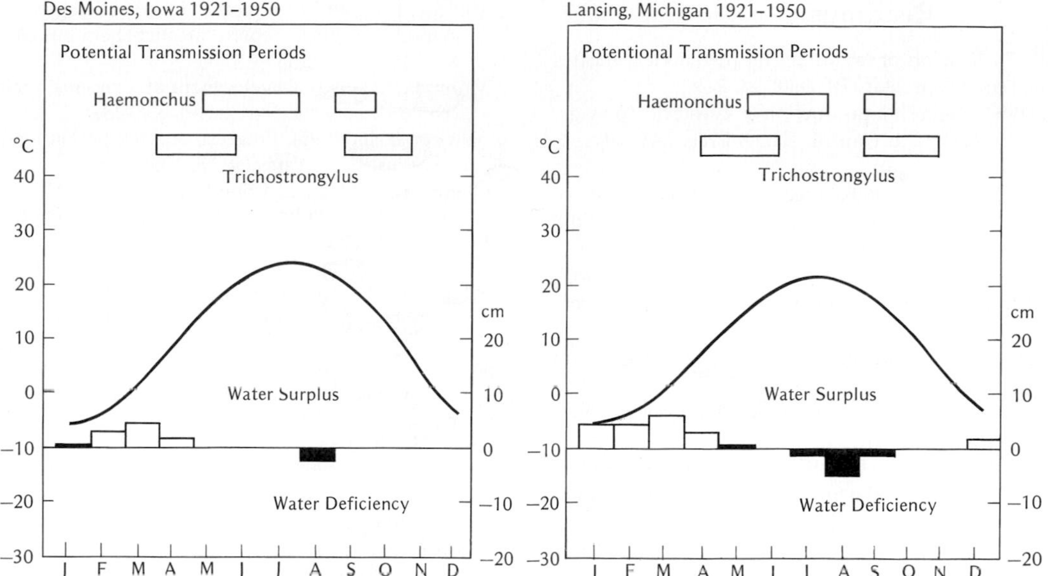

FIGURE 30.6 Times of the year when transmission of gastrointestinal nematodes can occur in various localities. These plots translate the data in Figure 30.5 to times of potential transmission. The temperature in degrees Celsius is along the left axis and is represented by the solid "bell curve" line. Available moisture is represented by the bar graph and the scale is along the right axis as cm of surplus or deficiency. Compare Lubbock, Texas, where there is never an excess of moisture in the soil and transmission of both *Haemonchus* and *Trichostrongylus* can occur only for short periods in spring and fall while at Beltsville *Haemonchus* can be transmitted for six months or more on pasture. The blackened boxes indicate the times when transmission can be especially high. ▩, Soil moisture utilization; □, soil moisture recharge; ▤, water deficiency; ■, water surplus.

the pasture would be well utilized because it would not be trampled or selectively grazed. Such a system might work where there is a long growing season with abundant rainfall and where both energy and labor costs are low. However, most ruminants are raised on the vast grasslands, savannas, and steppes that comprise the largest biomes in the world in Asia, North America, South America, Africa, and Australia. The zero-grazing proposal ignores the facts of life for the greater part of animal husbandry on earth.

As knowledge has progressed on infectious diseases, attempts have been made to develop mathematical relationships among the factors involved in disease transmission. In this book, some attention has been given to schistosomes of humans and fascioliasis of ruminants. Success has been moderate with *Nematodirus* spp.; the beginnings of methods exist for the other trichostrongyles, but little has been done for lungworms of ruminants.

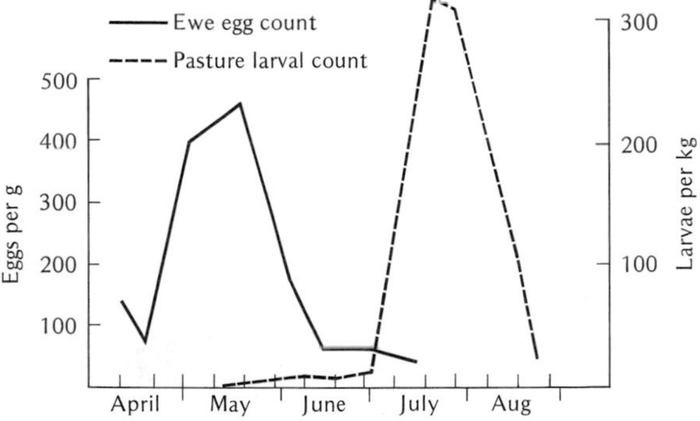

FIGURE 30.7 Gastrointestinal nematode infections in sheep: egg counts in ewes and pasture contamination with larvae. [Redrawn from Thomas, 1974.]

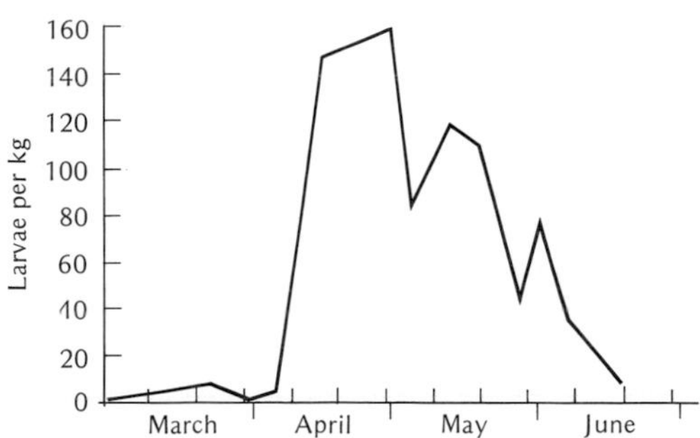

FIGURE 30.8 Occurrence of third-stage larvae of *Nematodirus battus* on pasture in Britain. [Redrawn from Thomas, 1974.]

Readings

Behnke, J. M. (1987). Evasion of immunity by nematode parasites causing chronic infections. *Adv. Parasitol.* **26,** 2–72.

Boughton, D. C. (1957). Helminth production in livestock: Tonnage, carrying capacity, costs and control. *Am. J. Trop. Med. Hyg.* **6,** 455–461.

Gibson, T. E. (1966). The ecology of the infective larvae of *Trichostrongylus colubriformis.* In *Biology of Parasites* (E. J. L. Soulsby, Ed.), pp. 2–13. Academic Press, New York.

Gordon, H. McL. (1948). The epidemiology of parasitic diseases with special reference to studies with nematode parasites of sheep. *Aust. Vet. J.* **24,** 17–44.

Levine, N. D. (1963). Weather, climate and the bionomics of ruminant nematode larvae. *Adv. Vet. Sci.* **8,** 215–261.

Levine, N. D. (1980). *Nematode Parasites of Domestic Animals and Man,* 2nd ed. Burgess, Minneapolis.

Lichtenfels, J. R., and Tromba, F. G. (1972). The morphogenesis of *Stephanurus dentatus* (Nematoda: Strongylina) in swine with observations on larval migration. *J. Parasitol.* **58,** 757–766.

Michel, J. F. (1969). The epidemiology and control of some nematode infections of grazing animals. *Adv. Parasitol.* **7,** 211–282.

Monroy, F. G., and Enriquez, F. J. (1992). *Heligmosomoides polygyrus:* A model for chronic gastrointestinal helminthosis. *Parasitol. Today* **8,** 49–54.

Munn, E. A. (1993). Development of a vaccine against *Haemonchius contortus. Parasitol. Today* **9**(9), 338–339.

Newton, S. E. (1995). Progress on vaccination against *Haemonchus contortus. Int. J. Parasitol.* **25,** 1281–1289.

Ollerenshaw, C. B., and Smith, L. P. (1969). Meteorological factors and forecasts of helminthic disease. *Adv. Parasitol.* **7,** 283–323.

Rogers, W. P. (1961). *The Nature of Parasitism: The Relationship of Some Metazoan Parasites to Their Hosts.* Academic Press, New York.

Rogers, W. P., and Sommerville, R. I. (1963). The infective stage of nematode parasites and its significance in parasitism. *Adv. Parasitol.* **1,** 109–177.

Rogers, W. P., and Sommerville, R. I. (1968). The infectious process, and its relations to the development of early parasitic stages of nematodes. *Adv. Parasitol.* **6,** 327–348.

Smith, G., and Granfell, B. T. (1985). The population biology of *Ostertagia ostertagi. Parasitol. Today* **1,** 76–81.

Thomas, R. T. (1974). The role of climate in the epidemiology of nematode parasitism in ruminants. In *The Effects of Meteorological Factors upon Parasites* (A. E. Taylor and R. Muller, Eds.), *Symp. Br. Soc. Parasitol.,* Vol. 12, pp. 13–32. Blackwell, London.

CHAPTER

31

Strongylid Lungworms

Among the bursate nematodes, the superfamily Metastrongyloidea contains the lungworms and some worms of blood vessels. They can be recognized superficially by the small buccal capsule similar to that of the trichostrongyles, a small bursa, and relatively short, uncomplicated spicules. There are a few worms in other groups of nematodes, which inhabit lungs such as the Strongyloidea and some of the spirurids, but nearly all of the metastrongyles are lungworms.

Most of the lungworms of economic importance parasitize ruminants or swine. Their life cycles are completed by ingestion of the L_3, but some have direct life cycles and some have invertebrate vectors. The effects on the host are often by direct damage, but there are some interesting interactions with other infectious agents that are discussed.

Since the L_3s are ingested, the larvae must migrate from the intestine to reach the lungs. As is true in a number of other instances, if larvae are ingested by a foreign host, migration may be abnormal. An example is eosinophilic meningitis in humans caused by *Angiostrongylus cantonensis*.

LUNGWORMS WITH DIRECT LIFE CYCLES

Name of Organism and Disease Associations

Dictyocaulus filaria and *D. viviparus* produce lungworm disease, husk, hoose, and lungworm pneumonia.

Hosts and Host Range

D. filaria is found principally in sheep and goats among domestic ruminants but also occurs in others such as camel and alpaca and some wild ruminants. *D. viviparus* is found principally in the ox but is also in other ruminants as well, both domestic and wild.

Geographic Distribution and Importance

Cosmopolitan, but lungworms usually cause problems in mild, wet climates.

In small numbers, these two species of lungworm cause no discernible damage to their hosts; however, in large numbers, or in connection with heavy infections with gastrointestinal nematodes, they can cause considerable economic loss.

Morphology

D. filaria females are from 43 to 112 mm long, with a conical posterior end and the vulva just posterior to the middle of the body. Males are from 25 to 80 mm long, with moderately heavy, bent spicules 400 to 500 μm long (Fig. 31.1).

D. viviparus females are from 23 to 80 mm long and have a short, pointed tail; the vulva is near the posterior of the body. Males are from 17 to 50 mm long, with moderately heavy, bent spicules 195 to 215 μm long.

Life Cycle

The cycles of both species are essentially the same. Adults lie in the air passages from the trachea down to the bronchioles. Eggs are coughed up, swallowed,

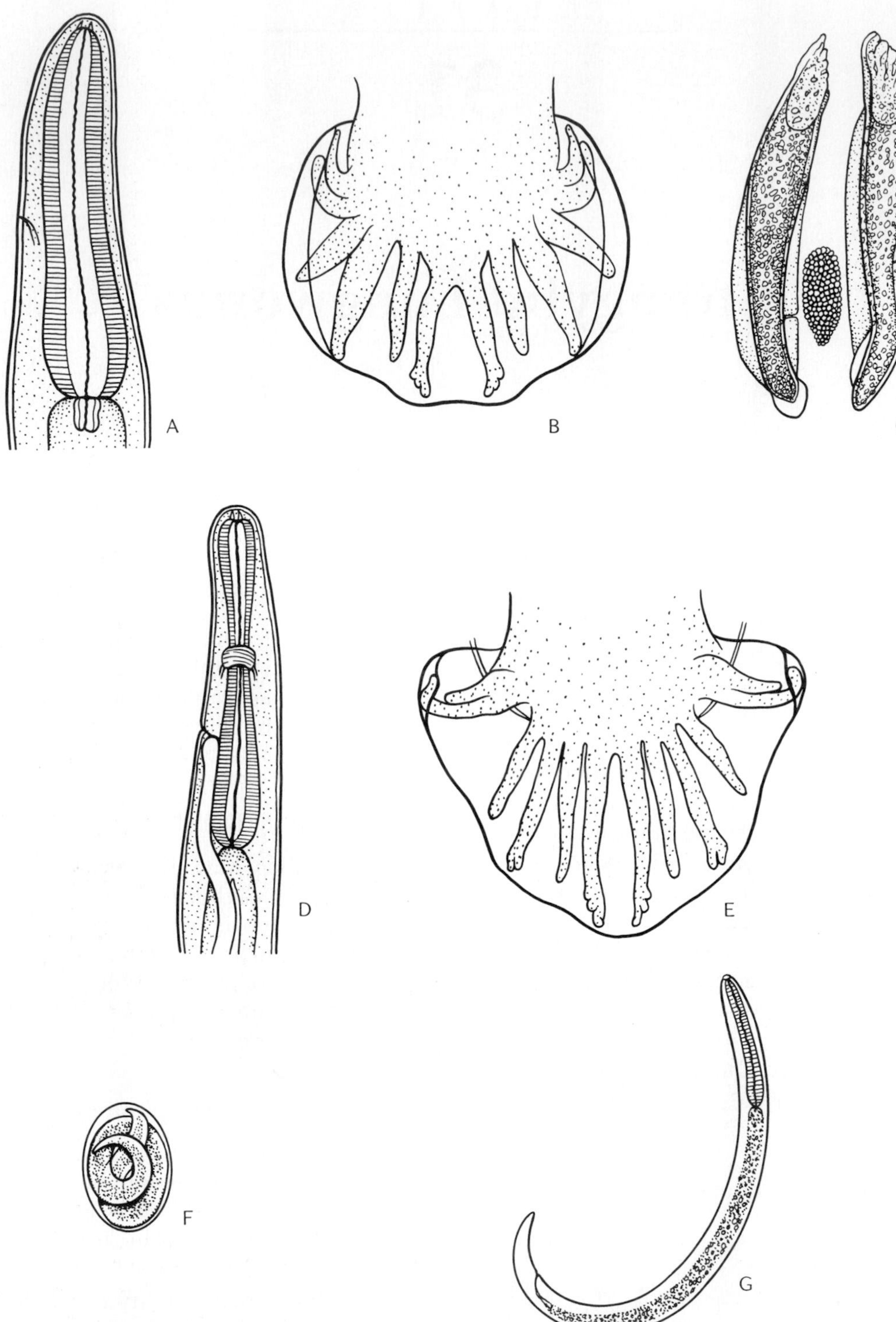

Figure 31.1 Two lungworms of large ruminants. *Dictyocaulus viviparus* of cattle: (A) head, (B) bursa, (C) spicules and (center) gubernaculum, (D) head and esophagus. *D. filaria* of sheep, (E) bursa, (F) egg with L_1 as passed in the feces, (G) newly hatched L_1.

and normally hatch in transit through the digestive tract. The free-living stages do not feed; the L_3 is encased in the cast cuticles of both the L_1 and L_2 and is reached in four to six days under optimal conditions of temperature and moisture.

The L_3s are ingested with the forage, escape from the cuticles in the small intestine, and penetrate the gut to enter mesenteric lymph nodes. The L_4 is reached about four days after infection, and the larvae then leave the lymph nodes to be carried by the vascular system to the lungs. They break out of the alveoli of the lungs and reach sexual maturity about eighteen days after infection.

Diagnosis

Determining whether a ruminant is infected with lungworms is based on the following:

1. Clinical signs of infection
2. Finding L_1s in the feces

Clinical signs of infection include rapid, labored breathing, pneumonia, and failure to gain properly. In an enzootic lungworm area, these signs are highly suggestive. The signs together with finding large numbers of L_1s in the feces give good evidence of clinical lungworm infection. A number of other infectious agents including viruses and bacteria also cause pneumonia in ruminants.

Larvae may often be found in feces examined following one of the standard fecal flotation methods; however, the usual method is to use the Baermann apparatus. Additional methods that can be used under some circumstances are examination of mucus from the respiratory tract for L_1s and finding L_3s on the herbage where animals are pastured.

Host–Parasite Interactions

A considerable part of the damage to the host occurs during the preadult stage of infection. Larvae are trapped in the capillaries of the air sacs (alveoli) of the lungs and then break out of the tissue into the alveoli themselves. Clinical signs are seen at this time, and the damage to the lung is both direct and indirect. Pneumonia is caused directly by the lungworms, and other infectious agents may also invade the lung tissue because of the damage to the endothelial surfaces. The adults cause production of excessive amounts of mucus from the lungs, leading to chronic coughing. Animals that die from lungworm infection have large, tangled masses of worms in the air passages as well as a large quantity of mucus. Portions of the lungs are purple and lack the usual spongy texture and pink color of the normal lung.

Animals that have been exposed to moderate numbers of larvae develop immunity against the preadult stages in the lymph nodes and lungs. Immunity affects not only the numbers of worms that may reach maturity but also the rate at which the worms develop. The prepatent period of about three weeks can be lengthened considerably in immune animals. Although some of the larvae are killed by the immunity, some survive, and these tend to accumulate in the lungs causing long-term, low-grade damage.

Epidemiology and Control

Since cattle are seriously affected by lungworms, a number of approaches are taken:

1. Treatment of animals with anthelmintics to cure the infections
2. Separation of age classes of animals
3. Treatment of patent infections to reduce pasture contamination
4. Avoidance of contaminated pastures
5. Promoting of immunity artificially

Chemotherapeutic drugs for lungworm infections in ruminants have shown variable efficacy. Some of the newer benzimidazoles and macrolide antibiotics are effective against both immature and adult worms. As noted, much of the damage caused by lungworms is in the preadult stage, and although there may be some beneficial effect from removing adults, it is a second-best solution.

The distribution of lungworm disease indicates the effect of external conditions on the free-living stages as discussed in Chapter 30 on trichostrongyles. Although lungworms are found nearly everywhere, they become serious pathogens in moist, moderate climates.

The larvae do not survive freezing or drying, and they survive a shorter time than the free-living stages of the trichostrongyles. Although larvae of *D. viviparus* have been found to survive for nearly 11 months on pasture in Britain, this is quite unusual, and they almost always die within a month after being deposited. Interestingly, the cast cuticle in the trichostrongyles is said to provide protection for the L_3; however, in the lungworms the L_3 is ensheathed in two cuticles and survives rather poorly.

As is true with gastrointestinal nematodes of ruminants, lungworm disease usually follows exposure to large numbers of L_3s over a short period. Thus, environmental conditions of moderate temperatures accompanied by moisture allow the accumulation of preinfective stages that become infective within a short time. If the animals on pasture are not immune, clinical disease results.

Studies in Britain on lungworm disease of cattle brought to light important aspects of transmission. For example, lush, tender grass tends to grow around the margins of a fecal deposit. One might think that this grass would be attractive to cattle, but they tend to avoid it. Without belaboring the point, it is well to remember that ruminants are not four-legged mowing machines. They select particular plants at particular stages of growth, and in this case somehow avoid the place where contamination with lungworm larvae may be greatest.

In opposition to this grazing behavior of the cattle, larvae are distributed widely through their association with the fungus, *Pilobolus*. This fungus is commonly found in manure and it has a sporangium with a cap that is explosively ejected when stimulated by dim light. Infective lungworm larvae curl up on the cap of the sporangium and are carried up to 2 m when the cap is ejected (Fig. 31.2). It appears that this worm-fungus association is a means of distributing the worms.

The general principle of separating age classes of animals is a useful one for controlling various parasitic diseases. On a dairy farm, say, replacement animals are likely to range in age from a few weeks to young heifers ready for breeding. If all of these animals are pastured together, the younger animals may be exposed to various parasites before they have the capacity to respond immunologically.

Points 2 and 4 attempt to do the same thing—that is, reduce exposure of animals to large numbers of larvae. Despite the relative sensitivity of the free-living stages, it is rare for a pasture to be vacant long enough for all the larvae to die (see Chapter 30).

Immunity has been exploited more successfully than other control measures, but it is not ideal. Lungworm disease in Britain had been a long-standing problem, and lack of adequate control measures stimulated an investigation on immunity at the School of Veterinary Medicine at the University of Glasgow in Scotland.

It was known that older animals developed resistance, and investigations found that a strong, specific immunity developed. Immunity was expressed against the preadults when they migrated to lymph nodes and lungs. The question posed was how to produce immunity against the larvae so that they would not cause damage. The answer lay in x-irradiation of the larvae. Larvae "attenuated" by x-irradiation developed partially in the lungs and then died due to radiation damage. The protocol finally developed calls for administering 1000 irradiated larvae by mouth on two occasions at an interval of one month. The immunity elicited reduces worm numbers by about 95% on challenge with 10,000 larvae shortly after immunization. Even after four months, there is still 89% immunity,

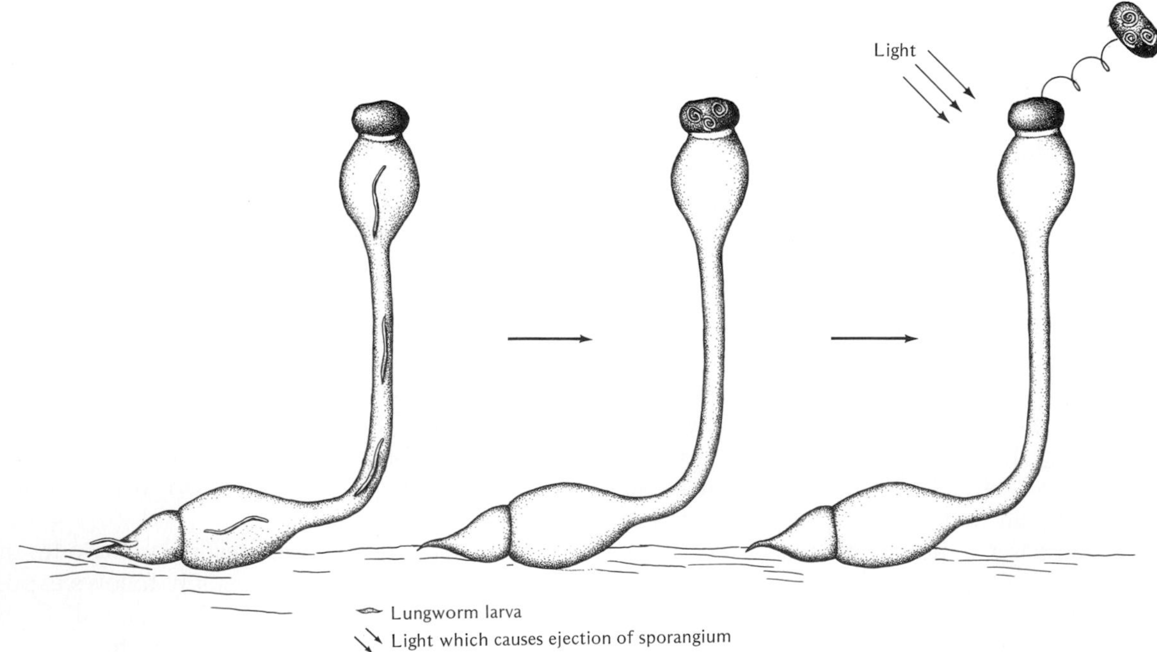

Figure 31.2 Sporangium of *Pilobolus* with *Dictyocaulus* larvae on it and their being ejected into the air under the influence of light falling on the sporanium.

as measured by the number of worms that mature upon challenge. This vaccine is marketed in Europe and has been useful in controlling lungworm disease in some situations.

The vaccine has two drawbacks: shelf life and occasional unexplained failures. It can be readily appreciated that x-irradiated larvae are not perfectly healthy, and one must use such a product soon after preparation. The difficulty of producing high-quality vaccine lots from fecal cultures cannot be overstated. Conditions of shipment and storage are crucial for successful vaccination. In large countries such as Canada and the United States, shipping time may and various regulatory requirements do present insurmountable problems. In the tropics, maintenance of temperature can be difficult. The fact that such effective vaccine immunity can be produced is encouraging. Application of modern vaccine tools could be used to overcome manufacturing, shelf-life, regulatory, and distribution problems.

LUNGWORMS WITH VECTORS

The lungworms with vectors are in the subfamily Protostrongylinae; these worms have life cycles that require an intermediate host, usually a snail or an oligochaete. Protostrongyline lungworms are common in ruminants and rabbits in all parts of the world.

Lungworms of Bighorn Sheep

The disease complex in Rocky Mountain bighorn sheep (*Ovis canadensis*) called lungworm pneumonia is of interest because its etiology involves both a number of biotic factors and human incursion into bighorn habitat. What impact lungworm pneumonia had on populations of bighorn sheep prior to the colonization of western North America is unknown. It is abundantly clear that the disease is now a controlling factor in populations of bighorn sheep and that further interference by humans is essential to the continued survival of herds in the Rocky Mountains. Having generated the problem, we now have to manage bighorn herds so as to minimize the effect of lungworm infections.

Name of Organism and Disease Association

Protostrongylus stilesi causes lungworm disease or verminous pneumonia. A synergistic relationship exists between three organisms in bringing about clinical disease: the lungworms, at least one virus, and a bacterium. *P. frosti* and *P. rushi* are also common in bighorn sheep, but they contribute less to the lungworm pneumonia complex than *P. stilesi*.

Hosts and Host Range

The principal host is the Rocky Mountain bighorn sheep (*Ovis canadensis*), but domestic sheep (*Ovis aries*) are infected occasionally.

Geographic Distribution and Importance

North America in the area contiguous with the distribution of bighorn sheep throughout the Rocky Mountain chain and in the plains east of the mountains. Prevalence of infection ranges from about 30% to nearly 100% in different herds.

In association with at least one virus and bacterium, lungworms cause debilitating and fatal pneumonia, principally in younger animals.

Before 1800 there were about 2 million bighorn sheep in North America. The current population is about 18,000, 1% of the original number. Individual herds have sometimes declined gradually over a period of years, but in other instances there have been spectacular die-offs over a short period

Outbreaks of verminous pneumonia in bighorn sheep were described starting in the early years of the 20th century. Mortalities have ranged widely, but in a few instances more than 50% of the animals in a herd have died. Lungworm disease contributes to the decline in the numbers of sheep through the deaths of lambs and attrition in the adults.

Morphology

Since *P. stilesi* adults are embedded in the parenchyma of the lung, the length of the adults is not known. The bursa and spicules of the male are used in identification (Fig. 31.3).

Life Cycle

Despite their lying in the tissue of the lung, eggs laid by the adults reach the alveoli, pass forward, are swallowed and carried out with the feces; the L_1s hatch some time during this early journey. The intermediate hosts are tiny terrestrial snails in the genera *Pupilla*, *Vertigo*, and *Euconulus*, but many terrestrial snails can be infected. L_1s enter the snail by being eaten. The larvae grow and molt twice to reach the infective L_3. Infectivity for sheep is reached about two weeks after infection depending on the temperature. When snails are ingested with the forage, the larvae leave the sheep

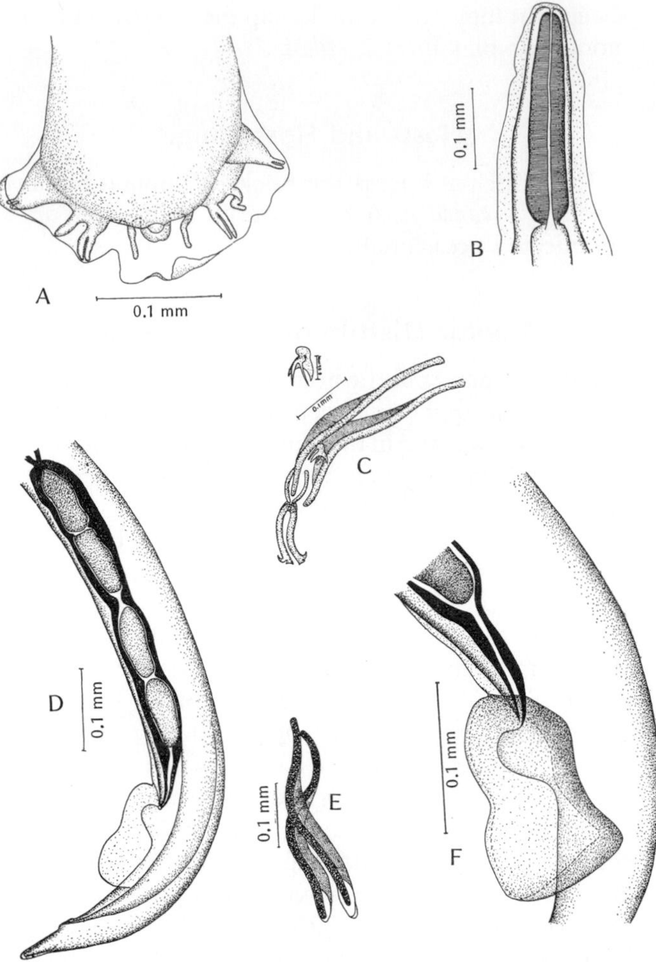

Figure 31.3 Structures used in the identification of *Protostrongylus stilesi.* (A) Bursa of the male; (B) esophagus; (C) spicules; gubernaculum and telemon; (D) tail end of the female; (E) spicules; (F) vulva and provagina of the female. [From Dikmans, 1931.]

intestine and migrate via the bloodstream to the lungs (Fig. 31.4).

The infection can be transferred transplacentally from the pregnant ewe to the lamb. This is an important mode of infection since a high proportion of lambs are infected and are often eliminated from the population.

Diagnosis

Infections with lungworms in bighorn sheep are determined by the following:

1. Finding larvae in the feces
2. Examining typical lesions in the lungs at postmortem examination

Larvae are readily found in the droppings of infected sheep by using the Baermann method, and this technique can be used for determining both whether an individual is infected and the prevalence of infection in a herd. At postmortem examination, lungworm lesions can usually be seen on the surface of the diaphragmatic lobes of the lungs. Portions of worms can be dissected out of the tissue for identification. The question of whether lungworm pneumonia may be the cause of illness and death is determined by herd history, examination of vectors, and isolation of the microbial agent(s) in the laboratory.

Host–Parasite Interactions

Protostrongylus stilesi lies in the parenchyma of the lung of the sheep (Fig. 31.5B) where adults (seen as large bodies) and developing eggs (smaller roundish bodies) cause considerable change in the lung tissue. A normal lung has an open, lacy appearance such that the red blood cells are close to the alveoli of the lung where gaseous exchange takes place (Fig. 31.5A).

The lungworms themselves cause damage to a relatively small proportion of the lung. However, their association with viruses and bacteria bring about pneumonia, which results in extensive damage to the lungs followed by debilitation and death.

Young animals are especially susceptible to infection and a large proportion of lambs are infected before birth. These young animals are removed from the population by the disease, leaving an aging population. In addition, animals that are not otherwise in good nutritional condition are likely to suffer from the effects of the combined agents and succumb to them or they are preyed upon by carnivores.

Epidemiology and Control

Control of diseases in wild, free-ranging animals presents some difficult problems, but some steps can be taken in the case of lungworm disease in bighorn sheep:

1. Management to allow normal migration
2. Maintenance of a high level of nutrition
3. Free-choice treatment with anthelmintics

Lungworm pneumonia in bighorn sheep is the result of interaction between two or three infectious agents combined with the general physical condition of the host. It should be recognized that a die-off of bighorn is merely the culmination of a series of other events that have worked indirectly to the detriment of the sheep.

Bighorn have been hunted, but they were not a staple food such as the buffalo and deer were for early settlers. Bighorn occupy high mountain areas that are harsh and inaccessible; this niche was where they were

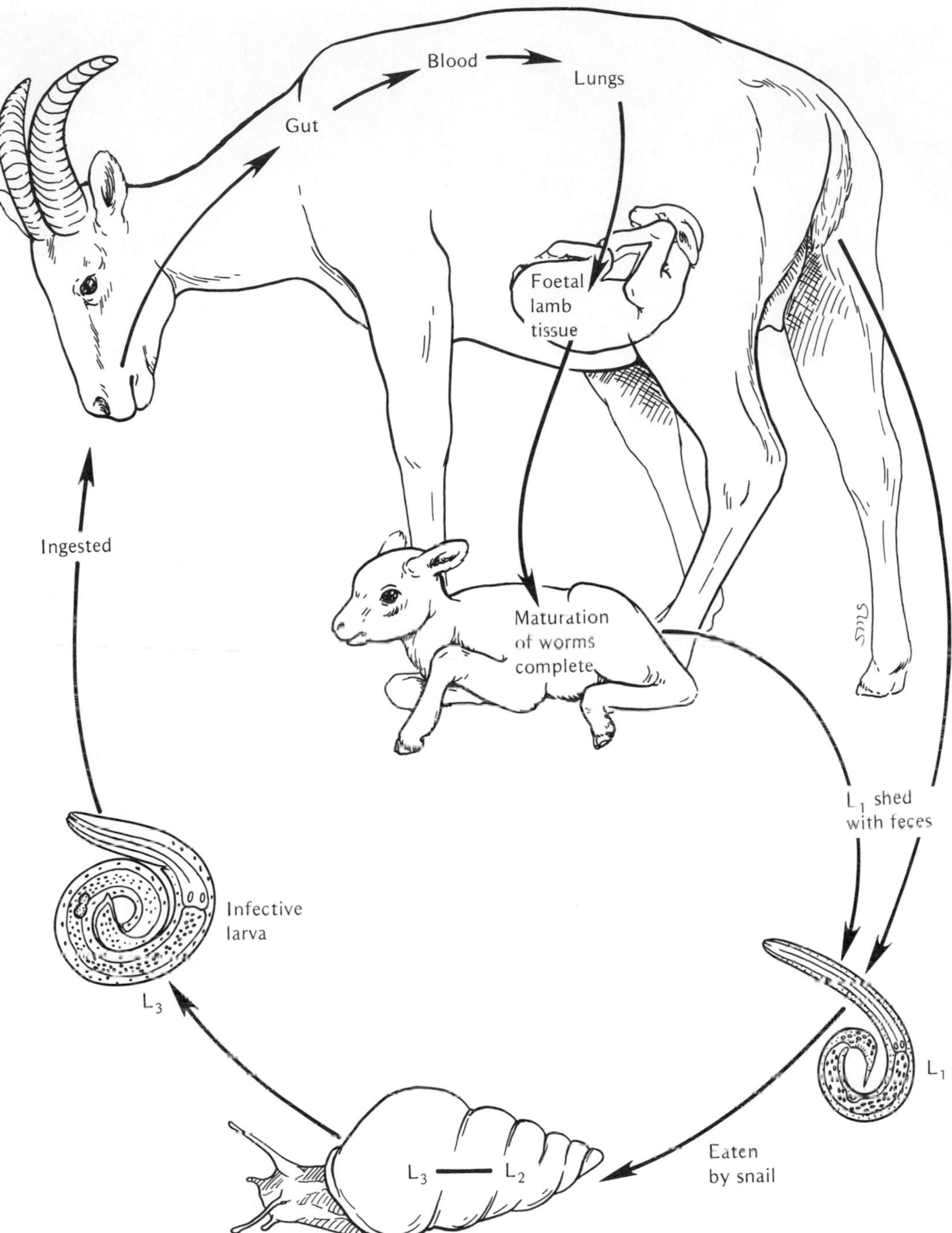

Figure 31.4 Diagram of the life cycle of lungworms of bighorn sheep. Infection of adults takes place by ingestion of infected snails. Lambs are often infected before birth, and mortality in this age group can be severe.

seen by early explorers and settlers, except for a population along portions of the Missouri River in Montana and the Dakotas. They are wary animals and drift away at the sight of humans. They also do not mix well with other species of ruminants such as domestic cattle and sheep.

Bighorn remain in herds; they migrate seasonally to lower elevations during the winter but still inhabit a harsh ecological niche. They also are creatures of habit, using certain bed grounds that are free of snow and are protected from the wind.

With the incursion of humans into the mountains

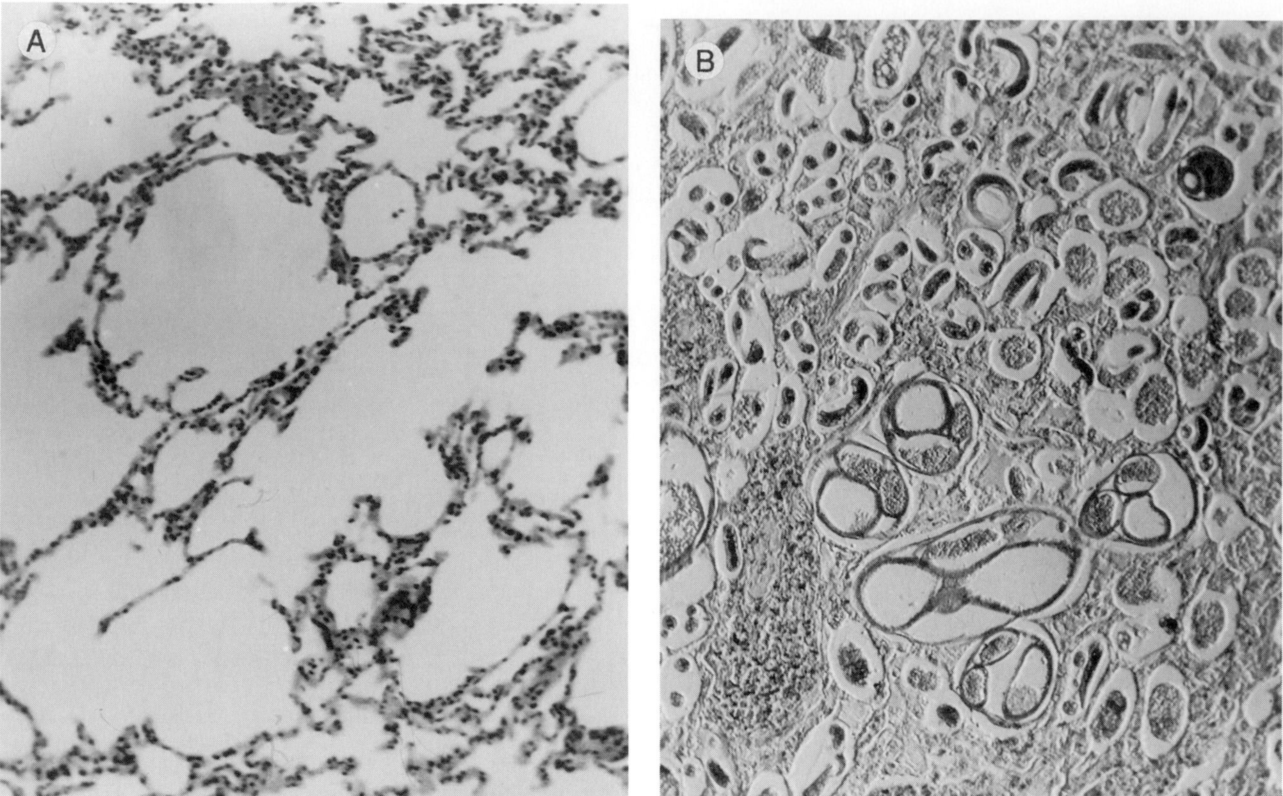

Figure 31.5 Normal lung from a mammal (A), and lung from a Rocky Mountain bighorn sheep infected with *Protostrongylus stilesi* (B). Note the open, lacy appearance of the normal lung so that gaseous exchange can easily take place and the consolidated character of the infected lung. In cases where infection is heavy, the lung becomes inflamed and gaseous exchange is reduced.

for travel, mining, settlement, and grazing of domestic animals, the habitat and the habits of the bighorn were altered. They drifted away to more restricted areas. Their traditional grazing areas were more and more occupied by domestic sheep and cattle and the forage deteriorated. Bed grounds became a solid mat of feces, and snails grazed on the feces as a source of food.

It is hard to conceive of these animals being crowded in the vast areas of the Rocky Mountains and subject to the pressure of parasitic diseases we associate with the intensive grazing practices used with domestic animals. But that is what happened. Human activities in the mountains restricted the habitat and movement of the sheep and reduced their level of nutrition. Lungworms were present and precipitated the pathologic condition.

Many human modifications of the world are irreversible, and the uses that are now made of high mountain areas for grazing of livestock, recreation, and other activities are not going to be stopped. The problem posed is how to maintain healthy populations of bighorn in the face of heavy pressure from humans. There have been partial solutions to the dilemma. For example, it has been found feasible to administer drugs to animals in a feed supplement with an anthelmintic that is made available in feeding grounds. In herds of central Colorado, this technique has reduced the level of infection so that young lambs survive through their first summer and winter. Unfortunately, the crux of the problem is not whether animals are infected with lungworms, but rather their general health and nutritional level. It is not feasible to return to the 18th century and abandon the high mountains. We are left with stopgap measures that buy time until better solutions can be devised.

LUNGWORMS IN SWINE

Name of Organism and Disease Associations

Metastrongylus apri, M. pudendotectus (syn. *Choerostrongylus p.*), and *M. salmi* cause lungworm disease.

Hosts and Host Range

The adult worms are in the air passages of the lungs of swine and other members of the family Suidae. Occasionally they are found in ruminants, dogs, and humans.

Geographic Distribution and Importance

The three species are cosmopolitan in swine, but their prevalences differ. *M. apri* is the most common; its prevalence in domestic swine in moist climates is 50 to 80%. *M. pudendotectus* is the next most frequent, and *M. salmi* has a prevalence of perhaps 4%.

Life Cycle

The development of all three species of lungworms in pigs is essentially the same. The adults lie in the air passages of the lungs, where copulation and egg laying occur. The eggs are passed up the respiratory tree by ciliary action, and when they reach the upper part, they are coughed up and swallowed. The eggs have L_1s in them when they are passed with the feces. They hatch when eaten by earthworms (*Lumbricus terrestris, Eisenia foetida,* among others), releasing the L_1, which penetrates the gut and develops in the coelom of the earthworm. In two to three weeks the L_3 stage is reached and it encysts in the gut.

The L_3s do not develop further until eaten by a susceptible animal, they can remain alive in the earthworm for as long as four years. If the earthworm dies, the exposed larvae probably live only for two weeks or so.

Pigs are infected usually by eating infected earthworms, but secondarily by eating the free L_3s. The L_3 is released in the small intestine and passes through the wall of the gut to the lymph system. The L_3 or L_4 moves by the circulatory system to the lungs, where it is filtered out in the capillaries. The L_4 breaks out of the alveoli of the lung, molts once more, and becomes mature about four weeks after infection. Egg production may continue for several months.

Host–Parasite Interactions

Swine lungworms are not generally considered to be highly pathogenic; however, they can cause significant damage on their own. During migration of the preadult worms, the greatest damage is to the alveoli of the lungs. Each L_4 causes a small hemorrhage (petechia) where it leaves the capillary to enter the air sac; the greater the number of worms, the greater the damage. As the worms mature, they irritate the air passages and may block some of the smaller ones. Pigs show labored breathing and cough to expel excess mucus.

Epidemiology and Control

Control of lungworms is based on the following:

1. Preventing infection by maintaining swine on pastures that are dry and well drained
2. Raising swine on concrete
3. Treating swine for the lungworms with an anthelmintic

It is not surprising that the prevalence of lungworm infection in swine exceeds 70% in many areas. The adult stages may persist for eight months in the pig, and the stages may live for years in the intermediate host.

An example of the hardiness of the eggs is contained in a study on the effect of freezing where temperatures between −8 and −20°C had little effect on viability until more than 49 days had passed. On the other hand, desiccation was detrimental to survival, especially at 37 to 39°C, at which fewer than 1% survived for 10 days. At 17 to 22°C, survival was better, but none lived longer than 25 days. At 1 to 2°C, about 10% lived 38 days.

Once they enter the earthworm, the larvae seem to be almost completely protected. In a study made on an abandoned pasture near the Beltsville Agricultural Research Center in Maryland, it was found that earthworms were still infected 4 years after any hogs had been on the land. Seventy-five sexually mature earthworms were found to have a prevalence of infection of 46.6% with levels of infection as high as 100 larvae, and these larvae were found to be infective for a pig. Immature earthworms from the same pasture were uninfected. Interestingly, although lumbricid earthworms have a potential longevity of 4 to 8 years, the life span is considered generally to be no more than a few months. Under protected cultural conditions, however, the following have been found to be maximal survival times: for *Allolobophora longa*, 10 1/4 years; for *Lumbricus terrestris*, 6 years; for *Eisenia foetida*, 4 1/2 years. If one assumes that most earthworms live only a few months and that the maximal life span is 6 years, only 5 to 10% of the original population of the worms would be alive at 4 years. The finding that nearly half of the worms were still infected at 4 years is startling.

The recommendations usually made for control of lungworms are that the animals be kept on areas that are dry or well drained, that temporary pastures be used, and that contaminated pastures be left for more than four years before allowing pigs on them. Since pigs will root in the soil if allowed, ringing their noses reduces that habit; they then are less likely to eat earthworms. In areas where swine are raised on concrete, the probability of lungworm infection is reduced nearly to insignificance.

Treating animals with one of the better anthelmintics benefits both the individual and the herd. Animals so heavily infected that they cough and have difficulty breathing benefit from removal of the worms. Since the adult worms continue to lay eggs for months, they also continue to contaminate the area; reduction in the amount of contamination is beneficial to the herd. Also, since contamination can persist for years, any measure to clean up the environment is desirable. Lung damage in the air-passage-dwelling lungworms takes place mainly when they break out of the alveoli. Therefore, much of the damage may be done to the individual by the time treatment is administered.

METASTRONGYLE INFECTIONS IN HUMANS

No metastrongyle is considered to be a normal inhabitant of humans. However, two species found in rodents cause disease: *Angiostrongylus cantonensis* and *A. costaricensis*, found in the Eastern and Western Hemispheres, respectively. Both of these nematodes are parasites of the arterial system, rather than the lungs, and the problems of pathogenesis for humans result to an extent from these parasites being in an abnormal host.

Name of Organism and Disease Associations

Angiostrongylus cantonensis causes angiostrongylosis, eosinophilic meningitis, meningitis, or tropical eosinophilia in humans.

Hosts and Host Range

Rattus spp., including the Norway and black rat, seem to be the principal hosts, but bandicoot rats (*Bandicota* spp.) are also included among the important hosts. The final site of the adult worms in the normal definitive host is the pulmonary arteries; in humans the worms are most often in the central nervous system but may also he found in other organ systems including the eye.

Geographic Distribution and Importance

Infections in rats are widespread in tropical areas of the Eastern Hemisphere such as the Malay Peninsula, Japan, the islands of both Melanesia and Micronesia, northern Australia, Hawaii, and East Africa including Madagascar. The original enzootic area of *A. cantonensis* probably was Madagascar, the large island off the southeastern coast of Africa, from which it spread northward to India and Sri Lanka, thence to the Malay Peninsula. Migration then took place in a number of directions: northward to China, eastward through the islands of the South Pacific, New Guinea and Australia (Fig. 31.6).

Infections in humans have been found in Southeast Asia, Japan, many islands of the South Pacific, and Hawaii. All well-documented infections have been found to be contiguous with the distribution of the infection in rats.

Although infections are widespread in rats, infections in humans are sporadic in the present enzootic area and they are related to the types of food eaten and their method of preparation. Infections in humans seldom result in death; it is therefore difficult to determine with certainty whether *A. cantonensis* is actually the cause of eosinophilic meningitis in any specific instance. Most often, only a few persons suffer from the infection at a particular location and time.

Morphology

The female worms (Fig. 31.7) are 18 to 33 long by 0.28 to 0.5 mm wide with the vulva about 0.25 mm from the posterior end. Males are 15 to 22 by 0.25 to 0.35 mm and have subequal spicules that are 490 and 1200 μm long (Fig. 31.7). Both sexes feed on blood and therefore have a red intestine around which the reproductive system winds; this gives a barber-pole appearance also noted in such worms as *Haemonchus*.

Life Cycle

The life cycle described here is that which occurs in the normal rat host, and in the invertebrate hosts. As is true with many other metastrongyles, the L_3s are ensheathed in the cast cuticles of the two previous stages. The L_3s are eaten by rats and within a day reach the central nervous system via the circulatory system. The early adult stage is reached in 11 to 13 days after infection, and migration then begins. The worms move to the meninges covering the brain and remain between the layers (subarachnoid space) for about two weeks. They then move to the venous system and are carried through the heart to the pulmonary arteries, where they remain and begin laying eggs. The unembryonated eggs are carried with the arterial blood to

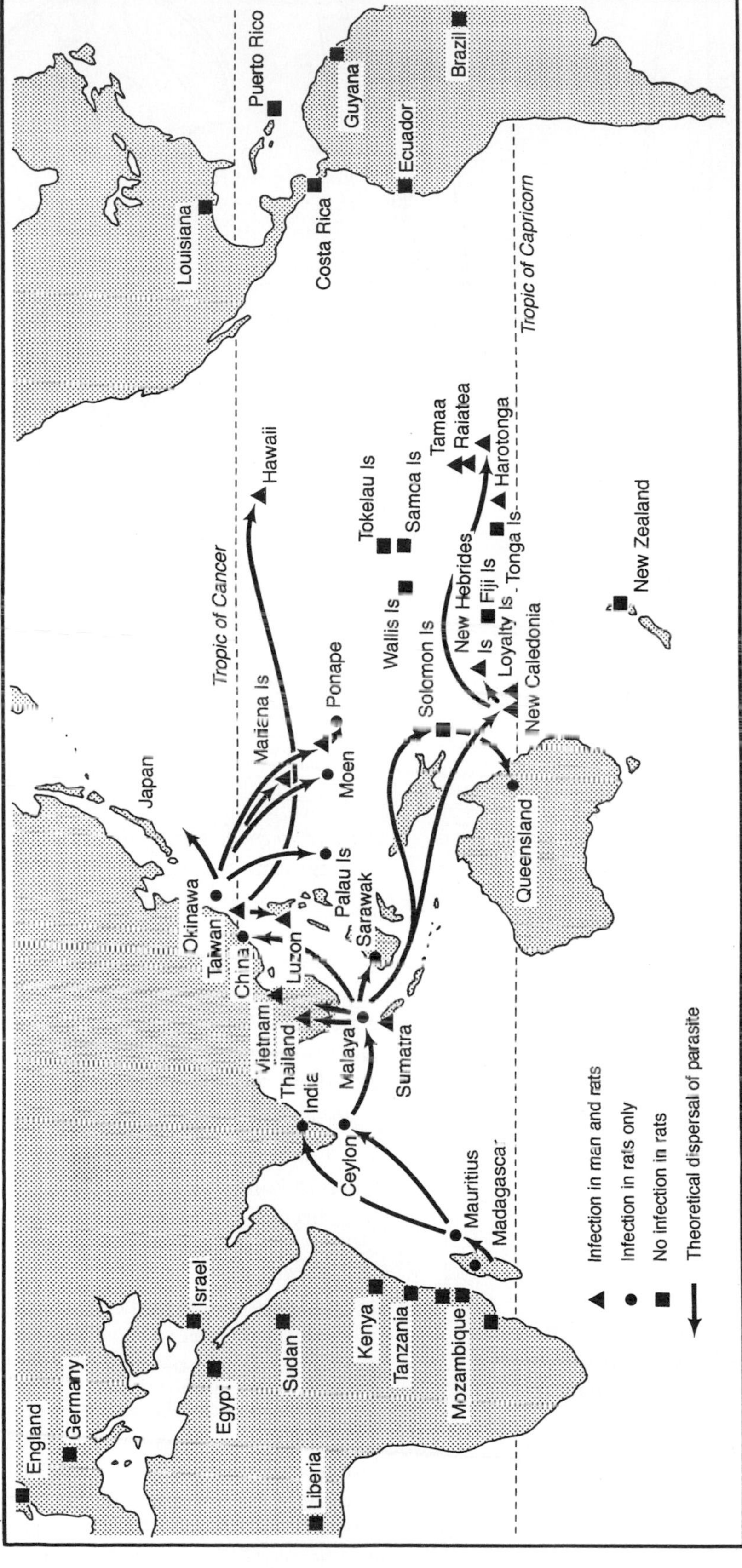

Figure 31.6 Probable dispersal of the rat lungworm, *Angiostrongylus cantonensis*, from the island of Madagascar through much of the Pacific Rim. [Redrawn from Alicata, J. E., and Jindrak, K., 1970.]

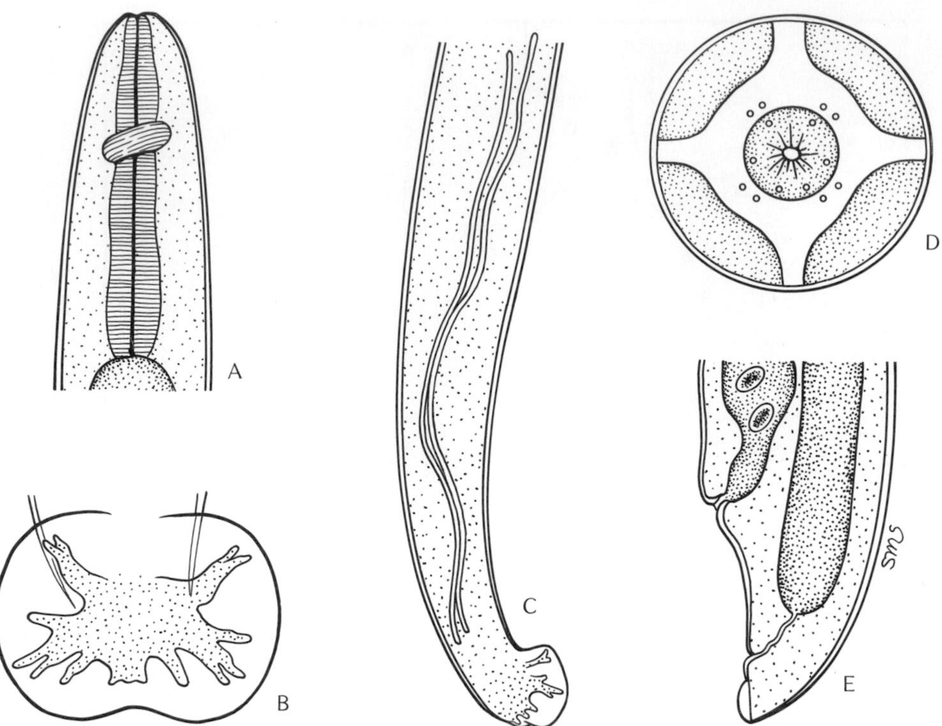

Figure 31.7 Structures used in the identification of *Angiostrongylus cantonensis*, the rat lungworm. (A) Anterior end; (B) bursa; (C) spicules of the male; (D) head and esophagus; (E) posterior of the female.

the capillaries in the alveoli of the lung, where they lodge. The L_1s hatch, break out of the alveoli, pass up the respiratory tree and are swallowed; the prepatent period is 42 to 45 days, with larvae appearing in the feces at that time (Fig. 31.8).

The first intermediate host is a snail or slug, usually a terrestrial one. The host range is quite broad, but development takes place more readily in some species than in others. The L_1s penetrate the foot of the mollusk and reach the L_3 in about 18 days at 21 to 25°C.

Having reached the infective stage, the L_3 can reach the definitive host by one of the following means:

1. The gastropod can be eaten.
2. The L_3s can escape from the gastropod and be eaten with food or with water.
3. A transport host can be infected by either of these routes and then it, in turn, may be eaten by the definitive host. The most important transport hosts seem to be freshwater crustacea such as prawns and crab, and land planaria. The most frequent mode of infection in wild rats is not known.

The life cycle in humans seems to be the same as in the rat except for the final site. In humans the worms remain in the brain, lying either between the meninges or migrating through the brain tissue itself.

Diagnosis

Diagnosis is difficult in humans; in the other hosts, a postmortem examination may be done to find the worms in the pulmonary arteries. Unless the person has died, the diagnosis of *A. cantonensis* infection is indirect and is based on the following:

1. Clinical signs and symptoms (Tab. 31.1)
2. Food habits and a history of having eaten a likely source of larvae about two weeks previously
3. The presence of eosinophils in the cerebrospinal fluid (CSF)
4. Evidence of antibody production
5. Finding worms in the CSF (rare; only two instances are on record)

There are many causes of meningitis; therefore both a skilled diagnostician and a laboratory capable of isolating and identifying various infectious agents are required to determine whether bacterial, viral, or other parasitic agents may be the cause of the disease. Skin and serological testing can indicate whether a nema-

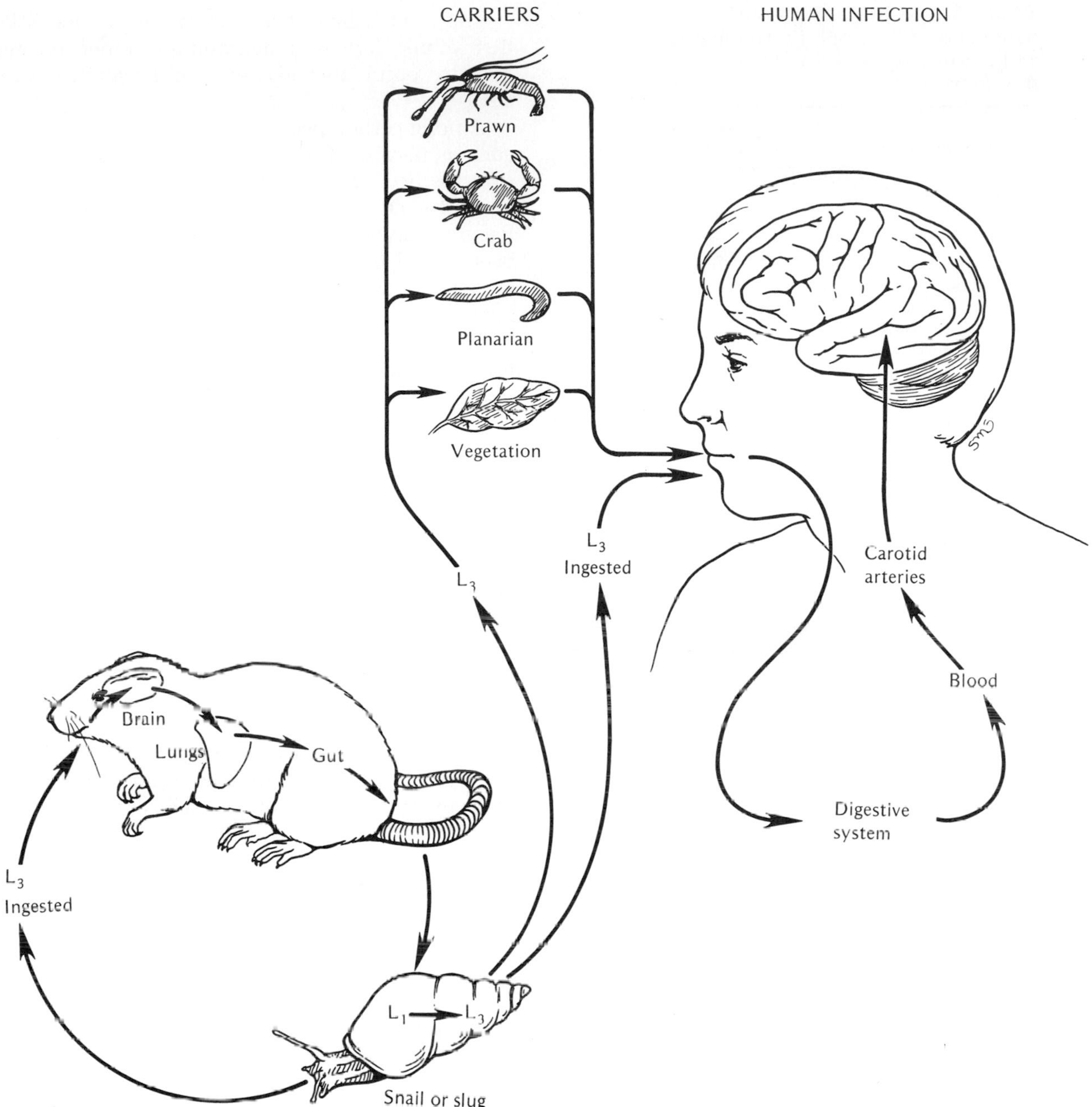

Figure 31.8 Diagram of the life cycle of the rat lungworm, *Angiostrongylus cantonensis*, and the modes of infection in humans.

tode may be involved in producing antibody. A further narrowing of the possible causes of meningitis comes from questioning of the patient. In an enzootic area, the typical symptoms coupled with suggestive laboratory tests and food habits consistent with becoming infected provide a good indication of infection with *A. cantonensis*.

Other infections with which *A. cantonensis* can be confused are *Taenia solium* cysticerci, *Paragonimus westermani*, and *Gnathostoma spinigerum*. Many other infectious or noninfectious processes may also be associated with an increase in eosinophils.

Host–Parasite Interactions

Frequently, but not invariably, *A. cantonensis* has a low degree of pathogenesis in the rat. On the other hand, in humans there is a full range of effects including severe damage to the central nervous system leading to death.

TABLE 31.1 Clinical Signs and Symptoms of Eosinophilic Meningitis and Presumably Infection with *A. cantonensis*

Sign or Symptom	Percentage Having
Headache	90
Stiff neck	56
Vomiting	56
Paresthesia (abnormal sensation)	54
Fever	41
Paralysis or tremors	9

[Modified from Kuberski and Wallace, 1979.]

In humans there no doubt are many inapparent infections and others in which there may be only mild symptoms of meningitis but with eosinophils in the CSF. Lesions are related to both the location and the number of the worms in the nervous tissue. Eosinophilia indicates an immune response to the worms and meningitis indicates that there is interference with normal nerve impulse propagation and probably swelling of the central nervous system. If damage is sufficient, paralysis of particular parts of the body or of areas served by the cranial nerves may result.

Epidemiology and Control

Since eosinophilic meningitis is usually a sporadic infection in small numbers of persons at any one time, control programs have not been developed. At the public health level, there are three approaches that might be considered:

1. Treatment of infected individuals
2. Changing food habits to avoid infection
3. Rat control

Anthelmintics along with anti-inflammatory drugs have been used with some success in treating laboratory animals. However, reservations have been expressed on the desirability of treatment. The concern is that a worm migrating through the brain tissue clearly causes damage, but a dead worm becomes a foreign body against which a strong inflammatory reaction is directed. The result is a large granuloma, which itself causes damage. Although some cases are on record in which persons have died from the infection, most recover completely without specific therapy. This is clearly as case where the treatment may be worse than the disease. The physician's cardinal principle pertains: first, do no harm.

The food habits of people in various localities or their ethnic derivation determine whether infection is likely to occur. In this case, food preferences are the key.

Among certain peoples of the Pacific islands, foods such as tiaro on Tahiti or keloguen on Guam consist principally of grated coconut mixed with the juice from ground or crushed freshwater prawns. On some of the Pacific islands, 5 to 10% of freshwater prawns have been found to be infected, mostly with two or three larvae of *A. cantonensis;* in one instance more than 3000 larvae were found in a single prawn.

The predilection of Europeans and North Americans for green salads leads to infection. Terrestrial gastropods, and planaria secondarily, shed infective larvae onto plants in the field and the larvae are then eaten with the salad. In some enzootic areas, eosinophilic meningitis occurs in visitors and not in the natives where the latter do not eat leafy salads.

Since the definitive host range is relatively narrow, rat control might be worthwhile, but in general rats are not restricted to areas of human habitation. Control is therefore likely to be unproductive.

Drinking untreated surface water is also a hazard since larvae escape from the intermediate host or from planaria and may be transmitted if this happens in small streams.

At the public health level, probably the best that can be done is to monitor the extent of the infection in the intermediate and transport hosts and make available information on the consequences and likelihood of infection. The responsibility then falls on the individual on whether to avoid infection or not.

RELATED ORGANISMS

Paraelaphostrongylus tenuis is a parasite of the white-tailed deer, *Odocoileus virginianus,* in North America. *P. tenuis* has an indirect life cycle with the intermediate host being any one of several terrestrial or semi-aquatic gastropods. The infected snails are eaten and the L_3s migrate from the intestine to the central nervous system. The adults are most often found in the brain of the definitive host where they lie in the dura mater or the veins of the dura; eggs or L_1s are carried via the circulatory system to the lungs where they break out of the alveoli and pass out with the feces. During about the past 100 years, the white-tailed deer expanded it range northward in the United States and into Canada. This gradual migration brought the deer into contact with typically northern ruminants: mule deer, moose, and woodland caribou, and the result has been the transfer of *P. tenuis* to these animals. The detrimental effect has been seen mostly in moose, which are severley affected by the worm. In the white-tailed deer, there is little or no discernible damage, but in the moose they cause inflammation and granuloma formation. The result is severe central nervous disease including blindness, incoordination, depression, and paralysis. *P. tenuis* has had a dentrimental effect on populations of moose in Ontario.

Readings

Alicata, J. E. (1991). The discovery of *Angiostrongylus cantonensis* as a cause of human eosinophilic meningitis. *Parasitol. Today* **7,** 151–153.

Alicata, J. E., and Jindrak, K. (1970). *Angiostrongylus in the Pacific and Southeast Asia.* Charles C Thomas, Springfield, IL.

Forrester, D. J. (1971). Bighorn sheep lungworm pneumonia complex. In *Parasitic Diseases of Wild Mammals* (J. W. Davis and R. C. Anderson, Eds.), pp. 158–173. Iowa State Univ. Press, Ames.

Loria-Cortes, R., and Lobo-Sanahuja, J. F. (1980). Clinical abdominal angiostrongylosis. A study of 116 children with intestinal eosinophilic granuloma caused by *Angiostrongylus costaricensis. Am. J. Trop. Med. Hyg.* **29,** 538–544.

Poynter, D. (1963). Parasitic bronchitis. *Adv. Parasitol.* **1,** 179–212.

Rose, J. H. (1973). Lungworms of the domestic pig and sheep. *Adv. Parasitol.* **11,** 559.

Ubelaker, J. (1986). Systematics of species referred to the genus *Angiostrongylus. J. Parasitol.* **72,** 237–244.

CHAPTER

32

Ascarids of Humans and Other Hosts

Members of the order Ascaridida are stout-bodied worms that are easily seen with the naked eye. Most of them have three prominent lips surrounding the mouth, but some have none and some have six (see Chapter 25 for a complete description). The posterior ends of the males are often curled ventrally, and most have two stout spicules.

All the members of the order are parasitic and many are of economic and medical importance. The adults are intestinal inhabitants of a wide array of vertebrates, both terrestrial and aquatic.

EVOLUTION OF THE ASCARID LIFE CYCLE

Students often have problems with the life cycle of an organism such as *Ascaris*, which enters the definitive host by mouth and then migrates through the body to reach the lungs from which the larvae are coughed up and swallowed only to end up in the small intestine where they started. This does not seem to be an entirely logical system, but in an evolutionary context, it can be seen that there is an underlying logic.

Ascaris lumbricoides and *A. suum* both have the type of life cycle just described. It appears that in *Ascaris* a multihost cycle is compressed into a single host; thus the same individual is both the intermediate and definitive host. Sprent (1954) set forth the following hypotheses:

1. The primitive ascarids were free-living marine worms.
2. The terrestrial forms arose secondarily.
3. The indirect (heteroxenous) life cycle pattern is a primitive and widespread feature of both marine and terrestrial species.

The rationale for these conclusions lies in the analysis of the life cycles of various members of the group:

1. The ancestors of the ascarids were marine bottom dwellers living on decaying organic matter.
2. Some completed the sexual portions of their life cycles in the bodies of decaying invertebrates.
3. The first stage of parasitism arose when these nematodes were ingested by carrion-feeding animals, perhaps shrimplike animals. The nematodes remained in the tissues of this first host.
4. The stage was then set for passing the incipient parasite up the food chain to small fish and then to large fish.
5. The gut of the large fish provides a good source of food for the parasites, and the movement of the fish in seeking food would disseminate eggs of the worms over a large area, thereby increasing the probability of completion of the cycle.

Sprent's theory best explains the transitions that have taken place in those ascarids that migrate in the host. Thus, one can see that the worms are not as irrational as they appear. We are merely seeing a snapshot in an evolutionary continuum.

ASCARIS LUMBRICOIDES OF HUMANS AND *A. SUUM* OF SWINE

Name of Organism and Disease Associations

Ascariosis or ascariasis in humans is caused by *Ascaris lumbricoides* and in swine by *A. suum.*

RUDOLF LEUCKART

One of the great parasitologists of the 19th century, Rudolf Leuckart (1822–1898) laid the groundwork in the life cycles and morphology of a number of parasites of humans. During Leuckart's lifetime, great strides were made in defining and finding the causative agents of many microbial and parasitic diseases. It was an exciting era in which many societal changes took place and when Charles Darwin published *The Origin of Species*, a book whose repercussions are still heard throughout the world.

Ascaris infections in humans were quite common in western Europe in the 19th century, and the worm was seen so frequently that it was not considered to be a serious pathogen. Nevertheless, Leuckart wanted to sort out the life cycle, so he infected a number of animals including swine, horses, dogs, and himself. He never found eggs from the mature worms in the animal inoculations and experienced no symptoms himself.

At Leuckart's suggestion, another German investigator, Mosler, inoculated himself with *Ascaris* eggs on 12 occasions without any ill effect. He then experimented on several children a few of whom showed pneumonia and fever after infection.

The Italian parasitologist, Giovanni Grassi, also inoculated himself with eggs derived from worms found in a corpse. He passed eggs 33 days later, a time too short to have come from the inoculation. He probably was already carrying an ascarid infection. However, one of his students then infected a boy who passed eggs starting 60 days after infection, about the proper prepatent period of *A. lumbricoides.*

At about the same time that Grassi was studying *A. lumbricoides* in Italy, 1887, Adolf Lutz was working in Brazil where he infected a volunteer with embryonated *Ascaris* eggs. This 32-year old man suffered from abdominal pain and bronchitis following infection and then passed ascarid eggs.

Here we are more than a hundred years later with a good conception of the life cycle and migratory pathway of *Ascaris* spp, a result of careful and repeated experiments done by many of the pioneering parasitologists. We are also aghast not only that they experimented on themselves, but worse yet, that they commandeered children as their experimental subjects. They justified the experiments on the basis that *A. lumbricoides* was so common that the children would become infected anyway. We find that unacceptable today, and our ethics give hope that our relations with one another will continue to become more humane.

Hosts and Host Range

Adults of *Ascaris lumbricoides* live in the small intestine of humans and in the chimpanzee, rhesus monkey, gorilla, and pigs. *Ascaris suum* is the common pig ascarid, but has also been reported from goats, cattle, sheep, and humans.

Geographic Distribution and Importance

Human ascariosis is cosmopolitan. Because of the number of infections plus the large size of the worms, numerous reports of human infections appeared in early literature. *Ascaris lumbricoides* was the first human helminth recorded in Chinese medical literature (about 300–200 B.C.). Descriptions also appear in early literature from India, Greece, and Rome.

In more modern times, it was estimated that there were about 4 million human ascarid infections in the United States in 1972, infecting about 20% of the rural southern population. Somewhat more recent surveys indicate that between 1 and 12% of persons in rural Georgia were infected. Estimates of worldwide human ascarid infections run as high as 1 billion, making *Ascaris* one of the most common human parasites.

A. suum is considered by many to be the single greatest cause of economic loss in the swine industry. Estimates in 1965 indicated that it caused $34 million loss annually in the United States. In North America, swine husbandry is generally a high-technology enterprise in which attempts are made to keep disease losses to a minimum. In many developing countries pigs are an essential source of protein, but little may be done to maintain their health and productivity.

Morphology

Adult *Ascaris* are large; adult males are up to 30 cm long and 3 mm in diameter, and adult females reach 35 cm in length and 5 mm in diameter. Compare these sizes with a standard lead pencil, which is about 18.5

cm long by 5 mm in diameter (Fig. 32.1). Males have a characteristic curved tail, two stout spicules about 2 mm long, but no gubernaculum. The vulva of the female is near the end of the anterior third of the body.

The mouth is surrounded by three large, fleshy lips, each with two basal papillae (Fig. 32.2). There are dentigerous ridges on each lip in the vicinity of the mouth opening. These ridges were used to distinguish between *Ascaris lumbricoides* and *A. suum*, but these ridges in *A. suum* may vary as the worms age. Thus, it appears that no single characteristic can be used to distinguish morphologically between *A. lumbricoides* and *A. suum*. There are, however, physiological differences so these two organisms are considered to be separate species.

Fertilized *Ascaris* eggs are 45 to 75 by 35 to 50 μm and have a thick, mammilated shell (Fig. 32.3). They are passed in feces in the one-cell stage. Unfertilized eggs are larger, 85 to 90 by 43 to 47 μm, and have thinner shells (Fig. 32.3). Occasionally eggs lack the characteristic mammilations (Fig. 32.3), which may cause problems in diagnosis.

Life Cycle

The life cycles of *A. lumbricoides* and *A. suum* are similar (Fig. 32.4). Eggs are shed in the feces in a one-celled stage. They develop within the egg capsules to the L_2 in 10 to 20 days; under less than optimal conditions, it may take much longer.

Eggs containing infective L_2s hatch in the stomach and small intestine. Larvae penetrate the wall of the small intestine and travel through the hepatic portal circulation, and occasionally the lymphatics, to the liver. The molt from L_2 to L_3 takes place within 18 to 96 hours after ingestion. A large number of larvae are in the liver two days after infection and they leave it between four and nine days. The L_3s migrate to the lungs by way of the circulatory system and are caught in the capillaries of the alveoli. They break out of the alveoli into the air spaces, are coughed up, swallowed, and reach the small intestine again. The molt to L_4 occurs at about 23 days; a month after ingestion, the final molt to the adult occurs. Copulation takes place and eggs are shed in the feces beginning 50 to 60 days after infection.

Diagnosis

Determining whether a host is infected with *Ascaris* involves the following:

1. Finding eggs in the feces by a concentration method
2. Observing clinical signs such as labored breathing and pneumonia
3. Observing stunting in growing hosts

In both humans and swine, finding eggs in the feces is the best evidence of infection. There is a correlation between the number of worms in the intestine and the

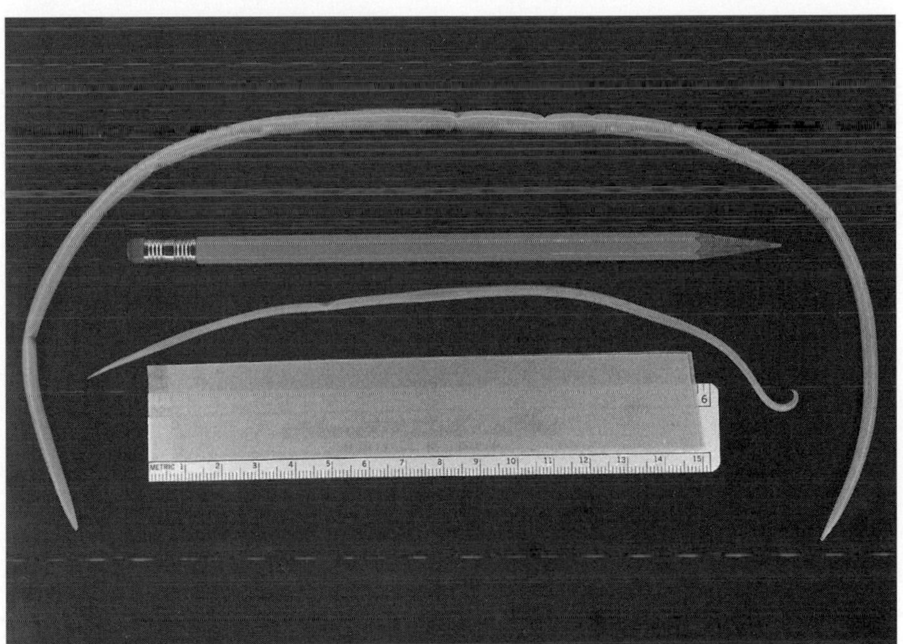

FIGURE 32.1 Comparison of a lead pencil (middle) with an *Ascaris* female (upper) and male (lower). (Metric scale on ruler)

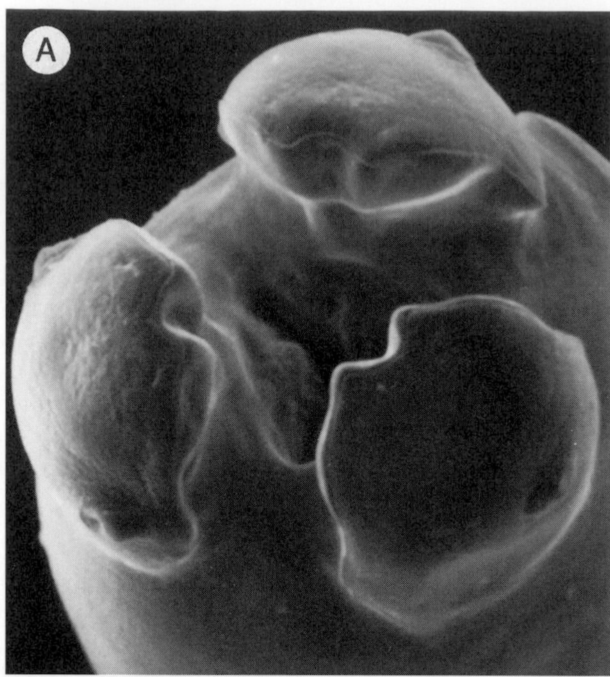

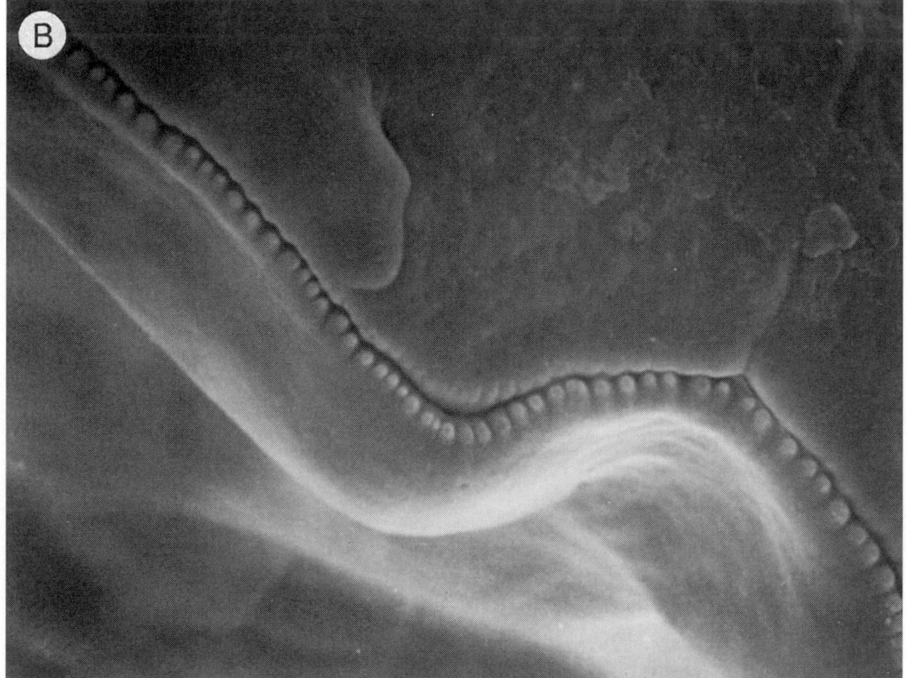

FIGURE 32.2 Head structures of *Ascaris suum* as seen in SEM. (A) The three lips are characteristic of members of this genus and several others in the order. (B) A dentigerous ridge located on the margin of a lip.

number of eggs passed with the feces; since *Ascaris* is a heavy egg producer, eggs are easily found by a flotation technique.

Before the worms mature, pigs may have pneumonia and show labored breathing when the worms reach the lungs; farmers recognize this breathing pattern where the pigs exhale forcefully and call it "the thumps." There are few other signs of infection before the worms reach the intestine, but after that weight gains may be less than expected.

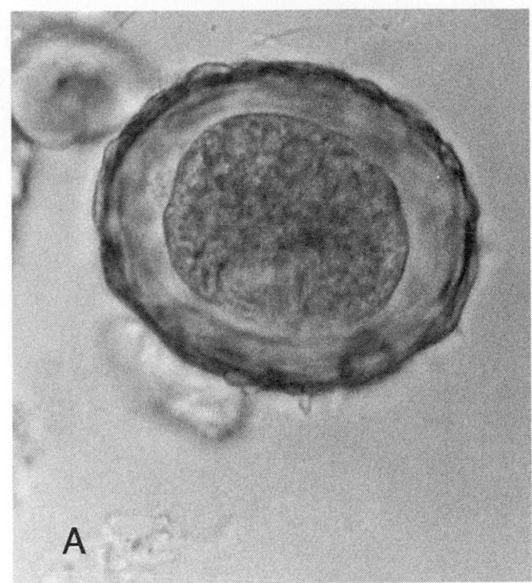

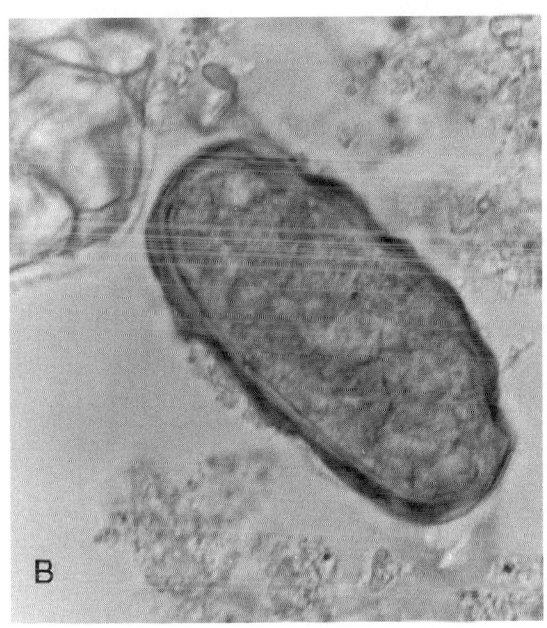

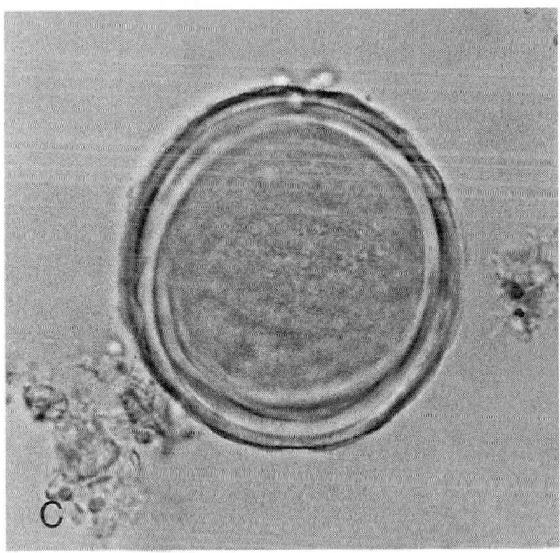

FIGURE 32.3 *Ascaris* eggs (A) A fertilized egg with the typical mammilated outer capsule or shell. (B) An unfertilized egg; these are usually rather elongate and lack a clearly defined zygote inside. (C) A fertilized egg lacking the characteristic mammilations.

There may also be respiratory problems in humans if a large number of eggs is ingested, but usually the signs and symptoms of infection occur after the worms reach the small intestine.

Host–Parasite Interactions

The symptoms and effects of *Ascaris* infection are directly related to worm burden. Light infections are often asymptomatic and cause little lasting damage, but heavy infections cause severe damage.

If we consider *A. suum* only, losses arise from the following:

1. Larvae may migrate through the lungs, where they may cause lung disease.
2. Exacerbation of other infections during migration. Viral and bacterial pneumonias may be triggered or made worse by the migration of the larvae through the lungs.
3. Scarring from larvae migrating in the liver. Such livers are condemned at slaughter because of "milk spot."
4. Reduced feed efficiency caused by adult worms. Adults feed on intestinal contents and thereby remove nutrients from the small intestine that would otherwise be absorbed.

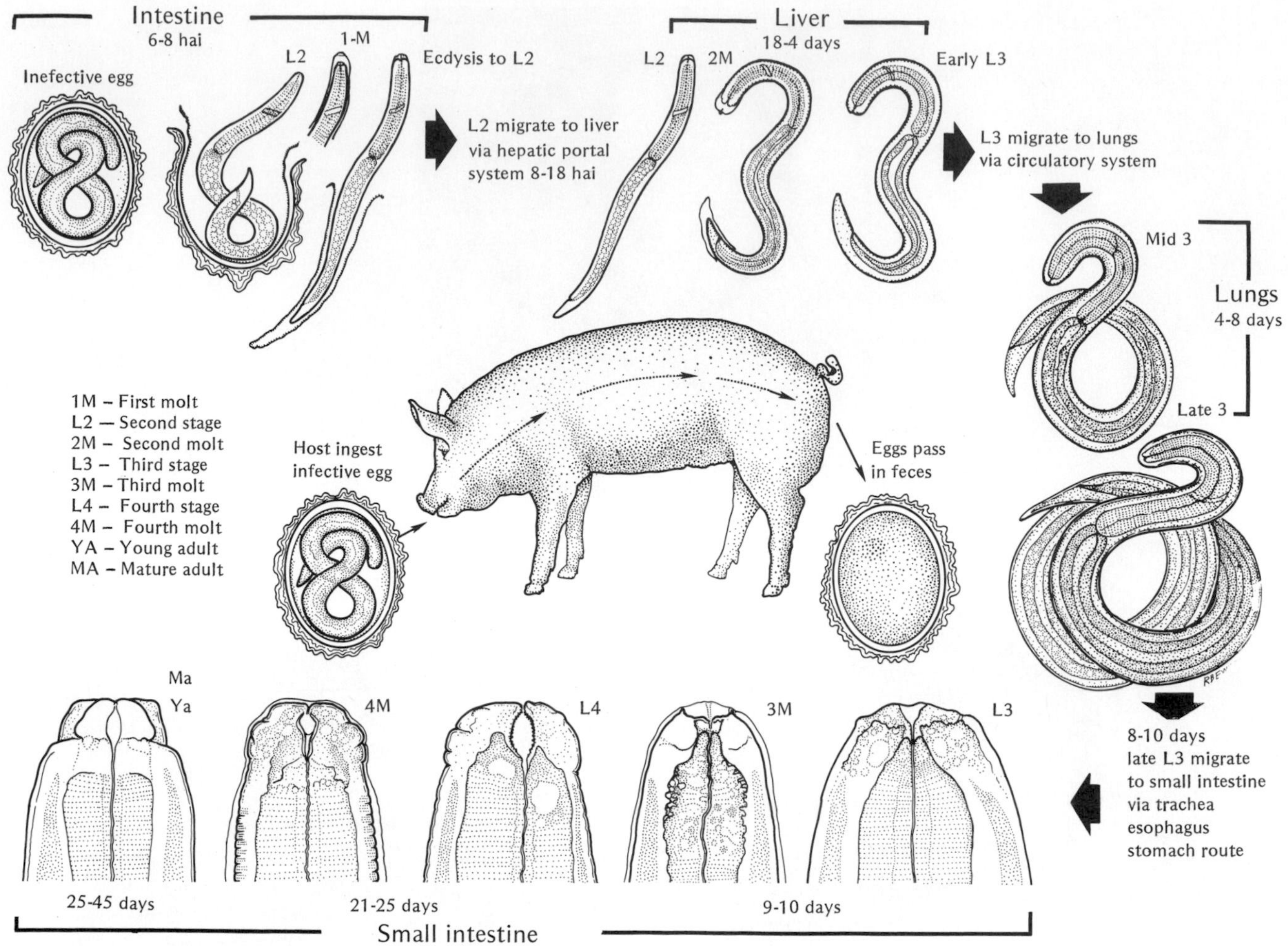

FIGURE 32.4 Life cycle of *Ascaris suum.* This pattern of development is also seen in the ascarid of human, *Ascaris lumbricoides.* Abbreviation: hai, hours after infection. [Courtesy of Dr. F. W. Douvres, Agricultural Research Service, USDA, Beltsville, MD.]

5. Blocking of the intestine. Worms sometimes occur in such large numbers that movement of the intestinal contents is impeded.
6. Migration into extraintestinal sites. Trucking of animals to market or having a fever, among other upsetting factors, may cause worms to migrate. They may move through the intestinal wall into the peritoneal cavity, or anteriorly so that they are coughed up, or they may move into the common bile duct and then to the smaller bile ducts of the liver. When the worms move into the bile ducts, they may become so tightly packed that the flow of bile is reduced. Movement into the peritoneal cavity can give rise to bacterial peritonitis, which may be fatal.

Humans can be infected by both *Ascaris lumbricoides* and *A. suum*. Similar lesions result; however, the physiology of the two species is markedly different in humans and pigs. An extensive study compared the development of *A. suum* and *A. lumbricoides* in specific pathogen-free pigs as well as rabbits and concluded that in the pig, *A. suum* "completes development in the lungs and migrates to the intestine earlier, it requires less time to reach the egg-laying stage, and when taken into man it develops to maturity less frequently and remains in the intestines for relatively short periods."

Five to six days after infection, larvae in the lungs cause fever, chills, and a paroxysmal cough. If large numbers of larvae are present, pneumonia associated with eosinophilic infiltration of the lungs may result. These symptoms last seven to ten days but improve progressively. During the initial phase of the lung pathology, the sputum often contains abundant eosinophils and, rarely, larvae.

A few adult worms usually cause no clinical disease, but severe disease results from heavy infections. The most severe complications result from parasites wrapping themselves around one another, leading to intestinal obstruction, abdominal pain, loss of weight, nausea, and several other symptoms.

On rare occasions, ascarids may perforate the intestines and cause peritonitis. Wandering ascarids occasionally enter bile ducts, pancreatic ducts, kidneys, or pass from the mouth, nose, anus, or umbilicus, causing physical as well as mental trauma. Female worms apparently seek the curved tail of a male and may pass through openings similar to those described here.

Information on immunity to *Ascaris* in humans is sketchy; however, there is a large body of knowledge on immunity in swine. There seems to be little effective immunity against the adult worms but good immunity against the migrating larvae. Most likely, the immunity acts at the molt from the second to the third stages. It should be noted that this immunity is manifested by the absence of adult worms following challenge and does not necessarily mean that larvae are destroyed. The immune response may simply preclude further development. In spite of a good deal of knowledge about immunity to *Ascaris* it has not yet been possible to develop a vaccine to prevent ascaridosis in pigs.

A high percentage of laboratory workers who have studied *Ascaris* have become allergic to it. Their hypersensitivity may become severe enough that some investigators have switched their interests to other less allergenic parasites.

Epidemiology and Control

Control of ascaridosis in humans is based on the following:

1. Treatment of individuals
2. Treatment of populations where the prevalence of infection is high
3. Sanitary disposal of human waste
4. Holding human waste for a period of time when it is to be used for fertilizer

Various drugs are available to treat ascaridosis in humans. If other helminths are present, the ascarids should be treated first so that they will not be stimulated to wander by ineffective drugs. There is no successful treatment for larval ascaridosis.

Ascaris infections are more common in humans in the tropics and subtropics than in the temperate zones. Eggs are extremely resistant and can survive up to six years in nature, up to six months in sewage sludge, and even on paper money. Egg production is truly prodigious in *Ascaris;* most estimates lie in the range of 200,000 or more eggs per day per female worm.

Sanitary disposal of feces plus education should prevent ascaridosis in humans. However, lack of adequate fertilizer in many parts of the undeveloped world means that night soil must be used to fertilize crops. Due to the resistance of *Ascaris* eggs to standard disinfectants, the situation is difficult at best.

A difficulty in control is preventing children from ingesting eggs with contaminated soil. Given the habits of children throughout the world, including pica (dirt eating), playing in the dirt and then placing their fingers or other contaminated objects in their mouths, ascaridosis will unfortunately be with us until adequate sanitation is accomplished. That prospect may be a long way off for many undeveloped nations.

Control of ascarid infections in domestic swine that are raised on soil is particularly difficult. High egg production coupled with the long survival of the embryonated eggs outside the host means that a farm can become heavily contaminated in a short time and remain contaminated for years. The systems that have been developed for mitigating the impact of ascaridosis are directed toward reducing infections in and on sows and protecting young pigs from being exposed to significant infections.

One of the early systems developed for control of diseases in swine is the McLean County system of swine sanitation; although we are concerned here with *Ascaris*, other soil and feces-borne infections are controlled as well. The method was first implemented by B. H. Ranson of the USDA in 1921 in McLean County in central Illinois. Where it was adopted and followed faithfully, swine production benefited.

The objective of the system is to allow young pigs no contact with anything contaminated with ascarid eggs. Even though the principles were laid down more than 70 years ago, they are still valid:

1. Prior to the birth of the pigs (farrowing), the quarters are cleaned. The floor should be concrete, but if not, all feces should be removed. The whole farrowing pen should be scrubbed with a brush and a strong detergent.
2. The sow is treated with an anthelmintic so as to reduce contamination of the area with helminth eggs.
3. Just prior to farrowing, the sow is washed so that all mud and adhering feces are removed from all parts of her body.
4. The sow and pigs are kept in the clean quarters until they are ready to be moved to pasture. When they are moved, they are carried by truck so that they have no opportunity of contacting eggs on the ground.
5. The pasture should not have been used by pigs

for several years, and the water supply should be built so as to be free of possible contamination with ascarid eggs.

Swine are treated for helminths by adding drugs to the feed or the water; individual handling of pigs is rather time-consuming, and a number of highly efficacious drugs are available.

OTHER ASCARIDS

Ascaris of humans and swine demonstrate the general principles that pertain to other members of the group, but some additional aspects of transmission and control are found in other ascarids of both humans and other hosts. The genera discussed in this section include *Toxocara, Toxascaris, Anisakis, Contracaecum, Phocanema, Ascaridia,* and *Heterakis.*

DOGS AND CATS

Name of Organism and Disease Associations

Toxocara canis is a parasite of canids: dogs, coyote, fox; it is a significant pathogen of puppies. It is also pathogenic in humans and is of particular concern when infecting children in which it causes toxocariosis, toxocariasis, or visceral larva migrans (VLM) as well as ocular larva migrans (OLM) in humans.

Hosts and Host Range

Adults are in the small intestine of canids. Humans, especially children, can be paratenic hosts; they harbor migrating infective larvae, which wander through deep body tissues, causing VLM, or into the eyes, causing granulomatous lesions called OLM. There is a wide variety of other paratenic hosts for *T. canis* including most animals commonly used for research. Larvae are found in most deep body tissues such as the liver and kidney.

Geographic Distribution and Importance

Cosmopolitan. Evidence from serological studies and fecal examinations suggests that nearly all dogs have been infected by *T. canis*, and most of these infections were contracted in utero or as young pups.

The potential contamination of the environment is mind boggling when one considers the estimate that the dogs and cats in the United States produce thousands of tons of feces per day. This high egg production coupled with long survival of larvae in the egg capsules points up the potential problem.

The risk of humans, especially children, accidentally becoming infected is substantial. The actual number of human infections may be far greater than realized, too. An enzyme-linked immunosorbent assay (ELISA) test employing larval antigens of *T. canis* showed that nearly 3% of more than 8000 healthy Americans had evidence of exposure to this parasite. Seroprevalence was higher for children 6 to 11 years of age.

Morphology

Toxocara canis, like *Ascaris*, has three prominent lips with sensory papillae and fine dentigerous ridges. Prominent long, slender cervical alae (Fig. 32.5) are present. The esophagus has a distinct muscular bulb and a prominent ventriculus (Fig. 32.6).

Males are 4 to 10 cm by 2 to 2.5 mm, have 20 to 30 preanal papillae, five postanal papillae, a narrow terminal appendage, and subequal spicules. Females are 5 to 18 cm by 2.5 to 3.0 mm, and have a vulva in the anterior fourth of the body. Eggs are subspherical, pitted, and are 85 to 90 by 75 μm (Fig. 32.7A).

Life Cycle

In the life cycle of *Toxocara canis* (Fig. 32.8), unembryonated eggs are shed in feces. Larvae molt once

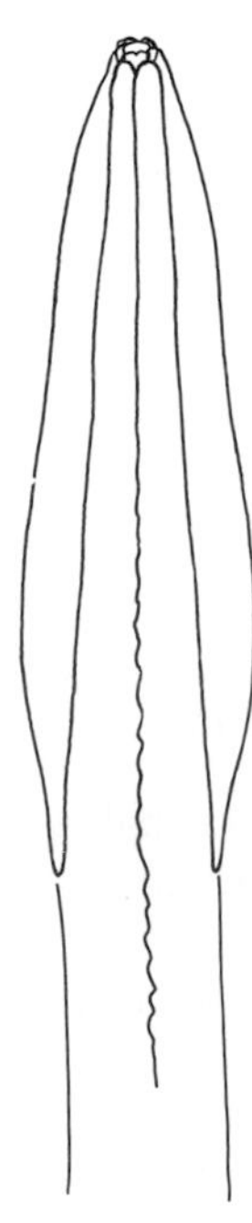

FIGURE 32.5 The anterior end of *Toxocara canis* showing the prominent cervical alae giving it the common name of "arrow worm." [Redrawn from Morgan & Hawkins, 1949.]

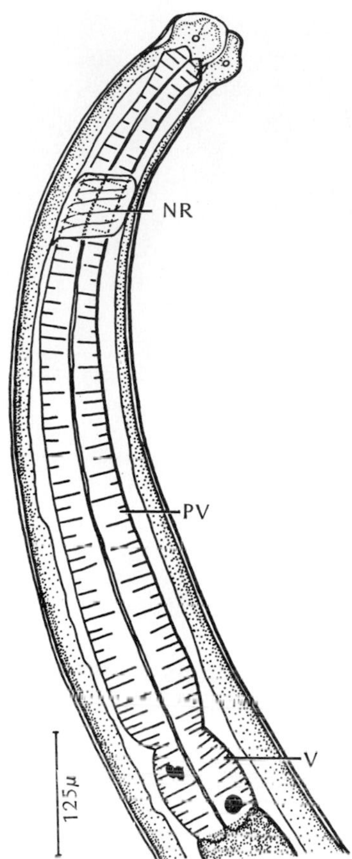

FIGURE 32.6 The esophageal region of *Toxocara canis* showing identifying structures. Abbreviations: NR—nerve ring; PV—proventriculus; V—ventriculus. [Redrawn from Schacher, J., 1957.]

to the infective stage in 9 to 15 days under optimal conditions. Dogs ingest ova containing infective larva; the larvae are released in the small intestine and penetrate the intestinal mucosa. At this point the life cycle can follow one of two paths, depending on the age of the dog.

If a dog less than three months old ingests infective ova, larvae hatch in the duodenum, penetrate the intestinal wall, and enter lymph vessels. They travel to the liver via the hepatic portal system, arriving there one to two days after infection. No molt occurs in the liver. Larvae then migrate to the heart through the hepatic vein or vena cava. Peak numbers of larvae in lungs are reached three to five days after infection. Two paths may be followed from the lungs. Most larvae in young dogs break out of the alveoli, travel up the trachea, are swallowed, and pass to the stomach by ten days postinfection. The molt to L_4 occurs in the stomach and small intestines. The molt to adult occurs in the intestines two to three weeks after infection. Adult worms mate and eggs are passed in the feces four to five weeks after infection.

The second route followed by larvae in lungs (especially larvae in dogs six months of age and older) is to travel by the pulmonary vein to the heart and then throughout the body through the arterial circulation; they leave small blood vessels and enter nearly every tissue. They can be found in greatest numbers in the liver, skeletal muscles, and kidney. This somatic tissue migration gives rise to visceral larva migrans in humans (discussed in Host–Parasite Interactions). There are aggressive immune responses and inflammation surrounding the larvae but no real evidence that larvae are killed. The larvae seem to continue to migrate away from the inflammatory processes of the host.

A third life cycle pattern is the most important method of infection in dogs—transplacental infection. Infective larvae that are disseminated in pregnant bitches somehow become activated, enter the circulatory system, and eventually pass through the placenta to go to the liver of developing pups. The usual migratory route in young dogs continues after birth, and pups can harbor adult worms by one week after birth and pass eggs when they are three weeks old. Transplacental infection can occur by activation of somatic larvae or by ingestion of infective ova during gestation. The former is probably the source of most infections.

Puppies are also infected with the milk, but this is probably a less important aspect of transmission than transplacental infection. Bitches cleaning puppy feces may be reinfected with additional somatic L_2s, ensuring infections in future generations of puppies.

T. canis can infect a wide variety of transport hosts including rodents and humans; somatic larvae can remain infectious for years probably the lifetime of the host. The infection in a rodent can be continued as a larval infection. Infected paratenic hosts can also be source of larvae, which will develop in dogs following the ingestion of a paratenic host.

Diagnosis

Toxocariosis is diagnosed by finding eggs (Fig. 32.7) or worms in the feces. Puppies that have been infected prenatally typically become potbellied and have a rough hair coat. Most dog raisers need only these signs of infection, and knowledge of the fact that most puppies are infected, to know when to institute treatment.

Visceral larva migrans in humans can be confirmed by finding larvae in biopsies, especially liver, but larvae are only rarely found. An enzyme-linked immunosorbent assay is a diagnostic test used by the Centers for Disease Control to identify both visceral larvae migrans and ocular larva migrans.

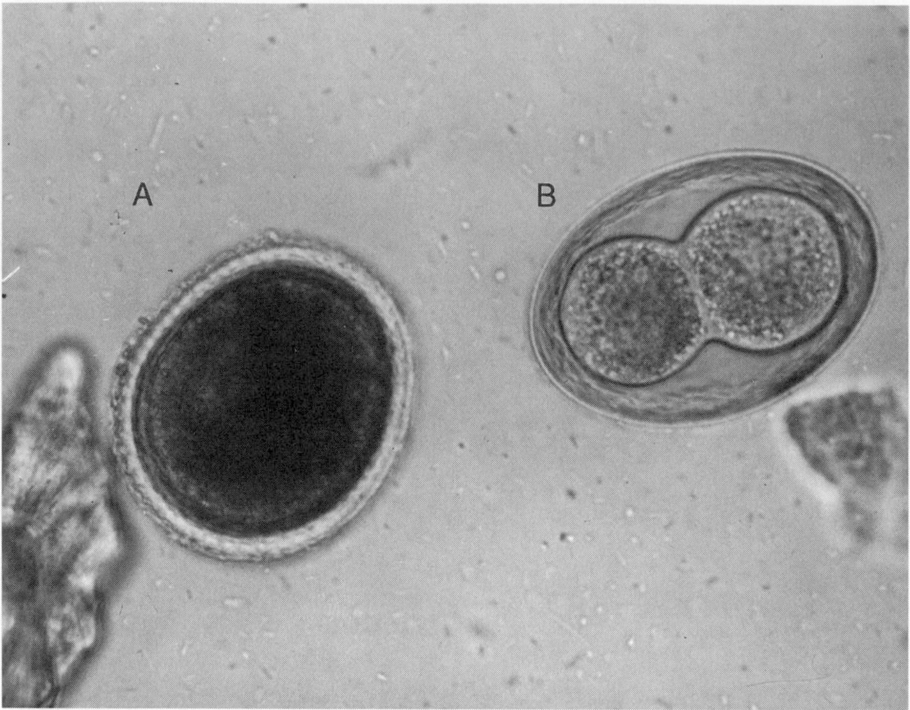

FIGURE 32.7. Eggs of *Toxocara canis* (A) and *Toxacaris leonina* (B). These eggs are about the same size, but *T. canis* has a mammilated outer capsule and *T leonina* is relatively smooth with a fibrous-appearing inner capsule.

Host–Parasite Interactions

Toxocara canis produces various responses in dogs, depending on the worm burden and the age of the dog. Infected puppies may have digestive disturbances, dull coat, and vomit often. Pneumonia is often present in infected young animals. Heavily infected animals may die two to three weeks after birth.

Adult dogs have granulomatous lesions caused by migrating larvae in almost any tissue or organ. Dogs are apparently afflicted with OLM similar to the human disease.

The term *visceral larva migrans* (VLM) is used for human infections with *T. canis* and some other helminths. The typical patient is a child one to five years old. Fatalities have occurred, but normally the disease is self-limiting. Pathogenesis in humans results from tissue damage (eosinophilic granulomata) caused by migrating larvae and a strong immune response. Early migration is often accompanied by abdominal pain, diarrhea, and hepatomegaly. Larvae cause pneumonia accompanied by eosinophilia during the lung migration. VLM sometimes occurs in the brain and has been associated with various neurologic symptoms.

Ocular larva migrans or OLM is the result of migrating *T. canis* larvae in the eyes and is seen typically in children from 3 to 13 years of age. OLM lesions look much like those of retinoblastoma, the most common eye tumor in children; this tumor is dangerous and requires an early decision on a course of action. This similarity has previously resulted in the needless removal of eyes from children. Serodiagnostic tests on ocular fluid and better ophthalmic medicine has helped to prevent such tragic losses.

Immunity to *T. canis* larvae is typical of immunity to many larval nematodes. That is, there is ample evidence of an immune response in the host, but there is no evidence that the immune response results in killing of larvae. In fact, immunity is either of no consequence or it is harmful. Larvae live and migrate in animals whose immune response probably exists for the life of the host. Clearly, puppies develop immunity that results in migrating larvae being shunted to various parts of the body rather than continuing maturation to the adult in the gut. Both in dogs and paratenic host, these somatically wandering larvae generate immune responses, and antibody attached to the surface coat of the parasite and leukocytes with potential to kill the parasite are bridged to the parasite surface with antibody. The larvae respond by shedding surface antigens and migrating away from the immunologically hostile environment much as a snake sheds it skin. New surface antigens are produced, and the cycle con-

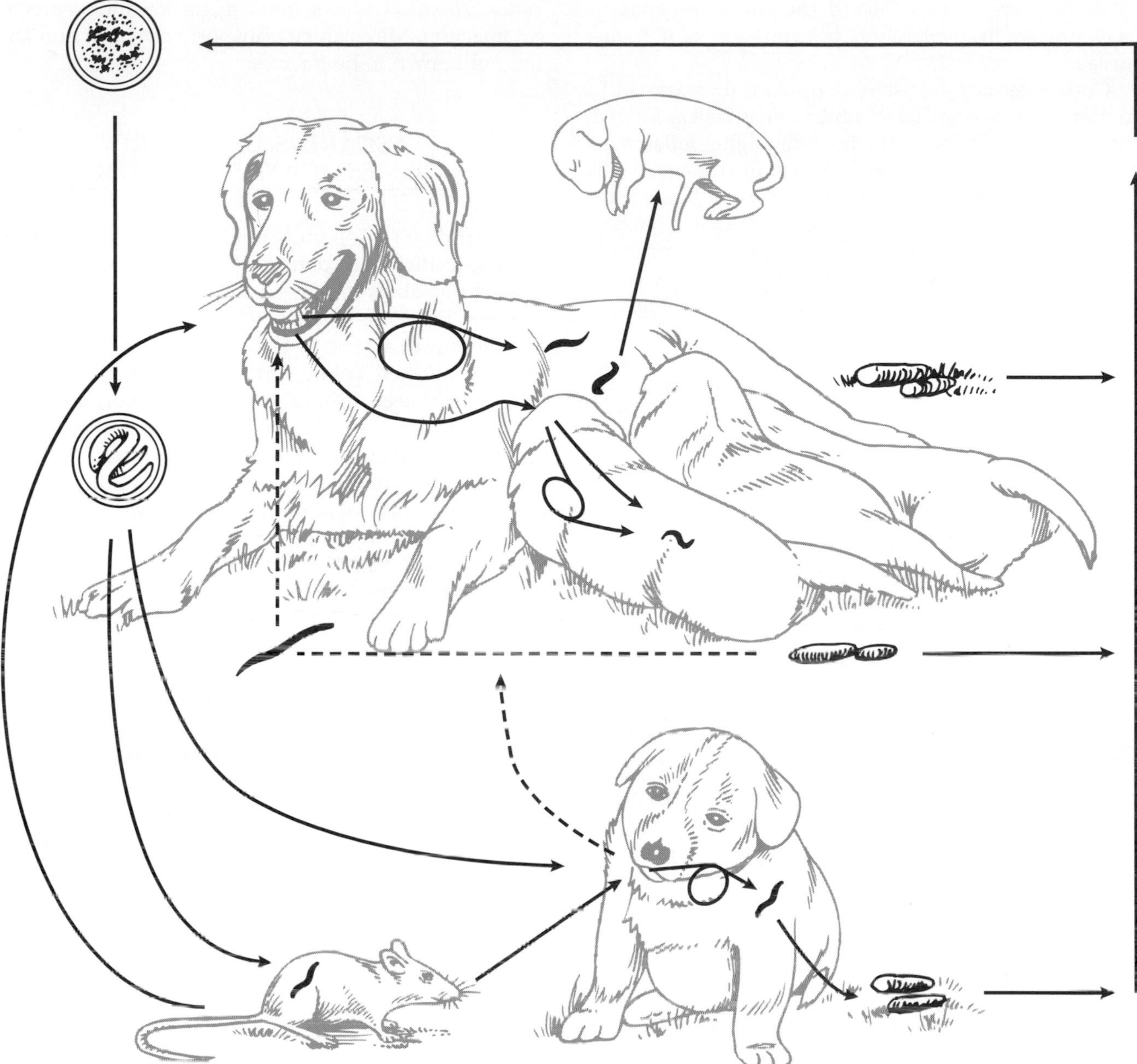

FIGURE 32.8 The life cycle and modes of transmission of *Topxocara canis*. There are three modes of transmission: by mouth, prenatally, and through the milk.

tinues. The result of this novel adaptation to host immunity is that the larvae continue to live and they leave, in their wake, tissue-destructive inflammatory disease and granulomas containing larval antigens.

Epidemiology and Control

Prevention should include the following:

1. Strategic anthelmintic treatment of dogs
2. Laws requiring owners to remove the feces of their animals from public places
3. Leash laws for controlling dogs
4. Excluding dogs from children's play areas
5. Education in order to change the habits of persons who may be in contact with dogs or their excreta

Intestinal worms in dogs are treated with any of a variety of modern anthelmintics. Certain of these drugs given at precise times toward the end of pregnancy may prevent transplacental transmission of *T. canis* larvae.

Corticosteroids are useful in humans for severe pulmonary and myocardial involvement as well as for eye inflammation. Quieting the host-damaging inflammatory responses may be the best overall strategy.

The timing of de-worming is important because of the parasite's biology. Young pups and nursing bitches should be treated as frequently as possible after parturition because pups can shed eggs at three weeks. Weanling pups can be de-wormed twice 10 to 14 days apart. The tendency for young puppies to see the veterinarian for the first time at six week of age works against effective treatment that can be provided. Better solutions are likely to be seen when the dog breeder involves the veterinarian shortly after birth. Older dogs should have fecal examinations once a year and be treated as needed, but dogs older than six to nine months of age rarely have patent infections with *T. canis.* In addition, puppy and bitch feces should be disposed of often so that eggs do not have a chance to embryonate and infect either dogs or humans. With adequate veterinary care and responsible owner behavior, the threat of toxocariasis (VLM and OLM) can be significantly reduced.

Infections in puppies approach 100%, but older dogs rarely have patent infections. The infection percentages are high in puppies because of the efficiency of transplacental infection. With 65 million to 70 million dogs in the United States, it is obvious that many households, parks, and playgrounds may be contaminated with *Toxocara* eggs, which potentially can cause either VLM or OLM in children. The problem is compounded by the fact that *Toxocara* eggs are extremely resistant to environmental insults and may survive for years.

Other Ascarids of Companion Animals

Toxocara cati occurs only in cats and has a migration similar to that of *T. canis* except that it lacks transplacental infection. Its cervical alae are short and broad. Eggs have a pitted surface and are 65 to 75 μm in diameter. Eggshell morphology in SEM is different for *T. canis* and *T. cati*. As many as 75% of cats are infected with *T. cati* , but this parasite rarely is implicated in VLM, but it must be regarded as an occasional human parasite.

The third ascarid found in both cats and dogs is *Toxascaris leonina*. *Toxascaris* has no esophageal ventriculus and its three lips differ slightly from those of *Toxocara*. *Toxascaris leonina* ova are smooth (Fig. 32.7B) and measure 75 to 85 by 60 to 75 μm. Adults have long, slender cervical alae resembling those of *Toxocara canis*. *T. leonina* has no somatic migration and no prenatal infection. Mice can be transport hosts, but humans are not known to be infected.

ASCARIDS OF OTHER DOMESTICATED ANIMALS

Ascarids of economic importance are found in horses, cattle, and poultry. *Neoascaris vitulorum* is passed prenatally to calves and is pathogenic in young animals. *Parascaris equorum* of horses is also pathogenic in colts up to a year of age, but the animals do not become infected before birth. Ascarid infections are not usually seen in adult cattle or horses, and it is therefore necessary to look for the signs of infection in young animals and for eggs in the feces. Prompt treatment to remove the adult worms is called for.

Chickens that are raised on the ground, as opposed to broiler or laying houses, are subject to infection with *Ascaridia galli* and *Heterakis gallinarum*. *A. galli* may affect growth rate in chicks when they average as few as 4.3 worms per bird. After about three months of age, birds become resistant to infection with *A. galli*.

H. gallinarum, the cecal worm, is usually found in small numbers. Its importance lies in its being a vector of *Histomonas meleagridis*, a trichomonad which is especially pathogenic for turkeys (Chapter 5).

ANISAKOSIS

The disease in humans called *anisakosis* or *anisakiasis* is caused by infections with nematodes of the subfamily Anisakinae. Two genera cause human disease—*Anisakis* and *Pseudoterrnova* (syns. *Phocanema, Terranova,* and *Porrocaecum*).

Adult anisakids resemble *Ascaris*. Three lips are present, usually with dentigerous ridges. The anterior diverticulum of the digestive tract is characteristic of the subfamily (Fig. 32.9). The esophagus is divided into a proventriculus and a ventriculus. Some genera have a ventricular appendix, and some also have an anterior, blind extension of the intestine, the intestinal cecum.

Definitive hosts of the Anisakinae are marine mammals and some fish, birds, reptiles, and amphibians. Life cycles are usually indirect. Eggs are passed in feces and the first molt occurs in the eggs. The second molt probably occurs in crustaceans such as the shrimp *Euphausia* spp. There is only a low infection rate in crustacea, but fish consume enormous numbers and thereby pass the infection up the food chain. Fish and squid

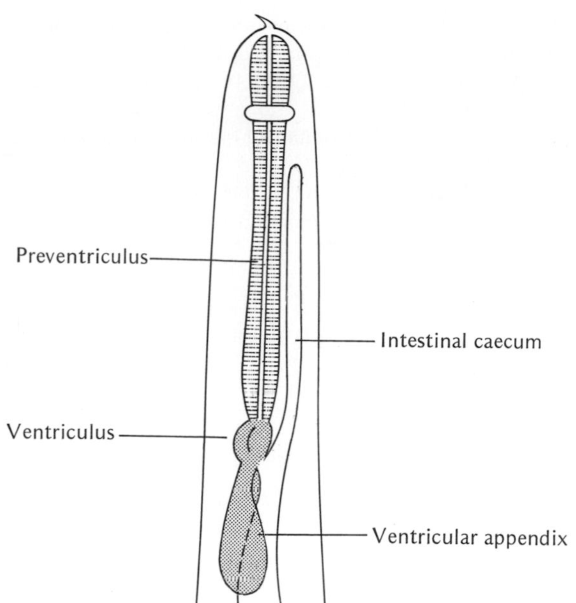

FIGURE 32.9 The esophageal region of the digestive tract of an anasakine nematode showing the cecum extending anteriorly. [Redrawn with modifications from Myers, B. J., 1976.]

harboring third-stage larvae are transport or paratenic hosts. The L_3s are infective for marine mammals and development to the adult occurs in their intestines.

Anisakosis has become recognized as a human disease because of two factors. First, the disease is usually diagnosed only after surgical removal or endoscopy of parasitized stomach or intestine. Second, recent changes in fishing methods probably have increased the incidence of infections. With modern factory ships, which process fish at sea, hours or even days may elapse before fish are eviscerated. Intestinal larvae (L_3s) move from intestines into other organs and muscles as the fish die. When humans then ingest uncooked fish, they are at risk. Identification of the species of larvae infecting humans is difficult.

Nematodes in the subfamily Anisakinae are found throughout the world. Human anisakosis has been reported in Japan, the Netherlands, Korea, Denmark, France, Belgium, and the United States—countries where marine fish and shellfish may be eaten raw, pickled, or lightly cooked.

Anisakosis in humans can produce either gastric or intestinal disturbances. Symptoms of gastric infection include sudden stomach pains, nausea, and vomiting four to six hours after eating raw fish. The larvae penetrate the tissue layers of the stomach and form tunnels of burrows in the mucosa and submucosa. This aggressive penetration is enabled by proteases that are secreted by the larvae which, in turn, cause destruction of the host tissue. Stomach lesions are typical showing a foreign-body responses with granulomata around the larvae. Intestinal infections cause severe abdominal pain, vomiting, fever, and blood in the stool within seven days after eating raw fish. Intestinal damage is an Arthus type reactions in acute cases, characterized by thickening of the intestinal wall along with eosinophilic infiltration. Later, eosinophilic granulomata form around the larvae.

Anisakosis will probably be seen more often with the change in fishing mentioned earlier and the trend toward "natural" foods, which are often uncooked or undercooked. Two surveys showed that commercially caught fish in Boston, San Francisco, and Los Angeles contained potential pathogens, especially on the West Coast, where 41.6% of the fish harbored *Anisakis* larvae.

Control includes not eating smoked, marinated, or raw fresh fish or squid. Heating fish to 60° C or freezing to −20°C for 24 hours kills the larvae.

Readings

Arean, V. M., and Crandall, C. A. (1971). Ascariasis. In *Pathology of Protozoal and Helminthic Diseases* (P. A. Marcial-Rojas, Ed.). Williams & Wilkins, Baltimore.

Badley, J. E., Grieve, R. B., and Glickman, L. T. (1987). Immune-mediated adherence of eosinophils to *Toxocara canis* infective larvae: The role of excretory–secretory antigens. *Parasite Immunol.* **9,** 133–143.

Beaver, P. C., Snyder, C. H., Carrera, G. M., Dent, J., and Lafferty, J. (1952). Chronic eosinophilia due to visceral larval migrans. *Pediatrics* **9,** 7–19.

Bier, J. W., Jackson, G. J., and Payne, W. L. (1980). Recovery of nematodes from Pacific and Atlantic pleuronectid fish, compared by sedimentation and digestion. *J. Parasitol.* **66**(Suppl.), 66. [Abstract]

Crompton, D. W. T. (1988). The prevalence of ascariasis. *Parasitol. Today* **4,** 162–169.

Crompton, D. W. T., Nesheim, M. C., and Pawlowski, Z. S. (1989). *Ascariasis and Its Prevention and Control.* Taylor & Francis, Bristol, PA.

Deardorff, T. L., Kayes, S. G., and Fukumura, T. (1991). Human anisakiniasis transmitted by marine food products. *Hawaii Med. J.* **50,** 9–16.

Gillespie, S. H. (1988). The epidemiology of *Toxocara canis*. *Parasitol. Today* **4,** 180–182.

Glickman, L. T., Schantz, P. M., and Grieve, R. B. (1986). Toxocariasis. In *Immunodiagnosis of Parasitic Diseases* (K. W. Walls and P. M. Schantz, Eds.),Vol. 1, pp. 201–231. Academic Press, New York.

Hoeppli, R. (1959). *Parasites and Parasitic Infections in Early Medicine and Science.* Univ. of Malaysia Press, Singapore.

Morgan, B. B., and Hawkins, P. A. (1949). *Veterinary Helminthology.* Burgess, Minneapolis, MN.

Myers, B. J. (1976). The nematodes that cause anisakiasis. *J. Milk Food Technol.* **38,** 774–782.

Parsons, J. C. (1987). Ascarid infections of cats and dogs. *Vet. Clin. North Am. Small Anim. Practice Parasitic Infect.* **17**(6), 1307–1339.

Sakanari, J. A. (1990). Anisakis—From platter to the microfuge. *Parasitol. Today* **6,** 232–237.

Sakanari, J. A., and McKerrow, J. H. (1989). Anisakiniasis. *Clin. Microbiol. Rev.* **2,** 278–284.

Sakanari, J. A., and McKerrow, J. H. (1990). Identification of the secreted neutral proteases form *Anisakis simplex. J. Parasitol.* **76,** 635–630.

Schacher, J. (1957). A contribution to the life history and larval morphology of *Toxocara canis. J. Parasitol.* **43,** 599–612.

Schantz, P. M., and Glickman, L. T. (1979). Canine and human toxocariasis: The public health problem and veterinarian's role in prevention. *J. Am. Vet. Med. Assoc.* **175,** 1270–1273.

Smith, J. W., and Wootten, R. (1978). *Anisakis* and anisakiasis. *Adv. Parasitol.* **16,** 93–163.

Sprent, J. F. A. (1962). The evolution of the Ascaridoidea. *J. Parasitol.* **48,** 818–824.

Williams, H. H., and Jones, A. (1976). *Marine Helminths and Human Health*, Misc. Publ. No. 3. Commonwealth Agricultural Bureaux, Farnham Royal, Bucks, UK.

CHAPTER

33

Pinworms

The pinworms (order Oxyurida) received their name because of the long, pointed tail of the female. Their other striking characteristic is the large bulb at the posterior of the esophagus (Figs. 33.1, 33.2). The females are stout-bodied, and the males, which have only a single spicule, are usually about half the size of the females. In an unusual kind of sex determination, males are haploid and females are diploid.

Pinworms are widely found in both vertebrates, especially mammals and reptiles, and in invertebrates such as millipedes and insects. They are often found in large numbers in the intestines of their hosts, but only a few species are of medical or economic importance. There are a number of species of *Skrjabinema* in ruminants, and laboratory rodents are frequently infected with *Aspiculuris tetraptera* or *Syphacia obvelata*. Striking species found in the cecum of the porcupine are *Evaginurus evaginata* and *Wellcomia evaginata*, in which the vulva of the female grows into an elegant, elongated structure (Fig. 33.3).

General principles of ecology and niche diversification can sometimes be elucidated with unlikely material, as was done by Schad (1963) with the pinworm, *Tachygonetra* spp. of turtles. Eight species of *Tachygonetra* occur in the large intestine of the turtle *Testudo graeca*, and they have different distributions not only along the length of the gut but radially as well. The result is that each species has its own niche and feeds on different food, as shown by different mouth structures.

OXYURIS EQUI OF HORSES

Name of Organism and Disease Caused

Oxyuris equi causes pinworm infection, oxyurosis, or oxyuriasis.

Hosts and Host Range

The organism is common in horses and other equids.

Geographic Distribution and Importance

Cosmopolitan. *O. equi* is a minor infection that can have secondary consequences of some importance in individual animals.

Morphology

The females are 40 to 150 mm long with pointed tails that vary considerably in length. Males are 9 to 12 mm long and have a single spicule about 140 μm long (Fig. 33.1). The operculate eggs are somewhat flattened on one side and are 85 to 95 by 40 to 45 μm.

Life Cycle

Eggs containing the infective larvae are ingested with contaminated food or water or upon grooming via the hair of an infected animal. The preadult stages develop in the paramucosal lumen and they return to the lumen when they become sexually mature. The prepatent period is about five months. Eggs are shed containing an L_1, and they reach infectivity as an L_2 within three days of leaving the host.

Diagnosis

The principal signs of infection are patches where hair has been rubbed off at the tailhead. Affected animals rub against a barn wall, fence, or even barbed wire to relieve itching.

Since it is more common to find eggs in the perianal region than in feces, diagnosis is often facilitated by impressing clear adhesive tape in the area and then

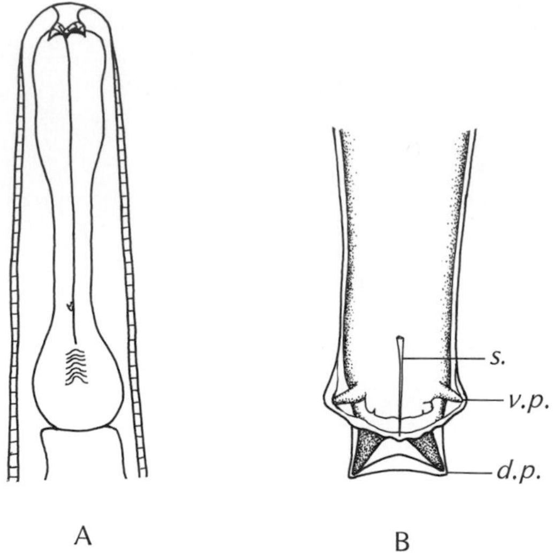

FIGURE 33.1 *Oxyuris equi.* (A) Anterior of a female worm; (B) Posterior of a male worm: s.—spicule; v.p.—subventral papilla; d.p.—dorsal papilla. [Redrawn with modifications from Yorke, W., and Maplestone, P. A., 1962.]

examining the tape microscopically for the characteristic eggs or fragments of adult worms.

Host–Parasite Interactions

The preadult stages do not generally cause any damage. When mature, the females migrate posteriorly to lay eggs in the perianal region. Material on the surface of the eggs is irritating and the anal region obviously itches, since animals then begin to scratch. Scratching can become so vigorous that the hair on the tail and tailhead area of the horse is pulled out and the skin becomes raw. There may be secondary invasion by bacteria, and flesh flies such as *Phormia* or *Cochliomyia* may oviposit in the wounds (Chapter 49).

Epidemiology and Control

Pinworm infection is not generally considered to be a herd problem; however, if a routine program of strongyle control has been established (Chapter 28), pinworms are automatically taken care of by anthelmintic treatment. A number of effective drugs are available.

ENTEROBIUS VERMICULARIS OF HUMANS

Name of Organism and Disease Caused

Enterobius vermicularis causes enterobiosis, enterobiasis, oxyurosis, oxyuriasis, pinworm, or seatworm infection.

Hosts and Host Range

Humans are the only host, for practical purposes; some other primates and rodents have been found to be infected, but these are rare infections that have no epidemiologic importance. *E. vermicularis* infections have never reliably been described from dogs and cats.

Geographic Distribution and Importance

The organism is cosmopolitan, with greater prevalence of infection in temperate and cold than in tropical climates. In North America and Western Europe, the prevalence of infection is about 30% overall and perhaps 50 to 60% in children. In the tropics, the prevalence is about 10%. Pinworms are a common childhood infection that may make a child nervous and irritable, but treatment is easy and effective.

Morphology

The females are 8 to 13 by 0.3 to 0.5 mm, and they have a pointed tail, which may reach 2 mm in length. The males have a curved tail with a single spicule and are 2 to 5 by 0.15 mm. Both sexes have an esophagus with a slender anterior portion and a large posterior bulb; there are small cephalic alae at the anterior tip (Fig. 33.2).

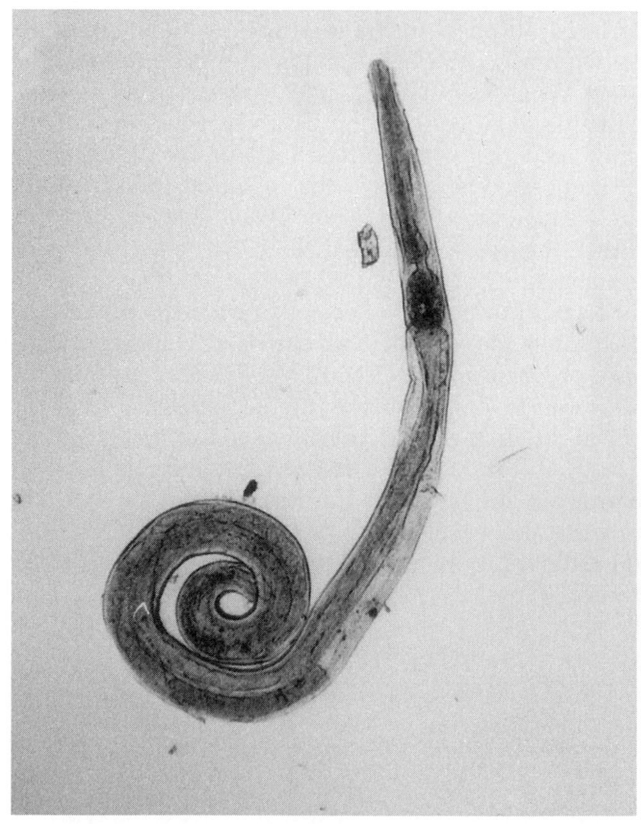

FIGURE 33.2 Adult male of *Enterobius vermicularis.*

The eggs are 50 to 60 by 20 to 32 μm, with a smooth, clear outer capsule; like many oxyurid eggs, they are flattened on one side, giving an asymmetric appearance (Fig. 33.4).

Life Cycle

The females oviposit, or actually burst, in the perianal region; eggs have infective larvae in them within 6 hours after release from the female. Eggs are carried to the mouth of a person on the fingers or are inhaled with dust. Eggs can also hatch within the body of the host giving rise to a type of infection called *retrofection* (or *autoinfection*). Most of the development takes place in the tissue of the large intestine; worms may be found rather superficially in the paramucosal lumen or as deep in the tissue as the serosa (the external covering of the intestine). The worms return to the lumen of the gut and move posteriorly as they mature. The prepatent period is 36 to 53 days. Retrofection may occur when eggs become infective in the perianal area and the hatched larvae reenter the anus.

Diagnosis

Pinworm infection are found by doing the following:

1. Observing clinical signs of nervousness, scratching, and so on
2. Finding eggs in the perianal region

The eggs and fluid from the body of the female worm are irritating and cause intense itching in the anal region. Nervousness, irritability, and scratching are signs often shown by infected children, and this should alert a parent or physician that pinworms may have entered the household.

Since the females oviposit outside the host, eggs are seldom found in the feces. The eggs are collected at the perianal region by swab when the person first arises in the morning. Different kinds of swabs have been developed, but the simplest and most effective is the Scotch tape swab. A piece of cellophane tape is placed sticky side out over the end of a tongue depressor. The tape is pressed into the folds around the anus to pick up the eggs or pieces of worm; it is then placed sticky side down on a microscope slide and a drop or two of toluene is allowed to run under it. The slide is examined under the 10× objective of a compound microscope for the typical asymmetric eggs (Fig. 33.4).

Host–Parasite Interactions

The preadult stages of *E. vermicularis* seldom cause significant damage to the intestine, but a few cases are on record in which they have. The signs and symptoms of infection are a result of the females ovipositing or breaking up in the perianal region. Although they primarily cause itching, there may also be skin eruptions and secondary invasion by bacteria. Vaginitis may occur in some girls from worms crawling from the anus into the genitalia.

Children are twice as likely as adults to be infected with *E. vermicularis*. It is uncertain whether the lower prevalence in adults is due to improved hygiene, age resistance, or to acquired immunity. The latter seems likely, because the preadult worms are in close contact

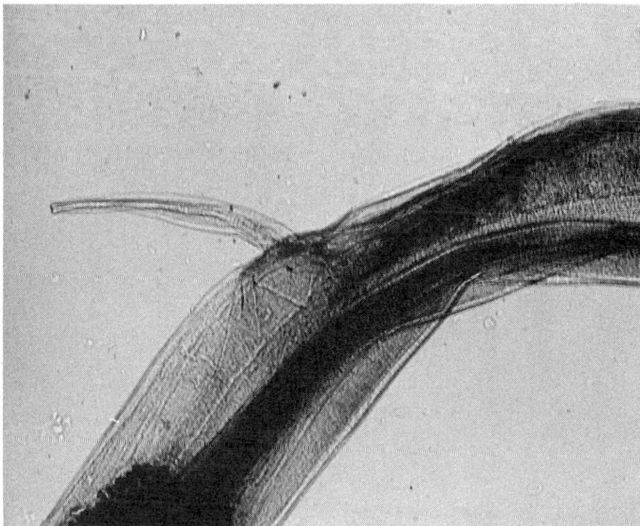

FIGURE 33.3 Pinworm, *Evaginurus* sp., of the porcupine; the large lateral extension is the vulva. Photographed in interference microscopy.

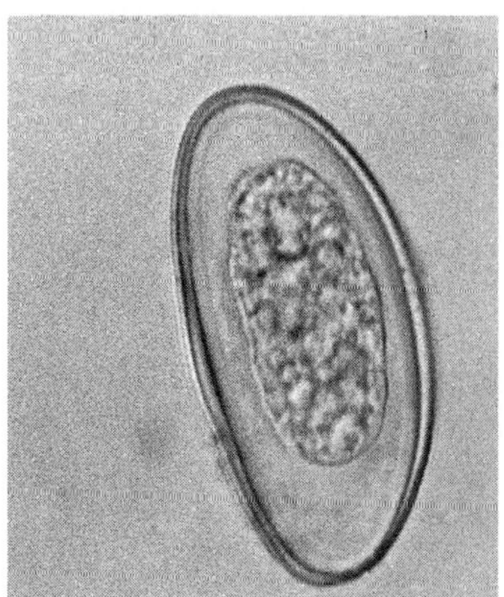

FIGURE 33.4 *Enterobius vermicularis* egg with characteristic flattening on one side.

with the intestinal tissue, but there is little direct evidence.

Epidemiology and Control

Enterobiosis is treated as a household infection by doing the following:

1. Treating both infected and uninfected members of the household
2. Scrupulous cleaning of the house, especially bed linens and blankets

Several good, safe drugs are available for use against pinworms. They are effective and seldom have side effects. Pinworm infection is a household disease; if one person in a family is found to be infected, usually other children and adults are also infected. Therefore, everyone in the family should be treated regardless of whether they have evidence of infection. More than one treatment may be necessary to eliminate the infection, because of the persistence of the infective eggs in the environment.

In addition to treating the people, scrupulous cleaning of the house and frequent washing of bed linens and underclothing are essential to ridding the house of infective eggs.

The high prevalence of *E. vermicularis* infection indicates both its ease of transmission and the hardiness of the free-living stages. Where the humidity is high, infective eggs can live for three weeks or more; low humidity is detrimental to survival. Transmission is principally from the fingers, contaminated clothing, or by inhalation of eggs with dust. Some eggs may be transmitted through contaminated food and water, but this mode is probably of minor importance. A female produces an average of about 11,000 eggs, so the contamination of a house can become heavy.

Children are usually the first to show signs of infection in a family. Because of their lack of fastidious habits, they are likely to have relatively high levels of infection. Perhaps an outbreak of oxyurosis in a family provides an occasion for teaching children not to put things in their mouths and to wash their hands after using the toilet. Pinworms can be exceedingly irritating to the host. The females oviposit or more often burst in the perianal region and they release body fluids. The eggs and the body fluid cause itching and irritation that may make children irritable and nervous.

Nearly every parasitologist or veterinarian has heard that a family dog or cat has brought pinworms into a household. Veterinarians are sometimes asked to euthanize a dog in order to eliminate the reservoir of infection. The host range of *E. vermicularis* is quite narrow and dogs and cats do not become infected. Ironically, it is often the veterinarian rather than the physician who brings proper insight into this common problem of children.

E. vermicularis is the vector of the intestinal protistan, *Dientamoeba fragilis* (Chapter 5). This fact may have implications for further investigation of any diarrheal disease in a household that also has persons infected with pinworms.

Readings

Adamson, M. L. (1989). Evolutionary biology of the Oxyurida (Nematoda)—Biofacies of a haplodiploid taxon. *Adv. Parasitol.* **28,** 175–228.

Cram, E. B. (1941). Studies on oxyuriasis. IX. The familial nature of pinworm infestation. *Med. Ann. District Columbia* **10,** 39–48.

Hugot, J. P., and Tourte-Schaffer, C. (1985). Étude morphologique des oxyures parasite de l'homme: *Enterobius vermicularis* et *E. gregorii. Ann. Parasitol. Hum. Comp.* **60,** 57–64.

Hulinska, D. (1968). The development of the female *Enterobius vermicularis* and the morphogenesis of its sexual organ. *Folia Parasitol.* **15,** 15–27.

Inglis, W. G. (1961). The oxyurid parasites (Nematoda) of primates. *Proc. Zool. Soc. London* **136,** 103–122.

Schad, G. A. (1959). A revision of the North American species of the genus *Skrjabinema* (Nematoda: Oxyuroidea). *Proc. Helm. Soc.* Washington **26,** 138–147.

Schad, G. A. (1963). Niche diversification in a parasite species flock. *Nature* **198,** 404–406.

Schüffner, W., and Swellengrebel, N. H. (1943). Retrofection in oxyuriasis. A newly discovered mode of infection with *Enterobius vermicularis. J. Parasitol.* **38,** 138–146.

Yorke, W., and Maplestone, P. A. (1962). *Nematode Parasites of Vertebrates.* Hafner, New York.

CHAPTER

34

Filarioid and Other Spirurid Nematodes

The nematodes in the order Spirurida include a diverse array of parasites, all of which have vectors in their life cycles. Their distinguishing features are a straight esophagus, with an anterior muscular portion and a posterior glandular portion, and unequal spicules in the males. The bodies vary from rather heavy, similar to the ascarids, to long and threadlike. Head structures range from elaborate looping cordons and buccal capsules supported by ringlike bands to tiny papillae that are almost invisible when studied under the light microscope.

Life cycles are all indirect. Most are passed by mouth through the food chain , but sometimes more than one intermediate host is required to complete the cycle. The filarioid nematodes, which are important to human health, are transmitted by bloodsucking arthropods including mosquitoes, black flies, and biting midges; a few nonhuman filarioids are transmitted by mites.

The 5 superfamilies in the order are separated by details of head structures that need not concern us here. A sampling of members from each of the families is given later, but the emphasis is on those worms that are important to humankind or illustrate certain principles of parasitism.

SUPERFAMILY SPIRUROIDEA

Name of Organism and Disease Associations

Habronema muscae and *Draschia megastoma* cause cataneous habronemosis, habronemiasis, draschiosis or draschiasis, or summer sore in horses.

Hosts and Host Range

Horses and other equids.

Geographic Distribution and Importance

Cosmopolitan. This infection can become serious at certain times and places, mostly warm climates. Individual horses may be seriously affected, and skin lesions may make it impossible to saddle a horse. Estimates of economic losses have not been made.

Morphology

H. muscae males are 8 to 14 mm long and have unequal spicules that are 500 and 2500 μm long. The females are 13 to 22 mm long and both sexes are rather stout. The complex mouth structures (Fig. 34.1) are 54 μm by 19 μm and the esophagus is 2.3 to 3.5 mm long. Eggs are 47 by 16 μm, and are embryonated when laid.

D. megastoma males are 7 to 10 mm long and have unequal spicules that are 280 and 460 μm long. The females are 10 to 13 mm long. The head structures are set off from the rest of the body by a deep groove and the mouth is 130 μm deep (Fig. 34.1). Eggs are 330 to 350 by 8 μm and are embryonated when laid.

Life Cycle

In both of these species, the adult worms lie in the intestine of the horse (Fig. 34.2), and the eggs, or newly hatched larvae, pass out with the feces where they are eaten by the larvae of various cyclorraphan flies (Chapter 48). They reach the L_3 in the fly larva and are carried over the adult stage during pupation. The L_3s

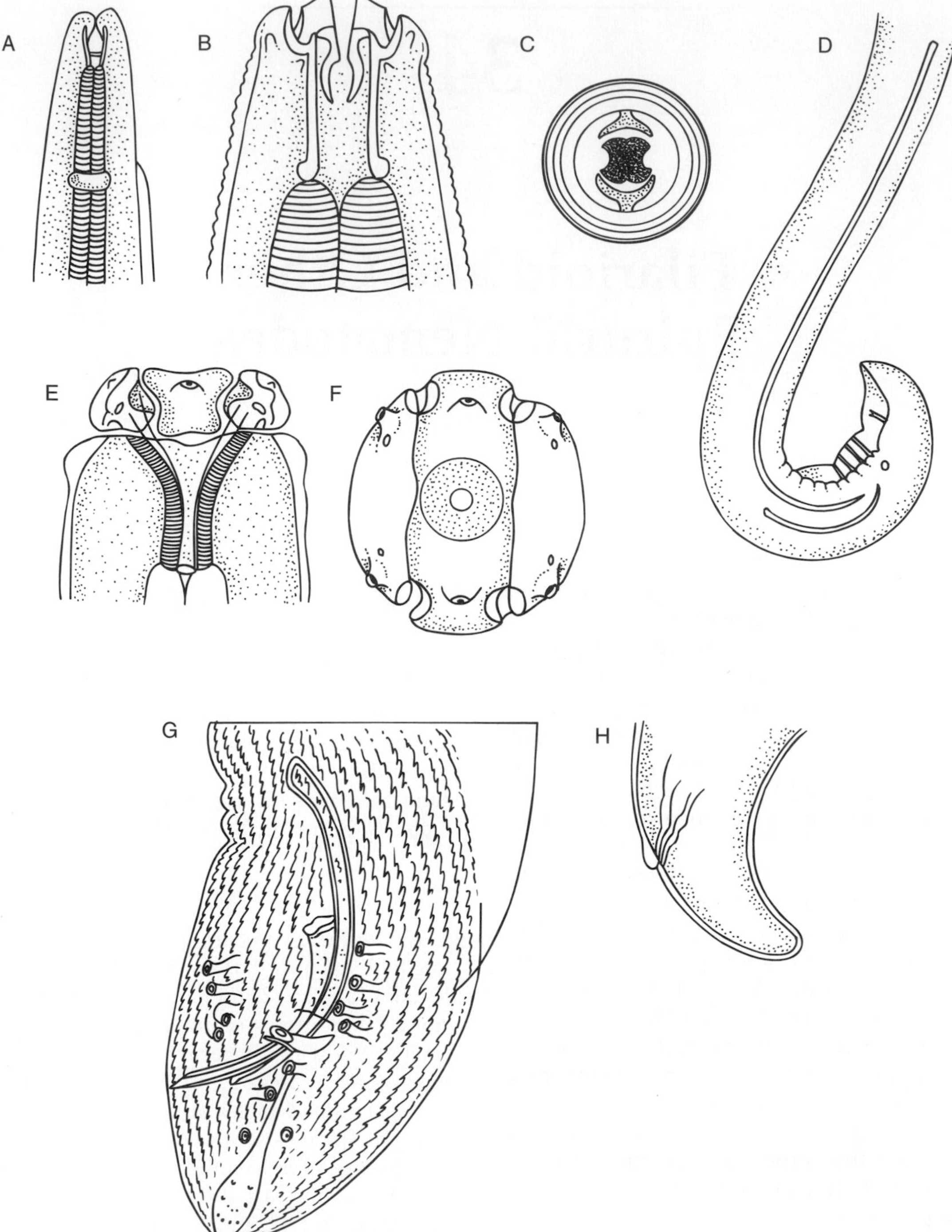

FIGURE 34.1 Head structures of *Habronema muscae* and *Draschia megastoma*. These two species have been placed in a single genus, but the mouth structures are quite dissimilar.(A–D) *Habronema muscae.* (E–H) *Draschia megastoma.* (A) Esophageal region of *H. muscae.* Compare head structures (A) and (E) in lateral view and (C) and *F en face.* Tail structures are also different; compare (D) with (G) and (H).

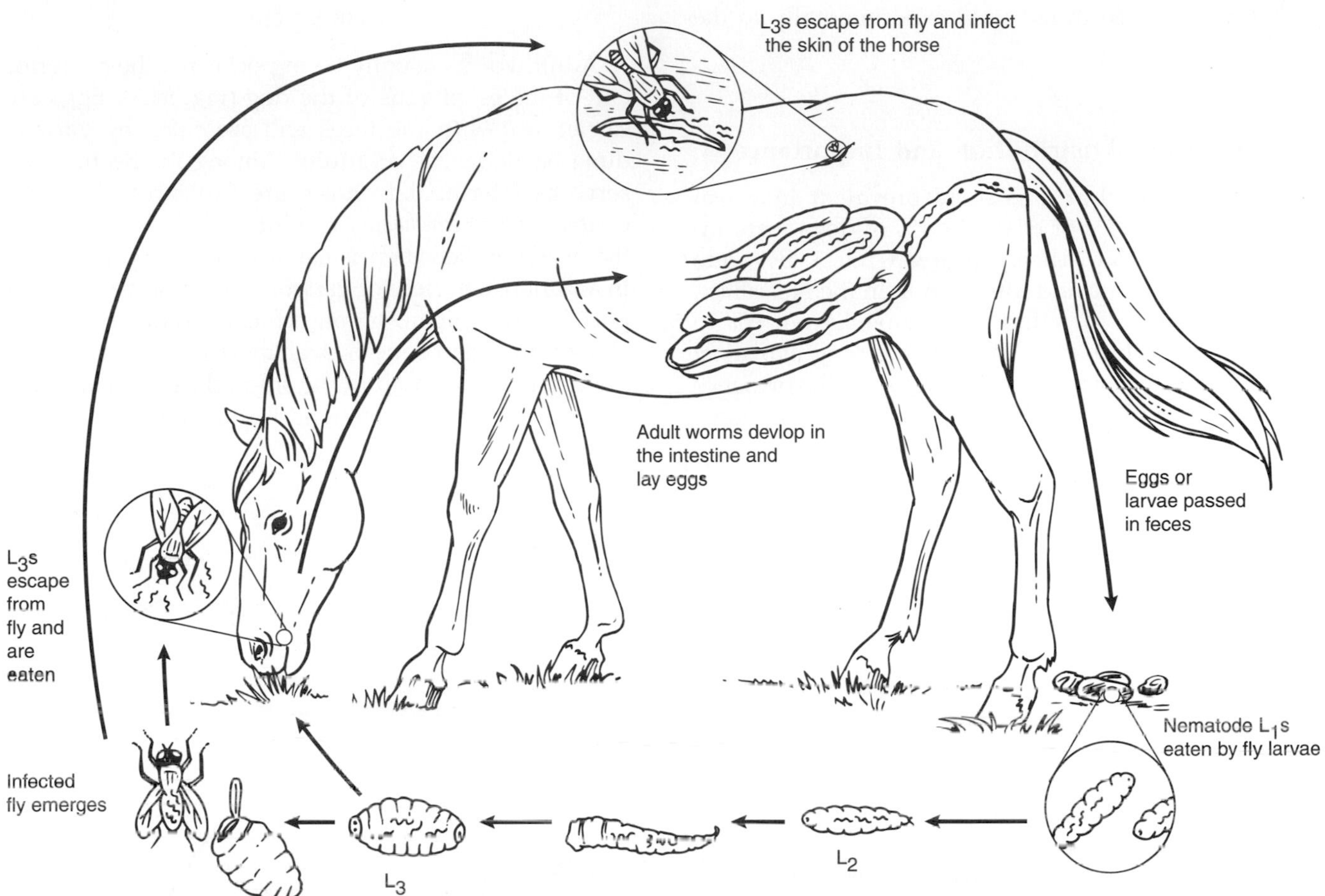

FIGURE 34.2 The life cycles of *Habronema muscae* and *Draschia megastoma*. The life cycles of these two parasites differ only slightly. Both are located in the intestine of the horse, cause summer sore on the skin, and have cyclorraphan flies as intermediate hosts.

escape from the mouthparts of the fly during feeding on a horse and are eaten, or flies themselves are eaten. The adults develop in the intestinal tract. Cutaneous infections result when larvae escape in the vicinity of sores on the skin.

Host–Parasite Interactions

When a few worms are present, there is no discernible damage to the host, but hundreds cause inflammation and ulceration of the intestinal tract. "Summer sore" occurs when larvae are deposited on the skin and enter lesions already present; larvae feed and cause spongy lesions that do not heal until temperatures moderate at the end of the warm months.

Epidemiology and Control

Fly control is the best method of making sure that infections are kept to a tolerable level. Sites of larval development for house flies, stable flies, and probably flesh flies (Chapter 48) should be eliminated. Spraying barns and sheds with a residual insecticide may also help to reduce the populations of adult flies.

SPIROCERCA LUPI

Name of Organism and Disease Associations

Spirocerca lupi is the cause of spirocercosis and indirectly gives rise to malignant neoplasms in the definitive host.

Hosts and Host Range

This worm is found in a number of canids such as the dog, fox, coyote, and jackal and felids such as the jaguar; it has been transmitted experimentally to the cat.

Geographic Distribution and Importance

Cosmopolitan, but it is more prevalent in warm climates than cold. For example, 1% of dogs were infected in the Detroit, Michigan, area while 33.5% were infected in Alabama and Mississippi. In the Near East, Asia, and Africa, infection rates ranged from 9% to 88% in various localities. There is a strong statistical association of *S. lupi* infections in dogs and the presence malignant tumors, usually in the esophageal region.

Life Cycle

Adult worms usually lie in pockets at the posterior end of the esophagus of the dog (Fig. 34.3). Eggs are carried out with the feces and are eaten by various dung beetle larvae or adults. Among the beetles that serve as intermediate hosts are *Geotrupes, Phanaeus, Canthon,* and *Scarabaeus.* The infective L_3 is reached in the beetle, which then is eaten by a susceptible host. In addition, a variety of vertebrates can serve as transport or paratenic hosts: pig, chicken, rodents, snakes, and so on. The beetle or transport host is eaten and the larvae are released in the stomach. The L_3s migrate via the circulatory system and ultimately come to lie

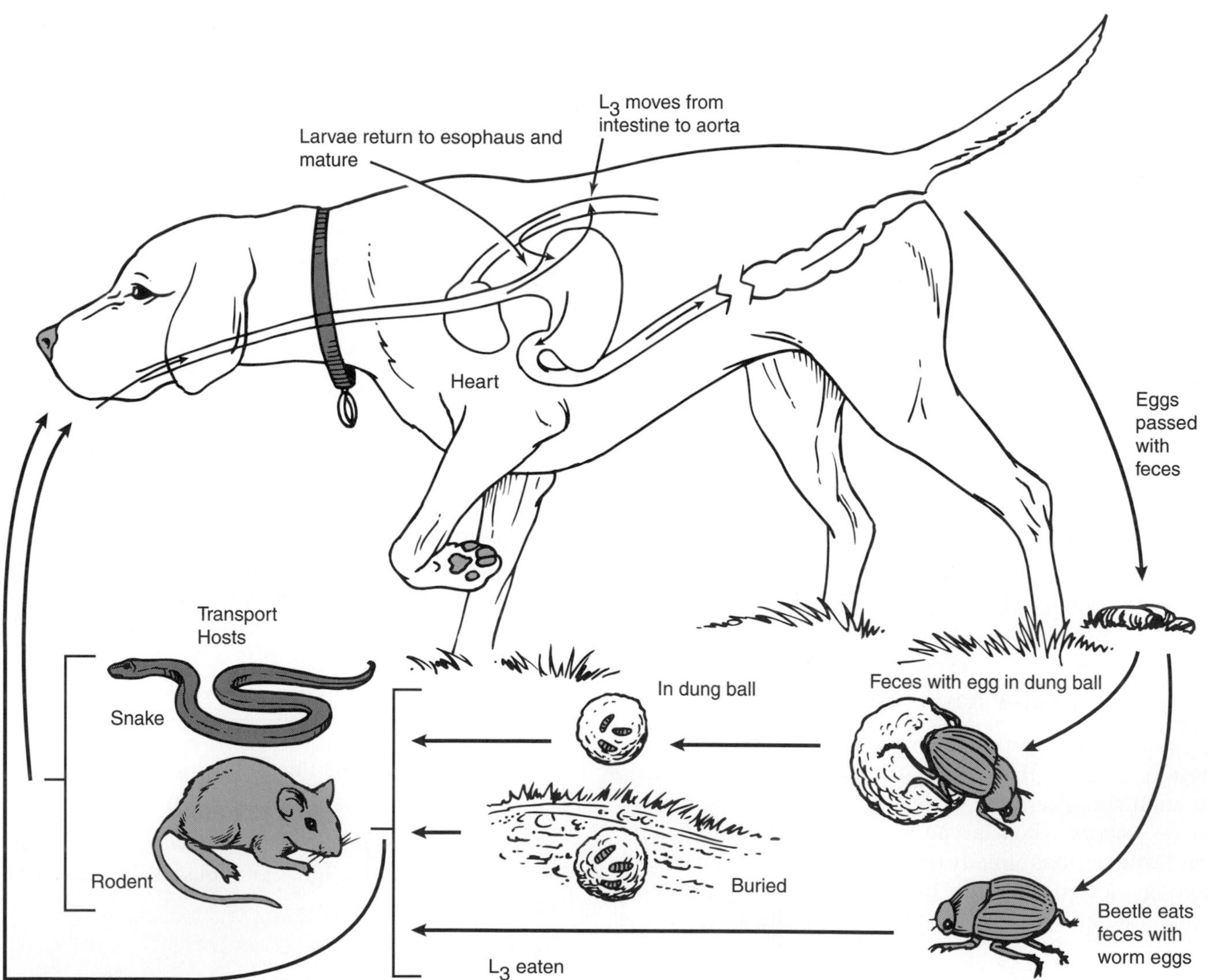

FIGURE 34.3 The life cycle of *Spirocerca lupi.* This parasite has a typical spirurid life cycle in that it is a food-chain based and insects serve as the first intermediate host. Paratenic or transport hosts include birds, mammals, and reptiles; these hosts are not essential but serve to move the parasite up the food chain.

in the proximal portion of the aorta. Some adults remain in nodules in the aorta, but others migrate to the esophagus where egg-laying begins.

Host–Parasite Interactions

Adult worms elicit an inflammatory reaction in either the blood vessels or the esophagus where they lie in nodules. An aneurysm (bulging of the blood vessel often with a clot) may form in the blood vessel and occlude its lumen. In the esophagus, there is growth of tissue that may partially block the esophagus and give rise to digestive problems.

Spirocerca lupi is among the few known carcinogenic helminth parasites. The worms cause a moderate amount of damage directly to the esophagus, but over a long period they somehow cause the tissue in the vicinity to become neoplastic. Most dogs that develop malignant tumors are three to seven years old, so probably a long-term association is necessary before the inflammation at the site of the worms becomes neoplastic. The molecular and cellular mechanisms underlying this tumor development are unknown.

Epidemiology and Control

Preventing dogs from running freely and attempting to control beetle populations in the vicinity of where they are kept may help to reduce infections.

HUMAN INFECTIONS

Infections of Humans with Food-Borne Spirurids

Humans occasionally become infected with spirurids such as *Gongylonema pulchrum*, *Gnathostoma spinigerum*, and *Thelazia californensis*. *G. spinigerum* is obtained by humans by accidentally ingesting infected insects. *G. pulchrum* has a more complex life cycle involving two intermediate hosts, a copepod, and a cold-blooded vertebrate. *Thelazia* has yet another life cycle variation in that it is transferred to the human eye from the mouthparts of muscoid flies such as *Fannia* spp. There are a few hundred case reports of spirurid infections in humans, but their prevalence is not well documented; all are zoonoses, with their normal hosts being ruminants, suids, and carnivores.

FROM FOOD CHAIN TO BLOOD-SUCKING INSECTS

The transition from a food-chain type of life cycle to one in which bloodsucking arthropods are intermediate hosts is exemplified by members of the family Diplotriaenidae, whose adults are found in the air sacs, lungs, and subcutaneous tissues of birds and some reptiles. *Diplotriaena bargusinica* lies in the air sacs of birds; the eggs pass from the lungs up the trachea and leave the host with the feces. Eggs are eaten by grasshoppers and develop to the infective L_3; birds eat infected grasshoppers and thereby obtain the infection. The preadult stages most likely migrate and develop in the vessels of the circulatory system before coming to lie in the lungs; thus, there is a transition from those worms that remain in the gut to those that lie deep in the tissues and, then, to those that use the circulatory system as a migratory route; loss of the food chain would come about when some of the larvae remaining in the tissues or blood vessels were ingested by a bloodsucking insect.

SUPERFAMILY FILARIOIDEA

Filarioid nematodes are generally long, slender worms that have little development of either head or tail structure. They are found in the blood, lymphatics, or extraintestinal tissues of the body and are transmitted by bloodsucking arthropods, mostly nematocerans such as mosquitoes, black flies, and biting midges. The filarioids are an especially important group of parasites for human, animal, and wildlife health.

WUCHERERIA AND *BRUGIA* INFECTIONS IN HUMANS

This section discusses those filarioid nematodes that cause the human disease known as lymphatic filariosis and elephantiasis. The important organisms are *Wuchereria bancrofti* and *Brugia malayi*. They are considered together because they have some common areas of distribution, but also because their differences point up the need for different approaches in control.

The lymphatic filarioses and onchocercosis (discussed later) are among the most distressing of the helminth infections in humans. They lead to gross disfigurement, irreversible changes in the skin, sexual dysfunction, and the affected individuals are often ostracized from their societies. In 1997, the World Health Organization (WHO) estimated that about one-fifth of the world's population lives in areas where they are at risk of infection with either *Wuchereria bancrofti* or *Brugia malayi*. These organisms are spread over 173 countries and there are 120 million human infection at any one time.

Name of Organisms and Disease Associations

Wuchereria bancrofti (syn. *W. pacifica* for the subperiodic form) and *Brugia malayi* (syn. *Wuchereria malayi*) cause lymphatic filariosis, Bancroftian filariasis, Brugian filariasis, periodic filariasis, subperiodic filariasis, and elephantiasis.

Hosts and Host Range

W. bancrofti is a parasite of humans; although it has been established in certain nonhuman primates, no reservoir host has been uncovered. On the other hand, *B. malayi* is partly a zoonotic infection; the reservoirs are monkeys, dogs, and cats.

Geographic Distribution and Importance

W. bancrofti is the more widespread of the two worms; it is found in both the Eastern and Western Hemispheres, principally in the tropics, but with some extension into subtropical climates and small pockets in temperate areas. The areas of greatest prevalence are in Southeast Asia, the islands of the South Pacific, Africa, the southern portion of the Arabian Peninsula, and India. Areas of lesser importance are in Japan and Korea, West Indies, South America, and areas fringing the Mediterranean Sea. (Fig. 34.4).

B. malayi has a limited distribution, principally in Southeast Asia, with more scattered distribution on the Indian subcontinent and on mainland China and Korea (Fig. 34.5).

In 1974 the WHO estimated that there were 250 million infections. In 1994, WHO figures were 106 million persons infected with *W. bancrofti* and for *B. malayi* 12.5 million. The estimate of infection by WHO in 1997, as indicated earlier, is 120 million human infections for both *W. bancrofti* and *B. malayi*. Hence, in 20 years, some progress has been made in reducing the prevalence of infection. As discussed later, there is optimism that at least *W. bancrofti* can be controlled in the foreseeable future. However, no one seriously discusses eradication of the parasite.

The notorious deformities that may be seen in longstanding infections with lymphatic filariae are those where the legs or genitalia are swollen and the skin has undergone mainly irreversible changes. The prevalence of infection in endemic areas may exceed 50%, as measured by microfilaremia, but the prevalence of elephantiasis is usually much lower. In some localities 10 to 20% of the population may be affected; however, in Puerto Rico, 24% of males were found to be infected, but the infection is nearly asymptomatic. Needless to say, when severe deformity occurs, it is a great burden to bear.

Morphology

W. bancrofti males are 28 to 40 long by 0.1 mm, with spicules of unequal length; females are 80 to 100 by 0.27 mm long. The head has eight small papillae. Microfilariae (mf) average 280 ± 8 μm long (Table 34.1; Fig. 34.6).

B. malayi males are 13.5 to 20.5 by 0.075 mm long; females are 43 to 52 long by 0.15 mm. The male spicules are unequal in length. The head has six small papillae. Mf average 220 μm long (Table 34.1; Fig. 34.6).

Life Cycle

The life cycles of *W. bancrofti* and *B. malayi* are similar; that of *W. bancrofti* is given here (Fig. 34.7). The mf circulate in the peripheral blood. The so-called nocturnally periodic forms of these parasites have the greatest numbers seen between 10 p.m. and 2 a.m.; during the daytime, they are seldom detected in the peripheral blood. The mf are ingested by mosquitoes during feeding. More than 60 species of mosquitoes in the genera *Culex*, *Aedes*, *Anopheles*, and *Mansonia* can support development.

The mf migrate from the gut of the mosquito into the hemocoel and penetrate muscle cells in the thorax, where they are found within a day after ingestion. They transform into sausage-shaped forms of about 190 by 14 μm and then begin to grow and molt. The L_3 is reached in 6 to 30 days, depending on temperature, and it measures about 1700 by 20 μm.

Transmission to humans takes place when the mosquito returns to take a second blood meal. The L_3s escape from the mouthparts of the mosquito, probably by sensing the bending of the labium, when the mosquito has its fascicle inserted deeply in the skin. The L_3s are not injected into the host but rather penetrate the wound made by the feeding mosquito after the mouthparts have been removed. There is usually a small pool of fluid at the site of feeding and the L_3s are able to survive for several minutes while the pool of hemolymph dries. When they penetrate, mf reach the tissue spaces and are carried by the flow of lymph to lymph nodes.

The worms remain in the lymphatic vessels and lymph nodes as they grow and reach sexual maturity. The prepatent period is 3 to 15 months, but hard data on the time of initial infection are understandably difficult to obtain. Adult worms may produce mf for 15 years or more.

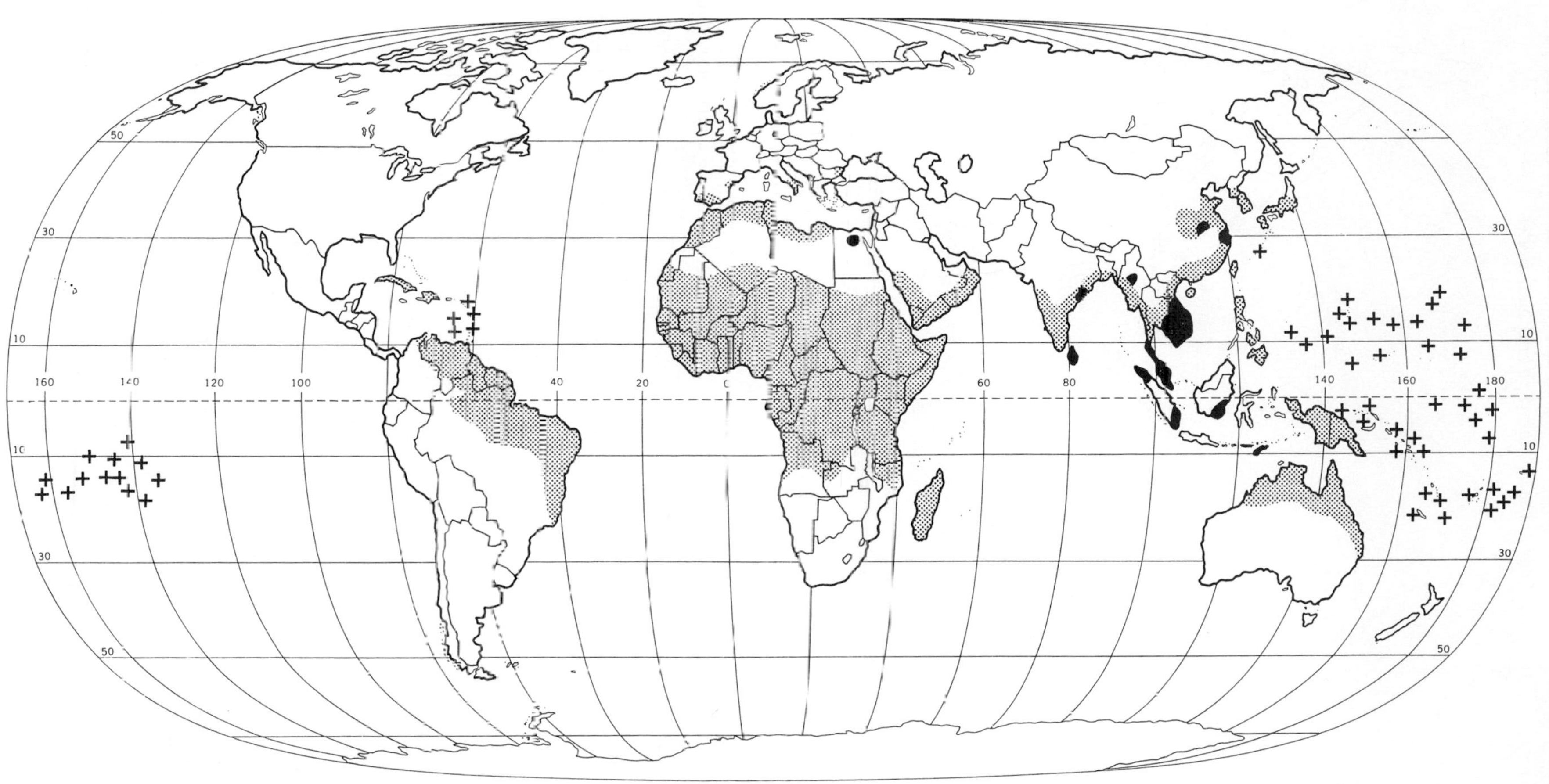

FIGURE 34.4 Geographic distribution of *Wuchereria bancrofti* and *Brugia malayi* (+ are island infections, and solid areas are *B. malayi*).

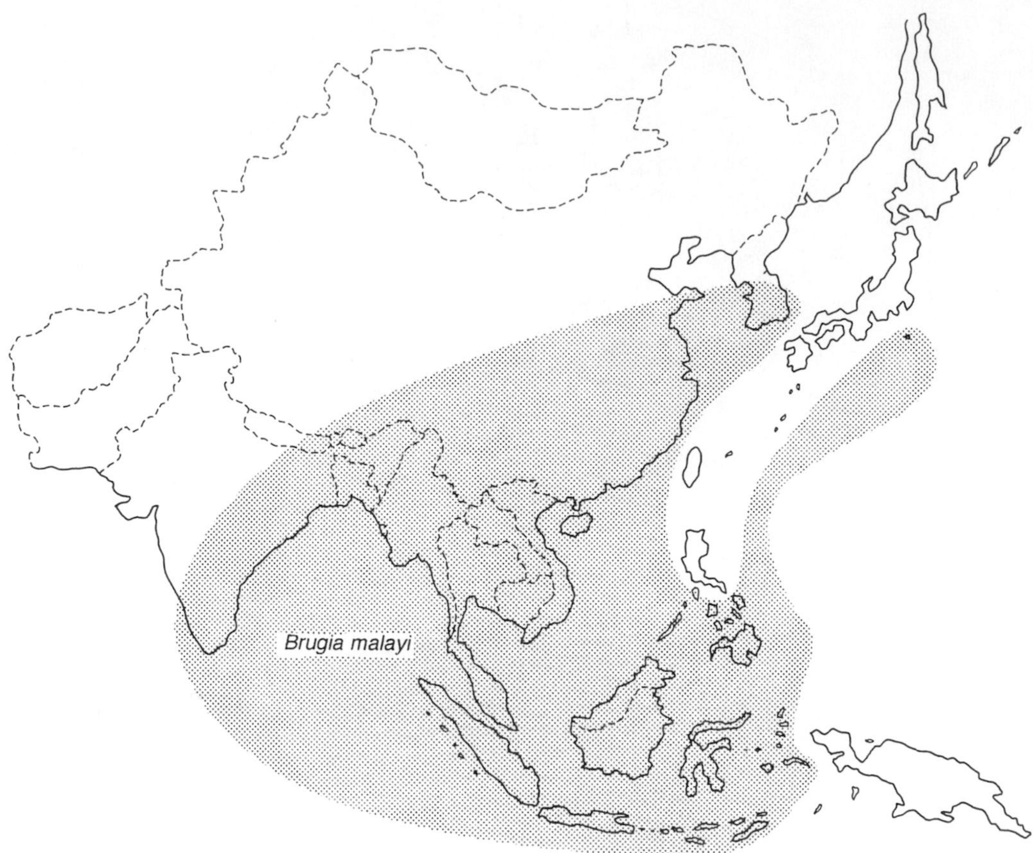

FIGURE 34.5 Geographic distribution of *Brugia malayi* in East Asia to show more detail than seen in Figure 34.4.

Diagnosis

Determining whether a person is infected with *W. bancrofti* or *B. malayi* depends on the following:

1. Clinical signs and symptoms
2. Living in or having visited an endemic area
3. Finding mf in the circulating blood
4. A positive test for circulating antigen; note that this is not antibody, but rather antigen shed by the parasite or the microfilariae themselves which are detected.

Early in the infection there is swelling of lymph nodes, skin rash, fever, and urine which has been made cloudy with lymph (chyluria). Such signs occur in a variety of infectious diseases and are not specific for filariasis.

TABLE 34.1 Characteristics of Microfilariae

	W. bancrofti	*B. malayi*	*L. loa*	*O. volvulus*	*D. perstans*	*D. streptocerca*	*M. ozzardi*
Length	200–300 μm	177–260 μm	250–300 μm	285–368 μm or 150–287 μm	150–200 μm	180–240 μm	150–200 μm
Sheath	Present	Present	Present	Absent	Absent	Absent	Absent
Location	Blood	Blood	Blood	Skin	Blood	Skin	Blood and skin
Vector	Mosquitoes	Mosquitoes	*Chrysops*	*Simulium*	*Culicoides*	*Culicoides*	*Culicoides*
Periodicity	Nocturnal or subperiodic	Nocturnal	Diurnal	Present	None	None	None
Tail end	No nuclei Pointed tip	Two widely spaced nuclei, blunt tip	Nuclei present, rounded tip	No nuclei, pointed tip	Nuclei present, rounded tip	Nuclei present, curved tip	No nuclei, pointed tip

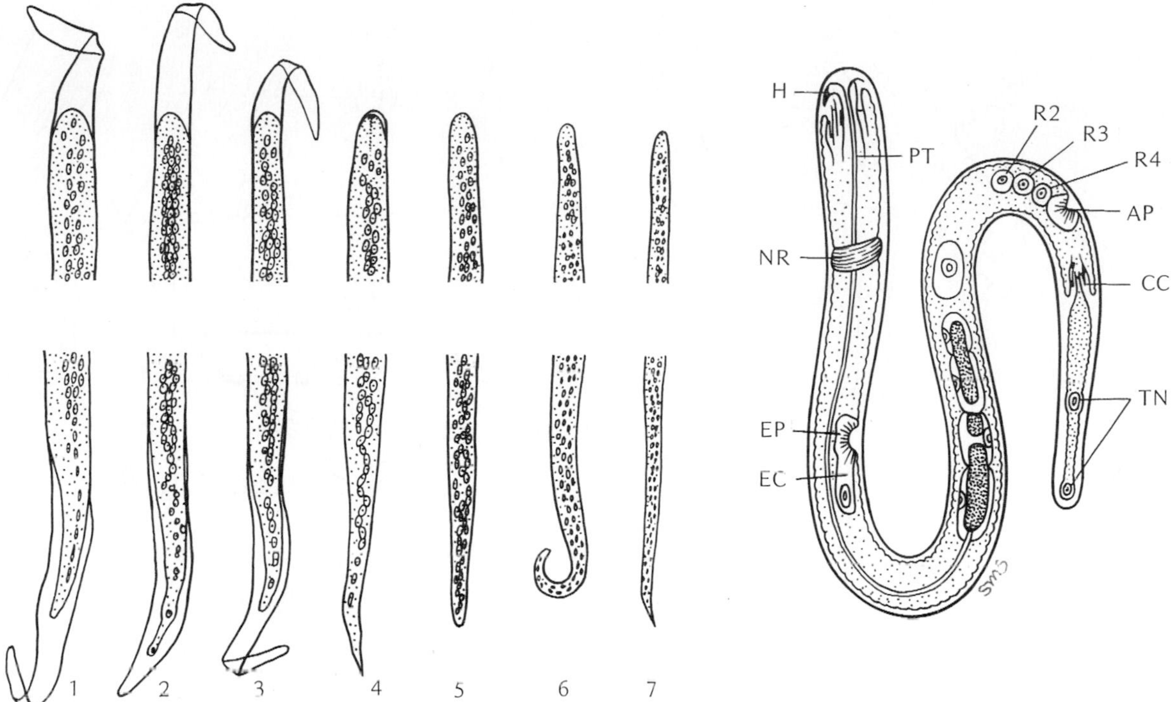

FIGURE 34.6 Morphology of microfilariae found in humans. (1) *Wuchereria bancrofti,* (2) *Brugia malayi,* (3) *Loa loa,* (4) *Onchocerca volvulus,* (5) *Dipetalonema perstans,* (6) *D. streptocerca,* (7) *Mansonella ozzardi.* Abbreviations: AP—anal pore; CC—caudal canal; EC—excretory pore; H—hook; NR—nerve ring; PT—pharyngeal thread; R2–R4—rectal cells; TN—terminal nuclei.

Finding the mf in the circulating blood is good evidence when combined with the clinical aspects and a high probability of having been exposed. Since there are a number of mf that may be found in humans, it is important to examine them with care and to identify them (Fig. 34.6 and Table 34.1).

Failure to find mf does not mean that the person is not infected with a filarioid; in periodic filariasis, mf are not seen in the peripheral blood during the daytime. As indicated previously, the peak of microfilaremia takes place between 10 p.m. and 2 a.m., and it is important to take a blood sample during that peak time, or at least close to it. If a patient is hospitalized, taking a blood sample in the middle of the night is feasible, but outpatients are not generally available. Epidemiologic studies as well are hampered by these factors. The DEC Provocative Test causes mf to appear in the blood 30 to 60 minutes after a patient has been given 100 mg of diethylcarbamazine (DEC); this eliminates the need for nighttime sampling. The DEC provocative test can be quite uncomfortable for the patient and is therefore seldom used at present. A small but significant percentage of infected individuals may not show a microfilaremia at any time.

Microfilariae are found by using a compound microscope and one of the following techniques:

1. Stained blood film
2. Counting chamber
3. Membrane filtration
4. Antigens in the blood

The stained blood film has been the traditional method of finding mf; a thick film is best so that a relatively large volume of blood can be examined easily. The counting chamber method allows one to examine up to 200 mm^3 of blood but does not allow identification of the species of mf.

In the membrane filter method, blood drawn from a vein is passed through a filter, which retains the mf. The membrane filter technique is generally considered to be the most sensitive.

Blood may be taken at any time of the day for a diagnostic test designed to find antigen in the blood. The test is based on using antibodies to specific circulating parasite antigens to both capture the antigens and to signal the presence of the captured antigen. This test can be done with a finger prick to obtain only a drop of blood. Thus, for both the individual patient and for a broader epidemiologic study, circulating antigen has advantages over all other diagnostic methods. In addition, the amount of antigen in the blood declines as the infection is eliminated and thereby provides a

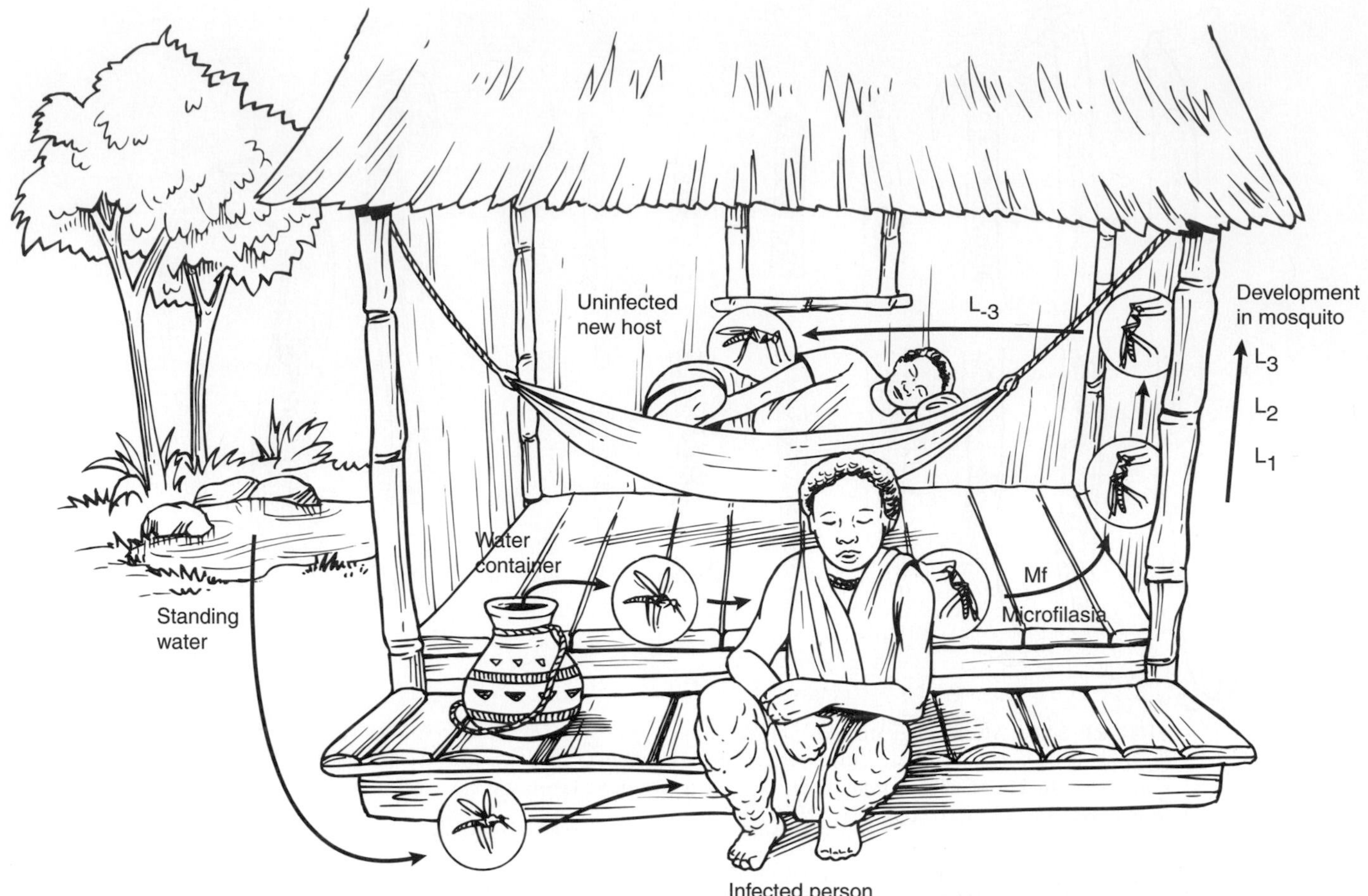

FIGURE 34.7 Life cycle of *Wuchereria bancrofti* and *Brugia malayi*. Both life cycles are much alike with the exception that some geographic strains of *B. malayi* are zoonotic and have reservoirs in various wild animals.

correlation between the amount of antigen and current infection.

Host–Parasite Interactions

The damage that either *W. bancrofti* or *B. malayi* causes is dependent on the length and intensity of exposure to infective larvae and the response of the individual person. For example, military personnel were exposed to infection on islands in the south Pacific during World War II for a period of a few months to two years. Many had signs and symptoms of infection, but the disease seldom progressed to the elephantoid stage.

For persons remaining in an endemic area, the disease progresses through four stages:

1. Incubation
2. Symptomless, but patent
3. Acute
4. Chronic

As noted, the L_3s are about 1 mm long when they enter the definitive host. They move through the lymph system and are trapped in lymph nodes or in the tissue spaces. There is a reaction around the growing worms giving rise to inflammation (pain, swelling, and tenderness) and usually fever. Seemingly at about the time the worms mature, the symptoms subside and mf are seen in the blood (stage 2). This stage may persist for more than a year or may never progress further. The acute phase (stage 3) is caused both by significant blockage of lymph vessels and by the reaction of the host to the worms. There is swelling due to obstruction of lymph vessels, and a complex of symptoms and signs indicate that hypersensitivity has developed.

After some years, the swelling and obstruction of vessels leads to the changes in the extremities and genitalia that characterize the disease. The sequence of events is basically blockage of the lymph vessels, causing retention of fluid distal to the blockage, a foreign body response, and an allergic reaction in the vicinity of the adult worms leading to additional swelling. The skin becomes progressively stretched and loses its normal structure (Fig. 34.8).

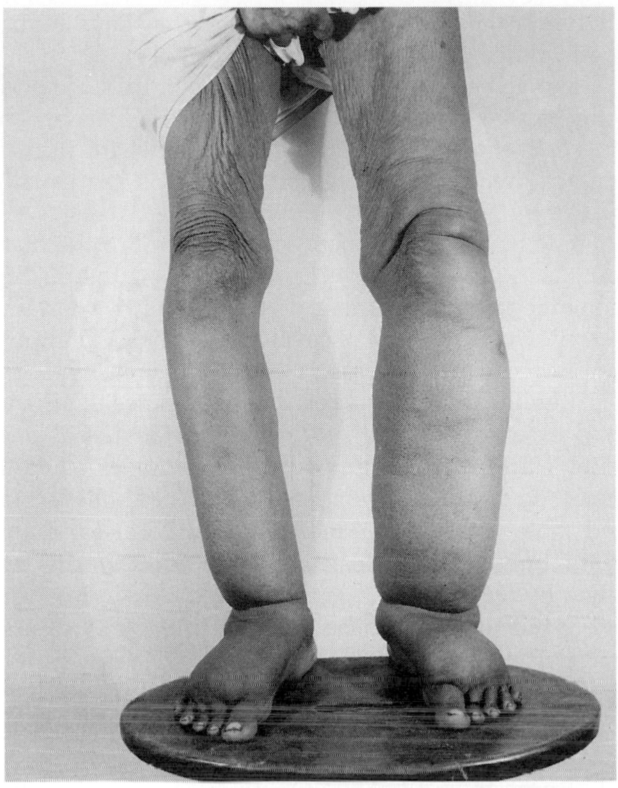

FIGURE 34.8 Elephantiasis of the legs of a human. [Courtesy of Armed Forces Institute of Pathology. AFIP Neg. No. 44430-1.]

The role of protective immunity in altering the course of lymphatic filariasis is unclear. Some persons living in endemic areas for long periods of time never demonstrate symptoms of disease, nor do they have evidence of either circulating mf or parasite antigens. It is theorized that these people have become immune to infection. Apart from this interesting subset of people there is no real evidence for any naturally occurring protective immunity. Typically vigorous immune responses contribute to disease such as elephantiasis and even pulmonary disease or, at a minimum, some immune responses actually aid the parasite in avoiding other potentially destructive immune responses.

Circadian periodicity is the typical pattern of microfilaremia in the definitive host. During the daytime, the microfilaremia is at such a low level that it is unlikely that any mf will be found in a sample of peripheral blood. During the evening, the mf begin to appear and peak usually between 10 p.m. and 2 a.m.; they then begin to decline and disappear around dawn.

The mf concentrate in the lungs during the daytime, and the mf appear in the peripheral blood at the time when there is greatest likelihood of their being ingested by those mosquitoes that normally feed from twilight till dawn. How the mf know it is nighttime is another issue, and most of the evidence points toward oxygen levels in the blood, which tend to decline when a person is asleep.

In some geographic areas, the nocturnal periodicity of microfilaremia is not as striking; originally this condition was referred to as *nonperiodic filariosis* but is more correctly called *subperiodic filariosis*, because the day-night alteration is damped so that there is about a twofold increase at night rather than nearly complete absence of periodicity. Subperiodic filariosis occurs with both *W. bancrofti* and *B. malayi* in localities where the principal vectors are day-biting mosquitoes. Subperiodic Bancroftian filariosis occurs in the Philippines, Fiji, Samoa, Tahiti, Tokelau, Wallis, and Ellice Islands. The localities of subperiodic Brugian filariasis are less well defined but seem to be based on the host in which it is principally found. The strains of *B. malayi* that cycle mostly in the human population are periodic, whereas those that cycle in feral animals with humans as an occasional host are subperiodic.

Epidemiology and Control

Control of lymphatic filariosis entails the following:

1. Vector control
2. Chemotherapy to reduce microfilaremia
3. Chemoprophylaxis to prevent infection
4. Integration of filariosis control with other public health problems such as intestinal helminth infection

Three drugs recommended for treatment of either Bancroftian or Brugian filariosis are diethylcarbamazine (hetrazan, DEC), ivermectin, and albendazole, a benzimidazole. All three are active against microfilariae, and DEC and albendazole have some action in killing adult worms.

The gross deformities seen in some cases of filariosis can be prevented by early drug treatment and by bandaging the legs so that fluid cannot accumulate. Keeping the affected limb clean and washing it frequently with soap and applying antibacterial and antifungal ointments to the skin have helped to reduce skin changes. When the part has been badly affected, the changes are irreversible; surgery may help to reduce elephantoid deformities.

In any control program aimed at infectious disease, it is essential to determine exactly what agents and vectors are involved, and filariosis in humans exemplifies that principle as well as any. One needs to know the following:

1. Whether the causative agent is *W. bancrofti* or *B. malayi*

2. Whether the filariosis is periodic or subperiodic
3. The identity of the vector(s)
4. The risk of a person becoming infected in any given period of time

Host range affects the design of a control program and determines whether control can be achieved. Either as the periodic or subperiodic form, *W. bancrofti* has only a single known host—humans. *B. malayi*, on the other hand, has humans as the principal host in the periodic form, but other animals in the subperiodic form. Therefore, after an identification has been made of the species of mf, it is necessary to determine the character of the periodicity. The investigator then knows whether it will be necessary to try to take into account the reservoirs of infection. In subperiodic Brugian filarioses, the worms probably circulate almost equally among humans, monkeys, and domestic dogs and cats. Whether it is possible implement control in hosts other than humans is problematic, but at least the infection there is known.

In any one locality there is usually a single principal vector, although development is possible in other vectors; Bancroftian filariosis can be transmitted by more than 60 species of mosquitoes in the genera *Culex*, *Aedes*, *Anopheles*, and *Mansonia*. *B. malayi* has not been studied as extensively, nor does it occur over as wide an area, but about a dozen species in the genera *Aedes*, *Anopheles*, and *Mansonia* are known to be vectors.

The risk of infection is determined by on-site studies in which female mosquitoes are captured by various means and dissected to determine the following:

1. Annual biting rate— ABR (no. of mosquito bites/person/year)
2. Annual infective biting rate— AIBR, (no. of infective mosquito bites/person/year)
3. Annual transmission potential—ATP (no of L_3s/person/year)

The ATP is the most informative of the three indices; it measures the number of L_3s/person/year. In two studies in Papua New Guinea, the ATP was found to range from 15 to 836 in one of them and as high as 1443 in the second. It can readily be seen that the number of worms potentially infecting a person over a period of several years can be quite significant.

Sites of larval development differ with the species of mosquito (Chapter 47); therefore, identifying the mosquito and knowing its biology are important. *Anopheles* vectors of *B. malayi* are usually found in clean water such as that of ditches and wells, but *Aedes togoi* larvae are found in water in small containers such as tin cans or rock holes. *Mansonia* larvae obtain oxygen by piercing plant tissues with their specially adapted air tubes; they are found in waters that have herbaceous plants growing in them.

Taking vector preferences one step farther, the periodic *B. malayi* is found in agricultural areas where *Anopheles* and *Aedes* spp. are associated with human artifacts, whereas the subperiodic forms are usually passed by *Mansonia* spp. in wet, forested areas.

A significant component of the control of the filarioses revolves around vector control, and the discussion in the chapter on mosquitoes (Chapter 47) pertains here; however, the role of chemotherapy is most important in reducing the probability of transmission.

Although DEC has been available since 1945 and used extensively since 1947, its characteristics as a filaricide are still being uncovered. It removes mf from the blood by killing them, and it sterilizes both female and male worms. Evidence was equivocal for many years, but now it is clear that some adult worms are killed by DEC.

Ivermectin also can be given in a single dose and microfilaremias are reduced 90% for two years. Single doses of both drugs have shown that two years later microfilaremias were only 5% of what they had been.

Albendazole has come into use in recent years, and it has been found that combinations of any two of the three drugs gives a 99% reduction in microfilariemia for at least a year. Albendazole also removes intestinal nematodes which are common in areas where the filarioses are prevalent. Thus, a carefully structured public health program can reduce the effects of both blood and intestinal helminths at the same time.

The rapid urbanization of cities in developing countries has resulted in the urbanization of lymphatic filariosis. It has generally been viewed as a disease of villages and rural areas, but conditions in cities which lack sewerage, vector control, and educational programs about filariosis lead to conditions where suitable vectors thrive and transmit the nematodes readily.

ONCHOCERCOSIS IN HUMANS

The genus *Onchocerca* represents filarioid nematodes that lie in tissues other than the vascular system. The adults are often found in subcutaneous areas, in connective tissue, and in some other internal organs.

Name of Organism and Disease Associations

Onchocerca volvulus causes a disease variously called onchocercosis, onchocerciasis, river blindness, Robles' disease, or blinding filariosis.

Hosts and Host Range

For practical purposes, humankind is the only host; a few infections have been established in some other higher primates, but they probably are not important in maintaining the infection.

Geographic Distribution and Importance

This parasite is distributed most heavily in subsaharan Africa from the west coast across the continent to Kenya and Tanzania. A few reports of infection have come from Saudi Arabia and Yemen. There are foci of infection in the Western Hemisphere in Guatemala, Mexico, Colombia, Venezuela, and Brazil (Fig. 34.5). Proper habitat for the black fly vector (Chapter 47) is the limiting element in distribution.

An estimated 17 million people are infected with *O volvulus* in Africa alone. In many localities in tropical Africa, 30 to 60% of people may be infected with *O. volvulus*. There are about 800,000 infections in the Western Hemisphere. Globally, about 85 million persons are at risk of infection and 1 to 2 million persons have been blinded or have severe visual impairment.

The figures for the prevalence of infection are not indicative of the catastrophic impact that onchocercosis has on the population in an endemic area. The term *river blindness* indicates where people become infected: along rivers and small streams where people live and where good farmland lies. In some areas one-fifth of the people in a village may be blind as a result of *O. volvulus* infection; the effect on the individual and the community in a subsistence farming economy can easily be appreciated. In many instances in Africa, the areas near rivers have been abandoned and people have tried to farm on less desirable land.

Morphology

Males are 19 to 42 long by 0.17 mm and have a ventrally curved tail; females are 335 to 500 long by 0.35 mm. The anterior end has eight small papillae and two large lateral ones. Although males may migrate, a male and a female are usually coiled together in a nodule. Microfilariae are found in two sizes—285 to 368 by 6 to 9 μm or 150 to 287 by 5 to 7 μm (Fig. 34.6 and Table 34.1).

Life Cycle

The mf do not circulate in the blood but are in the skin, where they are picked up when black flies feed (Fig. 47.6). The cycle is much like that of *W. bancrofti*, with development to the L_3 taking place within the thoracic flight muscles of the fly. Infectivity for humans is reached in a week or so after ingestion of the mf. When the black fly takes another blood meal, the L_3s escape from mouthparts and invade the host directly by entering the wound made by the vector. The route of migration in the definitive host is not known with certainty, but the adults come to lie in the subcutaneous tissues and begin to produce mf within six months to a year.

Diagnosis

Onchocercal infections are found by the following:

1. Observing clinical signs and symptoms of the disease
2. A history of living in or visiting an endemic area of onchocercosis
3. Finding mf in skin snips
4. Finding parasite antigen or antiparasite antibodies in the blood

The presence of nodules under the skin of persons living in endemic areas is good evidence of infection, especially if a nodule is opened surgically when the adult worms are easily observed (Fig. 34.9). Skin changes such as wrinkling, depigmentation, and so-called hanging groin are all signs of onchocercosis.

Since the mf do not circulate in the peripheral blood, skin snips are usually examined for evidence of infection. Small snips of skin are shaved or nipped from the skin surface in such a way that little or no bleeding occurs, and when placed in physiological salt solution, the mf migrate out and can be found under a microscope. In the absence of nodules, or where surveys for infection are done, the skin snip method is used. In moderate to severe infections, 40 to 245 mf/mg of skin have been found.

Early infections can be found by using an ELISA test for antibodies against *O. volvulus*. Parasite antigen can also be detected, as in the case of lymphatic filariasis.

Host–Parasite Interactions

The effects on the host are in the following:

1. Nodule formation, in which adult worms are encapsulated in fibrous tissue
2. Long-term skin changes
3. Damage to lymph nodes,
4. Damage to the eye eventually resulting in blindness.

The causes of the damage are complex, but many are directly related to immunity.

Early in an infection, the adult worms seem to move about under the skin, but about the time the infection

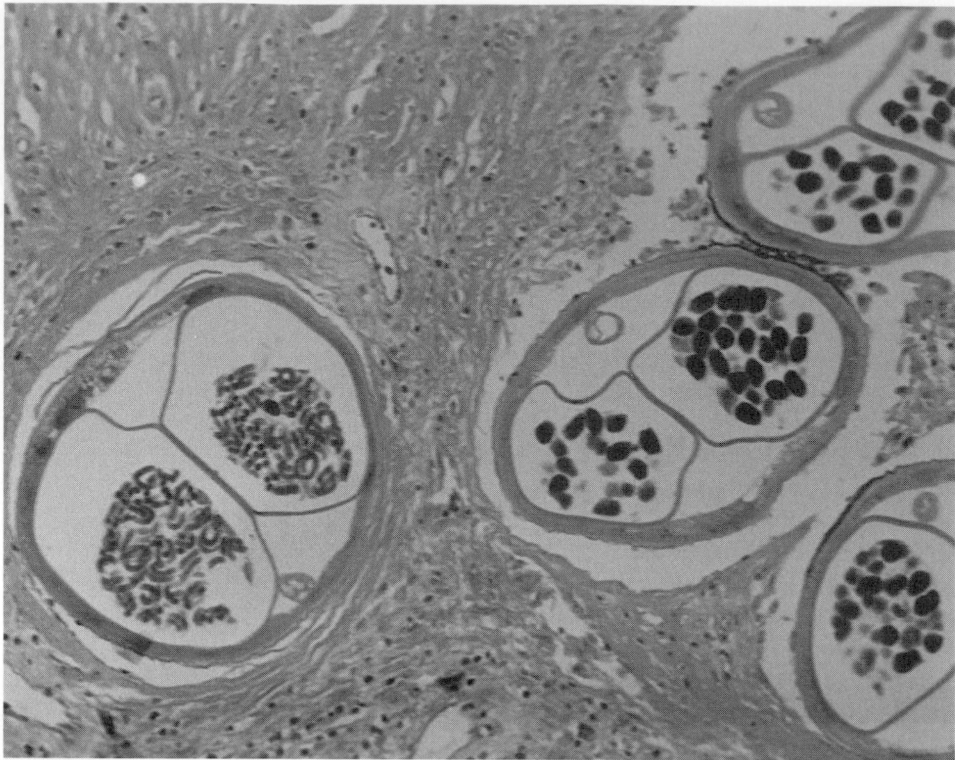

FIGURE 34.9 Histologic section of a nodule taken from a person infected with *Onchocerca volvulus*. The adults worms are a tangled mass of males and females in the nodule that is encapsulated with connective tissue. The two full sections of female worms show embryonating eggs in the worm on the right and microfilariae in the worm on the left.

becomes patent, the adults become encapsulated in fibrous connective tissue. These nodules are of no great consequence in themselves unless they mechanically effect certain tissues. But the adults are responsible for continuing microfilaremia.

The damage to the eye is related to the mf, most likely to direct damage by the mf and to an immune response to them. Greatest eye damage occurs when most mf are present. Damage is in the cornea, iris, retina, and optic nerve. The latter two structures are probably most important in the complete loss of sight. Blindness is not inevitable; for example, in a survey of 1015 persons in West Africa, 52% had nodules and of those, 9% were blind, 10% had lesions in the retina, 19% had lesions of the cornea, and 4% had involvement of the iris.

Skin changes are related to the breakdown and destruction of connective tissue in the epidermal and dermal layers; the skin sags and appears prematurely aged. In a few instances, elephantoid changes reminiscent of *W. bancrofti* infections have been seen. Skin disease may be equally important to blindness in onchocercosis patients. Itching becomes so severe that it leads to insomnia and fatigue as well as damage to the skin through scratching it with sticks or other instruments. Affected persons may be ostracized socially and many are unable to work productively.

Immunopathology may be important in causing some of the harmful effects of onchocercosis. Deposition of immune complexes may trigger inflammation, leading to irreversible changes in the lymph nodes and other organs.

The role of natural immunity in protecting a person against reinfection seems to be similar to the case with lymphatic filariosis. It is known that infections can last for 11 years or more and that the encapsulation of the adult worms does not lead to their demise, at least not within a short period. Again, there are a group of patients that live in endemic areas that are neither infected nor symptomatic and are putatively immune to the infection.

Although mf are found in the skin, they are probably normally distributed in a number of other organ systems. They are often found in urine and other secretions and excretions. Some investigators have attempted to determine whether there is a periodicity in the mf, as in *W. bancrofti* and *B. malayi*. The investigations have given equivocal answers, but it is important to note that mf are not merely trapped in the skin, passively awaiting a black fly to arrive and feed, but that they do move about.

In the preceding discussion, some generalizations have been made that may not hold in all localities. There are variations in the place on the body where the nodules are found, for example. In the Western Hemisphere, nodules are most common on the head, whereas in Africa, nodules are more common on the trunk. The pathologic aspects of onchocercosis vary geographically; for example, there seems to be a greater incidence of blindness in the savanna of Africa by contrast to the forest of Africa (Fig. 34.10).

Epidemiology and Control

Control of *O. volvulus* is directed toward reduction in the following:

1. Skin nodules containing adult worms
2. Microfilarial numbers
3. Populations of the black fly vectors

The objectives of treatment for *O. volvulus* infection relate to both the individual and the health of the community, and both surgery and chemotherapy are used. Obvious nodules under the skin of a person can be opened under local anesthesia and the adult worms removed. In addition to surgically removing adults, mf must be killed with Imervectin to eliminate the potential for transmission and the disease attributable to mf.

With the foregoing as a prelude, we are obviously left with black fly control as the principal means of controlling onchocerciasis. The larvae of these tiny insects are associated with running water (see Chapter 47 for details of black fly biology). They are found in well-aerated water, where they feed on small bits of organic matter; they are among many small stream invertebrates that process leaf litter. Most often larvae are found in cascading streams or shallow riffles where the rocks are partly out of the water. Some species adhere to rooted aquatic plants, and *Simulium neavei* attaches to freshwater crabs.

Despite their small size, adult simuliids are strong fliers and may migrate several kilometers from their sites of larval development. Interestingly, those insects that have relatively heavy infections with *O. volvulus* tend to migrate only short distances.

Relatively few species of black flies on a global basis are good vectors of *O. volvulus*. In Africa there are two principal species: *Simulium damnosum* and *S. neavei*. In Central and South America there are three species: *S. ochraceum* (the most important vector), *S. metallicum*, and *S. callidum*. Since there are relatively few vectors, the problem of control would seem to be simple because the bionomics of any one species is usually fairly circumscribed. Success in reducing fly populations has been difficult to achieve, because the habitats of the larvae are usually inaccessible and some species of flies have long flight ranges. *S. damnosum* has a flight range of at least 100 km (60 miles).

Reducing black fly numbers has involved the following:

1. Source reduction or habitat management
2. Killing larvae by putting insecticides in streams
3. Aerial spraying of insecticides to kill adults

Source reduction has been applied in two ways:

1. Cleaning streams of rooted plants
2. Water control

Removing plants eliminates the substrate to which larvae attach. Such a system was used in East Africa, but two problems presented themselves: the cost was high, and the larvae of *S. neavei* are phoretic on freshwater crabs; however, it appears that *S. neavei* has been eradicated.

Water control has come about more or less inadvertently with the construction of dams for irrigation and power production. Upstream from a dam, the cascades and riffles that provide substrate and maintain well-oxygenated water are covered up and the habitat of the larvae is reduced greatly; however, downstream from the dam there may be a better habitat than before.

Water control allows year-round availability of water for irrigation and other uses, so streams do not dry out seasonally. In addition, dam outlets are constructed of concrete and usually engineered in such a way that the energy is taken out of the water with drops and baffles. Such manufactured structures may provide excellent larval black fly habitat and increase fly numbers. Controlling the release of water to dry out the stream or to flood the steam may kill larvae.

Most control programs rely on second-generation insecticides, currently carbamates and organophosphates. Early larviciding programs in Kenya starting in 1947 relied on large concentrations of DDT applied frequently; by this method and by meticulous monitoring, *S. neavei* was eradicated from an area of 15,000 square miles. Later, aerial spraying also reduced fly populations significantly, but it was found that insecticide supposedly directed against the adults was actually killing larvae, because of their extreme sensitivity to DDT. Clearly DDT is no longer a sensible or viable approach.

Success of a control program requires the following:

1. Monitoring fly populations, including the appearance of insecticide resistance, which occurs with disturbing frequency

2. Monitoring transmission, that is, the incidence of infection during a given period of time
3. Continuing the program for many years
4. Placing most of the available resources in areas of highest potential impact

It is essential to continue a program of surveillance until the focus has been completely eliminated. Adult worms may live longer than 11 years, and as long as mf are present, the possibility of transmission exists. Given the long time required for surveillance and control, what is the probability of success in developing countries? At this point the answer must be equivocal. Good success against *O. volvulus* has been achieved in parts of West Africa where widespread insecticide use and Imervectin treatment have been used. In many areas of Africa entire populations of teenage children in endemic areas are free of infection. However, in Central America, the inaccessibility of sites of larva development has hampered control. But even if initial success is realized, will hard-pressed governments allow the public health personnel to continue to fight a battle that seems to have been won? If malaria eradication programs are an indicator, the most optimistic answer is probably not.

An aid in developing an effective control program is Rapid Epidemiologic Monitoring of Onchocercosis (REMO) in order to attack those areas of greatest hazard. A country (usually) is divided in regions based on river drainages; each drainage is examined using detailed maps and on-site investigations for likely sites of black fly habitat. The human population is then sampled for *O. volvulus* infection. On a country-wide basis, public health authorities can set priorities in developing an effective control program. It should be pointed out that REMO may be an efficient means of determining the distribution and severity of other infections that are vector-borne, especially those that are tied to an aquatic ecosytem.

In many instances, undesirable results occur in control programs against various diseases. It is worth quoting Nelson (1970) in this regard:

> Onchocercosis is an economically important disease, but not a killing disease. It incapacitates large sections of the community and makes them an economic burden. Control of the parasites can do nothing but good; it will not increase the birth rate and produce more mouths to feed, but it will release whole communities from an intolerable burden of misery. Also, by ridding the countryside of biting simuliids, vast fertile areas will be freed for agricultural development.

OTHER FILARIAL INFECTIONS IN HUMANS

In addition to the three filarial infections of humans discussed earlier in this chapter, there are four others that commonly occur in humans and several others that occur sporadically.

Loa loa is the eye worm; it occurs in subsaharan Africa principally in rain forest areas (Fig. 34.11), where it is transmitted by *Chrysops* spp. (Diptera, Tabanidae) (Chapter 47). Although found first in the eye of a West African in 1770, the adults lie in subcutaneous tissues as well, where they cause inflammation and swelling.

Dipetalonema perstans occurs in North Africa and widely in subsaharan Africa, but is of only minor medical importance. Its vectors are *Culicoides* spp. (Diptera, Ceratopogonidae). *D. streptocerca* and *D. semiclarum* are also found in humans.

Mansonella ozzardi is a New World parasite that occurs in tropical areas, where it is transmitted by *Culicoides* and *Simulium* spp. Although the prevalence of infection in some Amerinds is as high as 96%, the damage to the host is minor or limited to pain in the joints.

FILARIOSIS IN DOGS

Name of Organism and Disease Associations

Dirofilaria immitis causes dirofilariosis, dirofilariasis, filariosis, and heartworm disease.

Hosts and Host Range

The principal host is the domestic dog; other canids also are good hosts. The domestic cat is also infected although with a lower prevalence; even the California sea lion has been found to be infected. There are a number of reports in higher primates, but humans are rarely infected. Some animals such as the ferret can serve as experimental hosts.

Geographic Distribution and Importance

Cosmopolitan. This worm was originally thought to be found only in warm, moist climates such as the southeastern United States, but in the late 1950s data began to accumulate showing that *D. immitis* also occurs in temperate and cold climates. There are enzootic areas in Canada and in semidesert locales such as parts of Colorado, where irrigation is practiced. It is likely that the organism has extended its range in the United States by American tendencies for increased travel and changing of residence and possibly parasite adaptation to colder climes. Surveys in the southeastern United States usually show from 10 to 70% prevalence, whereas that in the northern part of the country is

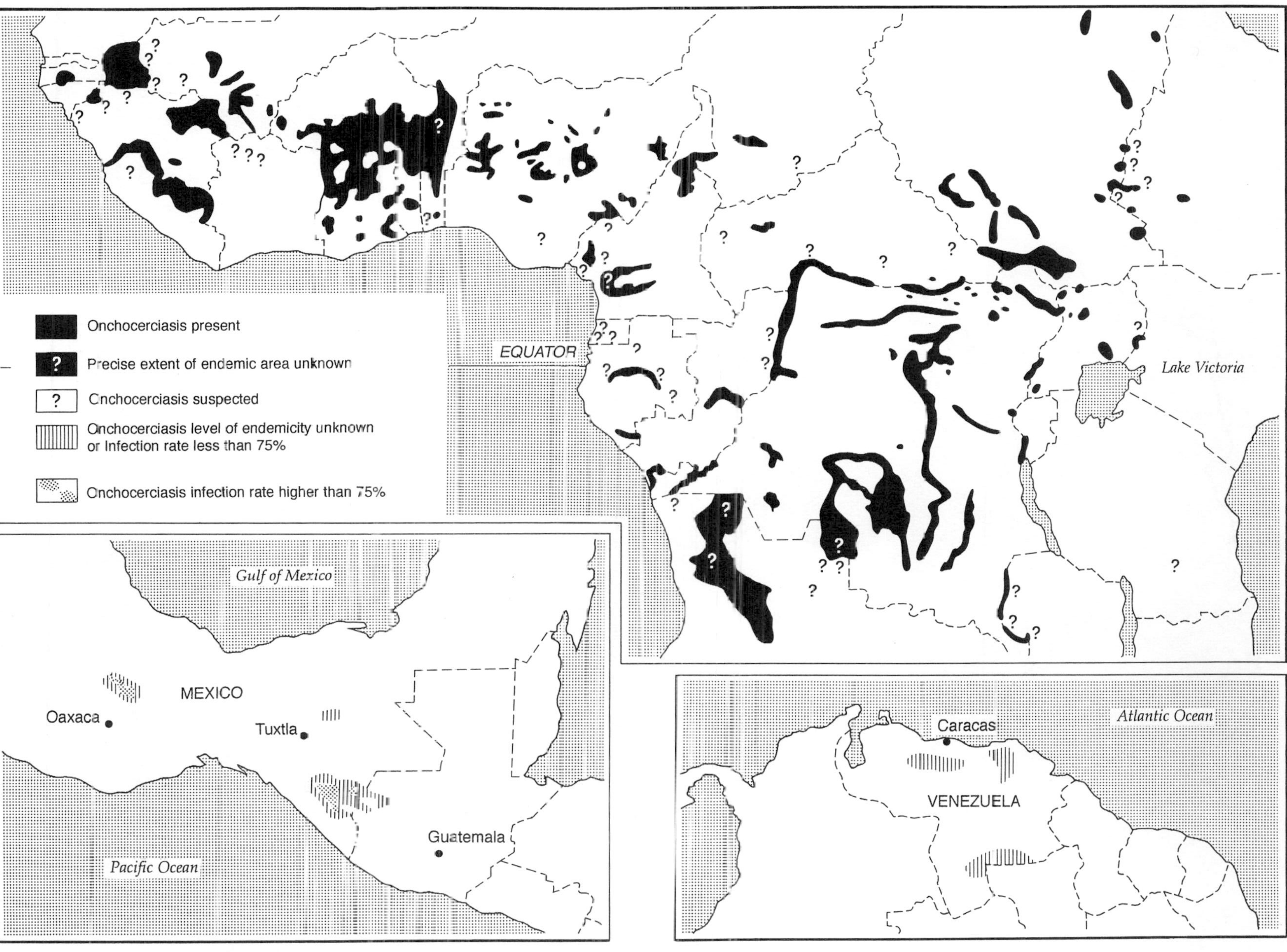

FIGURE 34.10 Distribution of *Onchocercia volvulus* in Africa and in the New World. [Redrawn from Sasa, 1978.]

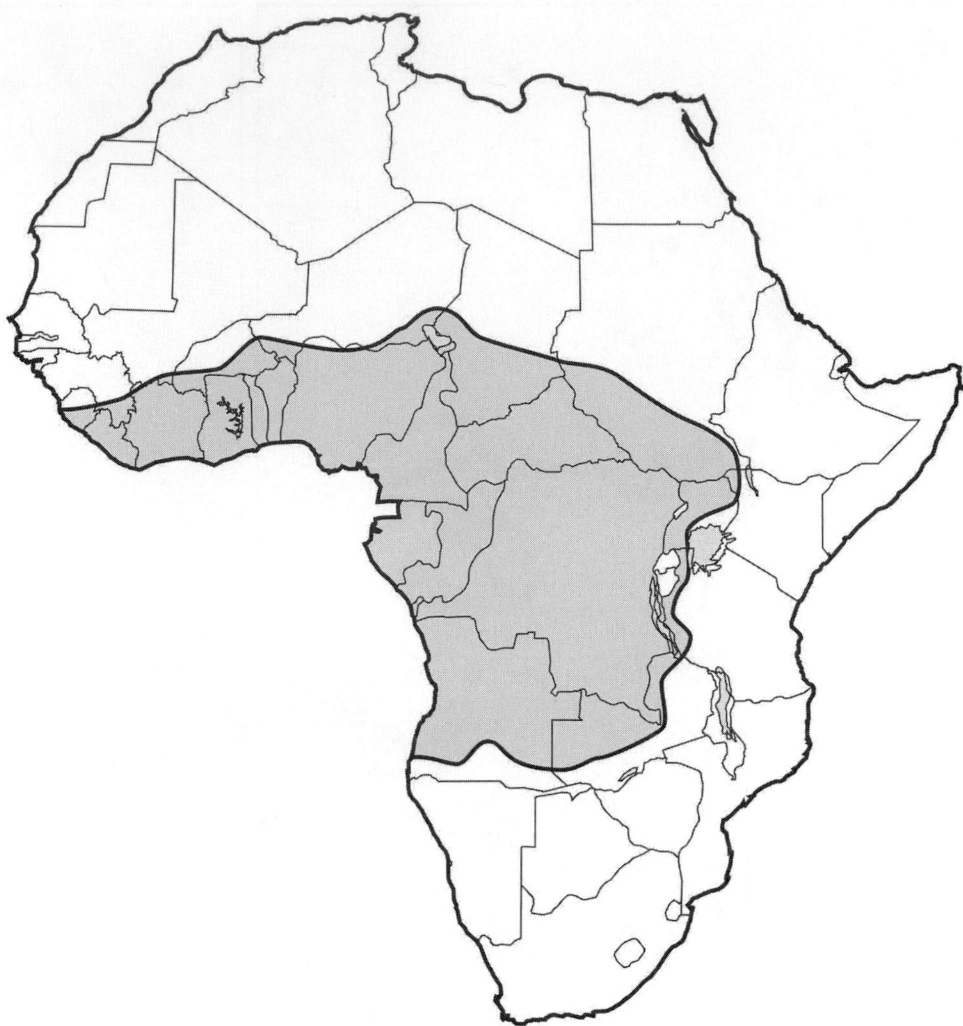

FIGURE 34.11 Distribution of *Loa loa* in Africa.

from 1 to 8%. These prevalence data vary widely depending on the population examined. Cats generally have a prevalence of infection about a tenth that of dogs in any one area.

Dirofilariosis is considered to be a major disease of dogs in North America, Japan, Australia, and parts of the Mediterranean region of Europe.

Morphology

The adult males are from 12 to 200 by 0.8 mm and the females are 250 to 310 by 1 mm (Fig. 34.12). Head structures are minimal, but six papillae surround the mouth. The male has 11 pairs of papillae in the anal region and a pair of unequal spicules 300 and 200 μm long, respectively.

Life Cycle

The infective stage, the L_3, develops in various genera of mosquitoes; about 70 species of mosquito have been implicated as vectors of dirofilariosis. The L_3s escape from the mouthparts of the mosquito during feeding and enter the wound made by the mosquito. (Fig. 34.13). Early in the infection the developing worms occur in subcutaneous, adipose, and muscular tissue. When the worms reach early L_5 at about 90 days postinfection (PI), they begin to locate in the heart. The prepatent period is about 200 days before microfilariae appear in the blood.

Mf are picked up by mosquitoes during blood feeding. They migrate from the gut and enter cells of the Malpighian tubules, where they become short, sausage-shaped organisms. They then begin to grow and molt twice to reach the L_3 10 to 16 days PI. The L_3s

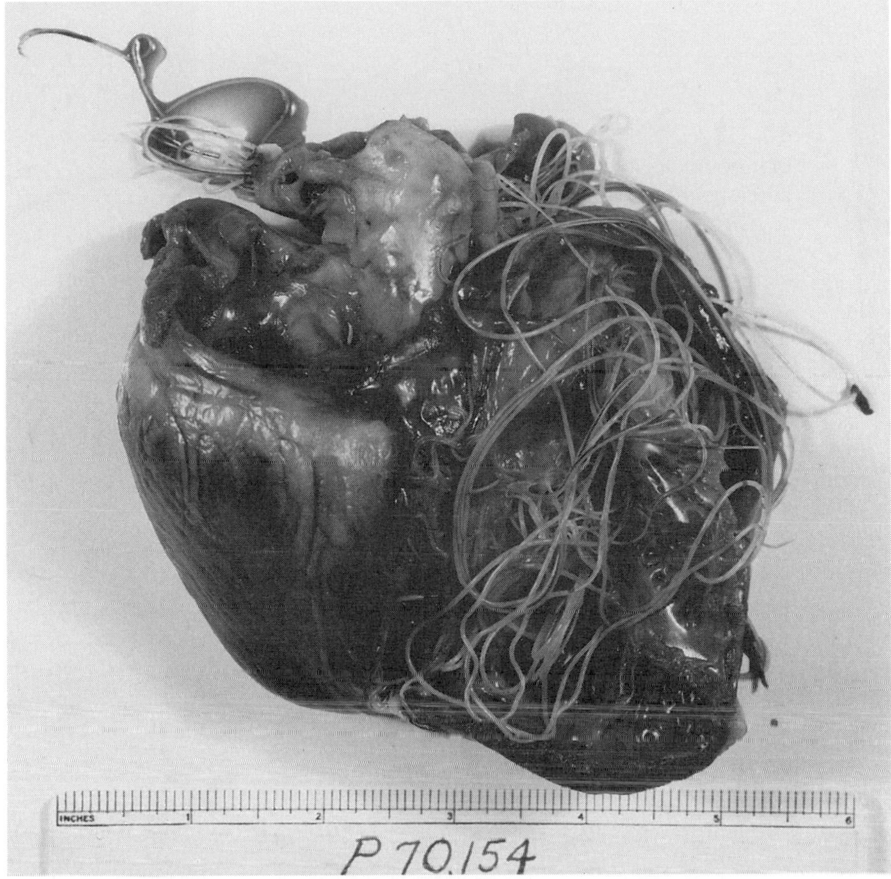

FIGURE 34.12 *Dirofilaria immitis* adults in the heart of a dog.

migrate to the head of the mosquito and escape when another blood meal is taken.

Diagnosis

The principal means of determining whether an animal is infected are the following:

1. By finding the mf in the circulating blood of dogs or cats
2. By finding parasite antigen in the blood of dogs or cats
3. By finding specific antibodies in the blood of infected cats

Finding the mf is done by drawing a small amount of blood into a weak formalin solution and then looking for them in the sediment after centrifugation. As indicated in the section on *Wuchereria* and *Brugia*, mf can be differentiated from one another, and it is sometimes important to do so. *Dipetalonema reconditum* of the raccoon is most often the filarioid that needs to be differentiated from *D. immitis*:

	Length	Width	Tail	Anterior
Dirofilaria immitis	286–340 μm	5–7 μm	Straight	Tapered
Dipetalonema reconditum	269–283 μm	4.3–4.8 μm	Hooked	Blunt

Other mf landmarks can also be used, but the overall dimensions and shape are most important for these two species.

Host–Parasite Interactions

Clinical signs typically appear in dogs as the worms become sexually mature. Given the size, location, and potential number of adult worms, the principal clinical signs relate to interference with blood flow. The worms locate in the right heart and pulmonary artery. They impede blood flow and prevent proper closure of the heart valves. There is back pressure from the lungs to the liver because the blood does not move through the right heart normally The heart works harder in an

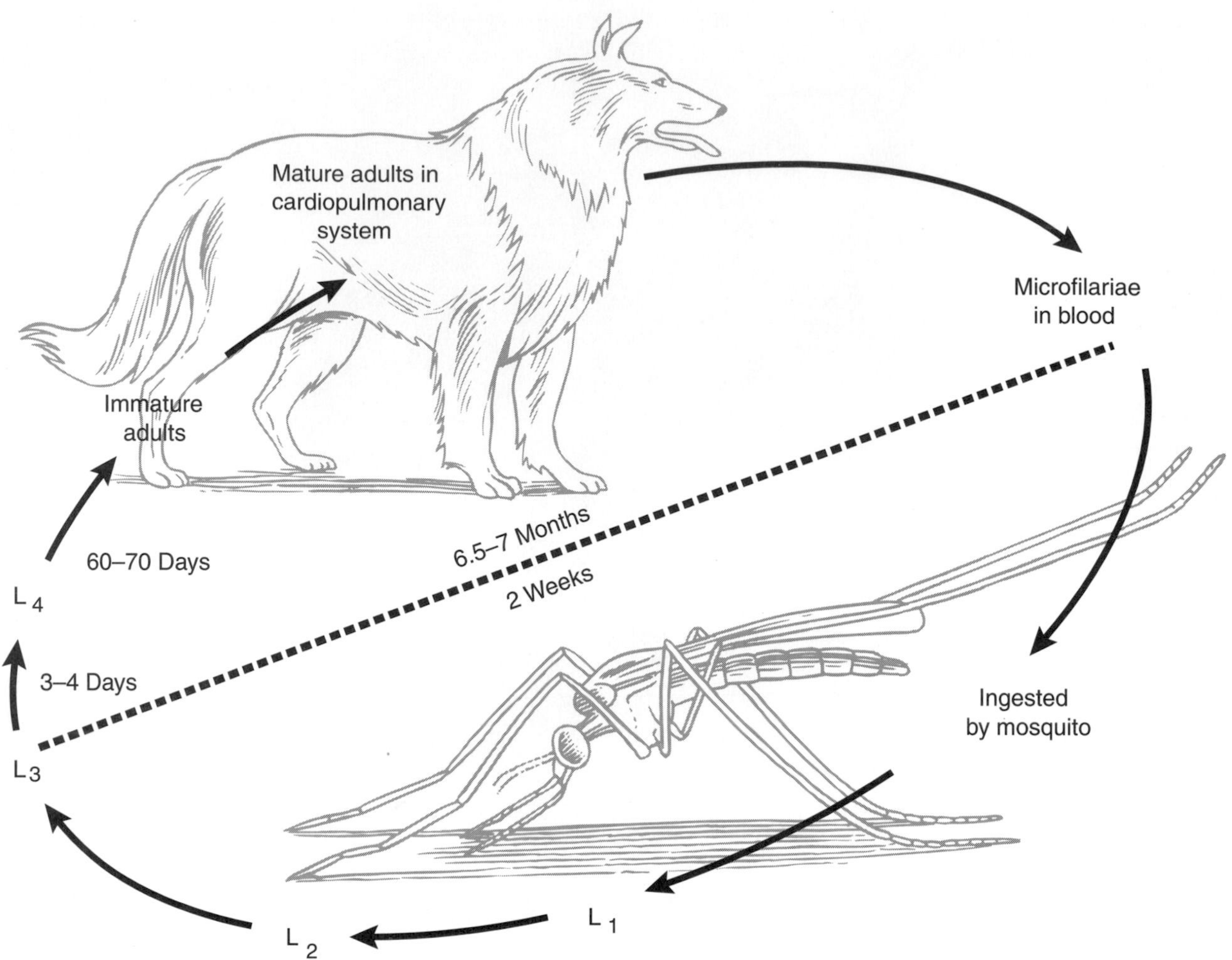

FIGURE 34.13 Life cycle of *Dirofilaria immitis* in the dog. Ten to sixteen days are required for development in the mosquito in order to reach the L_3. The prepatent period in the dog is about 180 days.

attempt to empty and also to meet the need to move blood from the heart to all organs of the body.

The results of this lesson in fluid mechanics are that the liver becomes enlarged as a result of engorgement with blood, the right heart becomes enlarged, and there is insufficient oxygenated blood for the animal to maintain strenuous activity.

There are effects on the host in addition to these mechanical ones. Lesions occur in the blood vessels such as the pulmonary artery due to the effects of parasite metabolites on the vessel surface. Immune complexes may also cause disease in the kidney.

As in the case of certain lymphatic human filarioses, there is pronounced subperiodicity of the mf. That is the mf numbers vary markedly over the course of the day but typically peak in association with the activity of the host animal and ebb with inactivity.

There is limited evidence of any naturally occurring immunity in canine filariosis. Clearly dogs in endemic areas do not demonstrate the enormous infections that would theoretically be possible given exposure to infective larvae. Curiously, an average infection in different areas and at different times is about 20 to 30 adult worms.

As in the case with other related nematodes, in most cases animals with ongoing adult worm infections have markedly dampened immune responses or, alternatively, immune responses can result in more disease. In the latter case a small, yet significant, percentage of dogs will make an overwhelmingly effective immune response that kills the mf as soon as they leave the female worm. The result is a tremendous amount of parasite debris and inflammation in the lungs, which results in unusually severe pulmonary disease.

Epidemiology and Control

Three principal aspects of control of heartworm infection are as follows:

1. Preventing development of worms in the dog
2. Killing the microfilariae
3. Killing or removing the adult worms

In enzootic areas, dogs can be given one of a variety of chemical preventatives before the start of the mosquito season and for about two months after it is over. These drugs prevent the development of the worms that may infect the dog.

If a patent infection develops, the adult worms may be killed with arsenical drugs. The treatment of adult worms can be dangerous due to both the inherent toxicity of the drugs and the fact that as worms die they are carried downstream and damage the lung so severely that the dog may die.

Surgical removal may be done in certain instances, but it involves surgery in which the worms are extracted by cutting into the major vessels. Special circumstances are required because surgery is both risky and expensive.

The mf may be killed by administering any of the various macrolide anthelminthics although none are officially licensed for that use.

Although dirofilariosis is more prevalent in warm than in cool climates, it can become a problem in almost any area where mosquitoes are abundant. The host range is quite broad in the vector, so the probability of its being able to establish in a given area is high. This is confirmed by the cosmopolitan distribution in the United States and in other countries such as Australia. *D. immitis* seems to have spread inexorably into areas such as California and Canada where it once was rare or nonexistent. The increased prevalence of infection in various parts of the United States and elsewhere is probably a result of the high mobility of the human population. People move from one part of the country readily and they travel long distances on vacation. Dogs are taken along and carry their infections back home or to their new homes. Finally, there is some evidence that the parasite may be adapting to cooler climates.

Once established in an area, the infection appears to remain enzootic. The reasons may relate to the long life of the adults, up to several years, and the high microfilaremia in even moderate infections. Hundreds of mf/mm^3 of blood are common in dirofilariosis. Dogs are seldom continuously protected from mosquitoes. The role of wild canids in perpetuating the infection has not been systematically investigated, but both foxes and coyotes have been found to be infected in enzootic localities.

No public health measures have been taken to reduce the incidence of *D. immitis* infection in dogs, but community mosquito control programs should reduce the probability of infection. The responsibility for control lies with the individual owner. In an enzootic area, the owner can take the following steps:

1. Protection of the dog from mosquitoes by providing screened quarters or by keeping the dog confined at times of day when mosquitoes most actively seek blood meals, usually at dusk and dawn.
2. Administration of chemoprophylactic drugs during and after the mosquito season. In areas where mosquitoes are active year round, chemoprophylaxis must be given continuously.
3. Periodic examination of the dog to determine whether it has a patent infection and to provide treatment of adult worms and mf if necessary.

As described earlier, dogs generate many different immune responses to *D. immitis* following infection. Most of these immune responses are either inconsequential or actually aid in the maintenance of the parasite in an otherwise immunologically competent host. Other immune responses actually contribute to the heartworm disease syndrome as in the case of the immune-mediated destruction of microfilariae or the creation of immune complexes in various tissues as previously described. Considerable data generated in the recent past show encouraging evidence of the possibility of protective immunity. That is, even though there is limited evidence of naturally-occurring, significant protective immunity, it has been possible to demonstrate that dogs can be made to be immune. This evidence has resulted in research toward the development of a commercially viable vaccine. Progress has been made in finding and molecularly cloning the antigens that may play a role in such a vaccine, yet the complexity of both the infection and the requisite immune responses provide formidable barriers to the creation of such a product.

This parasite will infect humans. Although finding adult worms in the cardiovascular system of humans is exceedingly rare, it is not unusual to find partially developed, decomposing immature adults in the lungs of people. The parasites seem to be able to partially develop in some cases, but they die before completing development due to the fact that they are in an unnatural host. This syndrome in humans is typically not associated with disease, but rather a "pulmonary coin lesion" is noted when chest X rays are done on certain patients. The lesion cannot be distinguished from a tumor. Surgery is done to remove the mass and dead worm fragments may be evident. Dozens of such cases have been described in the past couple of decades.

FILARIAL INFECTION OF RUMINANTS AND HORSES

Five genera of filarioid nematodes have been found in domestic herbivores in temperate and warm climates throughout the world. Where systematic studies have been done, the prevalence rate sometimes exceeds 75%. Nearly all species cause at least minor damage to the host and a few cause serious losses in some populations of animals. Some species that are representative or are of interest because of their impact on populations are the following:

Stephanofilaria stilesi occurs in the skin of the belly of cattle in the United States; it seems to be most common in cattle in the western United States, where it occurs in up to 90% of animals at slaughter. The skin where the adults and mf are found becomes thickened, inflamed, and leaks blood and serum; such lesions may reach 15 cm (6 inches) in diameter. Horn flies, *Haematobia irritans* (Diptera: Muscoidea), are the intermediate hosts. Losses from this parasite lie principally in trimming of small parts of the hide at slaughter, not a major loss.

A number of species of *Onchocerca* lie in ligaments, where they cause inflammation and significant discomfort to the host. For example, *Onchocerca cervicalis* occurs in the ligamentum nuchae, the large ligament that inserts at the back of the head and supports it. About 50% of horses in the United States are infected, and up to 80% of horses in both temperate and warm climates in other parts of the world have been found to be infected. The parasite causes inflammation of the ligament and then necrosis of the connective tissue fibers and calcification later in the infection. Vectors are biting midges of the genus *Culicoides* (Diptera, Ceratopogonidae). Eight zoonotic infections with *Onchocerca* have been found in humans in the United States

The normal hosts of *Elaeophora schneideri* are mule deer (*Odocoileus hemionis*) and white-tailed deer (*Dama virgiana*) in the United States. In the normal host the parasite causes little damage, but there can be considerable damage in domestic sheep and in elk (*Cervus canadensis*). We have discussed some instances in which migratory patterns are altered in a foreign host and a few in which the infection is more severe than in the normal host. *E. schneideri* is a good example of the latter: Sheep suffer from a severe allergic dermatitis and elk are often blinded. The infection in sheep was first described by Dr. H. E. Kemper of the United States Department of Agriculture in 1938 in sheep in southern Colorado and northern New Mexico that had grazed on pastures above 2000 m (6000 feet) during the summer. It was later found that elk in the Gila National Forest of north central New Mexico were blinded because of infection.

LABORATORY MODELS OF FILARIOID INFECTIONS

It is evident that there is a good deal of conjecture and partial knowledge of nearly all aspects of filarioid infections in humans and other animals. Although filarioids may infect many hosts, some have a narrow host range or develop abnormally in other hosts. *W. bancrofti*, for example, develops only in humans and certain nonhuman primates; on the other hand, the subperiodic form of *B. malayi* develops fairly readily in primates other than humans and in cats. Thus, we have better descriptions of the course of the disease in *B. malayi* than in *W. bancrofti*. An ideal situation is one in which a parasite can be propagated in its normal hosts in the laboratory and studied in a controlled way. *Dirofilaria immitis* has been studied in the dog , but its long prepatent period and the expense of keeping dogs preclude its use as a widespread laboratory model. One of the best models found to date is *Litosomoides carinii* of the cotton rat; it has been used for a variety of studies on transmission, immunity, and other aspects of host–parasite interactions. A great deal has been learned with *L. carinii*, but it is of limited usefulness; for example, it can be used as a drug screening system, but with reservations. In none of these cases is it possible to study infections in genetically identical hosts, a real limitation on immunological studies. Better models would allow knowledge to advance more rapidly.

Readings

Adcock, J. L., and Hibler, C. P. (1969). Vascular and neuroophthalmic pathology of elaeophorosis in elk. *Pathol. Vet.* **6**, 185–213.

Anderson, R. C. (1959). Possible steps in the evolution of filarial life cycles. *Proc. 6th Int. Congr. Trop. Med. Malariol.* **2**, 444–449.

Bailey, W. S. (1971). *Spirocerca lupi*: A continuing enquiry. *J. Parasitol.* **58**, 3–22.

Bertram, D. S. (1966). Dynamics of parasitic equilibrium in cotton rat filariasis. *Adv. Parasitol.* **4**, 255–319.

Conder, G. A., and Williams, J. F. (Eds.) (1986). *Onchocerciasis/Filariasis. Proceedings of a Symposium April 8–10, 1986.* Upjohn, Kalamazoo, MI.

Day, K. P. (1991). The endemic normal in lymphatic filariasis: As static concept. *Parasitol. Today* **7**, 341–343.

Denham, D. A., and McGreevy, P. B. (1977). Brugian filariasis: Epidemiological and experimental studies. *Adv. Parasitol.* **15**, 243–309.

Duke, B. O. L. (1990). Onchocerciasis (river blindness)—Can it be eradicated? *Parasitol. Today* **6**, 82–84.

Eberhard, M. L. (1979). Studies on the *Onchocerca* (Nematoda: Filarioidea) found in cattle in the United States. 1. Systematics of *O.*

gutterosa and *O. lienalis* with a description of *O. stilesi* sp. n. *J. Parasitol.* **65,** 379–388.

Gibson, C. L. (1952). Comparative morphology of skin inhabiting microfilariae of man, cattle and equines in Guatemala. *Am. J. Trop. Med. Hyg.* **1,** 250–262.

Grieve, R. B., Lok, J. B., and Glickman, L. T. (1983). Epidemiology of canine heartworm infection. *Epidemiol. Rev.* **5,** 220–246.

Grieve, R. B., Wisnewski, N., Frank, G. R., and Tripp, C. A. (1995). Vaccine research and development for the prevention of filarial nematode infections. In *Vaccine Design: The Subunit and Adjuvant Approach* (M. F. Powell and M. J. Newman, Eds.), pp. 737–768. Plenum, New York.

Hibler, C. P. (1966). Development of *Stephanofilaria stilesi* in the horn fly. *J. Parasitol.* **52,** 890–898.

Hibler, C. P., and Metzger, C. J. (1974). Morphology of the larval stages of *Elaeophora schneideri* in the intermediate and definitive hosts with some observations on their pathogenesis in abnormal definitive hosts. *J. Wildlife Dis.* **10,** 361–369.

Kartman, L. (1953). Factors influencing infection of the mosquito with *Dirofilaria immitis* (Leidy, 1856). *Exp. Parasitol.* **2,** 27–78.

Knight, D. H. (1987). Heartworm infection. *Vet. Clin. North Am. Small Anim. Practice Parasitic infect.* **17**(6), 1463–1518.

Nelson, G. S. (1970). Onchocerciasis. *Adv. Parasitol:* **8,** 173–224.

Nutman, T. B., Kumaraswami, V., and Ottesen, E. A. (1987). Parasite-specific anergy in human filariasis: Insights after analysis of parasite antigen-driven lymphokine production. *J. Clin. Invest.* **79,** 1516–1523.

Orihel, T. C., Ash, L. R., Ramachandran, C. P., and Otteson, E. A. (Eds.) (1997). *Bench Aids for the Diagnosis of Filarial Infections.* World Health Organization, Geneva.

Otteson, E. A. (1992). Infection and disease in lymphatic filariasis: An immunological perspective. *Parasitology* **104,** 571–579.

Sasa, M. (1976). *Human filariasis. A global survey of epidemiology and control.* Univ. Park Press, Baltimore.

Shoop, W. L. (1992). Ivermectin resistance. *Parasitol. Today* **9,** 154–159.

Southgate, B. A. (1974). A quantitative approach to parasitological techniques in Bancroftian filariasis and its effect on epidemiological understanding. *Trans. R. Soc. Trop. Med. Hyg.* **68,** 177–186.

Taylor, H., Pacque, R. M., Muñoz, B., and Greene, B. R. (1990). Impact of mass treatment of onchocerciasis with Ivermectin on the transmission of infection. *Science* **250,** 116–118.

Worms, M. J. (1972). Circadian and seasonal rhythms in blood parasites. In *Behavioral Aspects of Parasite Transmission* (E. U. Canning and C. A. Wright, Eds.), pp. 53–67. Academic Press, New York.

CHAPTER

35

GUINEA WORM

The worms discussed in this chapter belong to the order Camallinida in the class Secerentea. They are typically long slender worms that have rather undistinguished morphologic features. The esophagus is usually cylindrical, but in the adult worms most of the intestinal tract is atrophied. Both the head end and the tail end have papillae which are used in classification and identification (Fig. 35.1). The life cycles involve arthropod intermediate hosts and the organisms are passed via the food chain. The adults inhabit the internal organs of their vertebrate hosts.

THE GUINEA WORM OF HUMANS

Name of Organism and Disease Association

Dracunculus medinensis is the guinea worm that causes a disease variously called dracunculiasis, dracunculosis, and dractoniasis. It is the fiery serpent of the Old Testament, and the scientific name translates as "the little dragon of Medina."

Hosts and Host Range

Humans and a wide range of other hosts include wild and domestic carnivores, herbivores, and primates.

Geographic Distribution and Importance

The organism has historically been distributed in the Sudan area of Africa, New Guinea, India, southern Asia, the Middle East, some Caribbean islands, and parts of Brazil. Currently the disease is still endemic in India, Yemen, and 16 African countries with 99% of infections reported from Africa.

In the late 1940s there were an estimated 47 million infections worldwide. By the early 1980s there were about 20 million infections in Africa, the Middle East, and the Indian subcontinent. The prevalence continues to decline through concerted control programs. For example, from 1986 to 1994 reported cases dropped from 3.6 million to 165,000. The number of endemic villages has decreased from more than 23,000 in 1992 to fewer than 8000 at the end of 1995. There is hope for eradication within the foreseeable future.

Infected persons are incapacitated for about three months when the worms are under the skin. Deaths are rare, but permanent physical disabilities may occur in some persons.

Morphology

Female worms are from 1.5 to 70 cm by 1 mm, but they may reach a length of 120 cm (47 in.) Males are 12 to 29 by 0.4 mm. The head and tail structures are rather poorly developed (Fig. 35.1).

Life Cycle

The ovoviviparous female worms lie in subcutaneous tissues and release L_1s through a break in the skin (Fig. 35.2). The L_1 is eaten by a copepod such as *Cyclops viridis* in which it develops to the L_3 in about two weeks. Infection is passed to the definitive host when

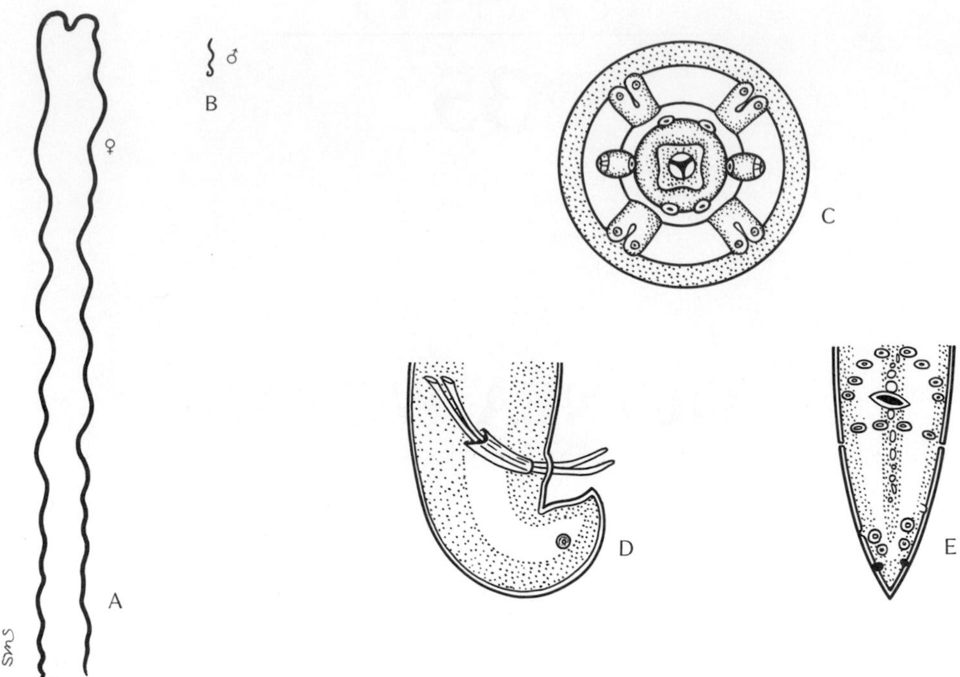

FIGURE 35.1 Adults of *Dracunculus medinensis*. (A *and* B) Relative sizes of the adult male and female worms; (C) anterior end of male showing papillae; (D) tail of male showing curved tip and spicules; (E) tail male showing papillae and anus. [Redrawn from Moorthy, V. N., 1937.]

drinking water contaminated with infected copepods. The prepatent period is nearly a year.

Details of the life cycle have been worked out in the dog, and the pattern fits well with observations made on naturally infected humans. When an infected copepod is ingested, the L_3s are released in the small intestine and they migrate probably via the lymphatics to various tissues throughout the body. The worms continue to migrate and reach the subcutaneous tissues about six weeks after infection. By three to four months after infection, equal numbers of male and female worms are present, but by six months males are absent; copulation must take place before six months after infection. It is possible, as with certain filarial nematodes, that male worms migrate from time to time. As sexual maturity approaches, nearly a year after infection, the females move to the connective tissue just under the skin.

About 20 species of copepods have been implicated as intermediate hosts of *D. medinensis.* The species vary, of course, in various parts of the world.

Diagnosis

Finding a portion of the body of the female worm protruding through a blisterlike break in the skin is the usual means of diagnosis.

Host–Parasite Interactions

The developing stages in the definitive host do not cause any known symptoms, but when the mature female reaches the subcutaneous area, both local and systemic reactions occur. As the female worm moves toward the surface to make a hole in the skin, there is extreme burning and itching at the site; thus the name "fiery serpent."

Joints such as the knees swell and make walking difficult or impossible. There is an allergic-like reaction in the area where the worm lies, and the person may suffer from a constellation of vague symptoms such as intestinal upset, difficulty in breathing, dizziness, and fainting. Worms sometimes lodge in tissues other than the skin where abscesses may form, and they may cause paralysis if in the central nervous system.

The area where the worms form an opening in the skin allows the entrance of bacteria, which may lead to a serious infection if left untreated. Apparently, little or no immunity is elicited by the infection.

Epidemiology and Control

Control of the guinea worm revolves around the following:

1. Providing a clean water supply to endemic areas

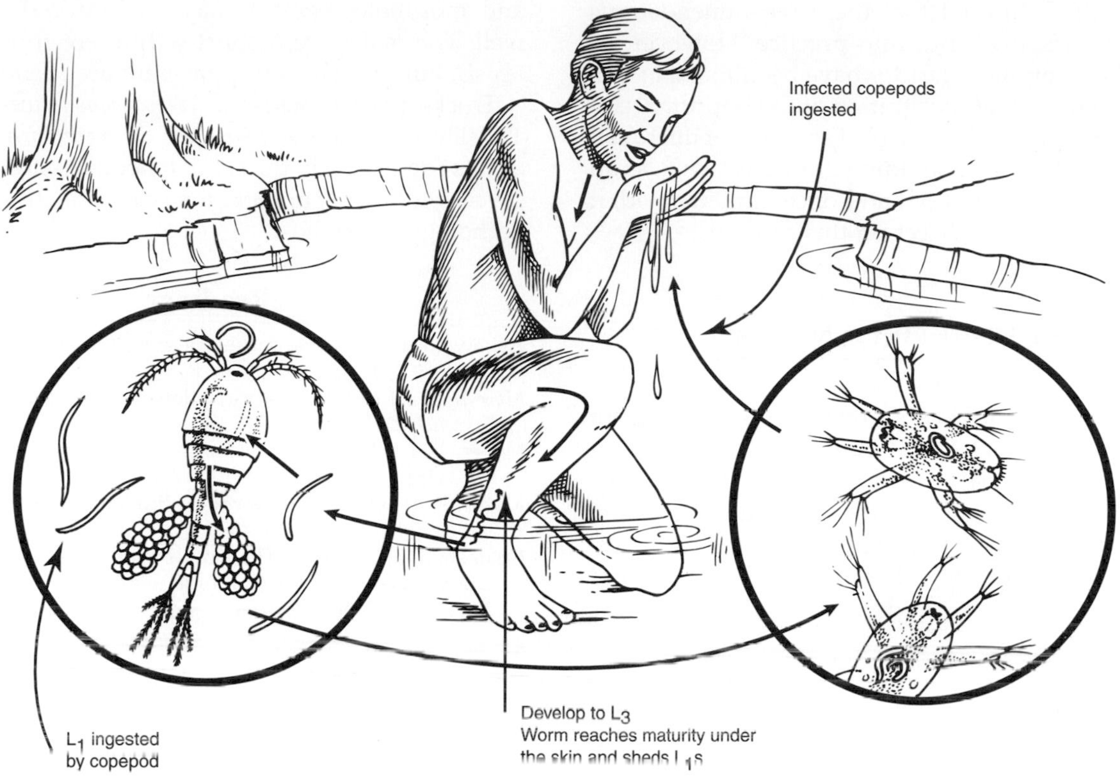

FIGURE 35.2 Life cycle of *Dracunculus medinensis.*

2. Treating water that may be contaminated
3. Preventing contact of persons who have active infections with the water supply

The treatment used for thousands of years has been to pull out a portion of the worm through the hole in the skin and to wind it up on a stick (Fig. 35.2). Care must be taken not to break the worm or it will retract, die, and cause a considerable foreign body or allergic reaction. The treatment is memorialized in the staff of Asclepius with a serpent wound around it. This is the symbol of the healer or physician commonly recognized in medical certification documents seen in physicians' offices.

Although some drugs have been used to kill or immobilize the worms, it is generally agreed that they should still be extracted by surgical or other means.

The 1980s were designated as the International Drinking Water Supply and Sanitation Decade by the World Health Organization, and the success of the program has had enormous beneficial impact on the health of millions of persons in areas where guinea worm is endemic. Programs of control show the simplicity of some solutions and the difficulty in achieving them. Although guinea worm has a broad host range, the mode of infection and the habitat of the intermediate hosts are such that safe drinking water will nearly eradicate the infection from a localized human population in a year.

Infections with *D. medinensis* are associated with standing water where copepods live. In India, step wells are typically the source of infection; a step well is a community water supply in which stone steps allow people to climb down easily to wherever the seasonal water level is. Particularly at low levels, the water has a high population of copepods and can be readily contaminated with L_1s from persons having contact with the water by carrying it, bathing in it, or washing clothes. As many as 95% of persons have been found to be infected in such communities.

In Africa, where water is often taken from streams, water levels drop during the dry season and water is often confined to pools before the rains begin again. The same factors pertain here as in India: water is concentrated, people have little choice where to obtain water, and exposure to guinea worm is almost inevitable.

Recommendations for prevention of guinea worm infection have been to keep people from drinking potentially contaminated water and to prevent those who are infected from having contact with the water supply. It is generally admitted that these recommendations have been difficult to put into practice. However, as described earlier, great strides have been made in this regard. The universal recognition of the importance of clean, safe water for the control of a variety of microbial and parasitic diseases, including guinea worm, was an idea too long in incubation, and once implemented, it has made a profound effect on this disease.

RELATED ORGANISMS

The order Camallanida is a relatively small one, but there are some species that should be noted. *Dracunculus insignis* is a parasite of carnivores such as the raccoon and rodents, especially those that are associated with water. *D. insignis* is widely distributed in North America in both warm and cold climates. It is found in the dog and other canids, mustelids such as the skunk and weasel, and in aquatic rodents such as the muskrat. Its life cycle is much the same as *D. medinensis* and morphologically it may be confused with it as well. The males are distinctly different from *D. medinensis,* but the females apparently are identical.

Ducks serve as hosts for *Avioserpens taiwana* in Asia. The life cycle is the same as *D. medinensis* and the adults come to lie in the subcutaneous tissues. Nodules 2.5 cm in diameter or more may cause relatively serious pathology to the host.

Readings

Anomymous (1996). Dracunculus near eradication. *Trop. Med. Hyg. News* **45**(1), 12.

Moorthy, V. N. (1937). A redescription of *Dracunculus medinensis. J. Parasitol.* **23,** 220–224.

Muller, R. (1971). *Dracunculus* and dracunculiasis. *Adv. Parasitol.* **9,** 73–151.

Muller, R. (1992). Guinea worm eradication—Four more years to go. *Parasitol. Today* **8,** 387–390.

Onamabiro, S. D. (1956). The early stages of the development of *Dracunculus medinensis* (L) in the mammalian host. *Ann. Trop. Med. Parasitol.* **5O,** 157–166.

CHAPTER

36

TRICHINELLA, TRICHURIS, AND *CAPILLARIA*

The members in this class of nematodes, the Adenophorea, are characterized as lacking both phasmids and lateral excretory canals. Both of these characters are difficult to see in specimens unless one has had experience in identifying nematodes. A number of adenophoreans are parasites of insects and are in the superfamily Mermithoidea; they are widespread and serve to modulate insect populations. An infected insect, such as a grasshopper, may have its hemocoel so packed with worms that they burst out in great profusion when the body wall is cut. We are concerned in this chapter with those adenophoreans that cause economic losses or are medically important.

TRICHINELLOSIS

From its discovery in 1835 until the present time, *Trichinella spiralis* has been the pivotal character in a series of dramas. The discovery of the worm by a medical student, James Paget, in the muscles of a cadaver in 1835 was overshadowed by the published description of his material by his teacher, the eminent zoologist Richard Owen (later a virulent critic of Charles Darwin's theory of evolution). At the time, there was only speculation whether this little worm was associated with a disease.

Infected meat shipped from the United States to continental Europe brought about strained international relations and an embargo on pork from the United States. In recent years, France declared an embargo on horse meat from the United States in the wake of an outbreak of trichinellosis most likely associated with eating horse meat.

Epidemiologic studies in the Arctic done under exceedingly difficult conditions led to a clarification on modes of transmission and the probable spread of the infection throughout the world. The efforts to supplant older ideas on transmission have only slowly been successful, a cultural inertia that demonstrates human unwillingness to shift viewpoints. All in all, the interaction of *T. spiralis* with humankind is a fascinating intertwining of the biology of the parasite with food habits, politics, and economics.

Name of Organism and Disease Associations

Trichinella spiralis causes trichinellosis; this term is now being used more widely, especially in Europe, but the less correct term, *trichinosis,* is embedded in the literature, and the minds of biologists, and may never be eradicated. *Trichinella pseudospiralis* was described from the raccoon (*Procyon lotor*) in Russia and differs from *T. spiralis* principally in that *T. pseudospiralis* larvae do not form a capsule in the muscle, and they continue to move in the muscle. The term *trichina (-ae)* refers to the larvae that are found in the muscles of the mammalian host.

Hosts and Host Range

Humans, pig, bear, canids, raccoon, skunks, opossum, seals, walrus, and rodents are hosts. With few exceptions, any mammal can be infected experimentally, and a wide array of omnivores and carnivores has been found to be naturally infected, including about 75 species of wild animals. Although the domestic chicken has been infected experimentally, birds in general are probably resistant.

Geographic Distribution and Importance

Cosmopolitan. *T. spiralis* was probably originally prevalent in the Arctic and has spread nearly through out the world (Fig. 36.1). Its importance lies exclusively in infections of humans; other animals do not seem to be significantly affected. Outbreaks of infection in humans result from eating poorly cooked pork, bear meat, aquatic mammals, or other carnivores. Although rodents can be infected, and are commonly used to maintain *T. spliralis* in the laboratory, they probably play little role in maintenance of the organism.

During the 1930s and 1940s the prevalence of human infections in the United States was 16%, as measured by trichinae in the diaphragms of persons examined postmortem. A more recent study (1966–1970) showed only 4.7% of diaphragms containing trichinae. From 1947 to 1971 an average of 244 infections per year were reported in the United States. From 1947 to 1953 there was an average of 12 deaths per year, but from 1954 to 1971 there were only 2.8 per year. Among 10,204 infections, the death rate was 1.25%. Instances of clinical disease are sporadic at present and usually are associated with home-butchered pork or eating inadequately cooked meat of wild animals, most often bear.

Human infection is rare in continental Europe. For example, no human infection has been seen in the Netherlands since 1926. In Romania, and some other European countries, pork is preferred well cooked and human infections are rare.

Morphology

Adults are tiny worms (Fig. 36.2); the females are 3 to 4 by 0.06 mm and the males 1.5 by 0.04 mm. Members of the superfamily Trichinelloidea have a stichosome, a row of glandular cells forming a portion of the esophagus (see classification of nematodes Chapter 25). In the male, the stichosome extends nearly half the length of the body, but only about one-sixth in the female. The male has a pair of lobed structures called a pseudobursa at the posterior tip; spicules are lacking.

The larvae in the tissues are coiled up in cysts 250 to 500 μm long (Figs. 36.3, 36.4, 1.12); the larva itself is about 1 mm long.

Life Cycle

The larvae in the muscles of a mammal are in an advanced state of development, but are probably still L_1s (several investigators have studied the life cycle of *T. spiralis* and do not agree whether the infective lava is an L_1 or an L_3). Transmission to a new host takes place when muscle of an infected animal is eaten by a susceptible host. Development to adult males and females takes place quite rapidly in the intestine of the host; sexual maturity is reached in about 40 hours. After copulation, the females burrow into the tissue of the small intestine and larviposit in the mucosal or even submucosal areas of the gut. The niche occupied by the adults in the intestine is a multi-intracellular one, a unique niche among helminths. Newborn larvae enter the blood and lymph vessels, from which they are carried throughout the body. Females live about six weeks and give birth to perhaps 1500 larvae. The larvae develop intracellularly, especially in striated muscles, and they reach infectivity about 17 days after reaching their final site.

Diagnosis

Diagnosis depends on different methods during different phases of the infection:

1. Clinical signs and symptoms
2. Biopsies of somatic muscle
3. Serology to look for antibodies produced against the worm

Determining whether a person has been infected is seldom done during the intestinal phase of the life cycle. Signs and symptoms of infection at that time include abdominal pain, diarrhea, and vomiting; any number of infectious agents can cause the same signs and symptoms.

Trichinosis is usually suspected during the second phase of the infection when the larvae are migrating to the muscles and is usually diagnosed by examining muscle biopsies or by serology. At this point there is muscle pain, which is proportional to the number of trichinae in the muscle.

In epidemiologic surveys, small portions of somatic, diaphragm, or tongue muscle are examined for trichinae. The tissue may be pressed between glass plates and examined under the low power of a compound microscope; alternatively it may be digested with pepsin-HCI and the sediment examined for the freed larvae.

A number of serologic tests have been developed, and some of the more recent ones have a high degree of accuracy. Such tests can be useful in surveys and in determining which persons might be infected in an outbreak of trichinosis or they are used in epidemiologic studies of infections in hosts other than humans.

An ELISA (enzyme-linked immunosorbent assay) test employing excretory-secretory antigens has been

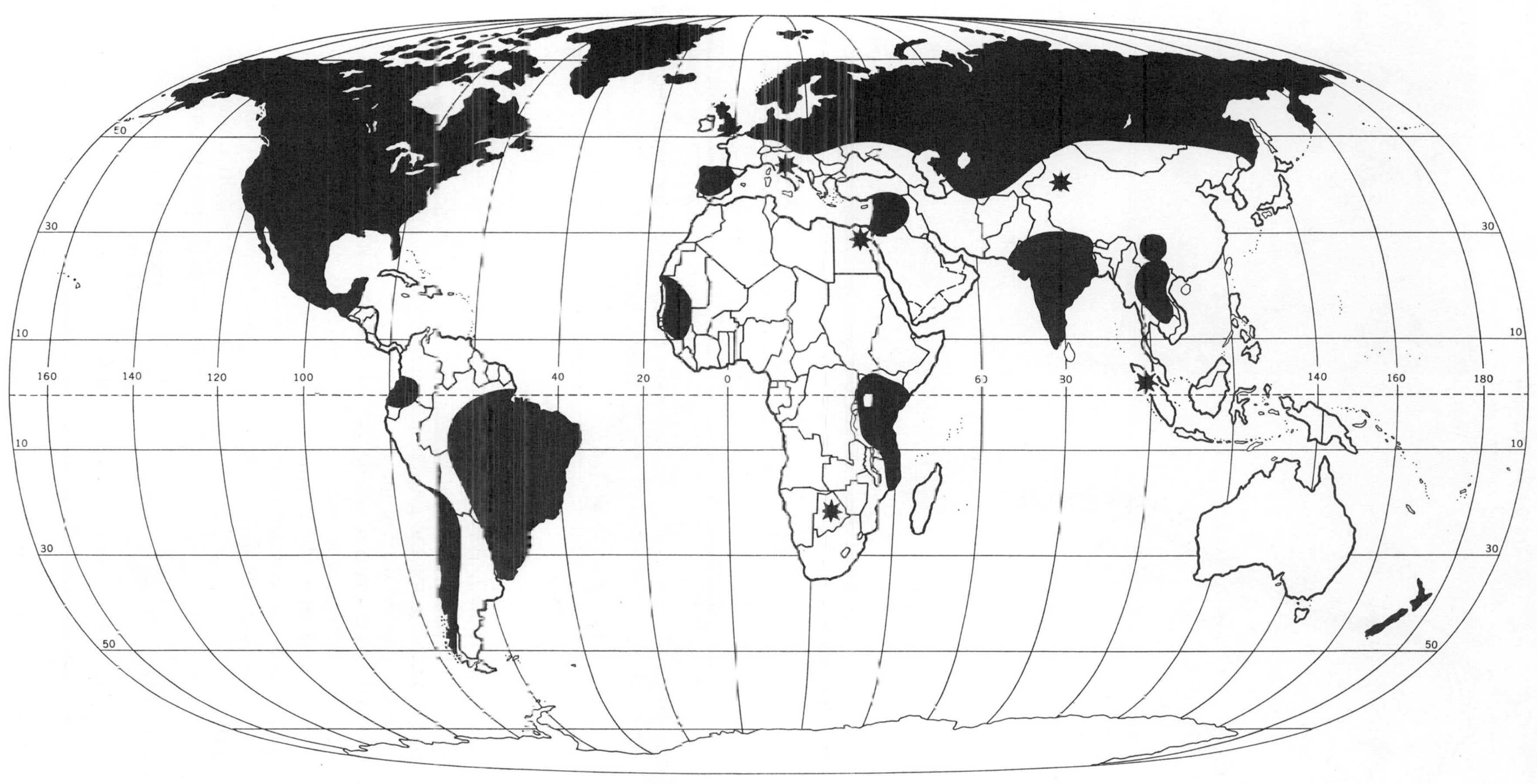

FIGURE 36.1 Geographic distribution of *Trichinella spiralis*.

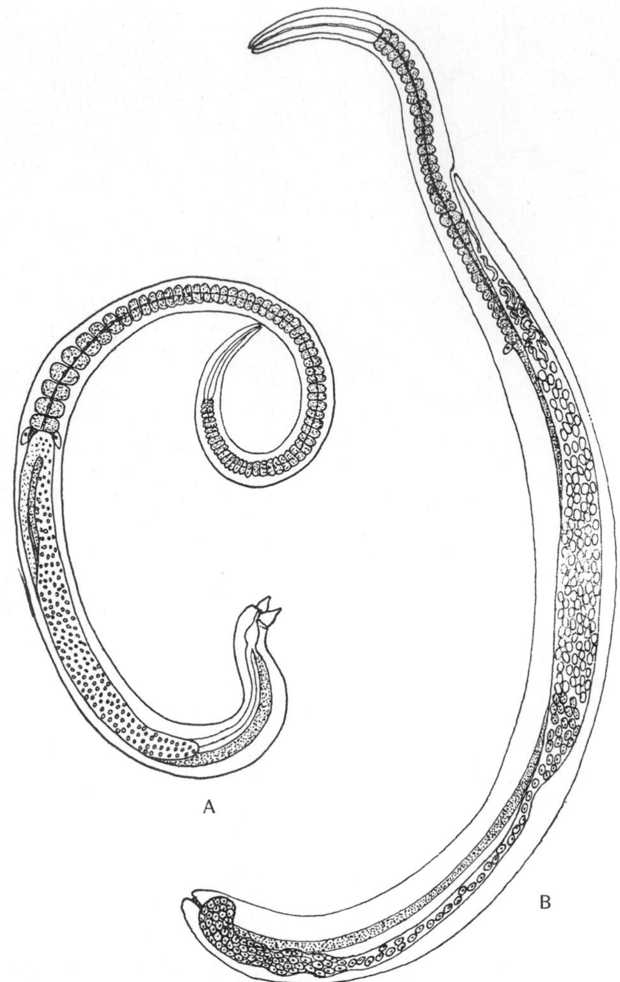

FIGURE 36.2 Male (A) and female (B) of *Trichinella spiralis.* [Redrawn from Yorke and Maplestone, 1962.]

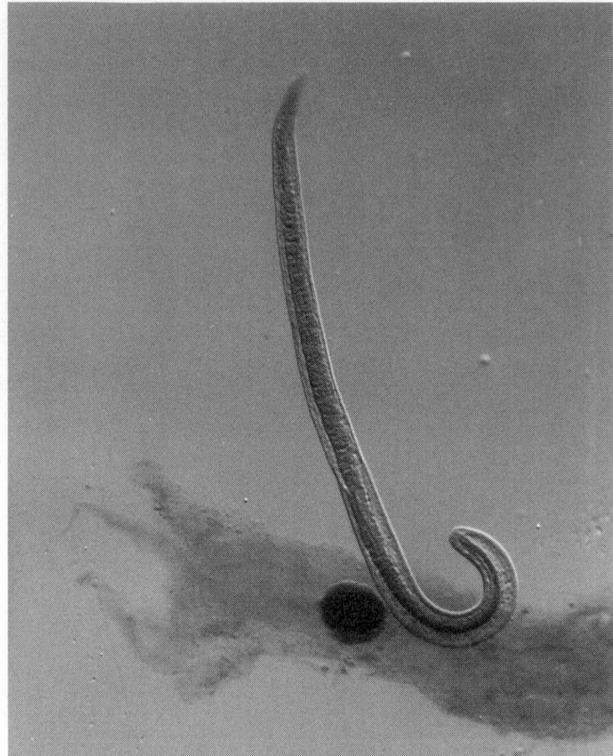

FIGURE 36.3 An infective larva of *Trichinella spiralis,* which has been released from a cyst in the muscle. See also Figure 1.12 for larvae encysted in muscle.

found to be both reliable and accurate and is widely used. The preferred ELISA now utilizes a unique carbohydrate, tyvelose, because it accounts for the greater part of the *Trichinella* antibody elicited during infection. It is interesting to note that tyvelose can be synthesized chemically and used as an alternative to complex parasite antigen mixtures to detect antibodies. While the significance of this highly unusual antigen is unclear in the context of host–parasite interactions, its use has great practical value.

Host–Parasite Interactions

As a general rule, hosts other than humans are not much affected by *T. spiralis.* In experimental studies in pigs, inocula of 100,000 larvae have not generally produce clinical disease, but in one study pigs showed decreased weight gains and probably muscle pain since they were reluctant to move at about three weeks after infection.

In humans, the infection has been divided into three phases:

1. *Intestinal.* Starting a few days after infection, there may be diarrhea, abdominal pain, and vomiting (Tab. 36.1).
2. *Migration.* About nine days after infection large numbers of larvae enter the circulatory system and begin to reach various organ systems. There is muscle pain, and difficulty in breathing, chewing, and swallowing. If death occurs, it usually takes place at this time.
3. *Inflammation.* About six weeks after infection, there is a strong reaction to the larvae in the tissues. There is pain and swelling of the tissues and fever. The symptoms resolve over time.

These signs and symptoms vary with the size of the inoculum. Data on the size of the inoculum in human infections are hard to come by. There can be a thousand-fold increase in tissue larvae over the number of worms ingested and that 100,000 larvae ingested by a pig might give 500 larvae per gram of pork loin. A poorly cooked quarter-pound pork tenderloin would

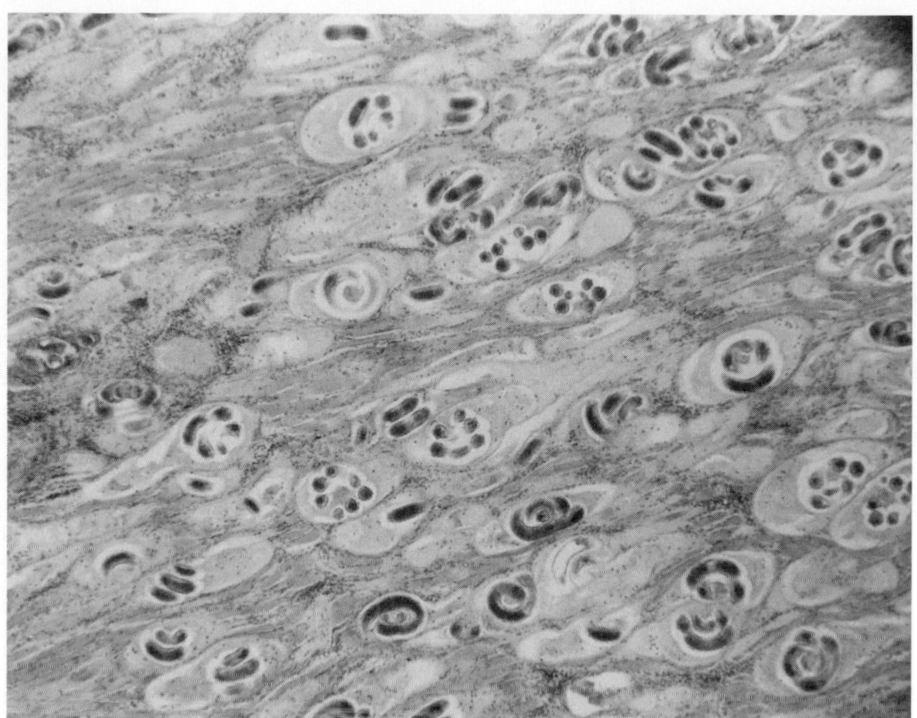

FIGURE 36.4 A histologic section of striated muscle showing a large number of *Trichinella spiralis* larvae in situ.

thereby constitute an inoculum of more than 56 million larvae in an a person or an average of 12,000 larvae/g of tissue in an average 68 kg (150 lb.) person. This inoculum could produce 56 × 10^6 larvae in a person or an average of 1.2 × 10^3 larvae/g of tissue in an average 68-kg (150 lb.) person. Larvae can be found in large numbers in histologic sections of infected hosts (Fig. 36.4).

TABLE 36.1 Clinical Features of Patients Who Had Eaten Bear Meat Containing *T. spiralis*

Signs or Symptoms	Percentage
Myalgia (muscle pain)	100
Fever	82
Diarrhea	76
Fatigue	65
Periorbital edema (swelling behind the eye)	47
Abdominal cramps	35
Visual disturbances	35
Nausea and vomiting	29
Skin lesions	18
Dyspnea (difficulty in breathing)	12

Larvae are not distributed randomly in the host and have a preferred site in each species of host. In humans, diaphragm and tongue have the largest numbers. In swine, using the diaphragm as 100%, other sites are tongue, 53%; shoulder, 44%; ham, 22%; loin, 14%. In cats, the intercostal muscles are preferred; in rodents it is the masseter mucles.

When the larvae reach their final sites in the muscles, they become encapsulated by a collagenous capsule elaborated by the muscle fiber (Fig. 36.4). Infected cells are referred to as nurse cells since the larvae elicit production of substances that they require. For further discussion of the larval cyst see Notable Features later in this chapter.

Infection with only moderate numbers of larvae confers immunity to reinfection. and the response results in a reduction in the number of adults. The stichosome forms a part of the esophagus and is secretory. Proteins have been isolated from the stichosomes of infective larvae that are 43 and 50/55 kD (kiloDaltons) in size and they are antigenic. Following immunization of mice with one of these proteins and challenge with 360 infective larvae each resulted in the following:

1. The number of female worms was reduced.
2. Fecundity of female worms was reduced.
3. The number of larvae in the muscles was a third to a half that of the nonimmunized control mice.

Adult *T. spiralis* also produce proteins from the stichosome cells, but these do not seem to protect mice on challenge. Thus, the antigens produced by infective larvae appear to have their protective effect against adult worms.

The immune response is directed toward the intestinal phase (adults) and is most likely T-cell dependent. When the larvae reach their final sites in the muscles, they become encapsulated by a collagenous capsule elaborated by the muscle fiber. It is generally agreed that larvae may live for 5 to 10 years in humans confirming the lack of significant response against larvae.

Larvae live within the muscle fiber; such infected cells are referred to as nurse cells since the larvae apparently elicit production of substances that they require. The larvae also take up nutrient across the body surface. Such a phenomenon is rather unusual in nematodes because the cuticle serves as a relatively impermeable barrier; this provides evidence that the larvae newly arrived in the muscle are pre-L_1s.

Epidemiology and Control

Control programs for the protection of the human population from trichinellosis have several aspects. Some of them are feasible in some times and places; others are not. The pattern of infection in any one locality must be taken into account (Fig. 36.5).

1. *Cooking potentially infected meat well.* Educational campaigns in the United States started early in the 20th century were partially successful. In parts of Europe, there probably was less success; among primitive northern peoples there was probably no impact.

2. *Inspecting pork for infection.* Modest laboratory facilities and a microscope with a magnification of about 60x are required. The cost per animal for examination is also important; inspection by trichinoscope in Europe has been used to determine which animals are infected and to remove them from the market. Using the trichinoscope in the United States has been considered to be cost-prohibitive, but digestion techniques have reduced the cost to about 9 cents per animal (1970 dollars).

3. *Freezing pork products.* If pork is frozen, the larvae can be killed. Regulations call for the following:

Temperature	**Time in Days**	
	6″ Thick or less	More than 6″ thick but less than 27″
−30°C or −20°F	20	30
−12°C or −10°F	10	20
−30°C or −20°F	6	12

This technique can be used for infected pork only

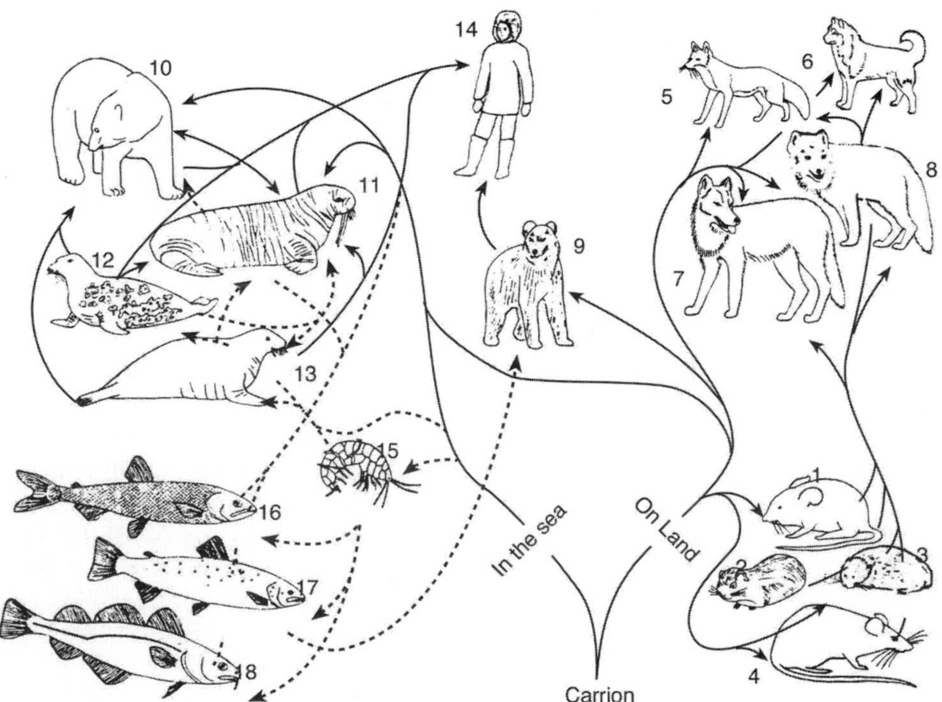

FIGURE 36.5 Epizootiology of *Trichinella spiralis* in the arctic. The organism is passed among terrestrial and aquatic mammals. The role of amphipods and fish remains uncertain. [From Williams, H. H., and Jones, A., 1976.]

or for all pork regardless of infection. It should be noted that there are some differences in the sensitivity of different isolates to freezing.

4. *Cooking garbage.* This method is clearly based on moderate affluence and low fuel costs, but it has been successful in the United States in controlling trichinosis and other infections.

5. *Eliminating wild reservoirs of infection.* Although there may be special local circumstances that will allow this method to be used, it is generally impractical.

Unless an astute physician has made a proper diagnosis, treatment of trichinellosis is not usually undertaken until late in the second or in the third phase of infection. At this time most of the adult worms have disappeared. If the infection has been recognized early, in the first or early second phase, anthelmintics may have some efficacy. The action of thiabendazole during the time when adult worms are in the intestine is temporarily to sterilize the female worms. The result is a reduction in the number of larvae invading the tissues in the late second and third phases of the disease. Other benzimidazoles in addition to thiabendazole are effective.

After the worms reach the tissues, anthelmintics have some effect, but usually symptomatic treatment is also given. For example, corticosteroids help to reduce inflammation of the tissues and thereby reduce discomfort.

T. spiralis originally occurred in the Holarctic region of the Northern Hemisphere. It was passed among various carnivore and carrion-eating hosts such as bear, seal, walrus, fox, and wolf (Fig. 36.5). We tend to think of the infection as being passed directly from one host to the next through predation, but some isolates of *T. spiralis* can survive for long periods outside the host. At or near the freezing point, larvae in muscle have survived up to a year. Thus, the original cycle in the Arctic involved both mammalian predators and scavengers. The role of fish and amphipods (Crustacea) is still not settled, but it is likely that they play only a minor role in maintaining the cycle of *T. spiralis.*

The organism spread from the Arctic to other regions of the world by increased travel and trade. For example, infected animals and people have been found in Kenya only since the early 1960s; the infection was previously unknown there. As a result of the dissemination of the *Trichinella,* three more or less distinct cycles are recognized:

1. *Feral.* This is the primeval cycle in the Arctic.

2. *Semidomestic.* This cycle occurs in temperate zones. Both wild and domesticated carnivores as well as some rodents are infected. Infection may spread from infected pork scraps in garbage dumps or from pigs dying in areas that make them accessible to scavengers. Once established, the cycle can continue through predation and scavenging.

3. *Domestic.* Pigs are the principal hosts in this cycle, and the cycle is perpetuated by garbage, carrion feeding, and cannibalism in pigs. Rats have been implicated in the cycle, because of their feeding habits, and recent evidence leads to the conclusions that rats can maintain the life cycle on pig farms in the absence of infected pigs, presumably through rat to rat cannibalism.

In all three cycles, humans are only an incidental host and for obvious reasons rarely contribute directly to the maintenance of the infection.

The pattern of transmission in *T. spiralis* is related to trade and technology. The original focus of infection in boreal regions spread into temperate and finally tropical climates. As the infection spread, it became established as a domestic cycle in swine. At that point, the infection became a more widespread public health problem and was undoubtedly promoted by certain methods of swine husbandry. At one time, many piggeries were located in the margins of cities, and the industry was based on feeding garbage. As a result, 5.7% of garbage-fed pigs were infected, whereas only 0.95% of farm-raised pigs were infected, a sixfold difference. At this same time, 16% of the U.S. human population was infected.

The relatively high prevalence of infection in swine in the United States led to outbreaks of trichinellosis in Germany from pork imported from the United States. Germans prefer rare pork and are therefore at some risk of infection, but pork is inspected at slaughter in Germany for trichinae, so the probability of infection is low. Because trichinellosis in Germany resulted from U.S. pork, embargoes have existed on pork from the United States.

In the United States, the main reliance for prevention of trichinellosis is currently placed on education of the populace to cook pork well. Inspection of pigs at slaughter is deemed to be too costly relative to the potential benefit, but digestion techniques or the ELISA test discussed earlier can be done at a small cost per animal and could be instituted if the risk were considered to be sufficiently high.

The prevalence of infection dropped to its present low level in the United States for reasons unrelated to trichinellosis. The crucial events were an outbreak of vesicular exanthema in swine and the campaign to eradicate hog cholera; both infections are caused by viruses that can be transmitted by ingestion of infected meat. Because of the seriousness of these infections in the swine industry, a federal law was passed in the early 1950s prohibiting feeding of raw garbage to pigs. All garbage had to be cooked to the point where the viruses were killed; fortunately, the trichinae were also killed. Recent studies in humans show a prevalence of infection of less than 5%; thus, human health has benefited from the need of swine producers to maintain the health of their herds.

It should be noted also that increasing use of high-technology in swine husbandry has had a significant impact on infection levels. Keeping swine on concrete and feeding them prepared food for maximal growth and feed conversion clearly make *T. spiralis* infection unlikely. Thus, the prevalence of infection in swine in the United States is now well below 1%.

In North America, most outbreaks of trichinellosis are now related to eating home-slaughtered pork from which uncooked sausage is made or from eating wild meat such as bear. Both types of outbreaks emphasize the importance of cooking meat well if there is even a minimal risk of infection.

Notable Features

The relationship of the larva to its host muscle cell in *Trichinella* is an example of an exquisite interaction between host and parasite. When the larva leaves the mother, it is carried throughout the body but ultimately comes to lie in the striated, somatic muscle. Interestingly, the larvae of *T. pseudospiralis* are found almost exclusively in slow-twitch fibers of the somatic muscle, but *T. spiralis* is found about equally in slow- and fast-twitch fibers. Cardiac muscle, even though striated, is not infected by *Trichinella.*

The larva enters the muscle fiber probably by mechanical means; there is a stylet at the entrance to the mouth which may allow it to penetrate the muscle cell. The larva moves away from the site of penetration, and the interaction begins. Over a period of about 19 days, the larva induces extreme changes in its host cell that provides it both protection and nutrient.

There is first a disappearance of the striations of the myocyte in the vicinity of the larva; then there is proliferation and movement of the nuclei of the host cell. There is a four- to ninefold increase in the number of nuclei and they move to the center of the fiber rather than their normal location at the sarcolemma. The nuclei become larger and the nucleoli increase dramatically as well, indicating an increase in protein synthesis.

Starting at day 4, the larva grows rapidly and probably uses host cell proteins as food. ATP and other sources of high energy phosphate decrease.

As development proceeds, there is an increase in the amount of RNA in the region of the larva, indicating that the host cell is providing the larva with crucial substances for its growth. Mitochondria increase and there are changes in citric acid (Krebs) cycle intermediates. Glutamate, malate, and pyruvate oxidation decrease and succinate oxidation increases. The glycogen content of the muscle fibers is elevated above normal, but as the larva reaches its final size, glycogen content declines to about a normal level.

At about 10 days after infection of the muscle cells, the capsule around the larva is formed. The capsule (Fig. 36.4) is formed entirely by the host but is somehow initiated by the larva. The capsule is almost entirely collagen, but it remains permeable and may allow nutrients to enter.

Remarkable as this host–parasite interaction may be, the complexity of the larva is further evidence that small organisms are not, in fact, so simple. The cephalic sense organs of two-day old larvae have been studied and 16 sensory structures were described using both SEM and TEM. Amphids are paired sensory structures at the anterior end of nematodes, and in *Trichinella* they each have 10 dendritic processes. What all of these sense organs do is still problematic, but they most likely are important for the larva in finding its way and settling in at a final site in a muscle fiber.

The entirety of the complex interaction in *Trichinella* infections, particularly its unusual cell biology, is the subject of considerable research. It is possible that the results of these investigations will help us to understand the host–parasite relationship. These insights may also be of extraordinary value in better describing cellular genetics in other animals, especially processes in differentiation.

WHIPWORMS

Name of Organisms and Disease Associations

The genus *Trichuris* contains a number of species that infect mammalian hosts and cause whipworm disease or trichurosis. The following are some common species and their hosts:

Trichuris	*Hosts*
trichiura	Humans and other primates
suis	Suids: domestic pig, peccary
vulpis	Canids: dog, fox, coyote
ovis	Artiodactyls: sheep, goat, ox, camelids, cervids

Morphology

The members of the genus *Trichuris* are called whipworms because they have relatively short, stout bodies and an extremely long esophageal area (Fig 36.6). The name means "hairlike tail"; it has been pointed out that the name should more correctly be *Trichocephalus*, that is "hairlike head," but the rules of zoological nomenclature call for retention of the original name even if it refers to the wrong end of the worm.

The female worms have some differences among species, but identifications are made from the genitalia of the male worms. Their copulatory structures vary and are easily differentiated from one another (Fig. 36.7A).

The eggs are brownish and have clear plugs at either end (Fig. 36.7B), which make them easily recognizable; they are passed in the feces in a one- to two-cell stage. They vary somewhat in size from species to species:

Trichuris	*Size range*
trichiura	50–54 × 22–32 μm
suis	50–56 × 21–25 μm
ovis	70–80 × 30–42 μm
vulpis	72–90 × 32–40 μm

Life Cycle

Whipworms live in the large intestines of their hosts, where they are found almost exclusively in the cecum. The long esophageal region is threaded through the mucosa of the gut with only the body in the lumen. Their life cycles are direct, with eggs (Fig. 36.7B) developing to the infective L_1 stage in about two weeks. The larvae hatch when the eggs are eaten and they enter the mucosa of the small intestine. After 10 days to two weeks they return to the lumen and move to the cecum, where they mature. The prepatent period may be as short as 30 days in some species or as long as 90 days in others.

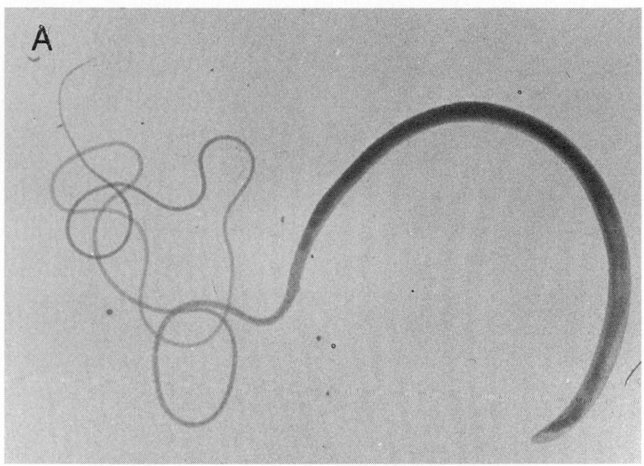

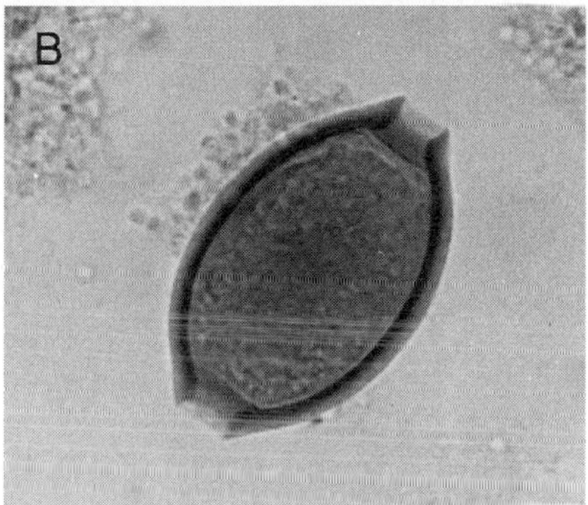

FIGURE 36.7 (A) While mount of a female *Trichuris*. (B) Egg of *Trichuris* sp.

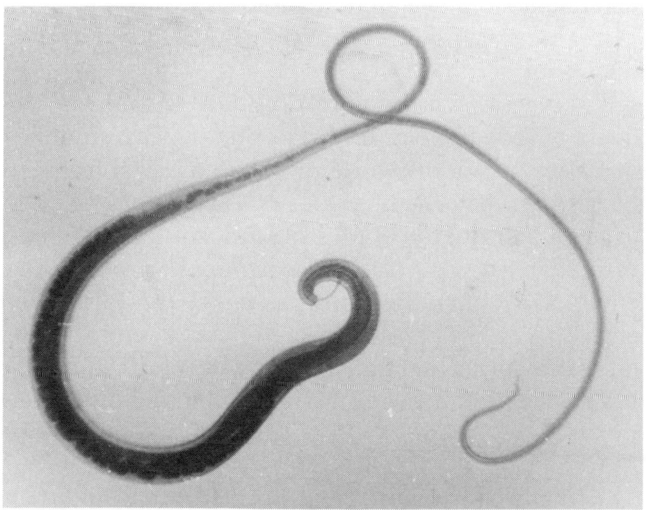

FIGURE 36.6 A whole mount of an adult male *Trichuris* sp. as seen under a low power LM.

Hosts and Importance

Although about 70 species are known from a wide range of mammals, only a few are of economic or medical importance. *Trichuris trichiura* is a cosmopolitan parasite of humans that has mild pathogenicity; *T. suis* is identical anatomically to *T. trichiura*, but they apparently do not cross-transmit and have a different chromosome number. *T. suis* has generally been considered to be benign, but enteric disorders have been found in both naturally and experimentally infected pigs. *T. vulpis* is a cosmopolitan parasite of dogs and other canids, and it can cause chronic colitis with severe disease in dogs. The whipworms of ruminants, such as *T. ovis* of sheep, cattle, and other ruminants, seem to be only slightly pathogenic, but they have not been studied extensively.

Epidemiology and Control

Removal of whipworms by anthelmintics has been erratic, at best, in the past. While effective drugs are available, the worms are refractory to many of the commonly used anthelmintics.

Trichuris has many of the same developmental characteristics as *Ascaris:* slow development outside the host, retention of the infective larva within the egg capsules, and extraordinary hardiness of the embryonated eggs (Chapter 32). Therefore, control programs that are effective for ascarids tend also to be effective for whipworms.

CAPILLARIA AND RELATED GENERA

A number of members of the superfamily Trichinelloidea in the subfamily Capillarinae are widespread parasites of the digestive tracts of higher vertebrates and a few of them are either of economic or medical importance. They are generally found threaded in the mucosa of the intestinal tract: in the esophagus or small intestine.

Morphology

The adults are 0.5 to 4 cm long and quite slender, so that special care is needed to find the worms in the tissue and then to dissect them out. The eggs are similar to those of whipworms; they are double-plugged and yellow or brownish (Fig. 36.7B), but the plugs are relatively small.

Fecal examinations of dogs and cats sometimes reveal *Capillaria* eggs which, at first glance, may be mistaken for *Trichuris* eggs. However, consideration should be given to the animals having preyed on small rodents or birds and merely temporarily be passing *Capillaria* eggs. Feces should be reexamined in a day or two to determine whether this is a true or a pseudoparasite.

Importance and Life Cycles

Capillaria philippinensis is the cause of severe intestinal disease in humans in the Philippines and parts of Southeast Asia. Humans are the only known definitive host, but evidence indicates that infection comes from eating insufficiently cooked fish. Pathogenesis can be severe, and a number of people have died from the infection.

In domestic birds, *C. caudinflata* and *C. contorta* require earthworms as an intermediate host, whereas *C. obsignata* has a direct life cycle. All three species are pathogenic for their definitive hosts and cause losses in free-ranging poultry because of damage to the intestinal tract.

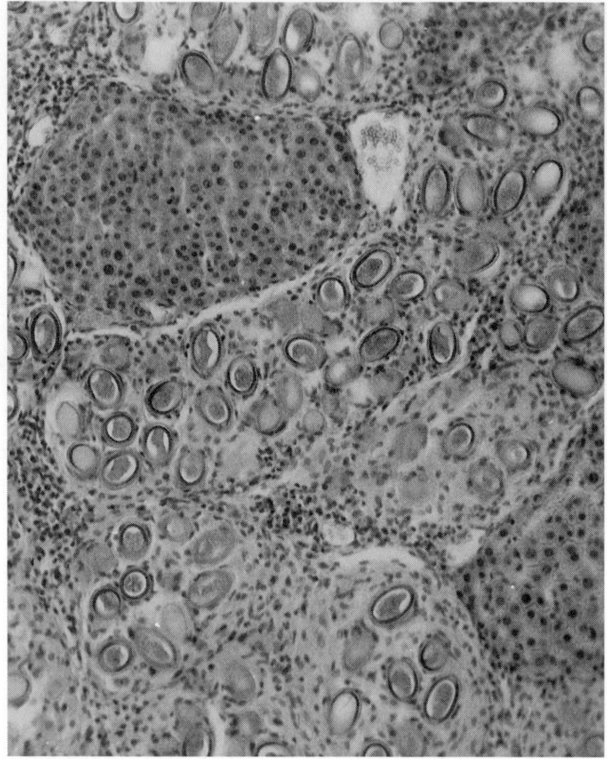

FIGURE 36.8 A tissue section of the liver of a rodent showing eggs of *Capillaria hepatica* in situ. A small island of normal liver tissue lies at the left side of the photograph; the eggs scattered through most of the tissue elicit a strong foreign body reaction. Adult worms (not seen in this section) and their eggs are retained in the liver and reach the outside only when the host is eaten or dies and disintegrates. [Rodent collected by Dr. Charles H. Calisher. Slide courtesy of Dr. Barbara E. Powers, Director, Diagnostic Laboratory, Colorado State University.]

C. hepatica (syn. *Hepaticola hepatica)* is found in the livers of rodents (Fig. 36.8) and sometimes in humans in many parts of the world. Eggs are released from the liver only when the host dies or is preyed upon. The eggs pass through the intestinal tract of the scavenger or predator, which may be a mammal or a bird, and embryonate after they are passed in the feces. The embronated eggs are then eaten by a rodent or other animal in order to transmit the infection again. If a rodent dies and the eggs are released into the environment, these eggs, also, will embryonate and become infective.

Rodents are found to be infected at postmortem examination. The liver is normal in size, but shows white streaks that run along the surface and in the parenchyma as well; these streaks represent the locations of the worms and their eggs (Fig. 36.8).

In most areas, the Norway rat, *Rattus norvegicus*, is the principal host. In urban locations along the east coast of the United States, 70% to 94% of Norway rats were found to be infected in several surveys done in Hartford Connecticut, Baltimore Maryland and New York City. In Malaysia only 10.5% of rats were infected. Infections in *Mus musculus* are generally low, being 4% or less in several surveys. In sylvatic habitats, infections in white footed mice and meadow voles have generally been less than 3%.

Human infections have been reported four times in South Africa, so there is some hazard to human health, but the risk is not high. Humans probably become infected when rodent droppings contaminate food.

Readings

Al Karmi, T. O., and Flaubert, G. M. (1981). Comparative analysis of mobility and ultrastructure of intramuscular larvae of *Trichinella spiralis* and *Trichinella pseudospiralis*. *J. Parasitol.* **67**, 685–691.

Bagheri, A., Ubelaker, J. E., Stewart, G. L., and Wood, B. (1986). Muscle fiber selectivity of *Trichinella spiralis* and *T. pseudospiralis*. *J. Parasitol.* **72**, 277–282.

Campbell, W. C. (1979). History of trichinosis; Paget, Owen and the discovery of *Trichinella spiralis*. *Bull. Hist. Med.* **53**, 520–552.

Campbell, W. C. (Ed.) (1983). *Trichinella and Trichinellosis*. Plenum, New York.

Campbell, W. C. (1988). Trichinosis revisited—Another look at modes of transmission. *Parasitol. Today* **4**, 83–86.

Childs, J. E., Glass, G. E., and Korch, G. W., Jr. (1988). The comparative epizootiology of *Capillaria hepatica* (Nematoda) in urban rodents from different habitats of Baltimore, Maryland. *Can. J. Zool.* **66**, 2769–2775.

Cooper, E. S., and Bundy, D. A. P. (1989). *Trichuris* is not trivial. *Parasitol. Today* **4**, 301–306.

Cross, J. H. (1990). Intestinal capillariasis. *Parasitol. Today* **6**, 26–28.

Despommier, D. D. (1990). *Trichinella spiralis*—The worm that would be virus. *Parasitol. Today* **6**, 193–196.

Despommier, D. D. (1993). *Trichinella spiralis* and the concept of niche. *J. Parasitol.* **79**, 472–482.

Despommier, D. E., and Muller, M. (1976). The stichosome and its secretion granules in the mature muscle larvae of *Trichinella spiralis*. *J. Parasitol.* **62**, 775–785.

Leiby, D. A., Duffy, C. H., Murrell, K. D., and Schad, G. A. (1990). *Trichinella spiralis* in an agricultural ecosystem: Transmission in the rat population. *J. Parasitol.* **76**, 360–364.

Murrell, K. D., Anderson, W. R., Schad, G. A., Hanbury, R. D., Kazacos, K. R., Gamble, H. R., and Brown, J. (1986). Field evaluation of the enzyme-linked immunosorbent assay for swine trichinosis: Efficacy of the excretory–secretory antigen. *Am. J. Vet. Res.* **47**, 1046–1049.

Pozio, E., La Rosa, G., Murrell, K. D., and Lichtenfels, J. R. (1992). Taxonomic revision of the genus *Trichinella*. *J. Parasitol.* **78**, 654–659.

Pozio, E., Varese, P., Gomez Morales, M. A., Croppo, G. P., Pelliccia, D., and Bruschi, F. (1993). Comparison of human trichinellosis caused by *Trichinella spiralis* and *Trichinella britovi*. *Am. J. Trop. Med. Hyg.* **48**, 568–575.

Reason, A. J., Ellis, L. A., Appleton, J. A., Wisnewski, N., Grieve, R. B., McNeil, M. M., Wassom, D. L., Morris, H. R., and Dell, A. (1994). Novel trevelose containing tri- and tetra-antennary N-glycans in the immunodominant antigens of the intracellular parasite *Trichinella spiralis*. *Glycobiology* **4**, 593–603.

Schad, G. A., Leiby, D. A., and Murrell, K. D. (1984). Distribution, prevalence and intensity of *Trichinella spiralis* infection in furbearing mammals of Pennsylvania. *J. Parasitol.* **70**, 372–377.

Schad, G. A., Leiby, D. A., Duffy, C. H., and Murrell, K. D. (1985). Swine trichinosis in New England slaughterhouses. *Am. J. Vet. Res.* **46**, 2008–2010.

Schad, G. A., Duffy, C. H., Leiby, D. A., Murrell, K. D., and Zirkle, E. W. (1987). *Trichinella spsiralis* in an agricultural ecosystem: Transmission under natural and experimentally modified on farm conditions. *J. Parasitol.* **73**, 95–102.

Shanta, C. S., and Meerovitch, E. (1967a). The life cycle of *Trichinella spiralis*. I. The intestinal phase of development. *Can. J. Zool.* **45**, 1255–1260.

Shanta, C. S., and Meerovitch, E. (1967b). The life cycle of *Trichinella spiralis*. II. The muscle phase of development and its possible evolution. *Can. J. Zool.* **45**, 1261–1267.

Silberstein, D. S., and Despommier, D. D. (1985). Effects of *Trichinella spiralis* on host responses to purified antigens. *Science* **227**, 948–950.

Steele, J. H., and Arumbolo, P. V., III (1975). Trichinosis: A world problem with extensive sylvatic reservoirs. *Int. J. Zoon.* **2**, 55–75.

Stewart, G. L. (1983). Pathophysiology of the muscle phase of *Trichinella* infection. In *Trichinella and Trichinosis* (W. C. Campbell, Ed.). Plenum, New York.

Wisnewski, N., McNeil, M. M., Grieve, R. B., and Wassom, D. L. (1993). Characterization of novel fucosyl- and tyveslosyl-containing glycoconjugates from *Trichinella spiralis* muscle stage larvae. *Mol. Biochem. Parasitol.* **61**, 25–36.

Williams, H. H., and Jones, A. (1976). *Marine Helminkths and Human Health*. Commonwealth Inst. of Helminthology, Commonwealth Agric. Bureau, Fanham Royal, Bucks, UK.

Yorke, W., and Maplestone, P. A. (1962). *Nematode Parasites of Vertebrates*. Hafner, New York.

PART

4

ACANTHOCEPHALA, NEMATOMORPHA, ANNELIDA, AND PENTASTOMIDA

CHAPTER

37

Acanthocephala: Spiny-Headed Worms

The phylum Acanthocephala (spiny-headed worms) is a small group of pseudocoelomate endoparasites with a number of unique structural and biological features. A few members are important economically and medically; however, they are commonly found as parasites of the intestinal tracts of fish, reptiles, birds, and, less often, mammals in the wild. There are only scattered reports of the effects of Acanthocephala on populations of nondomesticated animals. Transmission of these worms depends on the food chain. Behavior of intermediate hosts of acanthocephalans is often altered to make them more likely to be eaten by the definitive host.

A prominent characteristic of the phylum, from which it receives its name, is a protrusible proboscis that is armed with recurved hooks (Fig. 37.1) by which the worm attaches to the wall of the intestine of the definitive host (Fig. 37.2). Hooks and spines are also present on other parts of the body: around the anterior part and the genital openings. The anterior part of the body is divided into the *presoma*, comprising the *proboscis* and the unarmed *neck*; the trunk or body contains the rest of the organs. Sexes are separate; there is no larval reproduction, such as occurs in the digenetic trematodes. There is no digestive tract, and all food is absorbed through the surface of the body. The internal organs lie in a body cavity, the pseudocoelom. Because of their many peculiarities, the Acanthocephala have been a puzzle for taxonomists since the first descriptions were given early in the 18th century. Hyman's (1951) review of the various taxa in which they have been placed is instructive and shows why there have been disagreements. Hyman had originally placed the Acanthocephala in the Aschelminthes in the first volume of her series on the invertebrates, but she later reconsidered and gave them phylum status because both their embryogenesis and adult structures did not allow them to be allied with any other group. It is said that she had planned to include the Acanthocephala in the Aschelminthes rather by default, but that Dr. Harley J. Van Cleave dissuaded her because he felt that phylum status was justified for the animals he had studied for so many years.

The fact that the Acanthocephala have no digestive tract has made the tegument of interest to many investigators. Light microscopic (LM) studies gave some information, but the advent of thin-sectioning techniques for transmission electron microscopy (TEM) revealed structures that had only been vaguely described. As in the tapeworms and digenetic trematodes, the tegument is a syncytium, that is, a multinucleate structure in which there are no cell membranes; however, unlike the flatworms, which have microvilli and microtriches, the Acanthocephala have pores that extend into the tegument (Fig. 37.3). It has been calculated that the pores increase the surface area as much as 44 times over that of a flat surface. The pores extend into the hypodermis, branch repeatedly, and end blindly. The tegument has a secreted glycocalyx, sometimes called an *epicuticle*, then deeper are the striped, felt and radial layers. Also in the tegument is the fluid-filled *lacunar system* (Fig. 37.4), which apparently serves as a circulatory system as well as a hydraulic system; the pattern of the lacunar system is used to separate the members of the phylum into classes. The *rete system* (Fig. 37.5) is a series of thin-walled tubes on the surface of longitudinal or longitudinal and circular muscles. It is not connected to the lacunar system. Even though it sits

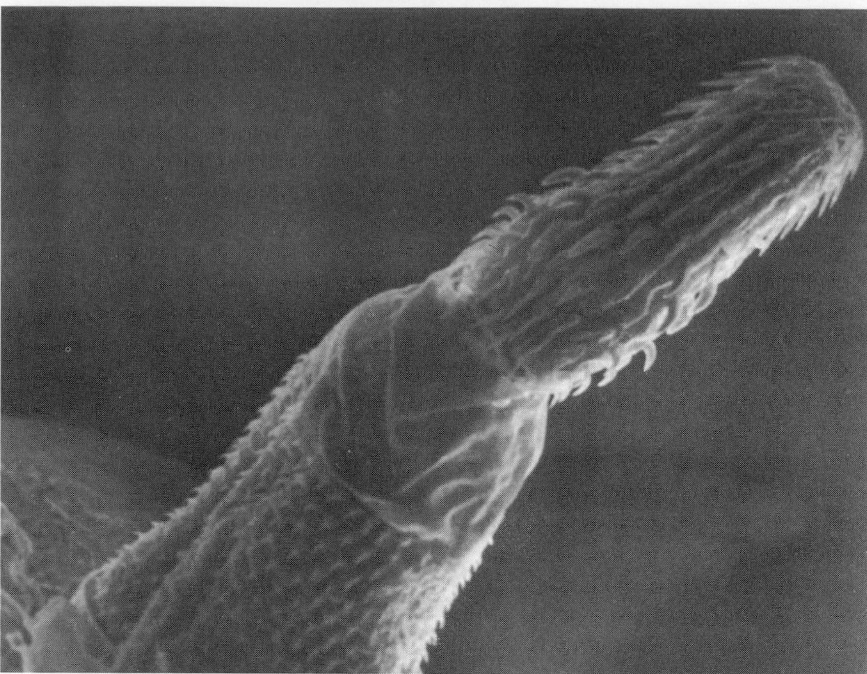

FIGURE 37.1 The proboscis of an acanthocephalan as seen in SEM.

on the surface of muscles, this system apparently is involved in electrical polarization-depolarization, similar to that seen in sarcoplasmic reticulum of "higher" animals.

Protonephridia (flame cells) containing multiple cilia have only been reported in the Family Oligoacanthorhynchidae of the Class Archiacanthocephala. Knowledge here is still fragmentary.

The sexes are separate; usually females are larger than males. Other than the tegument and proboscis, acanthocephalans are largely given over to the reproductive system. In both males and females the reproductive organs are attached to a ligament that extends from the base of the proboscis receptacle to the posterior end of the body. Usually the ligament is composed of two *ligament sacs*; in some males only one sac develops; in females both sacs often rupture as ova develop. The males have two testes, sperm ducts, and cement glands (Fig. 37.6). The cement glands produce a proteinaceous secretion that forms a fertilization or copulatory cap in the vulva of the female; the cap probably prevent additional fertilization. Males have a posterior, reversible copulatory bursa, with which they grasp the female, and a penis to facilitate transfer of sperm.

Initially, the ovary of the female is attached to the ligament, but as she matures, the ovary breaks up into a number of ovarian balls that float free in the ligament sacs. The uterine bell, which serves as an egg-sorting mechanism, is located at the posterior end of the body (Fig. 37.7); immature eggs pass into the bell and then back to the body cavity, and mature eggs pass out of the genital pore. Females that have been mated frequently have a characteristic constriction where they were clasped by a male; the copulatory cap in the vulva of the female dissolves before the release of ova (Fig. 37.8).

Early in embryonation, between the 4- and 32-cell stages, an acanthocephalan becomes syncytial; this pattern is similar to that of members of the Aschelminthes. Nuclei continue to divide and sometimes become so large that they are referred to as giant nuclei. The ova passed from the female contain a developing larva called an acanthor (Fig. 37.9). When fully developed, the acanthor has bladelike hooks at its anterior end, the aclid organ or rostellum. An ovum containing one acanthor develops into an acanthella when ingested by the proper intermediate host. The acanthor penetrates the gut of the host and develops to the acanthella in the hemocoel. The features of the adult worm are apparent in the acanthella, but the reproductive system is immature. The acanthella becomes infective for the definitive host when it has been encapsulated as a cystacanth, that is, surrounded by a hyaline envelope produced by host cells. Cystacanths can be ingested and remain alive in transport or paratenic hosts. The cystacanth is released in the gut of the definitive host, attaches to the gut wall, and matures sexually.

The physiology of the Acanthocephala has not been studied extensively, but some studies give information

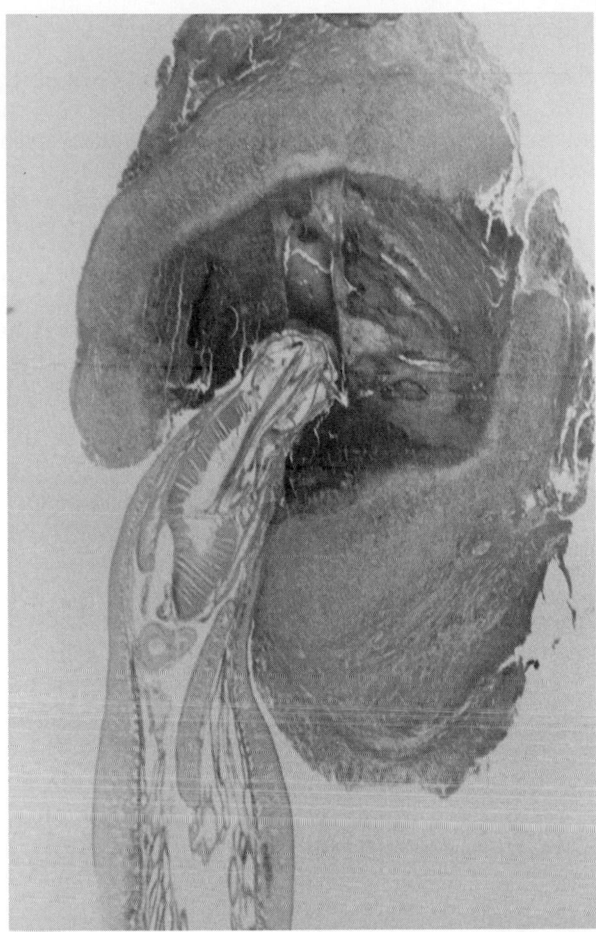

FIGURE 37.2 A histologic section of swine intestine with the proboscis of *Macranthorhynchus hirudinaceus* embedded in it. Note the large dark area indicating hemorrhage around the proboscis.

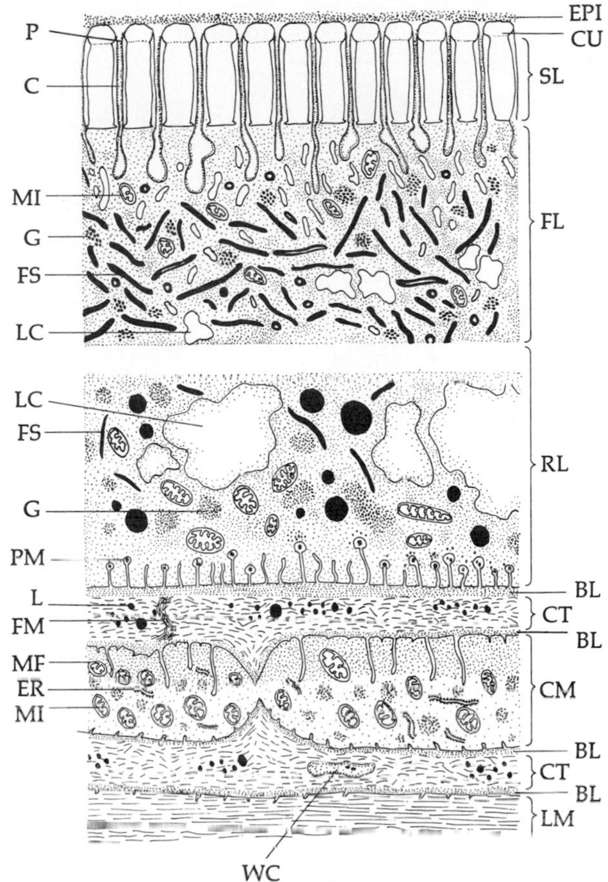

FIGURE 37.3 Diagram of the body wall of an acanthocephalan. Abbreviations: BL basal lamella; C canal; CM circular muscle; CT connective tissue; CU cuticle; EPI epicuticle; ER endoplasmic reticulum; FL felt layer; FM fibers attaching muscles to the body wall; FS fibrous strands; G glycogen; L lipid; LC lacunar canal; LM longitudinal muscle; MI mitochondrion; MY myofilaments. P pore; PM plasma membrane; RL radial layer; SL striped layer; WC wandering cell. [From Cheng, T. C.]

on the way in which they interact with the host. For example, if the intestine of a host is infected with an acanthocephalan, it appears at first that the worms embed in the gut and remain attached at that spot; however, they do move periodically, one of the influences being other parasites in the gut. The proboscis and the neck are hollow and fluid filled. The proboscis can be both everted and withdrawn into the body by a combination of muscular movement and hydraulics. The proboscis is pushed into the wall of the intestine so that the hooks catch; then the neck retractor muscles force fluid out of two lateral sacs, the *lemnisci*, into the lacunar system of the proboscis, causing it to expand, thus firmly anchoring the worm (Fig. 37.10).

As is true of the tapeworms, acanthocephalans obtain all of their nutrient by absorption across the body surface; the digenetic flukes also obtain a significant portion of their food in the same means despite having an intestine. Substances are picked up at specific sites on the surface of the worm and transported to the interior. Amino acids are absorbed at the surface of the body after being enzymatically released from protein. Sugars are absorbed at two or more sites and then energy is obtained by glycolysis.

Name of Organism and Disease Associations

Macracanthorhynchus hirudinaceus is an intestinal parasite.

Hosts and Host Range

Swine, occasionally humans, and a variety of other animals such as wild pigs, cattle, monkeys, dogs, rodents, and moles are the hosts.

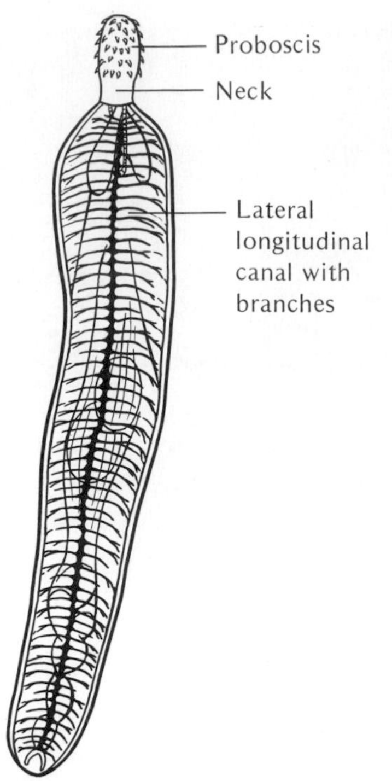

FIGURE 37.4 Diagram of the lacunar system of *Acanthocephalus ranae.*

Geographic Distribution and Importance

The organism is cosmopolitan in pigs. Although serious intestinal pathology and even death may occur, mild infections causing few lesions and little or no economic loss are typical.

Morphology

Females may exceed 35 cm in length; males are about 10 cm long. In life, the worms are usually rather flattened and wrinkled; their large size makes them appear, at first glance, like the large hog ascarid. The proboscis is small and bears only five or six rows of hooks. The eggs are brownish with a sculptured shell and 80 to 100 by 45 to 60 μm (Fig. 37.11).

Life Cycle

The adult worms are attached to the wall of the small intestine; eggs containing acanthors are passed in the feces and are infective when passed. Intermediate hosts are a number of species of beetle larvae including "June bugs," *Phyllophaga* spp. The acanthor migrates through the gut wall into the hemocoel and develops into an acanthella. By 60 to 95 days after infection, the acanthella develops into a cystacanth. When eaten by

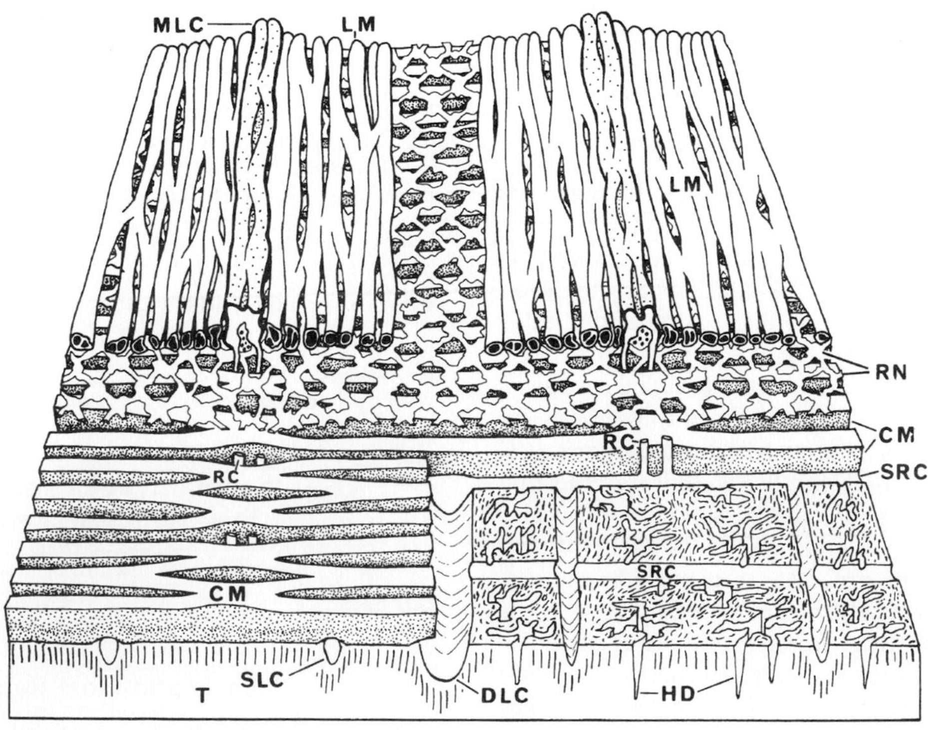

FIGURE 37.5 Diagram of the body wall of *Oligoacanthorhynchus tortuosa.* The rete network (RN) is located between circular (CM) and longitudinal (LM) muscles. Abbreviations: DLC dorsal lacunar channel; hypodermal ducts; MLC median longitudinal channels; RC radial channels; VLC ventral lacunar channels. [From Miller, D. M., and Dunagan, T. T., 1978.]

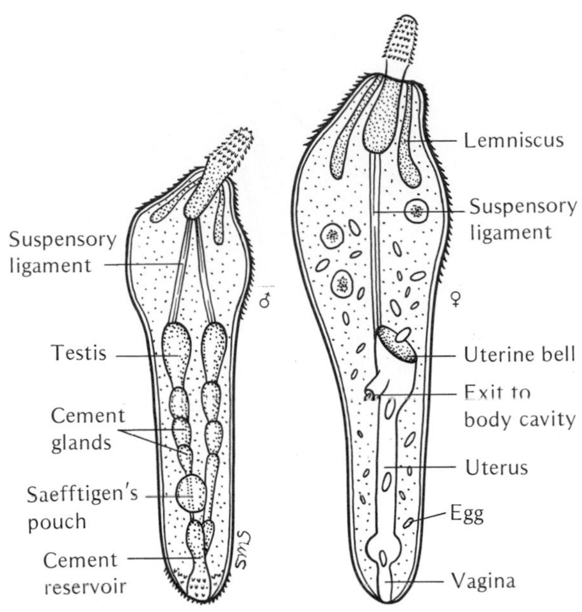

FIGURE 37.6 Diagram of the reproductive systems of a male and female *Corynosoma* sp.

a definitive host, it is released in the small intestine, attaches, and develops to sexual maturity in two to three months.

Diagnosis

Finding the characteristic eggs in the feces is the means of diagnosis; worms may also be found in the feces after successful drug treatment.

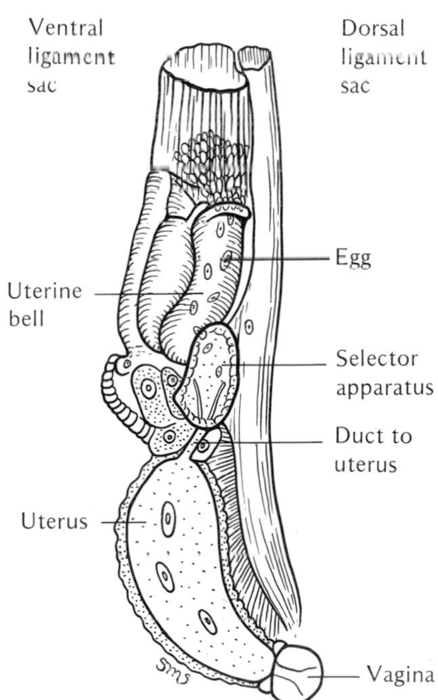

FIGURE 37.7 Diagram of the uterine bell of an acanthocephalan.

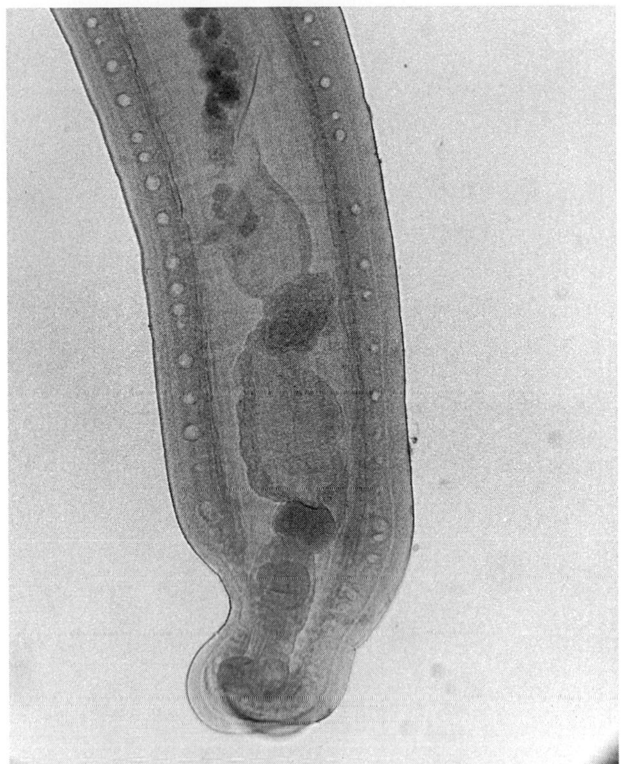

FIGURE 37.8 Female acanthocephalan that had been mated; there is a characteristic constriction at the posterior portion of the body where she had been clasped by the male.

Host–Parasite Interactions

Most infections produce no clinical signs; however, weight loss, diarrhea, and abdominal pain may occur in heavy infections. Usually, there is an inflammatory response where the proboscis is embedded in the gut (Fig. 37.2). If the gut wall is perforated, bacteria may leak into the abdominal cavity and cause peritonitis.

Epidemiology and Control

Options for control of *M. hirudinaceus* are minimal. The hardiness of the eggs and the fact that there is an intermediate host in the life cycle make control of infection in swine rather difficult. The eggs remain infective in soil for up to 3-1/2 years in Maryland; they tolerate both desiccation and temperatures below −18°C (0°F). A female worm may produce more than 250,000 eggs per day, so even a moderate infection can lead to heavy contamination of pastures or hog lots. Beetle control has not been successful in controlling infections. Humans become infected by eating infected beetle grubs. One would think that avoiding infection would be simple.

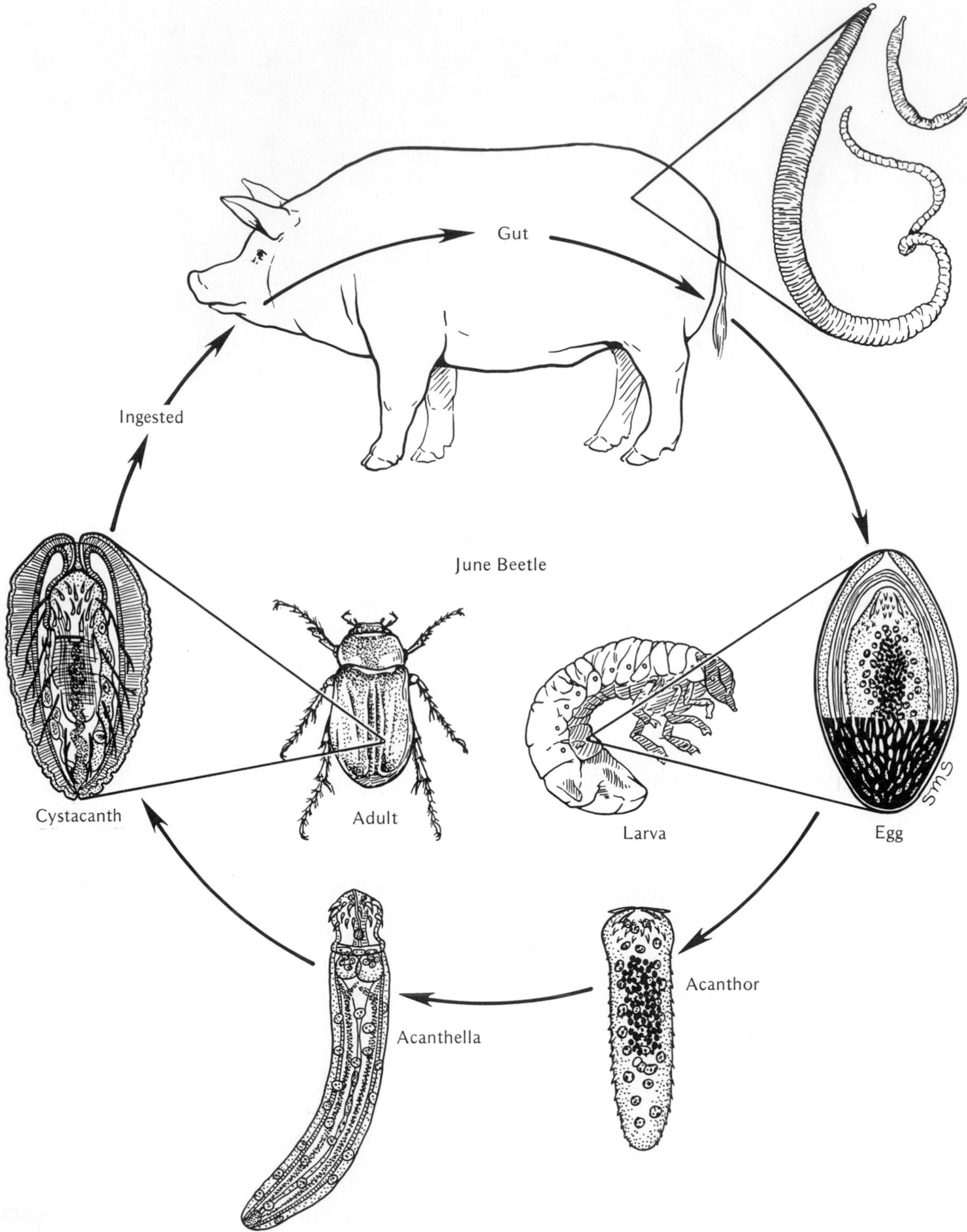

FIGURE 37.9 Diagram of the life cycle of *Macracanthorhynchus hirudinaceus.*

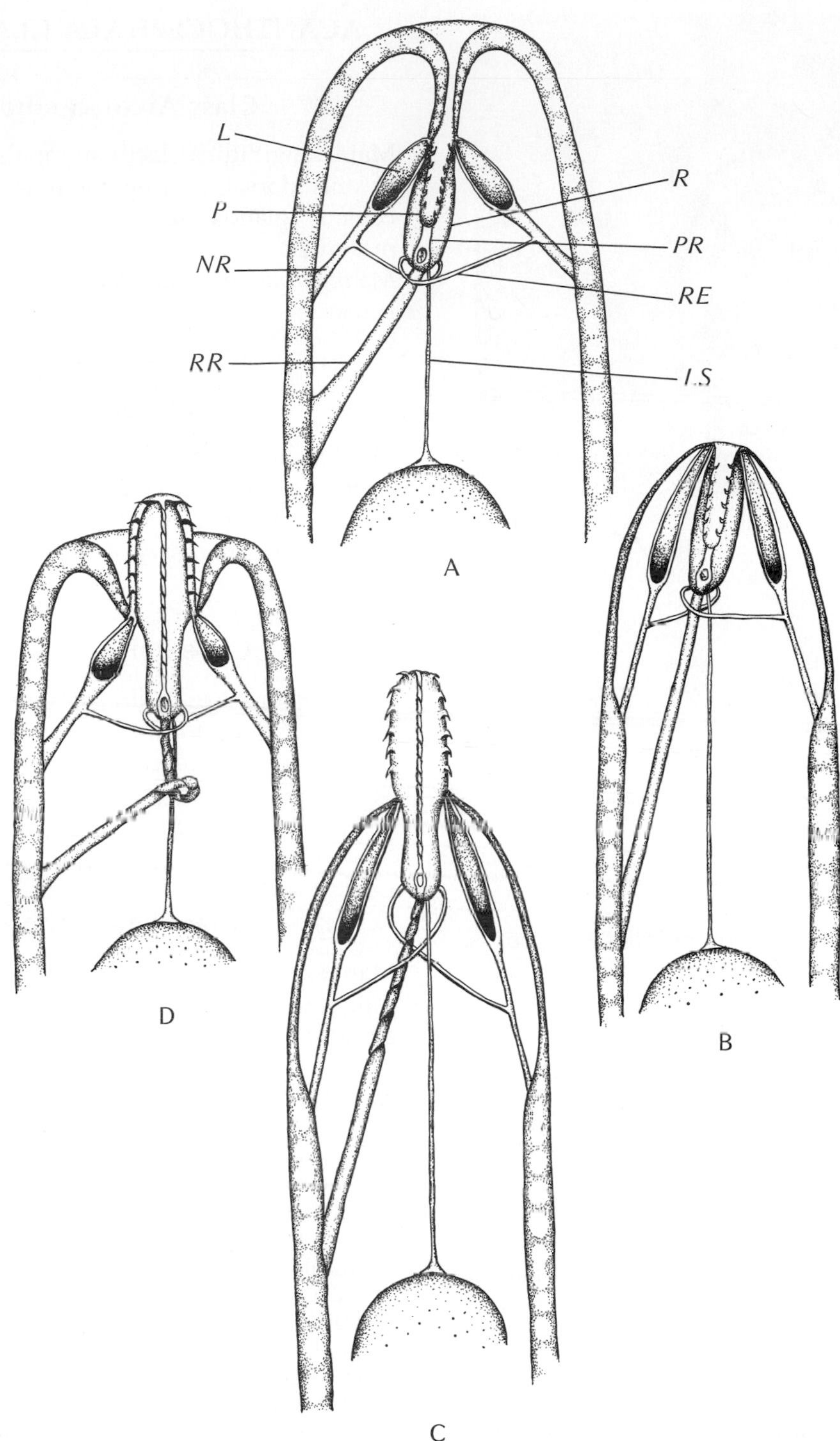

FIGURE 37.10 Diagram of the mechanism of eversion of the proboscis of an acanthocephalan. The sequence of the process is as follows: (A) proboscis withdrawn; (B) trunk extended and proboscis withdrawn; (C) trunk extended, proboscis beginning to be everted; (D) proboscis everted, neck muscles contracted. Abbreviations: L—lemniscus; LS—ligament sac; NR—neck retractor muscles; P—proboscis; PR—proboscis retractor muscles; r—receptacle; RR—receptacle retractor muscles. [Redrawn with modifications from Hammond, 1966. The Company of Biologists.]

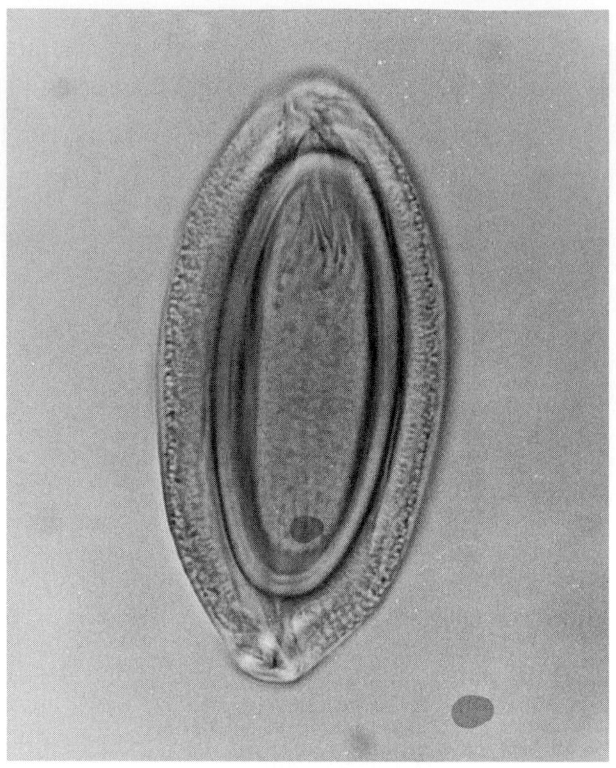

FIGURE 37.11 Egg of *Macracanthorhynchus hirudinaceus* contaning an acanthor larva as seen in LM.

Treatment with modern anthelmintics such as the macrolide antibiotics may be effective.

Other Acanthocephalan Infections

Humans have been reported to be infected with *Acanthocephalus bufonis, A. rauschi, Bolbosoma sp., Corynosoma stromosum*, and *Moniliformis moniliformis*, in addition to *Macracanthorhynchus hirudinaceus*. Intermediate hosts for *Acanthocephalus* and *Corynosoma* are crustaceans, and cockroaches serve for *Moniliformis*. Juvenile *Bolbosoma* were found in fish and sashimi. These foods pose a risk for both anisakosis and acanthocephalosis.

In Texas, dogs and coyotes are infected with *Oncicola canis*, a species that can produce serious disease. Infection probably occurs by eating armadillo (*Dasypus novencinctus*), the transport host; the intermediate host is not known.

Prosthenorchis elegans sometimes becomes a problem in caged primates; the intermediate hosts are cockroaches. A cycle can be established under conditions in which cockroach control is difficult. Infections build up in monkeys; sometimes the proboscis penetrates the gut wall, allowing bacterial peritonitis to develop.

ACANTHOCEPHALA CLASSIFICATION

Class Archiacanthocephala

Main longitudinal lacunar canals dorsal and ventral or only dorsal; two ligament sacs persist in females; cement glands separate. Parasites of birds and mammals.
Moniliformis moniliformis, Macracanthorhynchus hirudinaceus

Class Palaeacanthocephala

Main lacunar canals lateral; single ligament sac in females degenerates; cement glands separate. Parasites of fish, amphibia, reptiles, birds, and mammals.
Corynosoma stromosum, Acanthocephalus

Class Polyacanthocephala

Main lacunar canals dorsal and ventral, double ligament sacs persist in females, cement glands multiple, proboscis with longitudinal rows of hooks. Parasites of fish and crocodillians.
Polyacanthorhynchus

Class Eoacanthocephala

Main longitudinal lacunar canals both dorsal and ventral; two persistent ligament sacs in females; cement gland single, proboscis with radial rows of hooks. Parasites of fish, amphibia, and reptiles.
Neoechinorhynchus emydis

Readings

Amin, O. M. (1987). Key to the families and subfamilies of Acanthocephala, with the erection of a new class (Polyacanthocephala) and a new order (Polyacanthorhynchida). *J. Parasitol.* **73,** 1216–1219.

Cheng, T. C. (1973). *Parasitology*. Academic Press, New York.

Crompton, D. W. T. (1970). *An Ecological Approach to Acanthocephalan Physiology*. Cambridge Univ. Press, Cambridge, UK.

Crompton, D. W. T., and Nickol, B. B. (Eds.) (1985). *Biology of the Acanthocephala*. Cambridge Univ. Press, Cambridge, UK.

Gotelli, N. J., and Moore, J. (1992). Altered host behavior in a cockroach–acanthocephalan association. *Anim. Behav.* **43,** 949–959.

Hammond, R. A. (1966). The proboscis mechanism of *Acanthocephala ranae*. *J. Exp. Biol.* **45,** 203–213.

Hammond, R. A. (1967). The mode of attachment within the host of *Acanthocephala ranae* (Shrank, 1788) Luehe, 1911. *J. Helminthol.* **41,** 321–328.

Holmes, J. C. (1973). Site selection by parasitic helminths: Interspecific interactions, site segregation and their importance to the development of helminth communities. *Can. J. Zool.* **51,** 333–347.

Hyman, L. H. (1951). *The Invertebrates Vol. 111. Acanthocephala, Aschelminthes and Ectoprocta*, pp. 1–52. McGraw-Hill, New York.

Miller, D. M., and Dunagan, T. T. (1978). Organization of the lacunar system in the acanthocephalan, *Oligoacanthorhynchus tortuosa. J. Parasitol.* **64,** *436–439.*

Moore, J. (1984). Parasites that change the behavior of their hosts. Sci. Am. **250,** *108–115.*

Neafie, R. C., and Marty, A. M. (1993). Unusual infections in humans. Clin. Microbiol. Rev. **6,** 34–56.

Nicholas, W. L. (1967). The biology of the Acanthocephala. *Adv. Parasitol.* **5,** 205–246.

Nicholas, W. L. (1973). The biology of the Acanthocephala. *Adv. Parasitol.* **11,** 671–706.

Parshad, V. R., and Crompton, D. W. T. (1981). Aspects of acanthocephalan reproduction. *Adv. Parasitol.* **19,** 73–138.

Whitfield, P. J. (1970). The egg sorting function of the uterine bell of *Polymorphus minutus* (Acanthocephala). *Parasitology* **61,** 111–126.

Yamaguti, S. (1963). *Systema Helminthum. Vol. 5. Acanthocephala.* Wiley-Interscience, New York.

CHAPTER

38

Phylum Nematomorpha: Horsehair Worms

The phylum Nematomorpha (thread form) is a small group of about 230 species of long, slender worms that superficially resemble nematodes. The long-believed myth was that these worms had transformed from horse hairs that had fallen into water, hence the common name. Also, because the free-living adults often become entangled with one another, they are sometimes called Gordiacea, gordian worms, or gordiids after the mythical Gordian knot.

The adults are free-living in fresh water or moist soil; one genus, *Nectonema*, is pelagic in marine environments as an adult and parasitic in hermit crabs and true crabs as a larva. The larvae of all other nematomorphs are endoparasites of arthropods, especially grasshoppers, crickets, and terrestrial beetles, and sometimes of leeches.

Geographic Distribution and Importance

Horsehair worms are found worldwide in temperate and tropical freshwater habitats; they have been found recently as far north as the Arctic Circle. Except for rare, accidental infections in humans or other mammals, they are of no medical or economic importance.

Morphology

The adult worms are quite slender, with diameters from 0.3 to 2.5 mm and lengths of sometimes 1 m, although most are perhaps 20 cm long. The sexes are separate; the males are shorter than females, except in the genus *Nectonema*, in which the males are longer. Their colors range from gray to black. The anterior end or calotte is usually white with a dark ring at its posterior limit. There is a terminal or subterminal mouth. Both sexes have a cloaca, and the posterior end is lobed in some species. Horsehair worms have a cuticle similar to that of the nematodes (Fig. 38.1) and have characteristic areoles that are contiguous, rounded, or polygonal areas often projecting above the cuticular surface as papillae with bristles or pores (Fig. 38.2); their function is unknown.

Nematomorphs have no excretory, circulatory, or respiratory structures. They are pseudocoelomate, but the body cavity is filled with parenchyma in most freshwater species, with only limited space remaining. Only the marine form, *Nectonema*, has a complete pseudocoelom. The digestive tract is degenerate and apparently without function. The mode of nutrition is unknown; some authors say that food is not ingested at any time during the life cycle, and others state that nutrients must be absorbed through the cuticle. The nervous system consists of an anterior nerve ring and a ventral nerve cord; little is known about specialized sensory structures.

In freshwater forms, the gonads are paired tubular organs that fill most of the pseudocoelom in mature worms. The ovaries are unique in that they transform into uteri by developing lateral diverticuli after producing the eggs. Sperm are rod shaped and apparently nonmotile. In *Nectonema* the gonads are single.

Life Cycle

In temperate climates, the worms escape from the host in the fall and remain near water until the following spring. A male swims to a female, coils the posterior end of its body around the female, and deposits sperm

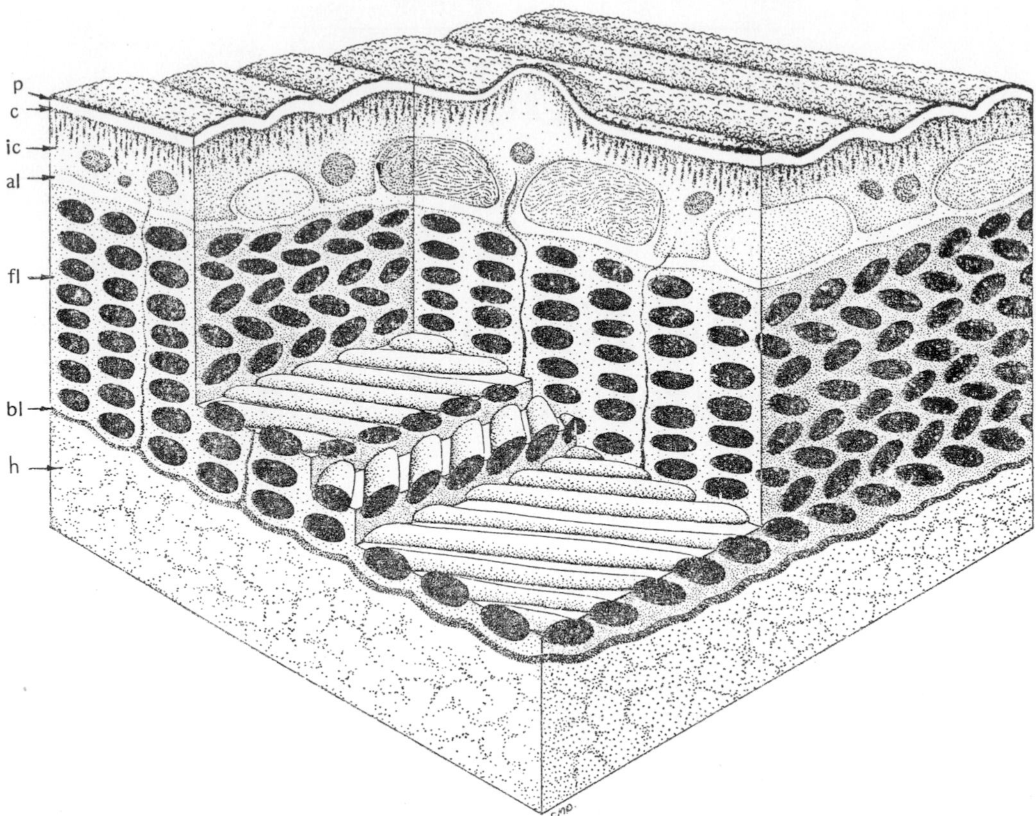

FIGURE 38.1 Diagram of the cuticle of *Paragordius varius*. Abbreviations: alalveolar layer; bl—basal layer; ec—external cortical layer; ep—ependymal layer; fl—fibrillar layer; h—hypodermis; ic—internal cortical layer. [From Zapatosky, J., 1971.]

in her cloaca. Fertilization apparently takes place inside the body of the female just before she extrudes the eggs in long, gelatinous strings. Embryonation requires 15 to 80 days. After hatching, the larvae (Fig. 38.3) either penetrate an arthropod host or, more likely, encyst on a substrate such as vegetation near the shoreline. Arthropods ingest the larvae along with the vegetation. The larvae encyst in the gut and then later burrow into the hemocoel and develop into adults. In transport hosts, including certain insects, snails, and fish, cyst walls are digested in the gut, but the freed larvae encyst again until ingested by a suitable host. After developing for two weeks to several months, young adults break through the exoskeleton of the arthropod (Fig. 38.4) and become free living. They survive only if they reach moist soil or water. Evidence shows that when the worms have reached their maximum size, the host becomes thirsty and dies near water, thereby releasing the worms in the environment they require. The worms typically emerge in late summer or fall.

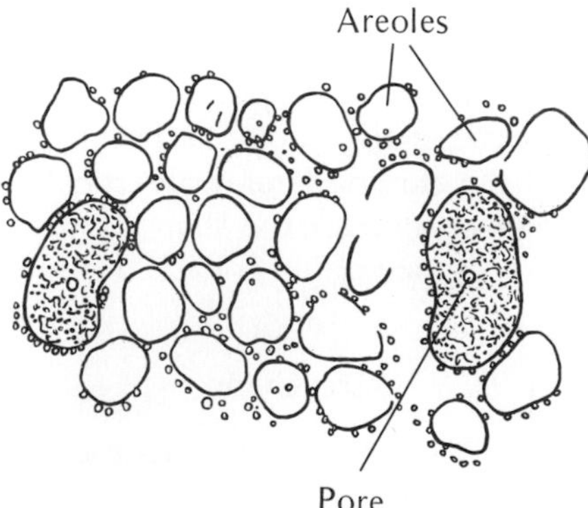

FIGURE 38.2 Diagram of the areoles of *Parachordodes*. [Redrawn with modifications from Hyman, L., 1951.]

NOTABLE FEATURES

Occasional human infections with horsehair worms have been reported. Most have been found when the worms were vomited or passed in the feces, but no serious illness has been associated with them. In one

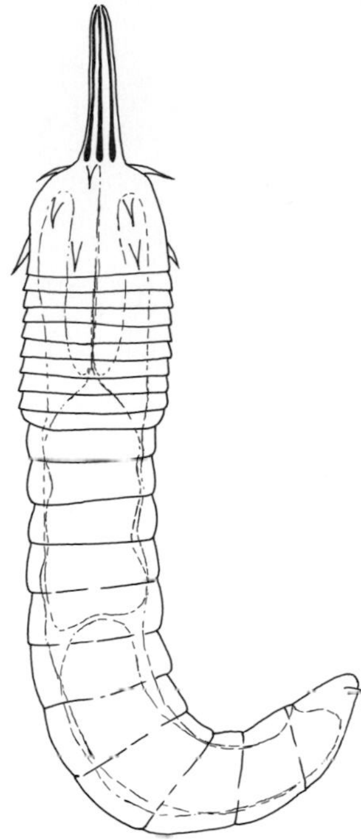

FIGURE 38.3 Diagram of a nematomorphan larva. [Redrawn from Pennak, R. W., 1989.]

case, an abscess in the orbit of the eye was associated with an infection with *Gordius robustus*. In another instance, *Paragorodius esavianus* was expelled from the urethra of a 23-year old woman with a history of urinary tract problems extending over three years. In both of these cases, it seems likely that infection was acquired while swimming. The rarity of human infection indicates that these worms are unlikely to become a widespread problem.

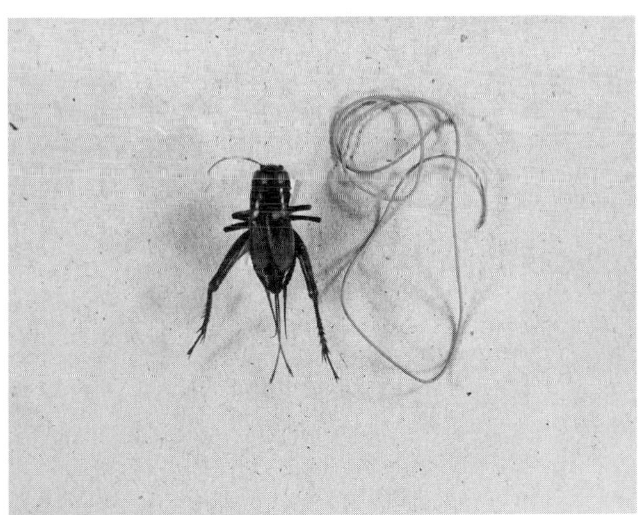

FIGURE 38.4 Young adult nematomorphans breaking out of a cricket.

At one time or another, nearly every parasitologist has had to deal with an excited parent carrying a bottle containing a horsehair worm and stating that his or her child had passed it. The conversation usually reveals that the worm was found in the toilet. In these cases, the source is most likely a cricket that sought water and died about the time it released the worm.

CLASSIFICATION: PHYLUM NEMATOMORPHA

Order Nectonematoidea

Pseudocoel open; both dorsal and ventral epidermal chords present; gonads single; marine. A single genus.
Nectonema

Order Gordioidea

Pseudocoel filled with parenchyma; only ventral epidermal chord present; gonads paired; freshwater and terrestrial.
Gordius, Paragordius

Readings

Burger, R. (1972). *Paragordius esavianus* passed per urethra. *J. Urol.* **108,** 469.

Donin, C. L. L., and Cotelli, F. (1977). The rod-shaped sperm of Gordioidea (Aschelminthes, Nematomorpha). *J. Ultrastruct. Res.* **61,** 193–200.

Hyman, L. H. (1951). *The Invertebrates: Acanthocephala, Aschelminthes, and Entoprocta. The Pseudocoelomate Bilateria.* McGraw–Hill, New York.

Pennak, R. W. (1989). *Freshwater Invertebrates of the United States,* 3rd ed. Wiley, New York.

Poinar, G. O., Jr. (1991). Nematoda and Nematomorpha. In *Ecology and Classification of North American Freshwater Invertebrates* (J. H. Thorpe and A. P. Covich, Eds.). Academic Press, New York.

Poinar, G. O., and Doelman, J. J. (1974). A reexamination of *Neochordodes occidentalis* (Mont.) comb. n. (Chordididae: Gordioidea): Larval penetration and defense reaction in *Culex pipiens* L. *J. Parasitol.* **60,** 327–335.

Sayad, W. Y., Johnson, V. M., and Faust, E. C. (1936). Human parasitization with *Gordius robustus*. *J. Am. Med. Assoc.* **106,** 461–462.

Zapotosky, J. E. (1971). The cuticular ultrastructure of *Paragordius varius* (Leidy, 1851) (Gordioidea: Chordodidae). *Proc. Helminthol. Soc. Washington* **38,** 228–236.

CHAPTER

39

Annelida

The phylum Annelida is composed of segmented worms, including the familiar earthworms or night crawlers. We see a few annelids in garden soil or on our lawns after a rain, but vast numbers are present as marine benthos. About 15,000 species have been described; most are free living, but there are examples of all types of symbioses, including parasitism.

Metamerism, the division of the body into similar segments or *metameres*, is characteristic of this phylum. Organs such as nephridia are present in most metameres. Annelids have a true coelom, closed circulatory system, complete digestive system, and chitinous setae often present on fleshy appendages called *parapodia*. They respire through the integument or the gills.

Most taxonomists accept two classes in the phylum Annelida: Polychaeta and Clitellata. In addition, three other groups have uncertain affinities. The enigmatic Archiannelida are sometimes placed in a separate phylum or class or are included in the class Polychaeta. No archiannelids are known to be parasitic. The branchiobdellids and acanthobdellids, which have parasitic species, are regarded by most systematists as primitive leeches and are included in the subclass Hirudinea.

CLASS POLYCHAETA

Polychaetes have paired appendages, parapods, which bear setae; they are used for locomotion and often for respiration. Parasitism is not common in the class Polychaeta, but there are examples of both ecto- and endoparasites. The ectoparasites are more modified for the parasitic lifestyle than are the endoparasites. One example is *Ichthyotomus sanguinarius*, which attaches to the fins of eels by means of protrusible stylets (Fig. 39.1). It has modifications for blood feeding including piercing stylets, an anticoagulant secretion, a sucking pharynx, and an enlarged gut extending into the parapods for storing large quantities of host blood. *Ichthyotomus* is a neotenic worm; except for the mature gonads, it resembles annelid larvae more than adults.

Endoparasitic polychaetes have surprisingly few modifications for parasitism, perhaps because they have only recently become parasites. Little is known about these organisms, most come from single reports.

CLASS CLITELLATA

Subclass Oligochaeta

Oligochaetes have no parapodia, but have well developed metamerism. Like the polychaetes, few oligochaetes are true parasites, and none are of medical or economic importance except for the few that are intermediate hosts for lungworms (Chapter 31). Members of the genus *Chaetogaster* (Fig. 39.2) are usually epicommensals or epiphoronts on freshwater mollusks, but some are true parasites. It is interesting to note that *Chaetogaster* eats both miracidia and cercaria. This should be detrimental to the reproductive success of the parasitic digenetic trematodes infecting the snail and thus advantageous to both the annelid and its host snail. This annelid is an example of the complete gamut of symbiotic relationships: (1) commensalism—the annelid eats detritus generated by the snail's feeding activities; (2) mutualism—the snail provides shelter and

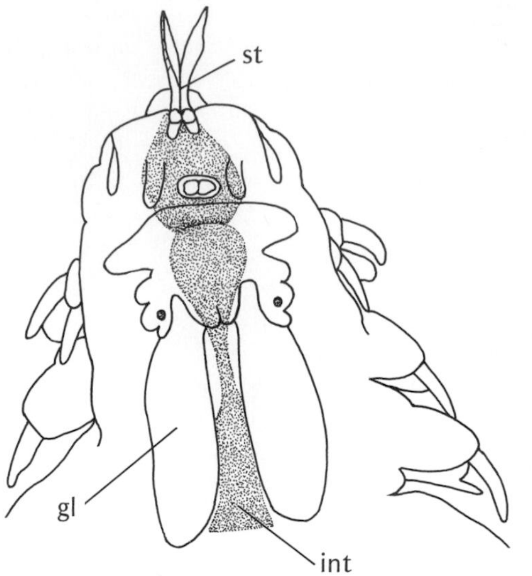

FIGURE 39.1 Diagram of the anterior end of *Ichthyotomus sanguinarius.* Abbreviations: gl—glands; st—stylets. [Redrawn from Baer, J. G., 1951.]

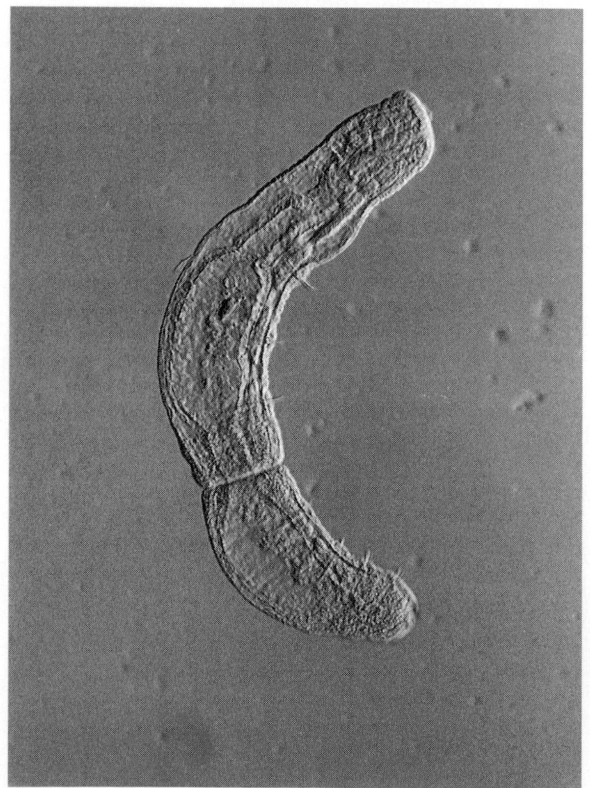

FIGURE 39.2 *Chaetogaster,* a small annelid as seen in the interference microscope.

the annelid reduces the number of digenetic trematodes infecting the snail; and (3) true parasitism—the annelid feeds on snail tissues.

Subclass Hirudinea

The subclass Hirudinea contains about 500 species of marine, freshwater, and terrestrial leeches. Only about 25% are parasitic, despite the notion that all leeches are bloodsuckers. Most leeches are predators or scavengers. Those that are true parasites are usually temporary; they abandon their hosts after engorgement with blood or tissue fluids. In Europe, North Africa, North America, and the Near East, leeches were used for bloodletting to cure headaches and a number of diseases. The early Greek and Roman medical writers provide detailed instructions on the techniques of bloodletting using leeches. In early Chinese medicine, ground-up leeches were used as a treatment for internal hemorrhaging. Probably this was done because it was thought that if living leeches could remove blood as ectoparasites, their powder should be helpful in removing internal blood; there is no scientific basis for this conclusion.

Leeches differ from other annelids in having (1) a well-developed posterior sucker and an anterior sucker or suckerlike depression; (2) a constant number of body segments, 34 in most leeches, 30 in acanthobdellids, and 14 or 15 in branchiobdellids; (3) no setae or parapodia except in acanthobdellids; and (4) a reduced coelom largely filled with muscle and connective tissue.

Name of Organism and Disease Associations

Hirudo medicinalis is the medicinal leech.

Hosts and Host Range

The medicinal leech is an ectoparasite that feeds on the blood of mammals, frogs, tadpoles, and small fish.

Geographic Distribution and Importance

This leech is native to Europe and Asia and has been imported into the United States. It was raised extensively for medicinal purposes in Europe and the United States, but that use has drastically declined in the past hundred years. However, anticoagulant proteins derived from leeches are used in treating patients with various vascular disorders.

Recently there has been a resurgence in the use of leeches, especially in microsurgery. When a finger is reattached, arteries can be joined, but veins are much more difficult to reattach. As a consequence, fluid accumulates and cannot be adequately drained. The medicinal leech can remove excess fluid and keep blood flowing by injecting the anticoagulant hirudin. Eventually the veins will reatttach by themselves and the leeches are no longer needed.

Morphology

A mature medicinal leech can extend to 12 cm long by 1.5 cm wide. The body has 102 annuli or external folds, not counting the posterior sucker. These annuli do not correspond to the 34 segments or metameres characteristic of most leeches; there may be one to five annuli per segment (Fig. 39.3A). The 34 segments are present in embryonic development; in the adult they are recognized as paired nerve ganglia, except for the seven that have fused into the large posterior sucker. The anterior sucker is a compression of segments I through IV on the ventral surface. Even though each annulus has sense organs, they are difficult to see, as are the five pairs of eyes on segments I through V.

The medicinal leech has a complete digestive tract. Inside the buccal cavity are three jaws (Fig. 39.3B) which make a Y-shaped incision in the skin of the host. Posterior to the buccal cavity is the muscular pharynx that pumps blood into the largest part of the digestive tract, the crop. It has 11 pairs of lateral branches and can store large quantities of blood. Following the crop is a thin-walled intestine and then a rectum leading to the terminal anus.

Hirudo is a hermaphrodite. The gonads are in the anterior part of the body (Fig. 39.3C). Ova are fertilized by sperm from another leech, coated with albumin in the oviduct, and passed through the female gonopore into a cocoon secreted by the clitellum. The leech then slips the cocoon containing developing eggs over its head.

The excretory system is composed of 17 pairs of nephridia. The circulatory system has no distinct blood vessels; instead, there are six blood sinuses. The two lateral sinuses have muscular walls and function as hearts to circulate the blood.

Life Cycle

There is an annual life cycle. Leeches mate in the spring; eggs in cocoons are deposited in damp soil. Young leeches develop and mate in the spring of the following year.

Other Human and Animal Leeches

In North America, *Macrobdella* and *Philobdella* are the only common leeches that regularly take human blood. Like the medicinal leech, they firmly attach by their oral suckers and move their jaws back and forth to make painless incisions in the host skin. They then secrete a small amount of an anticoagulant, hirudin, which remains in host tissues. Bloodsucking leeches feed infrequently, but take an enormous amount of blood when they do feed. They normally take two to ten times their own body weight and need feed only twice a year. They secrete only exopeptidases and need the help of gut bacteria such as *Pseudomonas hirudinicola* to aid digestion.

Members of the terrestrial genus *Haemadipsa* are important parasites of humans and domestic animals throughout tropical and- temperate regions in Asia and the Far East. A number of other aquatic and terrestrial leeches attach to almost any mammal.

A potentially serious problem is *internal hirudiniasis*, caused by the accidental ingestion of aquatic leeches of the genus *Limnatis*, commonly known as the horse leech. They are common in fresh water in Europe, northern Africa, and Asia. There are numerous case reports of horse and human upper respiratory tract infections and an occasional upper digestive tract infection. Many infections self-cure, but occasionally severe blood loss and secondary infections result, sometimes leading to death.

Fishes are often parasitized by leeches belonging to the family Piscicolidae, but species of *Actinobdella* and *Placobdella* are also found on fishes. The amount of injury is related to the number of parasites present and the amount of blood removed.

Leeches are also vectors for protozoa such as *Trypanosoma, Cryptobia,* and *Haemogregarina* and are intermediate or final hosts for some digenetic trematodes (Fig. 39.4) as well as cestode cysticerci.

CLASSIFICATION: PHYLUM ANNELIDA

Class Polychaeta

Body of numerous segments with lateral parapodia bearing setae; head distinct; no clitellum; trochophore larva usually; mostly marine.
Nereis, Ichthyotomus

Class Clitellata

Clitellum used to secrete a cocoon for eggs; direct development.

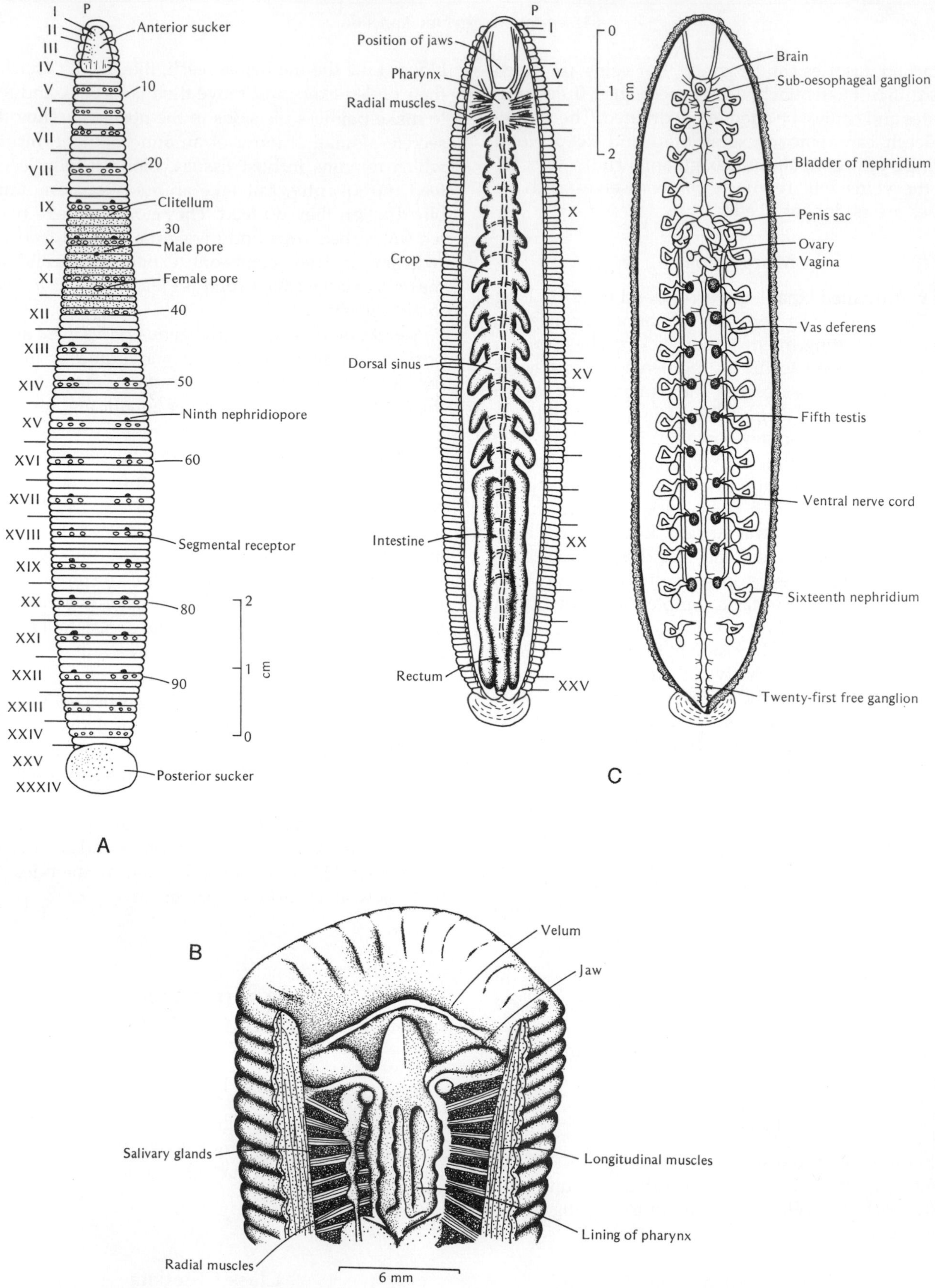

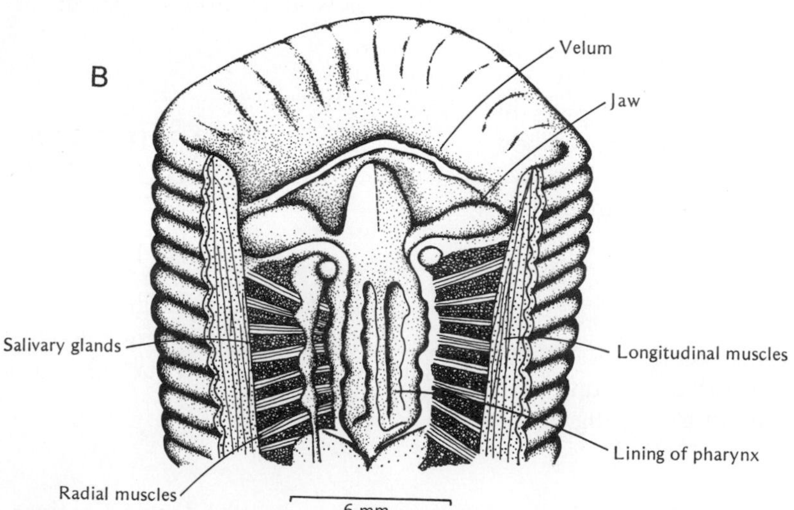

FIGURE 39.3 Diagrams of the medicinal leech, *Hirudo medicinalis.* (A) ventral view, (B) ventral dissection of the head, and (C) internal organs. [Redrawn with modifications from Mann, K. H., 1962.]

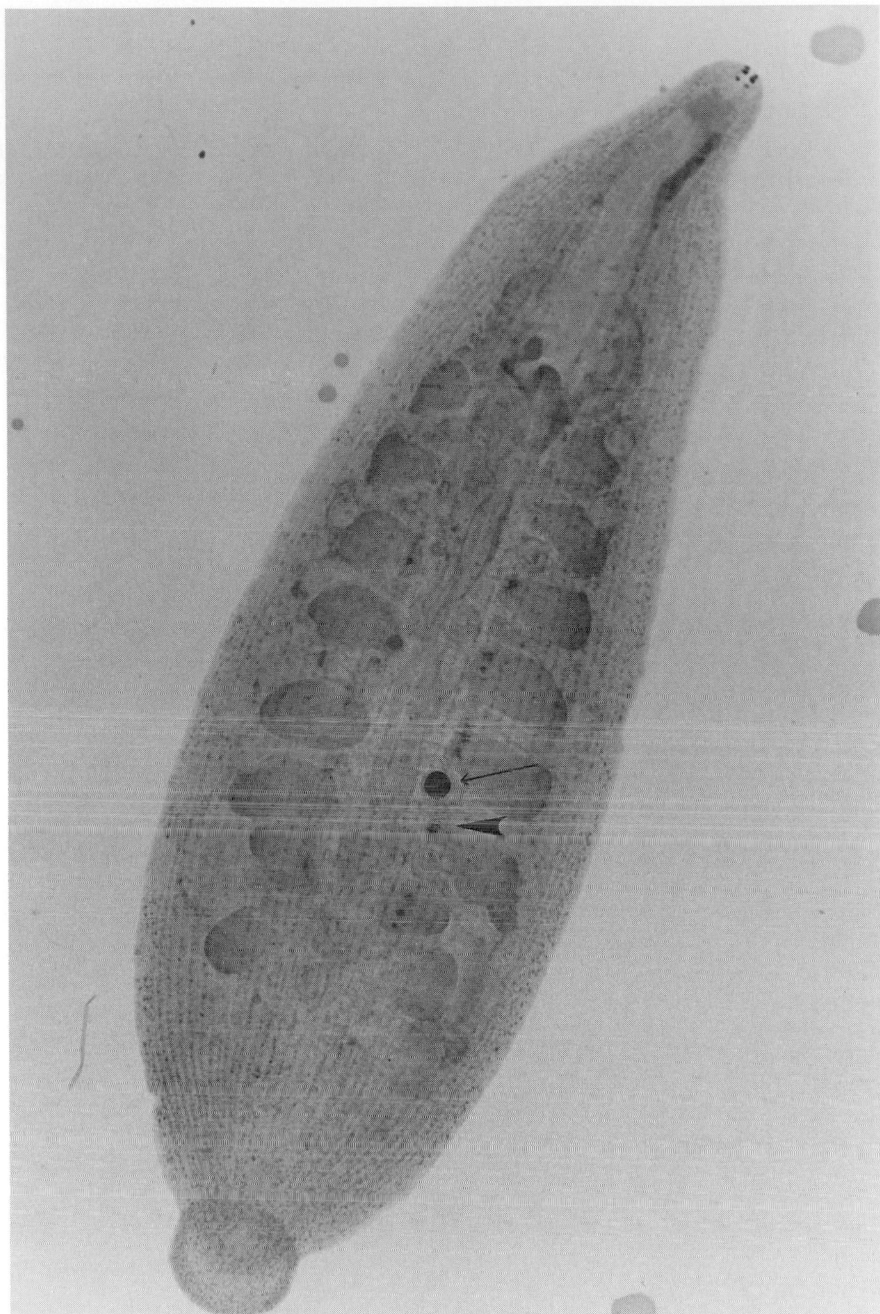

FIGURE 39.4 Leeches serve as intermediate hosts for some digenetic flukes. Note the dark, circular metacercaria.

Subclass Oligochaeta

Body of numerous segments with few setae per metamere; head absent; clitellum present; no larva; mostly terrestrial and freshwater. *Lumbricus, Eisenia.*

Subclass Hirudinea

Body usually with 33 or 34 segments; setae usually absent, clitellum present; anterior and posterior sucker usually present; terrestrial, freshwater and marine.

Order Hirudinea

Leeches; 34 body segments, anterior and posterior sucker. *Hirudo, Macrobdella, Placobdella.*

Order Branchiobdellida

Body with 15 segments; anterior and posterior suckers; ectocommensal or ectoparasitic on freshwater crayfishes.

Order Acanthobdellida

Body with 30 segments; no anterior sucker; ectoparasitic on freshwater fishes. *Acanthobdella*.

Readings

Baer, J. G. (1951). *Ecology of Animal Parasites.* Univ. of Illinois Press, Urbana.

Davies, R. W. (1987). All about leeches. *Nature (London)* **325,** 585.

Fauchauld, K. (1977). The Polychaete worms. Definitions and keys to the orders, families and genera. *Nat. History Mus. Los Angeles Sci. Ser.* **28,** 1–190.

Gelder, S. R., and Brinkhurst, R. O. (1990). As assessment of the phylogeny of the Branchiobdellida (Annelida: Clitellata) using PAUP. *Can. J. Zool.* **68,** 1318–1326.

Hoffman, G. L. (1967). *Parasites of North American Freshwater Fishes.* Univ. of California Press, Berkeley.

Holmquist, C. (1974). A fish-leech of the genus *Acanthobdellida* found in North America. *Hydrobiologica* **44,** 241–245.

Holt, P. C. (1965). The systematic position of the Branchiobdellida. *Syst. Zool.* **14,** 25–32.

Mann, K. H. (1962). *Leeches (Hirudinea). Their Structure, Physiology, Ecology and Embryology.* Pergamon, New York.

Sawyer, R. T. (1986). *Leech Biology and Behavior.* Clarendon, Oxford, UK.

Thorp, J. H., and Covich, A. P. (Eds.) (1991). *Ecology and Classification of North American Freshwater Invertebrates.* Academic Press, New York.

CHAPTER

40

Pentastomida

The phylum Pentastomida consists of about 100 species of endoparasites of the respiratory tract of vertebrates. The name pentastome or "five mouth" is derived from the four anterior leglike protuberances, plus a fifth median projection that actually bears the mouth (Fig. 40.1). Often the "legs" are reduced to little more than the terminal hooks used for clinging to the host tissues. Pentastomes are also called linguatulids or tongue worms because some, such as *Linguatula serrata*, are found in the nasopharynx of the host. Most adults are found in reptiles such as snakes and crocodiles, but a few are in birds and mammals.

These unusual parasites have been particularly puzzling to biologists. Most parasites have adults in more highly evolved animals and larvae in less highly evolved animals, suggesting that they evolved along with their hosts. However, in pentastomids this situation is sometimes reversed, sometimes not; for example, fish are intermediate hosts for crocodile pentastomids and mammals are intermediate hosts for snake pentastomids.

The unusual structure of pentastomids has made determination of evolutionary affinities difficult. They have no circulatory or excretory systems, nor do they have a distinct respiratory system. Similarities to annelids and arthropods have been suggested, but the evidence more strongly supports an arthropod affinity. The outer covering is a chitinous cuticle (Fig. 40.2) similar to that of arthropods, muscles are striated like those of arthropods; the molting sequence from primary larva to adult is similar; embryological development and especially spermatozoan characteristics resemble those of crustacea, and biochemical data suggest that there is affinity with crustaceans. Recognizing the arthropod affinities, but realizing that the evolutionary and taxonomic position of the pentastomes is still uncertain, we take a conservative approach and retain them in their own phylum, immediately adjacent to the phylum Arthropoda.

The pentastome digestive tract is a straight tube from a subterminal mouth to a terminal anus. The mouth is surrounded by a chitinous ring called a *cadre*; the muscular pharynx and frontal or head glands have secretions that apparently liquefy host tissue and prevent coagulation of blood.

The nervous system has paired, metamerically arranged ganglia along a ventral nerve cord much like those of annelids and arthropods. There are also specialized sense organs in the tegument.

Sexes are separate; males are usually smaller than females. Males have a single testis connected to a seminal vesicle, which is joined by lateral ducts to a pair of ejaculatory organs. The latter connect to a muscular cirrus, which fits into the groove of a dilator organ that may serve as a guide for the cirrus, just as the nematode gubernaculum does, or may actually be an intromittent organ in some species.

Females (Fig. 40.3) have a single ovary that sometimes branches into two lobes with joined oviducts. The single or double oviducts connect with a single, highly coiled uterus leading to the vagina and gonopore. The gonopore is in the anterior end of the abdomen in the Order Cephalobaenida and at the posterior end in the Order Porocephalida.

Fertilization is internal; embryonated eggs leave the definitive host through nasal and oral secretions, or are swallowed and passed in feces. Eggs hatch, releasing primary larvae which have four claw-bearing, stumpy

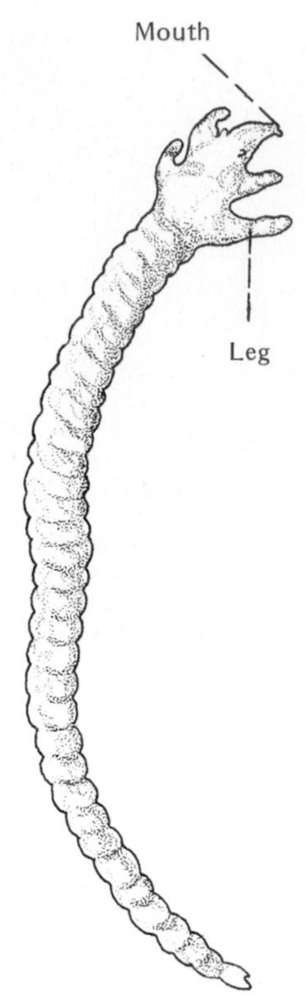

FIGURE 40.1 Diagram of an adult *Cephalobaenia tetrapoda* from the lung of a snake. [Redrawn from Barnes, 1987.]

appendages (Fig. 40.4). Primary larvae molt several times, becoming nymphs (Fig. 40.5). Infective nymphs in intermediate hosts are ingested by definitive hosts, molt several times, and become adults (Fig. 40.1)

Name of Organism and Disease Associations

Porocephalus spp. cause pentastomosis, porocephalosis, and visceral pentastomosis.

Hosts and Host Range

Adults commonly occur in the lungs of various snakes, whereas nymphs are found in the mesenteries and internal organs in many mammals, including monkeys and humans.

Geographic Distribution and Importance

The genus *Porocephalus* occurs worldwide in tropical and temperate zones. Adults usually cause little damage in snakes, and visceral infections in humans with nymphs are often incidental findings at autopsy. Human infections are common in some parts of Africa and have been reported worldwide, including in the United States.

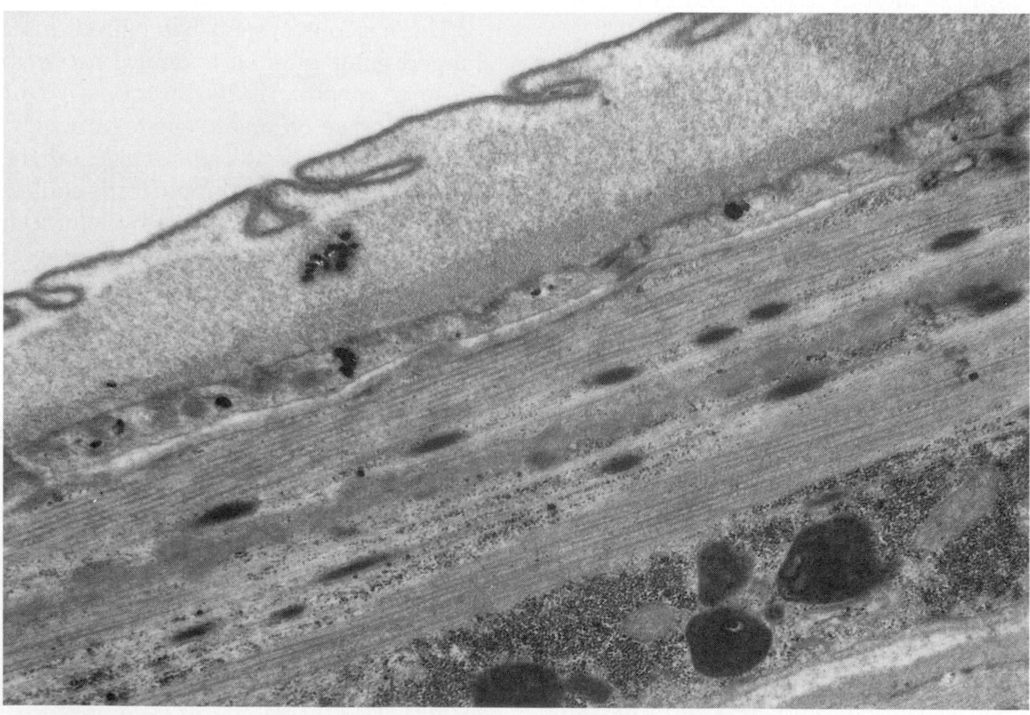

FIGURE 40.2 The nymphal cuticle and muscular layer of *Porocephalus* as seen in TEM.

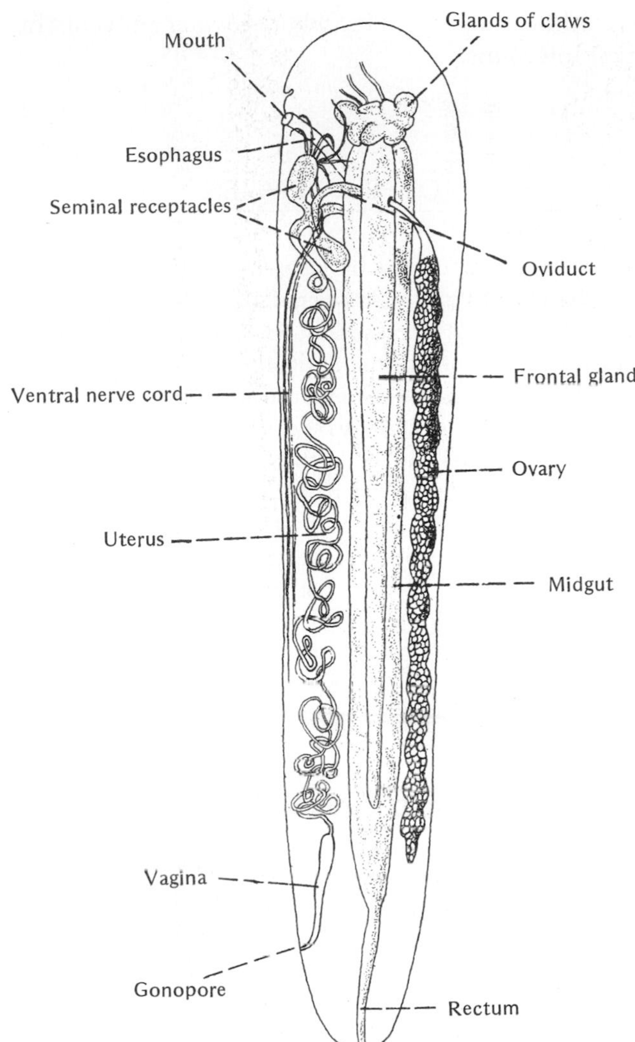

FIGURE 40.3 Diagram of the internal organs of a female *Waddycephalus teretiusculus*. [Redrawn from Barnes, 1987.]

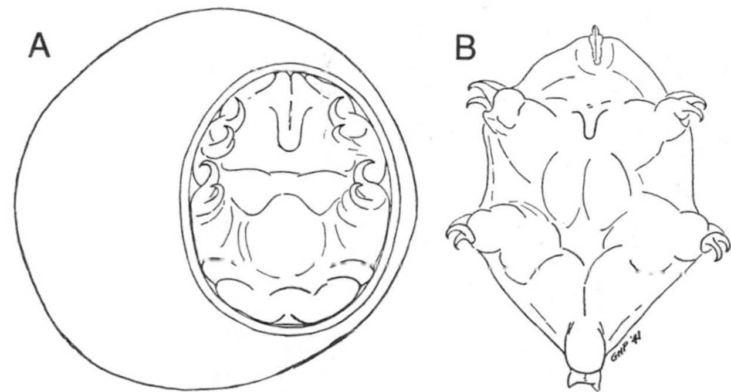

FIGURE 40.4 Diagram of the larva of *Porocephalus crotali*. [Redrawn from Penn, 1942.]

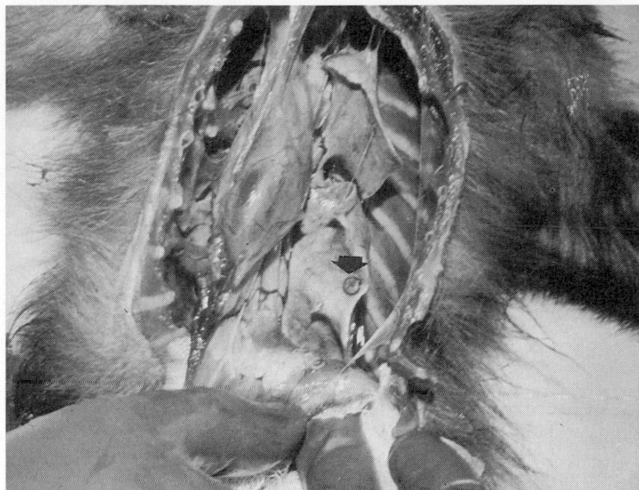

FIGURE 40.5 A nymph of *Porocephalus* encapsulated in viscera of a monkey (see arrow).

Life Cycle

The best-known life cycle is that of *P. crotuli* of rattlesnakes. Eggs are ingested by mammals such as mice; they hatch, releasing primary larvae, which penetrate intestines. The larvae wander about in the peritoneal cavity and molt six times to become infective nymphs. The nymphs then become encapsulated in the host tissues (Fig. 40.5). When a rattlesnake ingests infective nymphs, they penetrate the intestine and adjacent lung, molt three more times, and become adults. After mating, eggs are passed in nasal secretions or are swallowed and pass in feces.

Host–Parasite Interactions

As mentioned, little damage occurs in either the intermediate or definitive hosts. There are three types of human lesions: encysted pentastomid nymphs, necrotic pentastomid nymphs, and "cuticle" granulomas. The first type is shown in Fig. 40.6; it is a nymph encysted in the mesenteries of a capuchin monkey, *Cebus apella*, from Colombia. Sometimes, however, visceral larva migrans reactions develop in the reptilian and mammalian hosts.

HUMAN INFECTIONS

Halzoun or marrara syndrome is a human disease caused by pentastomids, principally *Linguatula serrata,* found in the Middle East, Turkey, Greece, Morocco, India, and Sudan. The onset of the disease is seen within minutes to half an hour after the ingestion

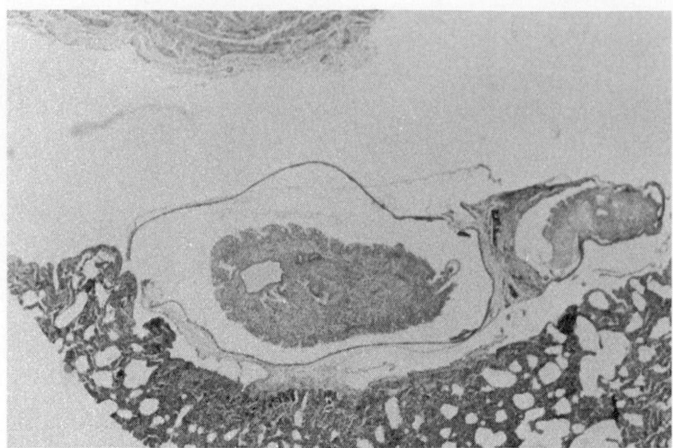

FIGURE 40.6 A histologic section of the lung of a monkey showing a nymph of *Porocephalus* encysted in it.

of raw liver or lymph nodes principally of sheep and goats. The signs and symptoms are usually restricted to the head and neck region, where there is swelling of the tissues of the throat, larynx, tonsils, nasal passages, and lips. The swelling can be so severe that the affected person may die of asphyxiation during the first few hours after onset. Later complications may include facial paralysis and bacterial abscesses in the throat. Not all persons ingesting infected tissues of sheep or goats are affected, but the same person may suffer repeated attacks The sudden onset and dramatic swelling of the throat tissues imply that halzoun is an immediate hypersensitivity or allergic reaction to the pentastomids.

A dish eaten in the Sudan and associated with marrara syndrome is made from raw stomach, liver, lung, and trachea of sheep, goats, cattle, or camels, seasoned with bile, lemon, spices, and sometimes onion and urine.

Epidemiology and Control

Control of halzoun in humans revolves around the following:

1. Changing food habits
2. Providing clean water for drinking and food preparation

Human infections are acquired in several ways. In Africa, where infections may be common, snakes are often eaten, and undercooked python meat is considered to be a delicacy. Water contaminated with eggs or vegetables washed with contaminated water may be sources of infection. In the United States the human visceral infections probably were acquired by eating inadequately cooked rattlesnake meat. Adequate cooking of meat and drinking filtered water prevents human infections.

OTHER SPECIES

Other pentastomes of interest include *Reighardia,* which is found in the air sacs of gulls and terns, *Armillifer* spp., which are similar to *Porocephalus* and can cause human infections, and *Linguatula.* The latter is found in nasal passages and frontal sinuses of canids and felids throughout the world. Intermediate hosts, including cattle, sheep, rabbits, and humans, ingest eggs from contaminated water or vegetation, leading to visceral pentastomiasis. Ingestion of infective nymphs is also a problem, see the preceding discussion on the epidemiology and control of halzoun.

CLASSIFICATION

Order Cephalobaenida

Mouth anterior to hooks; hooks without fulcrum; female gonopore at anterior end of abdomen.
Cephalobaena, Reighardia

Order Porocephalida

Mouth between hooks; hooks with fulcrum; female gonopore near posterior end of body.
Armillifer, Linguatula, Porocephalus

Readings

Abele, L. G., Kim, W., and Felgenhauer, B. E. (1989). Molecular evidence for inclusion of the phylum Pentastomida in the Crustacea. *Mol. Biol. Evol.* **6,** 685–691.

Barnes, R. D. (1987). *Invertebrate Zoology,* 5th ed. Saunders, Philadelphia.

Demaree, R. S., Jr. (1973). Ultrastructure of pentastome nymph integument. *Proc. 31st Annu. Mtg. Electron Microsc. Soc. Am.,* 502–503.

Esslinger, J. H. (1962a). Development of *Porocephalus crotali* (Humboldt, 1908) (Pentastomida) in experimental intermediate hosts. *J. Parasitol.* **48,** 452–456.

Esslinger, J. H. (1962b). Morphology of the egg and larva of *Porocephalus crotali* (Pentastomida). *J. Parasitol.* **48,** 457–462.

Fain, A. (1975). The Pentastomida parasitic in man. *Ann. Soc. Belg. Med. Trop.* **55,** 59–64.

Hangerud, R. E. (1989). Evolution in the pentastomids. *Parasitol. Today* **5,** 126–132.

Khalil, G., and Schacher, J. F. (1965). *Linguatula serrata* in relation to halzoun and the marrara syndrome. *Am. J. Trop. Med. Hyg.* **14,** 736–746.

Penn, G. H., Jr. (1942). The life history of *Porocephalus crotali,* a parasite of the Louisiana muskrat. *J. Parasitol.* **28,** 277–283.

Riley, J. (1986). The biology of the pentastomids. *Adv. Parasitol.* **25,** 45–128.

Self, J. T. (1969). Biological relationships of the Pentastomida. A bibliography on the Pentastomida. *Exp. Parasitol.* **24,** 63–119.

Self, J. T., Hopps, H. C., and Williams, A. O. (1972). Porocephaliasis in man and experimental mice. *Exp. Parasitol.* **32,** 117–126.

Storch, V., and Jamieson, B. G. M. (1992). Further spermatological evidence for the inclusion of the Pentastomida (tongue worms) in the Crustacea. *Int. J. Parasitol.* **22,** 95–108.

PART

5

ARTHROPODA

CHAPTER

41

Introduction to the Arthropods

The arthropods are so ubiquitous that they surround us and impinge on nearly every aspect of our lives. When we consider that there are over 1,000,000 described species in water, on land, and in the air, it can be appreciated that we live in a cloud of insects, mites, crustacea, and spiders. We depend on these creatures for food, pollination of crops, and control of unwanted pests, as well as for disposing of various kinds of dejecta in our environment. In this book, we are concerned with those arthropods that are harmful to humans either directly or indirectly, or with those that demonstrate some principles of symbiosis. Despite our limited view of arthropods here, most are not harmful, and many serve beneficial roles in recycling, controlling populations of other organisms, or as food. As we have discussed in connection with other organisms, arthropods often become problems when the environment is somehow altered by human activities.

PHYLOGENY, MORPHOLOGY, MOLTING, AND DEVELOPMENT

The organisms in the phylum Arthropoda belong to diverse groups, but they have some features in common:

1. Bilateral symmetry.
2. Chitinous exoskeleton with jointed legs.
3. Growth by molting, which is controlled by hormones.
4. A complete digestive tract extending from an anterior mouth to a posterior anus.
5. A nervous system consisting of an anterior set of ganglia and commissures, which extend around the esophagus and pass posteriorly as two fused chains of ventral ganglia.
6. True segmentation or metamerism. Primitively, each segment had a pair of legs, neural ganglia, probably an excretory unit, and a set of muscles. In primitive arthropods there is little difference among the segments along the length of the animal (homonymous metamerism), but in more advanced forms, there is movement toward specialized changes in segments (heteronomous metamerism) or the merging of segments into distinct body parts (tagmatosis).
7. The body cavity is a hemocoel and the circulatory system is open. In an open circulatory system, blood moves into the heart through openings or ostia and is pumped out to various parts of the body, where it leaves the vessels and bathes the tissues directly.

Let us consider the consequences of some of the characteristics of the arthropods. The *exoskeleton* and mode of growth are fundamental influences on what arthropods are and do. Chitin (an acetylated glucosamine) occurs principally in arthropods but also occurs in various other animal groups and fungi. It is a tough, flexible compound that is remarkably resistant to bacterial action but is eventually recycled. The hard exoskeleton associated with animals such as crab and lobster is chitin impregnated with calcium salts added for rigidity. In many small arthropods or insect larvae, the exoskeleton is tough but not rigid because of the presence of tanned proteins.

There are two areas in which problems are associated with an exoskeleton: size and growth. The largest arthropods, such as the king crab, are marine. The terrestrial arthropods do not have seawater to support the body and are generally rather small; some tropical insects may approach 15 cm in length, but they are exceptional.

The exoskeleton is a complex structure; exquisite control is required in the formation of a new one at molting. All of the new external structures (Fig. 41.1, parts A, B, and C) must be formed below the old exoskeleton and produced in such a way that the next stage can be larger (Fig. 41.2). The molt must be controlled so that it is coordinated and occurs relatively quickly. During the molt, the animal struggles to shed the old exoskeleton; because the new exoskeleton is soft for a short time, the animal is more susceptible to predation than at other times.

Hormones control molting and also differentiation of the body as it matures sexually. Hormonal systems differ in various groups of arthropods; insects are rep-

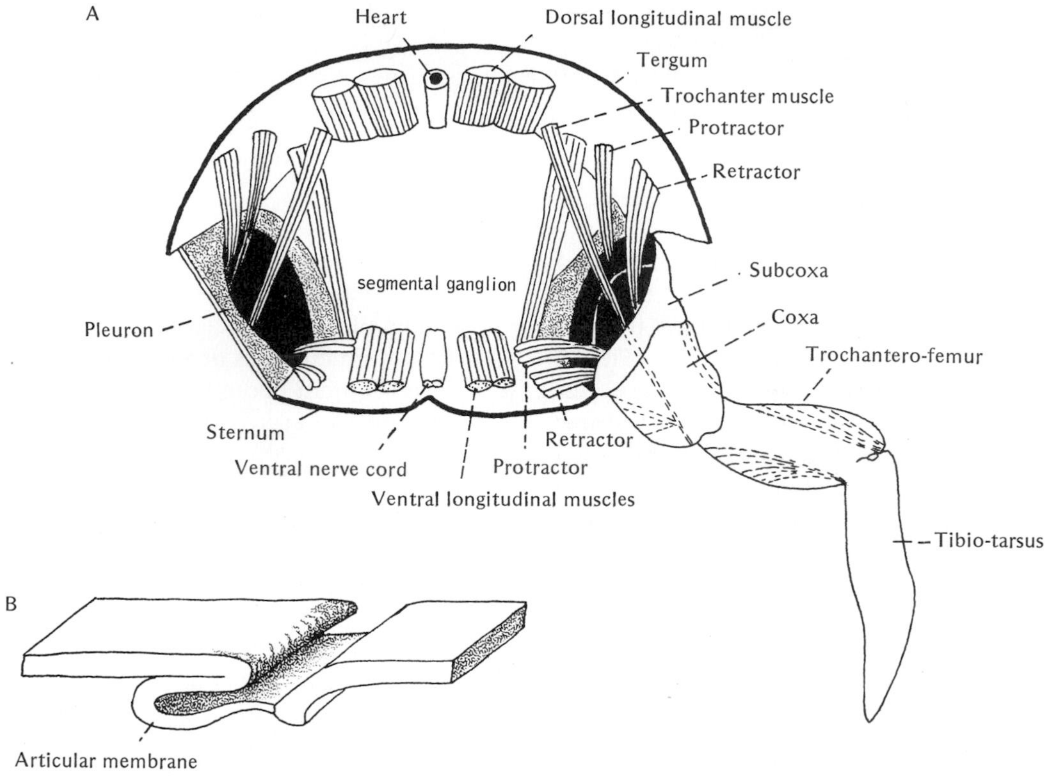

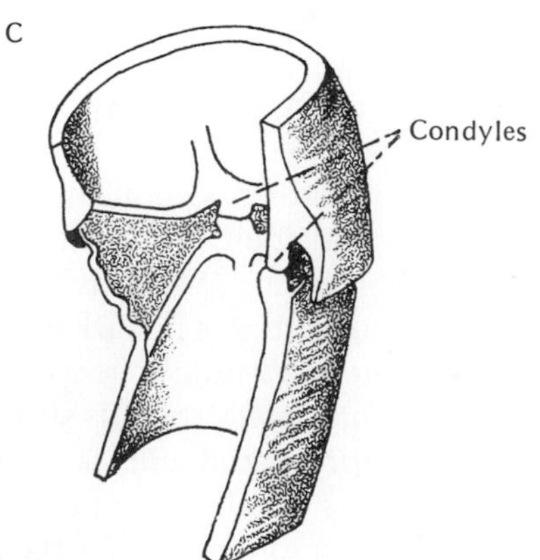

FIGURE 41.1 General body structure of arthropods: (A) a transverse section, (B) intersegmental articulation, (C) appendicular articulation. [Redrawn with modifications from Barnes, 1987.]

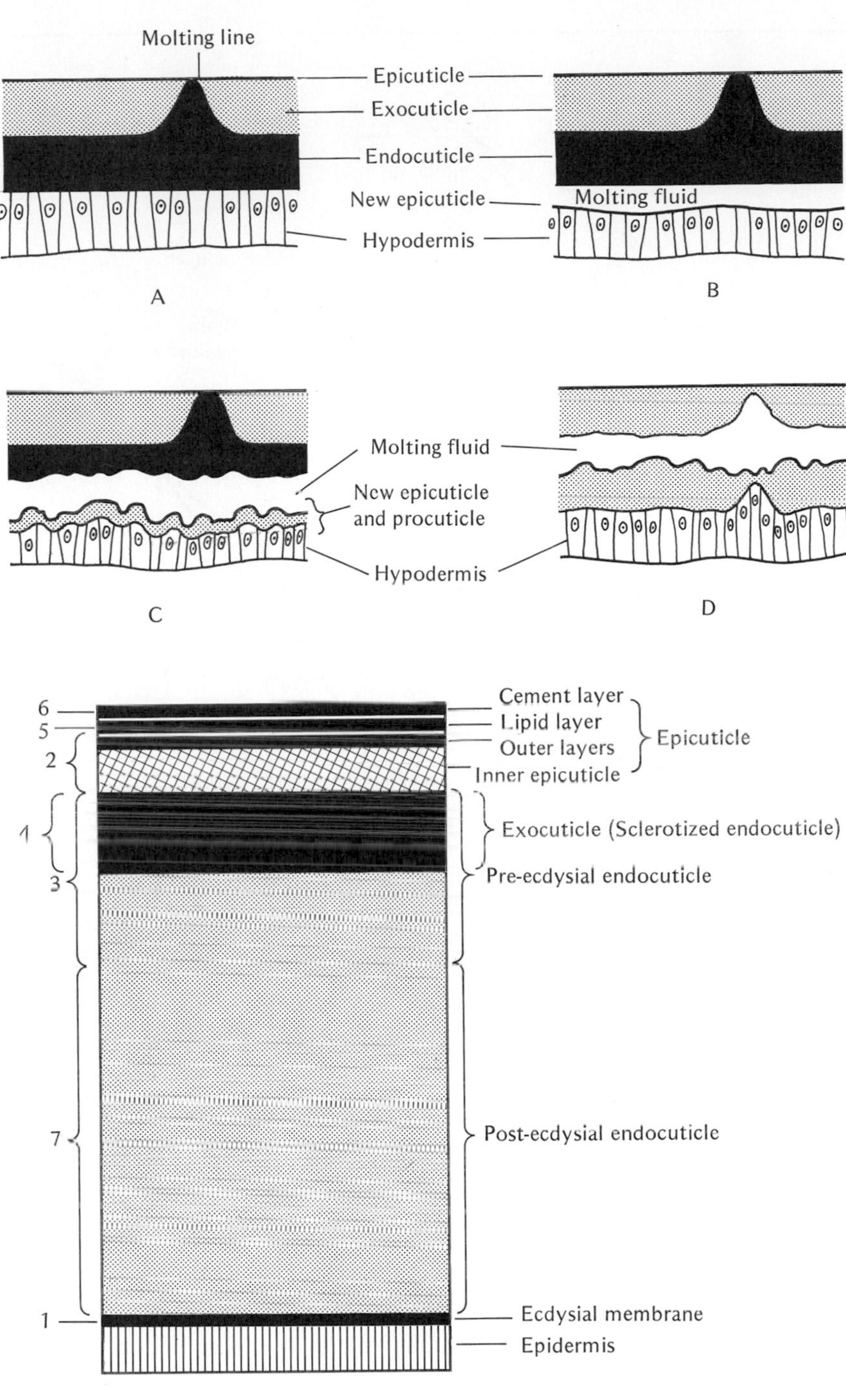

FIGURE 41.2 Stages in the molting process of an arthropod: (A) the cuticle and epidermis between molts, (B) accumulation of molting fluid beneath the old cuticle and the formation of a new epicuticle, (C) breakdown of the old epicuticle and the formation of a procuticle beneath the new epicuticle, (D) secretion of new procuticle nearing completion; the old procuticle is now reduced to exocuticle and is ready to be shed. (E) Details of the layers formed during molt. [Redrawn from Kozloff, E. N., 1990.]

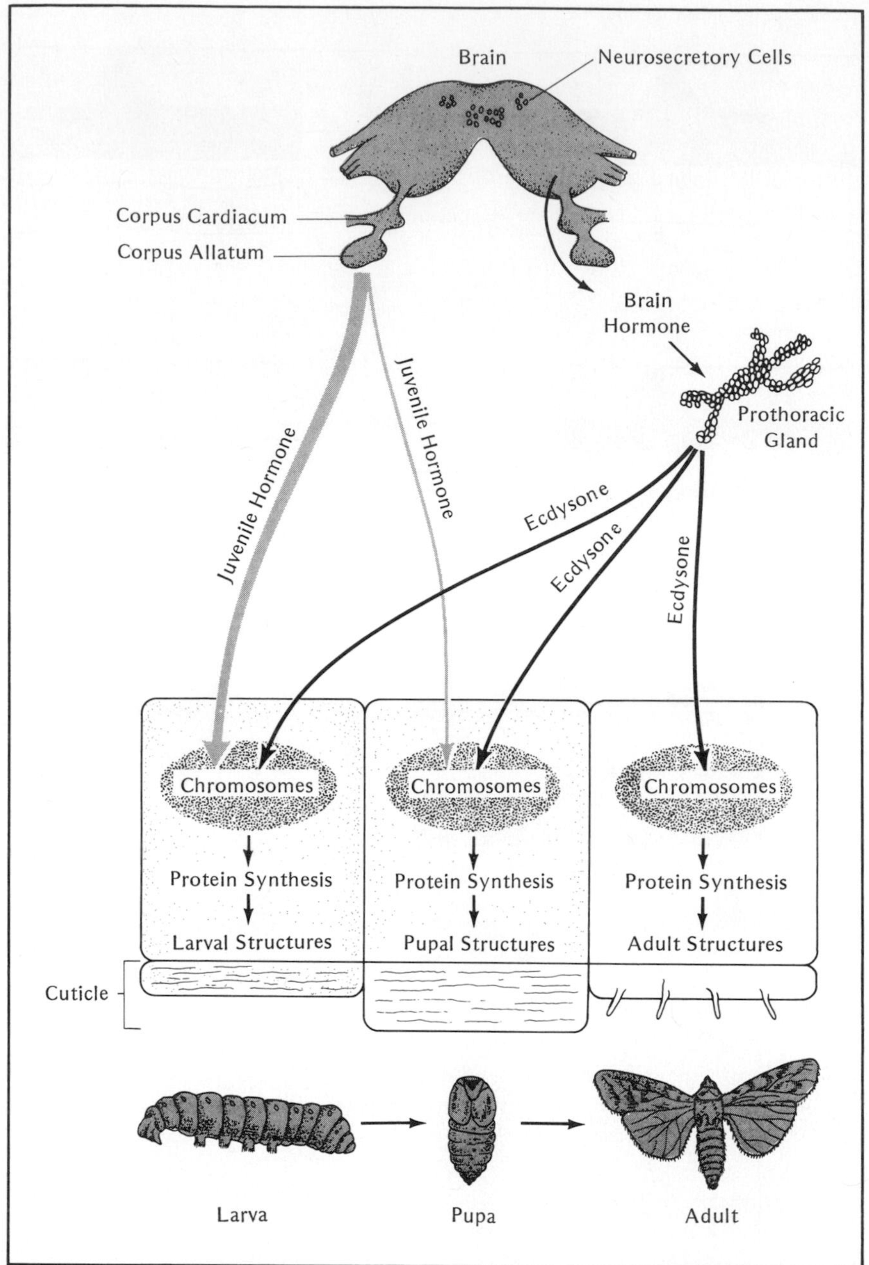

FIGURE 41.3 Control of molting and maturation in insects. [From Herried, C. F., 1977.]

resentative of the way control is effected. One hormonal system in insects controls molting and another controls sexual maturity. The stimuli to molt and to mature originate in the brain of the insect (Fig. 41.3). Brain hormone has the prothoracic gland as its target; this gland secretes *ecdysone*, which causes the new exoskeleton to form and the old one to be shed. Juvenile hormone (JH), secreted by the corpora allata, maintains the insect in a preadult stage. As the amount of JH decreases, the insect moves to the next stage of its life cycle. In the example given of a moth, the caterpillar moves to the pupal stage; when JH is almost gone, the pupa becomes an adult moth.

Much of the basic work on the control of molting and maturation of insects was done by V. B. Wigglesworth in Britain with *Rhodnius prolixus*, a vector of *Trypanosoma cruzi*, and by Carroll Williams at Harvard in the United States with the cecropia moth. The puzzle was fitted together by these two investigators and their students in a series of experiments done mostly in the 1940s. Their aim was to describe the mechanisms by which these extraordinarily complex processes of molting and maturation were controlled. They succeeded in what appeared to be solely an exercise in academic research, but the practical values are now being realized. Some of the third-generation insecticides are based on JH mimetics. JH is a terpene with a chain of 15 carbon atoms; its synthesis led to the synthesis of JH mimetics, compounds sufficiently similar to JH that they have some hormonal activity. A JH mimetic (methoprene) is now used to control some insects; its effect is to prevent development in the insect beyond a preadult stage and to cause maldevelopment.

Metamerism is associated with the exoskeleton and with most of the internal organs; it is fundamental to arthropod structure. The arthropods probably arose from wormlike forms intermediate between the arthropods and the annelids (earthworms, polychaetes, leeches) such as *Peripatus* (phylum Onychophora). Considerable modification has occurred in structure and development; however, segmentation is retained in a number of systems:

1. The nervous system has a pair of ganglia in each segment.
2. Muscles are associated with each segment.
3. Openings to the respiratory system are often present in each segment.
4. The exoskeleton usually retains its segmentation, which can be seen in its primitive condition during embryogenesis.

The digestive tract of arthropods is complete and has regional differentiation. There are various specialized structures in the gut, depending on the type of food the animal takes, but the basic plan is the same in all. If we go beyond these basic similarities, there is a great deal of diversity in the structures and modes of development in various arthropod groups. Excretory systems are associated with the gut (insects), the antennae (crustacea), or the legs (arachnids). Respiration, that is, gaseous exchange, takes place through the whole body surface in many small species, through a tracheal system (insects), wet gills (crustacea), or book gills or a dry surface (arachnids), among others. Light receptors also vary from simple eyes in spiders to compound eyes in the crustacea, and both in the insects. Other sense organs allow the reception of air movement (such as hairs in insects), orientation (statocysts in crustacea), or carbon dioxide (ticks and some insects).

Development is even more diverse and its patterns bear little relationship to each other. Copulatory and reproductive structures aside, embryogenesis and preadult patterns of development in the various groups are quite different. The crustacea have seven different larval forms (Fig. 42.3), but these do not occur in all life cycles and a few additional forms occur in some groups. The general pattern is for the organism to become more complex and more like the adult at each molt. However, in spiders the body form in the early molts is about the same as in the adults, and the adults continue to molt and to grow larger. The insects, on the other hand, reach the winged adult stage and do not molt again (Fig. 43.10). Taking into account both adult structures and the patterns of development, it is generally agreed that the arthropods are polyphyletic—that is, they arose from more than a single stem form, most likely as many as four. The classification generally used (see end of this chapter) contains four subphyla, representing the concept of four different origins of the phylum. This matter is by no means resolved, and there are almost as many proposals for higher level classification as there are experts in the field. Until detailed cladistic analyses have been completed, we will continue use the above mentioned scheme.

VENOMOUS ARTHROPODS AND ALLERGIC REACTIONS TO ARTHROPODS

A wide array of arthropods causes toxic reactions in vertebrates. The cause of intoxication may be direct (bites, stings, defensive secretions) or indirect because of hypersensitivity (allergy). The effect of such contact with arthropods may be a mild wheal, such as results from a mosquito bite, or a moderately severe reaction, such as occurs following the bite of a black widow spider, or death due to an anaphylactic reaction, such as in a person hypersensitive to bee stings. Although we are principally concerned with the responses in humans or in animals important to humans, the same effects occur in other vertebrates or (except for hypersensitivity) invertebrates.

Arthropods use various secretions in the process of obtaining food or in defending themselves from predators. Toxicants are found all through the phylum, but those of greatest importance are in the insects, arachnids, and centipedes. Local reactions often occur in animals bitten by bloodsucking arthropods such as insects and ticks. A bloodsucking arthropod must have mouthparts capable of penetrating or lacerating the skin. The clotting mechanism would immediately close the wound and stop the flow of blood unless there were some mechanism to prevent it. Organisms such as mosquitoes, blackflies, fleas, ticks, and mites inject salivary fluid into the wound in order to prevent clotting or to liquefy the tissues. These arthropods' mouthparts differ in origin and function, but all of them inject fluid to keep the blood from clotting or to liquefy the tissue. Such secretions are mixtures of substances, but they contain proteins, some of which are enzymatic. They produce an inflammatory response and an itching papule on the skin. If there are only a few bites, the host may be uncomfortable but not significantly affected. If there is massive attack by, say, black flies (Chapter 47), there may be severe intoxication from the injection of salivary fluid causing prostration or even death. Such occurrences fortunately are rare.

Predaceous arthropods have a number of mechanisms for capturing and immobilizing prey. Beetles often have strong mandibles, which they use to crush their prey; the effect is essentially mechanical. Alternatively, piercing mouthparts (Hemiptera, spiders, centipedes) or stingers at the posterior end (Hymenoptera, scorpions) are specifically constructed to pierce the integument of the prey and to inject an immobilizing toxin. These same structures and toxins are used defensively against people who handle or inadvertently come in contact with these animals. Usually, when a mammal is bitten or stung, the damage and the pain remain localized. This is true when a person is bitten by an insect such as the wheel bug (*Arilus*), which is common in gardens in temperate and warm climates; the pain is likely to be severe, but there is no long-term effect. Occasionally, plant-feeding insects such as thrips, leafhoppers, or boxelder bugs will bite humans, and considerable discomfort together with skin irritation may result, but serious effects are lacking. On the other hand, severe skin lesions can be seen following the bites of some bloodsuckers, such as soft ticks or kissing bugs, but is seen most dramatically in the case of the brown recluse spider, *Loxosceles reclusa*, and several related species (Chapter 50). The bite of the brown recluse may be so minor that it is not noticed initially, but within a few hours the site of the bite blisters; there may be systemic reactions causing the person to become prostrated. Death is unlikely except in small children. The long-lasting effects result from extensive tissue destruction in the vicinity of the bite; necrosis of cutaneous and subcutaneous tissue causes extensive scarring, which may require skin grafting.

The black widow spider, *Lactrodectus mactans*, and several related species, produce severe systemic reactions caused by injected neurotoxins. There is swelling at the site of the bite, but more severe effects are generalized: muscular pain, nausea, difficulty in speech and breathing, and sweating. The kidneys, liver, and spleen may be damaged. In adults, the effects may last two or three days; death, if it occurs, is usually in children, aged persons, or those who have cardiovascular disease. The probability of death resulting from a black widow bite is less than 4%.

A peculiar type of systemic intoxication is tick paralysis, discussed in detail in Chapter 51. Generally associated with hard ticks, tick paralysis affects mammals by causing a flaccid paralysis that may lead to death if the breathing center in the brain is involved. A few ticks may paralyze even a fully grown animal as large as a domestic ox.

Many arthropods have defensive secretions that serve to fend off would-be predators; often these chemicals are exuded from one of the body openings, from between the joints of the skeleton, or from the tips of body hairs. In a few instances, such as in the millipedes or whipscorpions and apparently a few Lepidoptera, there is forcible ejection of secretions. *Rhinocrichus latespargor*, a millipede found in Haiti, is said to eject fluid up to 82 cm. Many Hymenoptera use their stings defensively in addition to capturing prey. Defensive secretions may have a bad odor, which serves to drive off the predator; they may cause local irritation of the skin, mucous membranes, or eyes, or in a few instances they may have systemic effects.

Some common insects that have defensive secretions are Lepidoptera larvae and beetles. The hairs or setae on the bodies of lepidopteran larvae are frequently defensive; they may be irritating in themselves, or they may be hollow and secrete a chemical from a gland at the base of the hair. Blister beetles (family Meloidae) exude a toxicant from between the joints on the legs when they are disturbed. This secretion produces a severe burning sensation on the skin and on the mucous membranes of the eye, mouth, or intestine; not only severe discomfort but blistering of the epithelial surface occurs. Large animals such as horses may be killed by ingesting blister beetles baled with hay; they die from severe ulceration of the digestive tract.

Some persons who have been stung by a bee or wasp may become allergic or hypersensitive to the venom. When such a hypersensitive individual is stung again, a violent allergic reaction or anaphylaxis may result. The person may lose consciousness within a few minutes of being stung and, in a very strong reaction, may die within minutes unless epinephrine is administered. About 200 deaths from anaphylactic reactions to stings of bees or wasps are reported annually in the United States.

Hypersensitivity is usually manifested by upper respiratory symptoms or by stronger than normal skin reactions. Children particularly may become allergic to mosquito bites and have excessive swelling of the skin at the site of bites. The housedust mite, *Dermatophagoides farinae*, is one cause of housedust allergy usually manifested as asthma. Insect scales from lepidopterans may also cause hay fever or asthma.

CLASSIFICATION OF ARTHROPODS

Phylum Arthropoda—arthropods

Subphylum Trilobitomorpha—trilobites (fossils only)
Subphylum Chelicerata
  Class Merostomata—horseshoe crabs
  Class Arachnida—arachnids, mites
  Class Pycnogonida—sea spiders
Subphylum Crustacea—crustaceans
  Class Branchiopoda
  Class Copepoda
  Class Ostracoda
  Class Branchiura
  Class Cirripedia
  Class Malacostraca
Subphylum Uniramia
  Class Myriapoda
    Subclass Diplopoda—millipedes
    Subclass Chilopoda—centipedes
    Subclass Pauropoda—pauropods
    Subclass Symphyla—symphylans
  Class (Insecta) Hexapoda—insects

Readings

Barnes, R. D. (1987). *Invertebrate Zoology*, 5th ed. Saunders, Philadelphia.

Briggs, D. E. G., and Fortey, R. A. (1989). The early radiation and relationships of the major arthropod groups. *Science* **246,** 241–243.

Chang, E. S. (1985). Hormonal control of molting in decapod Crustacea. *Am. Zool.* **25,** 179–185.

Clarke, K. U. (1973). *The Biology of Arthropoda*. Elsevier, New York.

Gupta, A. P. (Ed.) (1979). *Arthropod Phylogeny*. Van Nostrand–Reinhold, New York.

Herried, C. F. (1977). *Biology*. Macmillan, New York.

Kozloff, E. N. (1990). *Invertebrates*. Saunders, Philadelphia.

Manton, S. M. (1977). *The Arthropoda: Habits, Functional Morphology, and Evolution*. Clarendon, Oxford.

Parker, S. P. (Ed.) (1982). *Synopsis and Classification of Living Organisms*, Vol. 2, pp. 71–728. McGraw–Hill, New York.

CHAPTER

42

Crustacea

Almost everyone has seen movies or still pictures of "cleaner fishes" busily removing "parasites" from various other fish species, including normally highly predatory ones. Many of the parasites being removed belong to the subphylum Crustacea. Because this cleaning behavior is so widespread, one can appreciate how important the removal of these pathogenic parasites must be to the infected hosts. As the world's population increases, aquaculture will play a greater role in meeting the need for more protein. Therefore, it is well to gain some information about the crustacean parasites that can have a significant impact on the aquacultural industry.

More than 45,000 species are known in the subphylum Crustacea, including the well-known and delicious lobster, crab, and shrimp, as well as the lesser known smaller species that form a significant part of the freshwater and marine food chains and the parasitic species. Indeed, many parasitic species have free-living larval stages that are part of the food chain.

The subphylum Crustacea (hard shell) has a number of features distinctive from those of the other arthropods; it is the only major subphylum that is primarily aquatic; has gills for breathing; has two pairs of antennae, one pair of mandibles, and two pairs of maxillae; and lacks Malpighian tubules. As with most higher-level classifications, there are various proposals in the literature, with experts still disagreeing. We choose to follow a conservative approach in which Crustacea is a subphylum in the phylum Arthropoda. The subphylum is divided into eight to ten classes. The class Malacostraca, contains the larger organisms such as lobsters and crabs, while the remaining classes contain the smaller organisms, including most of the important parasitic species.

Crustaceans typically have three tagmata, or body divisions: head, thorax, and abdomen. Often these regions are difficult to distinguish because of fusion of various parts. The head typically bears five pairs of appendages: two pairs of antennae, one pair of mandibles, and two pairs of maxillae. In addition, two types of eyes may be present; the median or *nauplius eye* is a central, relatively simple structure probably used primarily for orientation, and the much more complex *compound* or lateral eyes have complex visual discrimination abilities.

Appendages on the thorax are for swimming, and some, such as the maxillipeds, may be modified for feeding. In the primitive state, crustacean appendages were *biramous* (two-branched), but numerous modifications to this basic plan are seen, especially among the parasites.

CLASS COPEPODA

The Copepoda (oar foot) is the second largest class with about 7500 species; they form an important part of aquatic food chains. In addition, both free-living and parasitic copepods are of interest to the parasitological world. Free-living copepods (Fig. 42.1) are intermediate hosts for tapeworms (*Diaptomus* and *Cyclops* for *Diphyllobothrium* spp.), nematodes (*Cyclops* for *Dracunculus medinensis*), and acanthocephalans. Several parasitic crustaceans are serious economic problems in commercial fish hatcheries.

The parasitic crustaceans are fascinating organisms with all sorts of modifications for the parasitic way of life. Little is known about their biology, which presents

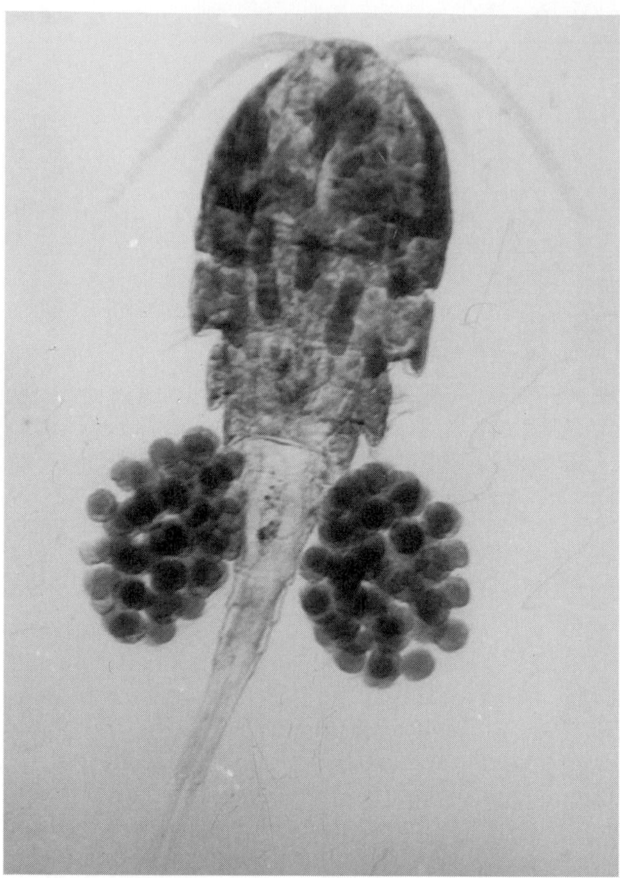

FIGURE 42.1 *Cyclops* female as seen in LM. Two large egg sacs are located toward the posterior of the cephalothorax.

numerous challenges to parasitologists of the future. We discuss only a few of the better known species to illustrate basic biological features typical of this diverse group.

Name of Organism and Disease Associations

Ergasilus spp. causes ergasilosis.

Hosts and Host Range

Ergasilids parasitize both freshwater and marine fishes. Freshwater hosts include game fishes such as bass, perch, catfish, and bluegill, as well as wild species such as sticklebacks.

Geographic Distribution and Importance

Ergasilus spp. are found worldwide; they are serious problems in fish culture and sometimes in nature as well.

Morphology

Parasitic female adult *Ergasilus* spp. have few modifications for a parasitic existence and greatly resemble free-living copepods. Their most obvious modification for parasitism is having greatly enlarged second antennae, which terminate in large claws (Fig. 42.2A); these antennae are used to grasp securely gill filaments. The mouthparts of ergasilids resemble those of free-swimming copepods rather than the highly modified mouthparts of many other parasitic copepods (Fig. 42.2B). Swimming legs are biramous (Fig. 42.2C); some species have stout spines on the first pair of swimming legs, presumably to dislodge tissue and move it toward the mouthparts.

Life Cycle

Complete life cycles have been worked out for only a few species. Probably the best-known life cycle is that of *Ergasilus sieboldi*. Copulation occurs while the males and females are free swimming; the males then die and the females attach to gills and embryonic development occurs in external egg sacs. There are three naupliar (Fig. 42.2D) and five copepodid stages, a single preadult stage, and then the adults. All except the fertilized adult are free swimming.

Diagnosis

Diagnosis is based on finding a parasitic adult female with greatly enlarged second antennae attached to the gills of fish.

Host–Parasite Interactions

Female ergasilids feed on gill tissue and mucus. Massive infections lead to emaciation, growth retardation, and even death, but infections with a single parasite may have no obvious detrimental effect.

Epidemiology and Control

Like most other parasitic copepods, *Ergasilus* spp. are problems only when crowding occurs, such as in fish farming. The best control method is not to introduce infected fish into lakes and ponds. Negatively phototropic larvae stay in the vegetation at the bottom; dispersal is reduced in vegetation-rich environments, resulting in only small numbers of copepod infections. A number of chemical treatments for *Ergasilus* spp. have been used with varying degrees of success.

Name of Organism and Disease Associations

Lernaea cyprinacea Linnaeus, 1761, causes anchor worm disease.

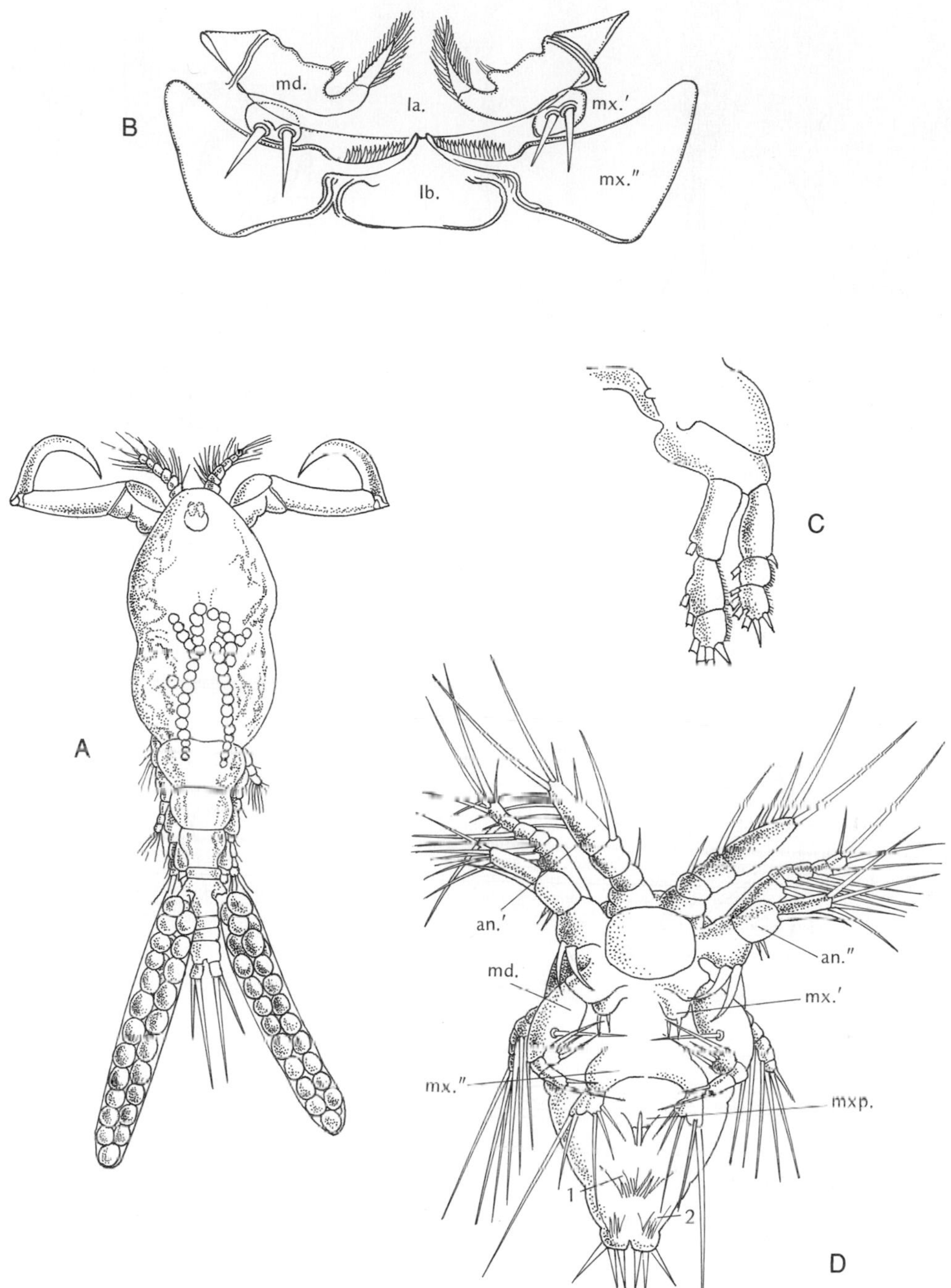

FIGURE 42.2 *Ergasilus* sp.: (A) adult female, (B) mouthparts, (C) swimming leg, (D) nauplius larva. Abbreviations: an', first antenna; an'', second antenna; la, labium, lb, labrum; md, mandible; mx', first maxilla; mx'', second maxilla; mxp, maxillary process. [Redrawn from Wilson, 1911.]

Hosts and Host Range

This copepod can probably infect any freshwater fish, as well as frog tadpoles and salamanders. Most adult females are embedded near fins, but they can be found almost anywhere on a fish that the copepod can penetrate.

Geographic Distribution and Importance

This parasite apparently has a worldwide distribution. *L. cyprinacea* may have been introduced into North America with the goldfish, *Carassius auratus*. This parasite is a serious problem in closed environments such as ponds and hatcheries and has been responsible for

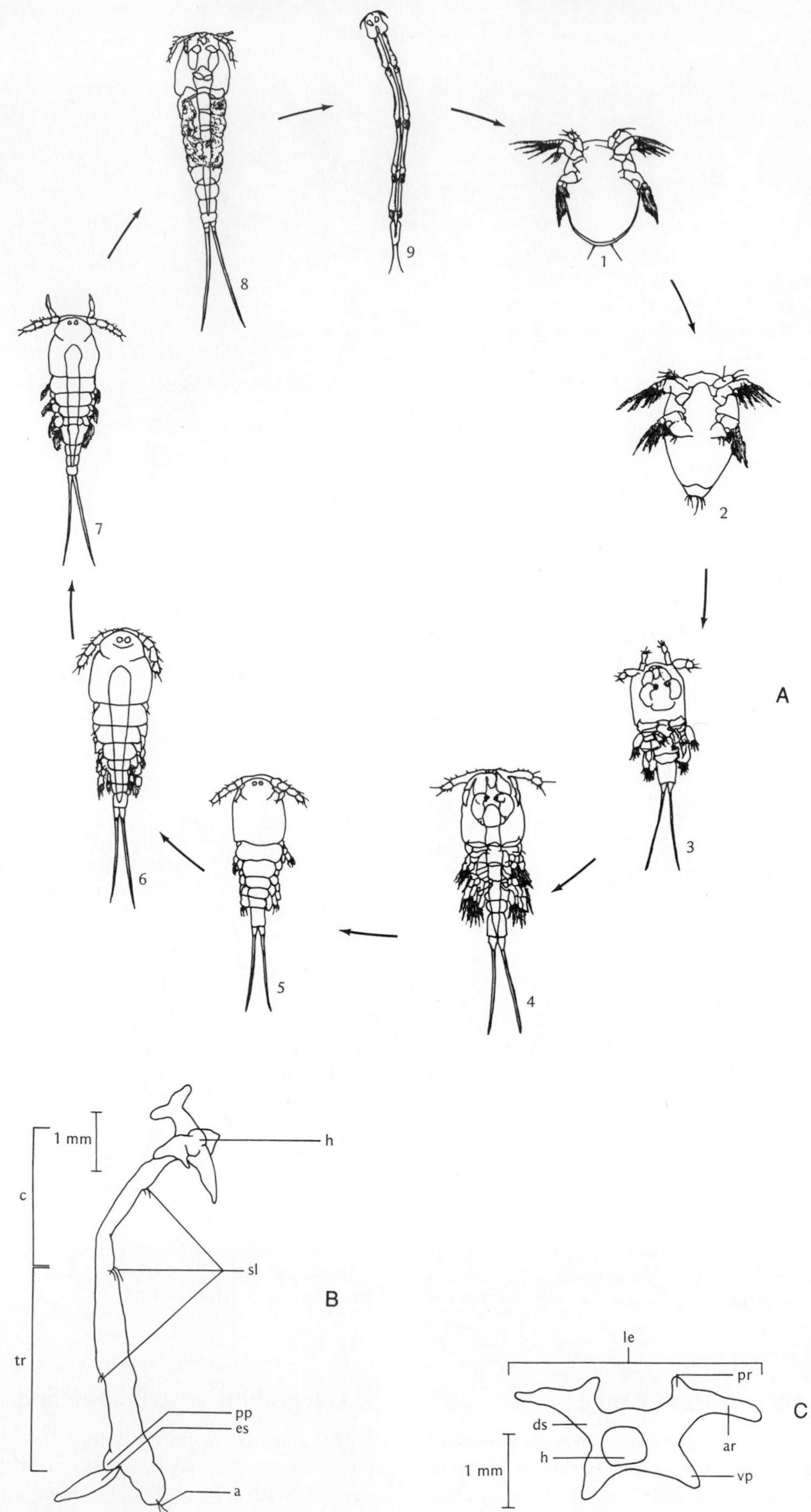
9
8
1
7
2
A
3
6
5
4
1 mm
h
c
sl
B
tr
pp
es
a
le
pr
ds
ar
C
h
1 mm
vp

massive fish kills; in one outbreak 18 tons of carp and 2 tons of goldfish were killed in a two-week period.

Morphology

All stages except the parasitic females have typical copepod structure (Fig. 42.3A) and are free living. The parasitic female embeds her anterior end in fish flesh and grows from about 1.5 mm to over 10 mm in length in about a week. Mature females (Fig. 42.3B) lose virtually all resemblance to copepods because growth does not involve mouthparts or swimming legs. The first thoracic segment enlarges greatly, forming the "anchor," which permanently secures the parasite in the host tissues. The anchor consists of two ventral processes and two branched dorsal processes (Fig. 42.3C). All thoracic segments enlarge greatly, but the swimming legs do not, so that the legs become difficult to see and the female takes on a wormlike appearance. Mature females have two egg sacs immediately posterior to the pregenital prominence.

Life Cycle

There are three naupliar stages, five copepod stages, a preadult, and an adult stage in the life cycle (Fig. 42.3). Earlier literature suggested that two hosts were needed to complete the life cycle, but in more recent studies both copepodid and adult females were found on the same host, suggesting that at least some can complete the life cycle on one host. In cooler climates there may be only a single generation per year, whereas in warmer climates the life cycle can be completed in 12 to 14 days.

Diagnosis

Anchor worms can be seen with the naked eye as they protrude from various sites on fishes.

Host–Parasite Interactions

Anchor worm infections produce lesions in fish and amphibia ranging from slight to fatal. The head and anchor of adult females are surrounded by host connective tissue. Hemorrhage and ulceration are common; major injury is caused by loss of blood and by secondary infection with bacteria, fungi, and other organisms. The degree of injury depends on the number of parasites and their attachment sites. Amphibian infections elicit similar responses, except that there is no integumental encapsulation.

Treatment, Epidemiology, and Control

Although control is not easy, some steps can be taken to reduce losses:

1. Chemical control
2. Inspection of introduced fish
3. Cleaning the environment once an outbreak has occurred

Anchor worm infections usually result in a single parasite per host fish in flowing rivers and streams and there is little damage, but in closed environments severe infections often result. A number of chemicals kill larvae, but there is no successful treatment for infections with adult females. Thus, prevention is most important; breeding stock should be examined carefully before introducing them into ponds or hatcheries, and stock fish should be isolated from contaminated waters. Once infections are present, waterways must be drained, chemically treated, and all parasitized fishes destroyed.

Name of Organism and Disease Associations

Salmincola edwardsi causes gill maggot.

Hosts and Host Range

The principal host in North America is the brook trout, *Salvelinus fontinalis*; infections of many other salmonid fishes are reported worldwide. Like other members of the genus, *S. edwardsi* is a parasite of freshwater fishes, but has been recovered from anadromous fishes when they migrate to salt water. The parasite is found on gills, in the gill cavity, and rarely in other sites.

Geographic Distribution and Importance

Most members of the genus *Salmincola* have little worldwide economic significance, but *S. edwardsi* causes serious damage and has forced the closure of fish hatcheries in the United States.

FIGURE 42.3 *Laernaea cyprinacea:* (A) larva, (B) adult female, (C) anchor of adult female. [(A) Redrawn from Bauer, 1962; (B, C) from Demaree, 1967.]

Morphology

Like *Lernaea*, the parasitic adult female of *Salmincola* bears little resemblance to a crustacean. She, too, is permanently anchored to her host. Her anchor, called a *bulla*, is secreted from glands in her head and maxillae. The enlarged maxillae then fuse with the bulla, creating the permanent attachment (Fig. 42.4). Only the bulla is inside the host; the remainder of the parasite is external, including the movable cephalothorax used for "grazing" on host tissues. There is no obvious external segmentation. The males are much smaller than the females, about 0.5 mm, and are not attached with bullae. The unique larva, called a chalimus, is described in the following section.

Life Cycle

The life cycle of *Salmincola edwardsi* consists of a nauplius, which develops inside the egg, several copepodid stages (chalimus), and the adult. After hatching, the nauplius molts to the free-swimming copepodid stage. This larva spends the daylight hours near the water surface and nighttime near the bottom, a behavior which coincides with that of the brook trout. Upon contact with a fish, the parasite crawls into the gill cavity, rasps a hole in the host tissues with its mouthparts, and then forces the end of the frontal or attachment filament into the cavity. Gluelike secretions of the filament together with the regenerating tissues of the host soon anchor the parasite. The attached larva, the chalimus larva (Fig. 42.5), undergoes several molts while attached by the frontal filament; it loses its segmentation and plumose swimming feet. It takes about 10 days to reach sexual maturity, at which time the males detach from their frontal filaments. A male grasps a female with second maxillae and maxillipeds, and transfers packets of sperm (spermatophores) to her. The male then drops off and dies, while the female breaks free from the frontal filament, secretes a bulla, places it in gill tissue, and attaches her second maxillae to it. The female then develops two egg sacs, which produce nauplii.

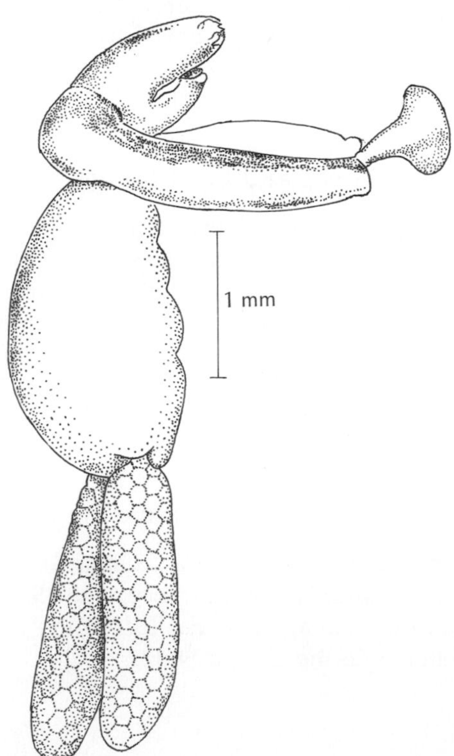

FIGURE 42.4 Female of *Salmincola* sp. with bulla. [Redrawn from Wilson, 1915.]

Epidemiology and Control

S. edwardsi usually presents problems only in restricted environments such as fish ponds and hatcheries. Recommendations for control include using sand filters to catch free copepods as the water enters the empoundment, washing the fish fry in salt solutions, destroying infected adult fish, and introducing small fish such as *Gambusia* and *Notropis* to feed on the free-swimming copepods. There is no satisfactory treatment for adult females, but a number of chemicals including formalin and copper sulfate kill larvae.

There are many other parasitic copepods, often with

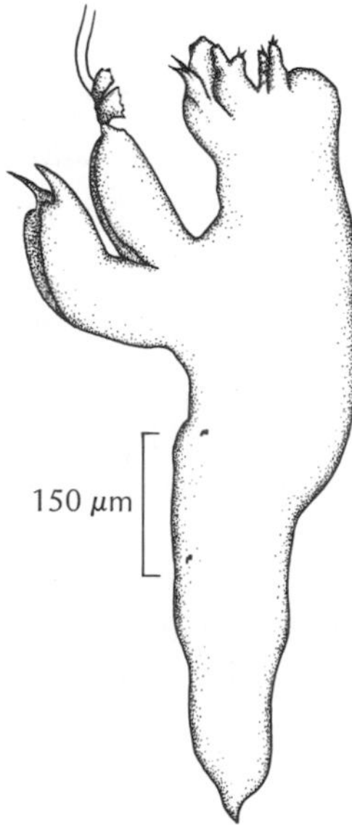

FIGURE 42.5 Chalimus larva attached to its host. [Redrawn with modifications from Kabata and Cousens, 1973.]

bizarre shapes, but the same principles apply to them as well.

CLASS BRANCHIURA

The class Branchiura is a group of about 150 species of bloodsucking ectoparasites that infect the skin and gills of freshwater and marine fishes as well as amphibians. Like the parasitic copepods just mentioned, some branchiurans, such as the cosmopolitan *Argulus* spp., cause serious disease and often death to fishes in hatcheries and ponds.

There are a number of differences between the class Copepoda and the class Branchiura. Branchiurans have compound eyes and a large, shieldlike carapace covering the head and thorax; they are not permanently attached to their host and continue to molt after sexual maturity.

The fish louse, *Argulus* spp., holds onto a host with two sucking disks, which are modifications of the second maxillae (Fig. 42.6). The proboscis penetrates the skin, and the parasite ingests host blood and also apparently injects toxic substances from glands near the stylet or sting (Fig. 42.6). After copulation, the *Argulus* female leaves the host and lays eggs on any submerged surface. Embryonic development lasts from 15 to 55 days, depending on the temperature. The newly hatched larva must find a host within three days or it dies.

Certain features of *Argulus* biology make control possible. The parasite cannot tolerate high oxygen tensions; thus a high rate of water flow through a rearing pond is a useful control measure. Placing removable boards as substrates for *Argulus* egg clutches also helps. Many antiparasitic chemicals have been employed successfully against *Argulus* spp.

CLASS CIRRIPEDIA

The class Cirripedia is the only group of sessile crustaceans, other than the various parasitic species in other classes. Best known are the barnacles that live

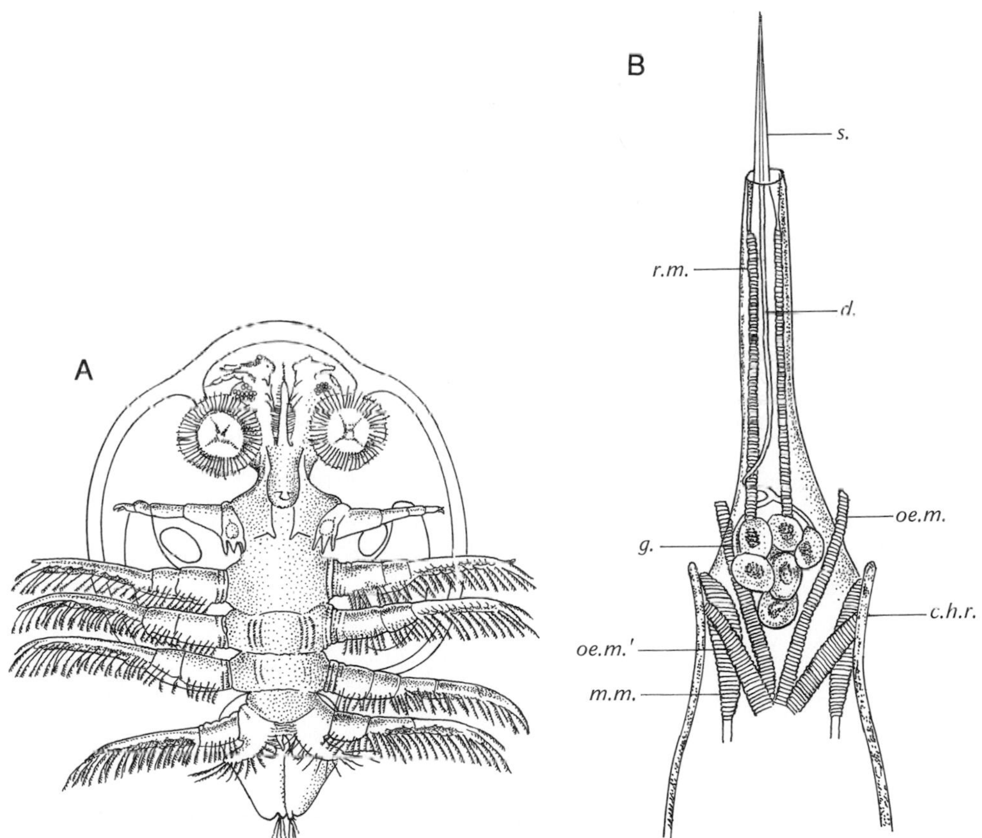

FIGURE 42.6 *Argulus versicolor:* (A) female, (B) sting. Abbreviations: c.h.r., chitin rib of proboscis; d, ducts of poison glands; g, poison gland; m.m, mandible muscle; oe.m, esophageal muscle; oe.m′, side esophageal muscle; r.m., retractor muscle; s, sting. [Redrawn from Wilson, 1904.]

attached to rocks and the undersides of ships. With their attached mode of existence, it is not surprising that a number of these organisms have evolved parasitic life-styles.

The cirripeds are attached to the substrate by their antennules; they literally stand on their heads. There are no compound eyes. The carapace is a fleshy covering or mantle that may have calcareous plates, as in the barnacles. The body usually has six pairs of biramous, jointed appendages, called the *cirri.* Most are hermaphroditic.

Some parasitic cirripeds such as *Sacculina*, a parasite of the shorecrab, lose all appendages and segmentation as adults. The larva, called a cypris (Fig. 42.7), attaches to a host using its first antennae, the host tegument is perforated, and a simple cell mass, the kentrogen, is injected into the host. This cell mass sends nutrient absorbing rhizoids throughout the crab's abdomen (Fig. 42.7). Then a male cyprid larva attaches and injects cells into the cell mass, thereby converting the female into a hermaphrodite. Because of the spread of parasite rhizoids, infected crabs often are unable to molt and their gonads are usually destroyed.

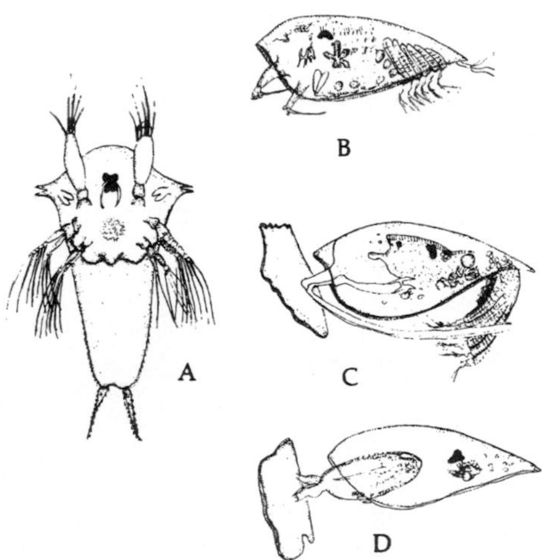

FIGURE 42.7 Early stages in the life cycle of the cirriped, *Sacculina* sp. (A) Nauplius larva; (B) Cypris larva; (C) Cypris attaching to a new host by means of its antennae and shedding its locomotory appendages; (D) Kentrogen stage and the beginning of invasion of its crustacean host. [Redrawn from Delage, Y., 1884.]

CLASS MALACOSTRACA

The large crustaceans of the class Malacostraca have only a few parasitic species. Most are isopods; a few are amphipods and decapods. Some cause economic losses to commercial fisheries, but as a group little is known about their biology and effects on their hosts.

Readings

Bauer, O. N. (1962). The ecology of parasites of freshwater fish, P. S. T. Cat. No. 622. Office of Tech. Services, U.S. Dept. of Commerce. [Translated from Russian; *Bull. State Sci. Res. Inst. Lake River Fish.* **49,** 3–216, 1959]

Bliss, D. E. (Ed.) (1982–1985). *The Biology of the Crustacea*, 10 Vols. Academic Press, New York.

Delage, Y. (1884). Évolution de la sacculine (*Sacculina carcini* Thomps.) crustacé endoparasite de l'ordře nouveau des rentrogonides. *Arch. Zool. Exp. Gen.* **2,** 417–736.

Demaree, R. S., Jr. (1967). Ecology and external morphology of *Lernaea cyprinacea. Am. Mid. Nat.* **78,** 416–427.

Emerson, M. J., and Schram, F. R. (1990). The origin of crustacean biramous appendages and the evolution of the Arthropoda. *Science* **250,** 667–669.

Hoffman, G. L., and Meyer, F. P. (1974). *Parasites of Freshwater Fishes.* T. F. H., Neptune City, NJ.

Kabata, Z. (1970). *Diseases of Fishes. Book 1: Crustacea as Enemies of Fishes.* T. F. H., Jersey City, NJ.

Kabata, Z. (1981). Copepoda (Crustacea) parasitic on fishes: Problems and perspectives. *Adv. Parasitol.* **19,** 1–71.

Kabata, Z., and Cousens, B. (1973). Life cycle of *Salmincola californiensis* (Dana, 1852) (Copepoda: Lernaeopodidae). *J. Fish. Res. Bd. Canada.* **30,** 881–903.

Reinhard, E. G. (1956). Parasitic castration of crustacea. *Exp. Parasitol.* **5,** 79–107.

Schram, F. R. (1986). *Crustacea.* Oxford Univ. Press, Oxford.

Wilson, C. B. (1904). A new species of *Argulus,* with a more complete account of two species already described. *Proc. U.S. Nat. Mus.* **27,** 627–655.

Wilson, C. B. (1911). North American parasitic copepods belonging to the family Ergasilidae. *Proc. U.S. Nat. Mus.* **39,** 263–400.

Wilson, C. B. (1915). North American parasitic copepods belonging to the Lernaeopodidae, with a revision of the entire family. *Proc. U.S. Nat. Mus.* **47,** 565–729.

Yamaguti, S. (1963). *Parasitic Copepoda and Branchiura of Fishes.* Interscience, New York.

CHAPTER

43

Introduction to the Insects

Insects comprise an important part of the biological world in all biomes. The tropics are oftentimes thought of as the typical biotope that has insects both large in size as well as numbers. Although this is true, by and large, insects also play an important role in the biology of the area at the other extreme, the Arctic. In cold climates, insects are especially opportunistic and develop in extraordinary numbers during a short summer season. In the Arctic, mosquitoes rise in hordes from the tundra making life for humans uncomfortable at best and unbearable at other times.

In the context of ways in which animals may use their resources in reproduction, insects are r-selected; there are only a few exceptions such as the tsetse, which transmit African trypanosomosis. Animals that are r-selected place their resources of energy and protein into a large number of rapidly growing, independent offspring. In opposition, K-selected animals produce a small number of large offspring, which may require extended parental nurture.

Mosquitoes are a good example of r-selection, because large numbers of eggs hatch to produce rapidly growing larvae and then adults become sexually mature within a few days of emergence, but they soon die. As a dramatic example, if one pair of houseflies were to reproduce and all of their offspring were to survive and reproduce during one summer in southern California, the earth would be 47 feet deep in houseflies (recounted in the 1961 edition of Herms and James). While this example results only from an interesting calculation, it does represent the potential of an r-selected species.

Insects are also clearly in a state of rapid evolution. They have invaded every free-living ecological niche imaginable as well as many parasitic niches. Except for birds and a few mammals, the insects have been the most successful group in the aerial niche. It is estimated that there are probably a million species of insects. Likewise, at the species level, many, such as in mosquitoes, are lumped into species complexes because they cannot readily be distinguished morphologically from one another.

Adaptable, opportunistic, ubiquitous, insects are both beneficial and harmful to human activities. We depend on them for pollination of many crops such as fruit trees and alfalfa grown for seed. Insects prey on other harmful insects, they serve as recycling centers for organic materials, and they are the principal food for many fish.

Even so, these beautiful creatures are generally thought of only for the direct or indirect harm that they do to humans. They destroy crops, transmit disease agents, and are pests that suck blood and invade households. In this book, we discuss those insects that are parasitic or are vectors of disease agents; however, whatever their importance, these harmful insects are only a small part of the biota.

MORPHOLOGY OF CLASS INSECTEA

The insects share with the other members of the phylum Arthopoda (1) a segmented exoskeleton with jointed legs, (2) an open circulatory system with a dorsal heart, and (3) paired, ventral nerve chords. They are differentiated from other members of the phylum by having (1) three distinct body segments: the head, thorax, and abdomen, (2) a single pair of antennae, and

(3) three pairs of legs (Fig. 43.1). Wings are present in most adults and they arise as extensions of the body wall on the meso- and metathorax. The legs all have the same parts, starting at the body: coxa, trochanter, femur, tibia, and tarsi.

Eyes and Sense Organs

The eyes of insects consist of a pair of compound eyes and as many as three simple eyes. The compound eyes are usually conspicuous and consist of a cluster of individual light-sensing units, the ommatidia. A pair of simple eyes are located near the medial margin of the compound eyes on the midline of the head; a third simple eye may be located on the midline of the head as in the grasshopper. Other sense organs that may be present are sound receptors, the tympanum on the first abdominal segment of the grasshopper; the halteres are modified hindwings in the Diptera. Insects rely not only on sight but also on air movement and the ability to detect tiny quantities of chemicals in the air and on the surface where they feed. Antennae and portions of the mouthparts are the organs principally used in these activities. Their ability to find one another for mating is dependent on an ability to detect minute quantities of pheromones.

Wings

Most of the highly evolved insects have two pairs of wings, and insects are the most successful of all animal groups in taking to the air. Wings of all insects arise on the meso- and metathorax (Fig. 43.1). Wings probably arose in stream insects such as the mayflies (order Ephemeroptera) or the stone flies (order Plecoptera) in which rudimentary extensions of the body wall served as stabilizers in the current of water. In extant species, functional wings occur only in the adult stage and once an insect has developed functional wings, it does not molt again (with the exception of a few Ephemeroptera). The wings are moved by muscles that deform the body wall and cause the wings to pivot in the exoskeleton (Fig. 43.2).

Mouthparts

Feeding structures in insects take many forms. A generalized type of mouthpart can be seen in the grasshopper (order Orthoptera) (Fig. 43.3). In this type of chewing mouthpart, there are strong laterally cutting mandibles and the principal food is plant material that is cut into small pieces and then passed to the mouth. This rather basic type has been modified into a variety

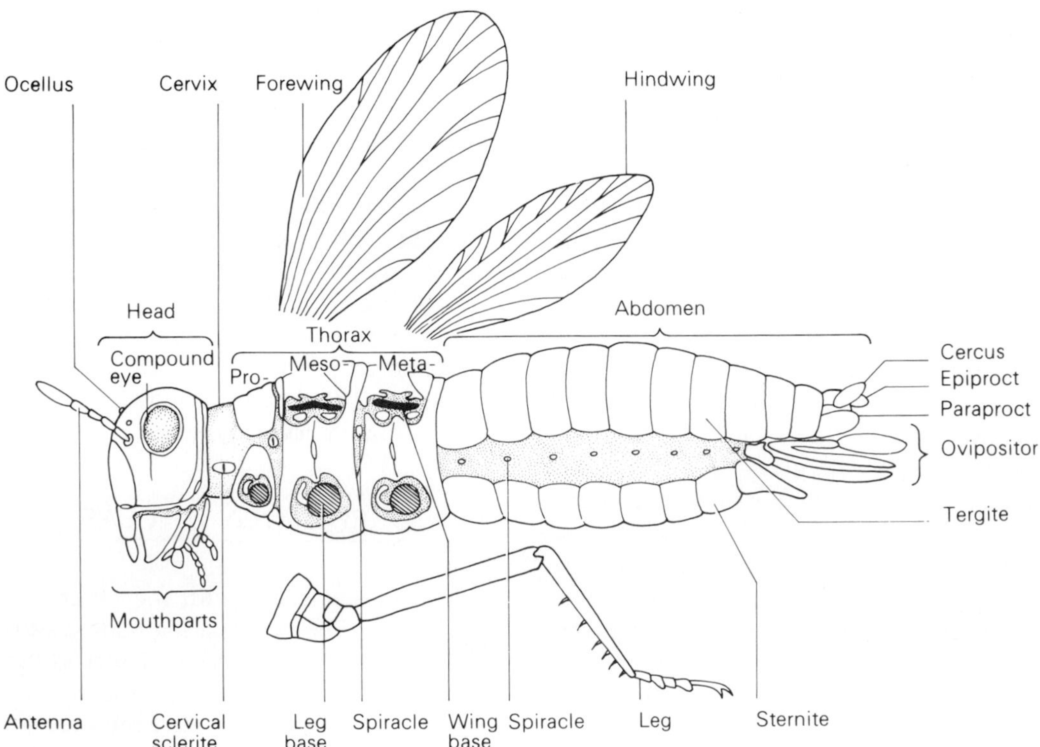

FIGURE 43.1 Generalized adult, winged insect. [From Romoser and Stofollano, 1994.]

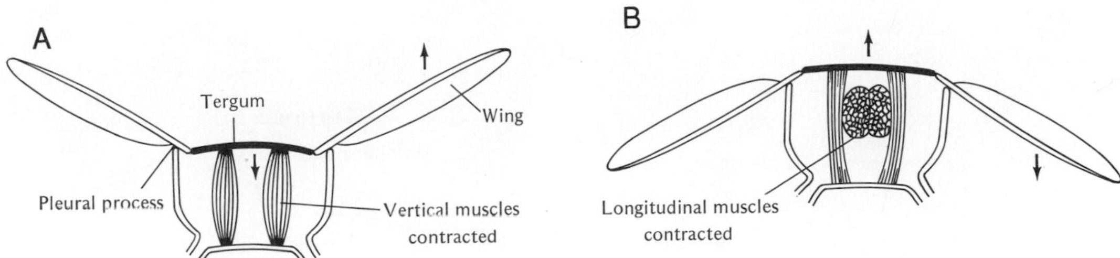

FIGURE 43.2 Simplified musculature and wing movement in an insect. The wings are extensions of the body wall and the muscles deform the exoskeleton to cause the wings to pivot upward or downward. [Redrawn with modifications from Snodgrass, 1935.]

of other types depending on the food of the taxonomic group.

In insects with sucking mouthparts such as the sucking lice, Hemiptera, and mosquitoes, the mouthparts become elongated so as to pierce the integument of the plant or animal on which they feed; however, there is elaboration of different elements in different groups. For example, in female mosquitoes, the mandibles and maxillae are designed for cutting and piercing (Fig. 43.4C and D). In the kissing bugs of the order Hemiptera, the mandibles are short and lock the mouthparts in the skin while the maxillae thrust deeply into the skin to tap a capillary (Fig. 43. 4A and B). In the sucking lice and male mosquitoes the mandibles are vestigial. In a few groups such as the mayflies, plecoptera, and cattle grubs, mouthparts are vestigial in the adults; they survive on stored food from the preadult stages.

Houseflies have a further modification for ob-

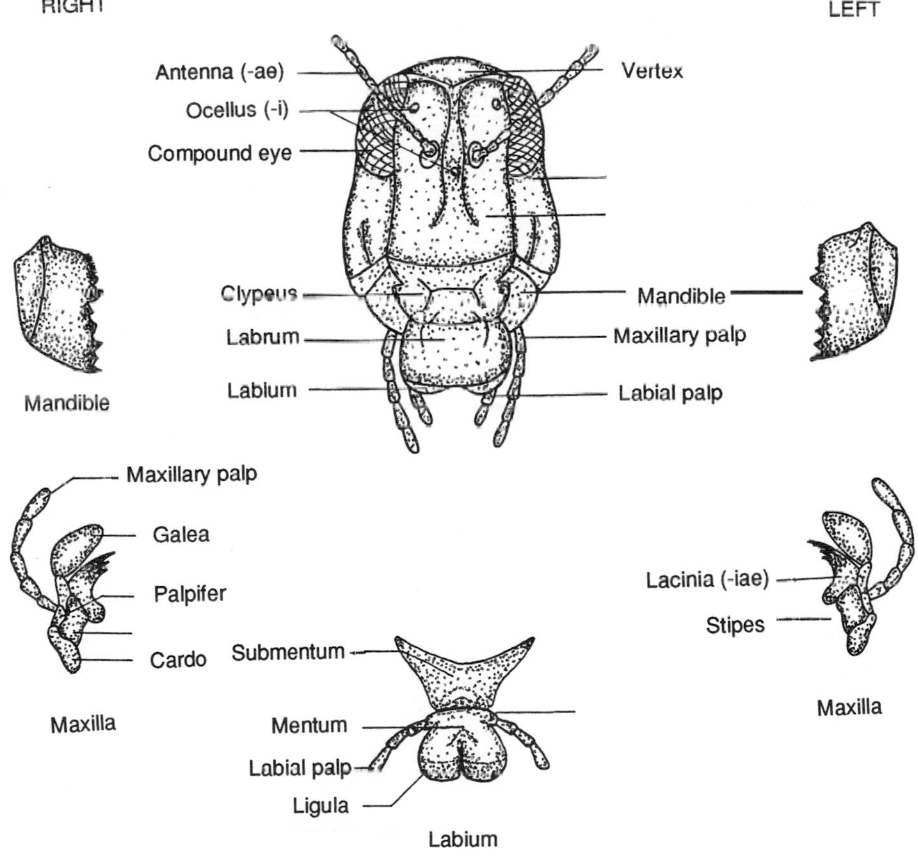

FIGURE 43.3 Mouthparts of a grasshopper. The grasshopper has rather generalized mouthparts; all of the parts shown here are retained in bloodsucking insects but are modified for piercing and taking liquid rather than cutting.

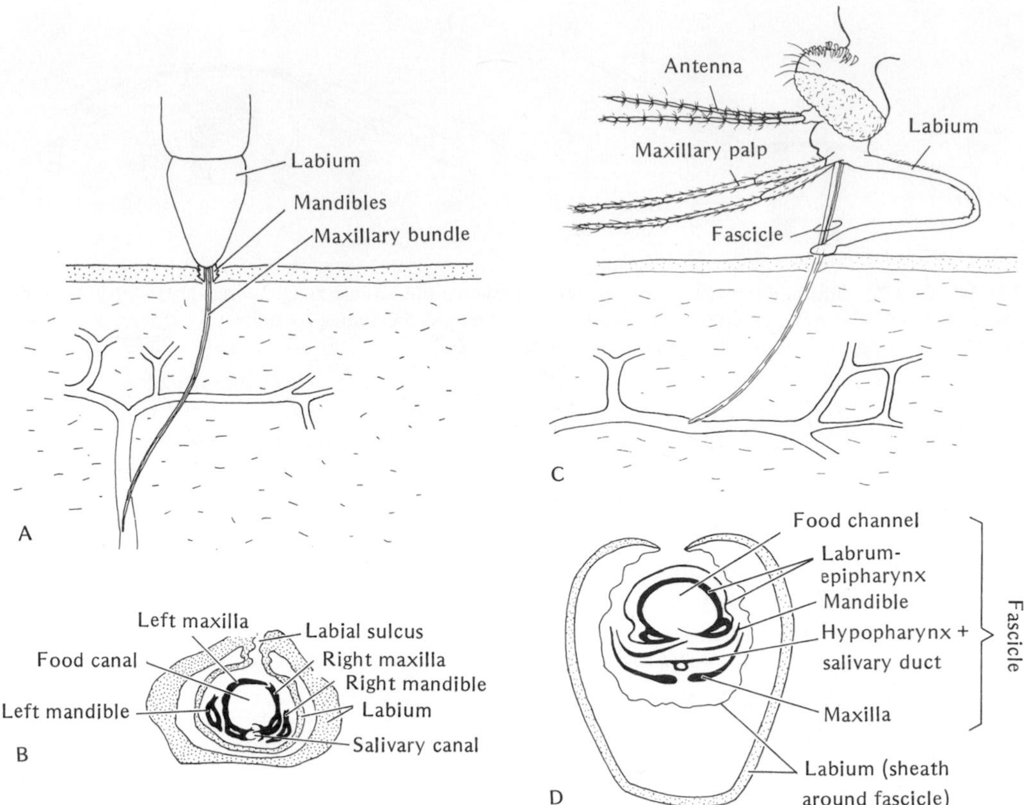

FIGURE 43.4 Mouthparts of two bloodsucking insects. (A and B) The kissing bug *Rhodnius.* (C and D) A mosquito. [Redrawn from Harwood & James, 1979.]

taining liquid food through the development of a large labellum (Fig. 43.5). The grooved lower portion of the labellum moves liquid food to the mouth by capillary action; these are sponging or mopping mouthparts.

Two main points should be kept in mind: (1) mouthparts and the type of food are inextricably bound together, and (2) convergent evolution has acted so that different groups of insects have achieved the same functional end by developing different portions of the basic mouthparts.

Intestinal Tract

The intestinal tracts of insects are all basically the same (Fig. 43.6). The gut has three sections:

1. Foregut, which includes the mouth, pharynx, esophagus, crop, and proventriculus
2. Midgut or stomach
3. Hindgut, which includes the ileum, colon, rectum, and anus

The foregut serves principally to store food for short period.

Digestion and absorption of food take place in the midgut. In the midgut, a peritrophic matrix (PM) (previously called the peritrophic membrane), containing chitin, protein, and carbohydrate, envelopes the food. In insects such as the grasshopper, which feed more or less continuously, the PM is formed continuously and is termed the PM2 (Fig. 43.7). The other type, the PM1, is found in insects such as bloodsucking Diptera, which feed to repletion and then do not feed again for some days. The PM1 is formed in response to distention of the midgut; it has been found that injection of a saline solution (or even air) rectally causes the formation of the PM.

The PM may begin to form in as few as two minutes in black flies or as long as 12 hours in *Anopheles stephensi*, an important vector of human malaria in India. It may require as long as 48 hours for the complete maturation of the PM, but in most bloodsucking insects it takes more or less a day.

The PM isolates the food bolus so that digestion can take place efficiently. Enzymes are induced by the presence of food and they enter the bolus to begin preliminary digestion. Partially digested nutrients move through the PM and are absorbed. As in verte-

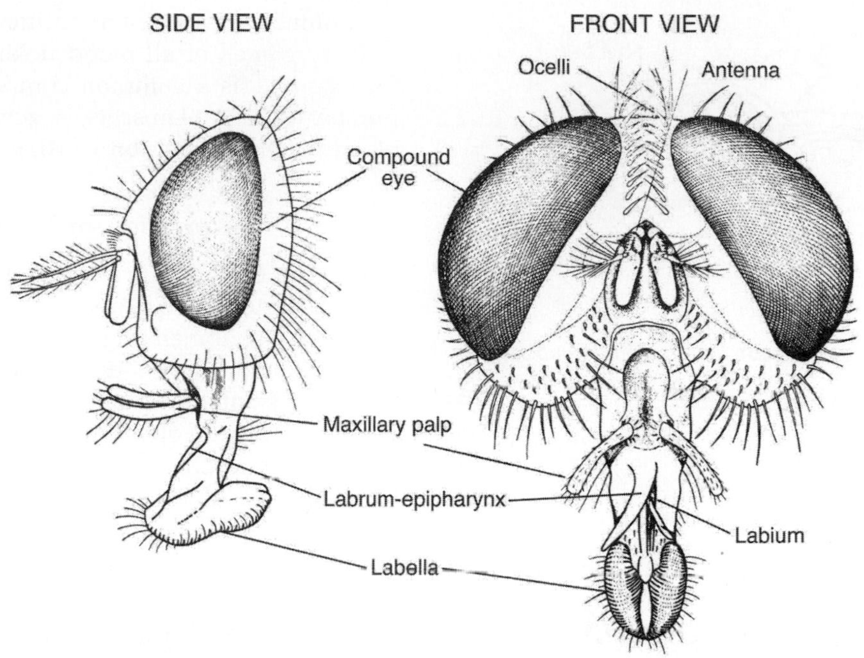

FIGURE 43.5 Head and mouthparts of a housefly. These are sponging type mouthparts; liquid is taken up by the labellum and passed to the mouth. [From Harwood and James, 1979.]

brates, a variety of hormones regulate intestinal function in insects.

In the context of vector biology, the PM is crucial in gaining an understanding of whether a particular agent will or will not infect the vector. The PM serves principally as a barrier to infection for those agents that are ingested with a blood meal. In a motile organism such as an L_3 of *Onchocerca volvulus*, the worm can escape from the food bolus before the PM forms. Viruses are small enough to move through the matrix and infect the cells of the intestine as soon as water is withdrawn from the blood meal. In the case of the ookinete of malaria, it must move on its own to the midgut cells where it squeezes between cells to form

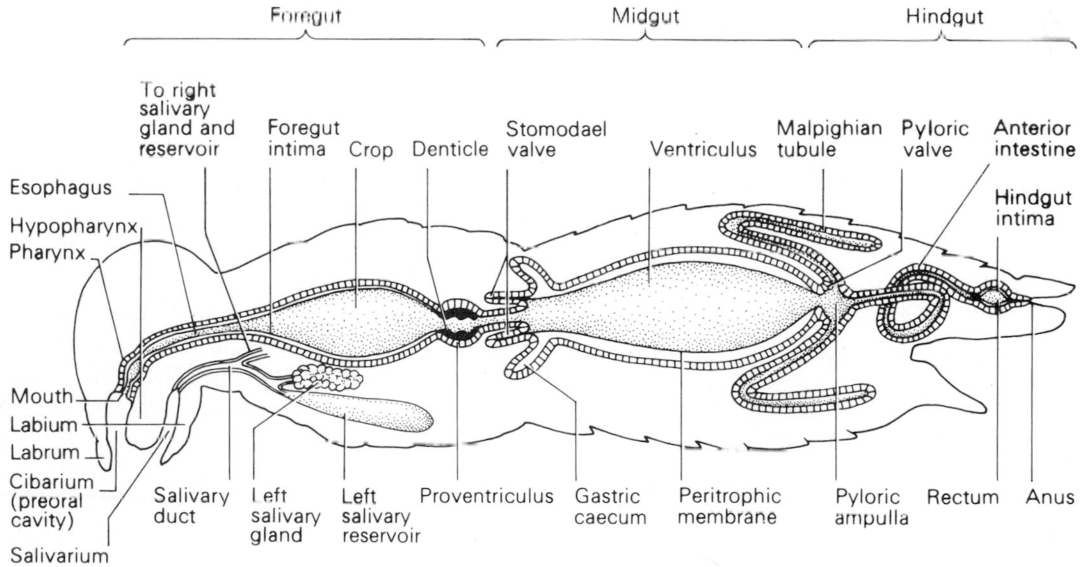

FIGURE 43.6 Intestinal tract of a generalized insect. [From Rosomer and Stofollano, 1994.]

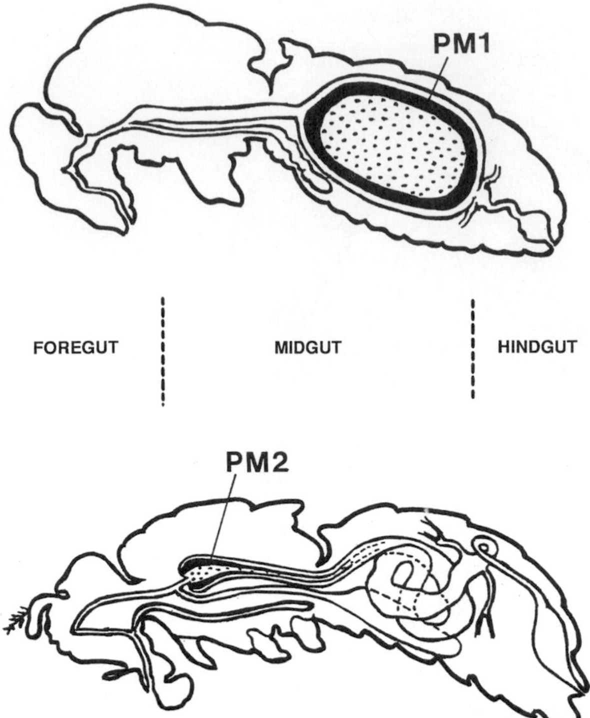

FIGURE 43.7 Outline drawings of insects showing the two types of peritrophic matrices. (A) is a peritrophic matrix type 1 or PM1 and (B) is a PM2. PM2 is probably the primitive type; it is formed from cells in the cardia of the stomach and is produced continuously. The PM1 is formed in those insects that take blood in response to distention of the midgut. [Drawings courtesy of Dr. Marcelo Jacobs-Lorena.]

the oocyst (Chapter14). (See Jacobs-Lorena and Oo in Beaty and Marquardt, 1996, for a detailed discussion of the PM.)

The hindgut, like the foregut, is lined with chitin and holds undigested food until it is evacuated. The Malpighian tubules, which are located at the junction of the midgut and the hindgut, serve in osmoregulation. A blood meal contains a great deal of water, and the Malpighian tubules eliminate water and concentrate the nutrients. The Malpighian tubules also excrete the end products of nitrogen metabolism. Uric acid is the most commonly formed, but other nitrogenous compounds are also excreted in certain insects.

Salivary Glands

The salivary glands of bloodsucking insects are of interest because of their role in transmission of infectious agents and in immunity developed by vertebrate hosts to the components of saliva. The obverse is that salivary components may inhibit the development of immunity to an introduced infectious agent as in hard ticks.

A number of molecular entities are secreted by the salivary glands of all bloodsucking insects. Apyrase, for example, is a common component of saliva in a number of taxa of insects; it acts at the level of the blood platelets to inhibit clotting.

Respiration or Ventilation

Gaseous exchange in insects takes place through the tracheal system, which opens through pores along the sides of the abdomen (Figs. 43.1 and 43.8). The tracheal system extends throughout the body of the insect ramifying into smaller and smaller tubules. In some larval forms, the tracheal openings are located at the posterior end, as in housefly larvae. In some preadult insects, such as naiads of mayflies or aquatic larvae of dobsonflies, gills serve in gaseous exchange. The so-called gills of mosquito larvae function in ionic regulation.

Reproduction

Insects are dioecious, although some, such as aphids, reproduce parthenogenetically during a portion of the life cycle. Sexual maturity is reached after the final molt.

Some insects copulate, oviposit, and die within a day or two of emerging as adults. This is striking the case with mayflies, which often emerge from the water in hordes and then are gone within a week or so. But others, such as tsetse, the vectors of African sleeping sickness, and the triatomins, which vector the agent causing Chagas' disease, produce offspring for many months. In the latter insect, the female dies after producing her last batch of eggs.

The female reproductive tract has two branches with the ovaries lying at the terminus of each branch. (Fig. 43.9B). Eggs pass down the oviduct and reach the outside through the vagina. The spermatheca stores sperm, and the female usually does not need to be inseminated each time a batch of eggs is laid. In some insects, such the primary screwworm (Chapter 49), females are inseminated only once. Other structures of the female system are the spermathecal gland and accessory glands.

The internal structures of the male system (Fig. 43.9A) are bilaterally symmetrical, with a pair of testes that produce tailed sperm. The sperm pass down the vasa deferentia and are stored temporarily in the seminal vesicles. Sperm are transferred to the female through the ejaculatory duct and the external genitalia. The external genitalia of the males are quite varied, but paired claspers to grasp the female and an intromittent organ to transfer sperm to the female are common. Each group of insects has distinctive structures that

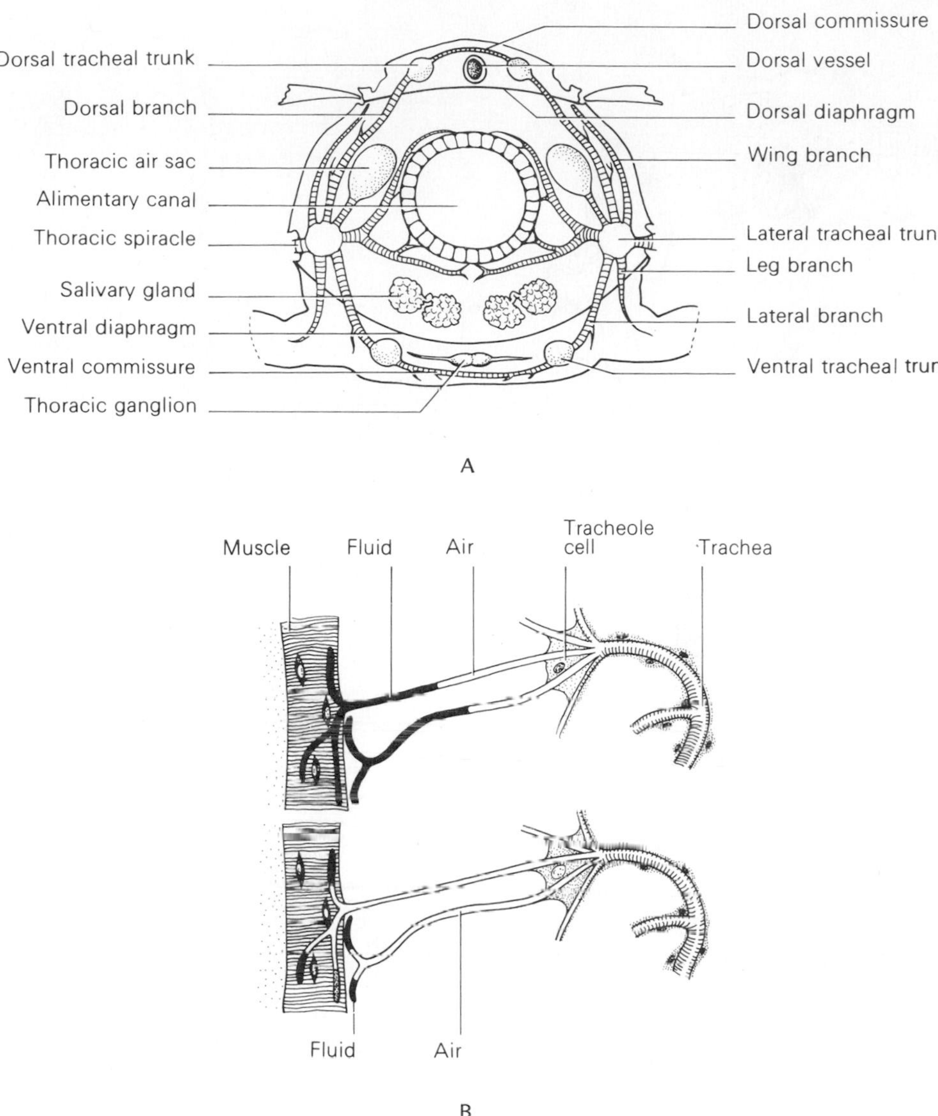

FIGURE 43.8 Tracheal system of a generalized insect. (A) A cross section of an insect body showing the spiracles in the body wall and the tracheae that ramify and extend to all of the body organs. (B) A detail of the close association of the distal tips of the tracheae at muscle cells. The fluid in the tracheoles moves back and forth implementing gaseous exchange. [From Romoser and Stofollano, 1994.]

are sometimes unique to a species. For example, in the *Culex pipiens* complex, the subspecies can be differentiated only on the basis of the male external genitalia. In the fleas, the males have long, elegant penile rods that can be seen coiled in the body of cleared specimens.

Nervous System

The nervous system of insects conforms to the segmental nature of the organisms. There are paired, ventral nerve chords with a large ganglion in each segment (Fig. 43.11). There is strong cephalization in insects and the eyes, antennae, and intestinal tract are well innervated with ganglia in the head (Fig. 43.12). As discussed later, nervous tissue may also produce hormones, and in this case, they indirectly control, molting, and maturation.

CLASSIFICATION AND GROWTH PATTERNS

Insects have three mains patterns of growth, and they are used to distinguish the highest divisions in

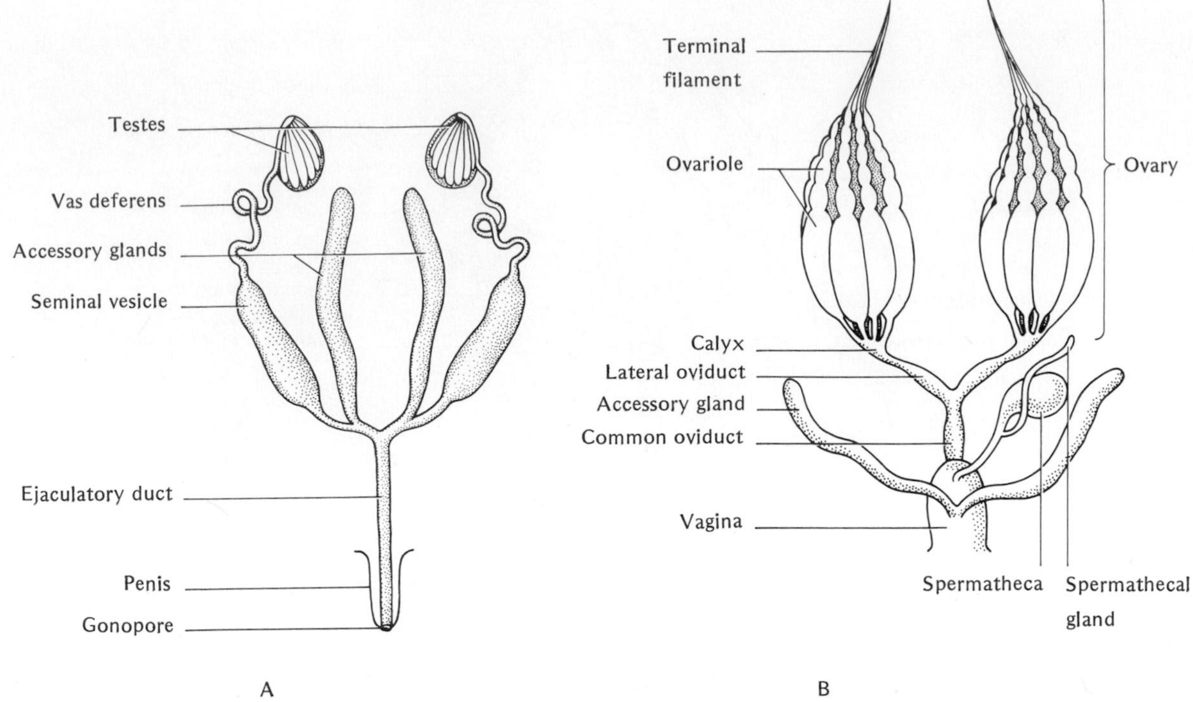

FIGURE 43.9 Reproductive systems of (A) male and (B) female insects. [From Snodgrass, R. E., 1935.]

the class although they are not taxa in the usual sense of the word:

1. *Ametabola.* The early instars are indistinguishable from the later ones except that the organism grows slightly larger with each molt (Fig. 43.10 and Tab. 43.1).
2. *Hemimetabola.* There is a gradual change from the early instars to the final one in which sexual maturity is reached and the wings (when present) are functional (Fig. 43.10 and Tab. 43.1). Body proportions change with each molt, and the wing buds appear some time before the final molt. This series is now often referred to as the Exopteryogota because the wings develop externally.
3. *Holometabola.* There is a striking change from the last larval instar to the adult, and reorganization of the body takes place in a pupa (Fig. 43.10 and Tab. 43.1). A well-known example is a butterfly, which has a series of larval instars during which it grows to the final size. It then forms a pupa (sometimes covered by a cocoon), in which it undergoes dramatic reorganization and emerges as the winged, sexually mature adult. This series is now often referred to as the Endopterygota because the wings develop internally.

At the level of taxonomic order, insects are differentiated on the following features:

1. *Type of metamorphosis.* This can be ametabolic, hemimetabolic, or holometabolic.
2. *Body proportions.* Usually within an order of insects, the proportions of the body are more or less the same and a specimen can be recognized simply by overall appearance.
3. *Wings.* Both the number of wings and their morphology are characteristic for an order. Pairs of wings are 0, 1, or 2 in number. The root "-ptera" often indicates the characteristic for the order. The grasshoppers are in the order Orthoptera and the wings are straight. Diptera have only two wings (one pair). Hymenoptera have membranous wings. In a few instances, some stages or individuals do not have wings, so there can be some inconsistency within an order.
4. *Mouthparts.* Feeding is accomplished by mouthparts that are categorized as (1) cutting, (2) sponging, or (3) sucking. In some orders there is a good deal of variation in mouthparts, as in the Diptera in which they may be sponging, or sucking, or both. In others, such as the Hemiptera and Siphonaptera, there is a remarkable degree of homogeneity and all members have sucking mouthparts.
5. *Antennae.* Insects have a single pair of antennae inserted near the eyes. The general character of the antennae gives an immediate clue to the order in which a specimen belongs. For example, some bees and cyclorraphan flies look much alike, but the bees have long antennae and the flies have short antennae that lie close to the head.

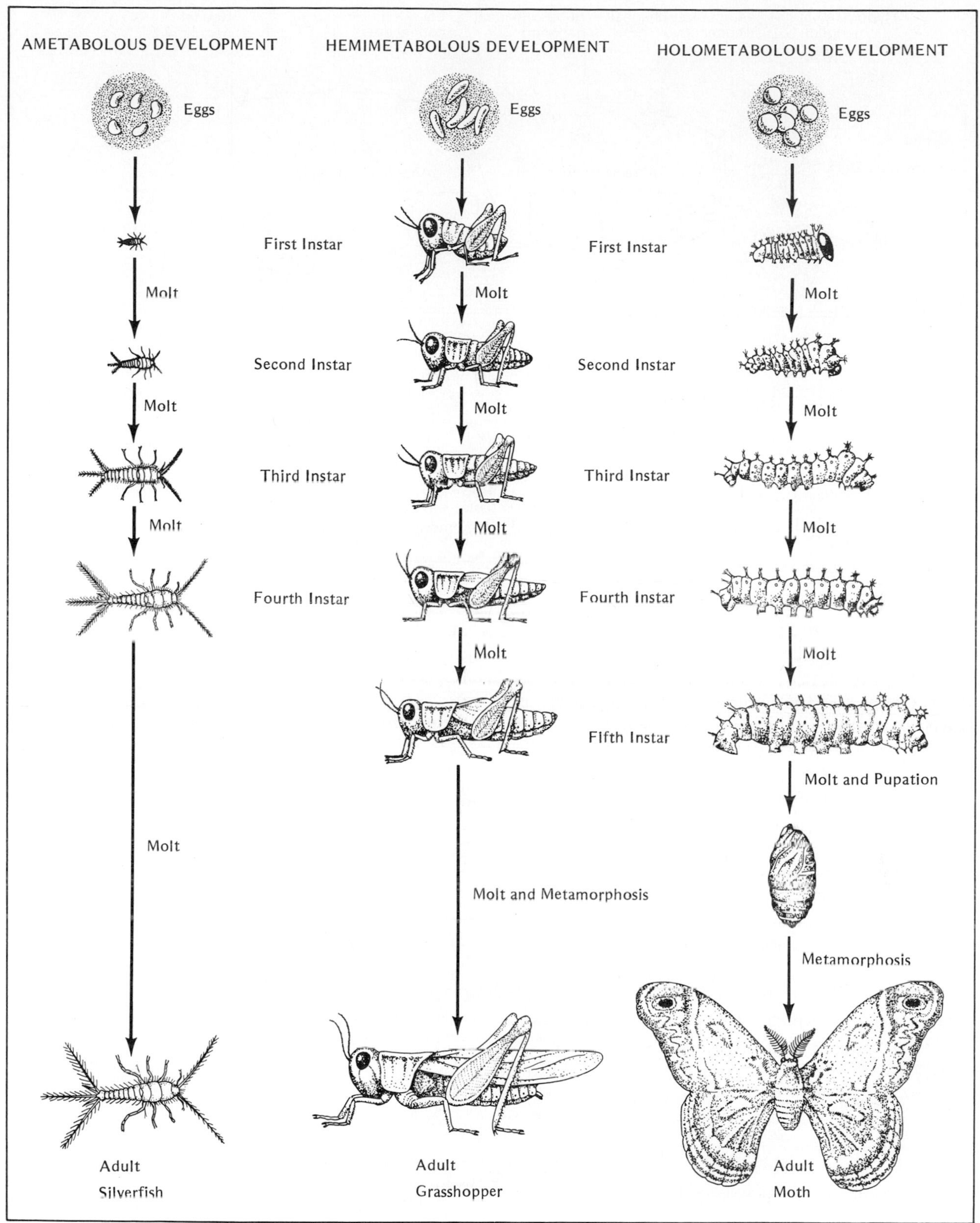

FIGURE 43.10 Patterns of development in insects. [From Herried, 1977.]

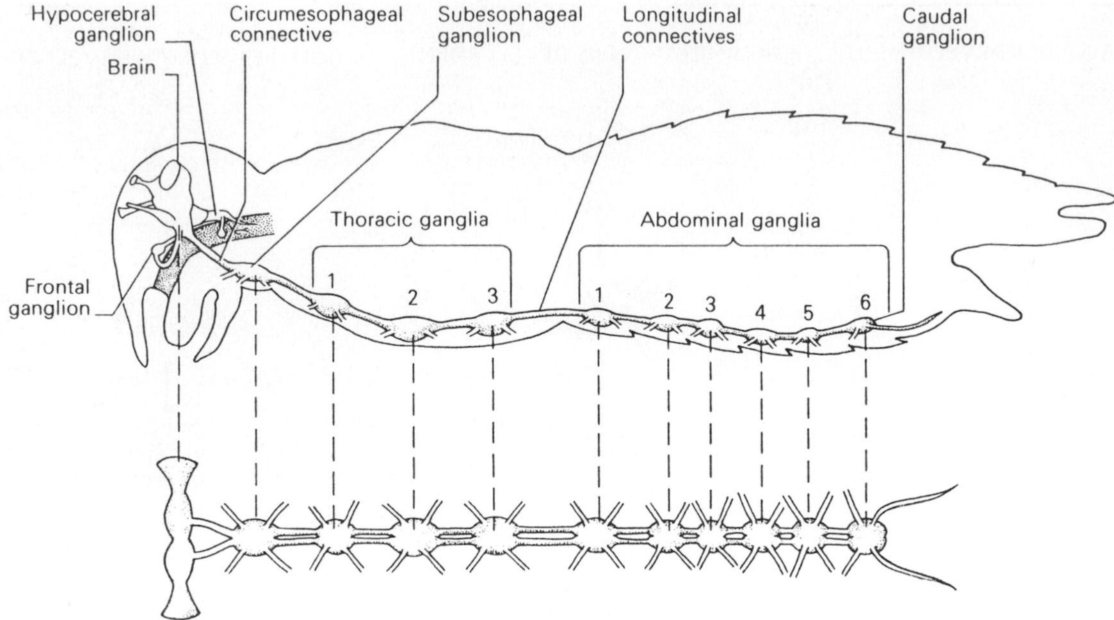

FIGURE 43.11 The nervous system of a generalized insect. A pair of ventral nerve trunks extend throughout the body and have ganglia in each segment. [From Romoser and Stoffolano, 1994.]

6. *Legs.* All insects have the same leg parts (Fig. 43.1). The parts starting proximally and extending distally are coxa, trochanter, femur, tibia, and tarsi. The proportions and some of the details may change from group to group and the number of tarsal segments is somewhat variable.

7. *Eyes.* Most insects have a pair of compound eyes and three simple eyes or ocelli (Fig. 43.1). The size of the eyes relates to the habits of the insect with the bigger one being found in fast-flying species that use their eyes to find prey or hosts on which to feed. Small eyes are found on parasites, such as the Mallophaga

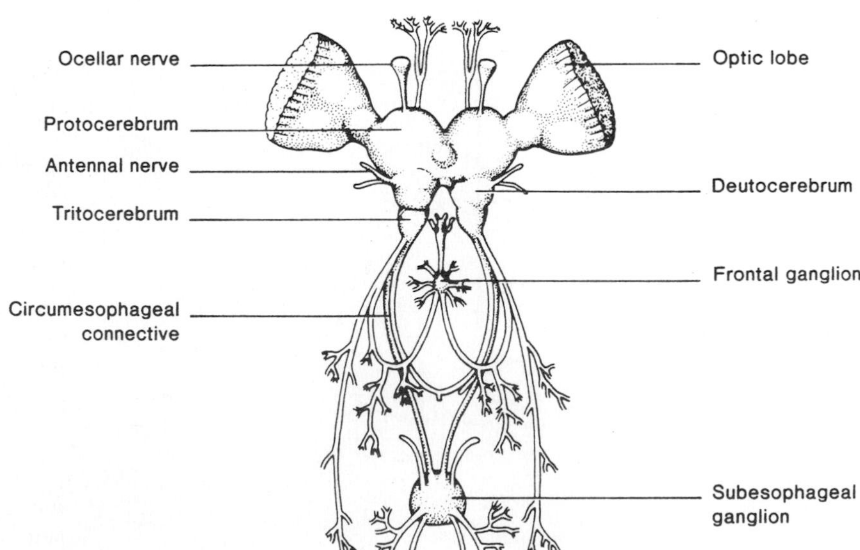

FIGURE 43.12. The brain of an insect. In an animal with strong cephalization, there is a concentration of ganglia associated with the sense organs such as the eyes, and this is the case with insects. Likewise, there are many ganglia and connectives associated with the intestinal system, another major system that requires control and monitoring. [From Romoser and Stoffolano, 1994.]

TABLE 43.1 Characters of Adult Insects at the Level of Taxonomic Order

Metamorphosis and formation of wings	Order and common name	Mouthparts—chewing (c), sucking (s), rasping (r), vestigial (v)	Wings: Fore (FW)	Wings: Hind (HW)	Other characteristics
Ametabola	Protura	C	None		No antennae or true eyes, 1 mm or less long
	Collembola springtail	C	None		Less than 5 mm long, furcula, a springing mechanism under abdomen
	Diplura	C	None		Long antennae, jointed cerci
	Thysanura silverfish bristletail	C	None		Long antennae, abdomen has 11 segments
Hemimetabola or Exopterygota	Odonata dragonfly damselfly	C	Membranous	Membranous	Eyes large, wings membranous with many cross veins, adults strong fliers and predaceous, aquatic nymphs, intermediate hosts of some helminths
			FW and HW nearly identical		
	Ephemeroptera mayfly	C or V	Membranous larger	Membranous smaller	Vestigial mouthparts, two or three long bristles on posterior of adult, aquatic naiads, intermediate hosts of some helminths
	Blattaria cockroach	C	Leathery	Membranous	Pronotum covers head, long antennae, flattened dorsoventrally, household pests, and vectors of disease agents
	Orthoptera grasshopper, cricket walking stick	C	Membranous straight	Membranous straight	Large eyes, variable body form, plant eaters and predators, intermediate hosts of some nematodes
	Dermaptera earwig	C	Hard, short	Membranous, fan-like	Forceps at posterior of abdomen, household pests
	Plecoptera stonefly	C or V	Membranous long, narrow	Membranous shorter, large anal lobe	Elongate, flat, soft body, nymphs aquatic
	Isoptera termite	C	Membranous straight	Membranous straight	Nearly colorless, sexual forms pigmented, colonial with castes, wood eaters
	Embioptera webspinner	C	Membranous	Membranous	Mostly subterranean, in colonies, silk spun from glands on basal segment of first tarsus
			Female wingless, males sometimes		
	Mallopohaga chewing louse	C	None	None	Parasitic, flat dorsoventrally, wide head, intermediate host of one nematode
	Anoplura sucking louse	S	None	None	Parasitic, flat dorso-ventrally, narrow head
	Psocoptera book/bark lice	C	Membranous	Membranous	Less than 5 mm, in debris or under bark; long, slender antennae
			Wings 0 or 4		
	Hemiptera bug	S	Half leathery	Membranous	Predators, plant parasites, hematophagous, base of beak on anterior part of head, triangular scutellum, vectors

(*Continues*)

TABLE 43.1 (*Continued*)

Metamorphosis and formation of wings	Order and common name	Mouthparts—chewing (c), sucking (s), rasping (r), vestigial (v)	Wings: Fore (FW)	Wings: Hind (HW)	Other characteristics
	Homoptera aphid, scale insect stink bug	S	Uniform texture 4,2, or 0		Plant parasites; base of beak near thorax, vectors of plant diseases
	Thysanoptera	R or S	Fringed with hairs, FW		In debris or harmful to plants
Holometabola or Endopterygota	Mecoptera scorpion fly	C Beaklike	Filmy, rooflike FW and HW about same size		Elongate beaklike head predators, scavengers
	Neuroptera lace wing, ant lion dobson fly	C	Filmy, many veins FW and HW about the same		On vegetation, near water, larvae predaceous
	Trichoptera caddis fly	C	Filmy, roofed FW and HW about the same hair coated		Aquatic larva, often in a case
	Lepidoptera moth, butterfly	S C in larva	Covered with scales FW larger		Larva caterpiller, maxilla a coiled proboscis
	Diptera fly, mosquito, midge	S or V	1 or 0 pairs	Halteres	Larva maggot, wide variation in mouthparts and food, vectors
	Siphonaptera flea	S C in larva	0		Adult laterally compressed, many bristles, feed on blood, vectors
	Coleoptera	C	Hard, veinless	Filmy, folded	80K spp., all habitats, intermediate hosts
	Strepsiptera stylops, twisted wing	C	0	In male 0 in female	Parasites of other insects, female maggotlike
	Hymenoptera bee, wasp, ant	C & S	Membranous or 0	Membranous or 0	Constriction between thorax and abdomen, often colonial

BLOOD MEALS

IT IS OBVIOUS THAT the size of an insect limits the size of its blood meal; however, the amount of blood taken between the smallest and the largest of the hematophagous insects is remarkable. This tabulation lists the volumes of blood taken by representatives of various groups of insects.

Taxon	Genus	Length of body in mm	Blood ingested in mg or μl
Psychodidae	*Phlebotomus*	2	0.3– 0.5
Ceratopogonidae	*Leptoconops*	2	0.23
Simuliidae		2–4	1.08–2.36
Anoplura	*Pediculus*	3	1.0
Hemiptera	*Cimex*	3	6.48
Culicidae		4	1–25
Hemiptera	*Triatoma*	5–20	307

It is obvious that the larger the blood meal, the more likely is the transmission of an infectious agent from the vertebrate host to the vector. Especially for those hematophagous arthropods at the lower end of the size spectrum, additional mechanisms have evolved to increase the probability of transmission. For example, in the phlebotomines, their saliva increases the probability of transmission of *Leishmania.* In the simuliids, microfilariae of *Onchocerca* are attracted to the site where the fly is feeding.

or bird lice, that remain on their hosts and do not need to search out a meal.

General evolutionary relations indicate that the insects probably arose from a common ancestor of a highly generalized type. They then diverged into several small side branches and three main stems giving the 26 orders presently accepted by most investigators. An excellent discussion of evolution in the arthropods and insects in particular may be found in Romoser and Stofollano, 1994.

TAXONOMY

A brief characterization the members of the class Insecta is given in Table 43.1. The Ametabola is composed of four orders of rather obscure organisms that seem to have only a tenuous connection to the other members of the class. They develop in such a way that the preadults have the same form as the adults, except for size; nearly all are tiny and usually secretive.

The Hemimetabola, also called the Exopterigota, all have development in which there is a gradual change from the newly hatched nymph (terrestrial) or naiad (aquatic) to the winged adult. Fourteen orders are included in this group. The Holometabola, also called the Endopterigota, contains those orders that have complete development, that is, there are several larval instars followed by a pupal stage in which a complete reorganization takes place before the winged adult emerges from the pupa. Nine orders are included in the Holometabola and many are the most evident and attractive of the insects such as the butterflies and beetles. Likewise, the Diptera and the fleas contain those insects that are most important to humans as vectors of disease agents.

Complete descriptions of the various taxa can be found in any of the general entomology textbooks cited in the Readings section.

Readings

Arnett, R. H. (1985). *American Insects: A Handbook of the Insects of North America.* Van Nostrand–Reinhold, New York.

Beaty, B. J., and Marquardt, W. C. (Eds.) (1996). *The Biology of Disease Vectors.* Univ. Press of Colorado, Niwot.

Borrer, D. J., and White, R. E. (1970). *A Field Guide to the Insects of North America North of Mexico.* Houghton Mifflin, Boston.

Borrer, D. J., Triplehorn, C. A., and Johnson, N. F. (1989). *An Introduction to the Study of Insects,* 6th ed. Saunders, Philadelphia.

Burgess, N. R. H., and Cowan, G. O. (1993). *A Colour Atlas of Medical Entomology.* Chapman & Hall, London.

Harwood, R. F., and James, M. T. (1979). *Entomology in Human and Animal Health,* 7th ed. Macmillan, New York.

Herms, W. B., and James, M. T. (1961). *Medical Entomology,* 5th ed., Macmillan, New York.

Herried, C. F. (1977). *Biology.* Macmillan, New York.

Kettle, D. S. (1995). *Medical and Veterinary Entomology.* CAB International, Wallingford, UK.

Lane, R. P., and Crosskey, R. W. (Eds.) (1993). *Medical Insects and Arachnids.* Chapman & Hall, London.

Lehane, M. J. (1993). *Biology of Blood-Sucking Insects.* Chapman & Hall, New York.

McCafferty, W. P. (1981). *Aquatic Entomology. The Fisherman's and Ecologist's' Illustrated Guide to Insects and Their Relatives.* Jones & Bartlett, Boston.

Romoser, W. S., and Stofollano, J. G. (1994). *The Science of Entomology,* 3rd ed. Brown, Dubuque, IA.

Snodgrass, R. E. (1935). *Principles of Insect Morphology.* McGraw–Hill, New York.

Wall, R., and Shearer, D. (1997). *Veterinary Entomology.* Chapman & Hall, London.

Wikel, S. K. (Ed.) (1996). *The Immunology of Host–Ectoparasite Arthropod Relationships.* CAB International, Wallingford, UK.

CHAPTER

44

Mallophaga and Anoplura: The Lice; and Blattaria: The Cockroaches

The organisms discussed in this chapter are hemimetabolic insects that often are nuisances but can also transmit important diseases of humans and other animals. The lice have a long history of living with humankind and with domestic animals. Their extreme host specificity indicates a long association with their hosts; they probably have been parasites of primates since the Eocene, about 50 million years ago. The cockroaches, likewise, are associates of humankind, but probably did not move in with early humans until they had established more or less permanent homes.

THE LICE

The lice, although quite similar to one another both morphologically and in their life cycles, are placed in two separate orders, the Mallophaga, called the chewing lice or bird lice and the Anoplura, the sucking lice.

Lice are small creatures usually less than 5mm long, and the first instar nymphs are less than 1mm long. They are flattened dorso-ventrally and have many short bristles or setae. Few have much color; they are generally off-white with a few being brownish or reddish. They ordinarily remain at or near the surface of the skin where they feed, copulate, and lay eggs. They have large claws on their tarsi, which they use to remain in place on the host. The Mallophaga have broad heads and strongly sclerotized mandibles, which they use to cut feathers, or skin (Fig 44.1). The Anoplura have elongated heads with the sucking mouthparts protruded from the anterior tip of the head.

The life cycles of both chewing and sucking lice are much the same. They have three nymphal instars and wingless adults. The operculated eggs are attached to hairs or feathers and hatch in about a week to release the first instar nymph. The adult stage is reached in two to three weeks after hatching. Females produce a single egg at a time, and it takes up much of the space in the abdomen while it is being formed. Transmission from one host to the next is by close bodily contact. Crowding, high humidity, and generally poor living conditions contribute to increasing louse populations regardless of the species of host. Lice seldom live longer than about ten days off of a host.

ORDER MALLOPHAGA

The chewing lice arose as parasites of birds. Of the 3000 described species, most are on birds. They are common on birds and only a relatively few species have colonized mammals. Among companion animals, for example, dogs have two species of Mallophaga, and cats have one. The ox, sheep, and goat each have one species.

CHEWING LICE OF POULTRY

The chewing lice of the domestic chicken are common and they illustrate certain hallmarks of all chewing lice: (1) the host specificty, (2) the site specificty on the host, and (3) the principles of identification of chewing lice. Among domestic animals, the greatest losses from chewing lice probably are seen in chickens. Chickens are raised under crowded conditions or are

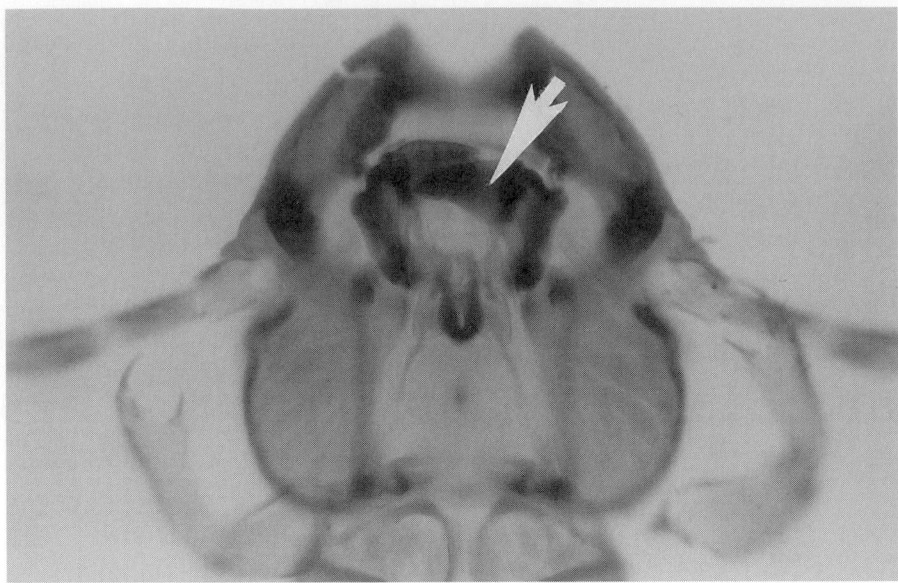

FIGURE 44.1 The head of a mallophagan, *Felicola,* showing the mandibles (arrow) that cut the feathers or skin. The muscles that move the mandibles can be seen as the diagonal strands in the lateral part of the head.

at least housed in coops at night where they are crowded and the humidity is high.

Name of Organisms, Host Range and Morphology

The following are the common chewing lice of chickens (Fig. 44.2):

Menacanthus stramineus—the body louse or little yellow louse
Menopon gallinae—the shaft louse
Cuclutogaster heterographus—the head louse
Goniocotes hologaster—the brown chicken louse
Lipeurus caponis—the wing louse
Goniodes gigas—the large chicken louse
Goniodes dissimilis

Not only are these lice limited to the chicken, but each species has it preferred location on the host, as indicated by some of the common names. As indicated in the key (Fig. 44.2), identification is based on antennal structure, head shape, setation, and markings on the body.

Geographic Distribution and Importance

Cosmopolitan. The threat of economic loss is always present wherever chickens are raised. Most Mallophaga feed on feathers and skin scurf, but the body louse may also feed on small feather shafts causing them to rupture; it may also cause the skin to bleed. Birds become restless, because the lice move about on the skin. They are especially bothered when the skin is bitten, and chickens fail to feed properly, which reduces weight gain or egg production.

Host–Parasite Interactions

Typical of lice in general, chicken lice remain on the host nearly all of the time. The transfer from one animal to another is usually by direct contact since they do not live long off of the host. Populations build up rapidly under moderate temperatures and high relative humidity such as might be found in chicken houses. When animals become restless, it can be determined whether lice are a problem by ruffling the feathers the wrong way and looking for lice on the skin. The head, vent, and undersides of the wings should be looked at with care.

Control

Chicken lice are typically controlled by insecticidal dusts. Care must be taken to ensure that the dust reaches the skin where the lice are.

Related Organisms

Turkeys have two chewing lice: *Chelopistes meleagridis,* the large turkey louse, and *Oxylipeurus polytrapezius,* the slender turkey louse. *Columbicola columbae* is a parasite of pigeons and is infrequently found on other species of birds.

As indicated earlier, mammals have mallophagans,

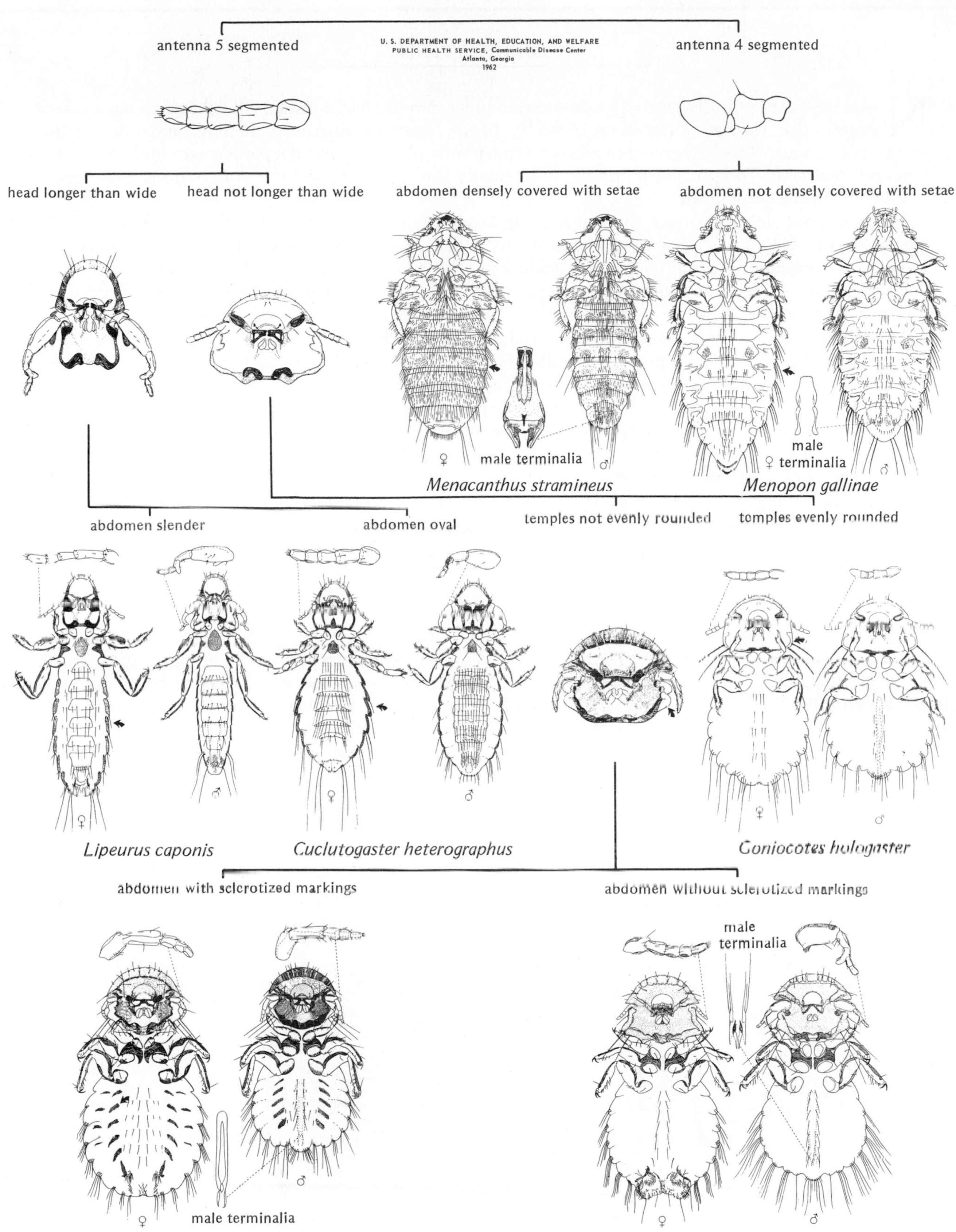

FIGURE 44.2 A pictorial key to the biting lice of chickens.

FORMICATION

NEARLY EVERY PARASITOLOGIST, ENTOMOLOGIST, or physician has had a visitor who claims to have insects, usually lice, on his or her head or body. These persons complain of itching, and find, to their satisfaction, insects. These fragments are taken to the family physician and the patient asks for an identification and treatment. The physician and his staff usually state that they do not find anything that appears to them to be entomological.

They are undoubtedly correct, but not wishing to sound overly emphatic, the patient believes that the diagnosis is only tentative. The next stop is the local college or university where an expert in insects is sought out. The identification usually is couched in tentative terms again, such as "I don't believe that these fragments are insects, I think that they probably are dandruff." The person is usually offended that his or her diagnosis has not been supported and asks for a third opinion.

The third expert renders the same opinion, and the victim of this insect attack concludes that the experts are really incompetents. These persons are often not put off completely by a failure to confirm their worst fears, and they continue to show up at our offices periodically for another attempt to hear what they want. The author was employed at a university where a woman periodically appeared with an envelope of dandruff and asked us to confirm that insects were crawling on her. We took turns patiently discussing with her the fact that this material was not insects. She would leave and return within a few months for another round of negative diagnoses.

The term usually used for this obsessive behavior is "formication" referring to ants. Whether this represents a serious mental illness is not in the purview of the authors.

but usually only one or two species. for example, dogs have two chewing lice, *Trichodectes canis* and *Heterodoxus spiniger* (Fig. 44.3). The cat has only one louse, *Felicola subrostratus* (Fig. 44.4). The mallophagans of dogs and cats can become quite irritating. Unlike fleas, lice remain on their hosts and once the infestation is eliminated, recolonization takes place only if there is contact with another lousy animal. Insecticidal shampoos are effective in treating companion animals.

Large domestic animals usually have only one or two chewing lice: *Bovicola bovis* on cattle; *B. pilosa* on horses; *B. ovis* on sheep. Studies on *B. bovis* in New York State showed that the numbers of lice fluctuated depending on the season. When populations were at a low level, lice were clustered on the head and at the base of the tail. As numbers increased, they moved out along the back and then downward to cover the whole body. Males constituted less than 10% of the population, and in some instances, less than 2%. It was possi-

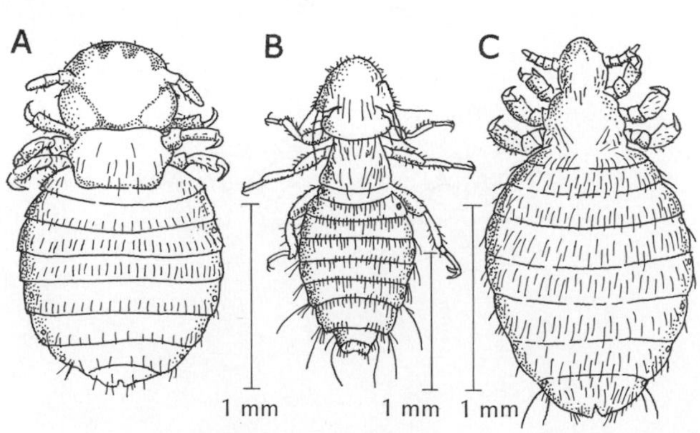

FIGURE 44.3 Lice of the dog. (A) *Trichodectes canis;* (B) *Heterodoxus longitarsus;* (C) *Linognathus setosus.*

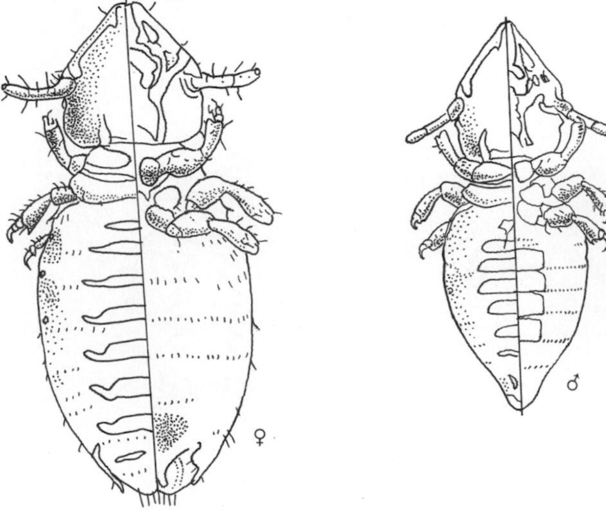

FIGURE 44.4 *Felicola subrostratus*, the biting louse of the cat.

ble to rear two generations without any males, and it was concluded that the reproduction might occur by parthenogenesis. The life cycle required 29 days from egg to egg.

Notable Features

Despite the fact that most mallophagans are rather superficially associated with their hosts, an unsuspected interaction has been uncovered. Foster(1969) studied museum specimens of certain tropical birds and found that the numbers of mallophagans fluctuated with the time of year and the breeding cycle of the bird. It appears that the reproduction of the lice is timed to coincide with the reproduction of their hosts so as to maximize the probability of transfer to new hosts. The mechanism of this phenomenon is not known.

ANOPLURA

Sucking lice are generally somewhat larger than chewing lice and they have narrow heads; another distinguishing feature is that the antennae of the sucking lice extend out from the head rather than pointing toward the posterior, as in many mallophagans. There are 500-odd described species on placental mammals, but probably only half of the extant species have been described. The chewing lice have been said to have a high level of host specificity, but the anoplurans are even more host specific. Members are vectors of important disease agents of humans, but not of domestic animals.

LICE AND LOUSE-BORNE DISEASES OF HUMANS

Name of Organisms and Disease Associations

There are three sucking lice on humans (Fig. 44.5):

Pediculus humanus, the body louse *Pediculus capitis*, the head louse *Pthirus pubis*, the crab louse

The names of the body and head lice have changed periodically. They are morphologically indistinguishable from one another, but they inhabit different ecological niches and have somewhat different habits. They are separate breeding populations and we therefore consider them to be separate species. Other investigators consider them to be subspecies.

The body louse is the vector of various disease agents.

Hosts and Host Range

The head and body lice are limited to humans, but the crab louse has been found on the gorilla.

Geographic Distribution and Importance

Cosmopolitan. All three species of lice can be extremely irritating. They crawl on the body, suck blood, and soil the clothing with their feces. The greater importance, however, is the transmission of the agents causing typhus, louse-borne relapsing fever, and trench fever.

Life Cycle

Body lice spend most of their time in clothing, and they oviposit there rather than on the body. When conditions are good, head and body louse populations can increase rapidly; a female head louse lays 50 to 150 eggs and a body louse 275 to 300 eggs during a lifetime. The time from egg to egg is about three weeks in both species; it has been estimated that there can be a 4000- to 5000-fold increase in the population in three months.

Crab lice (papillon d'amour) are often thought of as being venereally transmitted, and this is usually the case, but as with other lice, it is mostly a matter of close personal contact between individuals. Its life cycle requires about a month from egg to egg, but females are not as prolific as the head and body lice, producing only about 30 eggs in a lifetime. This species feeds almost continuously and causes considerable itching and skin irritation.

Host–Parasite Interactions

Head and body lice tend to feed frequently and to cause a good deal of irritation of the skin. There is some evidence that persons become tolerant to lice over a period of time. Whether immunity develops is still problematic, but circumstantial evidence indicates that it does. In feeding, lice pump blood through the intestinal tract and soil the skin and clothing of the host.

Epidemiology and Control

Lice do not live long off a host; unfed lice can survive about 10 days. The nits (eggs) are quite resistant, however, and constitute a reservoir for reinfestation when control measures are undertaken.

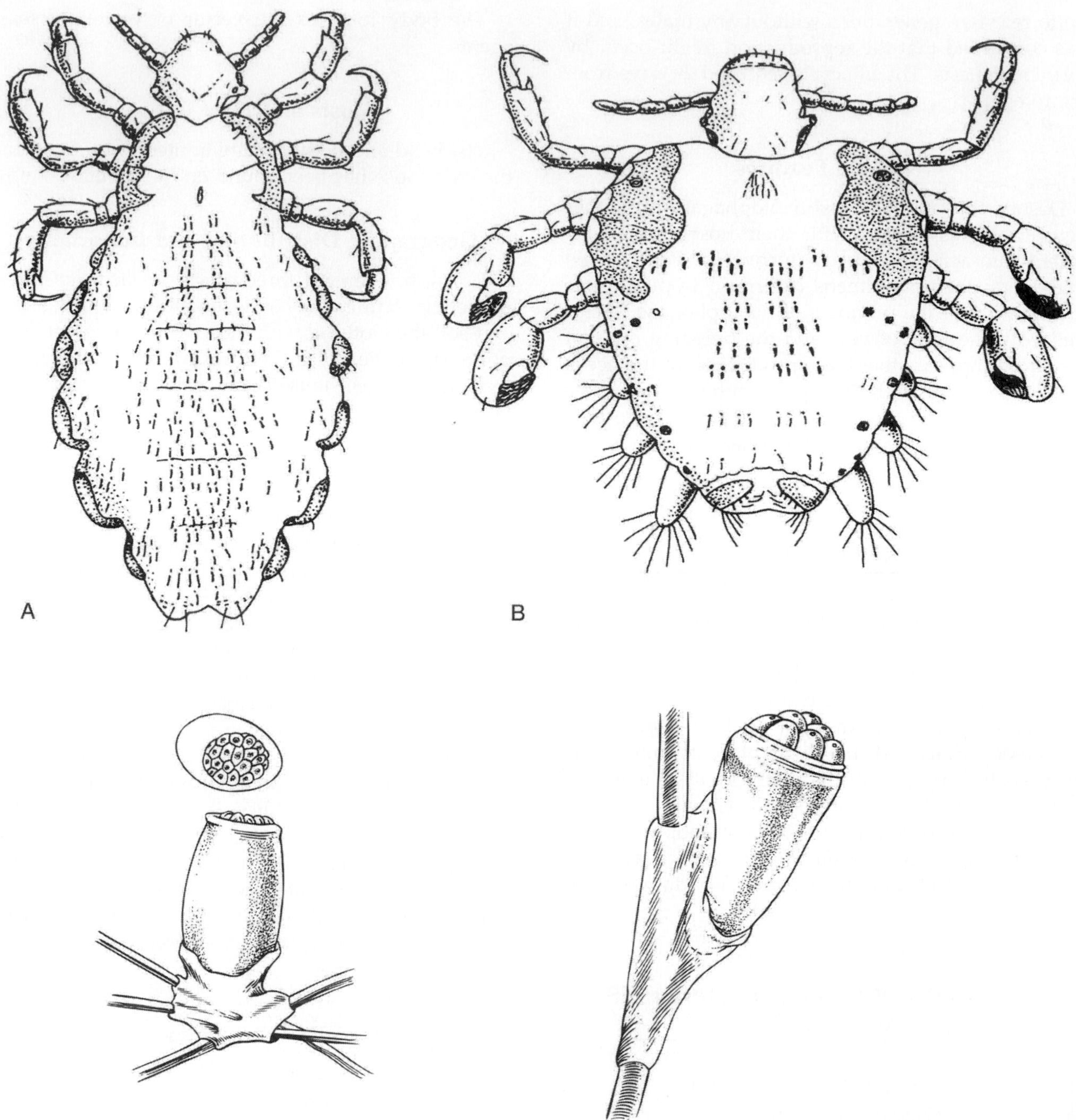

FIGURE 44.5 Lice of humans. (A) *Pediculus humanus,* the body louse and *P. capitis,* the head louse, and their egg; (B) *Pthirus pubis,* the pubic louse, and its egg.

When body lice are recognized as being present, both the person and the clothing must be treated. Reduction in populations can be achieved by dusting the inside of the clothing with an organochlorine insecticide. A better approach is to wash and heat-treat all clothing and to treat the person with an insecticide. A single treatment of the person and clothing is seldom sufficient to eliminate lice; a second treatment is usually given routinely a week or so after the first one. The second treatment eliminates the newly hatched nymphs.

Pediculus capitis infestions are endemic in children, and epidemics recur frequently in schools. The following procedures can be applied in the face of an outbreak of head lice:

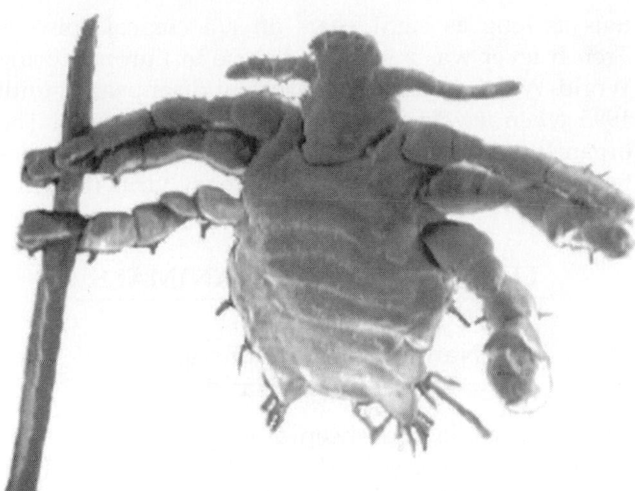

FIGURE 44.6 The crab louse, *Phthirus pubis* of human as seen in SEM.

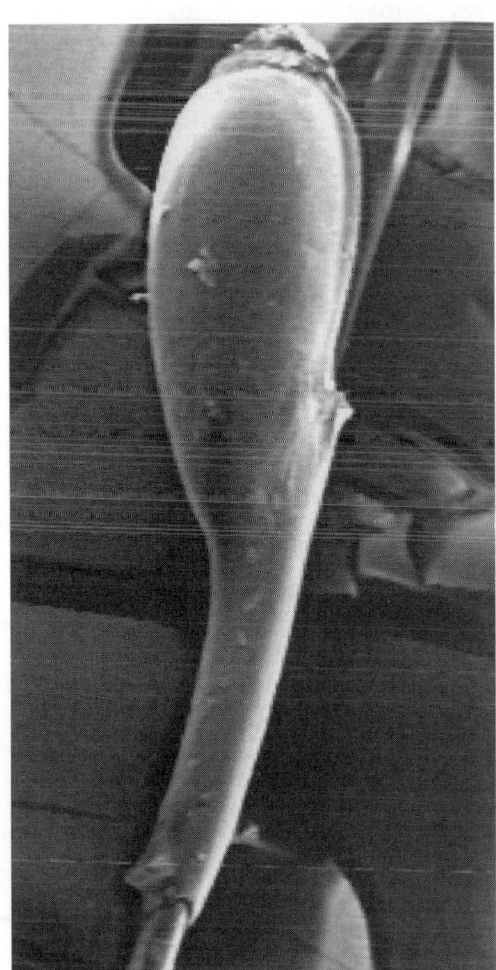

FIGURE 44.7 The egg of the crab louse, *Phthirus pubis*, as seen in SEM.

1. Determine the prevalence of infestation by inspecting all students or a representative sample of them.
2. Inform parents that there has been an outbreak of head lice, and try to explain to them that ultimate catastrophe has not descended.
3. Recommend a shampoo that parents can use on children. Recommendations from public health entities change from time to time, because of new products coming on the market and older ones being considered to be toxic. Two treatments are usually necessary. Since a few lice may have been missed on some children, all children should be treated.
4. Require children to come to school with the box or box top from the shampoo showing that they have been treated. Follow up, if needed.
5. Reinspect children two weeks to a month after treatment to ensure that none are infested.
6. Educate children not to wear one another's hats, or scarves, and make certain that the parents also receive this information in print form.

EPIDEMIC TYPHUS

Typhus is a rickettsial disease caused by *Rickettsia prowazeki*. This disease, along with a few others such as malaria, has had a decisive effect on human welfare and activities through history. Hans Zinsser's *Rats, Lice and History* is both a readable and informative history of the impact of human diseases. He discusses typhus in some detail and shows that it follows poverty, war, and natural disasters. Wherever there is crowding, interruption of sanitary services or displacement of people, typhus appears.

The impact of typhus can be appreciated when it is considered that in World War I there were 3 million typhus-related deaths in Europe, and in WWII there were 100,000 typhus-related deaths in North Africa. Another serious epidemic on the continent of Europe was aborted in Naples, Italy, in 1943–1944 by the use of DDT dust applied to the clothing of every person that could be reached.

Humans are the only host of this rickettsia and lice which vector the agent do not normally live on any host other than humans, thus we have a situation in which a low-grade infection in a population erupts when conditions are favorable for it. Infection seemingly is maintained in a few individuals for years; when they are placed under stressful living conditions, the infection becomes active and transmission is possible.

When a person has a rickettsemia, a louse becomes

infected and the organisms then multiply in the cells of its gut. The infected cells rupture releasing large numbers of rickettsiae; transmission takes place to a human through the feces of the louse or when a louse is crushed on the skin. The agent enters the body either through a break in the skin or through the unbroken mucous membranes of the eye, nose, or mouth. The rickettsiae can remain alive for up to 60 days in louse feces, so a contaminated area can remain a hazard for some time.

Mortality from epidemic typhus ranges from 10 to 100% in any one outbreak. There is a generalized infection in the body, with the organisms multiplying in endothelial cells of the smaller blood vessels. When the blood vessels break down, blood leaks into the skin and a skin rash composed of small hemorrhages appears. There is a good chance of recovery if broad-spectrum antibiotics are given. A good vaccine protects persons at risk.

EPIDEMIC OR LOUSE-BORNE RELAPSING FEVER

Epidemic relapsing fever, caused by *Borellia recurrentis,* is not as severe a disease as typhus, but it occurs under much the same circumstances. Death rates are less than 5%; currently the known focus of infection is in Ethiopia, but an epidemic occurred in Asia in the 1970s.

Transmission from louse to humans is through the feces of an infected louse or by a louse being crushed on the skin and releasing organisms onto the skin or mucous membranes. Relapsing fever tends to run a long course with recurring episodes of fever and prostration. Antibiotics are effective. Tick-borne relapsing fever is related (Chapter 51), but that agent is adapted to transmission by soft ticks.

TRENCH FEVER

Trench fever is a short-lived, acute disease with a low mortality and is caused by the bacterium, *Bartonella quintana* (syn. *Rochalimaea quintana).* An affected person is incapacitated and in a great deal of physical discomfort for about 48 hours, seemingly recovers, and then is clinically affected about five days later; additional attacks ensue with diminished severity.

The disease follows war and other human tragedies and has been seen in Europe, Africa, Asia, and South America. As with typhus, humans seem to be the only host, and organisms have been recovered from individuals as long as eight years after a clinical episode. Trench fever was a serious disease in Europe during World War I, but it then virtually disappeared until 1995 when it was found in Seattle, Washington. The organism was associated with persons who were infected with human immunodeficiency virus (HIV).

LICE OF DOMESTIC ANIMALS

Name of Organisms and Disease Associations

Lice on cattle and sheep are herd problems, and although there are several species on each host (Fig. 44.8, Fig. 44.9), they are controlled by the similar measures.

It is estimated that there is between $50 million and $110 million annual loss due to lice in domestic animals, mostly sheep and cattle, in the United States. Losses are due to decreased weight gains and damage to fleeces. Animals become anemic from bloodsucking and probably become susceptible to other infections.

Host–Parasite Interactions

Louse infestations of range cattle can be particularly devastating. The cumulative effects of anemia, nutritional distress, adverse weather, and pregnancy in late winter can lead to severe losses. Louse control can help to mitigate these stresses on cattle.

In any cattle herd there are always a few animals that are carriers, that is, animals especially susceptible to lice. They maintain infections at a higher level than other animals in the herd and serve as a reservoir of lice at a time when their numbers are likely to increase. A number of explanations have been proposed for the high susceptibility of carrier animals, but none has survived experimental scrutiny. With advances in molecular genetic characterization, it may be possible to show relative resistance and susceptibility among individuals in a herd.

It has been shown experimentally that antigens prepared from sucking lice can elicit an immunity in a mammalian host. If a vaccine were to be developed commercially, it would further simplify administration of a product and reduce environmental contamination with possibly hazardous chemicals.

Epidemiology and Control

Louse populations fluctuate with the seasons and are greater problems in temperate than in warm climates. Populations are generally low during the sum-

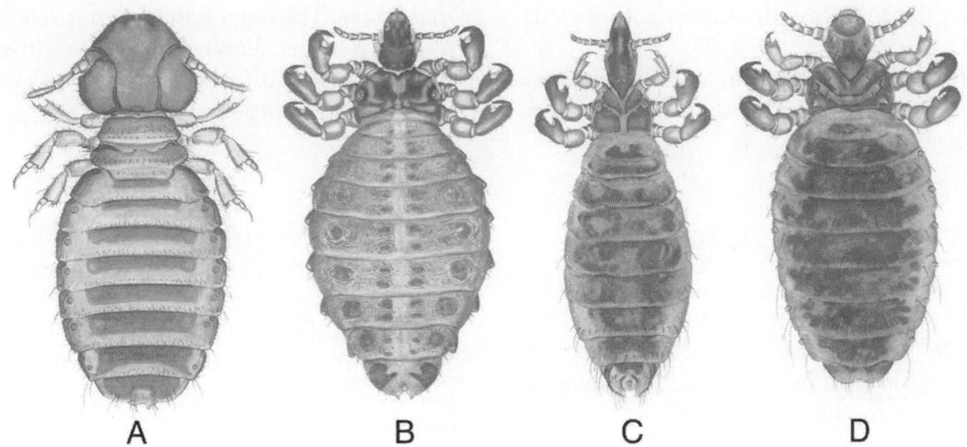

FIGURE 44.8 The lice of cattle. (A) *Bovicola bovis;* (B) *Haematopinus eurysternus;* (C) *Linognathus vituli; (D) Solenopotes capillatus.* [From Mathysse, J. G., 1946.]

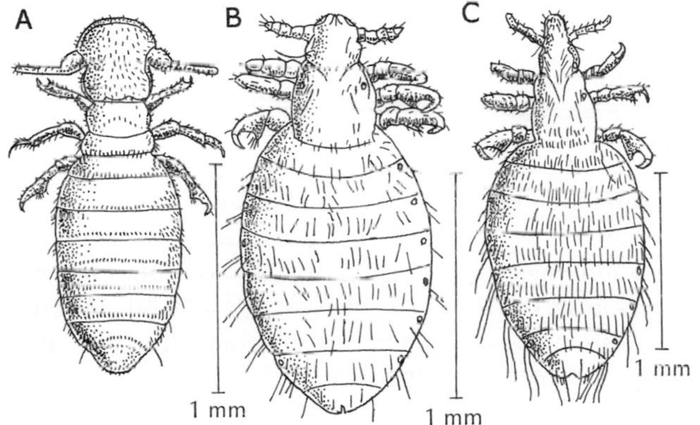

FIGURE 44.9 Lice of sheep. (A) *Bovicola ovis,* the biting louse; (B) *Linognathus pedalis,* the foot louse; (C) *Linognathus ovillus,* the body louse.

mer when skin temperatures are high; lice usually cannot survive long at temperatures above 38°C (100°F). When animals are on pasture during the summer and spread out, lice are not normally a problem. When the temperature declines in the fall and animals are gathered together, transfer among animals is facilitated and populations increase.

Treatment should be applied before louse populations become high for two reasons: (1) losses will not occur if treatment is given early, and (2) treating animals in the cold months is stressful. With animals such as sheep and cattle, which are raised in relatively large herds, individual treatment is not generally given. A number of kinds of treatment have been developed for large ruminants:

1. Dipping in a contact insecticide
2. Spraying with a contact or systemic insecticide
3. Pour-on with a concentrated insecticide
4. Injection parenterally with an insecticide

Before the development of the organophosphate systemic insecticides, it was essential that animals be wetted all over with the liquid insecticide; therefore, they were dipped in a large vat containing hundreds of gallons of insecticide. This is a labor-intensive method that is difficult for both the dipper and the dippee. Spraying is somewhat less laborious, but animals must be well wetted and every animal the in herd must be carefully treated.

The systemic insecticides allow the use of a concentrated insecticide which can be administered to the animal as a pour-on down the midline of the back or given by hypodermic needle. These procedures (1) reduce labor and (2) eliminate waste of expensive chemicals, (3) reach the lice through the bloodstream, and (4) mitigate environmental contamination with insecticide.

Macrolide antibiotics, such as ivermectin, administered in relatively low doses by subcutaneous inoculation are not only convenient to administer, but are efficacious as well.

Other Domestic and Companion Animals

Horses, swine, and companion animals are all susceptible to lice and often harbor unacceptably large populations of them. Unlike ruminants, these animals are treated individually, usually by hand. Horses, dogs, and cats, are usually trained to allow humans to do a variety of things to them and are easily hand treated. Cats are unusually susceptible to insecticides and may die, especially from organophosphate insecticides, so it is essential to follow the manufacturer's directions.

Swine are difficult animals to treat and require both patience and perseverance to ensure that they are properly treated for lice.

THE BLATTARIA—COCKROACHES

The cockroaches have often been classified with the grasshoppers (order Orthoptera), but their morphologies and life cycles justify their being placed in a separate order, the Blattaria (sometimes Cursoria).

Name of Organisms and Disease Associations

There are five main species of cockroach that are likely to be encountered in the temperate and warm climates of North America (Fig. 44.10). Cockroaches are likely to serve as mechanical vectors of a number of bacterial agents, especially enteric species. They have also been implicated as being paratenic hosts of hookworm larvae (Chapter 27).

They serve as biological vectors of a number of acanthocephalans (Chapter 37). Among them are *Prosthenorchis elegans* of monkeys, *Moniliformis moniliformis* of rodents, and *Oncicola canis* of canids.

Aside from transmitting some infectious agents, cockroaches have been implicated as causing asthma in children. About 37% of inner city children tested positive for cockroach allergens, and they were likely to require hospitalization for asthma.

Morphology

Cockroaches range up to 5 cm (2 in.) or more in length, are generally soft bodied and flattened dorsoventrally. They have chewing mouthparts much like a grasshopper, large eyes, and long flexible antennae (Fig. 44.10). The forewings are leathery and the hindwings membranous. A large pronotum covers the head.

Life Cycle

In keeping with their being hemimetabolic insects, cockroaches have a series of nymphs, which grow successively larger as they approach the winged adult. The adults have functional wings, except in the oriental cockroach, *Blatta orientalis,* which has only wing pads in the male and no wings at all in the female.

Females lay eggs which are attached to one another in packets. The eggs hatch giving rise to tiny, soft first-instar nymphs. Development is slow with the time from egg to adult requiring several weeks or months at moderate temperatures.

Diagnosis

Cockroaches are typically pests in houses, grocery stores, restaurants, and animal quarters such as zoological gardens and stables. Cockroaches are mostly nocturnal and they are seen when one enters a room and turns on the light; they then scurry back to their hiding places. Their droppings can often be seen on kitchen counters in the morning.

Roaches are said to have a characteristic odor and the experienced blattariologist can detect them upon entering a dwelling. In our experience with laboratory colonies of the American cockroach, a terrarium with fifty or a hundred of them does have a characteristic aroma.

Epidemiology and Control

Cockroaches are a concern mostly when they enter human dwellings or are associated with caged animals. In houses, they tend to remain out of sight during the day and come out at night from cabinets, behind loose baseboards, or from pipe chases. They search for food, enter cereal boxes which have loose lids, and they search in waste baskets for delicacies on which to feed. In fact, any scrap of food left out draws roaches in numbers that are sometimes startling.

In warm climates, such as the southeastern United States or the tropics, roaches live outside and enter houses because they are a source of easy food. In this circumstance, it is difficult to control roaches since it is not feasible to effect control out of doors.

In houses and other buildings, control is attempted by the following measures:

1. Insecticide application
2. Removal of any possible food sources
3. Preventing migration of roaches from one dwelling to another

A variety of insecticides are effective including organochlorines, organophosphates, and silicone dust. These are applied where roaches are likely to hide and paths that they take in moving about the building. So-called "roach motels" gather roaches but cannot usually reduce the populations to an acceptable level.

In a house or apartment, keeping all potential food away from roaches is the first line of defense. This means having containers of food that have tight lids or keeping whatever will fit there in the refrigerator.

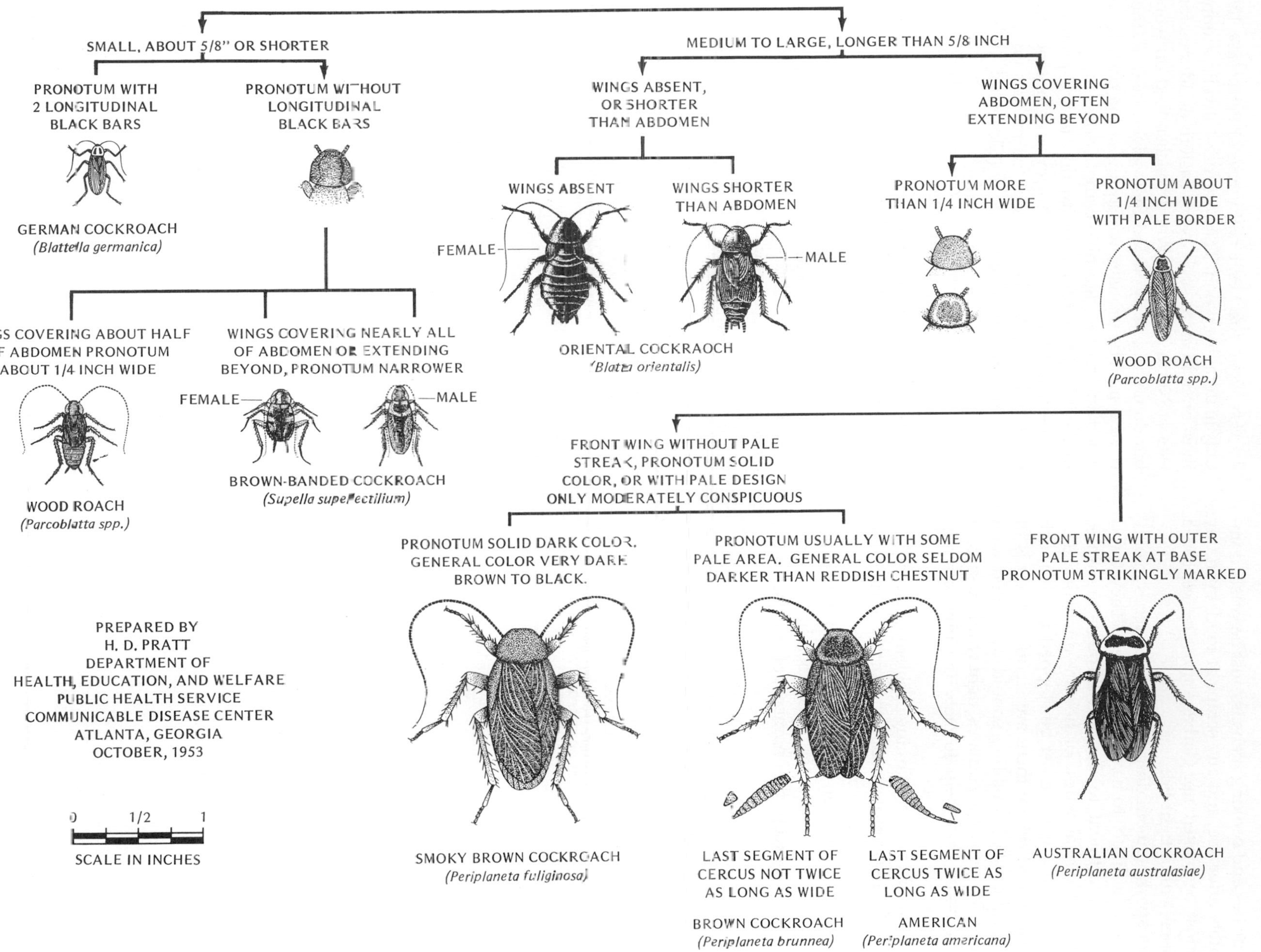

FIGURE 44.10 Pictorial key to some common adult cockroaches.

Dirty dishes and cooking utensils must be washed immediately after use, and any scraps of food, even tiny bits, must be picked up. Garbage must be kept in a container with a tight lid.

In an apartment building, control of roaches in only one unit is unlikely to have much effect. They travel from one apartment to the next through the walls, or follow electrical wires, or heating ductwork. The apertures in the walls must be stopped up as much as possible, and where there are significant levels of infestion, the whole building should be treated with an insecticide. In warm climates, tight window screening and doors may help to slow the invaders' encroachment.

Cockroaches are a continuing problem in zoological gardens. There is ample food in the form of scraps and feces, and there are many places to hide. The same level of tidiness that can be achieved in a home is not possible in a zoo. However, most zoos have control programs that keep the number of roaches at a minimum.

Notable Features

The previous discussion relates principally to roaches that invade human habitation and animal quarters, but some species do not become domiciliated. The oriental cockroach generally remains outside of houses, for example.

Also, wood roaches, *Cryptocercus* or *Parcoblatta*, live only in decaying wood. They are forest-dwellers found most often in areas such as the eastern deciduous forests of North America. Wood roaches feed on wood but do not digest the wood themselves. Instead, they have symbiotic protists, which ingest the particles of wood and return digestible carbohydrate and protein to their hosts. Sexual reproduction in the protistan symbionts is tuned to the molting cycle of the roach and when ecdysone levels are high, the protists undergo sexual fusion, a type of syngamy (Cleveland, 1956).

Readings

Busvine, J. R. (1978). Evidence from double infestations for the specific status of head lice and body lice (Anoplura). *Syst. Entomol.* **3,** 1–8.

Cleveland, L. R. (1956). Brief accounts of the sexual cycles of the flagellates of *Cryptocercus. J. Protozool.* **3,** 161–180.

Ferris, G. F. (1951). *The Sucking Lice,* Memoir No. 1. Pacific Coast Entomology Society.

Foster, M. S. (1969). Synchronized life cycle in the orange-crowned warbler and its mallophagan parasites. *Ecology* **50,** 315–323.

Kim, K. C. (Ed.) (1985). *Coevolution of Parasitic Arthropods and Mammals.* Wiley, New York. [Three chapters concern Mallophaga and Anoplura]

Kim, K. C., and Ludwig, H. W. (1978). The family classification of the Anoplura. *System. Entomol.* **3,** 249–284.

Mathysse, J. G. (1946). *Cattle lice: their biology and control.* Ag. Exp. Stat. Bull. No. 832. Cornell Agricultural Experiment Station, Ithaca, NY.

Zinsser, H. (1935). *Rats, Lice and History.* Little, Brown, Boston.

CHAPTER

45

The Bugs: Order Hemiptera

The ordinal name, Hemiptera, translates into "half wing" and refers to the fact that the forewings of these insects have leathery basal portions and membranous distal portions (Fig. 45.1, 45.2); the second pair of wings is membranous. Both pairs of wings are held over the abdomen at rest. They all have piercing-sucking mouthparts well adapted for feeding on plants, small arthropods, and vertebrate blood. There is usually a distinct pronotum and a pronounced scutellum between the bases of the forewings. The eyes are generally well developed. Antennae are straight with four to five segments. The sizes of adults range from a few mm to more than 2 cm in length.

The members of the Hemiptera comprise one of the largest orders of insects and is the largest among the Hemimetabola. More than 35,000 species have been described worldwide and more than 4500 have been described in the United States.

Most hemipterans are predaceous or feed on plant juices. Many are beneficial insects insofar as they prey on various small arthropods and are part of the natural biota that serve to modulate insect populations. They also provide useful products such as the dye cochineal, which is derived from members of the family Dactylopiidae. Members of the family Lacciferidae provide lac from which shellac is made. It should be noted that nearly any hemipteran will bite humans if provoked. Some of these are the giant water bugs (family Belostomatidae), backswimmers (family Notonectidae), the wheel bug (*Arilus cristatus*), and the masked hunter (family Reduviidae). Unlike the triatomins, the bites of these other bugs are painful.

Two families are of importance in medical entomology: the Cimicidae (bedbugs) and the Reduviidae (assassin bugs, kissing bugs). Reduviids are both predaceous and hematophagous, and members of the subfamily Triatominae are the ones that take blood and serve as vectors of disease agents. A number of species of triatomins serve as vectors of *Trypanosoma cruzi*, the cause of Chagas' disease in the Western Hemisphere (Chapter 3).

SUBFAMILY TRIATOMINAE—KISSING BUGS

Name of Organisms and Disease Associations

There are several genera in this subfamily that are of medical importance. Some of the important species are *Triatoma dimidiata*, *T. sanguisuga*, *T. protracta*, *T. infestans*, *Rhodnius prolixus*, and *Panstrongylus megistus*. Triatomins have various common names among them are kissing bugs, benchuca, vinchuca, cone-nosed bugs, giant bedbugs, and chinche de monte.

Triatomins are important because they serve as vectors of *Trypanosoma cruzi*, the cause of Chagas' disease. Kissing bugs can also be serious pests in households because of their bloodsucking proclivities.

Hosts and Host Range

Considering the triatomins generally, they exhibit mostly host preferences rather than specificities. In the wild, many are associated with burrowing animals such as rodents and the armadillo, but others live in trees and feed on lizards and birds. In houses, they

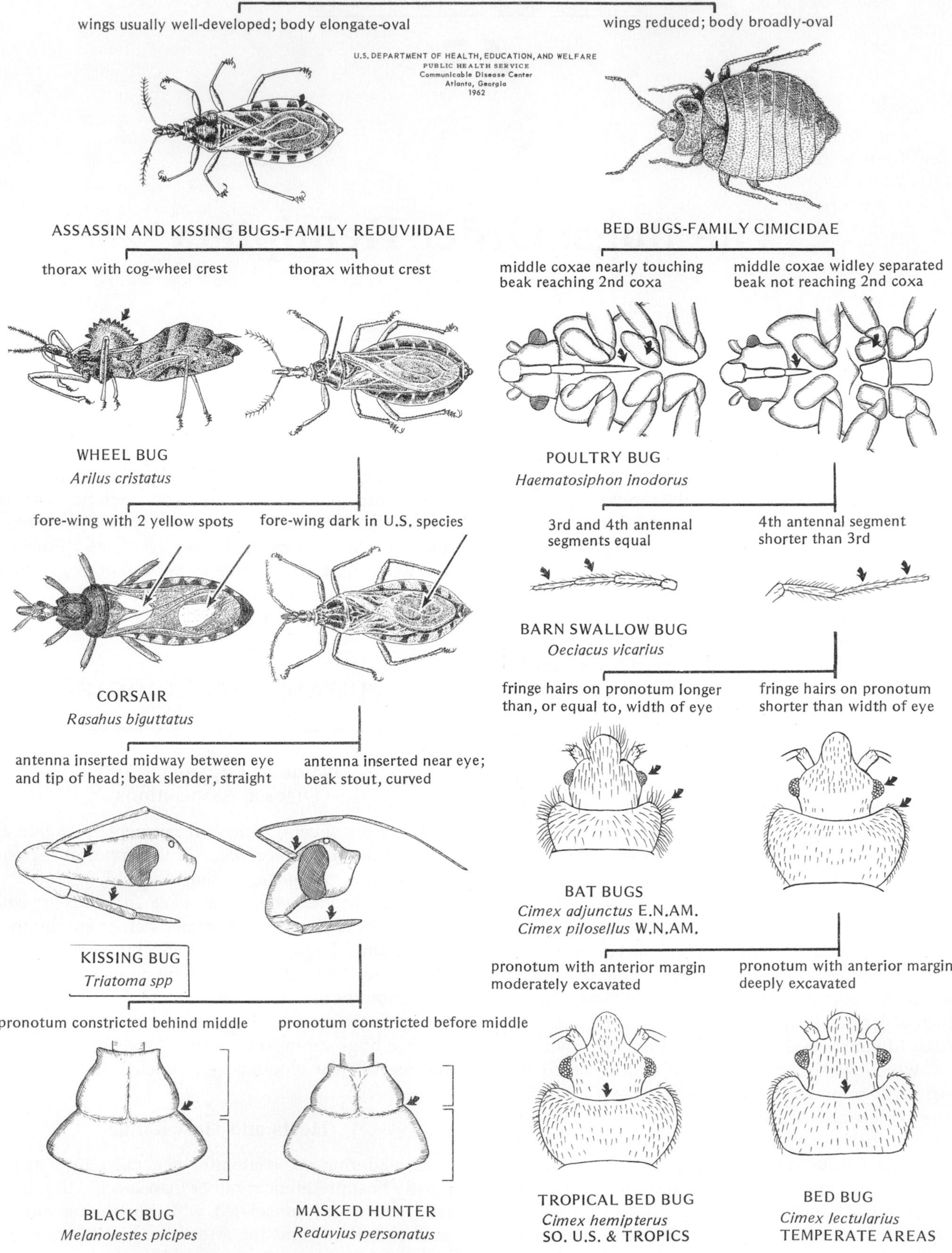

FIGURE 45.1 Pictorial key to some adult hemipterans that may bite humans.

feed on what is available, usually humans, dogs, and farm animals.

Geographic Distribution and Importance

Triatomins are distributed in the Western Hemisphere from warm temperate climates in the United States (40° north latitude) southward about three-fifths of the length of South America (45° south latitude) (Fig. 3.10). The five taxonomic tribes currently recognized are based on both morphology and habitat. Habitat ranges from warm-temperate to tropical climates and from desert habitat to tropical rain forest. They are found more or less contiguously with the distribution of Chagas' disease. The importance of Chagas' disease is detailed in Chapter 3.

Morphology

Members of the subfamily Triatominae are generally large insects with the adults ranging from about 5 mm to nearly 30 mm (Fig. 45.2). The eggs are operculated and while appearing smooth at the LM level, are somewhat textured in the SEM (Fig. 45.3). Newly hatched nymphs are 2 to 3 mm long. The head is long and narrow with prominent eyes, and the filiform antennae insert anterior to the eyes. The beak, which contains the mouthparts, has three segments and is held back under the head (Fig. 45.1). The thorax typically has a constriction at about its middle, and the abdomen is concave often with patterning on its margin. The wings fold over one another and fit down into this concavity. The long legs are well adapted for running, and there are three tarsi. The nymphs look much like the adults but lack wings and their abdominal patterning is less striking (Fig. 45.5).

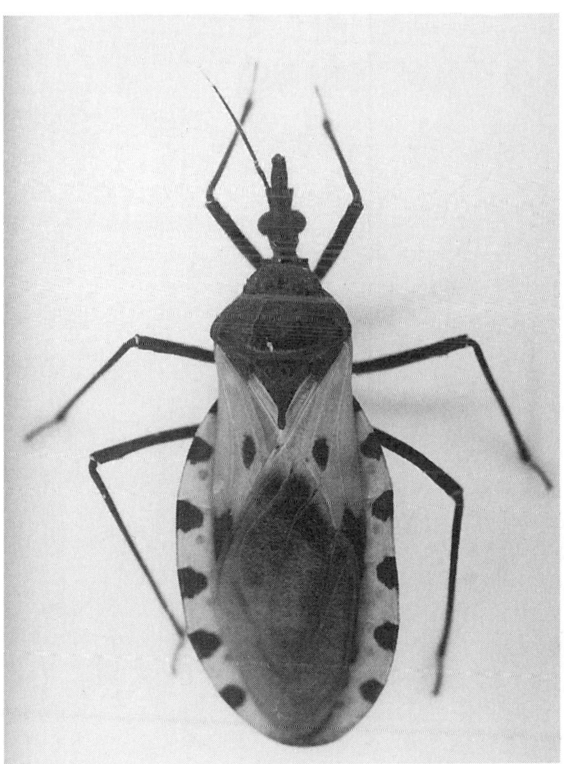

FIGURE 45.2. Adult *Triatoma dimidiata.* Note the membranous portion of the forewings and the striking pattern at the margin of the abdomen.

Life Cycle

Rhodnius prolixus is an important vector of *Trypanosoma cruzi* in South America and serves as an example of development in the group (Fig. 45.6). The operculated eggs are 2.5 mm in length (Fig. 45.3) and while white when laid, they turn bright red within a few hours. Development of the eggs is relatively long requiring about a month at 22°C, and 12 days at 32°C. The first instar nymph is, of course, about the size of the egg, 2.7 mm. Each of the five nymphal instars feeds and molts increasing in size approximately 1.5X at each molt. The life cycle in the laboratory requires about 80 days from egg to adult.

Other species vary in the length of the life cycle. For example, *Triatoma infestans* requires about 180 days to develop from the egg to the adult.

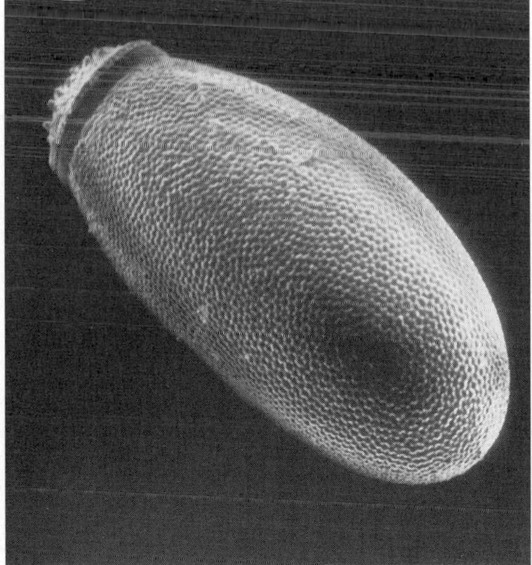

FIGURE 45.3 Egg of *Rhodnius prolixus* as seen in the SEM. Note the operculum, which has openings that allow gaseous exchange while the egg is embryonating.

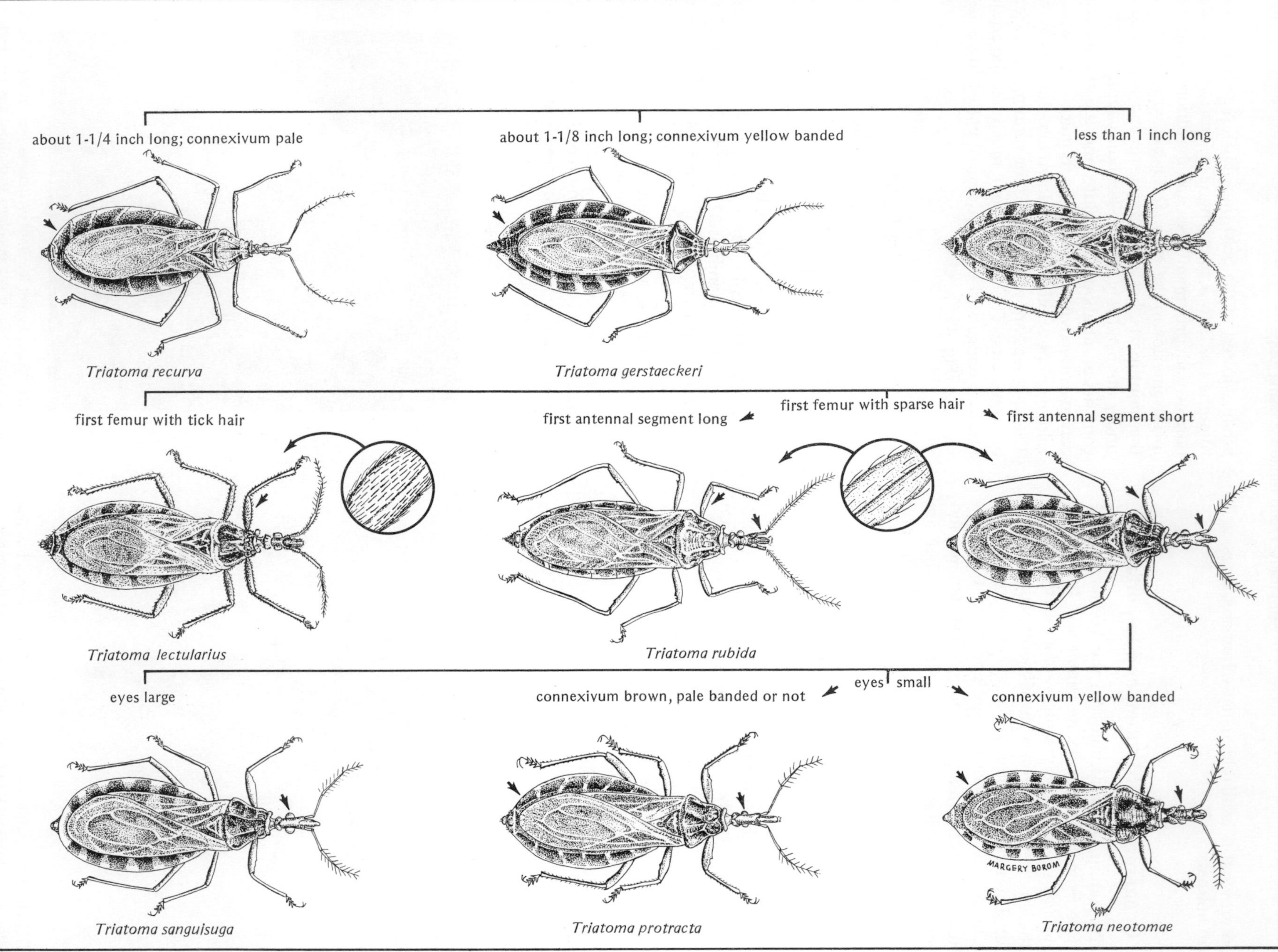

FIGURE 45.4 Pictorial key to some common adult kissing bugs in the United States.

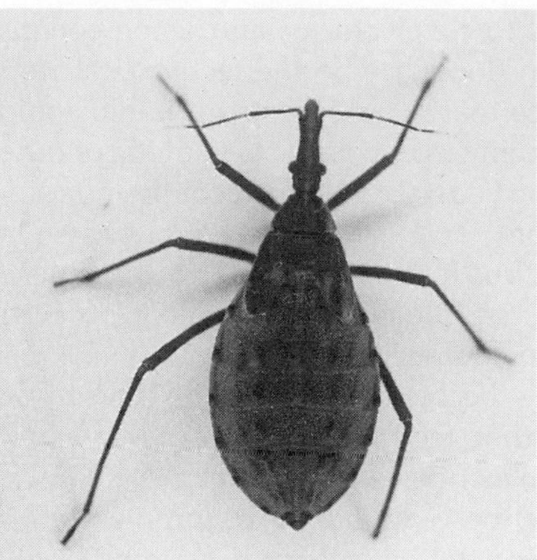

FIGURE 45.5 Nymph of *Triatoma dimidiata.* Proportions of the body are somehat different from the adult and the patterning on the abdomen is not as striking.

Kissing bugs lay their eggs off of the host in rodent burrows or, if domiciliated, in cracks and crevices in the house or in areas such as a thatched roof. Those that live in trees oviposit in bird nests, the crowns of palm trees, or in epiphytes. The rate of development of the eggs varies with temperature, and they do well over a range of 16 to 34°C. They are resistant to desiccation with 50% of eggs hatching at a humidity as low as 20%.

In the wild, bugs associate with burrowing animals such as rodents, or they may be found in epiphytes in a rain forest where they feed on both birds and reptiles. Many species become domiciliated by moving from habitats in the wild to human dwellings. Food is plentiful and readily available in houses. When they move into houses, they usually hide during the day in the walls or the roof. The poorer the quality of the housing, the more bugs are likely to be found in it. In South

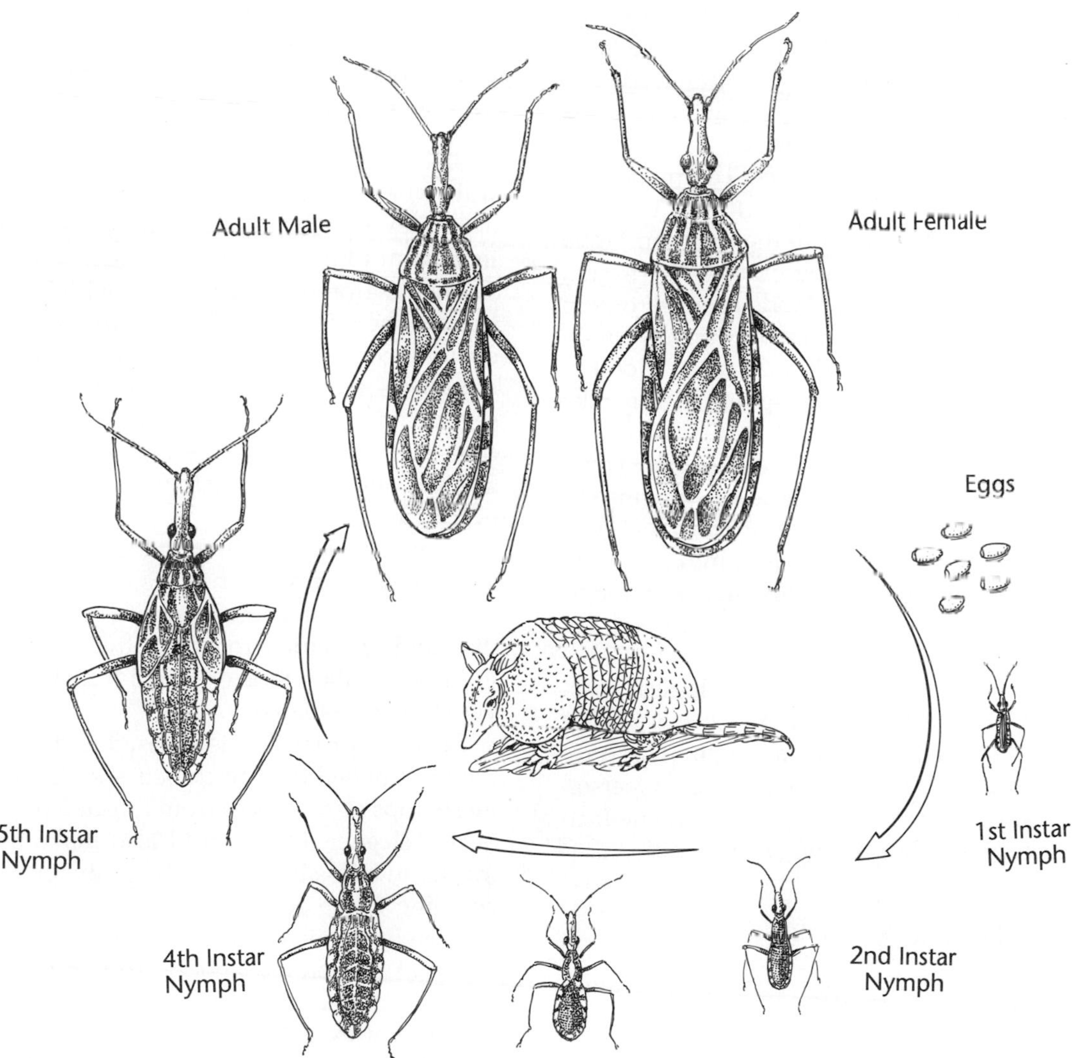

FIGURE 45.6 The morphology and life cycle of *Rhodnius prolixus,* an important vector of *Trypanosoma cruzi.*

America, as many as 8500 bugs have been found in a single poorly maintained adobe house.

Adults lay eggs in relatively small batches but egg laying continues over a period of several months. *Rhodnius prolixus* lays eggs in batches of up to 14, and may lay 30 to 50 batches of them. Thus, one female may lay 300 eggs in a lifetime. A blood meal is usually taken between laying batches of eggs. But at some point the female lays a final batch of eggs and dies. The life span is about six months, unusually long for an adult insect.

Host–Parasite Interactions

The term kissing bug comes from the predeliction of the bugs for feeding on areas of the face where the skin is thin: near the lips, around the eyes. Except for a few species, triatomins feed at night. They congregate in bedrooms in houses and come out of the walls and ceilings when people are asleep. They are attracted to their hosts by warmth and carbon dioxide; odor also seems to play a role in their being attracted to a host. They do not usually cause pain when they feed, and it is assumed that they produce an anesthetic with the saliva that is injected into the wound.

Kissing bugs are capillary feeders. The mandibles are short (Fig. 43.4) and lock in the surface of the skin. The maxillae then are inserted into the skin and probe until a capillary is found. Feeding times range from 3 to 30 minutes. The volume of blood taken by one of the smaller nymphal instars is relatively small, but an adult *R. prolixus* may take nearly 0.25 ml of blood at one feeding. Over the life of a kissing bug, it may take from 4 to 10 ml of vertebrate blood.

Although triatomins cause little or no pain while feeding, their bites are likely to cause at least an uncomfortable lesion at the site of feeding. In addition, they often elicit hypersensitivity, which, in some cases, may cause serious illness. *T. protracta* bites have been found to cause nausea, heartbeat irregularity, shortness of breath, and severe itching.

Some persons develop strong psychological reactions to having kissing bugs in the house and having them come out to feed on them at night. These responses have been termed psychoses, but a person who shows a strong emotional response to a one-inch bug feeding on him or her hardly seems irrational.

Epidemiology and Control

Most control methods for triatomins revolve around source reduction:

1. Attempt to eliminate places in the house where the bugs can hide during the daytime. Plastering interior walls to cover cracks, and using concrete instead of earthen floors are both effective first steps.

2. Since thatch becomes a veritable zoological garden, replacing thatch with sheet metal or other material with a hard surface is also recommended.

3. Doors and windows of houses should be screened, but in tropical climates that may meet with resistance on the part of people who wish to have maximum cool air at night.

4. Bugs become peridomestic and in addition to humans, they feed on domestic animals and companion animals such as dogs and cats. Removing resting sites near these animals is recommended. If there is habitat near the house that maintains small wild animals, that should be eliminated. In principle, a buffer zone should be established between the reservoir in the wild and houses.

5. Residual insecticides have been found to be effective against triatomins. DDT and dieldrin both can give good control, but they are now prohibited in some countries and discouraged in others. Silicone dusts were found to be effective in control of triatomins in the crawl spaces of houses in southern California.

Since only the adults have wings, the nymphs must walk to their source of food. It should be noted that even though many species are good flyers as adults, they seem to prefer to walk to their potential hosts.

Most triatomins that associate with humans are nocturnal. They remain hidden in the house during the day and come out at night to seek food. As indicated, the bite is seldom painful, but after being fed upon several times, certain individuals become hypersensitive to the bites and develop red, swollen areas at the site and they may show systemic responses, as noted earlier.

Nearly all kissing bugs have a broad host range. They feed readily on reptiles, birds, and mammals. Thatched roofs become homes to various kinds of animals and triatomins frequently live in such niches (Fig. 3.15) where they feed on small lizards and any other vertebrates available.

Personal protection is advised and it usually takes the form of bed nets. Such nets should have solid, not mesh, tops so that feces from infected bugs cannot fall on the sleeper. One should also make beds or hammocks inaccessible to the bugs by preventing their crawling to the occupant.

Novel methods of control are needed, because so much of prevention and control of Chagas' disease rests on eliminating contact between humans and triatomins. For example, symbiotic bacteria in the intestinal cells of triatomins provide essential nutrients. As discussed elsewhere, blood is rich in protein, but is far from being a perfect food. Therefore, energy sources from carbohydrate must be obtained somehow, and certain vitamins must also be synthesized. Intestinal symbionts provide some of these essential nutrients in haematophagous insects. A method for eliminating the bacteria could result in the death of the triatomins.

FAMILY CIMICIDAE—BEDBUGS

Name of Organisms and Disease Associations

Cimex lectularius is the so-called human bedbug and *C. hemipterus* is the tropical bedbug; there are seven species associated with humans in various parts of the world, but these two are the most common. Some other genera found on birds are *Leptocimex, Haematosiphon, Oeciacus,* and *Ornithocoris*. Cimicids are not vectors of disease agents, but a virus, Fort Morgan virus, has been isolated from cimicids in nests of swallows; its significance is still unknown.

Hosts and Host Range

Members of this family are associated mainly with birds and remain in their nests transeasonally. Some are associated with mammals, and two species live with humans in their dwellings. In sum, there is usually a moderately high degree of host specificity.

Geographic Distribution and Importance

Cosmopolitan. Cimicids are important as bloodsuckers on certain hosts including humans.

Morphology

Bedbugs are brownish, dorsoventrally flattened insects that lack functional wings as adults (Fig. 45.1). The adults have wing pads, but the earlier instars do not. The body is covered with many small hairs or setae. The three-segmented beak is held back under the head.

Life Cycle

The human bedbug, *C. lectularius*, is about 3 x 5 mm as adult, and it is typical of many members of the group. When the adult stage is reached, copulation occurs. It is interesting to note that the male inserts the copulatory apparatus through the exoskeleton of the female and deposits the sperm into her hemocoel. The female deposits her yellowish eggs in hiding places in a house. The eggs hatch in about 10 days. There are three nymphal instars, each of which takes up to three blood meals between molts. Development is fairly slow and requires from one to four months from egg to adult.

Host–Parasite Interactions

Bedbugs are intermittent feeders and remain off of the host most of the time. In the case of those that associate with humans, they find resting sites in the bed, behind torn wallpaper, or behind loose baseboards. Those cimicids that feed on birds remain in the nests and feed on brooding adults and especially naked nestlings.

Although bedbugs are not usually seen, they emit a characteristic aroma that can be detected when they are present in large numbers in a dwelling.

They do not usually cause any pain when feeding, and most persons do not know bedbugs are present until morning. A line of two or three reddened wheals on the skin of a person is usually the first evidence of bedbugs in a house.

Bedbugs sensitize the host to the saliva, which they inject while feeding. Over a period of time, many, but not all, persons become hypersensitive to the bites of bedbugs. The feeding sites develop raised, red, itching papules. Interestingly, some persons are not bothered at all by bugs and do not develop skin reactions.

Bedbugs have all of the characteristics of a good vector: (1) they suck blood, (2) they have host preferences but feed on a variety of species, (3) they live a long time, and (4) they are patient. Oddly enough, they are not known to serve as vectors of any infectious agents of humans. Laboratory studies have generally shown that a variety of agents may survive for a short period of time in the gut of a bedbug, but the agents do not replicate and are not transmitted.

Epidemiology and Control

When bedbugs are detected in a home, all of the following must be done to give good control:

1. Laundering all clothing and bedding that might have eggs or bugs in it
2. Eliminating hiding places around the room or house
3. Treating the house and all furniture with an insecticide

Readings

Barrett, T. (1991). Advances in triatomine bug ecology in relation to Chagas' disease. *Adv. Dis. Vect. Res.* **8,** 143–176.

Brenner, R. R., and de la M. Stoka, A. (1987). *Chagas' Disease Vectors,* 3 Vols. CRC Press, Boca Raton, FL.

Henry, T. J., and Froeschner, R. C. (1988). *Catalog of the Heteroptera, or True Bugs, of Canada and the Continental United States.* Sandhill Crane, Gainesville, FL.

Lent, H., and Wygodzinsky, P. (1979). Revision of the Triatominae (Hemiptera, Reduviidae) and their significance as vectors of Chagas' disease. *Bull. Am. Mus. Nat. Hist.* **163,** 123–520.

Usinger, R. L. (1944). The Triatominae of North and Central America and the West Indies and their public health significance, Bull. No. 288. U.S. Public Health Dept., Washington, DC.

Usinger, R. L. (1966). *Monograph of the Cimicidae (Hemiptera– Heteroptera),* Vol. 7. Thomas Say Foundation, College Park, MD.

Usinger, R. L., Wygodzinsky, P., and Ryckman, R. E. (1966). The biosystematics of the Triatominae. *Annu. Rev. Entomol.* **11,** 309–330.

Wood, S. F. (1953). Conenose bug annoyance and *Trypanosoma cruzi* Chagas in Griffith Park, Los Angeles, California. *Bull. Southern California Acad. Sci.* **52,** 105–109.

CHAPTER

46

Fleas and Flea-Borne Diseases

The fleas (order Siphonaptera) are highly specialized holometabolic insects that are adapted structurally and physiologically for a symbiotic life. All fleas consume blood as adults; birds and mammals are their hosts, and more than 2000 species are known. Approximately 95% of fleas have mammals as their host, leaving only about 5% on birds. Their phylogenetic relations to other insects groups are not known with certainty, but during formation of the adult in the pupal cocoon, wing buds appear and then are resorbed. It is likely that they were derived from a primitive mecopteran (Tab. 43.1).

The adults are wingless, generally less than 4 mm long and are laterally compressed. The body is well supplied with bristles, which are directly posterior (Figs. 46.1, 46.2), and the amount and kind of setation (bristles) indicates the kinds hosts on which they are found. The third legs are stout and adapted for jumping; mouthparts are of the piercing-sucking type adapted for capillary feeding (solenophagy) (Figs. 46.3 and 46.4), although some are pool feeders (telamatophagy).

The larvae are detritus feeders, and they have chewing mouthparts. They are assumed to have a dietary requirement for blood, which is derived from adult fecal blood.

As holometabolic insects, fleas have the egg, three larval instars, pupa, and adult stages (Fig. 46.5). Under optimal conditions, the life cycle may be completed in as short a time as two weeks, but it may extend over two years or more under adverse environmental conditions or when there are no hosts on which to feed. The crucial stage in long-term survival is the pupa.

It is interesting to note the characteristics of fleas that make them successful parasites and vectors of disease agents:

1. Bristles on the body, which keep them from being easily dislodged.
2. Mouthparts adapted for sucking blood.
3. Jumping ability. Despite their lacking wings, fleas can leap as much as 45 cm vertically. If a host appears in its vicinity, a flea can reach it quickly by leaping onto it.
4. Flexibility in the rate of development. When conditions are optimal, the life cycle of *Pulex irritans* requires about 60 days, but when a host is not available it may take 125 days. When fed, the adult has been observed to live 513 days.
5. Response to the presence of a potential host. Fleas may remain in the protective pupal cocoon for long periods before emerging. They are sensitive to vibration, heat, CO_2, and direct pressure. When stimulated, they emerge quickly and leap to reach a host. The leaping stimulus is not known for all fleas, but when the light is suddenly reduced, *Ceratophyllus gallinae* responds as if a chicken were passing by.
6. Low host specificity. Fleas readily feed on many species of hosts although they prefer one or a few species. Some have a high degree of host specificity, but these are not vectors of disease agents.
7. Reproduction is cued to the reproductive state of the host, at least in some species.

Name of Organism and Disease Associations

Ctenocephalides felis felis, the cat flea, and *C. canis*, the dog flea. Four subspecies of *C. felis* are recognized:

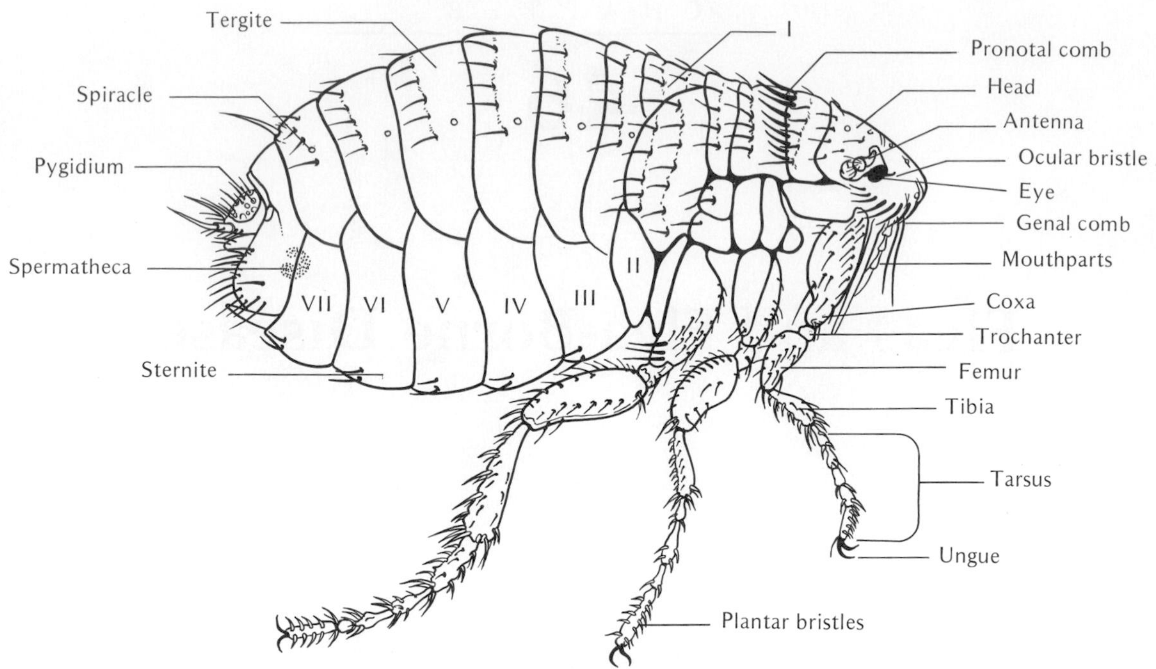

FIGURE 46.1 The external anatomy of an adult flea.

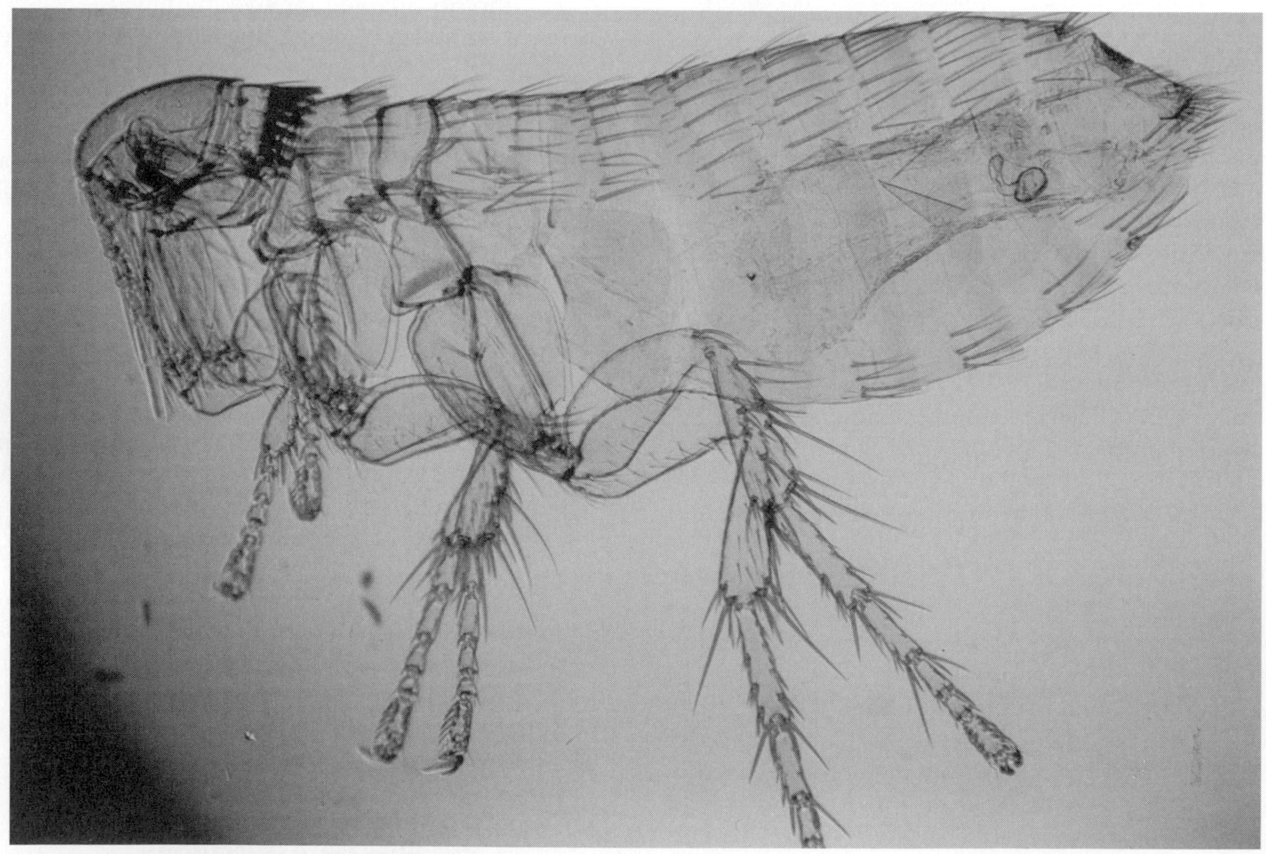

FIGURE 46.2 An adult female *Pleochaetus exiles* as seen under a low power microscope. Note the abundance of bristles on the body and that this species has only a pronotal comb. The spermatheca can be seen clearly in the seventh abdominal segment. [Courtesy of Dr. Rex Thomas.]

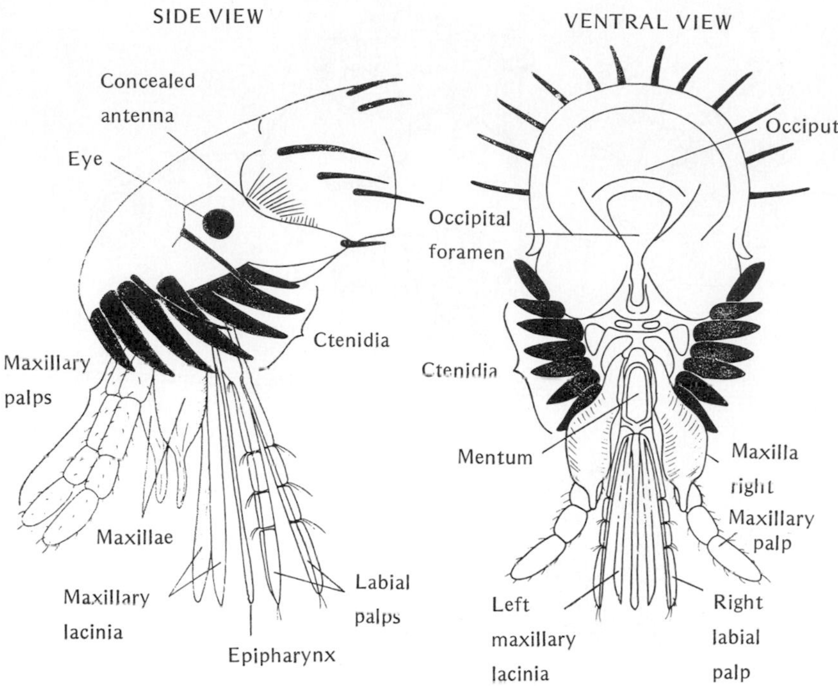

FIGURE 46.3 Mouthparts of a flea. [From Harwood and James, 1979.]

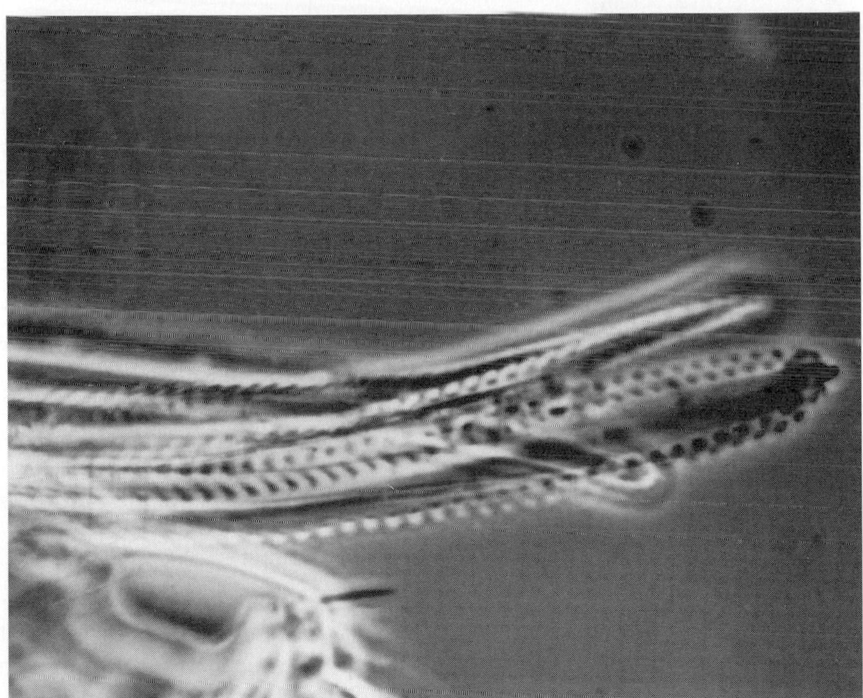

FIGURE 46.4 Photomicrograph of the mouthparts of *Ctenocephalides* showing the cutting surfaces of the laciniae and epipharynx.

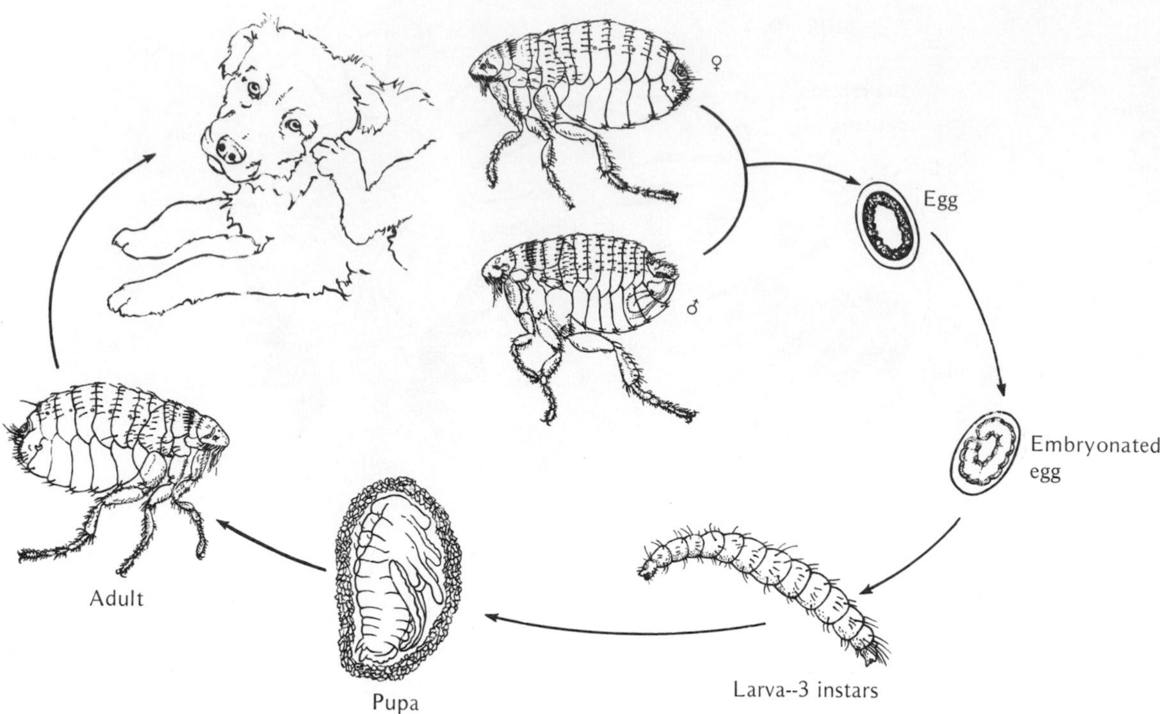

FIGURE 46.5 The life cycle of *Ctenocephalides.*

Name	Distribution
C. felis felis	Cosmopolitan
C. f. strongylus	Africa
C. f. damarensis	Africa
C. f. orientis	India, Pacific Rim, Australia

These organisms transmit the tapeworms *Hymenolepis nana* and *Dipylidium caninum* (Chapter 24) and the filarioid nematode, *Dipetalonema reconditum* (Chapter 34) (Tab. 46.1).

The discussion below is mostly about *C. felis* since it is most important and we have the most reliable information on it.

Hosts and Host Range

The hosts are dogs and cats, as well as on many other mammals, and humans occasionally.

Geographic Distribution and Importance

The common flea on dogs and cats in North America is *C. felis felis. C. canis* is seldom found in North America; the other subspecies are limited to the Eastern Hemisphere (see the previous discussion).

Fleas on dogs and cats can give rise to a severe skin condition called flea allergic dermatitis. The total cost of controlling fleas including antiflea preparations and veterinary services approximates $300 million annually in the United States.

Finally, the transmission of *D. caninum* or *H. nana* to humans, especially children, can become a fairly serious illness. The recent association of *C. felis* in the transmission of *Bartonella hensalae*, the cause of cat scratch fever, from cat to cat also has implications for this zoonotic disease of emerging importance.

Morphology

The body length of the adults is from 1.5 to 2 mm. Members of the genus *Ctenocephalides* have well-developed genal and pronotal combs. The head of the dog flea is proportionally shorter than the cat flea, and the genal spine I of the dog flea is shorter than genal spine II of the cat flea (Fig. 46.6, presented later).

Life Cycle

The life cycle of the *C. felis* is typical of nearly all fleas and is used here as representative of the group (Fig. 46.5). Eggs are laid on the host, but they fall off to develop usually in an area where the host rests. The eggs are 0.5 mm long, glistening, white and translucent. They hatch in 1.5 days at 35°C (95°F) and in 6 days at 13°C (55°F) ; the first instar larva leaves the egg by expanding an egg burster on the head.

TABLE 46.1 Disease Agents Transmitted by Fleas

Disease	Causative Agent	Normal Host	Vectors	Human or Animal Infections
Plague	*Yersinia pestis*	Rodents	*Xenopsylla cheopis* *Oropsylla montanus* *Nosopsylla fasciatus* *Opiscrostis labis*, etc.	Human, dog, cat
Murine typhus, endemic typhus	*Rickettsia typhi* (*R. mooseri*)	Rats and other rodents	*Xenopsylla cheopis* *Nosopsylla fasciatus* Louse: *Polyplax spinulosa* Mite: *Ornithonyssus bacoti*	Human
Myxomatosis	Myxoma virus	Rabbit: *Oryctolagus cuniculi*	*Spillopsyllus cuniculi* Mosquitoes	No
Dipylidium infection	*Dipylidium caninum*	Dog, cat	*Ctenocephalides felis*, *C. canis*	Human
Dwarf Tapeworm infection	*Hymenolepis nana* (syn. *Vampirolepis nana*)	Human, rodent Unknown	*Xenopsylla cheopis* *Nosopsylla fasciatus* *Pulex irritans*, etc.	Human
Hymenolepis infection	*Hymenolepis diminuta*	Rodents	*Nosopsylla fasciatus* *Xenopsylla cheopis* Other insects: beetles	Human
Dipetalonema infection	*Dipetalonema reconditum*	Raccoon	*Ctenocephalides felis*, *C. canis* and possibly others	Dog

The first instar larvae are about 2 mm long and they grow to about 5 mm through three larval instars. Larval development requires from 5 to 11 days, depending on temperature. The third instar larva spins a loose cocoon of silk, which picks up a good deal of debris from the environment. Pupal development may be completed in as few as 3 days, but may take as long as 174 days, depending on temperature and relative humidity. Most adults emerge from the cocoon in 8 to 9 days at a temperature of 27°C (81°F) and 80% relative humidity (RH).

Both males and females seek a host immediately upon emerging from the cocoon, and they both blood feed. The male has a plug in the genital tract, which is dissolved upon taking blood, and it can then copulate successfully. After taking a blood meal they copulate on the host. Females begin laying eggs about 36 hours after feeding and reach a peak of 40 to 50 eggs per day about a week later. Female *C. felis* can live as long as 113 days and therefore produce more than 3000 eggs in a lifetime, but the life span of a female flea is usually much shorter.

Diagnosis

The first sign of a flea infestation is seeing the dog or cat scratching and biting at the skin. When fleas are suspected, the fur can be ruffled the wrong way and one can see the fleas moving through the fur or on the skin. Also, dried adult flea fecal blood, called "flea dirt" can be seen in the fur. In some animals, the skin is also likely to become inflamed in patches indicating flea allergy dermatitis.

Host–Parasite Interactions

Ctenocephalides spp. are intermittent feeders; they feed for a period of time on the mammalian host, but remain on the host most of the time; some investigators state that *C. felis* does not leave the host.

In a significant percentage of *C. felis*-parasitized dogs and cats, an allergic response to flea bites occurs. The allergy is best described in dogs where certain proteins present in the saliva of the fleas are associated with hypersensitivity resulting in the allergic dermatitis. This is a serious, chronic skin disease, which is probably the leading dermatologic disorder of dogs.

Epidemiology and Control

Control of fleas on companion animals currently is directed toward the following:

1. Insecticidal treatment of individual animals
2. Reducing the number of eggs, larvae, pupae and adults off of the host

With companion animals, treatment is usually directed toward the individual except in a situation such as a dog kennel or cattery where a large number of animals may be housed; in that case more of a herd health approach is used. The animal may be dusted with a powdered insecticide; tick and flea collars are generally ineffective, because of the short residual life of the insecticides that they contain. Cats are especially susceptible to insecticide poisoning, and they should be treated with care and kept under observation after treatment.

Areas where eggs and adults are likely to be found should be vacuumed and bedding replaced. In mild climates, large numbers of fleas are found out of doors and may continually be brought into the house. It is not feasible to eliminate the larvae and adults outside of the house unless dogs and cats are confined to a relatively small area, and this makes continual control essential.

A third-generation insecticide, Lefenuron, is given by mouth to dogs and cats for flea control. This product is an insect development inhibitor, specifically a chitin synthase inhibitor, and it prevents normal egg formation in the female thus reducing the population of fleas in the home. The adult fleas are not affected, or perhaps only slightly.

Juvenile hormone (JH) mimetics are effective in controlling dog and cat fleas. Some of the forms of these products are sprayed in the house where preadult fleas are likely to hide and outside the house in small areas. Other compounds can be effective in collars. The current, most popular compound that interferes with larval development is lufenuron; it is given orally to dogs and cats once a month. In general, drugs that interfere with larval development are safe and they can be effective particularly when the animal is kept in a restricted environment. JH mimetics do not act with the speed of the typical second-generation insecticide, and it takes a while before their effects are recognized.

It is now feasible to vaccinate for fleas on companion animals. Although the saliva itself is immunogenic, it is also irritating and gives rise to flea allergy dermatitis; saliva is therefore not now a prime candidate for use as a vaccine. The approach that has recently been taken is to vaccinate against a tissue or protein that the host never contacts. For example, antigens can be isolated from the intestinal tissue of the flea and used in a vaccine. The resultant antibodies in the blood of the immunized host combine with the gut antigens. Death of fleas has been reported as well as reduced fecundity, measured by the number of eggs laid. This concept, the so-called *hidden* or *cryptic* or *concealed* antigen strategy, has been used successfully with other hematophagous parasites such as ticks (Chapter 51) and the stomach worm of sheep and cattle, *Haemonchus* (Chapter 30).

Name of Organism and Disease Associations

Pulex irritans, the human flea. This is one of many species that transmits the bacillus, *Yersinia pestis*, which causes plague, but is not a major vector. *P. irritans* transmits murine typhus, caused by *Rickettsia typhi.*

Hosts and Host Range

Humans, swine, dogs, rodents, and domestic animals are hosts; this flea has little or no host specificity.

Geographic Distribution and Importance

Cosmopolitan in warm, moist climates. Adults irritate and sometimes cause hypersensitivity in the hosts on which they feed. *P. irritans* is a vector of plague (occasionally) and murine typhus (Tab. 46.1).

Morphology

Adults are as large as 2 mm long. Females are slightly larger than the males. They lack both genal and pronotal combs (Fig. 46.6).

Life Cycle

The glistening, white eggs are usually laid off of the host; a female may lay as many as 448 eggs over a 196-day period. Eggs hatch in 7 to 10 days at an optimal temperature of 25°C (77°F). At 35° to 37°C (95° to 98°F) or at 11° to 15°C (52° to 59°F), development is slower. A relative humidity of 65% to 95% is required for development and survival.

The larvae are elongate, legless, and have sparse bristles. There are three larval stages that may be completed in 9 to 15 days under optimal conditions but may extend over as many as 200 days when food is scarce or the temperature is low. The larvae feed on organic matter that has a high protein content: dried blood passed as feces from adult fleas and animal feces. The third larval instar spins a loose cocoon and the adult may emerge in as few as 7 days or as many as 300 days, depending on the environmental temperatures. The time from egg to adult is usually 63 to 77 days.

Diagnosis

Most often, fleas are not seen, but rather their presence is recognized by people having small, reddened

Blocking, Virulence, and Toxins

In the transmission of *Yersinia pestis,* the cause of plague, the proventriculus of the flea becomes "blocked" with a mass of plague-causing organisms. Certain species of flea tend to block more readily than others, but blocking is also a quality of the bacterium. Likewise, virulence is an attribute of the bacillus, and the key to both lies in plasmids.

Plasmids are extrachromosomal, circular double-stranded DNA molecules found in most bacteria. They also occur in a number of other kinds of organisms including yeasts, protists, and plants. They replicate along with the other DNA in the cell, often code for antibiotic resistance, and they produce various proteins.

In *Y. pestis,* there are three plasmids, a 72-kilobase pair (kbp), a 90– 110 kbp, and 9.5 kbp plasmid. The 9.5 kbp plasmid controls blocking by producing two different enzymes at low and high temperatures. When the flea feeds, it takes in warm blood and then detaches from its host; as it cools below 27.5°C, the 9.5 kbp plasmid produces a coagulase, which causes the red cells to stick together and form the mass of bacteria that clog the proventriculus.

When the flea returns to a host to feed again, the same gene that codes for coagulase then switches on at temperatures above 27.5°C to produce fibrinolysin, which breaks down the mass of bacilli. The bacteria are then more readily introduced into the host.

When the bacterium is introduced into a mammalian host, it lacks a capsule, but at 37°C, the 90– 110 kbp plasmid becomes active and produces the glycoprotein that serves as a protective coat for the organism. When *Y. pestis* is ingested by a macrophage, the glycoprotein capsule confers resistance to digestion by the macrophage; it blocks a portion of the complement cascade and probably buffers against pH changes in the macrophage. These three functions allow the plague bacillus to replicate unimpeded in the phagolysosomes of the macrophage and then break out to cause a septicemia.

The 90–110 kbp plasmid also produces a toxin, which is lethal to mice. When bacteria are lysed, they release an endotoxin, which reacts specifically with the β-adrenergic receptors of the mouse. It is extremely potent being lethal at a dose of less than a microgram.

Virulence, or invasiveness, is a characteristic of pathogenic bacteria, and in the case of *Y. pestis,* the 72 kbp codes for number of outer membrane proteins that allow the invasion of the bacilli. If one or more of these proteins is not produced, virulence is decreased.

With knowledge of these molecular characters , we now can devise methods of combating intractable diseases such as plague.

areas on the skin where fleas have fed. A careful search then usually turns up larvae, pupae, and adults in the furniture, under the bed, or in cracks in the woodwork.

Host–Parasite Interactions

P. irritans, an occasional feeder, takes a blood meal and then returns to a hiding place. The bites cause skin irritation in the form of raised, itching papules, and hypersensitivity may occur in some persons.

Epidemiology and Control

Control of *P. irritans* is directed at those fleas that are in houses and attack humans. Vacuuming rugs, furniture, and cracks where fleas hide should be the first action. If a dog has a place in the house where it lies, the bedding should be thrown out and new bedding provided.

Insecticides such as an organophosphate or carbamate powder can be sprinkled in areas where the fleas are likely to lurk. A flea collar for the dog may help to reduce numbers further.

Name of Organism and Disease Associations

Tunga penetrans, the chigoe or jigger flea. This flea does not transmit any vector-borne agents, but it does cause sufficient skin damage to allow secondary invasion by bacteria.

Hosts and Host Range

The normal hosts are probably burrowing animals such as rodents and some owls; however, the chigoe

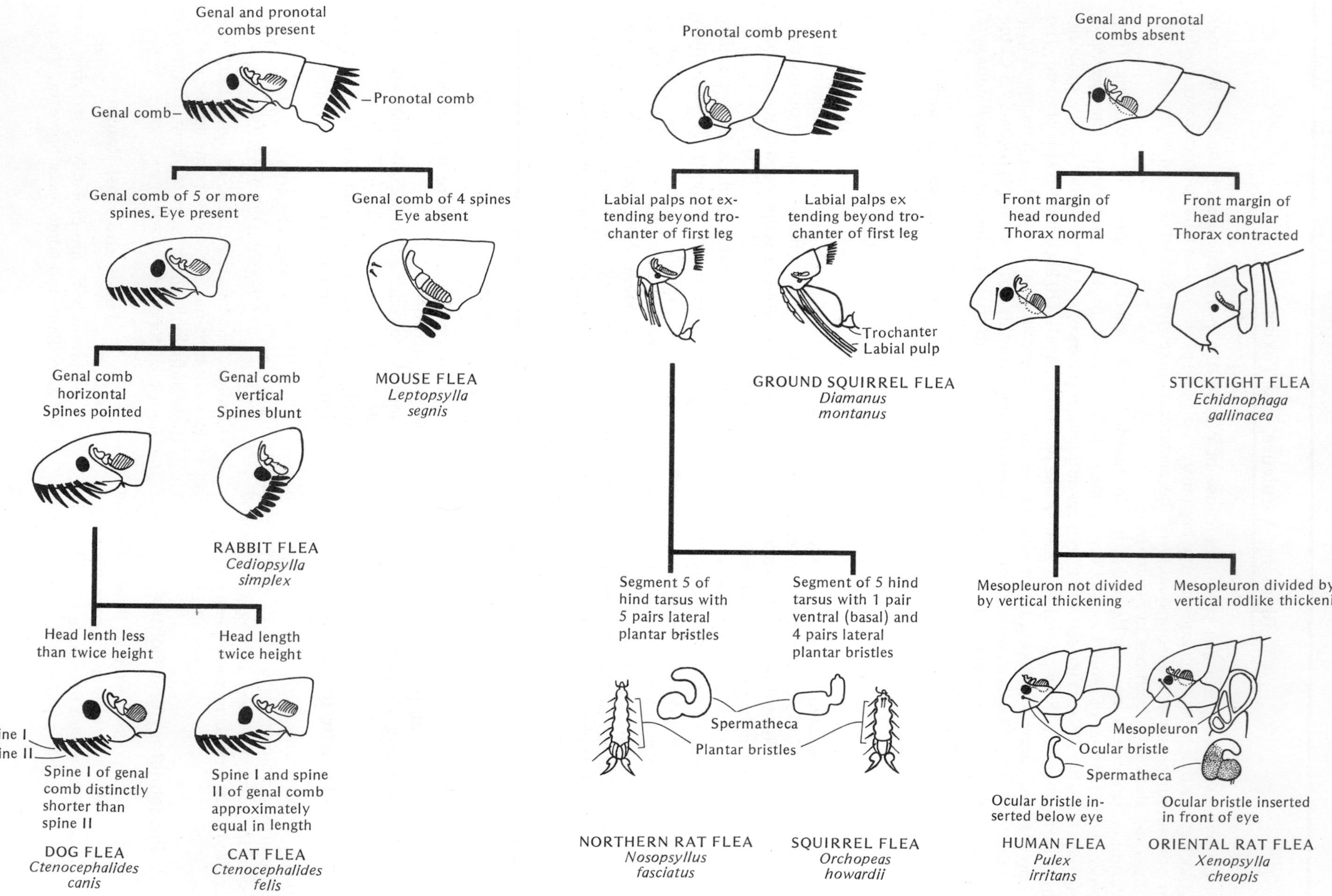

FIGURE 46.6 Pictorial key to some common fleas of North America.

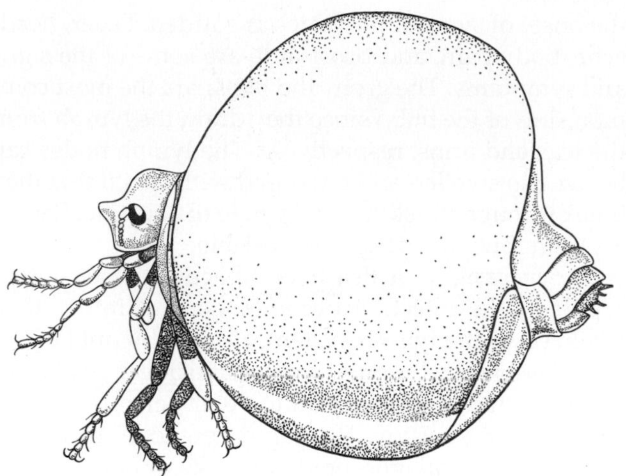

FIGURE 46.7 Female *Tunga penetrans,* the chigoe.

infects a wide range of other hosts such as swine, dogs, and humans.

Geographic Distribution and Importance

The distribution of this flea was originally in tropical South America, but it was carried to Africa in the 19th century. It is seen sporadically in almost any part of the world because of travelers becoming infected. Most concern relates to infestations of humans in which the flea often embeds near a toenail and allows serious secondary bacterial infections to develop.

Morphology

The female has a sharply angled head and a globular abdomen (Fig. 46.7). The engorged ovigerous female may reach 5 mm or more in diameter.

Life Cycle

The female enters the skin by slashing it with the mouthparts and then it burrows in until only the last two segments of the abdomen are at the surface. Copulation takes place after the female has penetrated the skin. Oviposition then takes place; eggs are sometimes retained in the skin. The mouthparts extend as deeply as the capillaries from which the female feeds. Both females and males feed on blood. The rest of the cycle takes place off of the host, as in other fleas.

Diagnosis

Once in the skin, considerable irritation takes place since the flea acts as a foreign body. A watery blister and localized inflammation are indications that a chigoe has entered the skin. In enzootic areas, this condition is recognized for what it is, but in travelers, the diagnosis may be missed. The best evidence of infestation with the chigoe is finding it in the lesion.

Host–Parasite Interactions

Having entered the skin, the inflammatory process progresses rapidly as the female feeds and engorges. The lesion becomes secondarily infected by bacteria and pain increases. Invasion of the wound with anaerobic, spore-forming bacteria may cause gangrene. Although any part of the body may be attacked, the feet and especially the area under the toenails are favored sites. If the flea is not removed, severe damage may result.

Epidemiology and Control

If the suspicion has been raised that a skin lesion is caused by *T. penetrans,* the treatment is simple: The flea is dug out with a clean needle and the wound is treated with a bactericidal solution. If the secondary infection has progressed, more extensive chemotherapy and other treatment may be required.

The original distribution of the chigoe was from the northern extremity of South America to about central Brazil (10° S. latitude), but it has been reported as far south as Uruguay (32° S). During the 19th century, this organism was imported into western Africa, probably the Congo drainage, as a by-product of the slave trade. It was probably carried in sand ballast from the New World.

The migration of the flea through tropical Africa was rapid; within a short time of its being taken to Africa in the 1870s or 1880s, it had been found 320 km (200 mi) from the coast at Stanley Pool. By the 1890s, it had extended its range to 2400 km (1500 mi) to the western Rift Valley and Lake Victoria. Unfortunately the local people did not know the cause of the foot infections, and they did not know how to treat them. There were instances in which so many people were disabled by the infection that whole villages starved because the crops were not tended or harvested.

Wearing shoes is usually recommended to prevent infection, and while this is good advice, people living in poor countries may not be able to comply. Persons visiting tropical enzootic areas should be aware of the likelihood of infection and either wear shoes or treat themselves at the first sign of infection. Vacationers from temperate climates are not likely to know about *T. penetrans* and neither are their physicians who may be faced with an infected toenail. This is another instance when the physician needs to ask the question, "Where have you been?"

Related Organisms

Laboratory rabbits and rodents are likely to have fleas, and they can become a nuisance as well as a factor that may confound experiments. *Spilopsyllus cuniculi* is the common flea on the laboratory rabbit, *Oryctolagus. Leptopsyllus segnis* is frequently found on mice and other laboratory rodents (Fig. 46.6).

Although birds have relatively few fleas, *Echidnophaga gallinacea,* the sticktight flea is often on chickens, as well as mammals such as the dog (Fig. 46.6). *E. gallinacea* is true to its common name and remains tenaciously applied to the skin of the host; on chickens it is usually seen in large numbers on the head, especially around the eyes.

PLAGUE

Plague is a flea-borne zoonosis caused by the bacterium *Yersinia pestis* (syn. *Pasteurella pestis*); the disease is referred to also as bubonic plague and the black death. Plague is one of the important diseases of human history. It has followed trade routes, decided the course of wars, and killed untold millions of people during historic times.

Plague is described in the Old Testament, and it seems likely that its original focus was in Africa. Its spread from North Africa and the Middle East to Europe did not take place until the 6th century. Four outbreaks were described by St. Bede in England in the 7th century. In the 14th century, Europe was struck with recurring epidemics of plague in which three-fourths of the people in some areas were killed. It has been estimated that 25 million persons died before the epidemics subsided. The impact of these epidemics brought enormous economic and social change and played a crucial role in the decline of the feudal system in Europe. Tuchman (1978) presented a fascinating account of the impact of plague on feudal Europe. The horror of one of the plague epidemics was graphically described by Samuel Pepys in 1664–1665 when the Great Plague of London killed 75,000 people out of a population of 450,000, about 17% of its inhabitants.

The manifestations of plague in humans range from mild, almost inapparent, infections to severe but nonfatal disease to rapid, fulminating infection resulting in death. There are three types:

1. *Bubonic.* The infection is transmitted by fleas into the skin. Swollen lymph nodes (bubos) are seen with the onset of symptoms, which is sudden. Fever, headache, body pain, and prostraton are some of the signs and symptoms. The groin and axilla are the most common sites of the bubo since they drain the lymph from the legs and arms, respectively. The lymph nodes can become so swollen and engorged with bacilli that they break through the skin and drain to the outside. Recovery from bubonic plague is possible.
2. *Septicemic.* If a flea injects bacilli directly into a capillary, the infection becomes general rather than localized in the lymph system. Recover is unlikely.
3. *Pneumonic.* In some persons, the infection reaches the lungs and is then spread to other persons through coughing or sputum. The rapid spread from person to person in a plague epidemic takes place through pneumonic plague rather than through fleas. Cats also spread plague to humans through pneumonic infections. Recovery is unlikely.

Recent outbreaks of plague have become pandemics, worldwide epidemics, because of rapid transport along trade routes (Fig. 46.8). Over the years 1894 to 1922, plague was spread from Chinese seaports, most likely with pelts of Siberian marmots. Plague was introduced into the United States in San Francisco in 1901, and it quickly spread throughout the western states. Attempts were made to contain the spread of the organism through rodent control, but to no avail. The organism is now enzootic in 15 western states (Fig. 46.9).

Plague remains a disease of worldwide concern. Where there is disruption of the social system, natural disaster, or poor living conditions, plague is likely to break out. A focus of infection of an especially pathogenic plague organism, which has not been satisfactorily controlled, exists in southeast Asia.

Y. pestis cycles in rodent populations in the wild or in urban areas. In most instances, plague is a disease of wild rodents such as prairie dogs, ground squirrels, rock squirrels, and members of the genus *Rattus.* On occasion it spills over into urban rodents and then into the human population.

Rodents not only become infected, but they also die from the disease. Certain rodents such as the Norway rat, *Rattus norvegicus,* can maintain a bacteremia for weeks. During the bacteremia, fleas feeding on the rat become infected and the bacteria multiply in their intestines.

Transmission takes place from the flea back to another rodent by so-called blocked fleas. In some species of flea, the bacteria multiply well and there are so many organisms that they tend to move into the anterior portion of the intestinal tract and to block the proventriculus. The bacteria make a sticky mass there forming

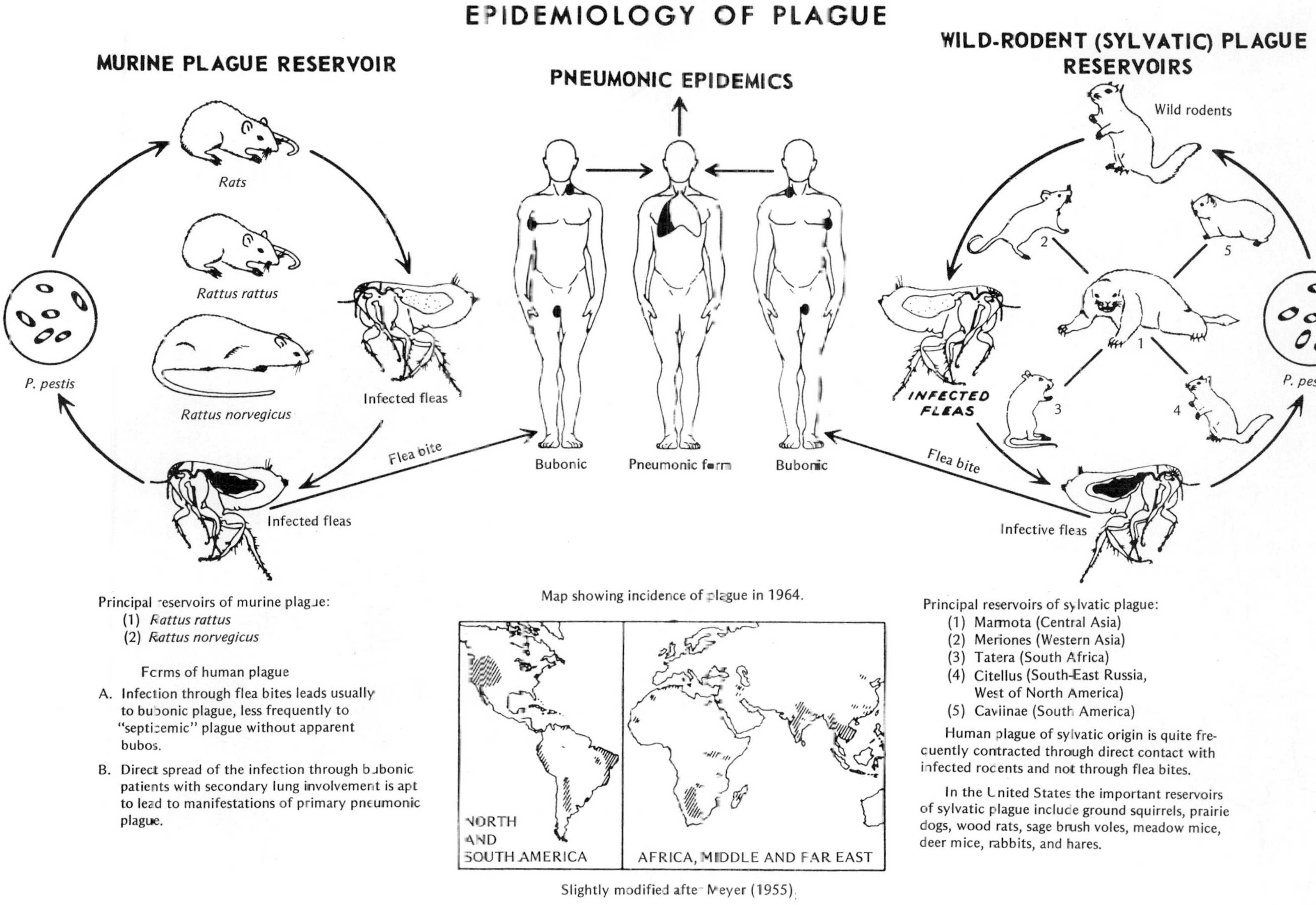

EPIDEMIOLOGY OF PLAGUE
MURINE PLAGUE RESERVOIR
PNEUMONIC EPIDEMICS
WILD-RODENT (SYLVATIC) PLAGUE RESERVOIRS
Rats
Rattus rattus
Rattus norvegicus
P. pestis
Infected fleas
Flea bite
Infected fleas
Bubonic
Pneumonic form
Bubonic
Wild rodents
INFECTED FLEAS
Flea bite
Infective fleas
P. pestis
1
2
3
4
5
Principal reservoirs of murine plague:
(1) Rattus rattus
(2) Rattus norvegicus
Forms of human plague
A. Infection through flea bites leads usually to bubonic plague, less frequently to "septicemic" plague without apparent bubos.
B. Direct spread of the infection through bubonic patients with secondary lung involvement is apt to lead to manifestations of primary pneumonic plague.
Map showing incidence of plague in 1964.
NORTH AND SOUTH AMERICA
AFRICA, MIDDLE AND FAR EAST
Slightly modified after Meyer (1955).
Principal reservoirs of sylvatic plague:
(1) Marmota (Central Asia)
(2) Meriones (Western Asia)
(3) Tatera (South Africa)
(4) Citellus (South-East Russia, West of North America)
(5) Caviinae (South America)
Human plague of sylvatic origin is quite frequently contracted through direct contact with infected rodents and not through flea bites.
In the United States the important reservoirs of sylvatic plague include ground squirrels, prairie dogs, wood rats, sage brush voles, meadow mice, deer mice, rabbits, and hares.

FIGURE 46.8 Epidemiology of plague.

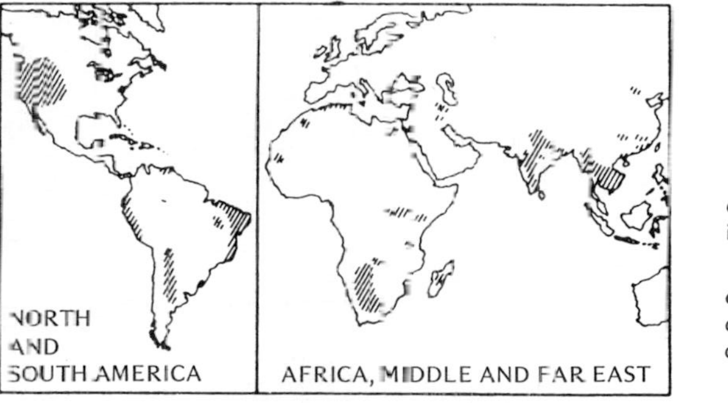

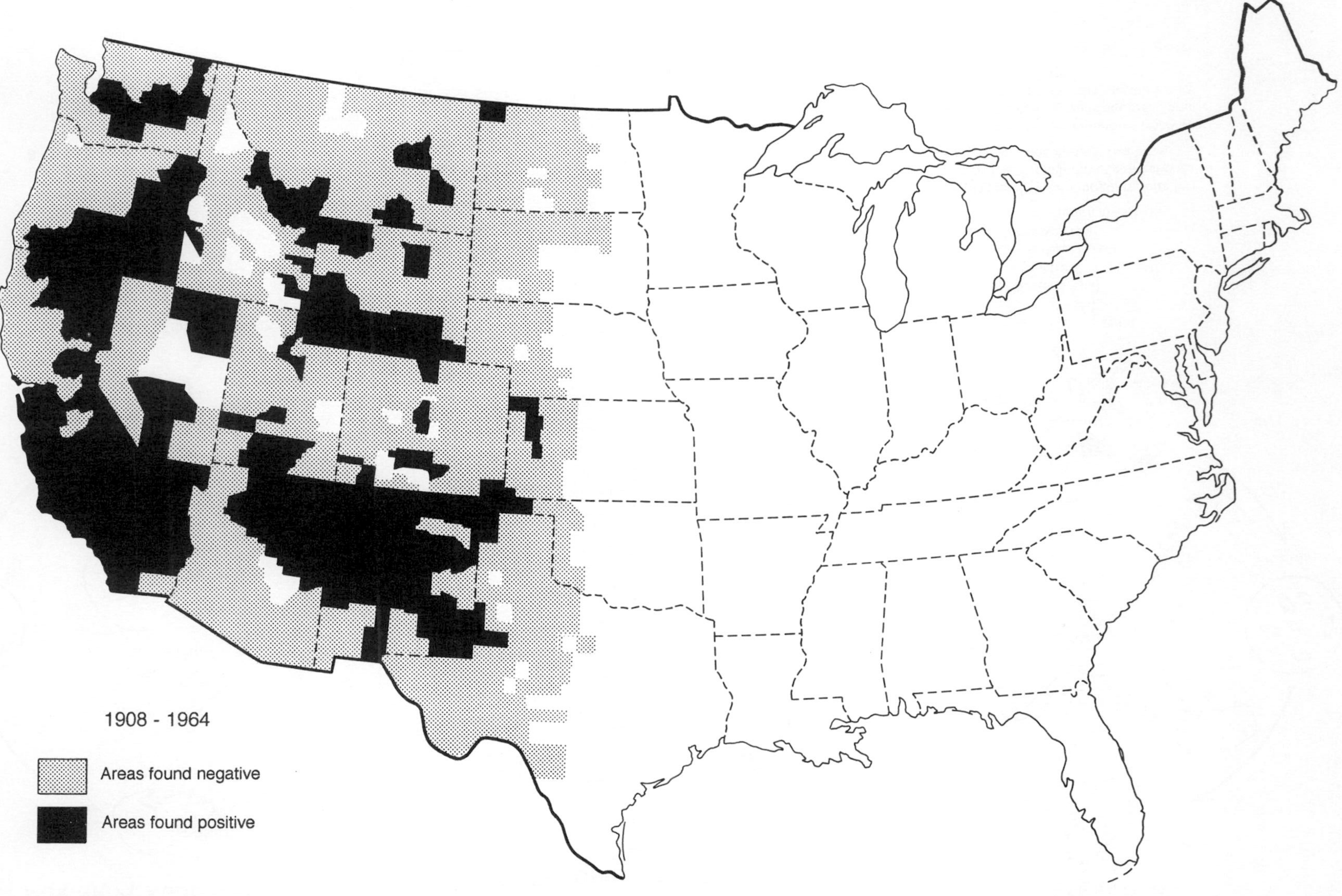

FIGURE 46.9 Distribution of *Yersinia pestis,* the cause of plague, in the United States.

a plug that prevents the esophageal pump from taking in blood. The flea attempts to suck blood, fails to do and, when it relaxes, ejects bacteria back into the wound. Transmission may also take place through fecal droplets contaminated with plague bacilli, which may be rubbed into the skin or enter through a break in the skin such as the wound made by a feeding flea. Handling infected rodents or rabbits is also a means of transmitting the infection.

Fleas differ in their capacity to transmit plague, and the concept of vector efficiency (VE) has been developed to give a quantitative estimate of how well a species may transmit an agent. VE is the made up of the following:

1. Blocking potential: the percentage of fleas with a blocked proventriculus
2. Length of the life of the flea
3. Population size
4. Host specificity, that is, the willingness of the flea to transfer to other species of hosts and to feed
5. Length of time the flea may carry an infection.

Of about 100 species of fleas known to transmit the plague bacillus, *Xenopsylla cheopis*, the Oriental rat flea (Fig. 46.6), is the most important vector on a global basis. It blocks well, and the infection remains in it for a long period., Other species of flea are also good vectors, but with the exception of the human flea, they are mostly found in particular geographic areas. For example, *Oropsylla montana* (syn. *Diamanus montanus*) is a common vector in the western United States.

The maintenance of plague in the wild between epidemics has been a continuing puzzle. It seems that there is a relatively low rate of transmission among rodents through fleas that remain blocked for months. Some fleas become infected, but remain unblocked for a long period, perhaps as long as six months. When they do become blocked, they are able to transmit the agent. This explains the continuing residue of infection in some areas, particularly in light of the observation that blocked fleas usually do not live longer than 30 days.

The following factors come together in plague epidemiology:

1. Susceptibility of the rodents in an area
2. A high population of susceptible rodents
3. The ability of the fleas to serve as vectors (VE)
4. The life cycle and behavior of the fleas

Campestral plague, sometimes called sylvatic plague, refers to the maintenance of plague in wild rodents, usually in grasslands or steppe. In the United States, plague is limited to the area west of the 100th meridian, about where the short-grass prairie begins (Fig. 46.9). On occasion, plague moves from these centers into the human population through infected fleas. When a rodent dies of plague its fleas tend to leave for any warm-blooded host that may be nearby. This may be another wild rodent, an urban rodent, or a human, among others.

Urban outbreaks take place primarily through urban rats, *Rattus norvegicus* or *R. rattus.* In major epidemics in humans, or pandemics spread across trade routes, rats have been the principal reservoirs. Subsidence of plague outbreaks occurs through the death of susceptible individuals to the point where transmission is unlikely, or by the development of immunity among the survivors.

Plague is treated by administering broad-spectrum antibiotics. It is important to ensure that a patient not be treated too aggressively. The bacteria contain an endotoxin, and it is likely that many of the symptoms of plague result from release of this toxin. If a high level of antibiotic is given over a short period of time, the patient may die as a result of the release of a large quantity of endotoxin.

Control of a plague outbreak requires a careful approach to ensure that the proper sequence of steps is carried out:

1. Quarantine. Persons are prevented from entering the area or from leaving it without some record of their whereabouts
2. Flea control
3. Rodent control
4. Isolation of human cases, especially of pneumonic plague
5. Vaccination of persons at high risk

It is important, early in the investigation, to determine what the extent is of the outbreak and to close off the area. Keeping people out is the first step, and then keeping track of those persons who are inside the area and who may leave. If they have been exposed, they should begin to show symptoms of infection within a week.

Flea control is done before rodent control. If rodents are controlled first, that leaves a large population of hungry, infected fleas which will attack any human walking nearby. Rodent control can be done by a variety of means; poisoning is the most effective, but trapping may also be done. Shooting them is ineffective.

A vaccine is available to protect against infection with *Y. pestis*, but it is usually given only to those persons, such as field or laboratory investigators, who are at risk of infection.

In rural outbreaks in prairie dogs, the first sign that plague has entered the area is that the rodents are not seen. Prairie dogs, *Cynomys* spp., are completely susceptible to *Y. pestis* and the whole colony is wiped out. If a humans enter, they are set upon by fleas, and if dogs enter the area, they carry home infected fleas that then may transfer to their owners.

Plague is enzootic in some areas of New Mexico and land use has contributed to maintenance of plague and its transfer to humans. Many people like the solitude of the desert and build in exurban areas in the rocky, rolling hills. It is usually necessary to flatten an area for the foundation of the house, so rocks are bulldozed over the edge of the hill and left to provide natural landscaping. Such rocks also provide new habitat for rock squirrels, and dogs like to harass these rodents. A number of cases are on record of dogs taking fleas home with them and transferring plague to their owners.

RICKETTSIAL INFECTIONS

Murine typhus, caused by *Rickettsia typhi*, is transmitted by the fleas *Xenospylla cheopis* and *Nosopsyllus fasciatus* as well as by the louse *Polyplax spinulos* and the mite *Ornithonyssus bacoti* (Tab. 46.1). Another rickettsial agent, *R. felis*, has been isolated from cats and fleas and has been determined to be the cause of at least one human infection.

Readings

Azad, A. F., Radulovic, S., Higgins, J. A., Noden, B. H., and Troyer, J. M. (1997). Flea-borne rickettsioses: Ecologic considerations. *Emerg. Infect. Dis.* **3,** 319–327.

Bahmanyar, M., and Cavanaugh, D. C. (1976). *Plague Manual*. World Health Organization, Geneva.

Barnes, A. M. (1982). The surveillance and control of bubonic plague in the United States. *Symp. Zool. Soc. London* **50,** 237–270.

Cohn, S. K., Jr. (Ed.) (1997). *The Black Death and the Transformation of the West.* Harvard Univ. Press, Cambridge, MA.

Dryden, M. W. (1989). Biology of the cat flea, *Ctenocephalides felis felis. Companion Anim. Practice Parasitol./Pathobiol.* **19,** 23–27.

Harwood, R. F., and James, M. T. (1979). *Entomology in Human and Animal Health,* 7th ed. Macmillan, New York.

Henderson, G., and Foil, L. F. (1993). Efficacy of diflubenzuron in simulated household and yard conditions against the cat flea *Ctenocephalides felis* (Bouche) (Siphonaptera): Pulicidae. *J. Med. Entomol.* **30,** 619–621.

Holland, G. P. (1949). The Siphonaptera of Canada, Tech. Bull. No. 70. Canadian Dept. of Agric.

Holland, G. P. (1964). Evolution, classification and host relationships of Siphonaptera. *Annu. Rev. Entomol.* **9,** 123–146.

Hopkins, G. H. E., and Rothschild, M. (1953, 1956, 1962, 1966, 1971). *An Illustrated Catalog of the Rothschild Collection of Fleas (Siphonaptera) in the British Museum (Natural History),* Vols. 1–5. British Museum, London.

Hubbard, C. A. (1947). *Fleas of Western North America.* Iowa State Univ. Press, Ames.

Kwochka, K. W. (1987). Fleas and related diseases. *Vet. Clin. North Am. Small Anim. Practice Parasitic Infect.* **17**(6), 1235–1262.

Langer, W. L. (1964). The black death. *Sci. Am.* **210**(2), 114–121.

Lewis, R. E. (1972–1975). Notes on the geographic distribution and host preferences in the order Siphonaptera. Parts 1–6. *J. Med. Entomol.* **9,** 511; **10,** 255; **11,** 147; **11,** 403; **11,** 525; **11,** 658.

Lewis, R. E. (1993). Fleas (Siphonaptera). In *Medical Insects and Arachnids* (R. P. Land and R. W. Crosskey, Eds.), pp. 529–575. Chapman & Hall, London.

Plama, K. G., Meola, S. M., and Meola, R. W. (1993). Mode of action of pyriproxyfen and methoprene on eggs of *Ctenocephalides felis* (Siphonaptera: Pulicidae). *J. Med. Entomol.* **30,** 421–426.

Rothschild, M. (1965). Fleas. *Sci. Am.* **213**(6), 44–53.

Rothschild, M., Schein, Y., Parker, K., Neville, C., and Sternberg, S. (1973). The flying leap of the flea. *Sci. Am.* **229**(5), 92–100.

Thomas, R. E. (1996). Fleas and the agents they transmit. In *The Biology of Disease Vectors* (B. J. Beaty and W. C. Marquardt, Eds.). Univ. Press of Colorado, Niwot.

Traub, R. (1985). Coevolution of fleas and mammals. In *Coevolution of Parasitic Arthropods and Mammals* (K. C. Kim, Ed.). Wiley, New York.

Traub, R., and Starcke, H. (Eds.) (1980). *Proceedings of a Conference at Ashton Wold, Peterborough, UK, June 1977.* Balkema, Rotterdam.

Trudeau, W. L., Caldas-Fernandez, E., Fox, W., Brenner, R., Bucholtz, G. A., and Lockey, R. F. (1993). Allergenicity of the cat flea (*Ctenocephalides felis*). *Clin. Exp. Allergy* **23,** 377–383.

Tuchman, B. W. (1978). *A Distant Mirror: The Calamitous 14th Century.* Knopf, New York.

CHAPTER

47

Diptera: Nematocera and Brachycera

Members of the order Diptera are a diverse group in both structure and development. Beyond their having a single pair of wings (the hind wings are reduced to balancing organs called halteres) and all being homometabolic, the suborders have quite different patterns of development and structures.

There are about 100,000 species of dipterans in 140 families, making it the third largest order of insects exceeded only by the beetles and lepidopterans (Tab. 43.1); diversity might well be expected in such a large taxon. Many important members are familiar: mosquitoes, house flies, flesh flies, deer flies, midges, black flies (Fig. 47.1).

Dipterans are important to humans for a variety of reasons. Many flies such as the house fly and face fly are pests. In addition, many serve as either mechanical or biological vectors of infectious agents. Tsetse transmit the agent causing African sleeping sickness; mosquitoes transmit malaria, lymphatic filariasis, and hundreds of viruses; biting midges transmit filarioid nematodes and viruses such as blue tongue virus; tabanids transmit tularemia. Since these flies are bloodsuckers, they can be serious pests regardless of whether they are vectors of infectious agents. Many flies are parasitic as larvae, and they can be serious medical and economic problems (Chapter 49).

Members of the order fall into three well-defined groups (Fig. 47.1) based first on antennal structure; however, additional characteristics define the suborders:

1. *Nematocera (thread horn).* Adult antennae with at least seven segments that are not fused; no arista; no ptilinum; larva with well-developed head; mandibles work horizontally; pupa not enclosed in the last larva skin (obtectate). Mosquitoes, midges, black flies, sand flies.

2. *Brachycera (short horn).* Adult antennae with three segments, although the third segment may appear to have additional segments so that there may appear to be as many as seven segments; no ptilinum; larval head incomplete and retractile; mandibles of larvae hooklike or knifelike and working vertically; pupa seldom enclosed in last larva skin; adults emerge from pupa through a straight or T-shaped slit. Deer flies, horse flies, snipe flies.

3. *Cyclorrapha (circular suture).* Adult antennae with three segments and an arista; ptilinum present; larva with vestigial head; larval mouthparts reduced to simple hooks, which work vertically; pupa enclosed in last larva skin (coarctate). House flies, flesh flies, bots, pigeon flies, tsetse.

SUBORDER NEMATOCERA: FAMILY CULICIDAE—THE MOSQUITOES

The family Culicidae contains more than 3500 described species that are divided into three subfamilies:

Anophelinae, Culicinae, and Toxorhynchitinae. Some of their recognition features are as follows:

1. *Toxorhynchitinae.* Larvae predaceous with large jaws for capturing other mosquito larvae on which they feed. Adults are relatively large with a long, curved proboscis; not blood feeders, but rather are plant feeders. *Toxorhynchites.*

TABLE 47.1 Some Disease Agents Transmitted by Mosquitoes

Disease agent and disease	Hosts		Vectors
	Natural	Tangential	
Virus			
Eastern equine encephalitis	Bird	Human	*Coquilletidia perturbans*
Venezuelan encephalitis	Small mammal	Human, horse	*Cx. pipiens*, etc.
Western equine encephalitis	Bird	Human, horse	*Cx. tarsalis*
Dengue	Human		*Ae. aegypti*, *Ae. albopictus*
Japanese encephalitis	Swine	Human	*Cx. tritaeniorhynchus*
St. Louis encephalitis	Bird	Human	*Cx. pipiens*, *Cx. nigripalpus*
Yellow fever	Primate	Human	*Ae. aegypti*, *Ae. africanus*
LaCrosse encephalitis	Rodent	Human	*Ae. triseriatus*
Apicomplexa			
Malaria	Human		*Anopheles* spp.
Malaria	Bird		*Culex* spp.
Filarioid Nematode			
Wuchereria bancrofti	Human		*Culex, Mansonia*
Brugia malayi	Cat	Human	*Culex, Mansonia*
Dirofilaria immitis	Canid	Human	*Culex, Aedes* spp.

2. *Anophelinae.* Larvae lack a breathing tube on the eighth abdominal segment; the body of the larva lies parallel to the surface of the water. Pupae have short, broad trumpets or breathing tubes, which have large openings that continue as a split down the front. Adult males and females both have maxillary palps at least as long as the proboscis, and in the males they are clubbed at the distal ends; the scutellum is often trilobed. Eggs are laid singly and have floats on their sides. Adults have a characteristic resting and feeding posture with the head down and the hind legs raised. *Anopheles, Chagasia, Bironella.*

3. *Culicinae.* Larvae have a long breathing tube on the eighth abdominal segment; the body of the larva hangs head down from the surface of the water. Pupae in *Culex* have long, slender breathing tubes that are not split, but other genera may have short trumpets some of which may be split. Adults have short maxillary palps in the females and long ones in the males. The scutellum is usually rounded. Eggs are laid in rafts and they lack floats. The resting and feeding positions of the adult females are with the body parallel to the surface and usually with all of the legs on the surface. Further subdivided into the tribes Culicini and Aedini. *Culex, Aedes, Mansonia, Culiseta, Wyeomyia, Psorophora,* and so on.

Morphology

Mosquitoes are generally 3 to 6 mm long, but a few exceed 9 mm. They have large numbers of flat scales on both the wings and to body; the scales on the wings are on the veins and the margins. The wings have an unforked vein between two forked veins on the distal margin (Figs. 47.1, 47.2). Mouthparts are a long proboscis or fascicle adapted for sucking blood and plant juices; the females have mandibles, but the males usually lack them and cannot take blood, only plant juices. The thorax is broader than the head, antennae are long and plumose in the males, but the females have only a few sparse hairs. Larvae are aquatic, and have a well-defined head, thorax, and abdomen; an air tube arises on abdominal segment 8 (Fig. 47.3, 47.5). A cluster of so-called gills arises on the anal segment, but these are actually osmoregulatory organs.

Geographic Distribution and Importance

Cosmopolitan. Ubiquitous might be a better term for mosquitoes since they are everywhere that has the tiniest amount of water in which the larvae can develop. It is difficult to overstate the importance of mosquitoes to human and animal welfare. Not only do they suck blood and make life intolerable at certain times and places, but they also transmit a huge number of disease agents of humans and other animals (Tab. 47.1). In addition to the few organism listed in the tabulation, mosquitoes transmit hundreds of arboviruses (arthropod-borne viruses) such as Cache Valley virus, Crimean Hemorrhagic Fever virus, and Japanese Encephalitis B virus; there are so many that it is not possible to give anything other than a brief glimpse of the agents. All of these agents (except dengue virus) cycle silently in the wild and may be transmitted to humans or livestock under certain conditions.

Life Cycle

All mosquitoes require water for the development of the larvae and pupae (Fig. 47.4). Eggs are laid in or near water but never in open water. Females respond to a number of environmental stimuli in choosing places to deposit their eggs. *Aedes* and *Psorophora* lay their eggs in damp or dry places, whereas *Anopheles*

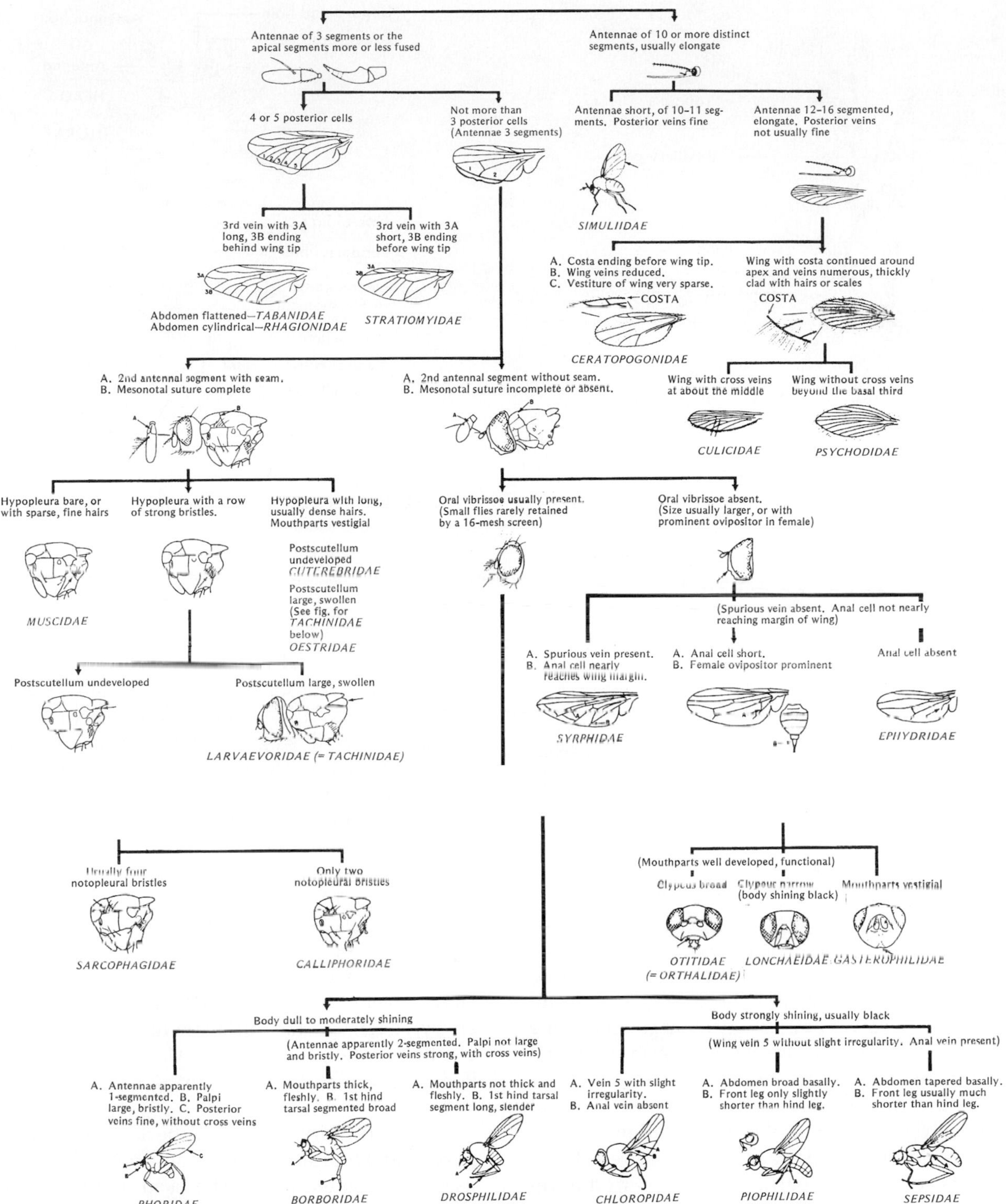

FIGURE 47.1 Pictorial key to the principal families of Diptera of importance in human health.

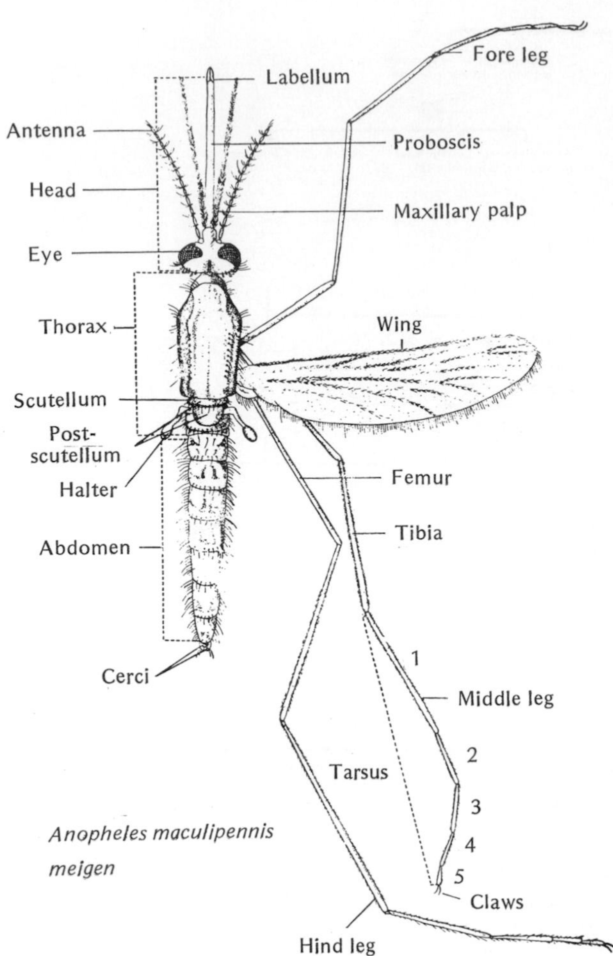

FIGURE 47.2 A diagram of a female anopheline mosquito, *Anopheles maculipennis,* to show major anatomical features.

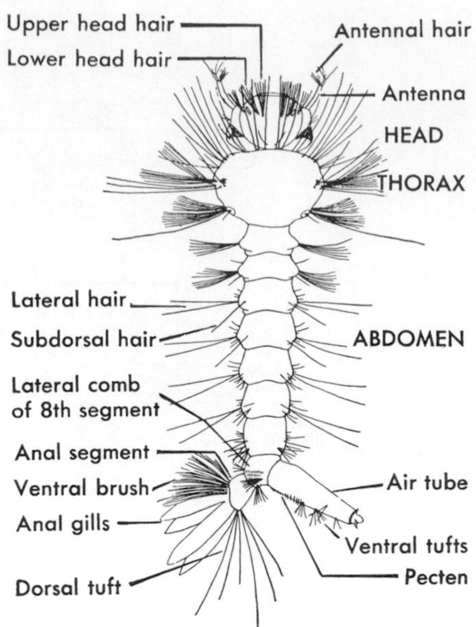

FIGURE 47.3 A diagram of a culicine mosquito larva to show major anatomical features.

lays its eggs in the water. *Culex* and *Culiseta* lay their eggs in rafts on the surface of the water, and *Mansonia* lays its eggs on the underside of leaves of submerged vegetation. *Aedes aegypti* is an example of a peridomestic mosquito that is a container breeder; eggs are laid in tin cans, tires, flower pots, or any other small volume of water near houses. *Ae. aegypti* is probably derived from a tree-hole mosquito.

Under the proper conditions, eggs develop and hatch quickly, often within 24 to 48 hours Some aedine mosquitoes develop partially and then require a stimulus such as cooling or a particular photoperiod to resume development. Floodwater mosquitoes, some members of the genera *Aedes* and *Psorophora,* lay their eggs in areas that flood periodically, and in temperate or cold climates, eggs laid during summer do not hatch until the following spring when the area is flooded. They typically come out in hordes at that time.

Most mosquito larvae trap little bits of food in their mouth fans; they are sometimes said to be filter feeders, but it is more accurately referred to as trapping. Food consists of bits of organic debris and microorganisms such as protists and rotifers. A few mosquito larvae, notably the larvae of *Toxorhynchites,* are predaceous and typically feed on other mosquito larvae.

The four larval stages may last for as short a time as three days to more than a month depending upon temperature and species. For example, *Psorophora confinnis* goes from egg to adult in three days at 46°C. (115°F.) in the California desert. *Culiseta inornata* requires 28 to 30 days to complete development at 14°C. (60°F.). The development of the yellow fever mosquito, *Ae. aegypti,* come almost to a standstill below about 26°C. (80°F.). Most culicine mosquitoes complete development in about seven days. Oxygen is required for larval development, and most larvae obtain it from the air by coming to the surface where they apply their breathing tubes; however, in *Mansonia* oxygen is obtained from plants by puncturing them with a posterior stylet.

The fourth larval stage is the last one before the pupa, and it typically does not feed but rather prepares itself to become a pupa. The head and thorax of the pupa are fused to form a cephalothorax. The pupa is free swimming but nonfeeding and usually lasts only two to three days. Pupae require oxygen and have breathing tubes, usually called trumpets, on the cephalothorax. In two genera, *Mansonia* and *Coquillettidia,* the trumpets are modified to penetrate plant tissue so as to obtain oxygen.

Adults emerge from the pupa at the surface of the

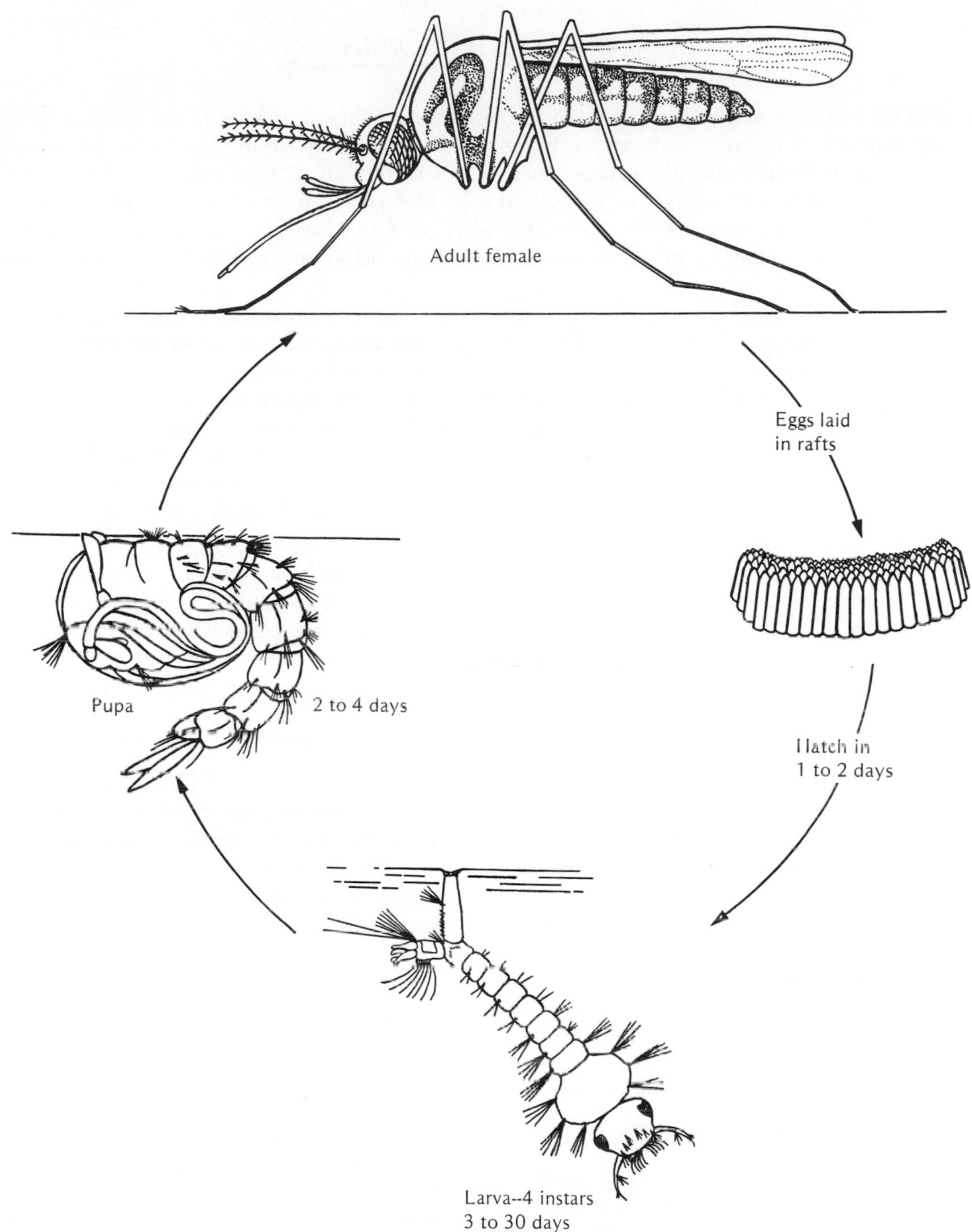

FIGURE 47.4 The life cycle of a culicine mosquito.

water; 10 to 15 minutes are required for emergence, drying of the body, and extension of the wings. During this time, mosquitoes are quite susceptible to predation.

Females are not ready to take a blood meal until one to three days after emergence. This is the beginning of the phase called the gonotrophic cycle. During this time the ovarian follicles develop. The females are then ready to mate, and it takes place in swarms of males. Females enter the swarm, pair up with a male, and they then probably leave the swarm, although this is difficult to determine. Males may mate several times, but females mate only once.

The next phase, host seeking, lasts for 3 to 10 days

OLD TIRES AND *Aedes*

An automobile tire is maniacally designed to hold water. There is no way that a tire can be oriented so that water will drain from it; trying to empty one is an exercise in frustration. In investigating the sporadic cases and outbreaks of LaCrosse encephalitis in Wisconsin, the vector was determined to be *Aedes triseriatus*, a tree-hole mosquito. A tree hole is a cavity likely to hold water for a period of time and in which the female mosquito oviposits. An old tire is as good as a tree-hole and females oviposit readily in them as well. In a number of instances, old tires were found to be the breeding sites of mosquitoes near houses.

Old tires were also determined to be the culprit in the importation of *Ae. albopictus* into the United States in 1985. Interestingly, in Asia used truck tires are not recapped but rather are sent in container ships to the United States where they are recapped and put back on the road. Old tires serve as oviposition sites for *Ae. albopictus* and the eggs withstand the sea voyage from eastern Asia to West Coast ports and to ports on the Gulf Coast. *Ae. albopictus* was first identified in the Houston, Texas, area, but it was later found to have been introduced into ports in California as well. This mosquito is an excellent vector of about 23 viruses. Of greatest interest to those living in the United States is that it is an efficient vector of the viruses causing St. Louis encephalitis, Dengue, and yellow fever. Fortunately *Ae. albopictus* has not been proven to have transmitted any disease agents in the United States—yet.

We see in these examples that economics, rapid transport, and the adaptability of potential vectors intersect both in the distribution of vectors and their likelihood of transmitting a pathogen to humans. If it were economical to recap truck tires in Asia, *Ae. albopictus* might not have been imported into the United States. Since it is now a resident here, a whole industry has sprung up to decipher the biology of the mosquito as well as to determine its potential as a vector and means of controlling it.

during which time they seek hosts, take a blood meal, and then rest somewhere while the eggs develop. Egg laying takes place over about a three-day period. The gonotrophic cycle, except for copulation, is then repeated, and one female may have as many as five cycles of egg laying. It should be noted that in the biological transmission of disease agents of all sorts, the female is infected at one feeding, lays eggs, and then must take another blood meal for transmission to occur.

Host–Parasite Interactions

Certain biological and behavioral characteristics of mosquitoes are important in relation to their ability to serve as vectors of disease agents (Figs. 47.5, 47.6). The categories are used principally in relation to humans, but the apply equally well to domestic animals:

1. Domiciliated species that have sites of larval development in or near houses readily enter dwellings and feed primarily on human blood; they usually rest in houses. They usually fly only a few hundred meters from the site of emergence. *Aedes aegypti* and *Culex pipiens* are examples of mosquitoes that transmit arboviruses. Several species of *Anopheles* that vector malaria fall into this group; *An. stephensi* is an example of a malaria vector that is a truly urban mosquito.

2. Species that regularly come into contact with humans outdoors and may enter houses but do not rest there. They breed in wet fields, irrigation ditches, swamps, and standing water that is either natural or made by humans such as tree holes, banana trees, tin cans, or old tires. *Culex tarsalis*, *Ae. albopictus*, and *Mansonia* are examples.

3. Salt- or freshwater marsh, temporary rain pool breeders, or floodwater breeders. Eggs are laid in dry or damp areas and adults emerge five days after rain or flooding or emerge the following season. Concentrations of preadults may be extraordinarily high: as many as 20 million larvae/hectare (50 million/acre). *Ae. sollicitans* and *An. taeniorhynchus* are examples; they may migrate 70 km (40 mi.) from the site of emergence. *Psorophora* spp. are also included since they are single-brood per year mosquitoes in the Arctic and high mountain areas.

4. Forest canopy mosquitoes breed in tree holes or water-holding portions of leaves such as the axils of bromeliads. These species come into contact with humans only under special circumstances such as lumbering where trees are cut and thereby carry mosquitoes down to the ground or when trees are planted for shade near dwellings. *Ae. africanus* is an example.

Another classification of mosquito habitat relies on

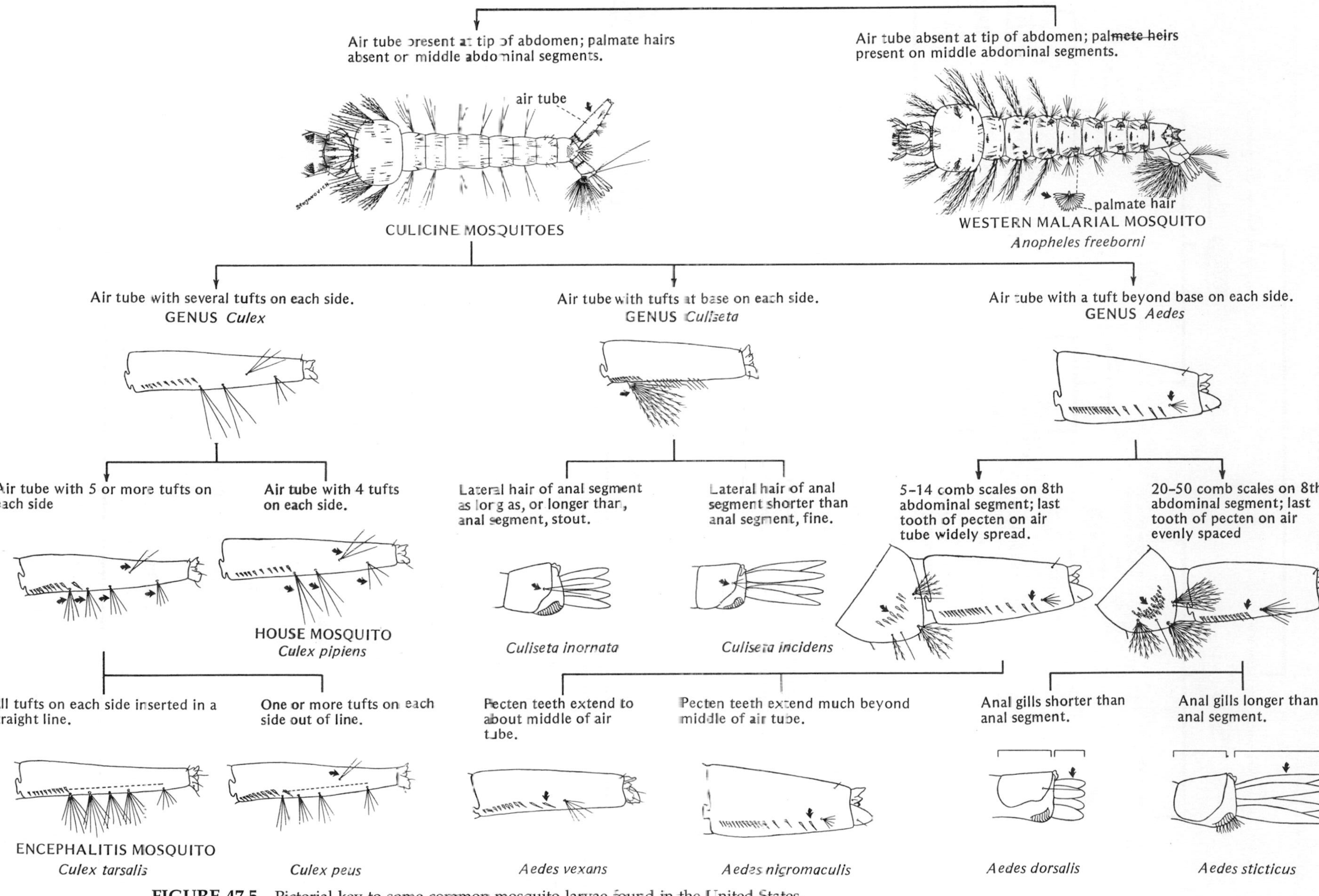

FIGURE 47.5 Pictorial key to some common mosquito larvae found in the United States.

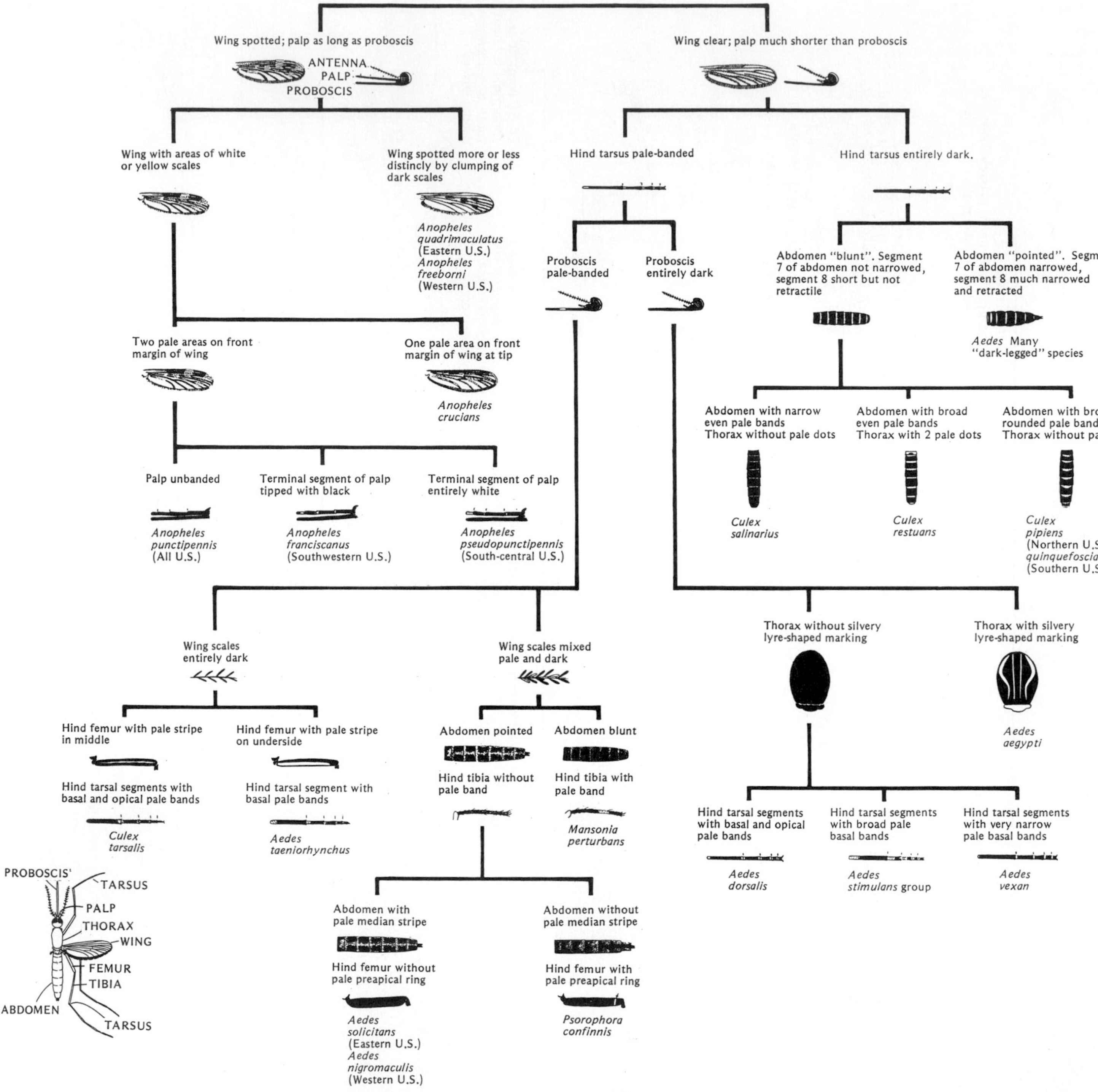

FIGURE 47.6 Pictorial key to some common female mosquitoes found in the United States.

the type of water rather than emphasizing the association with humans: flowing stream, ponded stream, lake edge, swamp and marsh, shallow permanent pond, intermittent ephemeral puddle, natural container, and artificial container.

The feeding preferences of mosquitoes are important in their abilities to serve as vectors as well as their being pests of humans and domesticated animals. Most mosquitoes have preferences for certain groups of vertebrates: birds, reptiles, amphibia, or mammals, but in some instances they switch hosts as the situation demands. Certain floodwater or marsh mosquitoes are

KNOWING WHEN TO QUIT

If left undisturbed, a mosquito will feed to repletion. A female mosquito may take up to four times her body weight in blood during two or three minutes of feeding. Blood, unlike other nutrients such as nectar, goes directly to the midgut. A fully fed mosquito is laden with an enormous quantity of fluid, and the meal is reduced in volume by excretion of water via the Malpighian tubules. Thus concentrated, the blood meal is then more manageable.

It is essential that a mosquito not take too much blood. The signal to terminate blood feeding comes from stretch receptors in the wall of the abdomen. This can be clearly demonstrated in a mosquito that has had its ventral nerve cords severed at the point where they enter the abdomen. Such a mosquito can feed, but it doesn't know when or how to quit. It continues to ingest blood until it literally explodes, showering the area with blood. It is not a pretty sight.

bird feeders and do not feed on humans. *Culex tarsalis* is the principal vector of St. Louis encephalitis (SLE) in the western United States. SLE has its reservoir in birds, and in the spring, *Cx. tarsalis* feeds on nestling birds, which are the amplifying hosts; as the summer progresses, nestlings fledge and are no longer readily available. *Cx. tarsalis* then switches to mammals for blood and may come to feed on humans thereby transmitting the virus. The anopheline vectors of malaria must have humans as their preferred hosts for transmission to be optimized.

We tend to think that blood feeding is essential for mosquitoes, and this is true in some species. However, some species and some demes can lay eggs without a blood meal; this capability is called autogeny. Usually only a few eggs are laid, perhaps 10% of the normal complement, but it is sufficient to keep the genetic line intact.

Notable Features

Both male and female mosquitoes take nectar as a source of energy, but only the females take blood. Nectar is an essential nutrient for the males both for the energy it provides as well as the water that is needed for survival. Although autogeny is a heritable trait, larvae that do not have good nutrition and do not carry over food reserves to the adult stage cannot produce eggs autogenously. Parenthetically, it should be noted that autogeny is not parthenogenesis, males are needed to fertilize the eggs.

Blood provides a good source of protein for production of eggs, but it is not by any means a perfect food. It is lacking in carbohydrate and fat so these sources of energy are not available. Energy must be sought from blood components such as proline. Also, blood has antibodies and leukocytes that may be harmful to a hematophagous insect. Blood also is low in vitamin content, and this lack is often made up by symbiotic bacteria in the cells of the intestine.

The female mosquito finds a host through a series of stereotyped maneuvers. The female flies at a right angle to the wind so that aromas drifting downwind cross its flight path. Once having encountered a plume of CO_2 or body odor from a potential host, the female turns upwind. As the mosquito approaches a host, it uses visual clues, heat, and moisture to decide that there is something worthwhile nearby.

Having reached a potential host, the female probes the skin to determine whether it should attempt to feed. Both lactic acid and octenol are stimulants to feeding. The mosquito salivates and probes searching for a capillary. When a capillary is found, or the mouthparts enter a hematoma formed by probing, the cibarial pump is activated and the midgut is filled. Stretch receptors in the midgut respond in order to stop feeding.

Epidemiology and Control

Control of mosquito populations requires an areawide program except in instances where the rooms of a dwelling might be sprayed to clear them of adults. The definition on an area depends on the particular mosquito(s) of concern as well as drainages, water courses, and prevailing winds. Different species of mosquito have different flight ranges, and as indicated earlier, different types of breeding sites. In short, the type of control program is determined by the species of mosquito that is the pest or vector.

Because their habitats and foods are so different, the control of larval and adult mosquitoes are also radically different.

Larval Control

1. Chemical
   a. No. 2 diesel oil may be applied to the surface of water. Larvae come to the surface of the water to obtain air (except for *Mansonia* and *Coquilletiddia*) and are killed by becoming covered in oil. Diesel oil also has a component that is directly toxic to larvae.
   b. Insecticide is placed in the water. The materials most often used now are second- and third-generaton insecticides. The organochlorine insecticides have been phased out in most countries, and organophosphates and carbamates are currently being used. Among third-generation insecticides, juvenile hormone (JH) mimetics can be used in waters where food products are not consumed by humans. JH mimetics have the advantage of not causing environmental contamination, and they are specific for insects; the second-generation insecticides may affect fish, birds, and mammals in addition to the target organisms.
2. Biological
   a. Predators
      (1) Fish such as *Gambusia*
      (2) *Toxorhynchites* larvae
      (3) Nematodes such as *Romanomermis petersoni*
      (4) Planaria that prey on larvae
   b. Disease agents
      (1) Microspora such as *Nosema algerae*
      (2) Bacteria such as *Bacillus thuringiensis israeliensis* (Bti) and *B. sphaericus*. Bti is a toxicant rather than a disease agent since it kills mosquito larvae when they ingest the spores that have a crystal of toxin; no reproduction of the bacterium takes place; that said, it is usually included among biological control agents.
3. Source reduction or habitat management. This method refers specifically to the techniques that do not use chemicals directly to kill insects and are not included under biological control; it can be thought of as physically altering the environment. For mosquitoes, the methods are as follows:
   a. Fill or drain swampy areas
   b. Remove aquatic plants that impede water flow or provide oviposition sites
   c. Remove manufactured sources of standing water such as tin cans, tires, and flower pots
   d. Use irrigation water properly so that ditches can be flushed or waste water does not accumulate in ditches or at the low ends of fields

Adult Control

1. Insecticides
   a. Direct action. Insecticide is sprayed into the air and kills mosquiitoes that fly into the spray. Compounds used are carbamates, organophosphates, and pyrethrins.
   b. Residual action. Insecticide is sprayed onto a surface or released from a carrier into a closed space. Organochlorine insecticides usually have a long residual action when sprayed onto surfaces in homes; because of environmental damage, organochlorines have been banned in many parts of the world. Organophosphates have only a short residual action but can be released slowly from a plastic carrier.
2. Personal protection
   a. Repellents or barriers.
      (1) Deet repels insects and may be placed on the skin or impregnated into clothing as has been developed for military personnel. A combination of Deet and a synthetic pyrethroid has been successful both spread on the skin or impregnated into clothing.
      (2) Screening of houses and use of mosquito netting at night. It is interesting to note that in areas of the United States where mosquitoes and mosquito-borne diseases have been historically important, they have become less so. Since the late 1940s both air conditioning and television have become common, and people spend less time in the cool evening air when mosquitoes are searching for a blood meal.
      (3) Use of barrier animals or zooprophylaxis. Since mosquitoes have feeding preferences, those which prefer animals other than humans may be kept away by providing an ox, say, as a diversion. Although possible to use, this method is not ordinarily purposefully employed.
   b. Traps. Various kinds of devices that emit ultraviolet light lure insects so that they are either electrocuted or drowned in a detergent solution. They may reduce mosquito populations as well as those of other harmless insects.
   c. Sound generators are sometimes marketed with the claim that certain frequencies drive away mosquitoes. These claims have not been substantiated.
   d. Birds. Purple martins are known to eat large numbers of insects, and some people provide houses to encourage their nesting near homes.

Whether the birds actually reduce mosquito populations is unknown.

Related Organisms

Some other families that have aquatic larvae and may be confused with the Culicidae are Chaoboridae, Dixidae, Tipulidae, and Chironomidae. None of these dipterans is hematophagous, but it is sometimes important to differentiate them from mosquitoes.

FAMILY SIMULIIDAE—THE BLACK FLIES

The black flies or buffalo gnats receive their common names from the fact that the bodies of the adults are nearly black or at least dark brown, and the thorax is enlarged in a way that the head seems to hang down from it (Fig. 47.7). They also have other names such as jejens, coffee flies, and no-see-ums (although this last name is also used for biting midges). Black flies are associated with well-aerated aquatic habitats in which the larvae and pupae develop and to which the females return to oviposit. They are important because of the aggressive feeding of the females and because they transmit several diseases of importance to humans as well as a number of viral, protistan, and helminthic organisms of zoological interest (Tab. 47.2).

Name of Organisms and Disease Associations

Simulium is the principal genus in the family, but other genera, *Australosimulium, Prosimulium, Parasimulium, Gigantodax,* and *Cnephia* are occasionally encountered in some locations. Some of the species that are vectors for *Onchocerca volvulus* of humans are *S. damnosum, S. neavei, S. metallicum, S. ochraceum, S. callidum,* and *S. exiguum.*

The agents known to be transmitted by black flies include viruses, apicomplexans, one or more trypanosomes of birds, and filarioid nematodes of both birds and mammals (Tab. 47.2). The most important of these organisms is *Onchocerca volvulus* of humans (Chapter 34), which has serious impact on human health in Africa, parts of the Middle East and Central America.

Hosts and Host Range

Black flies feed on warm-blooded hosts, mammals and birds, and they usually have host preferences. Those, for example, that transmit *Onchocerca volvulus* are anthropophilic. Certain of them feed on birds and can become the cause of economic loss in chickens.

Geographic Distribution and Importance

Cosmopolitan. Simuliids are found in all climates where there is water for the developing larvae. In arctic and temperate climates they are univoltine (one brood per year) and emerge in spring or early summer in hordes that make life unbearable. Several instances are on record where black flies have occurred in such numbers that cattle have been smothered and exsanguinated by them. One such disaster took place in Saskatchewan, Canada, in the 1940s.

Their serving as vectors of various infectious agents has been alluded to (Tab. 47.2).

Morphology

The members of the family are small flies ranging in size from 1 to 5 mm. They usually have dark bodies, and the thorax is quite convex dorsally. The eyes are large, actually holoptic in the males, and they have relatively short, filiform antennae (Fig. 47.7); the body is short and compact. The mouthparts are short and the females are pool feeders (telmatophagous).

Life Cycle

The females lay eggs, which are up to 0.5 mm long, on plants in or at the water's edge in gelatinous masses. In fact, there seems to be an aggregation pheromone that causes females to gather and lay eggs at the same time and place. They may deposit so many eggs on plants that they bend over into the water.

The eggs develop rapidly and the first stage larvae emerge within a day or two. There follow six to nine larval instars, with the usual number being seven. The larvae have glands that produce a silken protein that they use to hold the abdomen onto the substrate with the head extending downstream. The cephalic fans curve back upstream and serve to catch small bits of food, which are then transferred to the mouth. Food consists of finely divided plant material, protists, and small invertebrates within the range of 10 to 150 μm. Black flies are one of the principal processors of plant debris in streams.

In temperate and cold climates, there is usually only a single brood of black flies each year; they overwinter as partially developed larvae. In the tropics, there may be more than 15 generations in a calendar year. In the Australian desert, eggs can remain quiescent for as long as three years in moist sand in a dry river bed.

At the end of larval growth and development, the

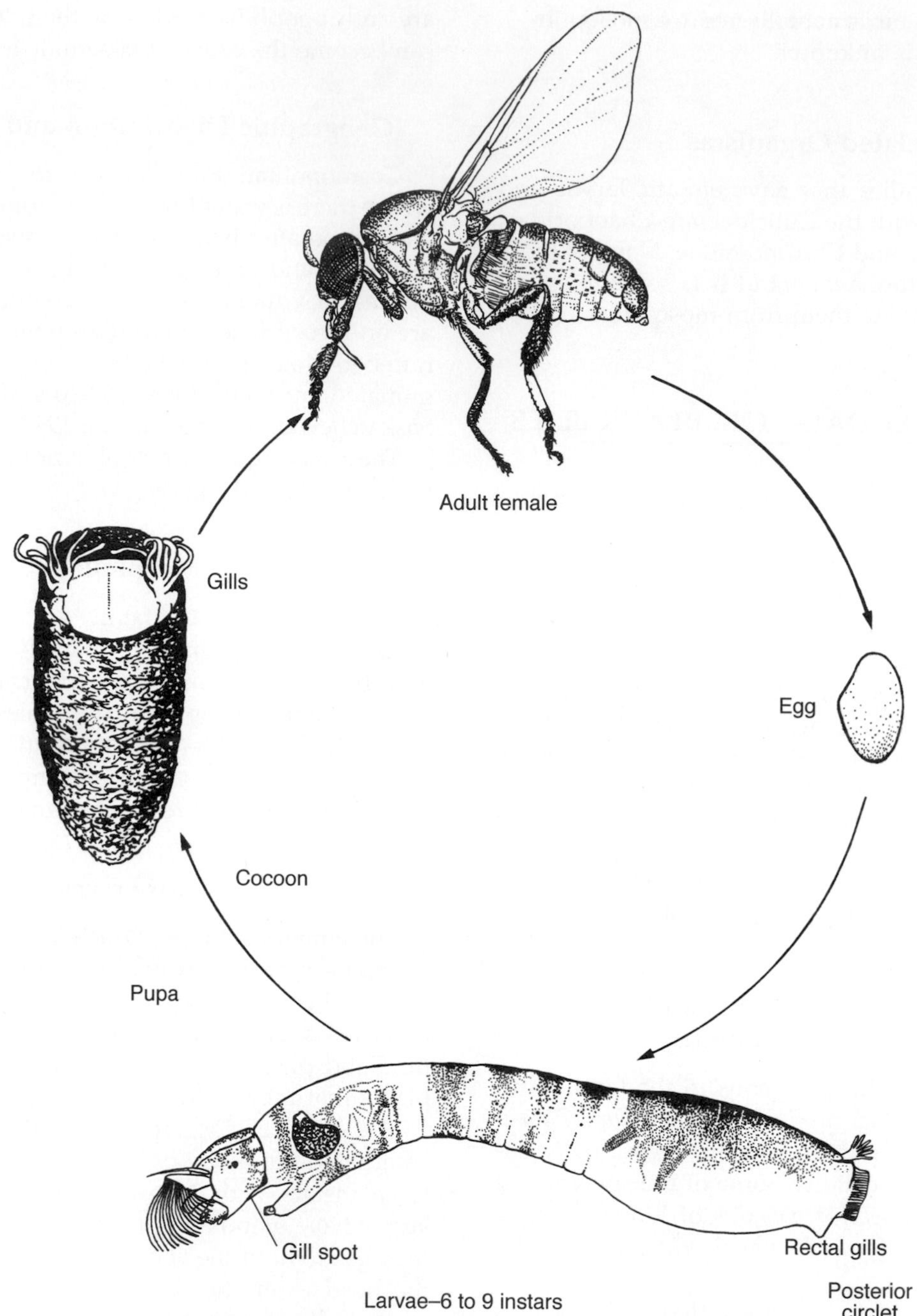

FIGURE 47.7 The structure and life cycle of a black fly.

pupal stage forms. A cocoon is formed, which is frequently open at one end and the pupal gills extend out into the water. Pupation is usually completed in a matter of days.

When the adult emerges, it remains in the cocoon trapped in a bubble of air that it has formed. The drying of the body and extension of the wings are completed in this bubble. The bubble rises to the surface of the water and releases the adult, which immediately flies away.

Host–Parasite Interactions

In any one area, males emerge before the females and aggregate in swarms at a prominent landmark such as a tree or post. The females are ready to mate

TABLE 47.2 Some Disease Agents Transmitted by Black Flies

Disease agent and disease	Hosts	Vectors
Virus		
Vesicular stomatitis virus	Ox, horse, swine	*S.* vitattum* *S. bivittatum*
Apicomplexan		
Leucocytozoon smithi	Turkey	*S. slossonae, S. aureum* *S. jenningsi*
L. simondi	Duck, goose	*S. ruggelsi, S. anatinum*
L. tawaki	Penguin	*Austrosimulium* spp.
L. sakharoffi	Corvid bird	*S. aureum, S. ruficorne*
Trypanosoma spp.	Passerine, Calliform, Falconiform bird	*S. ruggelsi, S. latipes*
Filarioid Nematode		
Dirofilaria ursi	Bear	*S. venustum*
Onchocerca cervipedia	Deer	*S. jenningsi, S. ornatum*
O. lienalis	Ox	*S. jenningsi, S. ornatum*
O. volvulus	Human	*S. damnosum, S. neavei, S. exiguum, S. ochraceum*
Mansonella ozzardi	Human	*S. amazonicum* *S. oyapockense*
Splendidofilaria fallisensis	Duck	*S. ruggelsi, S. anatinum*

* = *Simulium*

almost as soon as they emerge from the water. A female enters the swarm and is inseminated by the male placing a spermatophore on her genital opening.

Both males and female take plant juices and nectar as a source of energy, but only the females take blood. The gonotrophic cycle is similar to that of mosquitoes with the blood meal providing protein for production of eggs. Females search for blood sometimes many kilometers from their site of emergence. Finding a host depends on the female receiving certain stimuli. The first is body aroma, usually sweat in the case of anthropophilic species. As they close in on the host, CO_2 and visual clues direct the fly toward the host. The shape, size, color, and probably movement of the host are the close-range cues. Sensillae on the tarsi indicate that a satisfactory host has been found and probing begins. Warmth and ATP serve as stimulants to feed.

In pool-feeding dipterans such as the black flies, transmission of filarioid nematodes takes place during feeding, but the third-stage larvae are not injected into the bloodstream. Probably the presence of warm blood stimulates the larvae; they escape from the tip of the mouthparts and enter the wound made by the feeding fly. The escape of the larvae from the fly requires a little time, and the fly needs to feed from five to ten minutes for the process to take place.

The saliva of black flies has much the same properties as that of mosquitoes (see the box titled "Spit").

Epidemiology and Control

Black flies require clean, flowing, well-aerated water for larval and pupal development. Their typical habitat is in a small stream that has a rocky substrate to which the larvae can attach. One species, *S. neavei,* attaches to freshwater crustacea, but its requirements remain that of a well-aerated environment.

Certain water control structures encourage populations of black flies. For example, in irrigation or other water control structures, energy is taken out of the water with concrete baffles. These serve the same function as a natural rocky cascade or riffle and the larvae develop there.

In instances where there is heavy organic contamination of a stream from human or animal waste, black flies disappear. In the southeastern United States, black flies disappeared from some areas but have now begun to return with the cleaning up of streams and rivers.

Flies may migrate many kilometers in search of a blood meal but must return to an aquatic habitat for oviposition. Because of this dispersal, control of adult flies is not feasible. Some control can be used around houses in the form of screening and local use of insecticide, but black flies can pass fly screen and a smaller mesh is required. Window screens can be painted with insecticide to kill flies that land there.

Control is directed almost entirely toward the larval stages. Insecticide is placed in the water, usually a second-generation insecticide such an organophosphate or Bti. Use of insecticides requires that bodies of water be accessible. This is the case in endemic areas of Africa, but not in, say, the coffee-growing areas of Guatemala. It should be possible to control black flies in water control systems by allowing outflows to dry out periodically.

CERATOPOGONIDAE—THE BITING MIDGES

The biting midges and the black flies are often spoken of as no-see-ums, tiny biting flies that attack with ferocity and leave wounds running with blood. This much is, in fact, similar between the two groups, but beyond superficial resemblances of the adults they are quite different.

SPIT

All bloodsucking arthropods produce saliva, which is introduced into the wound during feeding. This saliva has a number of different functions such as preventing clotting and keeping blood vessels from closing when they are damaged. Although each group of arthropods has approached the development of a suitable saliva somewhat differently, all have had to solve the same problems. We can discuss mosquitoes as an example of the ways in which any bloodsucking insect has solved the problem of obtaining a meal from an unwilling host.

The salivary glands of mosquitoes lie in the thorax as paired structures whose products leave by ducts that join as they approach the mouthparts. In addition to the functions discussed later, saliva lubricates the mouthparts and holds the separate elements together in the feeding fasicle; in some instances, saliva has hygroscopic properties allowing the arthropod to maintain proper body osmotic concentration. There is a continual low-level flow of saliva to the tip of the mouthparts, and it is reingested and recycled. The flow of saliva when feeding is under control of both chemical and nervous factors. Serotonin and dopamine both stimulate the production of saliva; this response is still not well described and is a fruitful area of investigation.

In both sexes of mosquitoes, the glands have three lobes, and they produce an alpha-amylase, an alpha-glucosidase, a bacteriostatic factor, and a nonspecific esterase. Male mosquitoes have long mouthparts, which form a sucking tube, but they feed only on plant juices such as nectar. The female glands, however, are five times larger than those of the males, and they produce additional substances:

1. Apyrase acts to prevent platelet aggregation by degrading both ATP and ADP to AMP and inorganic phosphate. ADP is found in granules in platelets and is released by damaged cells such as capillaries during feeding by an insect. Platelet aggregation does not take place thus preventing that part of the coagulation cascade.
2. Tachykinin-like protein is secreted by the median lobe of the salivary gland and it has the effect of dilating the capillaries. This molecule and maxadilin (explained below) cause reddening of the skin when a mosquito feeds.
3. Anti-thrombin is involved in preventing coagulation but may also inhibit platelet aggregation.
4. Maxadilin is a protein that causes vasodilation in the same way that calcitonin gene-related peptide (CGRP) acts.
5. Anticoagulants such as fXa, an element of the clotting cascade, acts as a serine protease inhibitor.
6. Tumor necrosis factor (TNF) may play a protective role during feeding.

Thus we see that there are at least ten discrete chemical elements that are secreted by the female mosquito during feeding. It is safe to say that more will be found and that those that are known will have their genes cloned and their functions further clarified.

Name of Organisms and Disease Associations

The family Ceratopogonidae has a fairly complex taxonomy: There are four subfamilies and the subfamily Cetraopogoninae is further subdivided into six tribes. Some of the principal genera in the family are *Culicoides, Dasyhelia, Forcipomyia,* and *Leptoconops.* Among their common names are no-see-ums, sand flies (different from phlebotomines), punkies, and flying teeth. We think of these flies as bloodsuckers, but some also prey on other insects and feed on their hemolymph.

Perhaps the most important species is *Culicoides variipennis,* which is the vector of Blue Tongue virus (BTV), the cause of blue tongue disease in large ruminants. Blue tongue (BT) is a widespread, important disease of livestock in southern Africa and North America.

In addition to BTV, biting midges also transmit about 22 viruses, seven apicomplexan protists, and about a dozen filarioid nematodes, some of which are listed in Table 47.3 (see Holbrook, 1996, for a complete listing).

Besides their serving as vectors, biting midges can be serious pests of both humans and livestock as well as other animals. They remove blood and are often painful when they feed, but they also can cause dermatitis and allergic reactions in sensitized individuals.

TABLE 47.3 Some Diseases and Disease Agents Transmitted by Biting Midges

Disease agent and disease	Hosts	Vector
Virus		
Buttonwillow	Rabbit, rodent, bat, ox, horse, pig, goat	*C.* variipennis*
Oropouche	Primate, human, bird	*C. paraensis*
Nairobi sheep disease	Sheep, goat, human	*C. toroensis*
Blue tongue	Sheep, ox, goat, & other ruminant	*C. variipennis, C. insignis, C. imicola, C. nebeculosus*
Epizootic hemorrhagic disease	Deer, ox, sheep	*C. schultzi, C. kingi*
Rift Valley fever	Sheep, ox, human	*C. variipennis*
Apicomplexa		
Haemoproteus meleagridis	*Turkey*	*C. edeni, C. hinmani*
H. velans	Woodpecker	*C. stillobezzoides*
Hepatocystis kochi	Primate	*C. aderi*
Leucocytozoon caulleryi	Chicken	*C. arakawae*
Filarioid Nematode		
Chandlerella chitwoodi	Crow	*C. stillobezzoides*
Mansonella ozzardi	Human	*C. furens*
M. perstans	Human	*C. grahami, C. inornatipennis*
Onchocerca cervicalis	Horse	*C. nubeculosis*
O. gibsoni	Ox	*C. pungens, C. shortii,* etc.
Splendidofilaria californiensis	California quail	*C. multidentatus*

* = *Culicoides*

Hosts and Host Range

The hematophagous species have host preferences, but most feed on a variety of species. Hosts are reptiles, birds, and mammals.

Geographic Distribution and Importance

Cosmopolitan. Ceratopogonids range from the Arctic to the Tropics and are found in all kinds of habitat from semiarid to tropical rain forest.

Culicoides variipennis ranges in North America from Florida through the southeastern states northward through about two-thirds of the western states. It is not found in the New England States. This wide distribution is exceptional since most species have a limited range and the larvae develop in rather specific ecological niches.

Biting midges are nearly as important as mosquitoes as pests of humans and of livestock. The females are persistent bloodsuckers and can make life difficult if not unbearable when they occur in large numbers. Allergic reactions are also observed in both humans and other animals who have been fed upon repeatedly.

As alluded to earlier, certatopogonids are vectors of a large number of transmissible agents, most of which are not of great economic or medical importance. However, among livestock, African horse sickness, blue tongue disease, epizootic hemorrhagic disease, and Rift Valley fever are among the important viral diseases transmitted by biting midges. *Haemoproteus meleagridis* of the turkey is a serious disease in Florida and the Southeast. Among filarioid nematodes, *Mansonella* spp. of humans and certain *Onchocerca* spp. of livestock are important agents vectored by midges (Tab. 47.3).

Morphology

Adult biting midges are similar in size and appearance to black flies. The adults are 1 to 3 mm long and have the same humpback appearance as black flies (Fig. 47.8). The bodies are typically more elongate than those of the black flies. Midges are usually brownish and there is overlap between the darker midges and the lighter black flies. The wings are often patterned with dark areas. The antennae are relatively long, rather like mosquitoes, and most have 14 segments; the male antennae are plumose and the females have relatively sparse setation. Mouthparts are of the short, pool-feeding type.

Eggs are about 0.25 mm long; they are white or yellowish when laid, but turn nearly black within a short period. The larvae are elongate without distinct body regions except for the head; most species have only sparse setation. They range in size from 0.5 to 3.0 mm in length. Pupae are comma-shaped and are similar to phlebotomines.

Life Cycle

Culicoides variipennis can serve as a typical ceratopogonid in describing the life cycle (Fig. 47.8). Eggs are laid in muddy areas that have a high organic content. At 25°C eggs hatch in 48 to 72 hours, and the four larval stages develop rather quickly, in 10 to 14 days, to reach the pupa. The pupa last only 48 to 72 hours and the adults then emerge at the surface of the mud or water.

Adults require about two days before they are ready to mate and for the females to seek a blood meal. Mating takes place in swarms that appear over promi-

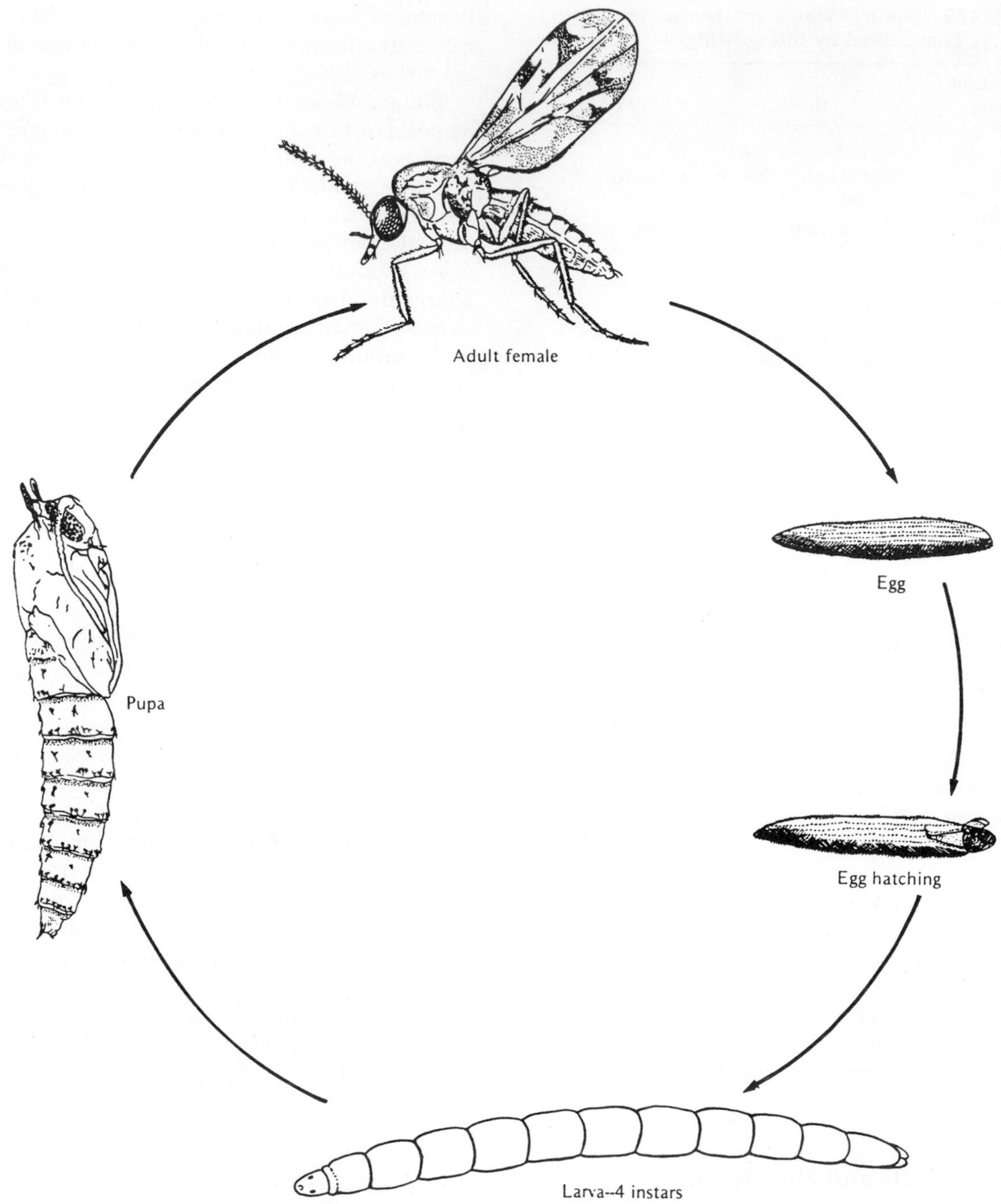

FIGURE 47.8 The structure and life cycle of a biting midge.

nent landmarks such as a fence post or tree, or sometimes a person. The gonotrophic cycle is completed in 48 to 72 hours after mating, and the females are ready to feed again shortly thereafter.

Host–Parasite Interactions

Only female ceratopogonids are blood feeders; the males feed on plant juices and nectar. Females are crepuscular (active at dawn and dusk) in their feeding activities. At these times of day there is usually little wind and the females do not fly when the wind is stronger than 7 m/sec (about 15 mi/h). They use the CO_2 plume to locate hosts and then animal odors, such as octenol, take them closer to the potential host. Similar to other nematocerans, biting midges have host preferences, and some feed only on birds, and others on mammals.

A few biting midges feed on other insects by either capturing them or attaching to them (when they are larger) and sucking hemolymph from them.

Epidemiology and Control

Females choose oviposition sites that are damp or wet and that have a high organic content. A typical site would be a cattle feed lot or an area near a stream where cattle water and then defecate. Larvae feed on bits of decaying organic matter near the surface of the mud.

When conditions become unfavorable, the larvae move downward and may be found near the frost line in winter or aggregated at the bottom of cracks in the mud when it is dry. They overwinter as larvae and develop to maturity in spring when the mud and water warms up.

In temperate climates there probably are four or so generations during spring and summer before declining temperatures slow down development in fall. In climates where there is little or no frost, development continues year round if water is available.

Resting sites of adult midges are not known. They certainly find hosts at dusk, but where they have been during the day is not known.

Control of ceratopogonids is directed mainly at the larval stages. The first step in a control program is finding the sites of larval development keeping in mind that adults of *C. variipennis* may migrate more than a kilometer when they emerge. Thus, it is necessary to search, mostly upwind, from the farm or home for breeding sites. If sufficiently defined, the breeding sites can be filled or otherwise dried out or treated with insecticide.

Some control or discouragement of adults can be achieved by screening, painting screens with insecticide, use of repellents, and, with livestock, using insecticide-impregnated ear tags.

Blue Tongue Disease

Blue tongue disease is caused by an orbivirus that infects a wide range of herbivorous hosts and occasionally infects humans. The virus is transmitted by ceratopogonids, mostly *C. variipennis*, in North America. Among domestic animals, BT disease is most important in sheep and cattle, but it also infects goats, wild sheep, the American antelope or pronghorn, among others.

The disease affects the mucous membranes, which results in hypoxia in some tissues, thus the blue tongue seen in infected sheep. Other tissues affected are the hooves of ruminants and the reproductive system. In cattle, the virus is transmitted from the infected cow to the calf in utero. Infected calves are born weak and often have skeletal problems that prevent them from walking normally. They may not be able to nurse and die unless they are given special care. Sheep are more severely affected than cattle and may die from the disease.

The greatest effect of BT disease is indirect. There are significant losses in the livestock industry from disease, but greater loss is felt from embargoes on shipping of cattle or semen of cattle to BT-free countries. Understandably, countries that do not have BT do not want it, and therefore they do not accept cattle or semen for artificial insemination from the United States. There is a vaccine that prevents the disease, but when these animals are tested, they show antibodies to BTV and it is not possible to determine whether they have been immunized or have been naturally infected. The result is a multimillion dollar annual loss to the cattle industry.

FAMILY PSYCHODIDAE—THE SAND FLIES

This family includes both hematophagous and nonhematophagous subfamilies. The Psychodinae are innocuous little flies often seen swarming over trickling filters at a sewage treatment plant. The Phlebotominae, on the other hand, are hematophagous and nearly ubiquitous. Probably the most obscure of the bloodsucking Diptera, the sand flies are vectors of leishmaniosis, one of the great scourges of humankind. Sand flies are tiny, hairy, secretive and those that are bloodsuckers are vicious. They have existed as a group since the Cretaceous, about 140 million years ago.

Name of Organism and Disease Associations

The sand flies fall neatly into two groups, the Eastern and Western Hemisphere genera. *Phlebotomus* and *Sergentomyia* are found in Europe, Asia, Africa, and Australia while *Lutzomyia, Brumptomyia* and *Warileya* are the New World species.

Although the phlebotomines are hematophagous, they are seldom serious pests of humans or domesticated animals. They do, however, transmit both protistan and viral diseases of humans. Leishmaniosis is caused by a kinetoplastid protistan (Chapter 4) and bartonellosis, a South American disease caused by the bacterium, *Bartonella bacilliformis*. Of the viral diseases transmitted by sand flies are sand fly fever of humans caused by a *Phlebovirus* and vesicular stomatitis of both herbivores and humans caused by a *Vesiculovirus*.

Because sand flies are so difficult to study in their natural habitat, much of the data on development and bionomics have been obtained from laboratory colonies, and only a few species have been successfully colonized.

Hosts and Host Range

There are general outlines as to the hosts on which phebotomines feed, but specific data are lacking in most instances. It is known that there are reptilian, avian, and mammalian feeders, but some feed on more than one group. The good vectors of human diseases must feed on the reservoir hosts and on humans in order for transmission to take place. *Sergentomyia* spp. probably feed only on lizards and perhaps other poikilothermal vertebrates. Certain species of *Lutzomyia* feed on humans, but other warm-blooded animals are probably their principal hosts.

Geographic Distribution and Disease Associations

The northern limit of sand fly distribution is about 50°N latitude and perhaps not quite that far south in the Southern Hemisphere. Interestingly, they do occur at least as high as 2300 m (7500 ft) in northern Colorado. Their habitats range from tropical rain forest to semiarid and arid regions.

As indicated earlier, sand flies serve as vectors of leishmaniosis, Carrión's disease, sand fly fever, and vesicular stomatitis. In addition, they vector several arboviruses seen occasionally in humans.

Morphology

Adult sand flies are only about 2 mm long and they may be recognized by their hairy bodies and wings that are held erect over the body (Fig. 47.9). They have short mouthparts and are pool feeders. The antennae are long, filiform and have sparse setation. Although they are tiny, sand flies can be recognized by their hopping type of flight; they make short bursts of flight, rest for a couple of seconds, and hop again. The wings are characteristic with about eight major veins that extend nearly the length of the wing and leave a number of open cells at the margin.

The eggs turn dark after being laid and have sculpted surfaces. The larvae are characteristic with a wormlike shape and have two tufts of erect hairs at the posterior end; there is also a distinct head capsule, but no other tagmatosis on the body. Larvae are quite active and scurry about as if they had someplace to go. Pupae are naked and similar to those of the biting midges.

Identificaiton of sand flies is based on adult characteristics and it is necessary to dissect and process them so that the spermathecae and esophageal structures of the females and the copulatory apparatus of the males can be studied.

Life Cycle

P. papatasi is one of the most important vectors of leishmaniosis in the Eastern Hemisphere and can serve as an example of a life cycle of a sand fly. Eggs are laid in protected areas where there is a good supply of organic material on which the larvae feed. There are four larval instars. Development is rather slow for a tiny insect and requires from 34 to 76 days from egg to adult at 28°C and 116 to 165 days at 18°C to go from egg to adult under laboratory conditions.

The gonotrophic cycle requires about six days after feeding to develop ova, and from 10 to 70 eggs are laid. Only females feed on blood, but both males and females take plant juices and nectar as a source of energy for flight and other activities.

Copulation appears to take place in swarms near hosts and a mating/aggregation pheromone has been reported. The pheromones obtained from *Lutozomyia longipalpis* are farnesene- and diterpenoid-like chemicals.

Host–Parasite Interactions

The mouthparts of sand flies are adapted for pool feeding (telmatophagy) and they take only a tiny quantity of blood at a feeding, from 0.3 to 0.5 μl (3 to 5 $\times$ 10^4 ml). *P. papatasi* is opportunistic; it takes blood from both birds and mammals and is anthropophilic. It is interesting to note that the saliva of a sand fly acts to increase the probability of infection of the host with *Leishmania* spp.

It is uncommon for sand flies to migrate more than a dozen meters or so from a breeding site, but they have been captured as many as 1500 m, probably having been carried by the wind. They approach their hosts in little hopping flights and are most likely attracted by CO_2 and warmth.

Epidemiology and Control

As indicated earlier, sand flies are found most commonly in warm climates, but they may range from tropical rain forest to outright desert. Eggs are laid in areas that have decaying organic matter on which the

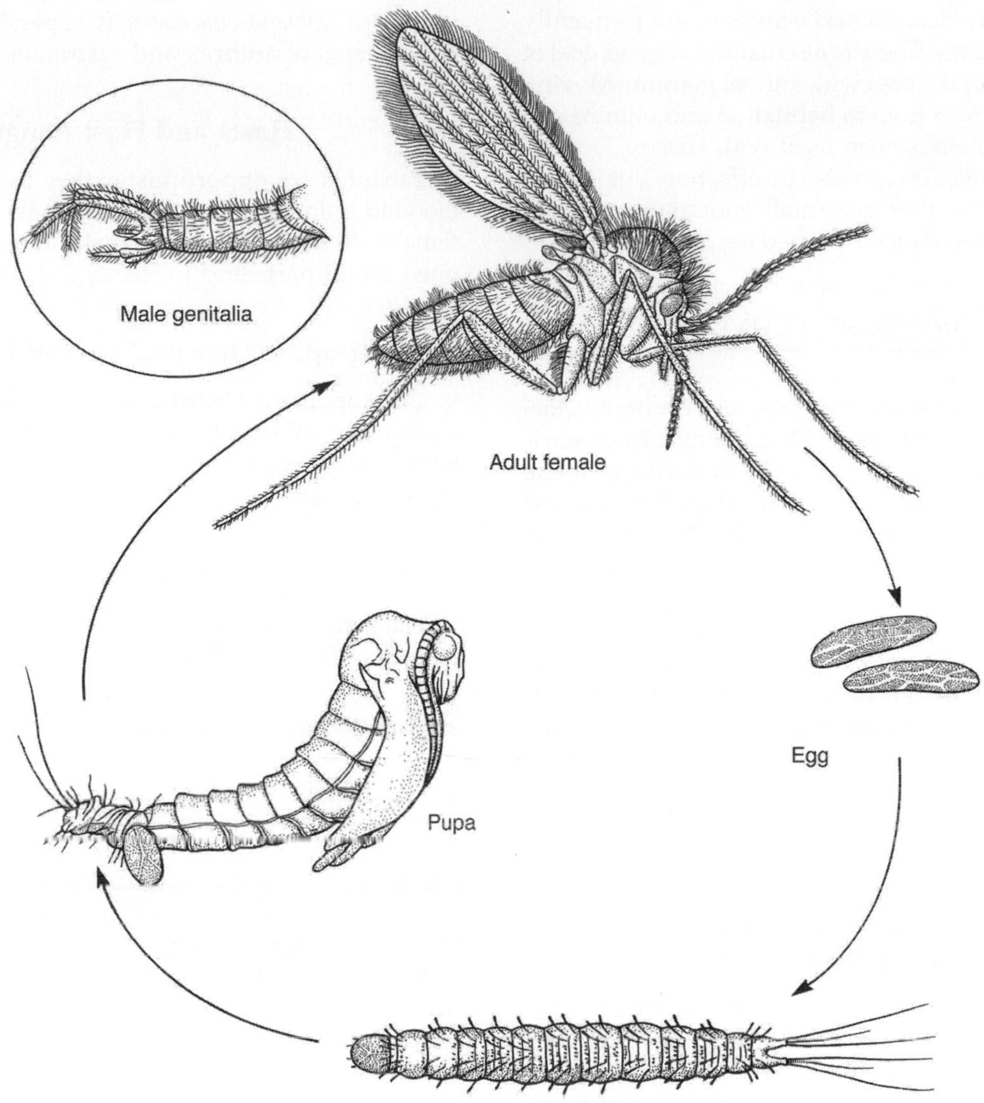

FIGURE 47.9 The structure and life cycle of a sand-fly.

larvae feed and, most often, where there are small animals on which the adults can feed. In many biotopes, these sites would be rodent burrows or rocky areas with deep fissures. In peridomestic situations, they breed in garbage or other organic material that lies around human dwellings. In Central America, they are found in large numbers in animal pens where the adults may be collected from spaces in the stone or stick walls.

Finding and collecting preadult stages of sand flies has been an exercise in futility. The adults, females mostly, can be trapped in or near likely sites of larval development, but few larvae have ever been obtained in collections of material from these areas. Larval stages are cultivated in a mixture of well-rotted rabbit manure and laboratory rodent food. Gravid females collected in the wild oviposit in this material and larvae of some species (*P. papatasi* and *L. longipalpis*, as examples) can be maintained in the laboratory on this unlikely food. In their natural habitats, quite similar to the laboratory medium, it is not possible to find larvae. In studies in Sudan in Africa, it was determined that *P. orientalis* is the most likely vector of visceral leishmaniosis, but during a five-year study, its breeding sites were never uncovered.

Because the larvae have been so elusive, efforts at control have been directed principally toward adults, and especially peridomestic species. Spraying of dwellings and areas near houses with insecticides has been moderately effective. In areas such as the Middle East and Central America, domestic animals are frequently kept at or in houses. There is also usually a good deal of contamination of the area with animal manure. Moving animals away from human habitation and eliminating the animal waste has been used with success.

Personal protection can also be effective, but it must be noted that the flies are small enough to pass fly screen and the usual mesh of a bed net or mosquito bar.

SUBORDER BRACHYCERA

This suborder is sometimes placed with the Cyclorrapha (Chapter 48), but we will consider it to be separate. The members are characterized as having grublike larvae (Fig. 47.10) with poorly developed heads and with mandibles that work vertically. The pupae are not enclosed and emerge from a straight or T-shaped slit. Adults are large, heavy bodied flies that fly well.

Two families in the Brachycera are hematophagous, Tabanidae and Rhagionidae, and the former is the most important. The tabanids have the characters of the suborder, and there is an open cell at the distal tip of the wing (between the divergent R4 and R5 veins).

FAMILY TABANIDAE

Name of Organism and Disease Associations

Some common tabanids are *Chrysops* (deer flies), *Tabanus* (horse flies), *Haematopota*, and *Hybomitra*. The eyes are large and holoptic in the males, and in keeping with the subordinal name, they have short antennae, usually with only three segments. The antennae usually extend away from the head unlike the cyclorraphans (Chapter 48), in which the antennae are short but are held close to the head. Tabanids are usually large flies that fly rapidly and noisily.

Tabanids are hematophagous and rather restless feeders that probe and take some blood, then move to another spot or another host and probe again. They cause pain when feeding and cause economic losses in livestock and misery for humans.

In addition to their being pests, horse flies and deer flies transmit a few diseases agents either mechanically or biologically. The best-known example of an agent that is transmitted biologically is *Loa loa*, the eye worm of humans, which is transmitted by *Chrysops silicea* in tropical Africa (Chapter 34). *Elaeophora schneideri*, a filarioid nematode of large, wild ruminants and domestic sheep, is transmitted by *Hybomitra* in the western United States. Tabanids also serve as mechanical vectors of *Trypanosoma evansi* (Chapter 3) and the causative agents of anthrax and tularemia.

Hosts and Host Range

Tabanids are opportunistic; they feed on all warm-blooded animals, birds and mammals alike. Only the females feed on blood; the males have poorly developed mouthparts and probably die after mating.

Geographic Distribution and Importance

Cosmopolitan. Distribution is limited only by the availability of larval habitat and hosts on which to feed. The disease agents that they vector were discussed earlier.

Morphology

The general characteristics of the tabanids were discussed earlier (Fig. 47.10).

Life Cycle

Ovigerous females deposit masses of eggs on plants near water or in marshy areas. The eggs hatch in two to three days. The grublike larvae (Fig. 47.10) are aquatic or live in muddy habitat. Some larvae, such as those of *Tabanus*, are predaceous whereas those of *Chrysops* are plant feeders. There are four to nine larval instars after which the pupa forms; the pupae normally leave wet areas to complete pupation in drier areas. Adults emerge from the pupa in a week to three weeks. The life cycle is rather slow; in temperate climates there is usually a single generation per year (univoltine) and sometimes two or three years are required to complete development.

Host–Parasite Interactions

Being bitten by a tabanid is a memorable experience. The bite is painful and there may be considerable swelling at the site of the wound. They are mostly pool feeders and lacerate the skin with their sharp mandibles so that the blood wells up at the surface. Tabanids are usually restless feeders in that they feed briefly and then move to another site or another host. They can take as much as 0.34 ml of blood, a large quantity compared to a midge or sand fly.

Tabanids find their hosts mainly by sight and they can be collected in traps that mimic the silhouette of a large domestic animal. They are mostly daytime feeders and harass both humans and livestock. The black horse fly, *Tabanus atratus*, is about 20 mm long and it

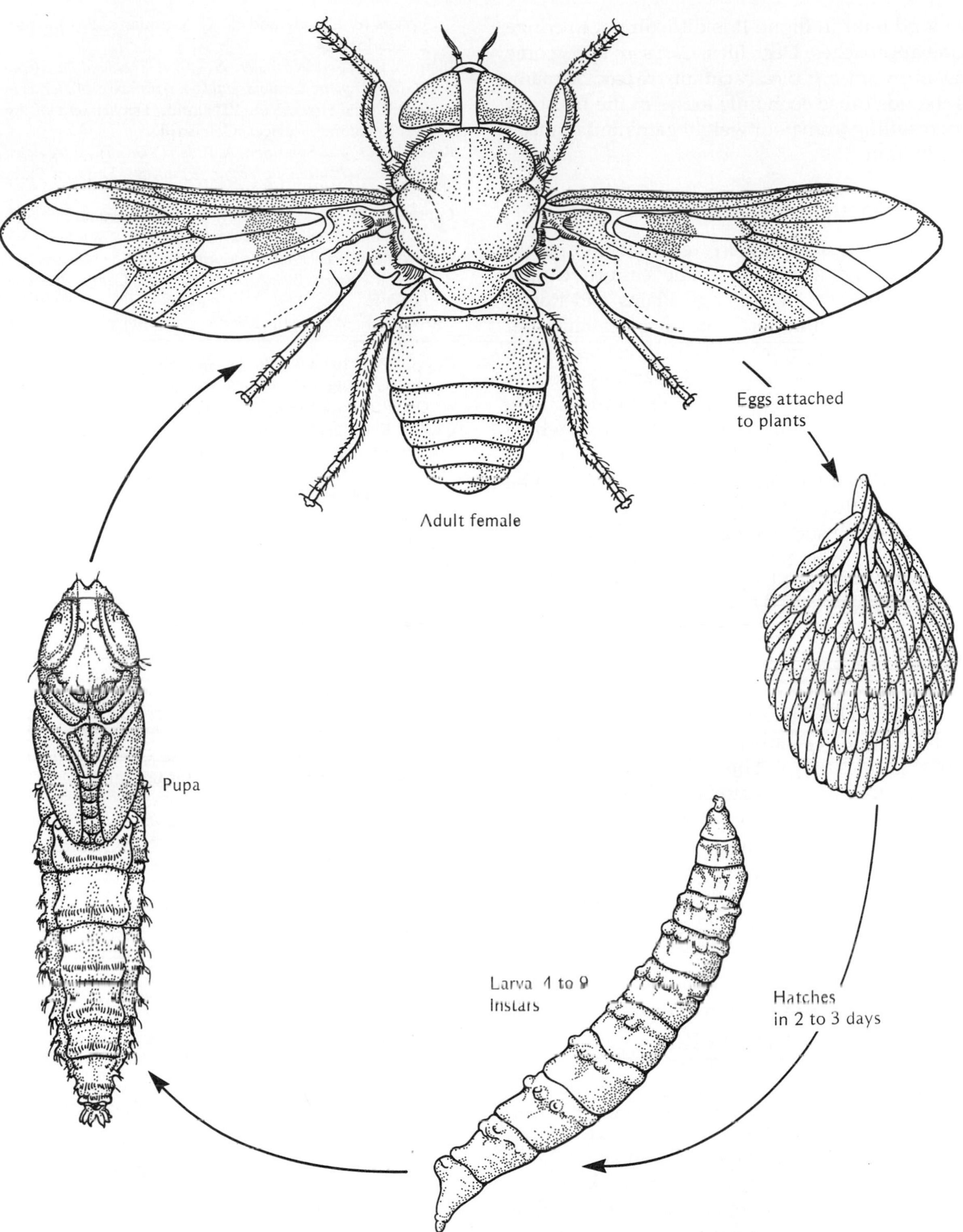

FIGURE 47.10 The structure and life cycle of a tabanid.

makes a loud buzz in flight. It is difficult not to cringe when one approaches. Deer flies, *Chrysops* spp., come out of swampy areas, typically cattails, to feed on mammals. Tabanids cause economic losses in the livestock industry resulting from poor weight gains and reduced milk production.

Epidemiology and Control

Tabanids are usually found in areas that have plenty of water. They are common in the eastern United States, and in pockets in the High Plains and Rocky Mountains. In mid-summer, a patch of cattails will almost always yield some tabanids if one comes near it.

Control of tabanids is usually only partially successful. Reducing the source by draining wet or boggy areas is sometimes feasible, but often the areas where the larvae develop are quite large. A few species require only muddy areas, and there is little that can be done to change those. Along the East Coast of the United States, some success was experienced in treating salt marshes from the area with organochlorine insecticides, but the problem of nontarget organisms being affected was a drawback.

Livestock can be protected by self-treatment with treadle sprayers or back rubbers containing insecticide, but animals must have access to such equipment at least once a day. Daily treatment is possible for dairy cattle or beef cattle in relatively small pastures, but in grasslands, animals may not be seen for days at a time, and they may not come to treatment centers very often.

Malaise traps, consisting of a large ball and CO_2 as attractants, have been used to trap tabanids, but they seem not to reduce populations sufficiently to make any difference. For personal protection, Deet may repel some tabanids, but apparently it is not effective against all species.

FAMILY RHAGIONIDAE—THE SNIPE FLIES

The members of this family are small to medium-sized and have small heads and large eyes. The antennae are short and some of them have an arista. Only a few are hematophagous, and they are not known to serve as vectors of disease agents. They can be vicious biters and feed repeatedly, so it is possible that they can be mechanical vectors of disease agents. Some genera are *Symphoromyia*, *Suragina*, and *Atrichops*.

Readings

Black, W. C., and Munsterman, L. E. (1996). Molecular taxonomy and systematics of arthropod vectors. In *The Biology of Disease Vectors* (B. J. Beaty and W. C. Marquardt, Eds.). Univ. Press of Colorado, Niwot.

Blanton, F. S., and Wirth, W. W. (1979). *The Sand Flies (Culicoides) of Florida (Diptera: Ceratopogonidae). Arthropods of Florida and Neighboring Land Areas*, Vol. 10. Florida Department of Agriculture and Consumer Services, Gainesville.

Borovsky, D., and Spielman, A. (Eds.) (1994). *Host Regulated Developmental Mechanisms in Vector Arthropods.* Univ. of Florida Press, Gainesville.

Calisher, C. H. (1994). Medically important arboviruses of the United States and Canada. *Clin. Microbiol. Rev.* **7,** 89–116.

Christophers, S. E. (1960). *Aedes aegypti (L.). The Yellow Fever Mosquito; Its Life History, Biology and Structure.* Cambridge Univ. Press, London.

Crosskey, R. W. (1990). *The Natural History of Black Flies.* Wiley, New York.

Cupp. E. W. (1996). Black flies and the agents they transmit. In *The Biology of Disease Vectors* (B. J. Beaty and W. C. Marquardt, Eds.). Univ. Press of Colorado, Niwot.

Gwadz, R. W. (1969). Regulation of blood meal size in the mosquito. *J. Insect Physiol.* **15,** 2039–2044.

Holbrook, F. R. (1996). Biting midges and the agents they transmit. In *The Biology of Disease Vectors* (B. J. Beaty and W. C. Marquardt, Eds.). Univ. Press of Colorado, Niwot.

Kim, D. C., and Merritt, R. W. (Eds.) (1986). *Black Flies.* Pennsylvania State Univ Press, University Park.

Kim, K. C. (Ed.) (1985). *Coevolution of Parasitic Arthropods and Mammals.* Wiley, New York.

Knight, K. L., and Stone, A. (1977). *A Catalog of the Mosquitoes of the World (Diptera: Culicidae)*, 2nd ed. Thomas Say Foundation/Entomol. Society of America, College Park, MD.

Knudson, D., Kafatos, F., Brown, S., and Zheng, L. (1996). Genomic organization of vectors. In *The Biology of Disease Vectors* (B. J. Beaty and W. C. Marquardt, Eds.). Univ. Press of Colorado, Niwot.

Krinsky, W. L. (1976). Animal disease agents transmitted by horse flies and deer flies (Diptera: Tabanidae). *J. Med. Entomol.* **13,** 225–275.

Laird, M. (Ed.) (1981). *Blackflies: The Future for Biological Methods in Integrated Control.* Academic Press, New York.

Laird, M. (1988). *The Natural History of Mosquito Larval Habitats.* Academic Press, London.

Lane, R. P., and Crosskey, R. W. (1992). *Medical Insects and Arachnids.* Chapman & Hall, New York.

McIver, S. B. (1980). Sensory aspects of mate-finding behavior in male mosquitoes. *J. Med. Entomol.* **17,** 54–57.

Monath, T. P. (1988). *The Arboviruses: Epidemiology and Ecology*, Vols. 1–5. CRC Press, Boca Raton, FL.

Moore, C. G., and Mitchell, C. J. (1997). *Aedes albopictus* in the United States: Ten-year presence and public health implications. *Emerg. Infect. Dis.* **3,** 329–334.

Muirhead-Thompson, E. C. (1982). *Behavior Patterns of Blood-Sucking Flies.* Pergamon, Oxford.

Post, R. J., and Flook, P. (1992). DNA probes for the identification of members of the *Simulium damnosum* complex (Diptera: Simuliidae). *Med. Vet. Entomol.* **6,** 379–384.

Ribeiro, J. M. C. (1987). Role of saliva in blood-feeding arthropods. *Annu. Rev. Entomol.* **32,** 463–478.

Spielman, A. (1971). Bionomics of autogenous mosquitoes. *Annu. Rev. Entomol.* **16,** 231–248.

Tesh, R. (1996). Sand flies and the agents they transmit. In *The Biology of Disease Vectors* (B. J. Beaty and W. C. Marquardt, Eds.). Univ. Press of Colorado, Niwot.

Wernsdorfer, W. H., and McGregor, I. (Eds.) (1988). *Malaria: Principles and Practices of Malariology*, Vols. 1 and 2. Churchill–Livingston, London.

CHAPTER

48

Diptera: Cyclorrapha

This suborder of dipterans contains those flies in which the pupa is enclosed in a case composed of the last larval skin. The adults are generally strong fliers and mostly rather heavy bodied such as the housefly. The mouthparts range from the sponging type of the housefly, *Musca domestica,* to the piercing type of the tsetse, *Glossina* spp., to a combination of the two types, as seen in the stable fly, *Stomoxys calcitrans.* Some flies, such as the cattle grubs, *Hypoderma* spp., have only vestigial mouthparts and do not feed as adults.

Larvae are maggots. The anterior end has only the remnants of a head and the mouthparts are hooklike structures referred to as the cephalopharyngeal skeleton (Fig. 48.3, presented later).The spiracles by which they obtain oxygen are at the posterior end, but some also have anterior gaseous exchange structures. The pupa is enclosed in the skin of the third larval instar and is therefore spoken of as being coarctate.

The classification and identification of cyclorraphan flies is based on the presence or absence of the ptilinum (by which they break out of the pupal case) between the eyes, on wing structure, antennal structure, and on setation especially on the head and thorax (Fig. 48.1). Since there are about 140 families in the order, most of them cyclorraphan, it can be appreciated that we can discuss only a few species.

Flies are important for the following reasons:

1. They are pests that often occur in large number and crawl over everything and everyone. Examples are houseflies, eye gnats, and fruit flies.
2. They suck blood from humans and other animals causing considerable discomfort and blood loss. Examples are louse flies and horn flies.
3. They are mechanical vectors of disease agents. Examples are houseflies, which transmit the agents causing amebic dysentery and typhoid fever, and eye gnats, which transmit the agents causing pink eye in cattle and yaws in humans.
4. They are biological vectors of disease agents. Examples are tsetse, which transmit the various African trypanosomes (Chapter 3), muscoid flies such as *Stomoxys calcitrans,* and the stable fly, which transmits the nematode causing summer sore in horses, *Habronema* spp. (Chapter 34).
5. They are parasitic as larvae and may cause extensive tissue damage to their hosts. Examples are blowflies of domestic animals such as *Phormia regina,* cattle grubs, *Hypoderma* spp., and *Dermatobia hominis,* the human bot fly or torsalo (Chapter 49).

Morphology and Life Cycle

The common blue bottle fly, *Calliphora vicina,* can serve as an example for both the morphology and life cycle of members of the suborder (Fig. 48.2). The blue bottle fly is somewhat larger than the housefly being 6 to 9 mm (3/8 in) long. The body is rather heavy and well covered with setae, although this characteristic varies widely among species. In the blue bottle fly and other Calliphoridae, the thorax and abdomen are a shiny, metallic blue; other species are green or copper or black. The head bears large eyes, and short antennae that are held close to the head most of the time. The eyes of the males are usually somewhat larger than those of the females (Fig. 48.1, near bottom). The wings are clear, lack scales, and have relatively few veins.

Cyclorraphans have small white eggs and three lar-

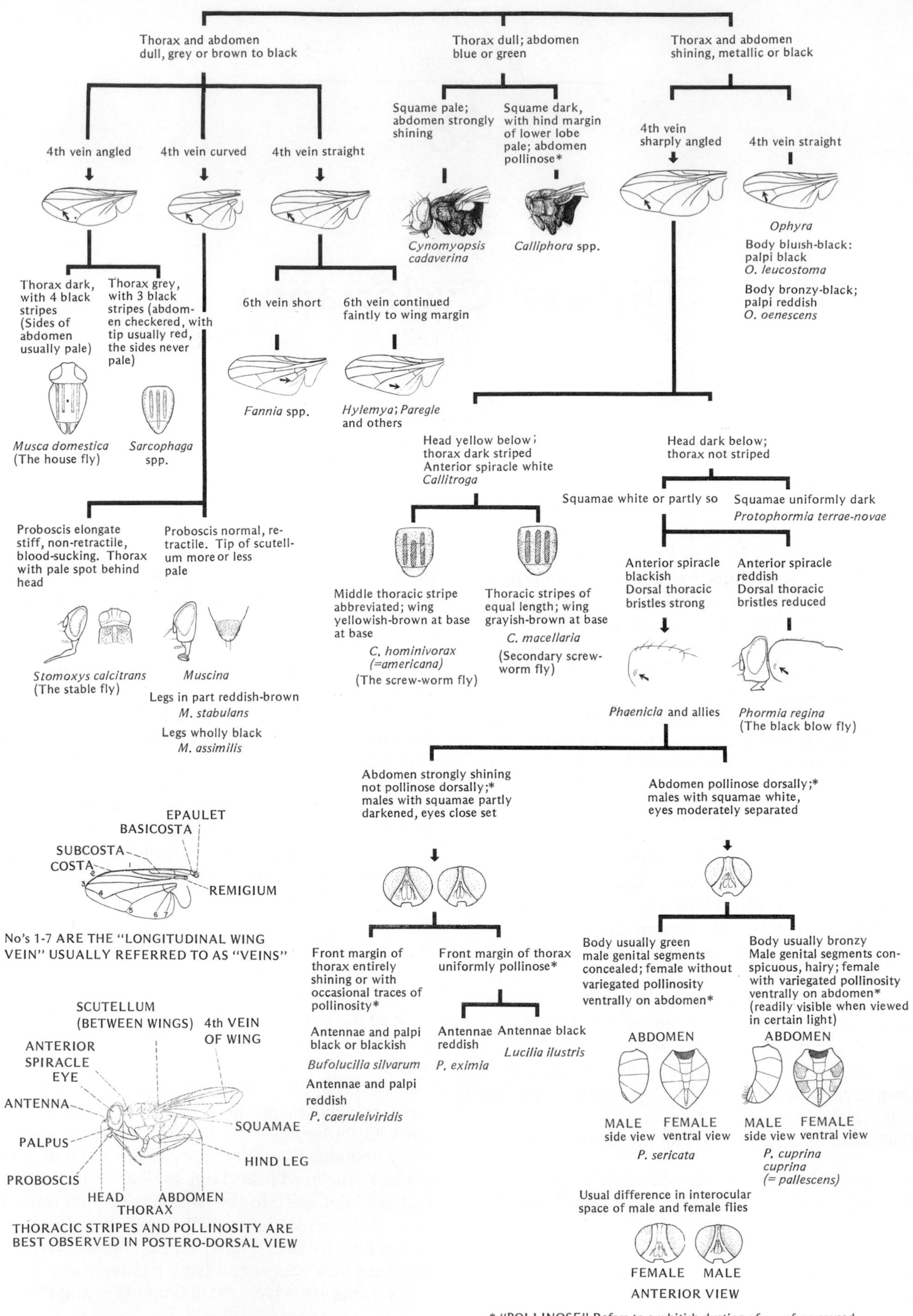

FIGURE 48.1 Pictorial key to some common domestic flies.

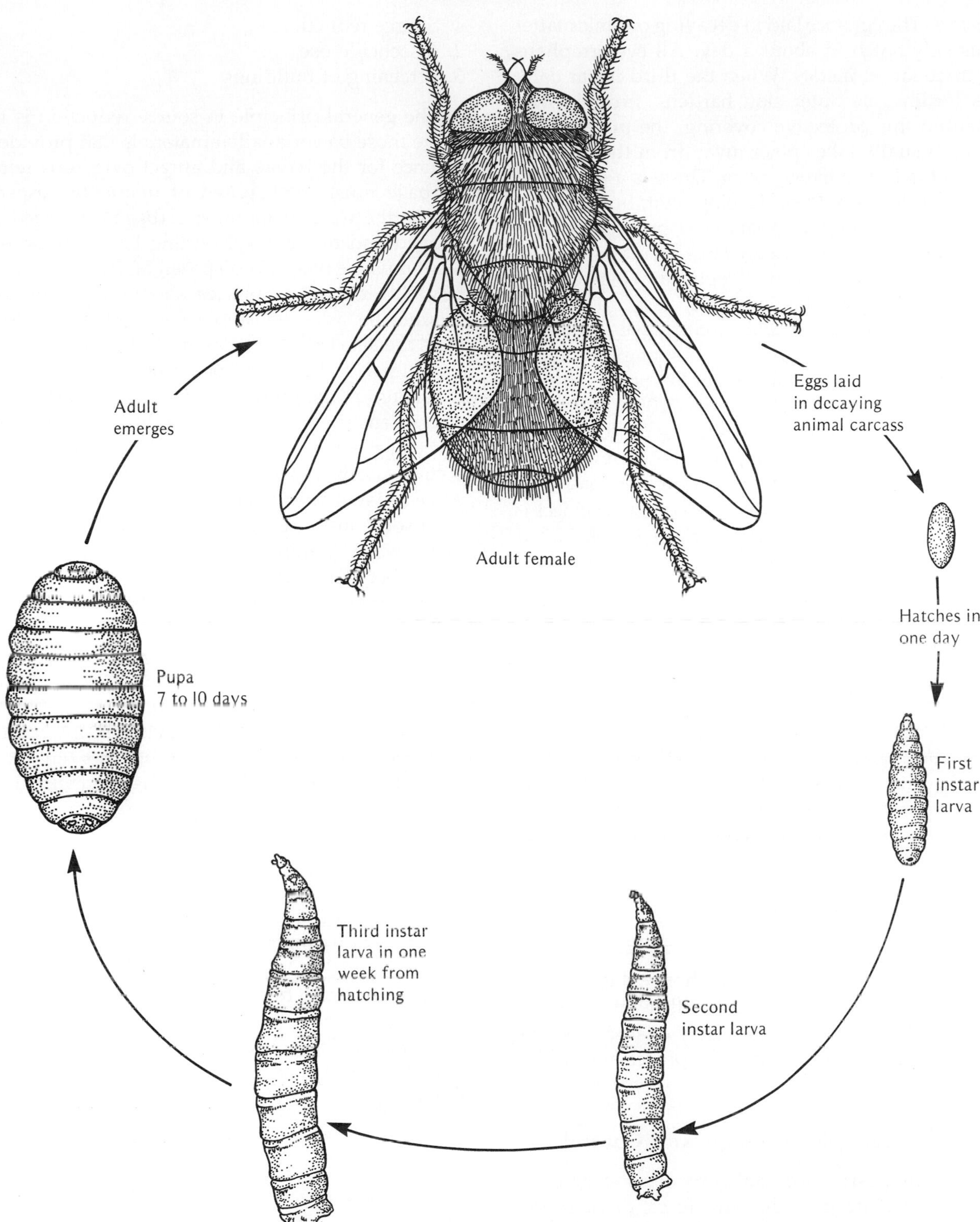

FIGURE 48.2 The life cycle of *Calliphora vicina*, the blue bottle fly. This fly is typical of nearly all cyclorraphan flies in that it oviposits and has three larval instars; the pupa is enclosed in the skin of the third instar. [Redrawn with modifications from Smart, 1948.]

val instars. The eggs are laid in decaying organic matter and usually hatch in about a day. All cyclorraphans have three larval instars. When the third instar completes feeding, its outer skin hardens, turns brown, and within this protective covering, the pupa forms. Pupation usually takes place away from the medium in which the larvae have grown. There is a good deal of variation in the rate of development, but *C. vicina* represents many cyclorraphans and progresses from egg to adult in two to three weeks. The adult leaves the pupal case by expanding the ptilinum between the eyes and pushing off the operculum.

Adults feed on various kinds of organic matter but are not hemataphagous; they have sponging mouthparts. After copulation, the females lay up to 180 eggs at a time and may lay as many as 720 in a lifetime. Transeasonality probably takes place in the pupal stage. *C. vicina* is a blowfly that ordinarily oviposits in decaying flesh, but it can become a problem as one of the blowflies or wool maggots of sheep; this subject is discussed in Chapter 49 where myiasis is considered in detail.

THE HOUSEFLY

Name of Organism and Disease Associations

Musca domestica, the housefly This fly serves as mechanical vector of various microbial agents such as the pathogenic enteric gram-negative bacteria exemplified by *Salmonella* spp., and the dysentery ameba, *Entamoeba histolytica*.

Morphology

The housefly is a medium-sized (4–6 mm) dark fly that has four black stripes on the thorax (Fig. 48.1). It also has a characteristic angled fourth wing vein that allows its differentiation from closely related flies. The larvae can be identified based on the posterior spiracles (Fig. 48.3).

Life Cycle, Epidemiology, and Control

Females oviposit in wet, decaying organic material. The usual sites are garbage cans, feces, or other decaying material. At summer temperatures, the life cycle is completed in about 10 days. A female lays up to 150 eggs during her lifetime.

Knowing the habits of the female and the kinds of material in which the larvae develop leads to methods of control through source reduction and use of insecticides. The main methods of control are as follows:

1. Source reduction
2. Insecticide use
3. Screening of buildings

The general principle in source reduction is to remove those bacteria-laden materials that provide sustenance for the larvae and attract ovigerous females. Garbage must be disposed of frequently, especially during the warmer months; garbage cans need to be cleaned and to have tight-fitting lids. Human excrement must be properly disposed of; if there is no sanitary sewer system, privies should be tight to the ground, be screened, and have tight doors. Animal feces are also breeding sites, and the feces of companion animals should be disposed of rather than allowed to remain on the ground. Feces of large farm animals or chickens present particularly difficult problems because of the sheer volume of material that is likely to accumulate in a short period of time in the face of present-day intensive animal husbandry methods.

In some instances, it is possible to scatter feces so that they dry rapidly, break down, and do not ferment. A number of natural biological agents such as mites, parasitiod wasps, and some nematodes have been used with some success in reducing fly numbers. In houses, barns, and milking parlors, screening to keep flies out is the first line of defense. In addition, insecticides can be used to kill those flies that do enter. Methoprene, a JH mimetic, can be fed to livestock to control fly larvae in their feces, but it also prevents the development of other beneficial arthropods that cause the material to break down quickly.

Related Organisms

A number of flies similar to the housefly are important in various times and places. *M. sorbens* fills the same niche in the Orient, Africa, and some of the Pacific islands. The lesser housefly is usually *Fannia canicularis* or *F. scalaris*; these flies have much the same habits as *M. domestica*. The legendary *M. vetustissima* of Australia migrates perhaps hundreds of miles to harass people in the southern part of the country.

THE FACE FLY

Name of Organism and Disease Associations

Musca autumnalis, the face fly of livestock. This fly mechanically transmits the causative agent of pink eye in cattle through its sponging mouthparts as it feeds around the eyes and nose of the ox.

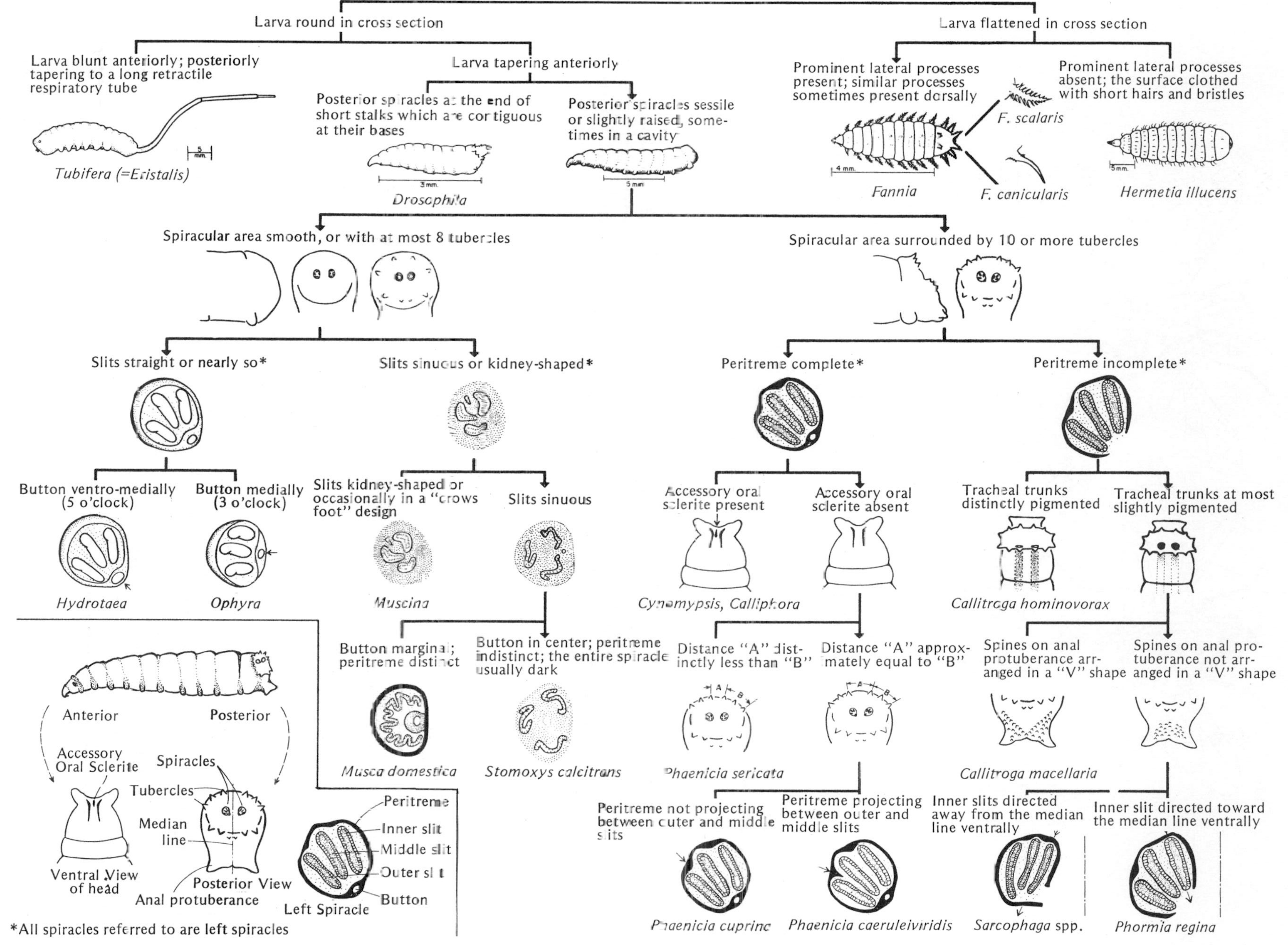

FIGURE 48.3 Pictorial key to the larvae of some common flies.

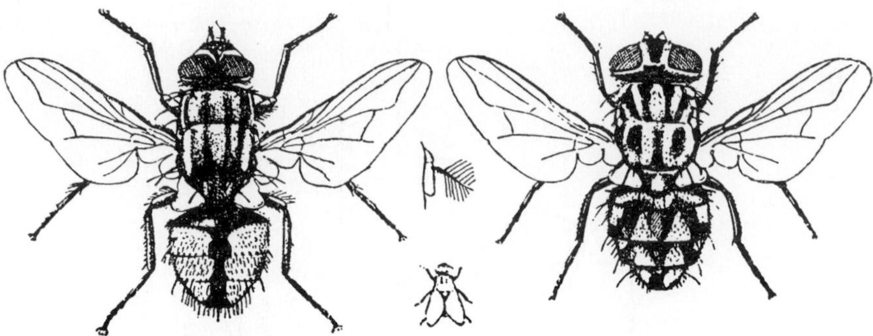

FIGURE 48.4 Adults of the face-fly, *Musca autumnalis.* Male on the left and female on the right. Note that this species is slightly smaller than the house-fly; the plumed antenna (inset) has longer, more regular bristles than the house-fly; wing venation is similar, but not identical, to that of the house-fly. [From Graham-Smith, G. S., 1913.]

Geographic Distribution and Importance

The face fly was originally a European native, but it was introduced into North America in about 1950, and it has since spread almost throughout the United States and Canada.

The fly is a summertime pest and it is estimated that annual losses are about $168 million.

Morphology

The face fly and the housefly are quite similar in appearance. Their size and coloration are nearly identical (Fig. 48.4). The usual feature used to distinguish between the two species is a white band between the eyes of the females, which is broader in the face fly than the housefly.

Life Cycle

Face flies develop in cattle feces and have about a 10-day cycle in summer. They probably overwinter as adults.

Host–Parasite Interactions

Face flies have sponging mouthparts, and they dab at secretions from the eyes, nose, and mouth of cattle. They also cluster around wounds on the skin. Cattle sometimes have their heads covered with hundreds of face flies and are understandably greatly annoyed by them. Cattle are so bothered by face flies that they fail to gain properly and milk production falls off. The mechanical transmission of the organism causing pink eye, or keratoconjunctivitis, in cattle can lead to serious damage to the eye if left untreated.

Epidemiology and Control

Since face flies breed in cattle feces, scattering of the feces helps to reduce populations. This technique is usually not feasible when cattle are on large pastures. Most often animals are allowed access to self-treatment devices, which puts an insecticide on their heads. Alternatively, their heads can be painted with an insecticidal preparation.

Because the face fly was imported into the Western Hemisphere, there are few or no natural enemies of it. It is probably this fact that has allowed the fly to spread almost unchecked over the continent. Efforts are being made to find biological control agents that will have an effect on the populations.

THE STABLE FLY

Name of Organism and Disease Associations

Stomoxys calcitrans is the stable fly. It is hemotaphagous and serves as a biological vector of *Habronema microstoma* of the horse (Chapter 34). It can also serve as a mechanical vector of various viral and bacterial agents of disease.

Hosts and Host Range

The stable fly primarily bites livestock, but it does feed on humans and usually tries to feed through the clothing.

Geographic Distribution and Importance

Cosmopolitan. The importance of this fly lies principally in its bloodsucking activities. It is a painful biter and livestock of all kinds are subject to its attention.

Morphology

The stable fly is similar to the housefly in appearance, but it has a curved fourth wing vein rather than an angled one, as in the housefly (Fig. 48.1). It also has a stiff proboscis, which is held down from the head and is not retractable. The stable fly is usually a little smaller than the housefly, and it has much the same coloration.

Life Cycle

The preferred breeding site of the stable fly is wet, rotting plant material, but it is found in feces, as well. The life cycle can be completed in as few as 12 days under optimal conditions; it requires 33 to 36 days at 21°C to go from egg to adult.

The females require blood to complete the gonotrophic cycle, and batches of 150 to 450 eggs are laid.

Epidemiology and Control

Source reduction and use of insecticides on surfaces are the means used to reduce stable fly populations. Eliminating their preferred breeding sites is the first step, and because they tend to rest on walls, these structures can be treated with an insecticide.

THE HORN FLY

Name of Organism and Disease Assocations

Haematobia irritans (syns. *Siphona irritans, Lyperosia irritans*) is the horn fly of cattle. The horn fly is a biological vector of the filarioid nematode, *Stephanofilaria stilesi*, a cause of minor losses in hides used for leather. It also transports the eggs of *Dermatobia hominis* (Chapter 49). This fly is suspected of serving as a mechanical vector of various microbial agents.

Hosts and Host Range

Although spoken of as the horn fly of cattle, *H. irritans* feeds on a variety of domestic animals such as equids, canids, and bovids in addition to the ox, humans, and probably other hosts as well.

Geographic Distribution and Importance

There are several species in the genera *Haematobia* and *Lyperosia*, which are closely related and have similar characteristics; they are found in the Nearctic region. Major regions of the world have their own fauna, but *H. irritans* has been accidentally introduced into Australia where it has spread unchecked because it has no natural enemies.

It is estimated that there is a $115 million loss annually in the United States from horn flies on cattle. Cattle may lose up to 0.25 kg per day and milk production may be reduced from 10 to 20% during fly season.

Morphology

The horn fly and the stable fly are similar in appearance. The horn fly is abour 4 mm long, but is somewhat more slender than the stable fly. Their mouthparts are also similar with the labium being somewhat heavier and the palps about as long as the proboscis. Wing venation in the two species is the same.

Life Cycle

Females deposit their eggs only in fresh cow droppings; after a matter of only a few minutes, they are not attracted to the dung. Only 20 to 24 eggs are deposited at a time, and usually near the edges of the dung. A female may produce as many as 400 eggs in a lifetime. Eggs hatch in about a day at 24° to 26°C (77°F), and larval development is completed in four to eight days. The pupal stage requires six to eight days and then the adults emerge. Overwintering is in the pupal stage.

Host–Parasite Interactions

The females remain on the host except to leave when they oviposit. It is interesting to note that horn flies feed with the heads down while stable flies feed with the heads up. It may require as many as 20 minutes for a fly to feed to repletion, and during this time, it feeds, withdraws the proboscis frequently, and reinserts it. Also, horn flies prefer to feed on the lower side of an ox, and the lesions of the filarioid nematode, *Stephalofilaria stilesi,* occur on the midline of the belly, the site where the flies feed and become infected with the L_1s of the nematode.

The numbers of flies on oxen during fly season stretch the imagination. Some estimates state that from 1000 to 4000 flies may occur on an animal. But from 10,000 to 20,000 flies have been estimated to feed on individual animals in Alberta, Canada.

Epidemiology and Control

Since horn flies cause considerable economic loss, a number of approaches have been taken to control their populations or reduce their effects on cattle:

1. Source reduction
2. Self-treatment
3. Biological control
4. Systemic insecticides
5. Switching breeds of cattle

Scattering of cattle feces reduces habitat for the larvae and pupae and when it is dry and scattered, manure does not support horn flies. This technique may be feasible in some instances, but not when cattle are on large pastures. Again, self-treatment devices are useful when animals can reach them on a daily basis. Where cattle are on range, systemic insecticides in feed supplements have been used experimentally, but supplemental feeding is not the norm in raising range cattle.

There is a whole range of inhabitants of cattle feces that not only interact in various ways but also serve to break down the dung pat. Attempts have been made to encourage certain species that compete with or parasitize horn fly larvae, but nothing has yet been developed to the point where it is useful.

Bos taurus, the ox, is quite susceptible to horn flies, but the zebu, *Bos indicus,* in its original and various cross-bred varieties is resistant to them. Since the zebu is well adapted to hot weather and horn flies are an especial nuisance there as well, switching breeds may be worthwhile.

THE CLUSTER FLY

Name of Organisms and Disease Associations

Pollenia rudis is the most common cluster fly, but several other species are found in various localities. These organisms are similar to houseflies insofar as they may transport microorganisms mechanically on their bodies or in the intestinal tract.

Morphology

Cluster flies are similar to the housefly; they are about the same size and coloration, but the body is dark overall. The thorax has yellowish, silky hairs on the side that can be seen without magnification. Cluster flies are sluggish fliers and are usually recognized because of their lazy flight.

Life Cycle

The larval cluster fly is either a parasitoid or a micropredator depending upon how one wishes to define its association. In any event, it uses earthworms for larval nutrition and housing. Females oviposit in the soil, and the first instar larvae seek out earthworms, which they enter through the male apertures (earthworms are monoecious). The larva then enters a quiescent period, which lasts eight months or more, in the coelomic cavity of the earthworm. The larva becomes surrounded by a foreign body reaction of the earthworm, and as the end of the first-larval instar approaches, it breaks out of its cyst and migrates toward the anterior end of the earthworm. The larva feeds, grows, and molts while feeding on earthworm tissue. By the time it reaches the third instar, the worm is nearly consumed and is, in fact, dead. Pupation takes place in the soil and the adult emerges. There is a single generation of flies per year.

The earthworm host/prey seems not to be an obligate association since cluster fly larvae can be raised on bits of earthworm tissue in the laboratory.

Epidemiology and Control

Cluster flies have received their name because they nearly always are seen in groups of a few to perhaps 50. They enter houses and fly lazily about the room. In fall, they tend to cluster on houses and to crawl into cracks around doors and windows. They somehow manage to penetrate houses and are seen at windows on warm winter days. How they manage to get into the house usually remains a mystery, but in some instances, they clearly crawl through slight cracks around windows.

Although cluster flies may transmit microbial agents mechanically, they are primarily a nuisance; some writers have even declared that they are an embarrassment. There is no satisfactory control that can be implemented. It is neither feasible nor desirable to attempt to eliminate earthworm populations. Spraying with an insecticide against the adults is possible but probably not worth the potential contamination. In most cases, the flies can be vacuumed up around the windows; the flies are slow enough to be readily sucked up by that low-tech device to which resistance has not yet been reported.

TSETSE—*GLOSSINA* SPP.

The tsetse, also called tsetse flies (although that is redundant) are limited to subsaharan Africa except for a report early in the 20th century from the Arabian peninsula. Their distribution at earlier geologic times was probably wider since fossil tsetse have been found in the Florissant fossil beds in central Colorado.

TABLE 48.1 Habitat and Groups of Some Vectors of African Trypanosomosis

Vector—*Glossina*	Habitat	Main Hosts	Transmits
	Fusca Group		
G. brevipalpis	Rivers and streams, thickets	Mammals, reptiles	Not a significant vector
	Palpalis Group		
G. palpalis	Forest, river thickets, savanna to an extent	Primates, reptiles, bovids	*T. b. gambiense* *T. b. rhodesniense*
G. tachinoides	Savanna, intermittent river areas	Primates, bovids, suids, reptiles	*T. b. gambiense* *T. b. rhodesniense*
	Morsitans Group		
G. morsitans	Savanna, grassland	Suids, bovids, primates	*T. b. rhodesiense* *T. b. brucei*
G. pallidipes	Rivers, thickets	Bovids, suids	*T. b. rhodesniense* *T. b. brucei*
G. swynnertoni	Dry, open areas, savanna	Suids, bovids	*T. b. brucei* *T. b. rhodesiense*

Name of Organisms and Disease Associations

The family Glossinidae (superfamily Muscoidea) contains only a single genus, *Glossina*, and 30-odd species or subspecies. Some of the important vectors are listed in Table 48.1; they fall fairly well into species groups and in habitat groups as well. Organisms such as *G. morsitans* and *G. palpalis* serve as good vectors of African trypanosomosis, and the role of tsetse as vectors of trypanosomosis make them one of the most important insect groups (Chapter 3).

The habitat and the taxonomic groupings of the species of *Glossina* correspond quite well (Tab. 48.1). The *palpalis* group has members that are mostly forest dwellers, but they extend along streams and are found along the shores of lakes. The *palpalis* group is among the most important as vectors of trypanosomes. The group includes *G. palpalis* (two subspecies), *G. tachinoides*, and *G. fuscipes* (three subspecies) all of which serve as vectors.

The *morsitans* group are mainly savanna dwellers ranging from forest margins to sahelian- or sudan-type habitats. *G. morisitans* and *G. swynnertoni* are examples of vectors in the group.

The *fusca* group occurs principally in lowland forest, but some species are found at forest edges where the microclimate is somewhat drier than the rain forest. This group does not have members that are important vectors of trypanosomiasis.

Hosts and Host Range

As indicated in Table 48.1, tsetse feed on various hosts, both mammalian and reptilian. They have host preferences and, in some instances, a moderate degree of host specificity. Those which transmit *T. brucei gambiense* and *T. b. rhodesiense* must be anthropophilic, even though they may feed on other hosts as well.

Geographic Distribution and Importance

Glossina are distributed only in Africa south of the Sahara Desert to about 25°S latitude. One species, *G. tachinoides,* was found in the Arabian peninsula in the early 1900s, but it is not known whether it is still there. Tsetse can be persistent feeders and make life for both animals and humans extremely unpleasant in the tsetse belt of Africa. Their greater importance, however, is in their serving as vectors of the *Trypanosoma* spp. that cause sleeping sickness in human, nagana in cattle, and other trypanosomoses in various domestic animals (Chapter 3).

Morphology

The adults vary from 6 to 14 mm long, depending upon the species. They have prominent eyes, and the wings overlap one another at rest (Fig. 48.5). A diagnostic character of the tsetse is the so-called *hatchet cell* in the center of the wing (Fig. 48.6). The proboscis extends straight forward from the head. The arista on the antenna has branching hairs.

The larvae are seen for only a brief period when they are deposited by the gravid female. The pupa (usually called the puparium) is characteristically dark brown, almost black, and has two lobes at the posterior end. These lobes represent the residua of the posterior spiracles but do not serve a respiratory function in the puparium.

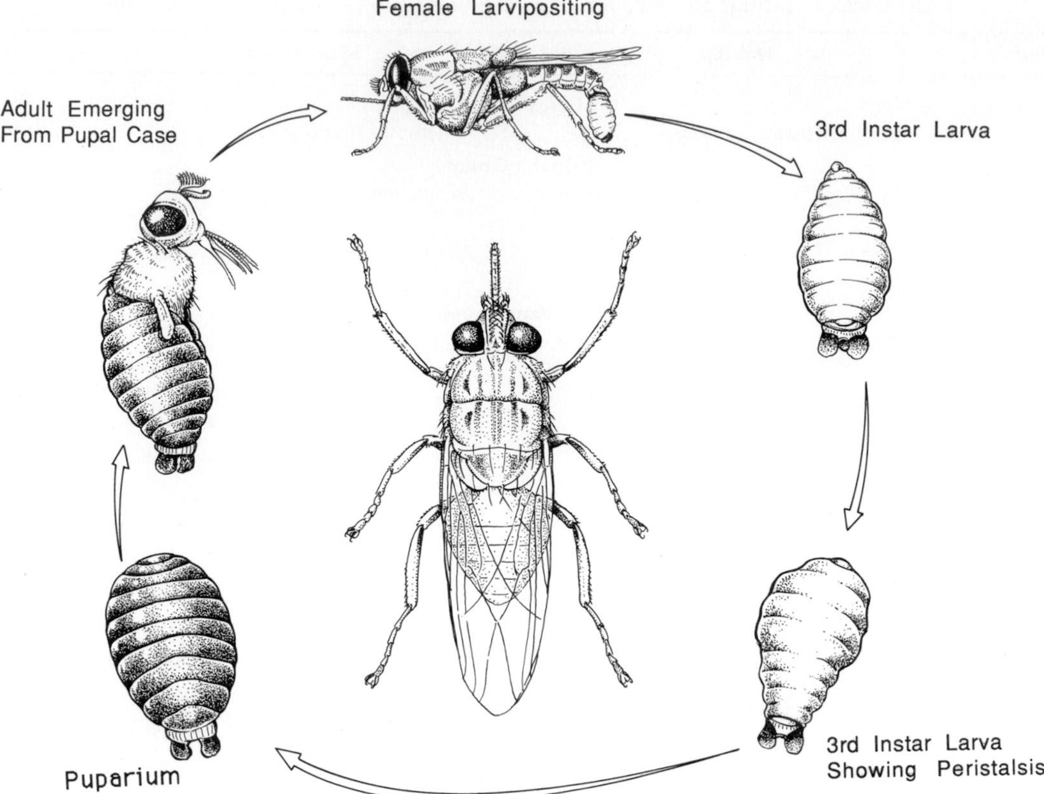

FIGURE 48.5 The life cycle and morphology of a tsetse, *Glossina*.

Life Cycle

Adult females mate only a single time, and the female produces an average of only nine offspring. The tsetse is probably the most highly selected "K" strategist among insects known. Unlike most flies, which lay eggs or sometimes first-stage larvae, the female tsetse retains the larva in the uterus and gives birth to a single, large third-instar larva at a time (Fig. 48.5). During gestation, the larva is fed from so-called milk glands that lie in the hemocoel and empty into the uterus. Three blood meals by the female fly are required for the maturation of the larva, and they are fully grown in from 8 to 25 days.

When the female larviposits, the larva burrows quickly into the soil and transforms within an hour into a pupa. Pupation requires at least two weeks and longer if soil temperature and moisture conditions are not optimal.

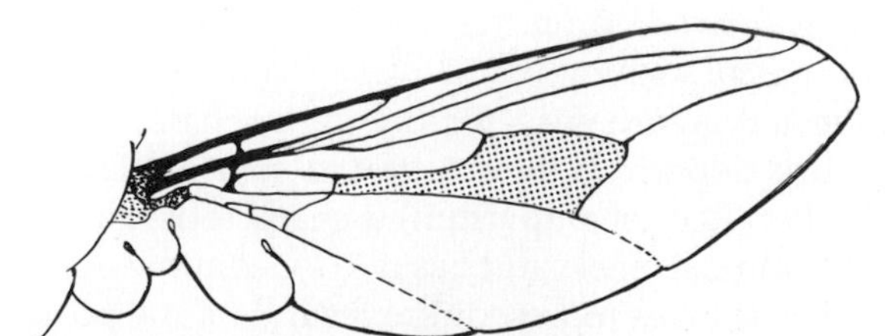

FIGURE 48.6 The wing of a tsetse to show the hatchet cell (stippled), which is characteristic of the family.

Host–Parasite Interactions

Both males and females are hematophagous, and tsetse are generally catholic in their tastes for blood They have host preferences, but normally feed on any available, warm-blooded, and sometimes reptilian, host. Most have large herbivores as their preferred hosts, and a few prefer to feed on reptiles such as crocodile. Relatively few have primates as their preferred hosts, but since they are opportunistic, in the main, humans are often fed on.

Glossina spp. find their hosts first by sight. They home in on large moving objects and tend to follow them. The CO_2 plume and body aromas then act to lure them closer to the potential host.

Epidemiology and Control

Tsetse do not ordinarily fly far; they typically remain within an area of a few hundred meters on a side.

Many species pursue moving objects such as animals, people, or vehicles. They are most likely seeking both mates and food sources. Since they cue in on dark, moving objects, one method of taking a census of tsetse is to have a team of collectors move through an area wearing dark clothing and vests with a sticky substance applied to the backs. The flies are later removed, counted, and identified. This census method is referred to as a "fly round."

In the case of riverine species, such as *G. palpalis*, the flies remain within about 10 meters of the shore; this area typically has a fairly dense growth of trees and shrubs that provide places for the adults to rest on the undersides of leaves. The females oviposit in loose soil in locations that are likely to retain some moisture such as under fallen logs or where plant growth is heavy.

G. swynnertoni, a savanna species, is more diffuse in its distribution but is found in brushy areas. It tolerates dryness better than the riverine species.

Tsetse are said to feed during the day, and that is true, but some individuals have been collected feeding at night. This diurnal feeding habit is used to keep livestock from being attacked by tsetse. Cattle are held in corrals during the day and then let out to graze at night. This has been an important method to keep animals from being infected in the tsetse belt of Africa.

At the turn of the 20th century, when the life cycle of the trypanosomes causing sleeping sickness in Africa was worked out, tsetse were found to be the vectors. At the time, there was no chemotherapeutic agent to treat the disease in either humans or domesticated animals, and control relied on reducing populations of tsetse. Biological studies showed that the flies did not move much, and for a time it was thought that they had home ranges. It was also observed that the pupae needed some moisture and moderate temperatures to survive. Therefore, the first control methods were based on source reduction.

For riverine and lacustrine species, the foliage within about ten meters of the water was completely removed thus denying the adult flies resting and larviposition sites. To prevent the flies from moving from one place to another, trees and brush were completely removed from lanes 2 km wide. This served to contain the flies since they do not readily cross broad, grassy areas. Such barriers are effective only temporarily and must be a part of a larger program that includes land use that eliminates breeding sites.

As insecticides were developed, they were applied so that resting sites had toxicants on them. Insecticides actually allowed the concept of selective clearing to be implemented. Low-growing plants were removed and limbs of trees were removed to a height of about 3 m. This left some desirable vegetation but eliminated resting sites on the branches of trees and shrubs and allowed hot, dry winds to desiccate the soil where the pupae were deposited.

After World War II, DDT was sprayed over huge areas in an attempt to reduce tsetse populations. In the mind-set of the time, a good tool in the form of organochlorine insecticides was available and should be used with great enthusiasm. Some success was achieved, but the costs, both short and long term turned out to be too great. Insecticidal use is now targeted to specific resting sites of tsetse.

Trapping of tsetse can be done relatively efficiently with the Harris trap that mimics the silhouette of an ox or with a biconical trap. Such traps are suspended from trees, and the flies, which tend to light on the underside, crawl through a narrow opening and are retained inside the screen body. Where financial resources and personnel are available, trapping can be effective in reducing the transmission of the trypanosomes.

The sterile male technique was developed for screwworm control in the early 1950s (Chapter 49), and it was thought that it could also be applied to tsetse since they, like the screwworm, mate only once. The development program has gone on for a number of years, but has not resulted in effective control in the field.

Tsetse, like many other insects, have symbiotic bacteria in the midgut, ovary, milk gland, and fat body. In general, these bacteria are considered to provide essential nutrients to their hosts. This is especially true of those insects that are hematophagous since blood is an incomplete food.

Tsetse have two species of bacteria in the gut and milk glands, and studies underway are attempting to bring about a genetic transformation in the bacteria. The concept is to introduce genes into the symbiotic bacteria that would interfere with the development and replication of the trypanosomes that they vector. Ideally, the bacteria would produce, say, a trypanostatic or trypanocidal compound that would not have a detrimental effect on the fly. The tsetse population would persist but not vector trypanosomes.

FAMILY HIPPOBOSCIDAE—THE LOUSE FLIES AND KED

Name of Organisms and Host Range

There are only about 120 described species of hippoboscids and they are parasites of birds and mammals. Some common species are listed in Table 48.2.

TABLE 48.2 Some Commonly Encountered Members of the Family Hippoboscidae[†]

Name	Wings + or −*	Hosts	Geographic distribution
Melophagus ovina	−	Sheep	Temperate and cold climates
Lipoptena despressa	−	Deer	North America
Neolipoptena ferrisi	−	Deer	North America
Lipoptena cervi	−	Deer	Europe, recently introduced to the United States
Hippobosca equina	+	Equids	Britain and Europe
H. longipennis	+	Dog	Asia, Mediterranean, possibly the United States
H. camelina	+	Camel	Eastern hemisphere
Pseudolynchia canariensis	+	Pigeon	Warm and tropical climates
Lynchia hirsuta	+	Quail	Warm climates

[†]Although a limited host range is given, hippoboscids are opportunistic and may be found feeding on a wide range of hosts, including humans.
*+ = Present, − = Absent

Morphology

Flies of the family Hippoboscidae are all hematophagous on warm-blooded vertebrates: birds and mammals. Most of them are medium-sized, being 2.5 to 10 mm long. They are flattened, rather hairy, and have inconspicuous antennae. Wings vary from well developed to shortened to absent (Fig. 48.7); in some species, the wings are shed (caducous) when the fly reaches a site in a nest where it will remain. Legs are relatively strong in keeping with their remaining on hosts and moving about in the hair or feathers.

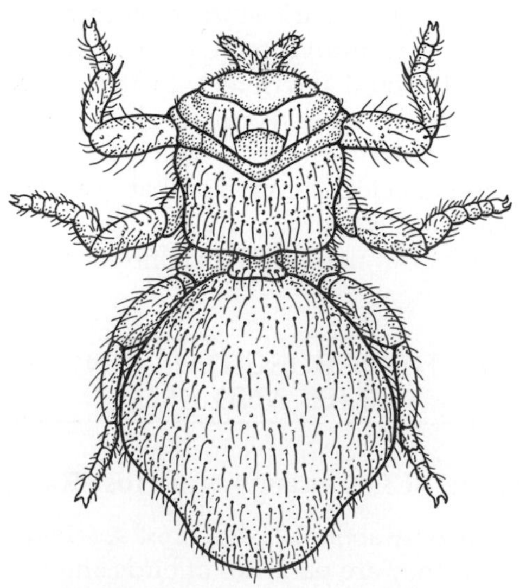

FIGURE 48.7 The sheep ked, *Melophagus ovinus*.

Life Cycle

The life cycles of these flies take place largely on or near a host. Similar to the tsetse, hippoboscids give birth to fully developed third-instar larvae that pupate immediately. The larvae are nourished by secretions from the body of the female. The life cycle of the sheep ked, *Melophagus ovinus*, requires about three weeks in summer and perhaps twice that long in winter. Those that do not have wings, such as the ked, remain on the host and are transferred by close contact. Those that have wings, such as many on birds, are usually strong fliers that seek out birds that are nesting and feed and larviposit there.

Host–Parasite Interactions

These flies serve as vectors of a few infectious agents. Most hippoboscids are parasites of birds, typically remaining in their nests, and thereby come some of the common names such as louse flies and pigeon flies. *Pseudolynchia canariensis* vectors the apicomplexan *Haemoproteus columbae* of columbiform birds. *Lynchia hirsuta* transmits *H. lophortyx* of quail (Chapter 14). The sheep ked, *Melophagus ovinus* (Fig. 48.7), transmits *Trypanosoma melophagium* to sheep, but the situation with this parasite of sheep is rather like the so-called *T. avium* of birds: the protistan does not multiply in the mammalian host. One might conclude that the sheep is a mechanical vector of *T. melophagium* for the fly.

The bites of louse flies are painful and may give rise to swelling and other damage to the skin.

Epidemiology and Control

The sheep ked or sheep tick is normally the only member of the group that is considered to be of economic importance and for which control methods have been developed. *M. ovinus* is common in temperate and cold climates but is not found in warm climates such as the southeastern United States or in the tropics. A few ked are not considered to be important, but when populations build up, sheep lose condition, become anemic, and may damage the fleece through rubbing and biting at it. Treatment is then justified.

The traditional treatment for sheep ked has been dipping or spraying of the animals. To eliminate the labor of spraying or dipping, a power duster has been developed that is quite effective when sheep are in short fleece. If a systemic insecticide, such as an organophosphate, were to be used, it probably would be necessary to treat animals more than once so that pupating insects would have time to emerge by the second treatment.

Readings

Baer, J. G. (1951). *Ecology of animal parasites.* Univ. of Illinois Press, Urbana.

Beard, C. B., O'Neil, S. L., Tesh, R. B., Richards, F. F., and Aksoy, S. (1993). Modification of arthropod vector competence via symbiotic bacteria. *Parasitol. Today* **9,** 179–183.

Cole, F. R. (1969). *The Flies of Western North America.* Univ. of California Press, Berkeley.

Dethier, V. (1962). *To Know a Fly.* Holden-Day, San Francisco.

Graham-Smith, G. S. (1913).

Jordan, A. M. (1993). Tsetse-flies (Glossinidae). In *Medical Insects and Arachnids* (R. P. Lane and R. W. Crosskey, Eds.). Chapman & Hall, London.

Lane, R. P., and Crosskey, R. W. (Eds.) (1993). *Medical Insects and Arachnids.* Chapman & Hall, London.

Pratt, H. D., Littig, K. S., and Scott, H. G. (1975). Flies o public health importance and their control, USDHEW, CDC, Publ. No. 77-8140. Centers for Disease Control, Washington, DC.

Smart, J. (1948). *Insects of medical importance, 2nd Ed.* British Museum, London.

CHAPTER

49

Myiasis

The larval stages of many insects develop in a range of animal tissues. Among Diptera the blue bottle fly, *Calliphora vicina* (Chapter 48), normally develops in decaying animal carcasses, but it can also develop in wounds on the bodies of mammals. Certain other members of the family Calliphoridae such as the primary screwworm, *Cochliomyia hominivorax* (Fig. 49.1), are active invaders of living tissue and are obligate parasites. A few flies such as the cluster fly, *Pollenia rudis*, are obligate parasites of invertebrates.

There are a few cases on record of beetle larvae parasitizing vertebrates, mostly humans. This association is termed canthariasis. A large number of families of beetles have been associated with canthariasis, and it is likely that they are facultative or accidental parasites. In some instances, people seem to have ingested stored food products, such as cereals, that have beetle larvae in them, and they have been found in the feces as pseudoparasites. In warm climates where dung beetles are common, adult beetles have occasionally been reported in the rectum of children probably having crawled in while the child was sleeping.

It is rare for the larvae of lepidopterans (moths and butterflies) to have what appears to be parasitic larvae, termed scolechiasis in this case. In the few cases on record, the larvae probably were ingested with raw vegetables or with stored cereal products. This relationship is not considered to be medically important. It is interesting to note that, although lepidopterans feed primarily on plants, a few families (Pyralidae, Geometridae, Noctuidae) have members that feed around the eyes of mammals where they ingest mucoid discharges. A noctuid, *Calyptera eustrigata*, pierces the skin of mammals to feed on blood, including that of humans. It is suggested that this moth may mechanically transmit some microbial diseases of the eye.

Parasitism by the larvae of dipterans is of greatest medical and economic importance and the other groups of insects will not be considered further.

CLASSIFICATIONS OF MYIASIS

Myiasis can be classified on the basis of host–parasite relations:

1. *Obligate parasitism.* The fly larvae require a living host for development. Examples are the stomach bots of horses, cattle grubs, and the human bot fly.
2. *Facultative parasitism.* Adults are attracted to foul aromas such as those caused by infected wounds or areas soiled by excrement; they oviposit and the larvae feed on softened or necrotic tissues. Examples are blow flies, which normally develop in decaying carcasses, and various members of the family Sarcophagidae.
3. *Accidental parasitism.* Larvae find their way into the body and live for a period of time but are poorly adapted to the habitat. Sometimes the larvae may be found in the intestinal tract having been eaten with contaminated food. Some flies in this category are fruit flies (family Drosophilidae), a number of domiciliated flies (family Muscidae), cluster flies (*Pollenia*), crane flies (family Tipulidae), and rat-tailed maggots (family Syrphidae).

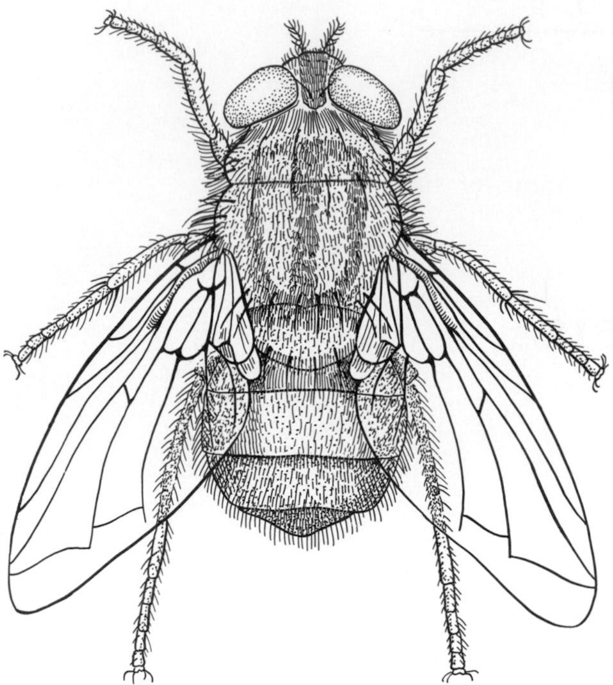

FIGURE 49.1 The primary screwworm, *Cochliomyia hominivorax*. [From James, 1947.]

FAMILY CALLIPHORIDAE

This group of flies contains organisms that are both facultative and obligate parasites. We discuss some important examples from the family as they represent particular situations to be addressed in their control.

FLY STRIKE IN SHEEP

Name of Organisms and Disease Associations

About a dozen genera of calliphorids or blow flies are associated with fly strike or wool maggots in sheep; the terms refer to females coming in to lay eggs on, usually, the hind quarters of sheep that are soiled with feces. Sheep are said to be "struck" or "fly blown" when the female flies oviposit and larvae develop. Some of the common flies in North America are *Phormia regina, Lucilia caesar, Phaenicia cuprina,* and *Calliphora vicina,* the blue bottle fly, whose life cycle is described in Chapter 48 as a generalized cyclorraphan fly. Since these flies often oviposit in carcasses, the association with the host is a facultative one.

Hosts and Host Range

The calliphorids have little or no host specificity.

Geographic Distribution and Importance

Cosmopolitan. Fly strike in sheep is an ever-present danger where sheep are on lush pastures, in feedlots, or in any situation where the animals may show diarrhea and become soiled on their hind quarters. A major economic loss lies in the labor and materials that are entailed in preventing fly strike and then treating the animals when it does occur. In Australia, there were, at one time, millions of dollars lost annually to fly strike in sheep. This motivated an intensive research program that brought about effective control.

Morphology

The calliphorids are those flies that are the same size and larger than house flies and that have shiny, metallic bodies (Fig. 48.2). Both the thorax and abdomen are usually the same color and they are likely to be blue, green, copper, or black, but they are always a strikingly beautiful color. On occasion it is necessary to identify either the adults or larvae and keys to some common forms are contained in Figures 48.1 and 48.3.

Life Cycle

Calliphora vicina (Fig. 48.2) serves an a model for all calliphorids, as well as other cyclorraphan flies. It is well to note that the life cycle is completed in two to three weeks, but can go faster at summertime temperatures.

Diagnosis

Sheep must be inspected closely to determine whether they have wool maggots. Usually this means restraining a few suspects and looking carefully at the hind quarters for maggots under the wool at soiled areas.

Host–Parasite Interactions

Flies are attracted by what we humans ordinarily consider to be foul odors. Adult flies both feed on such material and the females oviposit there. The larvae need a nutritious diet, and that is to be found in a decaying carcass or in a feces- and urine-stained hindquarters of a sheep. When the skin of an animal remains wet for several days, the skin becomes soft and

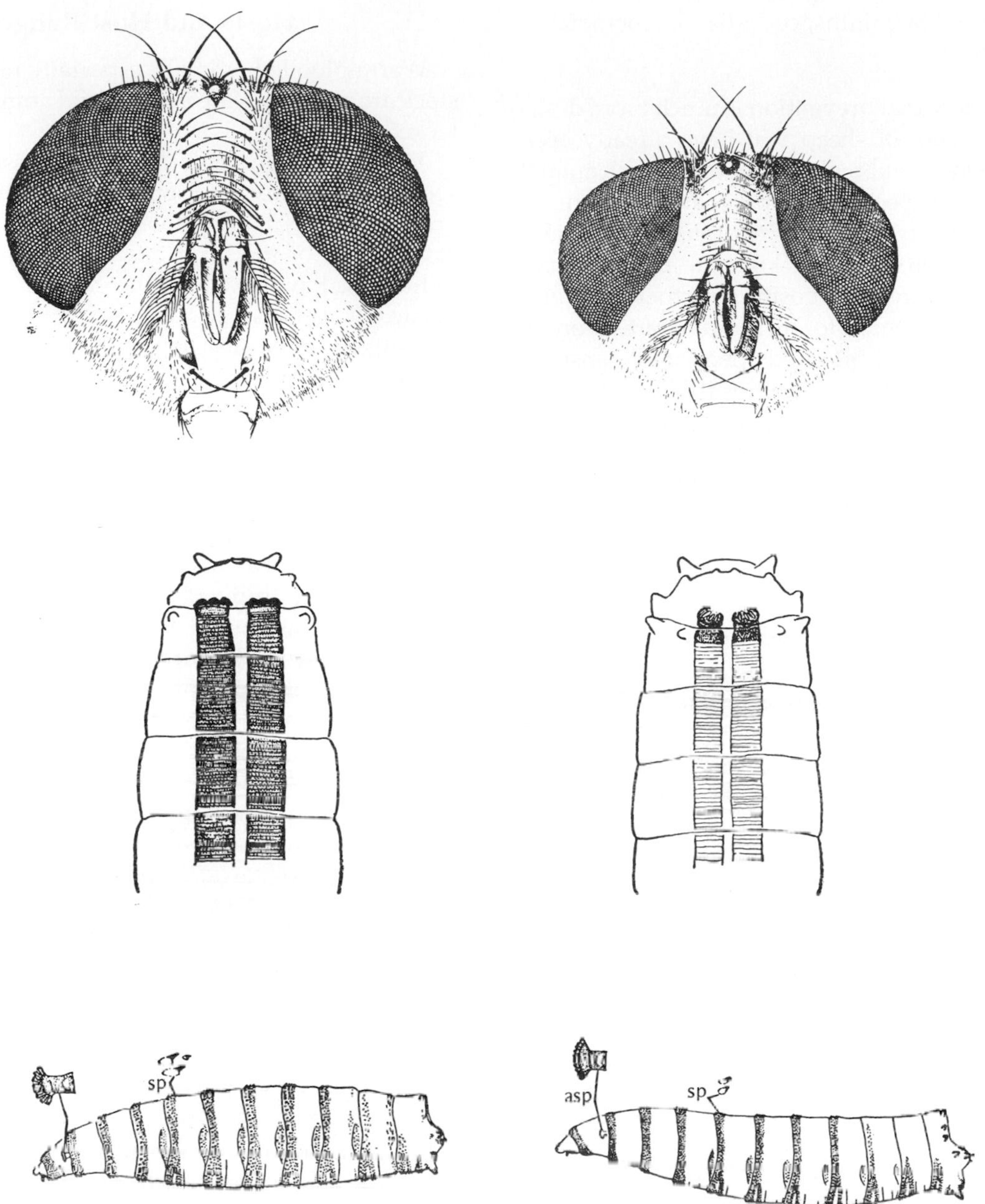

FIGURE 49.2 The differences between *Cochliomyia hominivorax* (left) and *C. macellaria* (right). Top to bottom: heads, tracheae of larvae, side view of larvae.

is subject to bacterial or fungal infection; certain of the fly larvae then abrade the skin with their mouth hooks. They consequently dig deeper into the skin which oozes and bleeds and becomes further contaminated with bacteria. The infestation then enters an uncontrolled cycle of larvae damaging the tissue, which attracts more flies that oviposit, and so on. If left untreated, the animal may die from extensive tissue damage, secondary bacterial infection, and probably intoxication from metabolic by-products of the flies.

Epidemiology and Control

Livestock producers are aware of the circumstances under which fly strike becomes a problem:

1. When pastures plants are growing rapidly, which means they have a lot of water in them and cause diarrhea
2. Around lambing time when lambs are castrated, docked, and have a little blood around the navel
3. When sheep are parasitized and show diarrhea

from intestinal helminths, coccidia, or microbial diseases

They also know that prevention is much more desirable than treatment of sheep that have already been fly blown. When an outbreak is underway, each animal must be caught, inspected, and treated. Treatment involves clipping the wool at the site of the maggots and then applying a product that kills the maggots and deters the females from ovipositing further. One animal may require from 5 to 10 minutes attention so even a small flock of a hundred sheep may consume a full eight-hour day to take care of it.

Prevention is based on the following steps:

1. Docking (amputating) the tails of lambs
2. Selective breeding for minimal wool on the hindquarters
3. Treating wounds such as the navel of newborn lambs with a repellent
4. Applying a residual insecticide/repellent on the hindquarters of all animals
5. Clipping wool from the hindquarters

All of these procedures are practiced in a well-run sheep operation. Docking of the tail is always done within a week or so of the birth of a lamb. When surgically castrated, the wound is treated with a repellent if flies are active at that season. During the pasture season, animals are inspected frequently and the wool may be clipped from the hindquarters of those that tend to soil themselves. In addition that area may also be treated with a residual insecticide/repellent if there is danger of fly strike. In fall, when lambs are weaned and sent to a feed lot, the sheep to be retained for breeding are examined for the characteristics that the owner considers to be desirable, and clean hindquarters may be one that is looked for.

THE PRIMARY SCREWWORM

Name of Organism and Disease Associations

Cochliomyia hominivorax (syn. *Callitroga h.*) is the primary screwworm and it may invade the unbroken skin of its hosts although it usually attacks wounds and sores. *Cochliomyia macellaria* (syn *Callitroga m.*) is the secondary screwworm. It is not as invasive as the primary screwworm. Both invade lesions on the skin of warm-blooded animals and cause serious damage and death of their hosts.

Hosts and Host Range

Warm-blooded animals, especially mammals. Livestock are severely affected, but wild animals are also attacked.

There are a number of human cases of primary screwworm infestation on record including an outbreak in Chile, South America, where there were 81 cases. Some of the lurid descriptions of screwworms in humans have involved the nasal passages and soft palate. In one case, it appeared that a man was thus parasitized while sleeping with his mouth open.

Geographic Distribution and Importance

Western Hemisphere. These flies were formerly distributed in the southern United States where there is little or no frost during the winter; each year they would move northward both by migration and with livestock being shipped. They are now virtually eradicated from the United States and northern Mexico. They are still prevalent in other countries of Latin America as far south as Argentina, and continue to threaten the United States through access from Mexico. Other species, such as *Chrysomyia bezziana*, the Old World screwworm, are comparable to *C. hominivorax* in southern Europe, the Orient, Africa, and islands of the Pacific Ocean.

In the United States, the primary screwworm caused severe economic losses all through the country, but especially in the warmer climates of Texas and the southeastern states. In the summer of 1935 in Texas there were an estimated 180,000 deaths in livestock from screwworms. It is likely also that they were a controlling factor in white-tailed deer populations in Texas and the Southeast. But the figures for dollar losses are rather pedestrian compared to the personal experiences of those who had to contend with screwworms on a daily basis. Richardson (1978) gives a moving description of the battle not usually seen in scientific writings:

> Every spring, as sure as the seasons, and for generations unknown, screwworms began their annual march northward from their overwintering sanctuaries in Mexico and South Texas. Pushed by an unknown force as inexorable as gravity, screwworms move north—ever moving, ever spreading, ever multiplying, ever destroying. No army ever advanced any more surely or methodically. No army was ever more destructive. Attacking, killing, maiming and destroying screwworms literally ate their way north. Reaching upper South Texas, they fanned east and west—all the while moving north—dotting the countryside with the dead carcasses of hapless wildlife, cattle, sheep, and goats. . . .
>
> There is no way to estimate the man-hours Southwesterners spent in search for and doctoring screwworm-infested animals. It undoubtedly reached into the billions of hours annually. . . .

Screwworm smear was shipped into Texas by the trainload. Most producers bought it by the case.

In effect, the screwworm ruled the livestock industry of the Southwest for a century and a half. Producers would not brand, dehorn or castrate animals during that season of the year when screwworms were severe.

People would not leave home for more than a day for fear of finding their animals had been eaten alive while they were away.

Morphology

Both species of screwworms in the Western Hemisphere are about the size of a house fly, but they have dark blue metallic bodies with striping on the thorax (Fig. 49.1). The two species are differentiated from one another by the interocular bristles, which overlap in *C. hominivorax* but not in *C. macellaria* (Fig. 49.2). The larvae are also quite similar but can be differentiated by the tracheae in the anterior part of the body, the spines, and the anterior spiracles (Fig. 49.2), but the posterior spiracles are not distinguishable (Fig. 48.3).

Life Cycle

The screwworms have typical cyclorraphan life cycles. In Texas, the life cycle is completed in 24 days in summer; the cycle is slower at the high summertime temperatures experienced there. The females lay from 10 to 400 eggs in a batch and may lay more than 2800 in a lifetime. Hatching seems to be completed in less than a day. The larvae feed from three to five days and then drop out to pupate.

Diagnosis

Direct inspection of animals is required to determine whether they have been infested with screwworms. Because the primary screwworm has been eradicated from the United States, it is sometimes essential to identify the larvae or adults to determine whether it has somehow been reintroduced.

Host–Parasite Interactions

C. hominivorax, the primary screwworm, is an obligate parasite and can invade the unbroken skin although it most often is attracted to, and oviposits in, wounds on the skin of its host. The secondary screwworm, *C. macellaria*, is a facultative parasite and is attracted to hosts once the primary screwworm has established a colony.

As with fly strike in sheep, once a beachhead has been established, additional flies are drawn in by the aroma of necrotic flesh, and a rapidly increasing number of maggots invade the host.

Epidemiology and Control

Prior to the eradication of the primary screwworm from the United States, and still in enzootic areas of the Americas, the following are the control methods in use:

1. Calving and procedures such as branding and castrating are done in the winter or when the weather is hot and dry.
2. Barbed wire is replaced with smooth wire to reduce the likelihood of wire cuts.
3. Animals are inspected regularly and treated. In fact, in the Southwest, cowboys rode continually among cattle looking for those that had been fly struck; those that had been were roped and treated immediately.

Where there was a concerted effort by all livestock producers, the impact of screwworms was reduced, but it was often a losing battle. The key to effective control lay in studies done in the middle 1930s by Drs. Knipling and Bushland of the United States Department of Agriculture on the basic biology of screwworms. They found that a female screwworm mated only a single time during her life, and they reasoned that if she could be mated with a sterile male, she would produce infertile eggs. It was finally possible to implement their theory in the period following World War II. That is, they sought to introduce sterile male flies to populations of females at levels adequate to control, and then eradicate, whole populations. The atomic age had arrived and sources of irradiation were at hand with which to sterilize flies. This came to be known as the "sterile male technique" or "autocidal control."

The theoretical base was well established, but there were technical problems to solve:

1. Raising millions, and then billions, of flies
2. Sterilizing large numbers of flies by ionizing radiation
3. Distributing the sterilized flies—how many?—how often—by what means?

Some of these stumbling blocks were overcome by inducing female flies to oviposit in a medium composed primarily of horse meat. The flies were irradiated at the proper time with ^{60}cobalt and then distributed by aircraft.

The first extensive field test was undertaken in 1952 on the island of Curaçao in the Caribbean. In 1954 as many as 68,000 sterile males were released each week. By the end of 1954, the island was declared to be screwworm-free. The technique had been shown to be effective and it was ready for further exploitation.

A screwworm factory was established at Sebring, Florida, and an eradication program was planned for the southeastern states. Between July 1958 and July 1959, 2.75 billion flies were released in the Southeast and screwworm infestations dropped from 40,000/year to zero. In 1962, the screwworm factory was moved to Texas and a campaign was initiated to push the screwworms southward. From 1963 to 1976 more than 140 million flies per week were released in Texas and southern Mexico. The total number from this one operation over the 14-year period was 1.44×10^{12}, or about 300 sterile males for every person on earth.

The total number of screwworm cases in the United States decreased overall from 1962 to 1971, and then began to increase again. The success that was achieved in the 1960s and early 1970s had obviously broken down. In response, the number of flies released per unit area was increased, but the number of cases was not reduced. The rearing system and its effects were analyzed, and it was found that flies had been selected for rapid development at a relatively high temperature and for short flight. The result was the establishment of a flight muscle enzyme (alpha-glycerol phosphate dehydrogenase) allele in such a high proportion of the captive population that males flew little and were unable to compete with the wild-type flies.

The solution was to reisolate wild-type flies and to establish them in culture. In addition the flies are now constantly monitored to ensure that noncompetitive alleles or mutants do not become established.

It had originally been thought that the sterile male technique would not have the same problems as the various organic insecticides. It is nonpolluting and resistance would not be a problem. Although the prediction has generally been true, this is a highly complex process that requires careful monitoring of all stages in the program, and there are ways in which it can break down, as we have seen.

The war against the screwworm has achieved a great deal, but it is not yet over. They have been eradicated from the United States, but a few reintroductions take place every year and careful surveillance is necessary to prevent widespread infestations from taking place. The screwworm factory has been relocated to southern Mexico with the area of eradication continually moving southward toward the Isthmus of Panama. A barrier of sterile flies is maintained and the line of attack is moved progressively farther south. Theoretically, when the Isthmus is reached, it will be relatively simple to keep a barrier of flies in that neck of land and flies will not be able to move northward.

The sterile male technique was put into practice just at a time when the costs of raising cattle were rising. Thus, some cattle raisers probably were able to remain in business because screwworms no longer took what would have been an insupportable toll. In summary, the implementation of the sterile male technique was brilliant conceptual biology; it was well orchestrated in its implementation and there was finally dramatic economic return for livestock producers.

HEMATOPHAGOUS CALLIPHORID LARVAE

Name of Organism and Disease Associations

Auchmeromyia luteola, the Congo floor maggot, is the only bloodsucking larva that is known to attack humans.

Hosts and Host Range

Although humans are the only known host, it is highly likely that other animals serve as hosts and maintain the organism in the wild. It has been found associated with the burrows of warthogs and associated with domestic swine.

Geographic Distribution and Importance

This fly occurs throughout much of subsaharan Africa to the Cape of Good Hope.

Morphology

The adults are robust flies are 9 to 13 mm long. The larvae lack spines and have two widely spaced spiracles with only a faint peritreme and three lateral slits.

Life Cycle

The adult fly oviposits in loose soil such as might be found in a village hut in Africa. The larvae are active at night and poke up through floor mats to take blood meals. The larval stages last about two weeks.

Host–Parasite Interactions

Only the larva is hematophagous. The adults feed on decaying organic material. The larvae are nocturnal and attach to the skin of the host with their mouth hooks. The larvae feed as long as 20 minutes and then withdraw to a hiding place until the next night. They seemingly do not cause enough discomfort to wake the victim. While the thought of a maggot sucking blood when one is asleep is distasteful, the Congo floor

INSECTS IN COURT

A subspecialty in entomology, referred to as forensic entomology, pertains most often to accidental death or murder in humans, but it is sometimes used in animal medicine as well. When a corpse is found, it is often important to determine not only the cause of death but the time also. The insects and other invertebrates feeding on the body can reveal with moderate certainty the time or date when death occurred.

This arcane, and some might say gruesome, branch of entomology is little more than a hundred years old. A. Megnin, a leader in medical entomology in the 19th century, laid out the general principles of forensic entomology in 1894 in an article titled "The Fauna of Cadavers" that he wrote for an encyclopedia. Although Megnin's work was done in central Europe, the successive waves of insects that occupy a body probably are relevant for any temperate climate taking into account that local fauna would be represented by different species. Megnin differentiated eight waves of insects starting with muscoid flies including calliphorids and muscids. Blow flies and peridomestic flies predominated. The second wave added sarcophagids, and at the third wave, dermestid beetles and pyralid lepidopterans showed attraction. By the eighth wave, the principal inhabitants were beetles in the families Dermestidae and Tenebrionidae, both of which clean up the remaining tissue on a skeleton.

One should note that this discussion pertains to an exposed body on the ground. If the body is buried, or is in the water the arthropodan inhabitants are different. Good bibliographies are found in Smith (1973) and De Jong (1994).

In Chapter 51 Ticks, we describe a case where it was clear that a moose was taken out of season, because the ticks remaining on the hide showed that the animal was shot outside of the hunting season.

You can learn a lot from the dead. They speak differently, but you can understand them if you know the language.

maggot is not considered to be a serious medical problem.

Epidemiology and Control

Only those persons who sleep almost directly on the ground are attacked by these larvae. If the bed is raised even a few centimeters off the ground, the individual is protected.

Related Organisms

In addition to four other species of *Auchmeromyia*, there are other species in the family Calliphoridae that are hematophagous as larvae. *Protocalliphora, Passeromyia, Philornis,* and *Noemusca* all feed on nestling birds and may weaken birds sufficiently so that they are preyed upon.

FAMILY SARCOPHAGIDAE

Name of Organisms and Disease Associations

Among the important, or common, members of this family are *Sarcophaga bullata, S. hemorrhoidalis, Wohlfahrtia vigil, W. opaca,* and *W. vigil.*

Hosts and Host Range

Although certain species are often associated with certain hosts, there is probably little or no host specificity among these organisms.

Geographic Distribution and Importance

Cosmopolitan. The sarcophagids are mostly parasites of wild animals, and are one of the many biocontrol agents in nature. They sometimes are found in young puppies and kittens. Human infestations are not unknown but are uncommon.

Morphology

The adults are 10 to 15 mm long with gray hairy bodies. *Sarcophaga* spp. have what appears to be a checker board pattern on the abdomen—alternating black and gray areas (Fig. 49.3). The thorax is usually a shiny black. The fully grown larvae are often quite large exceeding 25 mm in length. They are dark brown and have short, stiff spines.

Life Cycle

The females larviposit near a wound on the skin of a host. The newly emerged larva makes its way into

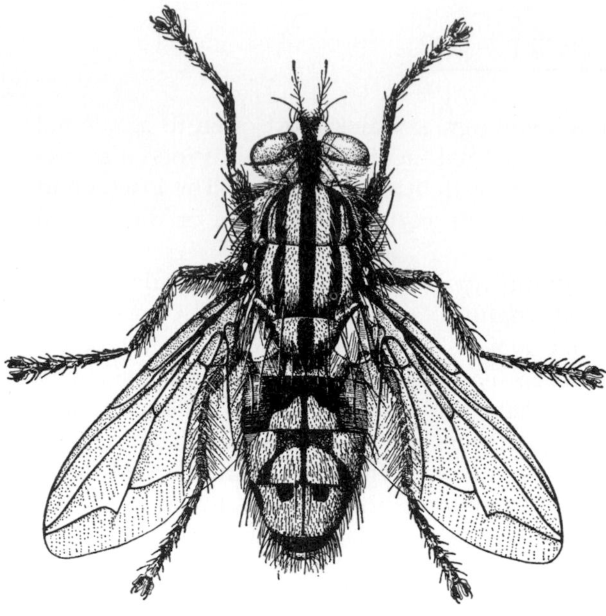

FIGURE 49.3 *Sarcophaga* sp.

the wound and feeds on the tissue. The two molts are often completed in as few as three to four days. They then drop out of the host tissue and pupate.

Host–Parasite Interactions

The sarcophagids range from facultative to obligate parasitism. Larvae of the genus *Sarcophaga* are frequently seen (along with calliphorids) in decaying carcasses of birds and mammals. They are also facultative parasites. Others, however, such as *Wohlfahrtia* are obligate parasites and usually attack newborn animals. They infest the navel or scrotal areas of mammals, and the full grown larvae may be nearly half the size of the host. *W. vigil* is an active invader of healthy tissue and does not require a break in the skin.

FAMILY CUTEREBRIDAE

These flies are usually 20 mm, or more, long and are often covered with short hairs; mouthparts are small or rudimentary. The larvae are often parasites of newborn animals, similar to some of the sarcophagids. The genus *Cephenemyia* includes a number of species that are parasites of the nasal passages and the upper respiratory tract of large ruminants such as deer and reindeer.

Name of Organisms and Disease Associations

Dermatobia hominis is the human bot. The larval stages cause considerable discomfort while they are in the skin, and secondary bacterial infections in the local area are common.

Hosts and Host Range

Although this is called the human bot fly, it is found in a wide range of other mammalian and avian hosts and is a particular problem in cattle in the Caribbean region, for example.

Geographic Distribution and Importance

Cosmpolitan in tropical areas of the Western Hemisphere.

Morphology

The adult fly is heavy-bodied and well covered with short hairs. It has some patterning on the thorax (Fig. 49.4). The fully grown third instar larva is from 18 to 24 mm long.

Life Cycle

The mode of transmission of the larvae of this fly is unique. The adult female captures a hematophagous insect such as a mosquito or stable fly and oviposits on it (Fig. 49.4). *Dermatobia* then turns the insect loose and it subsequently seeks a host on which to feed. The eggs embryonate in 5 to 15 days and the larvae hatch when the phoretic host takes a blood meal; it is unclear how the first instar larva is aware that it has reached a possible host, but one might speculate that it senses heat.

Larval development in the skin is relatively slow. The third instar larva does not drop out to pupate for 6 to 10 weeks after infection, and they have been known to remain in the skin for as long as three months.

Diagnosis

In human infections, there is little or no pain when the first instar larva penetrates the skin, but later there can be some discomfort. Since the larvae require oxygen, they place the posterior spiracles near the surface of the skin, and they can be seen at the point where there may be discomfort or the sensation that something is in the skin.

Host–Parasite Interactions

The larvae feed in the skin with their heads down and the spiracles near the surface. The mouth hooks

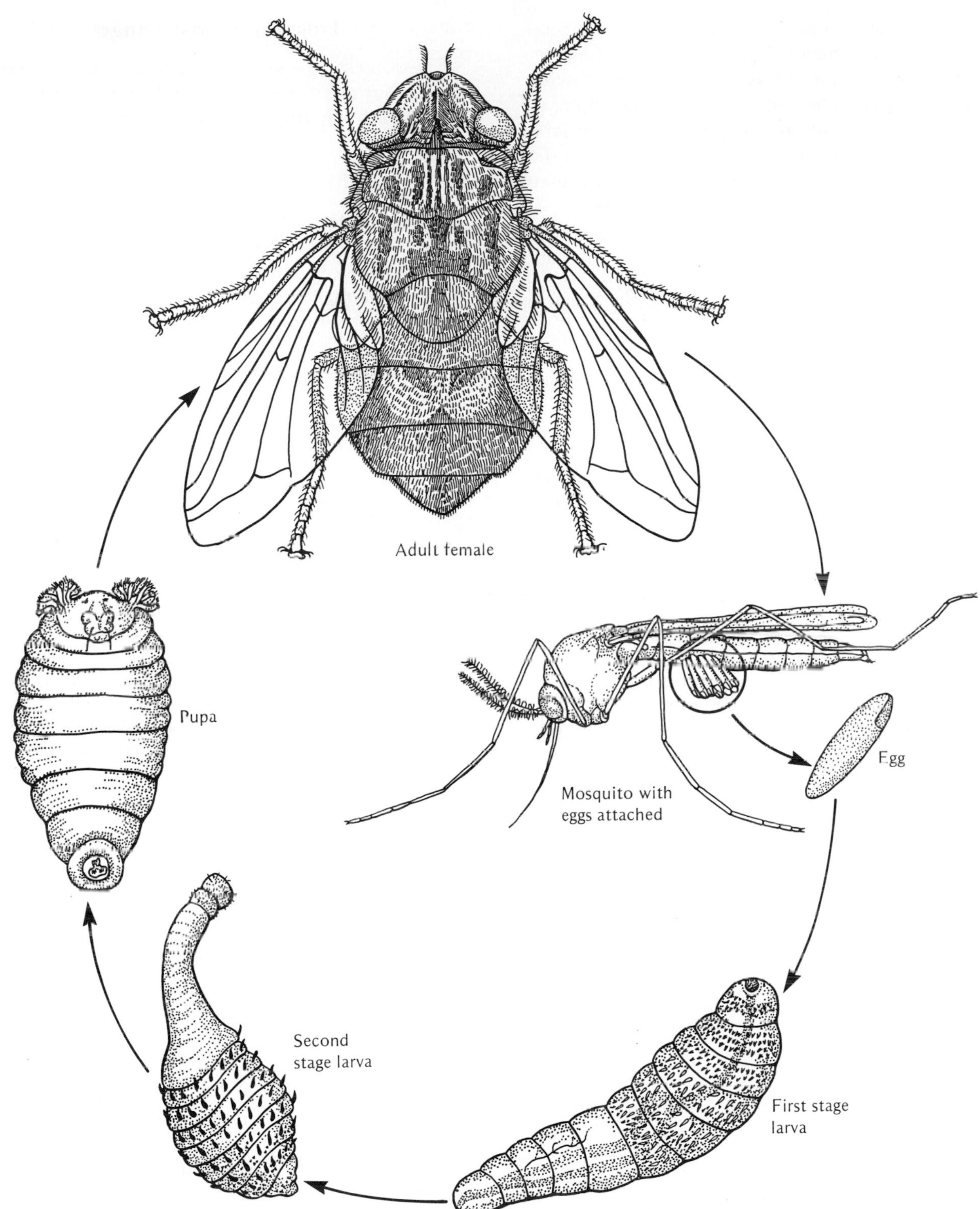

FIGURE 49.4 Life cycle of *Dermatobia hominis*, the human bot fly.

abrade the tissue and the larvae ingest liquefied food. Those persons who have been infected with *D. hominis* report some discomfort while the larvae are growing, but not much pain. There seems to be some difference in reports of the sensation when the third instar larva leaves the skin. In one instance, the person stated that there was little or no pain, and the other said that there was a sharp, piercing pain when the larva left.

The relationship of the adult fly to its surrogate egg carrier, the phoretic host, is an unique one, and although it has been described for *D. hominis* and some other closely related species, a number of physiological issues remain unsolved.

Epidemiology and Control

Control of *D. hominis* is at least difficult. There are many hosts for the larvae, which makes it a diffuse system to try to attack. Among domestic animals, cattle are the most affected and show the greatest economic loss. Cattle can be sprayed to kill the larvae as they hatch, or systemic insecticides can be administered to kill them when they get into the skin. None of this is likely to be highly effective.

D. hominis is frequently a parasite of well-to-do persons from temperate climates. Physicians and parasitologists frequently are consulted by those people who have taken a winter vacation in an idyllic tropical paradise and come home with "something funny" in the skin. Not infrequently it is the human bot whose spiracles greet the inspector when he or she looks at the spot in question. The bot can be removed by pulling up a fold of skin and squeezing gently. Killing the larvae in situ is probably ill advised since it would result in a foreign body reaction. Among parasitic organisms, "something funny" can also be a hookworm larva (Chapter 27) or *Tunga penetrans* (Chapter 46).

FAMILY OESTRIDAE—CATTLE GRUBS AND NOSE BOTS

Name of Organisms and Disease Associations

Two species of cattle grubs are of principal interest: *Hypoderma lineatum*, the common cattle grub, and *H. bovis*, the northern cattle grub. These organisms damage the host by penetrating the hides of cattle and through secondary bacterial infections.

Hosts and Host Range

The domestic ox is the principal host of both of these insects, but other hosts, such as bison and the horse, and occasionally humans, are known.

Geographic Distribution and Importance

Cosmopolitan in North America. The common cattle grub is found from the northern Great Plains to some tropical areas of Central America.

The northern cattle grub is found in about the northern three tiers of the United States and in Canada, but is seen occasionally in some southern locations such as the Carolinas. In the Eastern Hemisphere, it is prevalent in northern Europe but also occurs in some warm areas such as North Africa.

A limiting factor in the distribution of cattle grubs is their requirement for relatively dry sites for pupation. If a locality has a spring climate in which there is a lot of standing water, grubs are usually absent.

Economic losses are seen mostly in cattle, and in hides damaged by the grubs. Hides represent a significant percentage of the value of feeder cattle at slaughter, and any downgrading of the hides represents a loss for the producer. During fly season, cattle seem to be terrified of the buzzing flies and either spend their time running or standing in water so that the flies cannot approach them to oviposit. Weight gains even in heavily parasitized cattle are probably not adversely affected. Various estimates of losses are in the many millions of dollars annually.

Morphology

Hyopoderma are hairy flies that are relatively large; *H. lineatum* is 13 mm long and *H. bovis* is slightly larger at 15 mm (Fig. 49.5) During development in the host, the larvae grow from 0.7 mm in length to a spiny, brown grub that may reach a length of 30 mm.

Life Cycle

The cycle of *H. lineatum* begins in the early warm days of spring when the adults emerge from the pupal cases; adults are then seen until about mid-summer. In temperate climates, the cycle is tied to the seasons and becomes synchronized in any one locality. Adult cattle grubs have only vestigial mouthparts and do not feed. They copulate and the female searches for a proper host on which to oviposit. After oviposition the females die. The adult *H. lineatum* oviposits on the hind legs of cattle by darting in quickly and attaching individual eggs to hairs on the legs (Fig. 49.5).

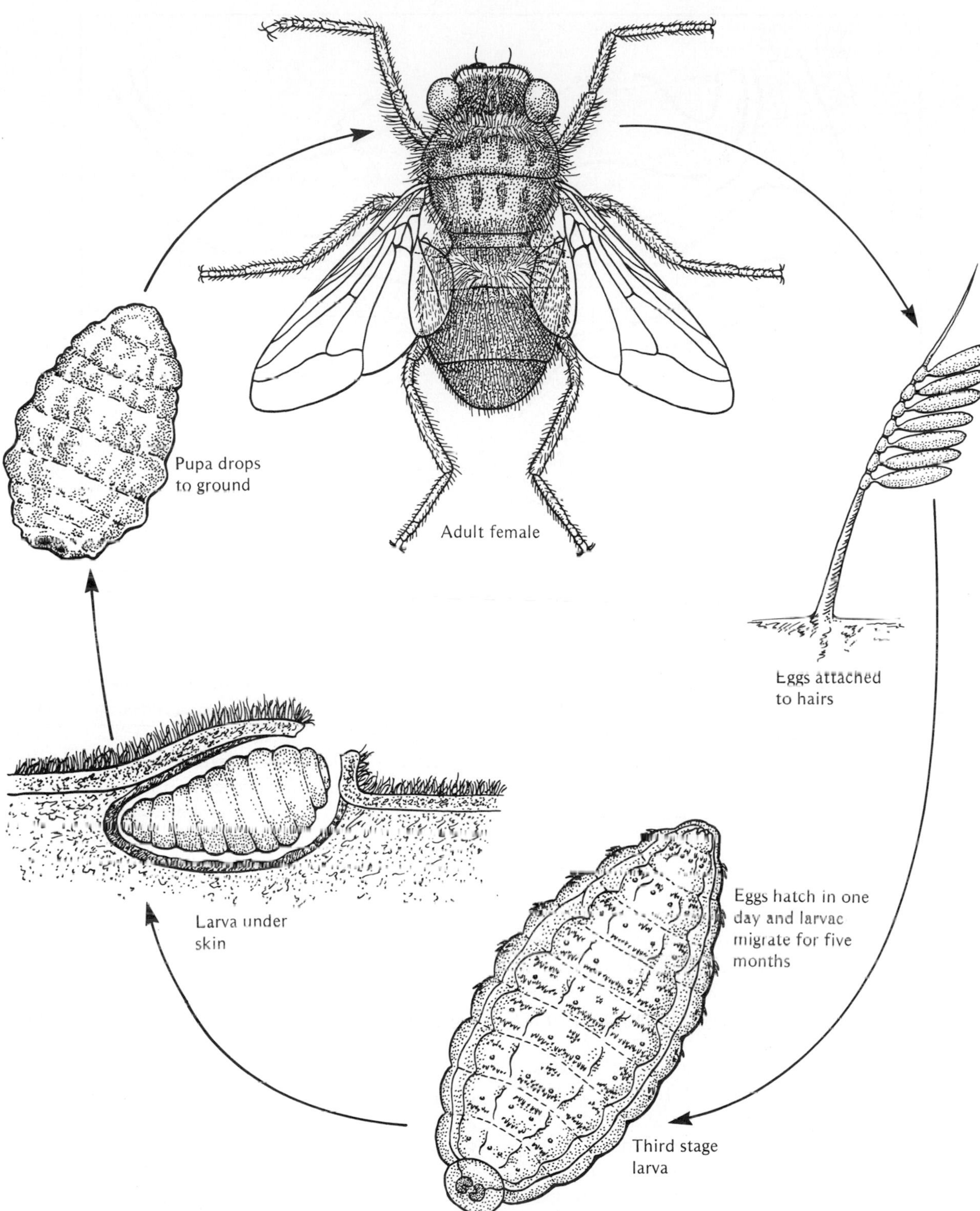

FIGURE 49.5 Life cycle of *Hypoderma lineatum*, the common cattle grub.

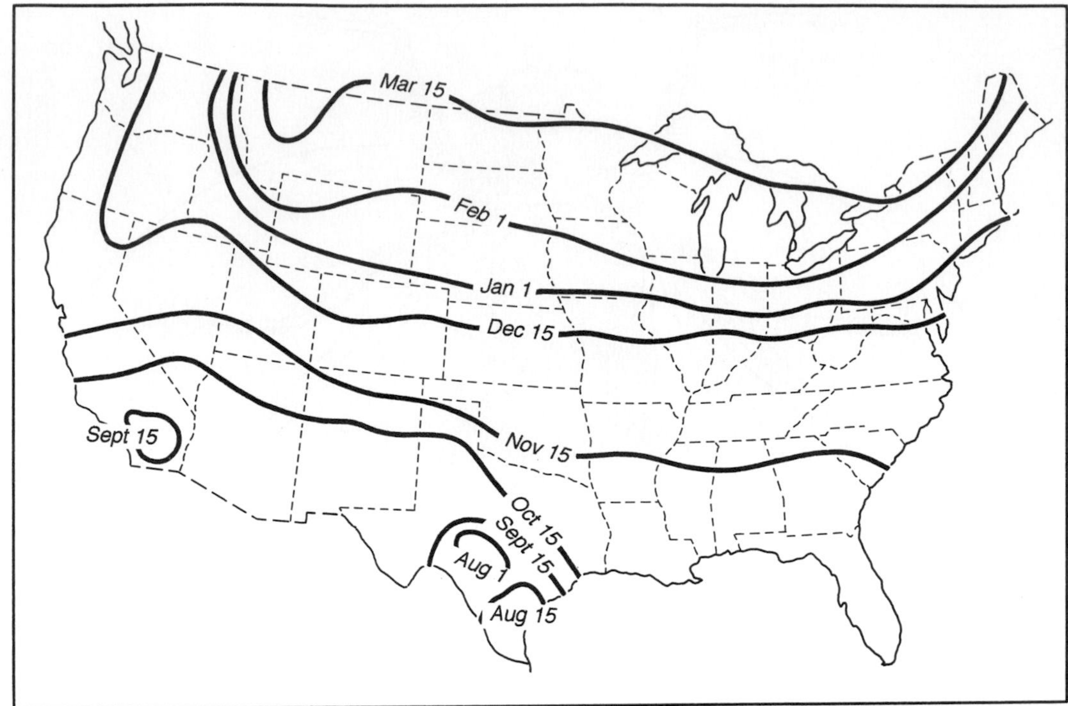

FIGURE 49.6 Time of first appearance of grubs in the backs of cattle in the United States.

Eggs hatch in three to seven days and the first stage larvae penetrate the skin, probably by entering hair follicles. At this time the larvae are about 0.7 mm long and are rather smooth. They migrate during the summer by passing through connective tissue planes and reach the connective tissue surrounding the esophagus in September or October. They are now about 10 mm long and look much like a large rice grain—smooth and rather translucent.

Starting in about November, the larvae begin to migrate again and move upward through connective tissue planes in the muscles, and come to lie under the skin along the midline of the back. They molt for the first time and begin to grow rapidly. The second instar larvae are about 15 mm long and they molt for the second time about 25 days later. In the back, the larvae cut holes in the hide with their mouth hooks and then apply the posterior spiracles to the hole so that they can obtain oxygen. The second and third instar grubs grow over a period of 50 to 100 days in the back of the host to reach their ultimate size of 30 mm. At this time the larvae shrink somewhat, crawl out of the hole, and drop to the ground where they pupate. Pupation requires from 18 to 77 days depending on soil temperature.

The cycle is very much tied to the climate (Fig. 49.6). In subtropical southern Texas, the grubs first appear in the back of cattle in August while in the northern states, they appear seven months later in March. The cycle in Texas is less synchronized than in more northerly climates.

The life cycle of the northern cattle grub is much like that of *H. lineatum* except that its stages are shifted about a month later, and there are some differences in its migratory pattern. Whereas the common cattle grub lies in the tissue surrounding the esophagus in fall, *H. bovis* lies in the subdural fat in the spinal canal.

Diagnosis

There are two phases of the life cycle during which a diagnosis can be made: (1) during fly season and (2) when grubs lie under the skin of the back and cut holes in it. Flies cause cattle to be agitated and their running with their tails raised is characteristic. When holes are cut in the hide, a warble, or bacteria-infected nodule forms and can be readily palpated.

Host–Parasite Interactions

Economic losses from cattle grubs come about from the following:

1. Activity of flies during egg-laying
2. Secondary bacterial infections when the hide is pierced by the second stage larvae

3. Trimming losses when animals go to slaughter with grubs under the skin
4. Leather losses because of holes in the hide or from scarring
5. Deaths due to anaphylaxis from crushed grubs

As was mentioned earlier, cattle seem to be terrified of the ovipositing females and either run or find a pond to stand in to keep them away. The adults do not bite and there is no pain associated with oviposition, nor is this a conditioned response since young calves run as do older animals. In some instances cattle have been stampeded by warble flies and have been injured or killed as a result. Those animals that stand in the water do not feed and fail to gain weight or give milk properly.

During migration no effect on the host has been discerned. However, when the grubs cut holes in the back, the cysts become infected with bacteria and grow to 2 to 3 cm (1 in.) in diameter.

Infected cattle develop immunity that is easily demonstrated by the decreasing number of grubs that are seen in the backs of animals one year of age and older. In addition, hypersensitivity (allergy) may be observed in some individuals. The result may be the death of an animal from anaphylaxis. It sometimes happens that the owner sees grubs in the back and squeezes a nodule to pop a grub out. If the grub instead is crushed, the hypersensitive animal may suffer from immediate anaphylaxis and die within minutes.

Following the observation of immunity associated with natural exposure to cattle grubs, research has been conducted on a vaccine. Although they are somewhat limited, early results have been encouraging. The focus of the research has been on the protease, which is produced by migrating larvae. This protease causes tissue degradation and facilitates migration of the larvae. The concept in producing the vaccine against the protease is that the larvae will be prevented from migrating and may be destroyed by various immune effector mechanisms.

Trimming losses are difficult to evaluate. When animals are slaughtered during the time when grubs are under the skin, there is a pus-laden area and usually a jelly-like area that extends a little ways from the grub. It is certainly unsightly and requires some trimming. Whether any prime meat is lost is a matter of debate; the back of an animal at slaughter usually has a layer of fat, and trimming that represents little or no economic loss.

Hides taken when grubs are in the back have holes in them when leather is made. However, if hides are taken after the grub season, the holes heal up, but there is a round scar where the hole had been. In either instance, the prime part of the hide loses value because it cannot be used for stylish leather goods. Such hides are downgraded.

It has been the conventional wisdom that cattle grubs have only a single host, the ox. This was never exactly true, but the horse seems to have become a more common host in recent decades. In some regions, horses are frequently infected, and the grubs appear along the midline of the back as in cattle. Thus, for several weeks in the spring, infected horses can not be ridden because they will not tolerate being saddled. Furthermore, because the horse is not a natural host, the grubs may have difficulty leaving the skin to pupate. In those cases, abscesses may form resulting in a long-standing lesion.

Epidemiology and Control

Control of cattle grubs is currently based almost entirely on use of insecticides. The concept of treatment is called "strategic treatment" and the term refers to treatment given after infection but before any significant damage to the host has taken place. The time of treatment varies with climate and is easiest to implement in temperate and warm-temperate climates rather than the subtropics. The cattle grub yearly cycle is relatively synchronized in temperate climates where treatment is given after fly season is over but before the grubs have appeared under the skin in the back.

Strategic treatment has generally worked well, but the presence of *H. bovis* in the spinal canal has allowed occasional severe pathology. If grubs are killed while in the spinal canal, they then become foreign bodies and a strong inflammatory response develops. Beyond the inflammatory response, the dying larvae have been shown to release a toxin, which may be directly neurotoxic. Some animals have become paraplegic following treatment, and they cannot be saved.

With the development of organophosphate systemic insecticides in the mid-1950s, a new era opened in the ability to control and possibly eradicate cattle grubs.

Systemic insecticides can be administered in several ways:

1. As a bolus or large pill
2. In the feed
3. As a spray
4. As a concentrated pour-on preparation

The early formulations of systemic insecticides were administered either by mouth or in a spray delivered by a high pressure machine that was certain to wet the skin of the animal. Both could be effective if properly used, but the labor involved was unnecessarily high.

The next alternative was to put the insecticide in a feed supplement and allow cattle to medicate themselves. This has the advantage of having little labor cost, except to deliver the feed where the animals are. The disadvantage is that not all animals take the same amount of supplemented feed— some take a lot and some avoid the feed trough. The results are therefore also spotty.

Finally, it was determined that a product with a highly concentrated insecticide could be administered with low labor cost and the expectation of nearly complete control of the grubs. The concentrated material is poured down the midline of the backs of animals while they are being handled for other reasons. In fall animals are collected for weaning of calves, vaccinations, and blood testing for certain infectious diseases. While the cattle are in a chute, one worker can treat many animals in a matter of a few minutes.

In recent years, the macrolide antibiotics, such as ivermectin, have been used successfully to kill *Hypoderma* sp. In general, these compounds are considered to be less toxic to the host than are the organophosphate compounds, which can be particularly toxic in *Bos indicus* breeds.

Eradication programs have been established in certain countries. When an eradication program is begun, all animals are treated and inspected. Second treatments may be necessary in any one year, but eventually the population of flies should be low enough that they fail to maintain themselves. These efforts have been successful in Denmark, Germany, the Netherlands, and the Republic of Ireland. In Great Britain, the incidence of grub infestations has been reduced from 38% in 1978 to virtually nil in the mid-1980s.

Name of Organism and Disease Associations

Oestrus ovis is called the nasal bot or head maggot of sheep. An infestation with this maggot is usually not life threatening, but occasionally there is a bacterial infection that causes encephalitis and the death of the host.

Hosts and Host Range

The domestic sheep is considered to be the primary host of this bot fly, but other hosts such as the goat and sometimes humans are also infected.

Geographic Distribution and Importance

Cosmopolitan wherever small ruminants are raised. Some direct damage is experienced by the host and results in failure to gain weight, or encephalitis, which may kill the host. Indirectly, sheep huddle to keep the flies from larvipositing and do not feed at that time.

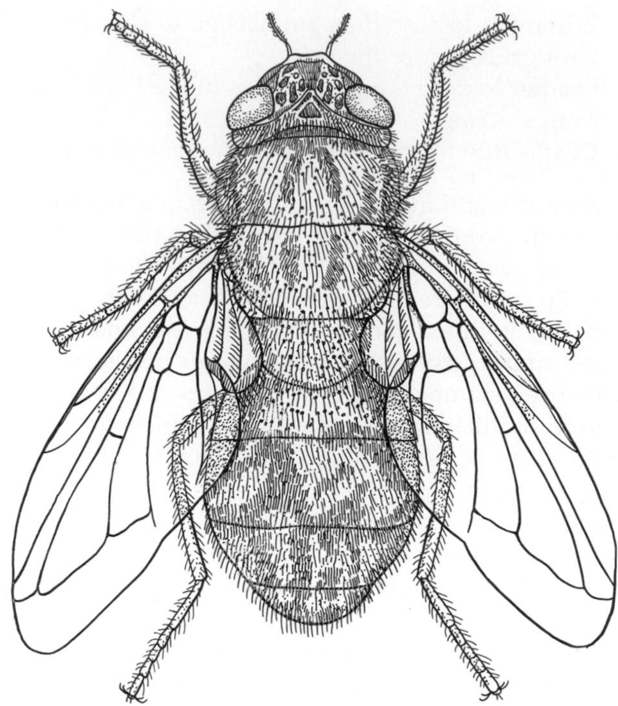

FIGURE 49.7 *Oestrus ovis*, the nasal bot fly of sheep.

Morphology

The adults are hairy flies (Fig. 49.7) that are beelike and 10 to 12 mm long. The mouthparts of the adults are vestigial and they do not feed. The larvae are white during most of their development, but turn dark brown during the third instar. The third instar is about 30 mm long.

Life Cycle

The female flies larviposit near the nostrils of sheep. The larvae enter the nasal passage where they remain and develop through the second instar. The third instar larvae enter the head sinuses and remain there for 8 to 10 months. The larvae usually attain full size in late winter or spring and leave the sinuses to pupate. Most often, when the third instar larva reaches the nasal passages, the host sneezes violently thus ejecting the larva with great force.

Pupation requires four to six weeks on the ground, and the adults die soon after larvipositing is completed. Overwintering is by the first and second stage larvae in the nasal passages.

Diagnosis

The presence of larvipositing flies is usually obvious because sheep will stand, often in a circle, with their noses close to the ground. After infection has taken place, the host shows a stringy, mucoid discharge from the nose.

Host–Parasite Interactions

It is obvious that nasal bots are irritating to the nasal mucosa because of the copious nasal discharge, but usually that is the greatest pathogenesis. It is interesting to note that one seldom sees more than a single third instar larva in a head sinus. It seems as though there is a feedback mechanism that limits the occupation of a relatively limited space.

Epidemiology and Control

Control of head maggots is limited to use of insecticides. Certain organophosphate insecticides and macrolide antibiotics can be administered with good results.

Notable Features

Although *O. ovis* is primarily a parasite of domestic sheep, humans are sometimes infected. The areas ringing the Mediterranean Sea as well as adjacent areas in the Middle East report the greater number of infections. Seemingly, where normal hosts are scattered, the flies oviposit on humans. In addition to the nares, the flies oviposit on the conjunctiva of the eye, the mouth and the ear canal. In general, the infection in humans is self-limiting, but a few cases have been recorded in which second and sometimes third instar larvae have been removed from the human head. In a case report from Spain, a 64-year-old man complained of nasal obstruction, but examination by two physicians failed to reveal any abnormality. An otolaryngologist had concluded that the man had mental illness, but a month later the man sneezed and forcibly ejected a total of five third-instar larvae of *O. ovis.*

FAMILY GASTEROPHILIDAE—STOMACH BOTS OF HORSES

Name of Organism and Disease Associations

On a global basis, there are six species of *Gasterophilus* in equids, but only three occur in North America: *G. intestinalis, G. nasalis,* and *G. haemorrhoidalis.* These larvae cause moderate to severe damage to the stomachs of horses or block the passage of food from the stomach to the small intestine.

Hosts and Host Range

The principal host of concern is the horse, but other equids are also infected.

Geographic Distribution and Importance

Cosmopolitan wherever horses are raised and kept. These flies are one of the important intestinal parasites of horses and are usually treated regularly.

Morphology

The adults are beelike with hairy bodies and large eyes (Fig. 49.8); they have vestigial mouthparts. The adults range in size from 10 to 17 mm. Larvae are fat maggots when seen in the stomach and are either white or red; they are 15 to 20 mm long.

Life Cycle

The cycles of the horse bots are similar and are tuned to the weather in temperate climates. the females oviposit on hairs around the muzzle of the horse (*G. nasalis, G. haemorrhoidalis)* or on the legs (*G. intestinalis* (Fig. 49.8). Larvae hatch in two to seven days when the larvae are licked off by the horse. The larvae penetrate the oral mucosa and tongue and move in the tissues locally. First instar larvae then reappear in three to four weeks and are swallowed. They attach to the lining of the stomach and probably remain in the same place for 10 to 12 months. They then detach and are carried in the feces to the outside where they pupate.

Host–Parasite Interactions

Although horses are annoyed when females oviposit, the principal damage is to the lining of the stomach where the bots bury their heads deeply in the tissue. Colonies of larvae are often seen that are 10 cm (4 in) in diameter. *G. nasalis* locates at the pyloric end of the stomach and oftentimes into the duodenum. They thereby impede the passage of food from the stomach to the small intestine. Larvae produce mucosal ulcers in the stomach and occasionally penetrate the stomach wall resulting in a life-threatening peritonitis.

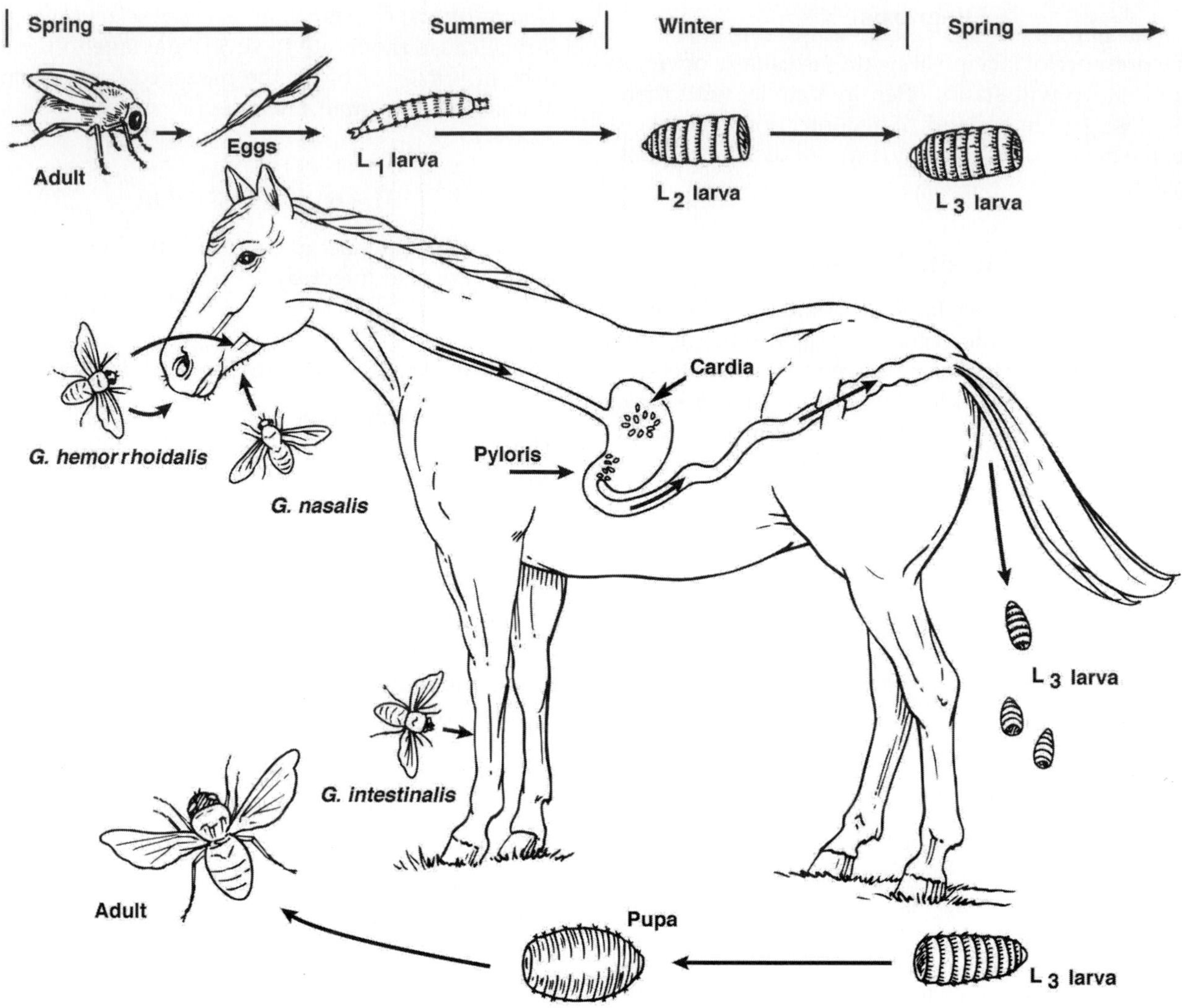

FIGURE 49.8 The life cycle of the stomach bots of horses: *Gasterophilus intestinalis, G. nasalis*, and *G. haemorrhoidalis*. In temperate climates, the life cycle begins in the spring when larvae leave the horse and pupate on the ground. The nonfeeding adults oviposit on the horse, the eggs are ingested and the larvae migrate to the stomach.

Epidemiology and Control

Stomach bots are controlled by the following:

1. Frequent removal of eggs from the hairs on the body and chin
2. Strategic treatment (see the discussion of cattle grubs)

Flies are active from spring through mid- to late summer and treatment is not ordinarily given until fly season is over. In some warm climates such as the southeastern United States, there may be two waves of fly populations. One wave of adults is seen in early to mid-summer and there is one in the autumn. Accordingly, two treatments per year may be necessary. When drug treatment is given, it is done in connection with treatment for gastrointestinal nematodes (Chapter 28). There are several effective drugs which are well tolerated.

In addition to drug treatment, prevention revolves around removing the eggs before they have embryonated and are capable of hatching. The eggs are visible to the naked eye as cream-colored specks almost 1 mm long attached to the hairs on the legs and around the muzzle. While it may be impractical under some circumstances, frequent removal of eggs with a pumice stone or sharp blade can be helpful.

Readings

Bush, G. L., Neck, R. W., and Kitto, G. B. (1976). Screwworm eradication: Inadvertent selection for noncompetitive ecotypes during mass rearing. *Science* **193,** 491–493.

De Jong, G. D. (1994). An annotated checklist of the Calliphoridae (Diptera) of Colorado, with notes on carrion associations and forensic importance. *J. Kansas Entomol. Soc.* **67,** 378–385.

Hall, M., and Wall, R. (1996). Myiasis of human and domestic animals. *Adv. Parasitol.* **35,** 257–334.

James, M. T. (1947). *The Flies That Cause Myiasis in Man*, Misc. Publ. No. 631. U.S. Dept. of Agriculture, Washington, DC.

Knipling, E. G. (1960). Eradication of the screwworm fly. *Sci. Am.* **203**(4), 54–61.

Richardson, R. H. (Ed.) (1978). *The Screwworm Problem: Evolution of Resistance to Biological Control.* Univ. of Texas Press, Austin.

Smith, K. G. V. (1973). Forensic entomology. In *Insects and Other Arthropods of Medical Importance* (K. G. V. Smith, Ed.). British Museum (Natural History), London.

Wilson, G. W. C. (1986). Control of warble fly in Great Britain and the European Community. *Vet. Rec.* **118,** 653–656.

Zumpt, F. (1965). *Myiasis in Man and Animals in the Old World.* Butterworth, London.

CHAPTER

50

Introduction to the Arachnids and the Mites

The subphylum Chelicerata contains those organisms that have piercing–cutting mouthparts called chelicerae, which contrast to the other principal groups that have mandibles (Crustacea, Insecta). There is no head, as such, because the segments are fused to form a cephalothorax and abdomen, which make up the body regions; in the mites, there is further fusion of body regions. Antennae are lacking and they have only simple eyes (not compound as in the crustaceans and insects). In addition to the chelicerae, the mouthparts have pedipalps and accessory structures that manipulate the food or have sensory functions, depending on the particular taxon. They have four pairs of legs and most members are terrestrial. Developmental patterns are such that the juvenile forms have much the same body form as the adults.

Chelicerates are predaceous (spiders, scorpions, some mites; Fig. 50.1), detritus feeders (some mites), or parasitic (ticks and some mites). Food is generally liquid, but some (scorpions) tear their prey apart with their pedipalps and then liquefy it near the mouth. The only group that sucks blood from vertebrates and serves as vectors of disease agents is the Acari (ticks and mites).

SUBCLASS SCORPIONINA

Scorpions are readily recognized, because their pedipalps are modified into pincers by which they grasp their prey (Fig. 50.1). The telson or tail is modified into a stinger. Their usual upper limit in length is about 10 cm, but one of the African species, *Pandinus,* reaches 20 cm. Their habitats are generally hot, dry climates, where they prey on small invertebrates. Their importance lies in the fact that they occasionally sting humans. The stings of most of the New World forms are only mildly toxic, but some of the African species are highly dangerous to humans, especially children. They do not seek humans to sting; humans are stung when they accidentally come into contact with scorpions. Keegan (1980) is an excellent source of information on the biology, identification, and hazards of scorpions.

SUBCLASS ARANEAE

Spiders (Fig. 50.1) are ubiquitous predators on other small arthropods. Most are harmless to humans, and many are distinctly beneficial by their feeding on insects. Further information may be found in Gertsch (1979) for general characteristics, Kaston (1972) for identification; Comstock (1940) provides an enormous fund of information on all aspects of spiders; Cloudsley-Thompson (1958) contains excellent descriptions of the natural history of spiders and some other taxa.

SUBCLASS ACARI—THE MITES AND TICKS

The Acari, whose members are commonly called mites or acarines, includes both mites and ticks. Ticks are actually giant mites and are spoken of separately primarily because they are much larger although they

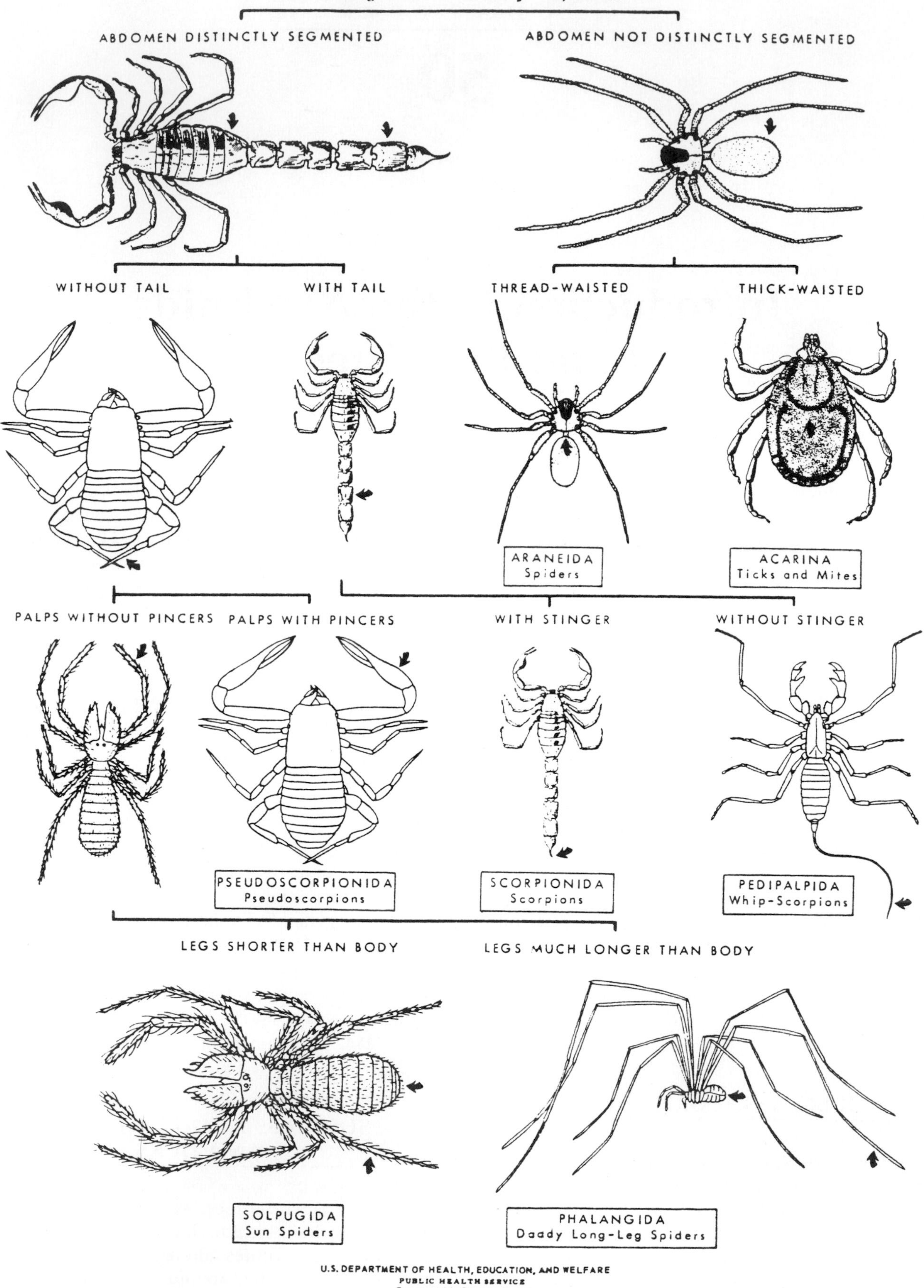

FIGURE 50.1 Pictorial key to the major groups in the class Arachnida.

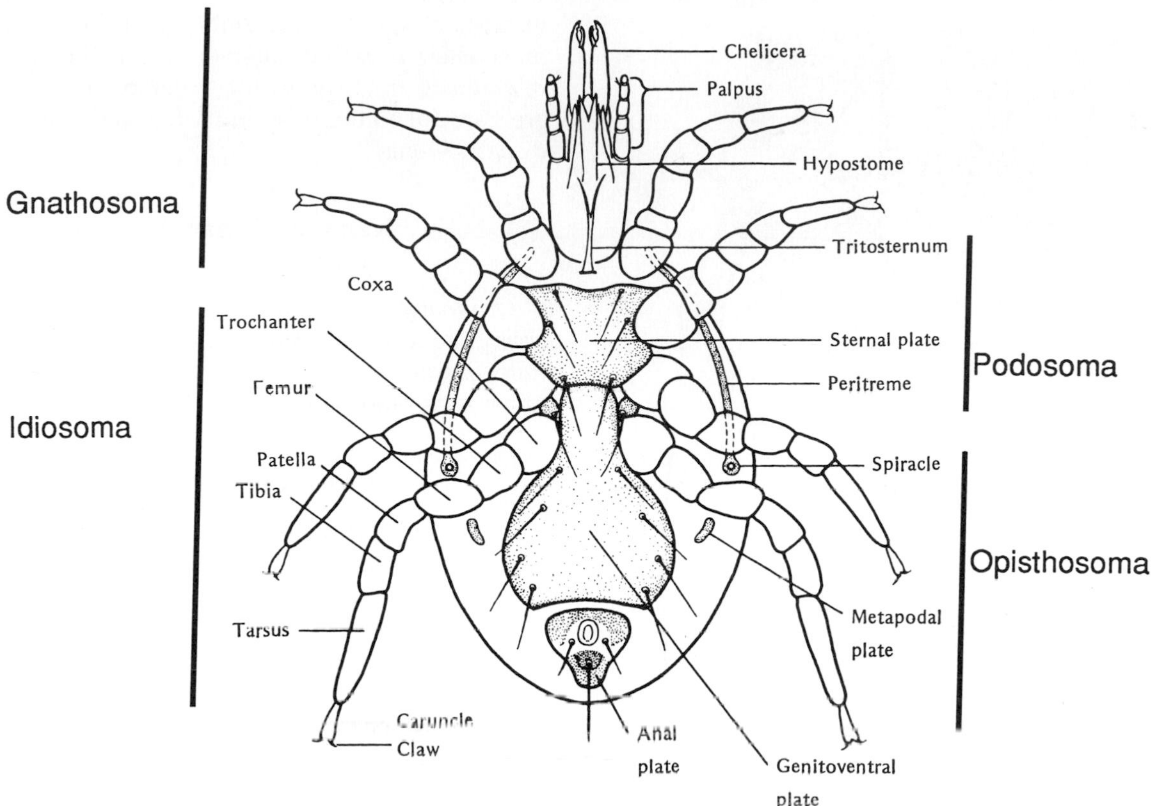

Figure 50.2 Diagram of the external anatomy of a mite.

do have anatomical characters that set them apart from the rest of the mites.

Mites are found in all habitats, terrestrial, aquatic, and parasitic. About 36,000 species are known and additional species are continually described in journals devoted to acarines, insects, plant pathology, parasitology, and medical entomology.

Mites are diverse both in structure and biology. The greatest number of species are free living and they are detritus feeders or predators. The parasitic forms feed on plants and animals by puncturing the tissues with their chelicerae and taking juices or blood. The parasites are important as vectors of disease agents of plants and animals as well as for the damage they produce directly through feeding.

Terminology for the body parts of mites and other arachnids takes into account the fusion of three segments. There is no head, but the gnathosoma or capitulum bears the mouthparts (Fig. 50.2). The chelicerae are derived from the first appendages and the pedipalps from the second. The other major body region is the idiosoma, which comprises everything except the gnathosoma. The terms employed for the subdivisions of the idiosoma are the podosoma, which bears the legs, and the opisthosoma, which is the region posterior to the legs. The hysterosoma includes the second and third pairs of legs and the opisthosoma. Leg terminology is similar that of the insects, but since the legs have more segments, the patella is an additional term for the fourth segment distal from the body. Although there is some variation, the anus is usually subterminal and the genital opening is at the level of the coxae of the fourth legs.

Classification of the mites is based principally on adult structures, and one of the first characteristics used at the ordinal level is the location and number of stigmata or spiracles, the opening to the respiratory system (Appendix 1). In many classifications (e.g. McDaniel, 1979; Woolley 1988), the ordinal names state either the number or the location of the stigmata, or both.

The developmental pattern is basically the same in all mites:

$$\text{egg} \rightarrow \text{larva} \rightarrow \text{nymph} \rightarrow \text{adult}$$

The stages are usually similar to one another in general form, but the larva has three pairs of legs and the nymph and adult have four pairs. The life cycle of the scab mite of humans is an example (Fig. 50.3). The life cycles vary in that there may be more than one

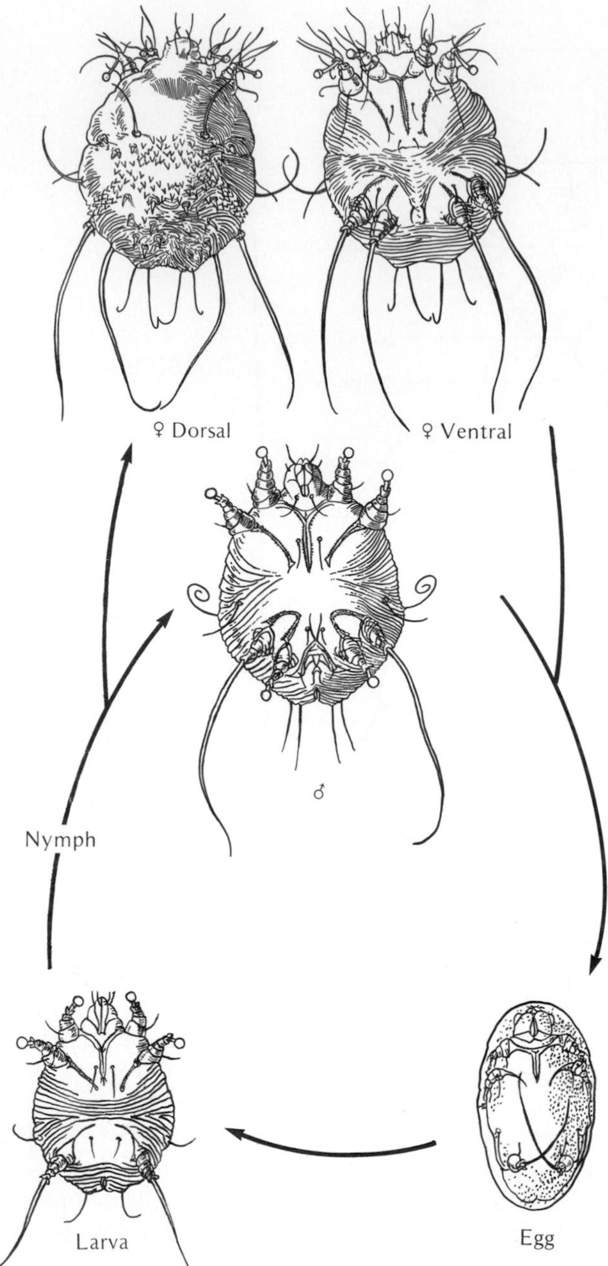

FIGURE 50.3 Life cycle of the scab mite, *Sarcoptes scabiei.*

nymphal stage and there may be quiescent stages such as the nymphochrysalis in the chiggers (Trombiculidae) (Fig. 50.11, presented later). In most cases, females die after laying eggs, but in a few instances such as the soft ticks (Argasidae), females may continue to lay batches of eggs for months.

COHORT PARASITIFORMES

Family Dermanyssidae

Members of this family (order Gamasida) are relatively long legged and have piercing chelicerae. A number of species are symbionts of birds and mammals Their parasitic habitats are on the skin, in the respiratory tract, or in the outer or inner ear; some are harmful to the host and a few serve as vectors of disease agents

Name of Organisms and Disease Associations

Ornithonyssus sylviarum, the northern fowl mite; *O. bacoti,* the tropical rat mite; *O. bursa,* the tropical fowl mite; *Dermanyssus gallinae,* the chicken mite. These mites suck blood and irritate the skin of their hosts.

Hosts and Host Range

These mites have host preferences, but are found feeding on an array of species. For example *O. sylviarum* occurs on chickens, but has been reported from 10 other species of birds and feeds on mammals such as humans for short periods. Because of their fairly broad host range and the fact that they occasionally feed on humans, these mites are considered here as a group.

Geographic Distribution and Importance

Cosmopolitan within the climatic zones indicated by their names. In poultry, heavily infested animals become fidgety, egg production drops, and the feathers may become discolored because of the large amount of blood-containing feces excreted by the mites. On any host, the skin irritation may be severe and there may be a rash as hypersensitivity develops.

Morphology

All of these mites are about the same size (Fig. 50.4); the females are about 0.5 to 1.0 mm long. The bodies have many bristles, the legs are long, and the chelicerae are styletlike.

Life Cycle

The pattern of development in these mites is as follows:

egg → larva → protonymph → deutonymph → adult

Eggs are deposited in nests or crevices in houses or buildings or in litter in poultry houses; they are sometimes laid on the host. Hatching may occur within a day releasing the larva; the larva does not feed, but molts to the protonymph, which does feed. After feeding, the protonymph molts to the deutonymph, which may or may not feed, depending on the species. The

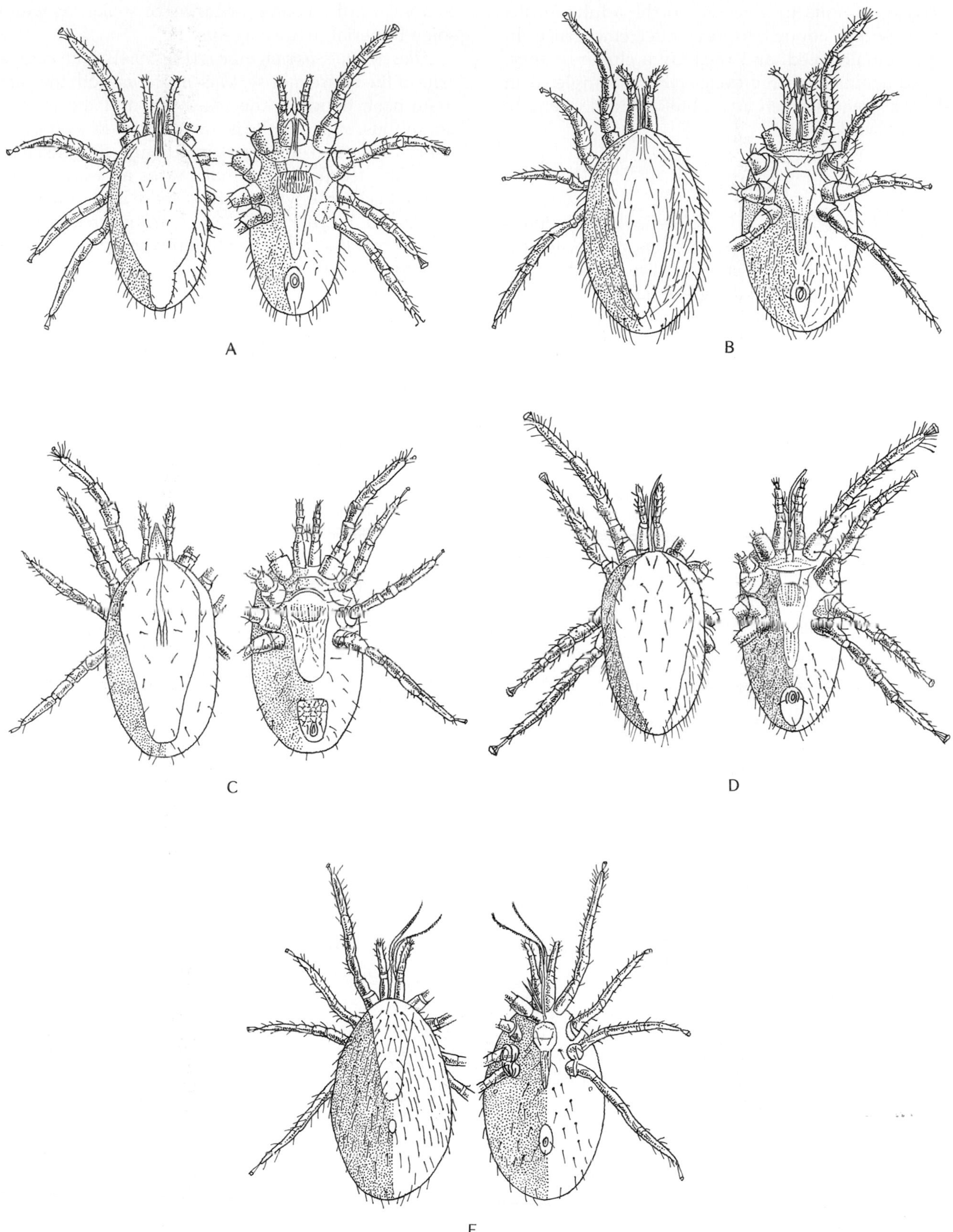

FIGURE 50.4 Some members of the family Dermanyssidae. (A) *Ornithonyssus sylviarum;* (B) *Ornithonyssus bacoti;* (C) *Dermanyssus gallinae;* (D) *Ornithonyssus bursa; (E) Allodermanyssus sanguineus.* [Redrawn from Baker et al., 1956.]

deutonymph molts to give rise to the adult. Adults copulate within about two days after emergence. In general, females feed, and then lay a clutch of eggs, and feed again. Their life cycles can be completed in as short a time as seven days, but ordinarily require about two weeks.

Diagnosis

Where poultry are raised, the owner usually looks for fidgety birds as a first sign of mites, but it can also mean an infestation with chewing lice (Chapter 44). Birds should be examined individually by looking carefully at the skin, particularly in the region of the vent. The person examining birds may well find mites on his or her own skin.

If a member of this family of mites is found on humans, its identification to species usually points to the source of the mites, whether birds or mammals.

Host–Parasite Interactions

Damage to the host involves feeding on blood, skin irritation, and development of hypersensitivity. Production losses in poultry result from decreases in egg production or failure to gain weight well. Animals may actually die from severe anemia.

Epidemiology and Control

Second-generation acaricides have been used successfully. They are usually applied to birds as a dust. Roosts of chickens may be painted with a liquid preparation.

Although mites spend most of their time on a host, they may also leave the host for fairly long periods. Some, such as *D. gallinae*, may survive four to five months off of a host without feeding. In considering a control program, it is essential not only to treat the affected birds, but also to clean out poultry houses and to apply an acaricide to the structure.

Related Organisms

A number of dermanyssids are found in the respiratory tracts of reptiles and mammals. For example. *Orthohalarachne attenuata* is found in the upper respiratory tract of the Alaskan fur seal, *Callorhinus ursinus,* and Stellar's sea lion, *Eumatopia jubata,* on the west coast of North America. *Pneumonyssus simicola* is commonly found in the nasal passages of rhesus monkeys. *Pneumonyssoides caninum* is in the dog and probably is widespread. *Ophionyssus natricis* is common on snakes in zoos, where it can cause serious blood loss. It serves as a vector of a haemogregarine of snakes as well as some bacterial disease agents.

Allodermanyssus sanguineus (Fig. 50.4E) is an ectoparasite of the house mouse, *Mus musculus.* Both the vertebrate host, which is the reservoir, and the mite are ubiquitous, and the mite is the vector of *Rickettsia akari,* which causes rickettsial pox in humans. Rickettsial pox is a mild, febrile illness that causes a rash similar to that of tick-borne typhus; the disease is not life threatening and usually does not warrant treatment, although broad-spectrum antibiotics are sometimes prescribed to hasten recovery.

FAMILY LAELAPIDAE

Name of Organism and Morphology

Echinolaelaps echidninus (Fig. 50.5A), the spiny rat mite, is representative of a number of closely related species; it is found principally on rodents, especially *Rattus norvegicus,* but it feeds on other rodents as well.

These mites bear a superficial resemblance to the dermanyssids; they have long legs and considerable setation on the body. There are both free-living and parasitic species in the family. The parasitic species are important as ectoparasites and as vectors of various disease agents, mostly those passed from rodents to humans.

Life Cycle

The life cycle of *E. echidninus* has the following:

egg → larva → protonymph → deutonymph → adult

The female gives birth to a larva that does not feed, but the nymphal and adult stages feed.

Host–Parasite Interactions

This mite is a vector of *Hepatozoon muris,* a common haemogregarine of rats. a related organism, *Haemogamasus pontiger,* has been implicated in causing skin rashes in soldiers who have used straw as bedding. Other species, such as *Eulaelaps stabularis* (Fig. 50.5B), may serve as vectors of the agents causing plague and tularemia.

Name of Organism and Disease Associations

Varroa jacobsoni is the cause of varroatosis or varroasis in the honeybee, *Apis mellifera.*

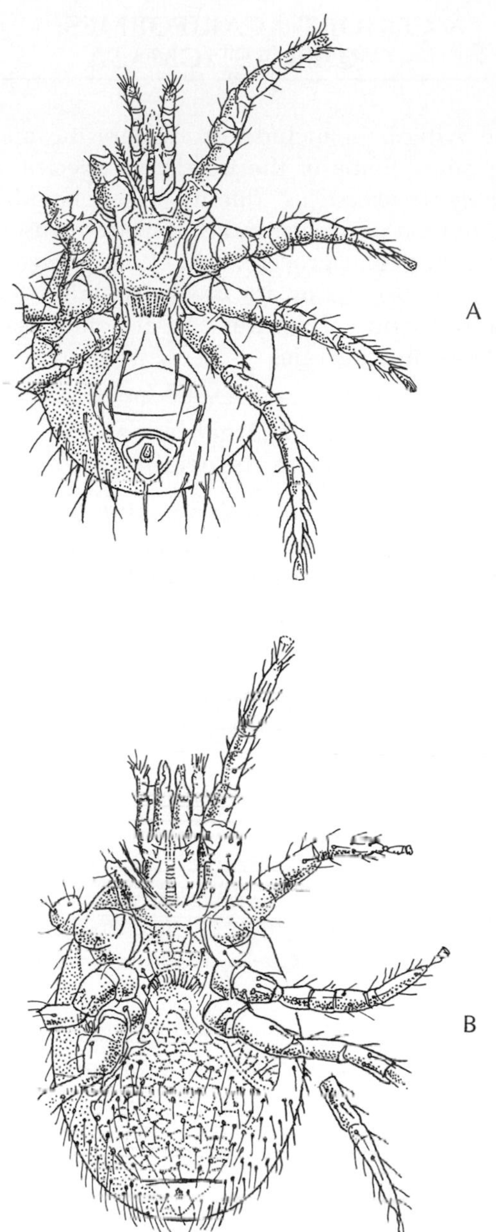

FIGURE 50.5 Two representative of the family Laelapidae. (A) *Echinolaelaps echidninus;* (B) *Eulaelaps stabularis.* [From Baker et al., 1956.]

Hosts and Host Range

The original host of *V. jacobsoni* was the eastern honey bee, *Apis cerana.* The mite also now parasitizes the honey bee, *A. mellifera.*

Geographic Distribution and Importance

A. cerana is kept in the Eurasian continent east of the Ural mountains and *V. jacobsoni* appears to be a commensal of that species of honey bee. At about the turn of the 20th century, the honey bee kept in most of the western world, *A. mellifera,* was moved to the Asian portion of Eurasia and to Japan. *A. mellifera* then became infested with *V. jacobsoni;* it can produce a devastating effect on colonies of that species of bee. The mite is now found essentially worldwide in honey bees.

Acarine parasites of honey bees have raised serious issues with respect to pollination of crops such as cucumbers, apples, and cantaloupes. Populations of both domestic and wild bees are declining, and there is concern that production of many crops will be affected. If wild bee populations are reduced beyond a certain level, domestic bees will have to be provided to ensure that certain crops are adequately pollinated.

Both *Varroa jacobsoni* and *Acarapis woodi,* discussed later, have beekeepers and farmers whose crops require pollination worried that these infestations will seriously affect production.

Morphology

These tiny mites are broader than long and are well supplied with setae especially on the dorsal surface.

Life Cycle

The life cycle consists of the following:

egg → larva → protonymph → deutonymph → adult

Development takes place in the hive and on the bodies of both larval and adult bees. A female invades the brood cell of the larva before it is sealed, and it feeds on the hemolymph of the developing larva.

Development to the adult female requires seven to eight days. The first egg is a female, the second a male, and the rest of the eggs are female. The mechanism of this phenomenon is not known, but similar situational sex determination occurs in other groups of animals as well, such as certain nematodes and mollusks.

Diagnosis

Worker bees can be caught and examined for the presence of mites feeding between the sclerites on the abdomen. A more definitive approach to diagnosis is to catch mite carcasses on cloth placed at the bottom of the hive. It is thereby possible to monitor the effect of treatment; when carcasses of mites are no longer found except in small numbers, treatment has been effective.

Host–Parasite Interactions

All stages of *V. jacobsoni* feed on hemolymph from both larvae and workers. The mites insert their mouthparts between the joints in the exoskeleton, and they may take as much as 0.1 mg of hemolymph in two hours. A larval bee infested with even two mites has its life span as an adult reduced from an average of 28 days to just 9 days.

Parasitized bees are subject to cold stress, and many of them die during the winter. They also are more susceptible to common bacterial and viral diseases of bees.

Epidemiology and Control

Control of varroatosis is based on the following:

1. Early diagnosis
2. Acaracidal treatment
3. Selection of resistant stocks of bees

Varroatosis is difficult to contain since it may be carried by foraging worker bees as much as 3 km in a season. In any one hive, the mites continue to reproduce during the foraging period, and toward the end of the season mites occur in such large numbers that there may be a mass die-off of workers and drones.

Some strains of *A. mellifera* are more resistant than others, but there seems not to have been an effort to select resistant bees.

Control is currently based on the use of an organophosphate systemic acaricide. The approved method of application is to hang strips, which are impregnated with the acaricide, in the hive. The time of year and duration of treatment must be followed explicitly.

Another type of treatment is also used; the diluted chemical is applied to the surface of the bees in all hives on a farm, but it is not necessary to treat all of the bees. Bees groom and feed one another, and since the acaricide finds its way to the hemolymph, the mites are killed. A few of the bees that were initially treated die probably because of an overdose of acaricide, but this does not affect the colony overall. More than one treatment is usually required to maintain good control through the stress of winter.

Related Organisms

A second pathogenic mite of bees is *Acarapis woodi*, a tiny mite, 150 μm, long, which lives in the larger tracheae of the bee. Infected bees are stressed and often die during the winter. Fumigation of the hives with menthol is the approved treatment. Programs are underway to develop mite-resistant strains of honeybees.

COHORT ACARIFORMES: ORDER ASTIGMATA

The Astigmata includes both parasitic and free-living mites. Some of the free-living species such as *Glyciphagus domesticus* (family Glyciphagidae) are found in food products, and this species causes a skin rash referred to as grocer's itch. *Dermatophagoides farinae* and *D. pteronyssus* are free-living mites that feed on various kinds of detritus and are often associated with host–dust allergies.

Name of Organism and Disease Associations

Sarcoptes scabiei is the scab mite. It causes sarcoptic mange or scabies, although the latter term is used for infestation with other mites, as well.

Hosts and Host Range

There is a single species in the genus with a number of varieties named for the hosts on which they occur. *S. scabiei* var. *humani* is on humans and *S. scabiei* var. *suis* is on swine, and so on. There is some cross-transmission possible with many varieties, but usually the ability of the mites to survive and reproduce on an abnormal host is limited. For example, *S. s.* var. *canis* remained on all eight common species of animals that were exposed to it for periods ranging from a day to 13 weeks.

Geographic Distribution and Importance

Cosmopolitan. *Sarcoptes* spp. are a significant medical problem in some circumstances, but they cause considerable economic loss in certain species of livestock and misery in companion animals if left untreated. Mites have a place in the history of modern medicine, because the mite that causes scabies in humans was the first infectious agent to be related to a specific disease. This finding was the result of investigations done by Bonomo and Cestoni in Italy in 1687.

Morphology

These are tiny mites, which are barely visible with the naked eye. All stages have stubby legs (Fig. 50.3), some of which terminate in long setae. The body has sculptured lines that are quite distinctive. The females are 300 to 504 μm long by 230 to 420 μm wide, and the males are 213 to 285 μm by 162 to 210 μm.

Among the varieties there are inconspicuous differences. Setae and bare areas on the opisthosoma vary.

Life Cycle

The pattern of development in *Sarcoptes* is as follows:

egg → larva → protonymph → tritonymph → adult

Transmission from one host to the next takes place through close contact or contamination of the environment, and any of the stages is capable of establishing an infection (Fig. 50.3). Entrance into the skin is accomplished by the mite secreting saliva onto the unbroken skin; the cells of the skin are lysed and the mite then eats it way into and burrows along under the keratinized layers of the skin.

The female burrows into the skin and lays eggs in a sinuous tunnel, which she forms as she oviposits. The eggs hatch in 50 to 53 hours releasing the larval stage. About half of the larvae molt to the protonymph within five days, but 15% require more than five days to molt. The protonymph lasts three to four days and molts to a tritonymph; this stage is slightly larger than the protonymph. The tritonymph lasts from two to three days and then molts to reach the adult. Most of the varieties which have been studied experimentally complete the life cycle in about 21 days.

The life cycle can take place entirely within the tunnel in the skin, but observations on the mites show that any stage can leave the tunnel and then reinvade the skin or is capable of transferring to another host. The female lays from one to three eggs a day and lives about a month; thus, a female lays from 30 to 90 eggs in a lifetime.

Diagnosis

Determining whether a host has been invaded by mites is based on the following:

1. Clinical signs and symptoms
2. Finding the mites in the skin

Sinuous tracks in the skin, inflammation, itching are all indicators of scab mites in humans or other hosts. Later in the infection, weeping, crusty patches are seen. A variety of other infectious agents and noninfectious processes can give about the same signs. The crux of the matter is finding the mites in the skin. They are not embedded deeply in the skin (Fig. 50.6), but it is necessary to scrape the skin somewhat nevertheless.

Scrapings are examined under a compound microscope for mites, parts of mites, eggs, and fecal pellets.

Host–Parasite Interactions

Most studies on *S. scabiei* have been done on those varieties that infest swine, humans, and the dog. The life cycles, location in the skin, and the responses of the hosts seem to be quite similar and it probably is safe to conclude that one can generalize from one variety to another on host–parasite interactions.

Studies in swine have shown that there is a sequence of stages in the development of lesions and of hypersensitivity. After an initial induction phase, there is a period of delayed hypersensitivity followed by immediate hypersensitivity and finally a desensitization. When hypersensitivity develops, the mites are burrowing in the skin and releasing their products and progeny. The itching becomes severe through the release of histamine and other cellular products. From this time onward the clinical manifestations of scabies are seen and felt.

In humans, relatively few mites can cause severe skin reactions. Some persons seem to tolerate the mites with little response, but most others have severe itching and allergic reactions. The irritation and hypersensitivity seem to result from excretions, which the females deposit in the skin as they burrow and oviposit. Secondary bacterial infections may also occur, probably as a result of scratching. Most of the mites live in places where the skin is thin, such as between the webbing of the fingers or in folds at the wrist, but other sites are invaded as well.

Those domestic animals that are often infected with sarcoptic mites are horses, swine, and dogs. In these hosts, the lesions are crusty, weeping patches corresponding to the final stage of desensitization.

Immunity develops in long-standing infections and is manifested by mites leaving their burrows and by a reduction in fecundity and survival time. Beyond these observations, little is known about the mechanisms or antigens associated with acquired immunity.

Epidemiology and Control

Mange is controlled by the following measures:

1. Use of acaricides
2. Quarantine and inspection of animals to be introduced

Regardless of the host, elimination of scabies is based on the use of acaricides. In humans, acaricides are applied to the skin after a hot, soapy bath. All clothing and bedding should also be laundered. Horses, dogs, and swine, in which most sarcoptic mange is seen, are treated individually by hand as opposed to herd treatment, despite the fact that a large proportion of them may be infected.

As is true with a number of transmissible diseases, scabies is usually prevalent when its hosts are crowded. In humans, crowded, disruptive conditions

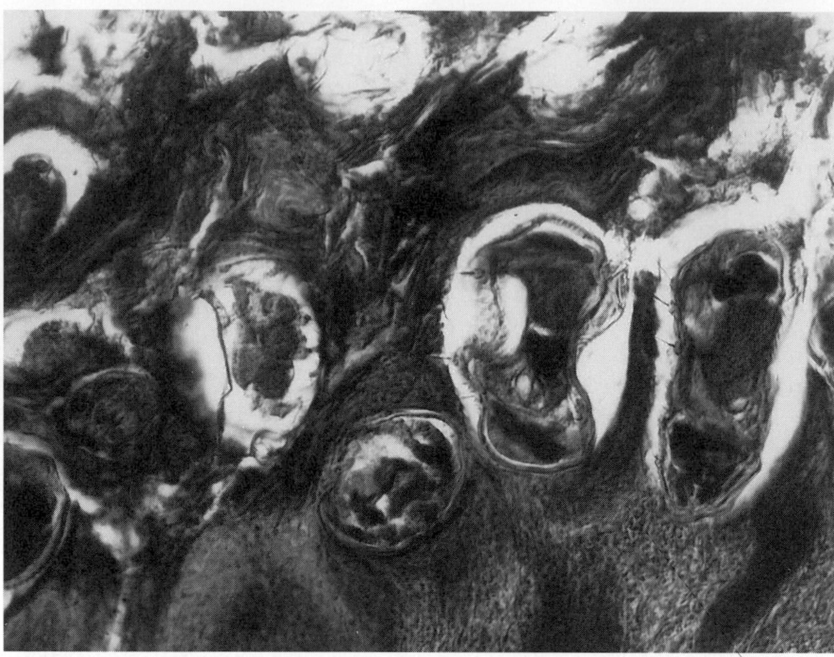

FIGURE 50.6 A histologic section showing *Sarcoptes scabiei* burrowing in the superficial cornified layer of the skin as seen in LM. The surface of the skin is at the top and the mites are distal to the germinative layer; they are the round objects.

such as those during a war, natural disaster, or generally poor living conditions are conducive to outbreaks of scabies.

Scabies is usually a household (in humans) or herd (in other animals) problem. If one host is infected, the others in contact with it also become infected. Even though the mites live for a period of time off of the host, the host is the main target for treatment.

In enzootic areas, before an animal such as a horse or dog is introduced into a paddock or kennel, quarantine and inspection are in order. Such measures are not ordinarily taken for humans, but it might be considered under some circumstances.

Moderation of *Sarcoptes* populations takes place in all hosts through grooming. The mites remain in a fairly superficial location and scratching removes some mites from the skin. It is not clear whether mites can be eliminated by this means, but at least reduction in the mites and their effects is achieved.

Sarcoptes can survive for many days off of the host. Most transmission undoubtedly takes place through close contact between hosts, but the surrounding area can be a source of living mites as well. They are found in the bedding, in rugs, and in dust. Where there is a high level of cleanliness in the living quarters, the probability of finding mites is quite low.

Cool temperatures and high relative humidity promote survival. At 97% RH and 10°C , 50% of female mites survived for eleven days, but at 25% RH, 50% survived only three days. At 20°C and higher, fewer than 50% survived even two days. Above 40°C, 50% died within a day.

Related Organisms

Two genera of sarcoptic mites that are important on birds or smaller mammals and sometimes humans are *Notoedres* and *Knemidocoptes* (alternate spelling *Cnemidocoptes*). *Notoedres cati* has been reported to cause mange in cats, rats, rabbits, squirrels, dogs, and humans. *N. muris* is sometimes a problem in laboratory rats and has been found on other rodents in the wild such as voles.

K. mutans, the scaly leg mite, also has a broad host range having been reported from pheasants, turkeys, partridges, parakeets, finches, and various other passeriform birds. They burrow into the skin beneath the scales on the legs and feet of birds and cause considerable damage. Birds may become lame, disabled, or even die from the infection. It may be necessary to differentiate this mite from other members of the genus. *K. laevis* is the depluming mite; it burrows into the skin at the base of the feathers so that feathers may be lost over a large portion of the body. *K. fossor*, on the other hand, is found at the base of the host's bill.

Name of Organisms and Disease Associations

Psoroptes spp. and *Chorioptes* spp. cause psoroptic and chorioptic mange, respectively, or, collectively, scabies or scab.

Hosts and Host Range

The genus *Psoroptes* has a single species, *P. equi*, and many varieties whose names are based on the host on which the mite is found. Thus, *P.e. bovis* is found on cattle, *P.e. cuniculi* on rabbits, *P. e. ovis* on sheep, and so forth.

The same terminology pertains to *Chorioptes bovis.* which has varietal designations depending on the host from which it is taken.

Geographic Distribution and Importance

Cosmopolitan. These two genera are important as parasites of both domestic and some wild animals. Of the two, *Psoroptes* is the more important economically. In North America, psoroptic mange continues to cause millions of dollars of losses annually.

Morphology

These are tiny mites, 0.5 mm or shorter in length. Their legs extend beyond the margins of the bodies and they have long setae on the body and some of the hind legs (Fig. 50.7). Differentiation between the two genera is usually based on the pedicels of the anterior two pairs of legs; the pedicels are at the distal tips of the legs and terminate at cuplike structures called suckers. The pedicels are long and jointed in *Psoroptes* and short and unjointed in *Chorioptes*

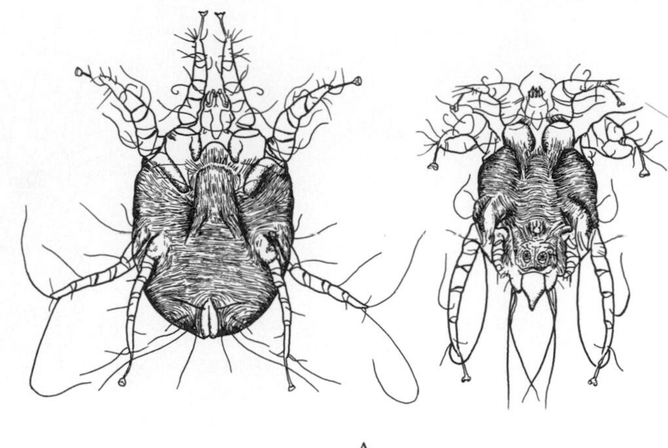

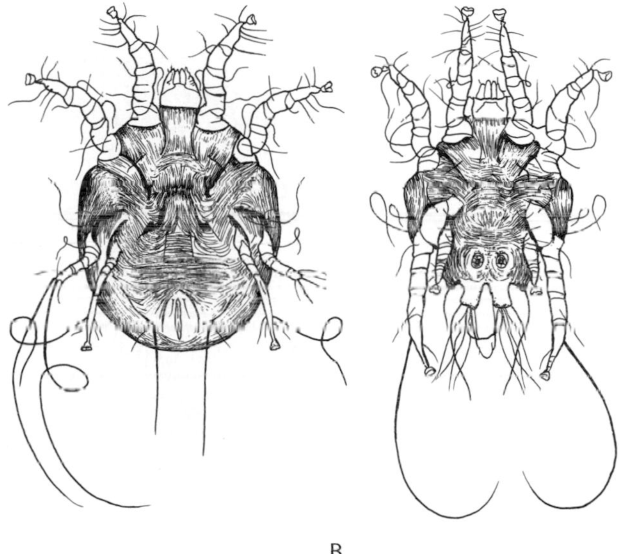

FIGURE 50.7 Adults of (A) *Psoroptes equi* and (B) *Chorioptes bovis*. [From Baker et al., 1956.]

Life Cycle

The stages of the life cycle are as follows:

egg → larva → nymph → adult

The whole life cycle (Fig. 50.8) is spent on the host and transmission takes place through close contact between animals.

Diagnosis

Skin scrapings taken in mineral oil or heated in KOH are required, as is a specific identification of any mites found under the microscope. Mites are generally at the margins of skin lesions. In sheep, the wool becomes ragged and has long tags of wool hanging down, because the sheep scratch against buildings, fences, even barbed wire.

Host–Parasite Interactions

Chorioptic mange is less severe than psoroptic, because the mites remain at the surface of the skin and do not cause either serious damage or much irritation. *Psoroptes*, on the other hand, cuts more deeply into the skin with its chelicerae and causes not only oozing lesions but a great deal of irritation. Infected animals scratch against posts or buildings, further damaging the skin. Sheep pull at the fleece in an attempt to reduce the itching and thereby make the fleece unmarketable.

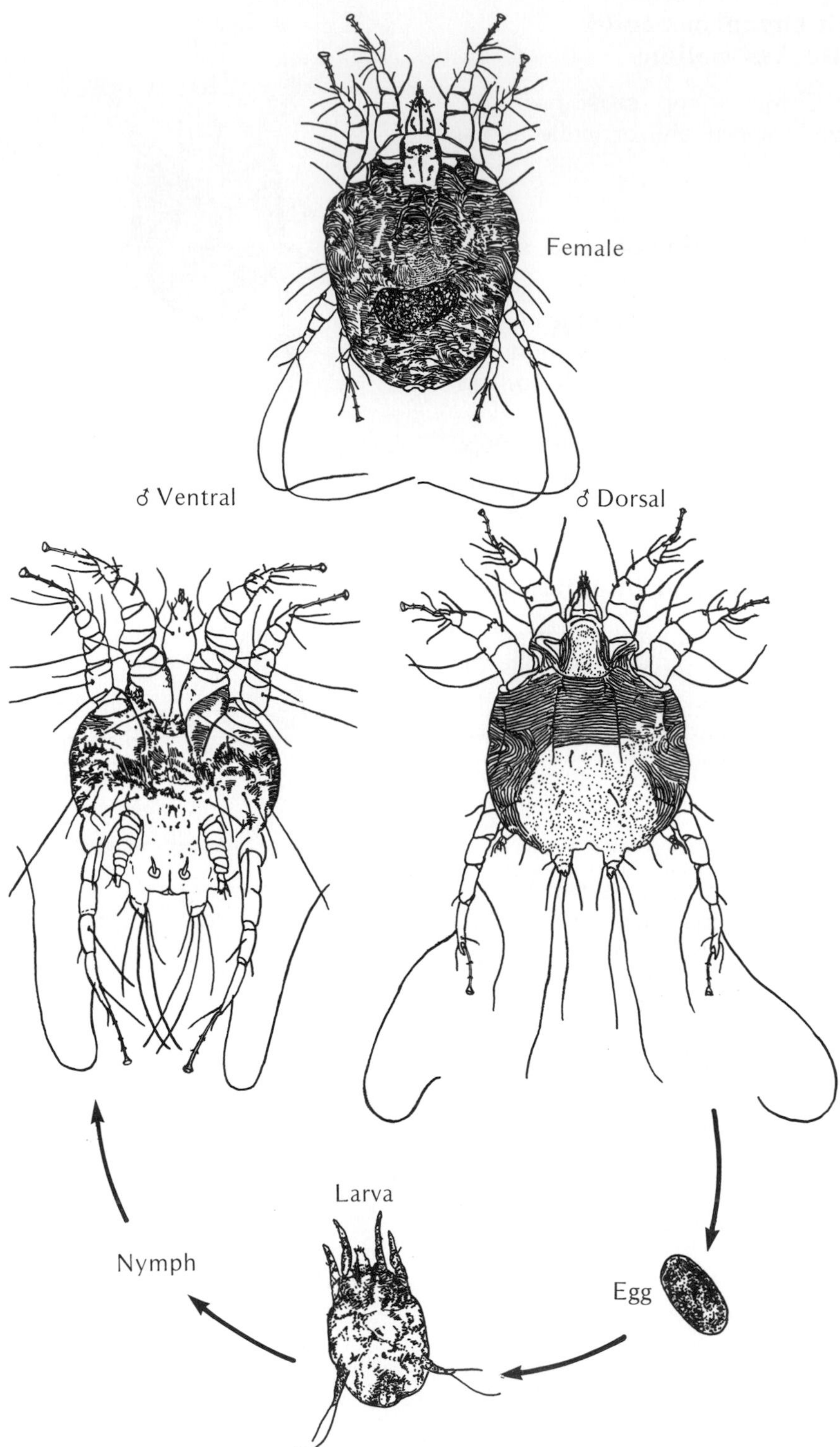

FIGURE 50.8 The life cycle of *Psoroptes equi.*

Epidemiology and Control

Control is based on the following:

1. Proper treatment with an acaricide
2. Inspection after treatment to ensure that all animals are clean
3. Inspection of animals to be introduced into a herd
4. Quarantine of infected animals, which should not be moved until they have been certified as being free of infection

Treatment for scabies in sheep, cattle, and goats almost always involves herd treatment with a second-generation acaricide. Most often animals are dipped or sprayed so as to be certain that they have become wet all over. Macrolide antibiotics such as ivermectin are also a effective acaricides; injectable formulations are available.

Mites spread readily from one animal to another by close contact. Therefore it is best to assume that all animals have been exposed and probably are infected.

Laws enabling the control of sheep scab have been on the books for 150 years. In the Australian state of New South Wales, laws were enacted in the 1850s to allow the destruction of scabby sheep; no other means of control were available at the time. By the turn of the 20th century, scabies had been eradicated in Australia, New Zealand, and some European countries by this drastic measure.

During the early part of the 20th century, sheep producers in the western United States experienced severe losses from psoroptic scabies, and there seemed to be no way that they could control the infections individually. As a result they requested help in setting up a control program, and both state and federal agencies cooperated in establishing and implementing a scabies eradication program. By 1943, eradication in the western states had been accomplished in the sheep industry and the producers in that part of the country were relieved of at least one economic burden.

Eradication was not achieved in the rest of the country until 1970 because sheep flocks outside of the West are typically small. For example, 8000 flocks of sheep existed in Wisconsin during the latter stages of the eradication program. All of the sheep had to be quarantined until they were inspected and declared scabies-free or treated and reinspected until free of mites. About 300 state and federal inspectors were assigned temporarily to the eradication program and all sheep in the state were inspected in about a month. The cost of the eradication program was high but was considered to be worthwhile since the mites have no alternate hosts and once they were eradicated from sheep, reinfestation could not occur.

A scabies eradication program is also in place for cattle, but it has not yet worked as well as that for sheep, in general. Cattle do not have a fleece that has economic value, and they may not be so obviously affected as sheep. Although many cattle producers recognize the benefits of eradication, a significant number do not appreciate the full economic impact of the infection. Some of the western states have effective aggressive, mandated control programs that have been successful.

ORDER ACTINETIDA

The order Actinetida includes both free-living and parasitic mites with quite diverse life cycles and structures. The stigmata, when present, are on the anterior part of the body, often at the base of the chelicerae. We consider a few families that are important to humans and domestic animals.

FAMILY PYEMOTIDAE

Many pyemotids are pests of stored food products and can cause significant losses. A secondary aspect of their being in foods is that they may cause skin irritation in persons coming into contact with them. Members of the genus *Pyemotes* (Fig. 50.9A) as well as other generas such as *Haemagamasus* (Fig. 50.9B) may be found in large numbers in foods, hay, or straw, and people handling such materials may suffer as a result of having the mites on the skin. The mites puncture the skin, and a wheal arises several hours later at the site of the puncture. In especially heavy attacks, persons may suffer from systemic reactions such as headache or intestinal symptoms and joint pain. Species in other families such as the Tetranychidae may also cause skin rashes.

FAMILY DEMODECIDAE

Name of Organism and Disease Associations

Demodex spp. are all parasites of mammals. They cause a disease usually called demodectic mange or demodecosis.

Hosts and Host Range

Members of the genus have a high degree of both host and site specificity. Humans have two species, *D.*

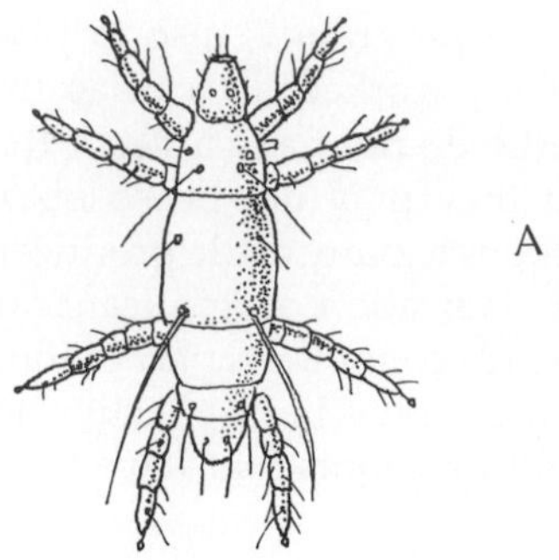

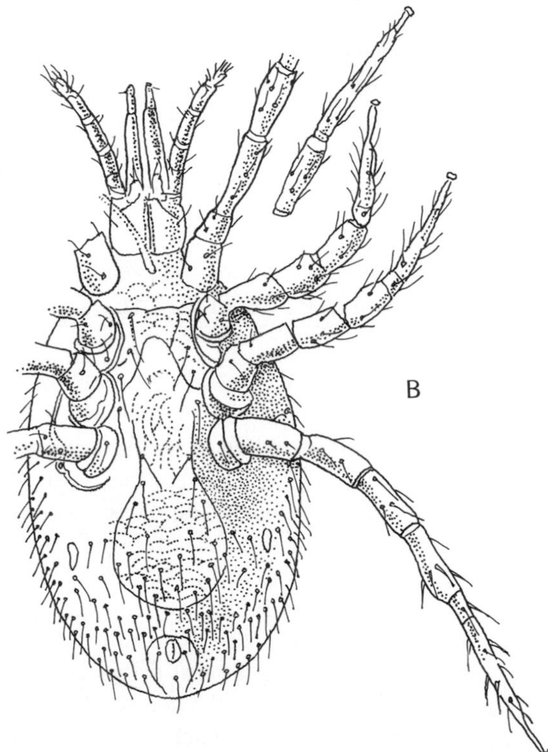

FIGURE 50.9 Two members of the family Pyemotidae. (A) *Pyemotes ventricosus;* (B) *Haemagamasus pontiger.* [From Baker et al., 1956.]

folliculorum, which lives in hair follicles, and *D. brevis,* which is found in sebaceous glands. Other species are typically named after the hosts on which they are found: *D. canis* on dogs, *D. bovis* on cattle, and so on.

Geographic Distribution and Importance

Cosmopolitan. One might say that these mites are ubiquitous rather than cosmopolitan since certain hosts have almost 100% prevalence. This is true in humans, and probably in dogs. An acarologist colleague has stated that only two species of animal have gone to the moon—humans and *Demodex*—since it is almost certain that at least one of the astronauts has carried mites there.

The importance of *Demodex* spp. is difficult to assess except in individual clinical cases in humans or other hosts. *D. folliculorum* has been cited as a culprit in causing acne in adolescents, but it may only be an incidental finding.

In dogs, demodectic mange is a common disease that can range from mild to life threatening. Therapy is usually successful but can fail with the result being that the animal is overwhelmed by the mites.

Morphology

Demodex spp. are elongate and have four pairs of stubby legs (Fig. 50.10). The mouthparts are not apparent and the hysterosoma is quite long. The species vary somewhat in size and proportions of the bodies.

Life Cycle

The mites live in hair follicles, sebaceous glands, and sweat glands depending on the species. The follicles or glands may become packed with mites. Transmission between hosts is by close bodily contact. The life cycle probably requires 20 to 35 days for completion.

In dogs, transmission takes place from the mother to the newborn pups during the first three days of life.

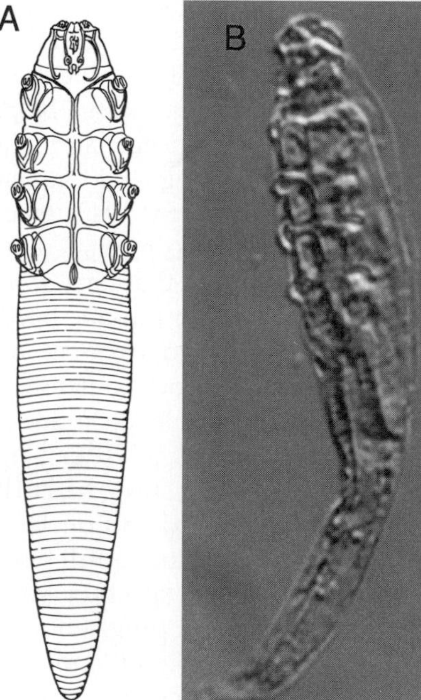

FIGURE 50.10 (A) The follicle mite, *Demodex folliculorum*, female. [From Baker et al., 1956.]. (B) A living mite as seen in interference contrast microscopy.

Transmission probably does not take place between healthy dogs later in life.

Diagnosis

In a host of nearly any species, the presence of *Demodex* can be determined by gently squeezing the skin and looking for the mites in the exudate. In humans, they are seen mostly on the face in oily areas, such as around the nose, or in the eyebrows and eyelashes which may be plucked and examined under a microscope.

In dogs, scrapings of the affected skin and squeezing suspect areas are the methods used to obtain material that can be examined microscopically. Hair loss, inflammation of the skin, and scratching are signs of demodecosis, but these can also be signs of other infections and noninfectious processes. The head, neck, and feet are sites of greatest infestation.

Host–Parasite Interactions

In dogs, clinical demodecosis is manifested in two forms:

1. Localized
2. Generalized

In the localized form, hair is lost in small areas and the skin becomes scaly and reddened. The animal also suffers from obvious itching. In some instances, only the feet or ears may be affected.

In the generalized form there is hair loss, inflammation and swelling of the skin and crusty, weeping lesions, among other signs. This is the severe form of the disease, which requires immediate treatment. Animals may develop a septicemia (generalized infection of the blood with bacteria). At this stage, dogs may die.

Evidence of cell-mediated immunity has been reported in dogs showing generalized demodecosis. It is not clear, however, how frequently dogs with depressed immunity due to other factors develop clinical demodecosis as opposed to how frequently generalized immunosuppression is the result of demodecosis.

Epidemiology and Control

In dogs, transmission occurs only within three days of birth, and usually only dogs younger than 18 months of age are affected. Mites die within a short period of time when they appear at the surface of the skin. Thus, contagion is not considered to be important in a control program.

Most dogs with a localized demodecosis clinically cure spontaneously. Only about 10% of dogs progress to the generalized form of the disease. When the disease does become generalized, weekly treatment with acaricides and other supportive means are necessary. Worse yet, treatment may need to continue as long as 20 weeks.

FAMILY TROMBICULIDAE

Name of Organism and Disease Associations

Among the common genera in this family are *Leptotrombidium, Euschoengastia, Trombidium,* and *Eutrombicula.* The common name is chigger, red bug, or harvest mite. These organisms cause chigger dermatitis or trombidiosis. The principal agent that they transmit causes scrub typhus or tsutsugamushi disease.

Hosts and Host Range

The parasitic stages have a low host specificity. They feed on birds, mammals, reptiles, and sometimes amphibia. Not all have such a broad host range, but they generally have catholic tastes in sources of food.

Geographic Distribution and Importance

Cosmopolitan in tropical and temperate climates. Chigger dermatitis is an uncomfortable consequence of coming into contact with these organisms, but it is not considered to be any more than a minor inconvenience except by persons in the midst of suffering with 50 or 100 chigger bites. In the Asian Pacific Rim, tsutsugamushi disease or scrub typhus is typically an epidemic disease that can have serious consequences for human health and productivity.

Morphology

Keys for identifying chiggers are based on the larvae (Fig. 50.11). They are tiny mites— 100 to 300 μm long— with three pairs of legs. They are typically reddish or orange, are well supplied with setation on the body, and the palps have five segments.

Life Cycle

The stages in the life cycle of trombiculids are as follows:

egg → deutovum → larva → nymphochrysalis
→ nymph → imagochrysalis → adult

The larva is the only parasitic stage (Fig. 50.11); it

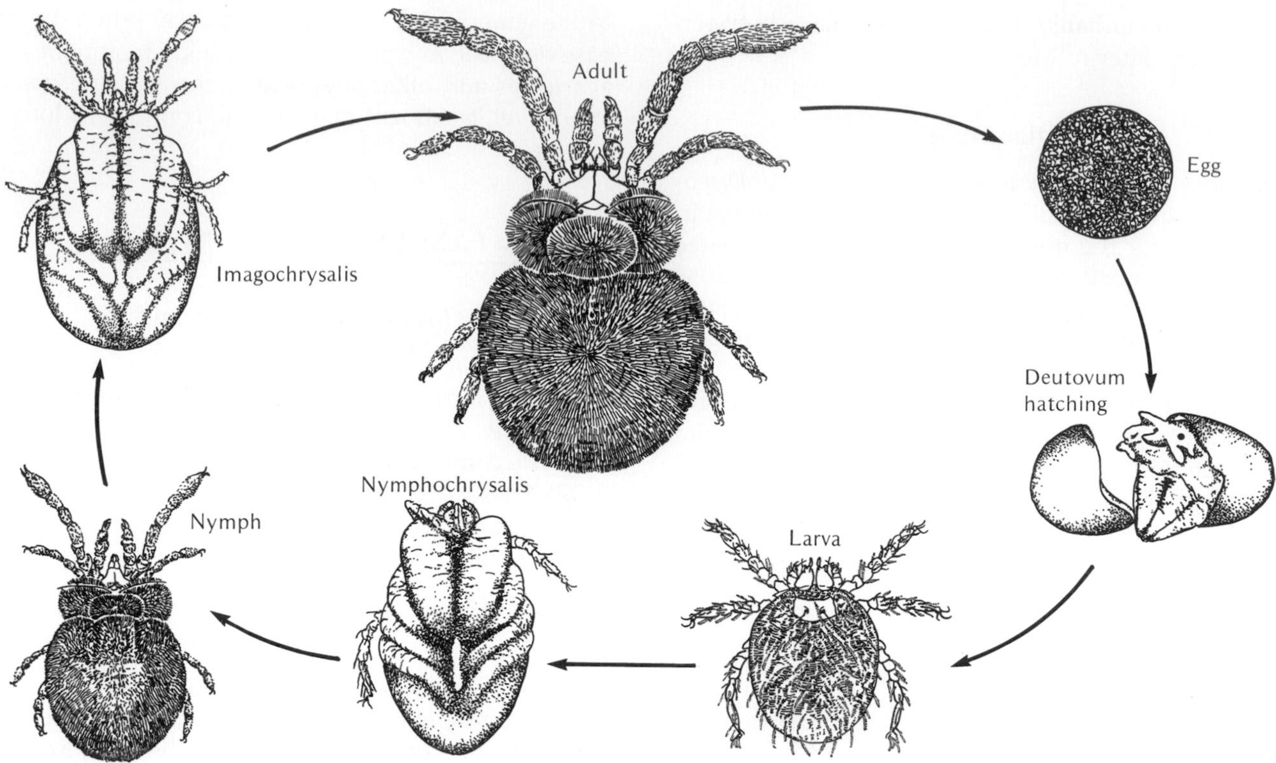

FIGURE 50.11 The life cycle and morphology of the chigger, *Leptotrombidium akamushi.* [Redrawn from Neal and Barnett, 1961.]

usually feeds on a wide range of hosts. The nymphochrysalis is a quiescent stage and is followed by the nymph, which is a free-living, feeding stage. Between the nymph and the adult is another quiescent stage, the imagochrysalis; adults are free living. Males deposit stalked spermatophores, which the females crawl over and take into the genital opening.

Life cycles of chiggers are dependent upon the weather. In cooler climates they may have three generations each year, but in tropical and semitropical climates, development takes place year-round. Forty days is about an average time for completion of the life cycle. The nymphs and adults probably feed on small invertebrates in the litter at or near the soil surface.

Diagnosis

Raised, itching papules and a history of having recently been in a grassy or forest edge area are usually adequate to determine that a persons has been attacked by chiggers. The papules are usually located where the clothing is tight: at the belt, at the top of the socks, and so on.

Livestock and poultry are often attacked during warm months, and diagnosis is usually based on recognizing the skin lesions that occur at certain times of the year.

Host–Parasite Interactions

Chiggers remain at the surface of the skin to feed. A few species such as *Hannemania* embed themselves in the skin of amphibia, but generally larvae insert their mouthparts into the skin and the body remains at the surface.

The chigger pierces the skin with its chelicerae, applies its mouth to the skin, and seals the margin of the wound. During feeding, the chigger alternately ejects salivary fluid, which liquefies the tissue, and then sucks up the liquid. A structure called a stylostome forms in response to the salivary fluid; there is proliferation of epidermal cells and inflammation resulting in a structure that has a well-defined morphology.

The inflammatory response of the host gives rise to the raised, reddened wheal with a depressed center characteristic of chigger bites. The initial response is usually seen within a day after the larva begins to feed and may continue as an intensely itching wheal for a week or more. The inflammatory response need only be initiated for there to be a strong response; even if the chigger begins to feed and then is removed, the inflammation and itching occur and are memorable. It is likely that there is an immune response on the part of the host after the initial attack. However, virtually nothing is known about the molecular pathophysiology of immunity associated with chigger bites.

Epidemiology and Control

Chiggers are unique mites insofar as only the larval stage is parasitic. The larvae typically feed on rodents and birds, animals that have burrows or nests. Humans are typically infested in areas where there are large numbers of rodents or nesting birds. Each species of trombiculid has its preferred habitat, but in general, shrubby areas, forest edges, grassy areas or those that have been cut for timber are most likely to have large numbers of larvae.

In temperate climates, chiggers are seasonal and have their largest numbers in spring. Thus, it is possible to avoid areas where the larvae are likely to be. If it is necessary to enter such an area, tick repellents such as deet should be applied and clothing tied tightly at the ankles and wrists. Area chigger control has been successful with organochlorine compounds, but these insecticides are no longer approved except for specific uses.

SCRUB TYPHUS—TSUTSUGAMUSHI DISEASE

Scrub typhus is caused by *Rickettsia tsutsugamushi,* which has a distribution in the Eastern Hemisphere in warm climates: Southeast Asia, India, the Pacific Islands, and Australia. The vectors are most often *Leptotrombidium akamushi* and *L. deliense.* The agent is transmitted transovarially in the mites since only the larvae feed on vertebrates. The signs and symptoms of scrub typhus include prostration, headache, fever, a body rash, and central nervous system abnormalities. The individual usually recovers in about a month.

Mortality in most outbreaks is 5 to 35%, but in a few instances it has reached 60%. It is estimated that there were nearly 18,000 cases in the Pacific theater during World War II, and that 150,000 workdays were lost in two outbreaks alone. Broad-spectrum antibiotics are effective in treating scrub typhus.

A second disease, epidemic hemorrhagic fever, is also suspected of being transmitted by chiggers. This disease occurs in Korea and was the cause of losses among American ground troops during the Korean War.

FAMILY CHEYLETIDAE

Name of Organism and Disease Associations

Cheyletiella parasitivorax is found on rabbits, *C. blakei* on cats, and *C. yasguri* on dogs. These organisms cause cheyletiosis or cheyletiellosis.

Hosts and Host Range

While it is indicated above that *Cheyletiella* is associated with certain hosts, they have host preferences rather than specificity. On dogs, for example, they prefer those breeds that have soft hair such as spaniels; the same species also infests rabbits. Humans are sometimes hosts.

Geographic Distribution and Importance

Cosmopolitan, but probably not in all localities or climates; systematic surveys seem not to have been done. Individual animals are bothered by cheyletids, but the infestations are not usually considered to cause serious disease.

Morphology

C. parasitivorax averages 266 by 368 μm and has a few long setae on the body. The palpal claw is strongly developed and the chelicerae are long, scissorlike instruments. The legs have a double row of hairs at their tips rather than claws. Eggs are 80 x 120 μm and are attached to hairs by a thread that wraps around it.

Life Cycle

The stages in the life cycle are as follows:

egg $\rightarrow$ larva $\rightarrow$ protonymph $\rightarrow$ deutonymph $\rightarrow$ adult

The life cycle is completed in about three weeks and all stages are found on the host.

Diagnosis

These mites cause a good deal of itching and production of a scaly dandruff. Mites remain more or less at the surface of the skin and can be found in the hair coat.

Host–Parasite Interactions

Unlike some of the other mites, cheyletids feed at the surface of the skin and cause a rather superficial irritation. The mites cause irritation of the skin so that the animal scratches and the skin becomes inflamed and shows small eruptions. The mites are most often on the back in greatest numbers, and younger animals are most likely to suffer from the infestation. Older animals may have mites, but the numbers are usually small.

Epidemiology and Control

A control program for companion animals involves the following:

1. Treating the animal(s)
2. Cleaning up the environment

Insecticides such as pyrethrins preceded by bathing to remove scaly exudates and scurf usually are sufficient to cure an animal. It may be necessary to treat animals weekly for as long as eight weeks. The mites live for some time off of the host, and it may be necessary to treat the house or building as well. The animal's bedding, as well as rugs, furniture, and so on, must be treated with an acaricide.

READINGS

Arlian, L. G. (1989). Biology, host relations, and epidemiology of *Sarcoptes scabiei*. *Annu. Rev. Entomol.* **34,** 139–161.

Arlian, L. G., and Vyszenski-Moher, D. L. (1988). Life cycle of *Sarcoptes scabiei* var *canis*. *J. Parasitol.* **74,** 427–430.

Arlian, L. G., Runyan, R. A., Achar, S., and Estes, S. A. (1984). Survival and infestivity of *Sarcoptes scabiei* var. *canis* and var. *hominis*. *J. Am. Acad. Dermatol.* **11,** 210–215.

Baker, E. W., Evans, T. M., and Gould, D. J. (1956). *A manual of parasitic mites of medical or economic importance.* Nat. Pest Control Assoc., New York.

Cloudsley-Thompson, J. L. (1958). *Spiders, Scorpions, Centipedes and Mites.* Pergamon, New York.

Comstock, J. H. (1940). *The Spider Book* (W. J. Gertsch, Ed.), Rev. ed. Comstock, Ithaca, NY.

Coddington, J. A., and Levi, W. H. (1991). Systematics and evolution of spiders (Araneae). *Annu. Rev. Ecol. Syst.* **22,** 565–592.

Duszynski, D. W., and Jones, K. L. (1973). The occurrence of intradermal mites, *Hannemania* spp. (Acarina: Trombiculidae), in anurans of New Mexico with a histological description of the tissue capsule. *J. Parasitol.* **59,** 531–538.

Estes, S. A., Kummel, B., and Arlian, L. (1982). Experimental canine scabies in humans. *J. Am. Acad. Dermatol.* **9,** 397–401.

Evans, G. W. (1992). *Principles of Acarology.* CAB International, London.

Gertsch, W. J. (1979). *American Spiders*, 2nd ed. Van Nostrand, New York.

Hase, T., Roberts, L. W., Hildebrandt, P. K., and Cavanaugh, D. C. (1978). Stylostome formation by *Leptotrombidium* mites (Acari: Trombiculidae). *J. Parasitol.* **64,** 712–718.

Houck, M. A. (Ed.) (1994). *Mites: Ecological and Evolutionary Analysis of Life History Patterns.* Chapman & Hall, New York.

Kaston, B. J. (1972). *How to Know the Spiders*, 2nd ed. Brown, Dubuque, IA.

Keegan, N. L. (1980). *Scorpions of Medical Importance.* Univ. Press of Mississippi, Jackson.

Kwochka, K. W. (1988). Mites and related disease. *Vet. Clin. North Am. Small Anim. Practice Parasitic Infect.* **17,** 1263–1284.

McDaniel, B. (1979). *How to Know the Mites and Ticks.* Brown, Dubuque, IA.

Neal, T. J., and Barnett, H. B. (1961). The life cycle of the scrub typhus chigger mite, *Trombicula akamushi. Ann. Ent. Soc. Am.* **54,** 196–207.

Polis, G. A. (Ed.) (1990). *The Biology of Scorpions.* Stanford Univ. Press, Palo Alto, CA.

Ritter, W. (1980). Varroatosis—A new disease of the honey bee *Apis mellifera. Bee World* **62,** 141–153.

Savory, T. (1977). *Arachnida*, 2nd ed. Academic Press, New York.

Schuster, R., and Murphy, P. W. (Eds.) (1991). *The Acari: Reproduction, Development and Life History Strategies.* Chapman & Hall, New York.

Varma, M. R. G. (1993). Ticks and mites (Acari). In *Medical Insects and Arachnids* (R. P. Lane and R. W. Crosskey, Eds.). Chapman & Hall, London.

Woolley, T. A. (1988). *Acarology: Mites and Human Welfare.* Wiley, New York.

The Cohorts and Orders of the Subclass Acari (Phylum Arthropoda, Class Arachnida)

COHORT PARASITIFORMES

Order Opilioacarida

Primitive mites that are purplish, violet-blue, or greenish-blue; they have the greatest number of primitive characters of members of the cohort; the podocephalic canal is absent; coxal glands are present and empty into sternal taenidia associated with the subcapitular groove; sometimes called "synthetic acarines" because of the combinations of characters that bridge the major groups, actinotrichid and anactinotrichid mites. Found mainly in warm, arid climates. *Opilioacarus, Panchaetes, Paracarus.*

Order Holothyrida

Large, (2–7 mm) strongly sclerotized mites; oval in outline and tortoiselike in shape; body has two regions: the gnathosoma and an unsegmented idiosoma; slight dorsal epistome is present near the anterior end; hairy in some families but hairless and glabrous in others; color ranges from bright red to dark brown; lack ocelli and tritosternum; two pairs of stigmata present; irritating to the mucous membranes of mammals and birds. Generally found in forests of tropical regions; predatory and detritovores. *Holothyrus, Allothyrus, Hammenius.*

Order Gamasida

Often referred to as Mesostigmata; lateral stigmata are located opposite coxae II and IV or between coxae III and IV; stigmata usually accompanied by an elongated peritreme, a groove or tube that extends anteriorly from the stigmata; no tracheal connections are associated with the peritreme; tracheae originate at the stigmata; the peritreme is reduced in some parasitic species; an epistome, or tectum capituli, covers the chelicerae; the gnathosoma is usually distinctly separated from the idiosoma so that the palps and chelicerae, the hypostome and gnathosomal base, are easily seen; chelicerae are usually chelate-dentate; palps are leglike with an apotele of two or three tines on the tarsus; usually heavily sclerotized with colors that are brown or reddish-brown; adults have an entire dorsal plate; the gonopore in the female is transverse and lies between the coxae. Free-living and parasitic forms. Parasitic forms are often hematophagous on the skin, in the nasal passages, or lungs; members of the family Varroaidae are found in honey bees in which they may cause economic losses. *Dermanyssus, Pneumonyssus, Ornithonyssus, Rhinonyssus, Varroa.*

Order Ixodida

Typically referred to as "ticks"; often classified as Metastigmata; stigmata are located posterior to coxae IV (Ixodidae or hard ticks) or anterodorsal to coxae IV (Argasidae or soft ticks); generally large, 2 mm to 2 cm in length; hypostome has recurved teeth; stigmata present but without sinuous peritreme; palps have three or four segments but without claws, leglike in Argasidae, and with knifelife edges and a fused tibiotarsus in Ixodidae; Haller's organ present and on leg 1; genital aperture intercoxal in both males and females usually between coxae I and II; anal valves are subterminal. Parasitic, hematophagous. *Dermacentor, Boophilus, Haemaphysalis, Amblyomma, Argas, Ornithodoros, Otobius.*

COHORT ACARIFORMES

Order Actinectidida

Body divided by a dorsosejugal suture with the gnathosoma distinct, but the rest of the body regions variable; genital and anal apertures dorsal in some groups; ocelli, when present, are propodosomal and lateral;

one or two pairs of stigmata are usually located in the region of the gnathosoma at or near its base or with the chelicerae; peritremes present or absent; chelicerae exposed or hidden; palps vary from simple free or adpressed forms to fanglike raptorial types; leg segments may be reduced or missing, and some forms may lack some legs; pronounced sexual dimorphism. Detritovores, predators, parasites. *Cheyletiella, Demodex, Tetranychus, Eriophyus, Pyemotes.*

Order Astigmata

Soft-skinned mites, usually colorless or light coloration; movable gnathosoma usually visible from above and sometimes covered by the propodosoma; infracapitulum bears two pairs of setae; chelicerae usually exposed and work in a vertical plane; palps are simple and have one segment; idiosoma oval without evidence of external segmentation and lacking overlapping sclerites; sparse setation; integument finely striated in many species; genital apertures ventral. Detritovores, predators, phoretic, parasites. *Psoroptes, Sarcoptes, Chorioptes, Pneumocoptes, Dermatophagoides.*

Order Oribatida

Distinguished by the presence of the trichobothrium (pseudostigmata) and its sensillium (pseudostigmatic organ) located at the posterolateral corners of the prodorsum, function not thoroughly known; body usually divided by dorsosejugal suture into the propodosoma and the hysterosoma; gnathosoma may be found in a camerostome because of the projection of a prodorsal sclerite over the chelicerae; sexual dimorphism is rare; openings to the tracheae are on the coxae of the legs, and no external stigmata are visible. Free living, some species serve as vectors of anoplocephalid tapeworms. *Liacarus, Camisia, Veloppia, Scheloribates, Galumna, Oribatula.*

CHAPTER

51

Ticks

Ticks are often looked on as being a group apart from the mites, but they are merely large mites and they have the same body plan (Figs. 50.2 and 51.1). The differences between the ticks and other groups of mites lies in (1) their large size, (2) a well-developed hypostome by which they attach to their hosts (Fig. 51.2), and (3) having Haller's organ, a complex receptor, located on the dorsal surface of tarsus I. The ticks are placed in the cohort Parasitiformes and, in the classification used here, in the order Ixodida. In some other classifications, they are placed in the order Metastigmata, because their stigmatal plates are located near coxa IV. The genera of ticks are separated on the basis of their mouthparts (Fig. 51.3); note the lengths of the pedipalps in the various genera and the shape of the basis capituli in the genera. *Ixodes scapularis*, a typical member of the genus, has relatively long pedipalps (Fig. 51.4), for example.

Ticks are important because they feed on blood and tissue fluids of humans and other animals and also because they transmit a large number of disease agents, including viruses, rickettsia, bacteria, apicomplexans, and filarioid nematodes (Tab. 51.1). Through hematophagy they cause a great deal of damage by removing blood from their hosts, damaging the skin at the site of feeding, and causing tick paralysis in humans and other animals. They are known to transmit more than 50 pathogenic agents and are suspected of being involved in the transmission of several others.

Ticks are divided into two families, the Ixodidae or hard ticks, and the Argasidae, or soft ticks. The division between the two families is based on the following characteristics:

Ixodidae. An inflexible, dorsal scutum covers the idiosoma of the male and the anterior part of the idiosoma of the female; mouthparts are terminal and visible from above; stigmata are located posterior to coxae IV; the body is usually smooth (Figs. 51.1 and 51.4).

Argasidae. The scutum is lacking; mouthparts are ventral and not visible from above; stigmata are usually located between coxae III and IV; the body is often wrinkled (Fig. 51.21, presented later).

FAMILY IXODIDAE— THE HARD TICKS

Adult hard ticks range from 3 to 10 mm long prior to feeding; the males do not increase much in size on feeding, but the females may be so engorged with blood that their legs are nearly useless. Engorged females may exceed 20 mm in length. The larvae are usually 1 mm or so long and the nymphs about twice that. The capitulum is the first structure to be examined in identification, and the genera of hard ticks have rather distinct structures (Fig. 51.3).

The life cycle of hard ticks fits the usual pattern seen in mites:

$$\text{egg} \rightarrow \text{larva} \rightarrow \text{nymph} \rightarrow \text{adult}$$

During development the tick feeds and molts, feeds and molts. The adults copulate while on the host, the females then drop off, lay eggs, and die. Although this pattern occurs throughout the ixodids, the number of hosts used by a tick in completing its life cycle is important both for planning control programs and for de-

HYPOTHETICAL MALE AND FEMALE IXODIDAE (HARD TICKS)
WITH KEY CHARACTERISTICS LABELED

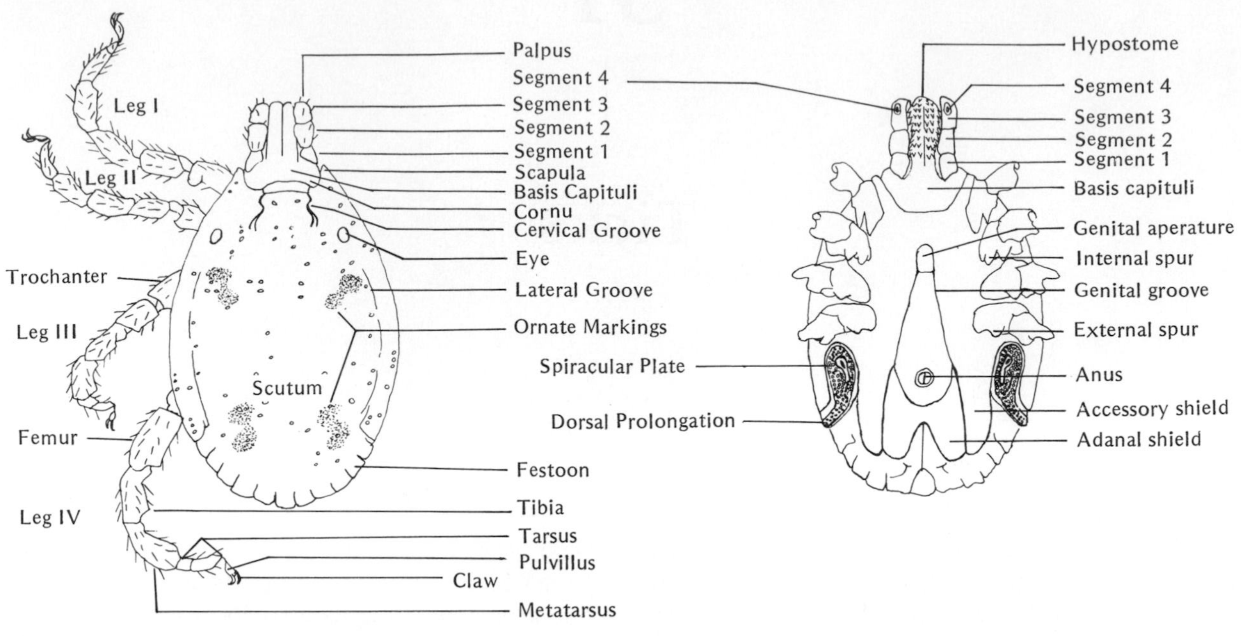

DORSUM OF MALE

VENTER OF MALE

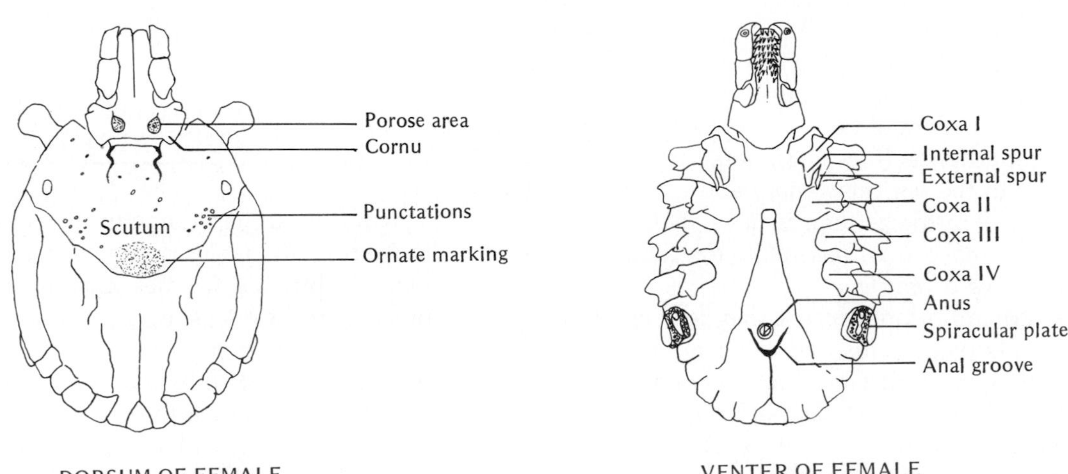

DORSUM OF FEMALE

VENTER OF FEMALE

FIGURE 51.1 External anatomy of male and female ticks.

scribing the epidemiology of a disease agent that is transmitted by a tick.

We speak of one-host, two-host, and three-host ticks. These terms refer to the number of different individual animals on which a ticks feeds during its life cycle. The simplest cycle is that of the one-host tick in which the tick reaches a host as a larva and remains on it until the female drops off to oviposit (Fig. 51. 5). *Boophilus annulatus,* the cattle fever tick, and *B. microplus* are both one-host ticks, as are other members of the genus. *Dermacentor albipictus,* the winter tick, is also a one-host tick.

Examples of two-host tick cycles are those of *Rhipicephalus evertsi, Dermacentor variabilis,* and *Hyalomma*

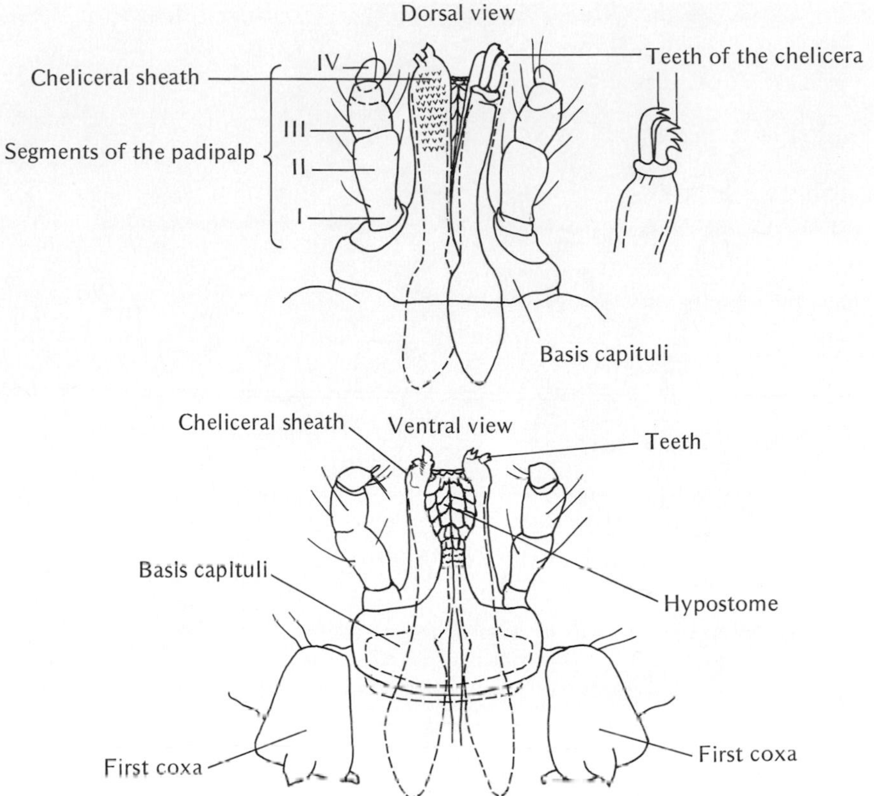

FIGURE 51.2 Capitulum and mouthparts of a tick.

aegypticum. In most instances, the larva and nymph feed on the same host (Fig. 51.6); the adults then seek the second host in the life cycle. In some species, the nymph and adult feed on the same host and the latter drops off to lay eggs. The hosts of the larvae and nymphs tend to be small rodents and birds, and those of the adults are large mammals such as canids or herbivores, and, in some cases, humans.

Three-host ticks utilize three different individuals during the life cycle. Some common three-host ticks are *Dermacentor andersoni, D. occidentalis, Ixodes ricinus, I. scapularis,* and *Rhipicephalus sanguineus.* In three-host cycles (Fig. 51.7), hosts tend to be larger as the ticks progress from the larva toward the adult. Larvae usually are on small rodents, nymphs on larger rodents, and adults on carnivores or larger herbivores.

Whether a species is a one- two-, or three-host tick is often important in the way it transmits infectious agents. A one-host tick typically remains on the same animal all during its life cycle, although some transfer to other animals may take place during close contact. Transovarial transmission (TOT) of vectored pathogens often takes place in one-host ticks because they have little probability of feeding on another host.

In a two-host tick, there can be either stage-to-stage transmission or TOT. In most three-host ticks, there is only stage-to-stage transmission.

Name of Organism and Disease Associations

Dermacentor andersoni (syn. *D. venustus)* is the Rocky Mountain wood tick, or the spotted fever tick. It is the

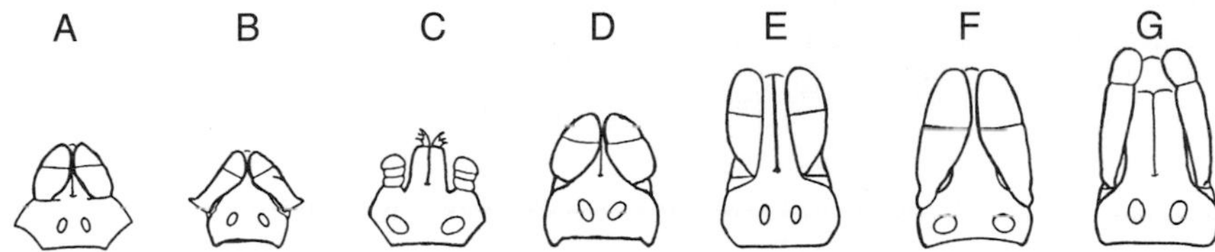

FIGURE 51.3 Capituli of the genera of hard ticks, family Ixodidae. (A) *Rhipicephalus;* (B) *Haemaphysalis;* (C) *Boophilus;* (D) *Dermacentor;* (E) *Ixodes;* (F) *Hyalomma;* (G) *Amblyomma.*

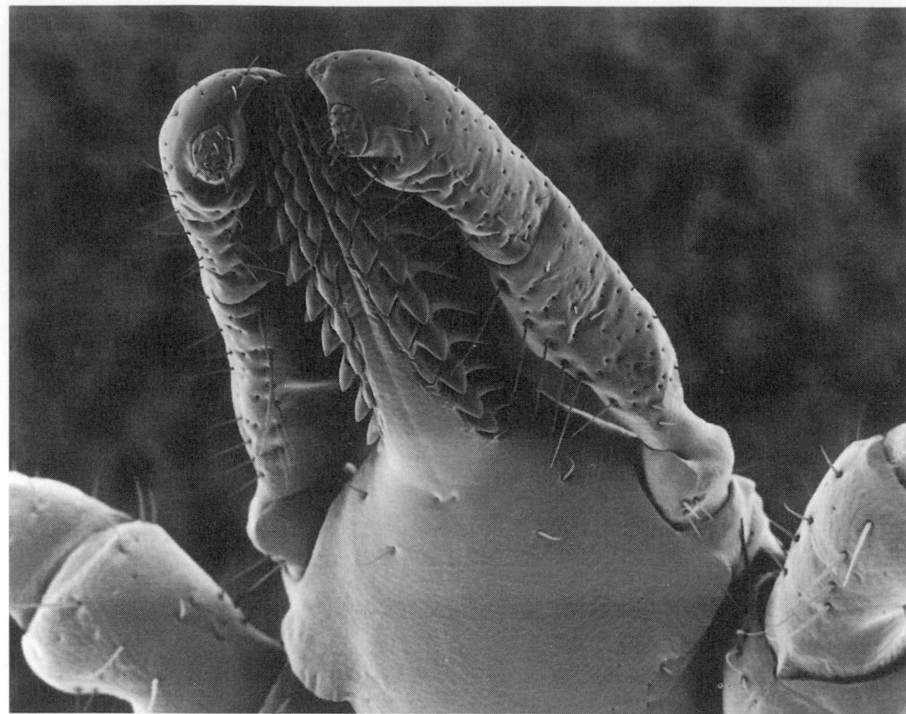

FIGURE 51.4 The capitulum of *Ixodes scapularis* (syn. *I. dammini)* as seen in SEM. Note the long pedipalps characteristic of this genus. The hypostome is typical of an ixodid tick, which has strong retorse teeth that keep it firmly fixed in the skin of the host. [Courtesy of Dr. David W. Dorward, Rocky Mountain Laboratory, USPHS, DHHS, Hamilton, Montana.]

vector for the causative agents of Colorado tick fever (CTF) and Rocky Mountain spotted fever (RMSF).

Hosts and Host Range

Mammals such as small rodents, lagomorphs, porcupine, large herbivores, canids and humans. *D. andersoni* shows what might be called ecological specificity: it feeds on those hosts that are in the places where the females oviposit.

Geographic Distribution and Importance

Western North America from northern New Mexico to British Columbia and nearly to the West Coast. Usually the ticks are found at elevations above 1800 m, but they live at lower elevations as one goes from the southern to the northern parts of the range (Fig. 51.8). Although the wood tick is a pest of humans and other hosts, it is of greatest importance as a vector of the agents that cause Rocky Mountain spotted fever and Colorado tick fever in humans.

Morphology

This is an ornate tick, a term which refers to the brown and white patterning on the scutum, most evident in the male (Fig 51.9). It also has festoons, boxlike markings on the posterior margin of the opisthosoma.

Life Cycle

The life cycle can be said to start in late winter or early spring when adults seek hosts such as canids, large herbivores, porcupine, or rabbits on which to feed. They attach and feed to repletion; aggregation pheromones cause the males and females to gather near one another and copulation takes place. After the female has engorged for about a week, she drops off and begins to oviposit in about another week. The female oviposits for about three weeks, produces 6400 eggs, on the average, and then dies.

The larva hatches in about 35 days and seeks a small rodent such as a deer mouse (*Peromyscus maniculatus*) to feed on. The six-legged larva feeds for three to five days, drops off, molts, and remains in the ground until the following spring. The nymph becomes active in late winter and seeks small rodents such as the golden mantled ground squirrel, *Citellus richardsoni* (syn. *Spermophilus richardsoni*). They feed for about a week, drop off, and molt to the adult stage.

The life cycle of *D. andersoni* is completed in one year in the southern and middle parts of its range. In

TABLE 51.1 Some Diseases and Disease Agents Transmitted by Ticks

Disease or disease agent	Vector(s)	Vertebrate Host(s)	Locality
Apicomplexa			
Babesia bigemina, Texas cattle fever	*Boophilus annulaltus*		Subtropics, tropics, not United States
B. bovis, bovine babesiosis	*B. calcaratus, B. microplus*	Ox, red deer, human	Cosmopolitan, not in United States
B. caballi, equine babesiosis	*Dermacentor, Hyalomma*	Equids	Cosmopolitan; southern United States
B. equi, equine babesiosis	*Dermacentor, Hyalomma*	Equids	Cosmopolitan
B. canis, canine babesiosis	*R. sanguineus, Dermacentor*	Canids, carnivores	Cosmopolitan
B. microti	*Ixodes scapularis*	*Microtus,* human	East coast, United States
Theileria parva, East Coast fever	*R. appendiculatus*	Ox, zebu, water buffalo	East coast of Africa
T. annulata, Tropical coast fever	*Hyalomma detritum*	Ox, zebu, water buffalo	North Africa, southern Europe
Rickettsiae			
Rickettsia rickettsi, Rocky Mountain spotted fever (RMSF)	*Dermacentor andersoni*	Rodent, rabbit, human	East coast and Rocky Mountains of United States
R. conorii, Boutonneuse fever	*R. sanguineus*	Rabbit, rodent, canid, etc.	Eastern Hemisphere
Ehrlichia chafeensis	*Dermacentor*	Human	United States
E. canis, canine erhlichiosis	*R. sanguineus*	Dog	Cosmopolitan
E. equi-like: human granulocytic ehrlichiosis	*Ixodes scapularis*	White-tailed deer *Peromyscus leucopus*	United States
Coxiella burneti	*Hyalomma*	Ruminants, human	Cosmopolitan
Bacteria			
Borellia burgdorferi, Lyme borreliosis	*I. scapularis, I pacificus*	*Peromyscus* spp.	United States, northern Europe, Asia
B. duttoni, relapsing fever	*Ornithodoros moubata*	Human	Africa, Mediterranean
B. recurrentis, relapsing fever	*O. hermsi*	Small rodent, human	North America
Francisella tularensis, tularemia	*Haemaphysalis*	Rabbit, rodent	Western North America
Viruses			
Colorado Tick fever (CTF)	*D. andersoni*	Rodent, human	Rocky Mountains of United States
Louping ill	*I. ricinus*	Sheep, other mammal	British Isles
Kyasanur Forest disease (KSD)	*Haemaphysalis*	Rodent, small mammal, human	India
Russian spring-summer encephalitis (RSSE)	*Ixodes, Haemaphysalis,* etc.	Small mammal, bird	Asia, central Europe

the northern part, or at high altitude, it may require two or even three years. In cold climates, the larva feeds, molts to the nymph in the first year and then the nymphal stage may not feed until late summer of the next year, thus putting off the adult stage until two years after the egg has hatched. All of the stages can survive a long time without feeding allowing the life cycle to be further stretched out if hosts are not available. Larvae and nymphs can survive for more than 500 days without feeding and the adults for more than 1000.

Host–Parasite Interactions

Some ticks have narrow host ranges, but the wood tick exemplifies many three-host ticks in that it has host preferences, controlled to a great extent by the hosts that are available. It tends to feed on larger animals as it moves from the larva to the nymph to the adult. The early stages are in rodent burrows and probably take the host that is close at hand. The adults seek out hosts by questing; they climb on vegetation and hang head down with the legs extended so as to catch a passing animal. Ticks sense warmth, CO_2, and odors from mammals; when they sense that an animal is nearby, they become agitated, and if on the ground, they crawl toward the potential source of food.

Ticks are pool feeders. Once attached and sealed to the host, they inject saliva into the wound, which liquefies the tissue and they suck up the liquid. This sequence of salivation and aspiration goes on the

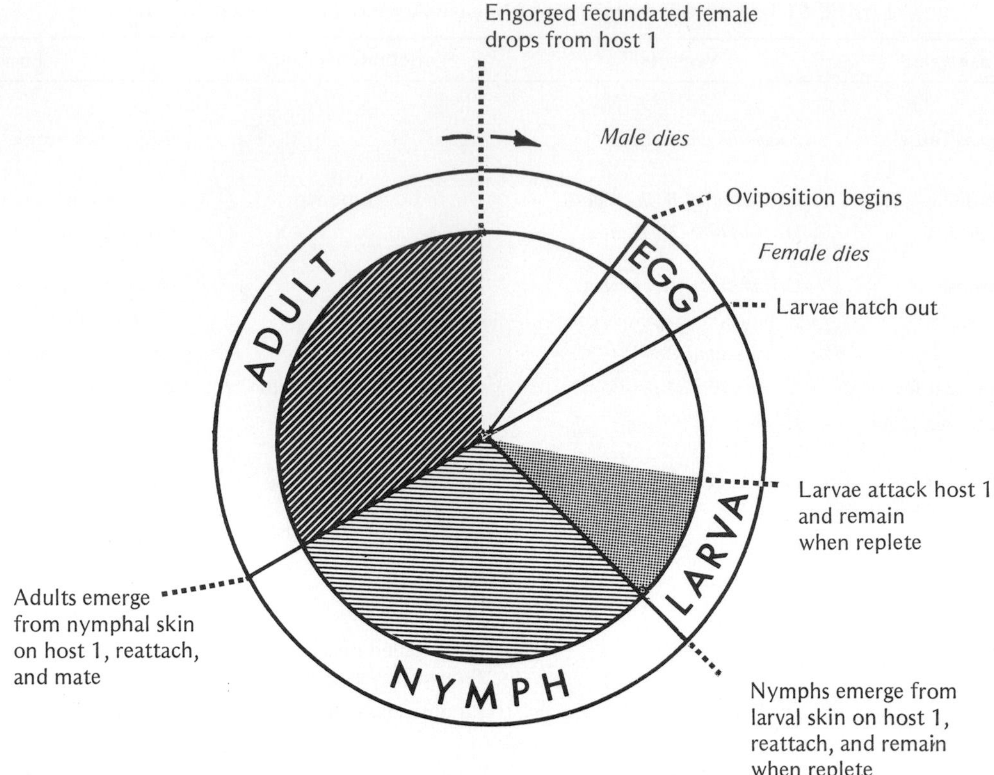

FIGURE 51.5 A one-host type of tick life cycle.

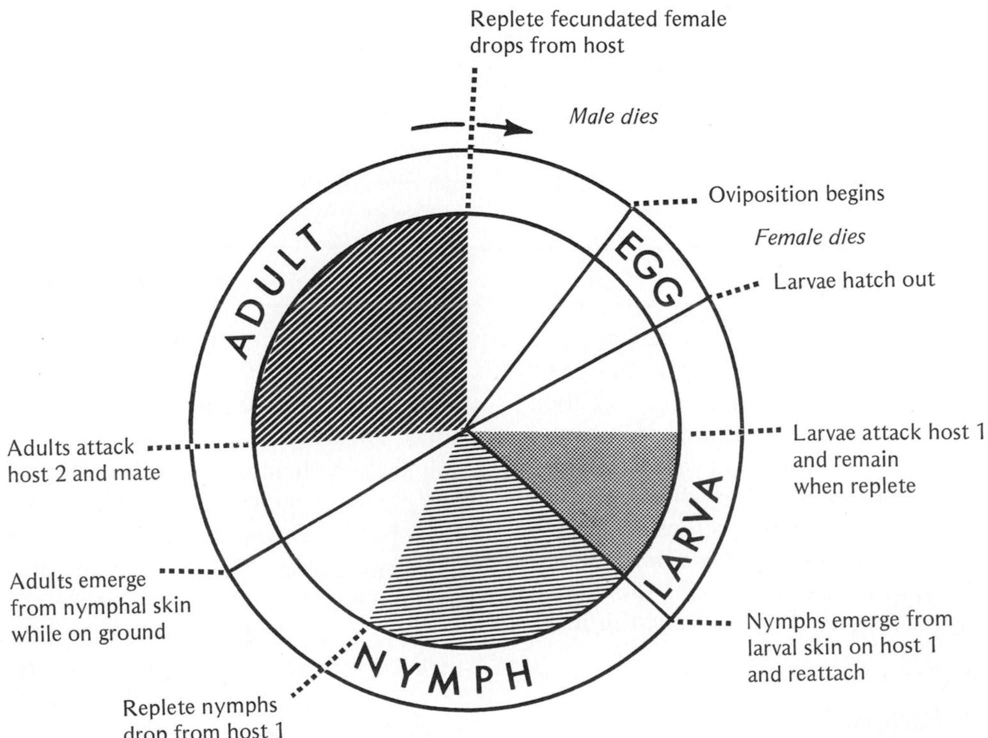

FIGURE 51.6 A two-host type of tick life cycle. Any two stages in the tick life cycle feed and remain on the same host.

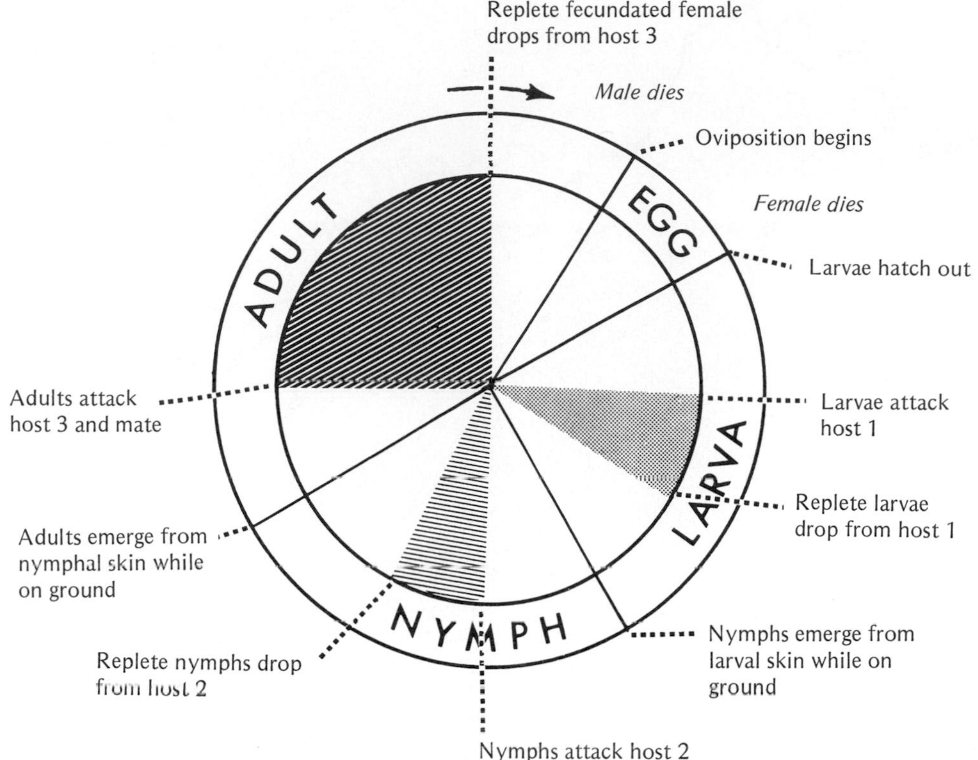

FIGURE 51.7 A three-host type of tick life cycle.

whole time that a tick is attached to the host. In hematophagous insects, there is a need to remove a great deal of water from the blood meal, which they do through the Malpighian tubules. But ticks reinject liquid into the wound and the host absorbs the excess water.

D. andersoni is one of the species that can cause tick paralysis (discussed later).

Epidemiology and Control

The wood tick is controlled by the following measures:

1. Acaricides applied to livestock or companion animals
2. Pulling off the ticks when they are embedded
3. Personal protection

The spotted fever tick is not usually found on livestock in large numbers and cattle are not usually treated for this tick. Owners sometimes treat horses individually with an acaricide as a spray or wash.

Wood ticks, as well as other ixodids, feeding on humans or companion animals can usually be removed by pulling them off. It is important to grasp the mouthparts of the tick at the surface of the skin so that nothing is left in the skin to serve as a site for bacterial infection. Removal is most efficiently done with forceps or tweezers and pulling steadily and firmly until the tick comes off. Many remedies have been suggested for removing ticks including burning them with a cigarette or painting them with nail polish, among others. These are not effective; pulling them off is the method of choice.

For humans, it is best to avoid allowing ticks to embed by using a repellent such as deet, tying clothing tightly at the ankles and wrists, and searching for ticks in the clothing and on the body after a day out of doors. The tick does not usually embed for about three hours, so one has a little time to procrastinate while the ticks wander about searching for a likely spot to dine.

Name of Organism and Disease Associations

Dermacentor albipictus, the winter tick.

Hosts and Host Range

The principal host seems to be the moose, *Alces alces*, but many other species are also infested: deer, elk, bighorn sheep, caribou, bear, equids, canids, and so on.

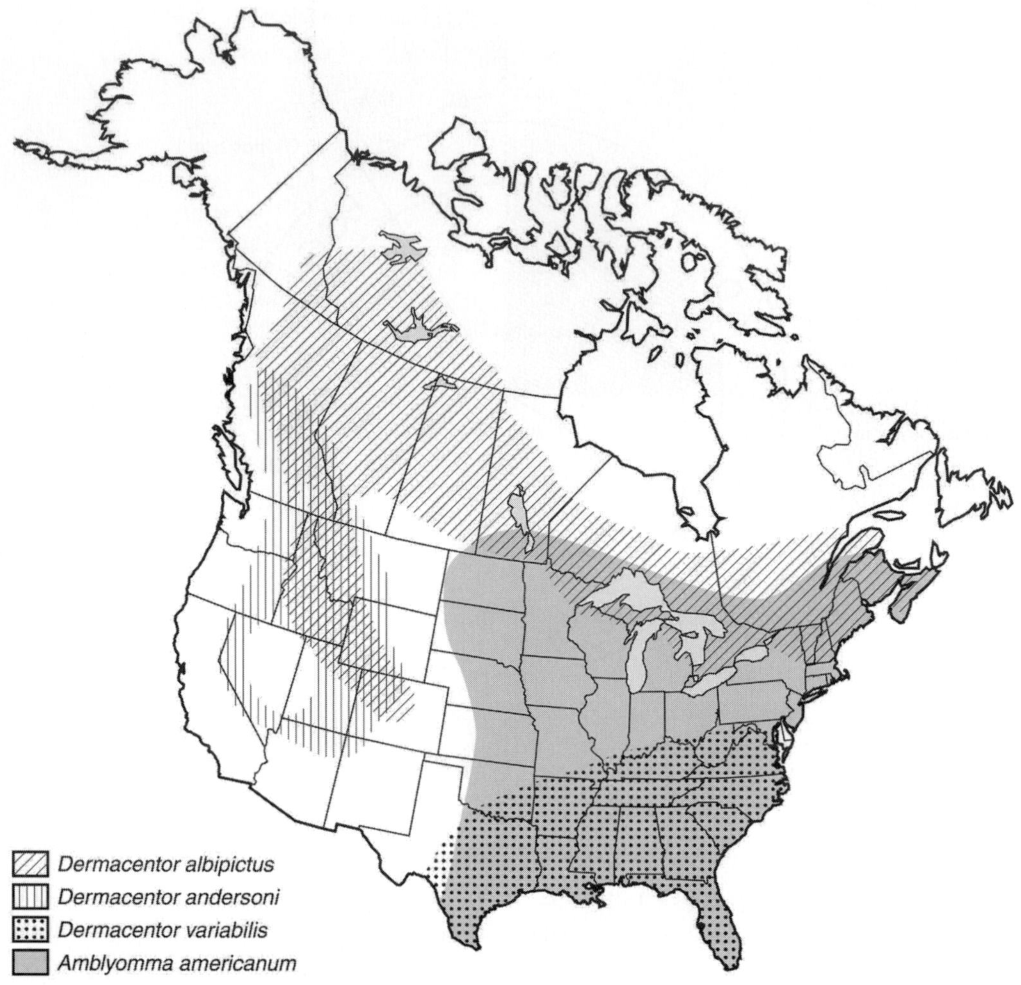

FIGURE 51.8 Approximate geographic distribution of some ticks in the United States and Canada: *Dermacentor andersoni, D. albipictus, D. variabilis,* and *Amblyomma americanum.*

Geographic Distribution and Importance

This tick has a montane and northern latitude distribution (Fig. 51.8). Even at its more southerly locations, *D. albipictus* is found above 1700 m. Its northernmost distribution is about 60°N. latitude. *D. albipictus* probably has a detrimental effect on the health of moose.

Morphology

This is an ornate tick (Fig. 51.10), which can be mistaken for *D. andersoni* since the patterning and size are much the same. The ticks increase dramatically in size, especially when the females engorge.

Life Cycle

D. albipictus is a one-host tick that has an annual cycle (Fig. 51.11). The timing of the life cycle is about the same regardless of the latitude where the tick occurs.

Larvae quest in fall by climbing on plants and awaiting a host; the larvae tend to cluster or aggregate on the upper reaches of grasses and larger plants so that a number of them are swept up by a passing moose or other mammal. All stages remain on the host with copulation taking place there and the females dropping off in early spring. The females do not oviposit immediately, and, in fact, do not oviposit until early June. Hatching does not take place until late August or early September.

Host–Parasite Interactions

Populations of ticks on moose can exceed 50,000, but other hosts usually do not have nearly this many ticks, except for a captive caribou, which had more

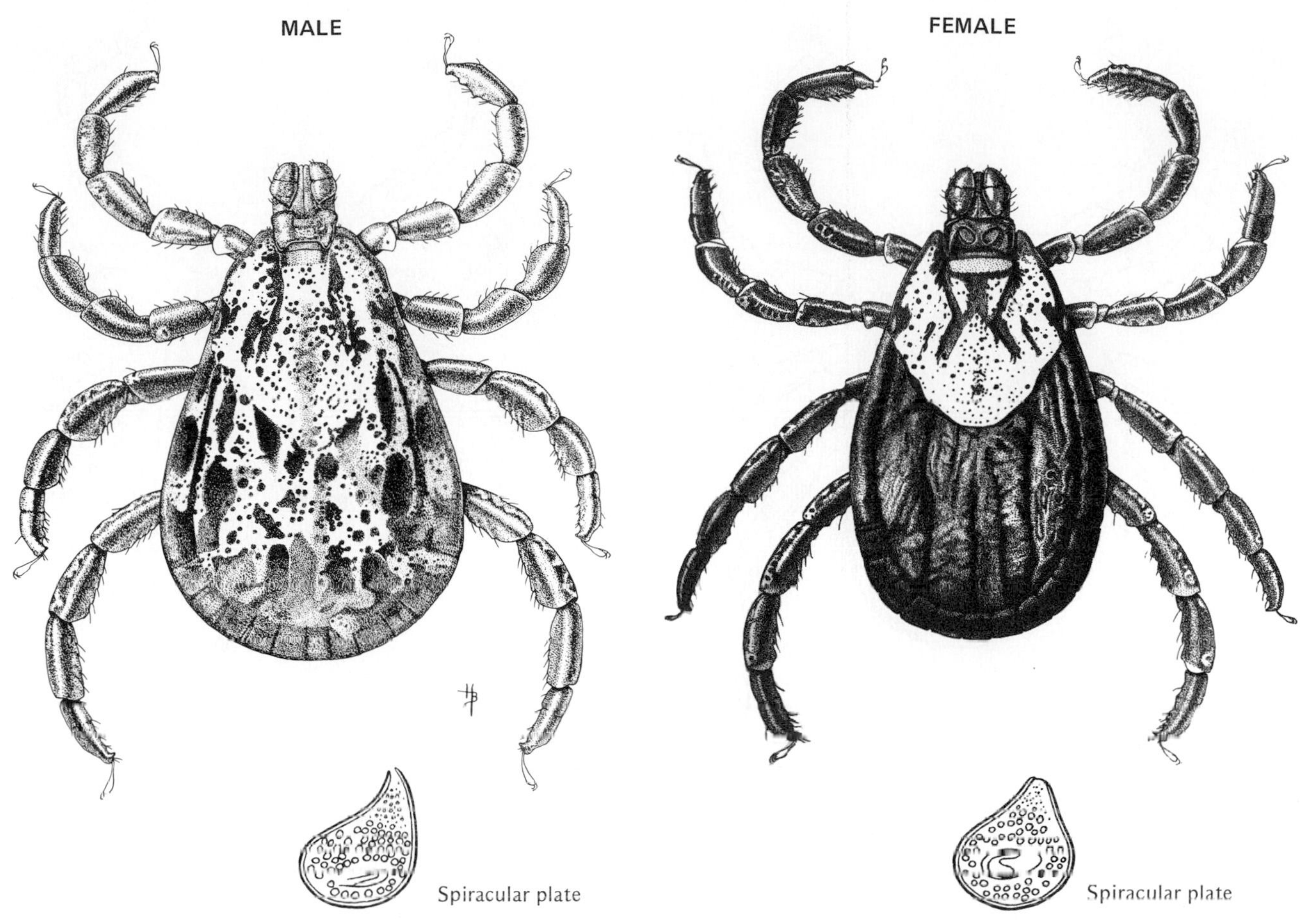

FIGURE 51.9 Male and female of *Dermacentor andersoni*, the Rocky Mountain spotted fever tick or wood tick.

than 400,000 ticks on it. Moose become anemic when heavily infested.

Moose that harbor a large number of ticks attempt to remove them by grooming. They rub against trees, scratch with the hind foot, and bite at the skin. They are successful in removing ticks, but they also remove large amounts of the thick winter coat. Seemingly, the ticks do not become seriously bothersome until late in the winter and the removal of the hair probably does not affect the host's ability to survive in the cold northern climates.

Epidemiology and Control

It remains unclear how detrimental ticks may be to the health of moose, and control programs have not been developed for the moose or, for that matter, for any other wild ruminant.

The ecology and epidemiology as well as a number of other aspects of *D. albipictus* on moose in Alberta and other locations have been studied intensively by Dr. W. M Samuel and his coworkers. This body of work gives an intimate view of how the ticks survive and prosper in a cold environment and the reader can appreciate the difficulty of carrying out the field studies as well.

A side benefit of these intensive studies was the apprehending and convicting a person who had taken a moose out of season. The person admitted to shooting a moose but claimed that it was taken during the hunting season in November. An examination of pieces of hide showed that it had been shot after hunting season was over, because there were no larvae present, only nymphs and adults, some of which were engorging. It was impossible for this population composition to be present in November, and the poacher was found guilty.

Related Organisms

The tropical horse tick, *D. nitens,* is distributed in Florida, southern Texas, the islands of the Caribbean,

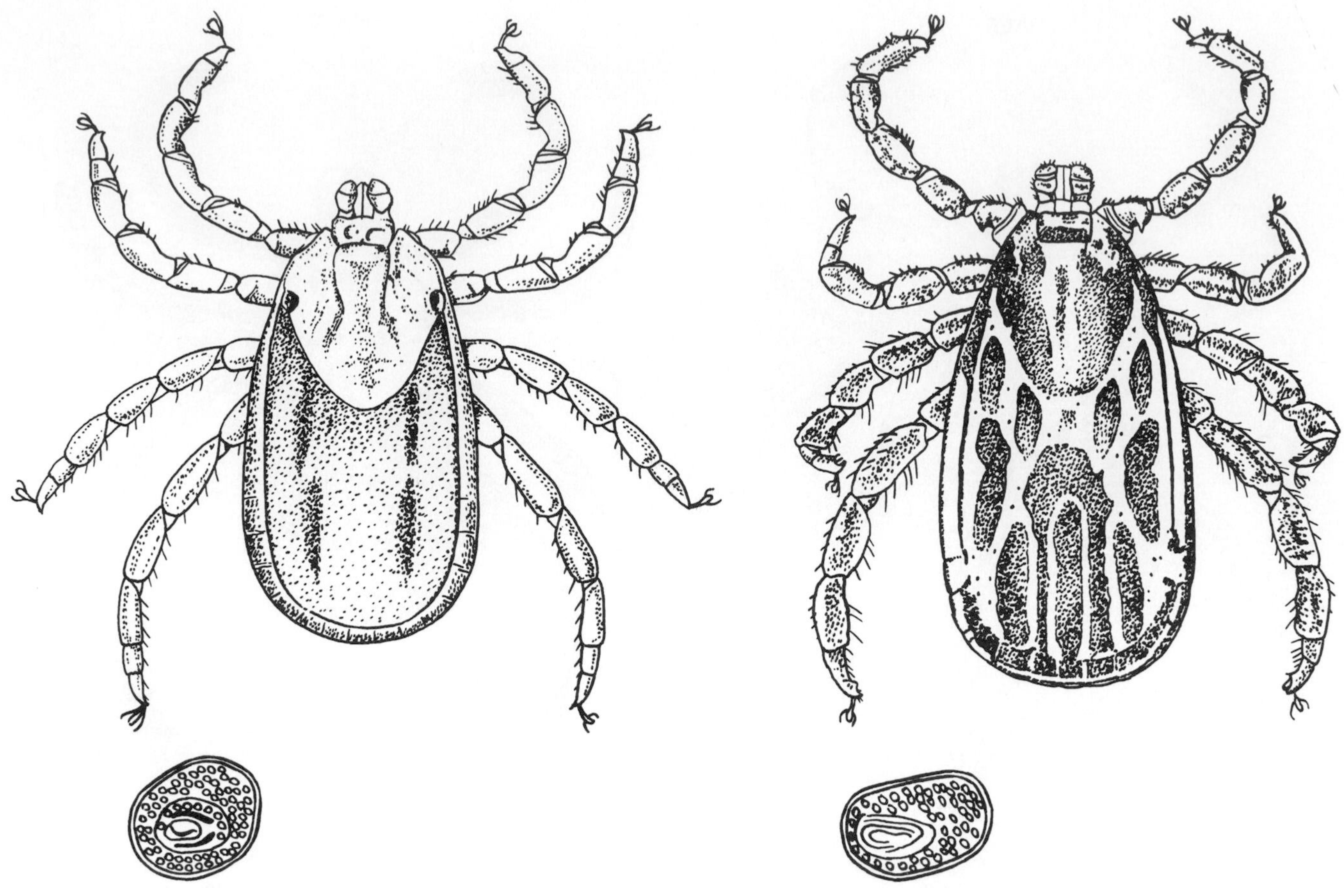

FIGURE 51.10 Male and female of *Dermacentor albipictus*, the winter tick.

Central America, and the northern part of South America. Although the name indicates that it has the horse as its host, it is common on many other large herbivores. *D. nitens* is a one-host tick that locates most often in the ears of the host and it may remain there as long as 99 days while feeding and molting. The auditory canal may become clogged with the bodies of the ticks, their excrement and cast skeletons leading to ear infections. *D. nitens* serves as the vector of equine piroplasmosis caused by *Babesia caballi* (Chapter 15).

D. variabilis, the American dog tick (Fig. 51.12), is a three-host tick that is distributed widely over the eastern two-thirds of North America from Labrador to Mexico (Fig. 51.8). Although its preferred host is the dog it is found on other carnivores, suids, some herbivores, rodents, lagomorphs, mustelids, and humans. In temperate climates it is found on dogs during the warmer months, but in warm climates it is active year-round. The dog tick is the principal vector of Rocky Mountain spotted fever in the eastern United States.

ROCKY MOUNTAIN SPOTTED FEVER (RMSF)

Spotted fever has a place in the history of vector-borne diseases that shows the ingenuity, perseverance, and outright heroism of many early workers. Late in the 19th century, a highly fatal disease had devastating effects on the settlers of the Bitterroot valley of western Montana. The cause and mode of transmission of the disease were unknown, and nothing seemingly could be done to stop its depredations. The U.S. Public Health Service sent Howard Taylor Rickets to the small town of Hamilton in the center of the valley and charged him with determining what caused the disease and doing something about it.

Rickets set up his laboratory (an exaggeration of the term) in a schoolhouse and went to work. Ultimately he determined that the tick *Dermacentor andersoni* transmitted an agent and that small mammals were the reservoirs of the infection. He also showed that there is both transtadial and transovarial transmission of the unknown agent. It was later determined that the

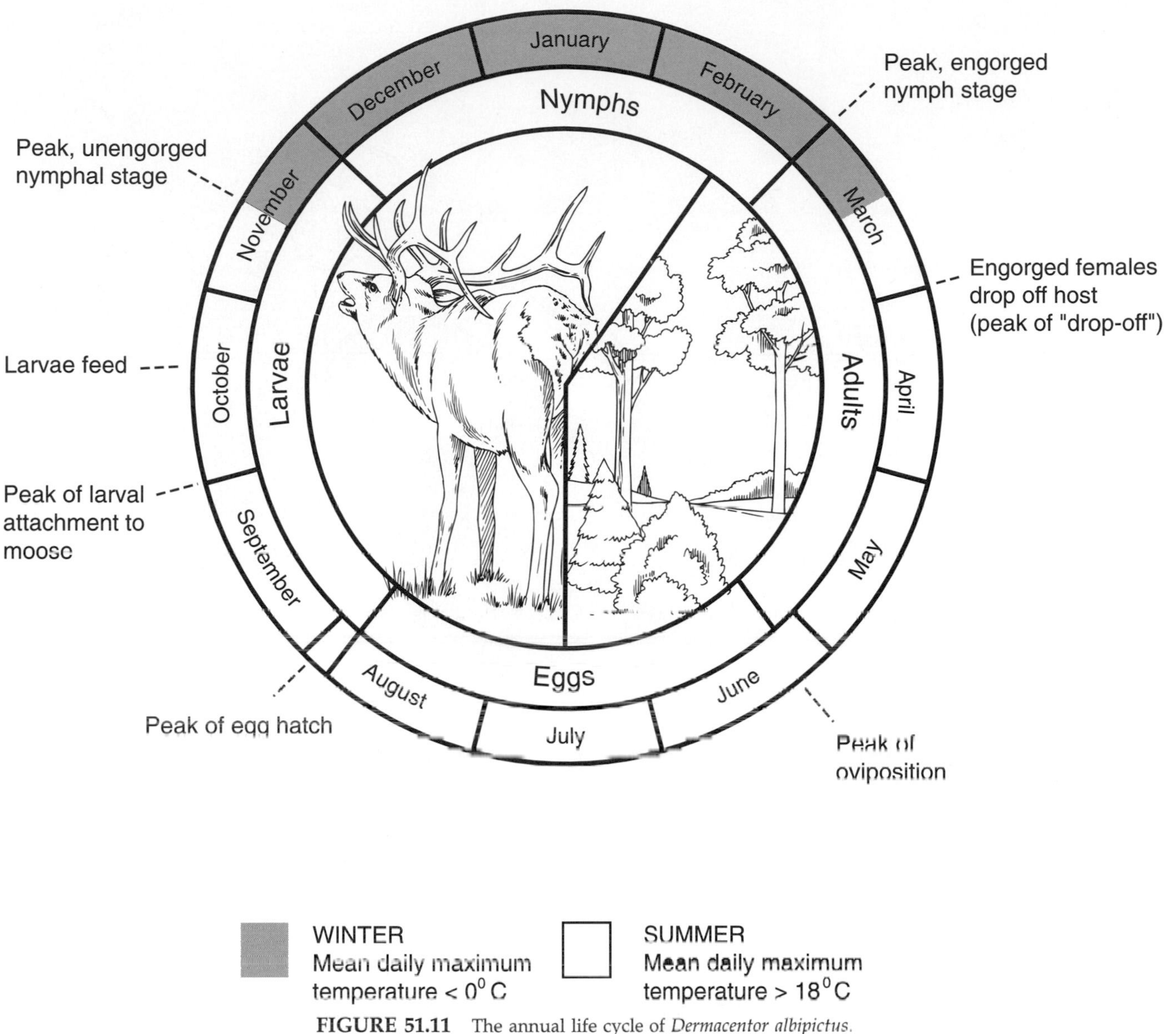

FIGURE 51.11 The annual life cycle of *Dermacentor albipictus.*

organism, named for Rickets, *Rickettsia rickettsi,* was the causative agent of RMSF. Both Rickets and Stanislas von Prowazek later died from louse-borne typhus caused by *Rickettsia prowazeki* (Chapter 44). The organism was named for both of these courageous men who investigated the very disease that killed them.

Many rickettsial diseases have much the same clinical pattern. There is a sudden onset of fever, which is accompanied by headache, aching muscles, mental confusion, and prostration. As the clinical phase progresses, a rash appears over much of the body, because the organisms replicate in the lining of the smaller blood vessels, which rupture releasing blood into the tissues. The worst of the disease lasts about two weeks. Mortality can reach 25% in an outbreak, but there is a good deal of variation in the virulence of isolates of *R. rickettsi.*

Early studies seemed to show that RMSF was confined to the Rocky Mountains, but in the middle of the 20th century, the disease almost died out in the western states and appeared in the Southeast. There are now a few scattered cases each year in the Rocky Mountain states, but several hundred in southeastern and some middle western states.

The reason for the decline in the West is not known, but the epidemiologic pattern in the East is well documented. As urban areas have expanded, more people have built houses in suburban and exurban areas

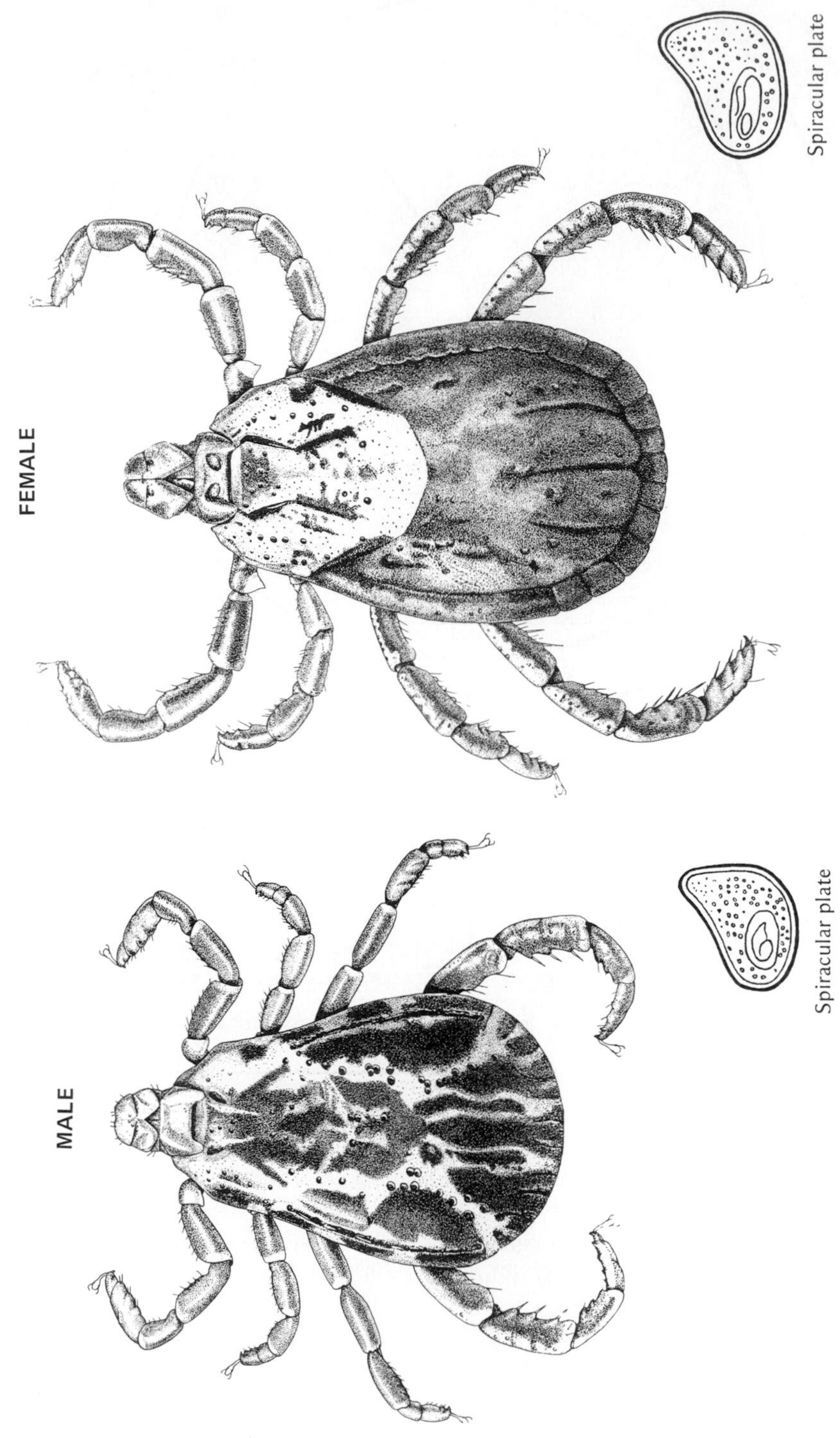

FIGURE 51.12 Male and female of *Dermacentor variabilis*, the American dog tick.

where there are trees and wildlife to enjoy. Clearings around homes make for good rodent and tick habitat and suburbanites also keep dogs that are often allowed to roam in the woods. This puts the infected ticks (*Dermacentor variabilis*) and humans in close proximity to one another and outbreaks have continued almost annually.

COLORADO TICK FEVER (CTF)

CTF is a viral disease that is transmitted by *Dermacentor andersoni* and that has a reservoir in small mammals in montane areas of the western states. CTF is acquired by picnickers and campers when they are fed upon by infected ticks. The incubation period is three to seven days. The disease has a flulike course in which there is fever, aching muscles, and prostration for a week to 10 days. Recovery is rapid in children, but the older the person, the longer the time for complete recovery. Although one might wish to die while in the midst of the disease, mortality is low; the few instances of deaths were in elderly persons.

The CTF ecosystem is an excellent example of landscape epidemiology as promulgated by the Russian epidemiologist Pavlovsky some years ago. The virus, the vector, the reservoirs, and the habitat are all tied in a Gordian knot and are inseparable from one another. The typical habitat for CTF is a south-facing slope that is warm and dry most of the year (Fig. 51.13). There are scattered coniferous trees, shrubs, and exposed rocks that have crevices extending below ground. In such a habitat 30% or more of ticks may carry CTF virus, and it has been calculated that there was one case of CTF for every 400 camper-days in Rocky Mountain National Park.

The virus cycles between small rodents and ticks, but is not transmitted transovarially, only transtadially, that is, from stage to stage in the tick life cycle. Since the adult ticks feed on animals (porcupine, canids, large ruminants) that are not part of the transmission cycle; maintenance of the virus depends on a mechanism at the rodent level (humans are dead-end or tangential hosts only). It has been shown that an infected nymph elicits a viremia in its rodent host and that the viremia lasts for a week or more. Then, a larva feeding on such a viremic host becomes infected; when the larva molts to the nymph and feeds the following spring, it transmits the virus to a young-of-the-year rodent. The virus, thus, cycles silently in the system probably without having any effect on its natural hosts. Susceptible rodents are provided each spring through the rapid turnover in their populations.

Name of Organism and Disease Associations

Haemaphysalis leporispalustris, the rabbit tick (syn. *H. leporis-palustris*; laws of zoological nomenclature do not allow hyphenated names; vernacular synonym is *Hlp*).

Hosts and Host Range

The rabbit tick prefers to feed on lagomorphs, but is found on many carnivores, rodents, opossum, and birds. About 60 species of birds are known to be hosts of the immature stages.

Geographic Distribution and Importance

Distribution is throughout North America from Alaska to South America. Heavy infestations are known to kill rabbits and birds. For example, snowshoe hare in Ontario were found to have as many as 2700 ticks in the summer. *H. leporispalustris* transmits the bacterial agent causing tularemia, *Francisella tularensis*.

Morphology

This is a small, inornate brown tick that has festoons at the posterior margin of the opisthosoma (Fig. 51.14).

Life Cycle

The preferred hosts for the adults *H. leporis palustris* are rabbits. *Hlp* is a three-host tick, and the larvae and nymphs are often found on birds, usually ground-nesting species such as grouse, quail, and meadowlark. The life cycle is completed in about 110 days; the adults remain on the host for about 17 days while engorging.

Host–Parasite Interactions

The rabbit tick is adapted for remaining in the vicinity of likely hosts by adjusting the time when it drops from the rabbit. Studies have shown that ticks leave the host in late afternoon, a time when rabbits are usually in their resting places or burrows.

H. leporispalustris is used widely in laboratory studies because it is relatively easy to maintain. It elicits immunity in the host and has been used to study this phenomenon.

Name of Organism and Disease Associations

Boophilus annulatus, the cattle fever tick.

Hosts and Host Range

Cattle are the principal hosts, but the cattle fever tick has been taken from deer and other large ruminants,

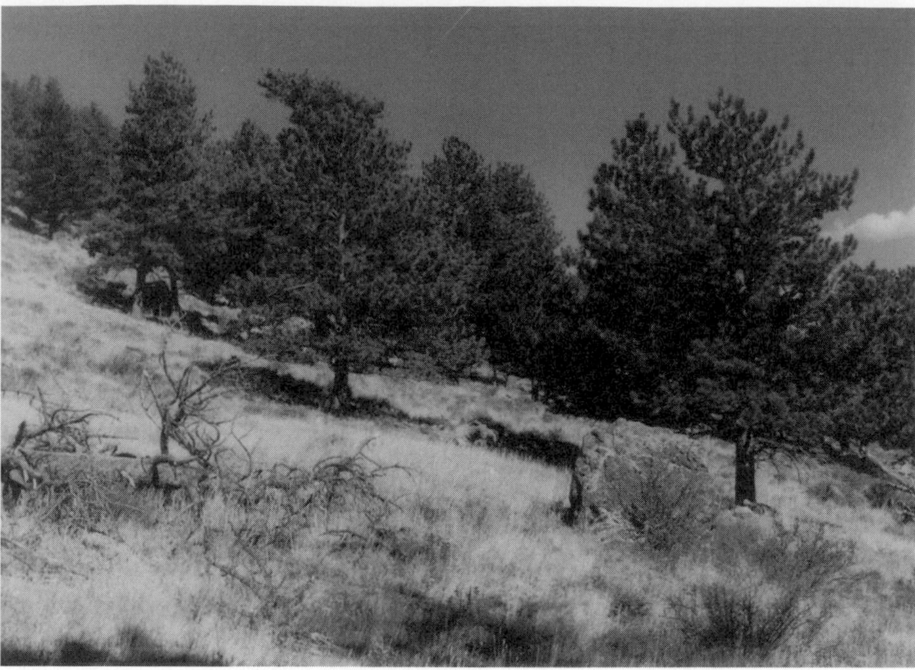

FIGURE 51.13 A typical habitat of Colorado Tick fever in Rocky Mountain National Park: a south-facing slope with scattered trees and shrubs; grasses and forbs also predominate. Protruding rocks with fissures provide underground habitat for both rodents and ticks. These slopes are occasionally snow covered but are generally clear and warm in the winter.

equids, and rarely dogs and humans. *B. annulatus* probably was originally a parasite of deer, but made the transition to cattle. Hosts other than cattle are probably not important in the maintenance of the tick.

Geographic Distribution and Importance

This tick is found in tropical and subtropical climates, but it may be carried into temperate climates during the warmer months. It occurs primarily in the Western Hemisphere south of the United States; distribution formerly included the southern United States, but it was eradicated from there. It is also found in tropical Africa, the Middle East, and the Mediterranean basin. The cattle fever tick is the vector of Texas cattle fever (Chapter 15).

Morphology

B. annulatus is a relatively large, inornate brown tick that lacks festoons; as is true with other members of the genus, the pedipalps are short (Figs. 51.3 and 51.15). Eyes are located on the margins of the scutum, and the spiracular plate is nearly round. The females swell to an enormous size when fully engorged.

Life Cycle

B. annulatus is a one-host tick (Fig. 51.5); it may complete development from the larva to the ovigerous female in as short a time as 20 days, but it usually takes longer and may extend to 66 days. Portions of the life cycle may be extended quite a bit; for example, females may begin to lay eggs as early as the first day after dropping from a host, but may not begin to lay for 98 days. Larvae may hatch in 17 days, at 30°C, but may require 202 days at low temperatures. Larvae can survive unfed for nearly eight months while awaiting a suitable host.

Epidemiology and Control

Although *B. annulatus* causes losses because of its hematophagous habit, the greatest danger to animal health revolves around its serving as a vector of *Babesia bigemina*, the cause of Texas cattle fever. Much of the biology and control of *B. annulatus* is discussed in Chapter 15.

Related Organisms

Other *Boophilus* spp. include *B.microplus*, the tropical cattle tick (Fig. 51.16), which is distributed widely in

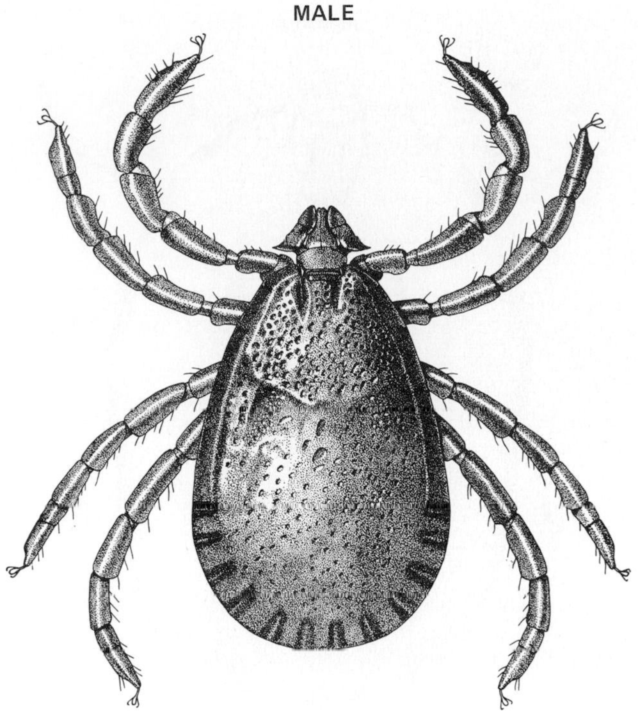

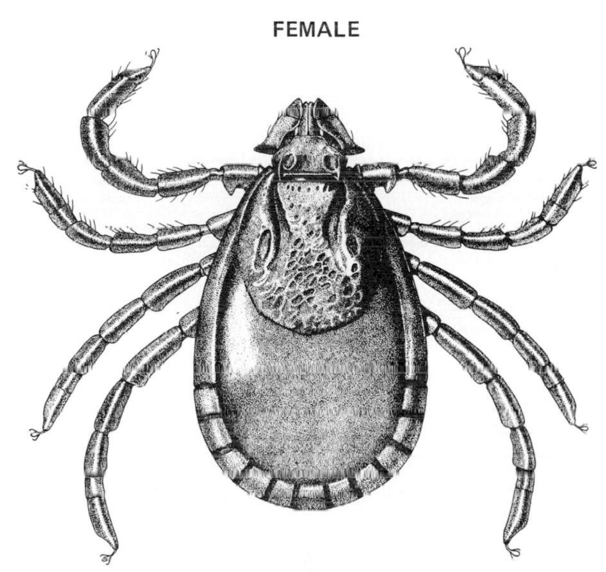

FIGURE 51.14 Male and female of *Haemaphysalis leporispalustris*, dorsal surface.

the warmer climates of the Western Hemisphere, Australia, Africa, and the Orient. Cattle are its principal hosts, but is found on other herbivores, some carnivores, marsupials, and suids. This is a one-host tick; the adult drops from the host about 23 days after the larva attaches. The larvae feed mostly in the ears of the host, but the nymphs and adults are found widely distributed on the body. *B. microplus* is a vector of *Babesia bigemina, B. ovis, B. caballi, Theileria mutans,* and *Anaplasma marginale* (Chapter 15).

In addition to being a vector of a variety of disease agents, it causes significant production losses, especially in cattle. In tropical areas, ticks are on cattle year-round and therefore are a continual drain on weight gain and milk production. An Australian study, for example, showed that there was a reduction in weight gain of 0.75 kg per tick per year in a growing animal (Tab. 51.2). This is not to say that a single tick would have such an effect, but the figure gives a way of calculating gains (or losses) when considering whether tick control is warranted.

Since *B. microplus* is so widespread in the warm climates of the world, global losses must be staggering. In Australia alone, losses have been estimated at $67 million (Australian) annually.

Complementing the usual methods of tick control through dipping in a second-generation acaricide and impregnated ear tags, a novel vaccine has been developed. The approach has been to produce antigens that the host would never "see" so to speak. In this case, a vaccine was produced against a proteins in the gut of the tick. This procedure has also been applied to fleas of companion animals (Chapter 46). The concept in such a vaccine is that the antibodies in the blood of an immunized animal combine with the intestinal proteins and have a detrimental effect on the tick. This, in fact, is what happens, and good control of ticks has been achieved.

The development of this vaccine by Willadsen and colleagues in Australia is fascinating. Through repeated empirical testing of protein fractions of the intestines of ticks with cattle challenge studies, a single antigen, Bm86, was selected as a vaccine candidate. The gene for Bm86 was molecularly cloned, overexpressed in *Escherichia coli* and used in the vaccine. A reformulated second-generation vaccine is also now available.

Name of Organism and Disease Associations

Ixodes ricinus is the sheep tick or castor bean tick. This tick serves as a vector of the disease agents causing louping ill in sheep, Bottonneuse fever, piroplasmosis, spring and summer encephalitis, and Lyme borreliosis

Geographic Distribution and Importance

The distribution of *I. ricinus* includes Great Britain, continental Europe, parts of the Middle East, Africa, and Japan. This is generally a cool climate tick; for example, in Iran it is found north of about 35° north

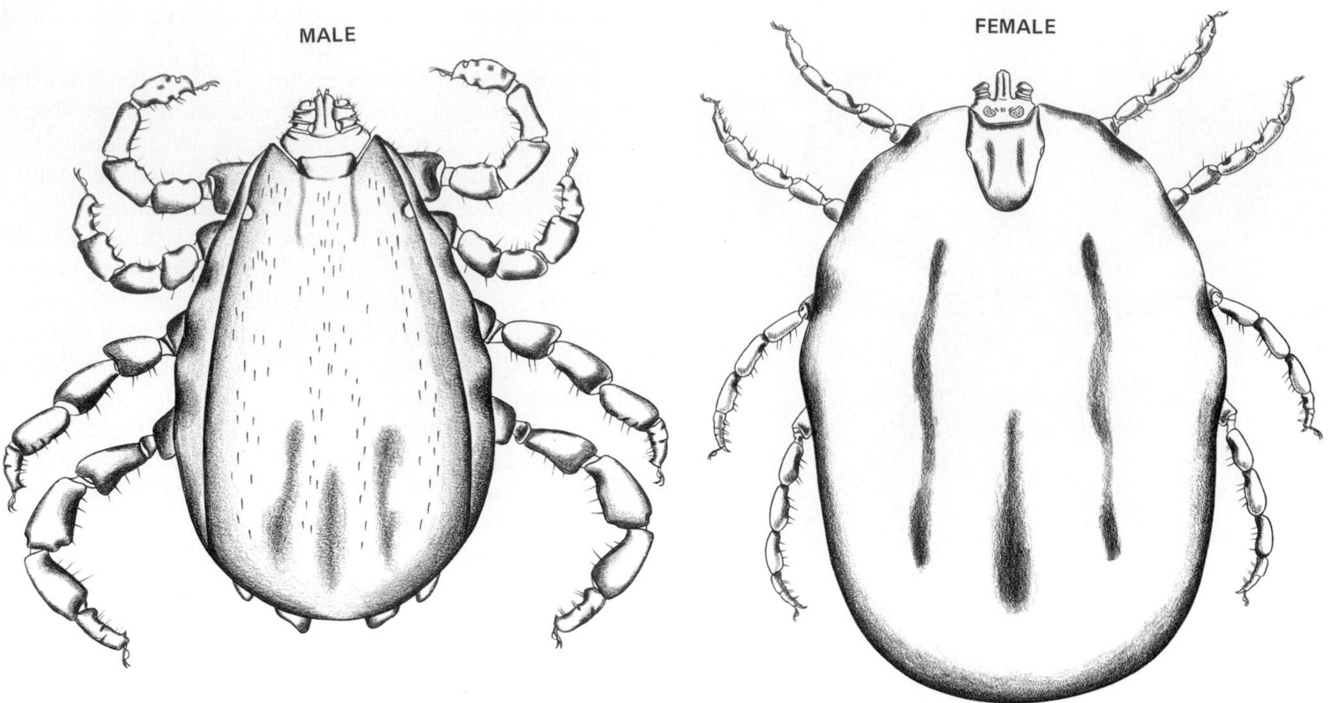

FIGURE 51.15 Male and female of *Boophilus annulatus,* the cattle fever tick.

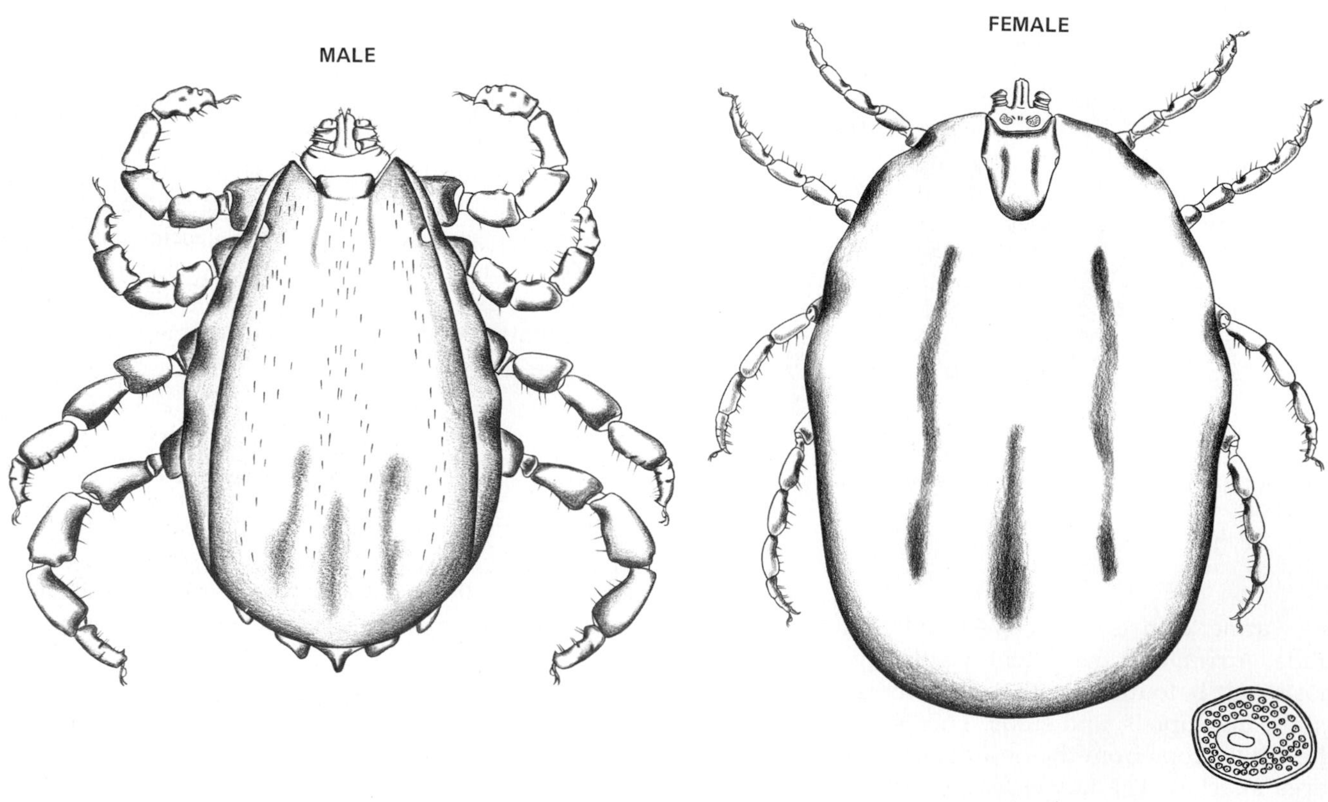

FIGURE 51.16 Male and female of *Boophilus microplus,* the tropical cattle tick.

TABLE 51.2 **Infestation of Cattle with *Boophilus Microplus* and Interference with Weight**

Retardation	Number of ticks				
	40	50	60	70	80
Pounds/Year	56 ± 19.8	82 ± 18.7	108 ± 19.5	134 ± 2.1	160 ± 25.9
Kilograms/Year	25 ± 8.9	37 ± 8.5	49 ± 8.8	61 ± 10.0	73 ± 11.6

latitude and may be found in other countries as far as 65° north latitude, not far from the Arctic Circle. *Ixodes* is one of the most widespread genera of hard ticks; there are 34 species in the United States and 9 species in Britain. In addition to the disease agents vectored, it also removes significant amounts of blood from its host when present in large numbers.

Morphology

Pedipalps of the gnathosoma are long, as are those of other members of the genus (Figs. 51.3, 51.4, 51.17). The body is reddish brown to black, inornate, and lacks festoons. A distinguishing characteristic of the genus is the anal groove, which curves around the anterior margin of the anus (Fig. 51.18). The male is 2.5 by 1.3 mm long and has scattered hairs on its body. The engorged female is 11 by 7 mm and while the body has hairs, they are shorter than those of the male. The hexapod larva is 0.6 to 1.5 mm long (Fig. 51.18).

Life Cycle

I. ricinus is a three-host tick but often uses the same species of host throughout its life cycle; larvae and nymphs are found on birds, but sheep may be the hosts for all three stages of the life cycle. The cycle in Britain requires three years for completion with each stage actively seeking a host during the spring of the year. Adults seek hosts in the spring and females engorge

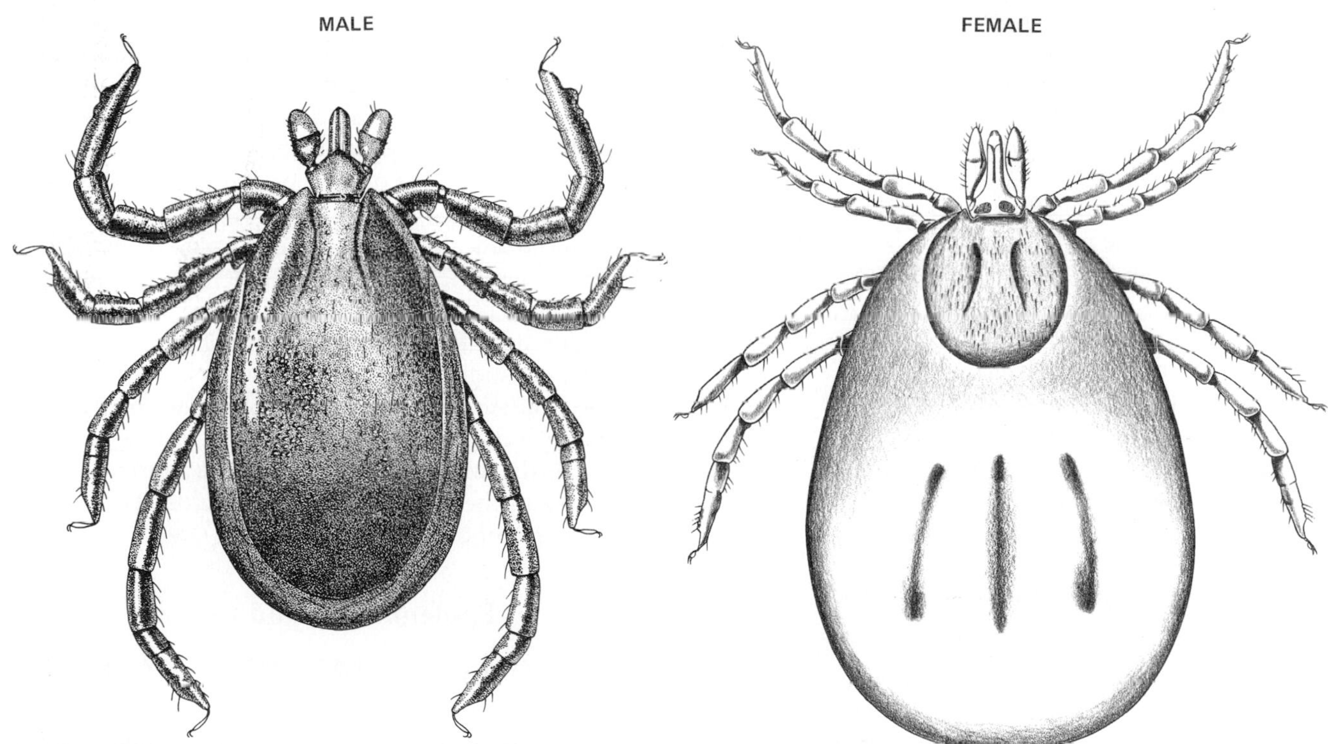

FIGURE 51.17 *Ixodes scapularis* (syn. *I. dammini),* the deer tick. The principal vector of the agent causing Lyme disease in the eastern United States.

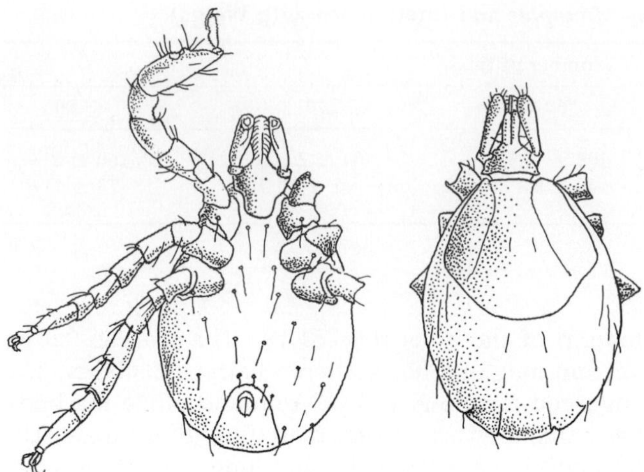

FIGURE 51.18 Larva of *Ixodes ricinus*. This larva is quite similar to that of *I. scapularis*.

for 5 to 14 days. The males inseminate females while they are engorging and may remain on the host to fertilize additional females. The females do not lay eggs until four to eight weeks after dropping from the host, and they continue to lay eggs over the next four to six weeks until early July. A female lays from 500 to 2000 eggs and then dies. Larval development proceeds slowly; the larvae hatch in late summer or fall, but they normally do not feed until the following spring.

In the spring, larvae climb up on plants and quest for a host. The larvae feed for three to six days, drop off, and molt during the summer. The nymphs also wait until the following spring to seek hosts. They feed for three to five days, drop off, and molt to the adult. The molt to the adult stage may not take place for seven months if the nymph has fed late in the season and cold weather has set in. There appears to be a diapause that must be broken so that development can proceed for each of the stages, because although development may have been completed during the summer, feeding does not occur until the following spring. In some parts of the British Isles, there are populations of *I. ricinus t*hat feed in the fall, and this appears to be a stable characteristic.

Host–Parasite Interactions

I. ricinus has been studied extensively in Britain, and many of the studies point up the exquisite adaptations of ticks as parasites. For example, despite poor or no eyesight, ticks can sense hosts and either prepare to be swept up by them or move toward them. They are sensitive to the following:

1. Vibrations of plants which they climb for questing. The swaying of the plant in the wind does not activate them, but more rapid vibration causes them to extend their legs so that they can catch onto the fleece or fur of a passing animal.
2. A reduction in light intensity also causes them to turn toward the shadow and extend their legs.
3. Warm air, as from the body or breath of a mammal, causes them to extend their legs in a questing attitude.
4. Aromas from the hair or wool of mammals also activate them.
5. Carbon dioxide is an attractant and may cause ticks to migrate some distance on the ground toward its source. CO_2 is used in many traps designed to capture ticks.

Ticks that begin to quest have about 30 days in which to find a host, or they use up their food reserves, and probably dehydrate, as well. Even so, the long time between feedings without questing activity, nearly a year, demonstrates a marvelous adaptation to survival while awaiting another meal. This ability of ticks to wait for long periods is seen in nearly all ticks and is even more remarkable in those found in hot, dry climates where retention of water is difficult and an elevated metabolic rate may exhaust food reserves.

Bloodsucking by *I. ricinus* may be a cause of reduced production in sheep. In a study in which it was assumed that a sheep would have 265 female ticks, 225 nymphs and 254,400 larvae on it over a four-month period, the animal would lose 1249 ml of blood or about 10 ml/day. For an animal on a good plane of nutrition, losing 1250 ml of blood may be tolerable, but if pasture is poor or if other disease agents or other stressors are present, there may be significant economic loss and death. In Britain, for example, the nematodes *Haemonchus, Trichostrongylus colubriformis, Oesophagostumum* spp., the digenetic trematode *Fasciola hepatica*, and the sheep ked, *Melophagus ovinus*, all cause anemia directly or indirectly and are likely to parasitize sheep, at least in small numbers. If animals are on marginal pasture and have a combination of parasites, as many animals do, another liter of blood loss from ticks could well mean the difference between profit and loss for the sheep producer.

Epidemiology and Control

Control of *I. ricinus* involves the following:

1. Use of acaricides
2. Avoiding pastures during the time when ticks are questing
3. Environmental management

As is true with most ectoparasites, a contact acaricide applied by dipping or spraying usually results in an immediate reduction in ticks. Sheep should be in short fleece when a toxicant is applied, because the fleece serves either as a barrier or a blotter for the toxicant.

The feeding habits of *I. ricinus* allow some measure of control; a tick feeds for a maximum of 25 days during its three-year life cycle. Although the ticks are active for three to four months in the spring and early summer, some demes feed in fall. Knowing the short time that they are active can be used to avoid areas where they are present. A questing tick has about 30 days in which to find a host or it perishes. If the tick does not come out to quest, it can survive for an extended period. Partial success in reducing tick populations has been achieved by burning, cultivating, or draining pastures in order to reduce habitat.

LYME BORELLIOSIS

In about 1975 an exceptionally high number of children were diagnosed with rheumatoid arthritis in the vicinity of Lyme, Connecticut. The observation that the number of cases was out of the ordinary was made by the mothers of some of the children. They called this to the attention of the public health authorities, and it was determined that there was a disease in the community that should be investigated.

Ultimately it was determined that the so-called Lyme disease was caused by a spirochete, *Borellia burgdorferi*, named for Willy Burgdorfer, the investigator who first saw the causative agent. *B. burgdorferi* is transmitted by an ixodid tick, *Ixodes scapularis* (syn. *I. dammini*) (Figs. 51.4, 51.17), a tiny tick usually referred to as the deer tick. This is a three-host tick that parasitizes small rodents such as the white-footed mouse, *Peromyscus leucopus*, during its larval and nymphal stages. The adults are on larger animals such as canids and deer. The vectors of Lyme borelliosis globally are ixodid ticks in the *I. ricinis* complex; these include *I. ricinus* in Europe, *I. scapularis* in the eastern United States, *I. pacificus* in the western United States, and *I. persulcatus* in Asia; all have much the same bionomics.

It became clear that *B. burgdorferi* was circulating between mice and ticks in wooded and forest-edge environments and that the relationship was commensal. Transmission of the spirochete was from stage to stage: A larva became infected and carried the infection to the nymph and then infected a clean mouse whose spirochetemia infected another larva. The hosts for the adult ticks, usually white-tailed deer, did not participate in the maintenance of the bacterium.

In the eastern United States, changes in both agricultural practices and housing patterns led to the epidemic. Large areas that were in crops were taken out of cultivation and in relatively few years returned to forest. White-tailed deer had been hunted to the point where their populations were extremely low and hunting of them was prohibited. As housing spread into suburban and rural areas in the 1950s and later, more forest-edge environment was created and the deer populations increased, sometimes dramatically. Exurbanites also keep dogs that are allowed to roam and to bring home ticks. The charm of suburban and rural life led to bringing this disease complex into contact with humans and precipitating a near epidemic.

Lyme disease, it turned out, was not a new disease. It was known as a distinct entity in Sweden early in the 20th century. Since its identification in the United States in the 1970s, more than 30,000 cases have been reported. It is the leading arthropod-borne disease in the United States.

Some of the signs of Lyme borreliosis are distinct, but most of them are rather general. There is, at first, a bull's-eye lesion usually at the site where the tick fed; this is a reddened area that spreads and for which the medical term is *erythema migrans* is used. Subsequently, arthritis, muscle pain, fever, headache, carditis, and neurologic disease are seen. The individual may be in considerable pain to begin with, but if treatment is given early, the arthritis is reversible. Broad spectrum antibiotics are effective.

Control of Lyme borelliosis requires the following:

1. Early diagnosis of the disease in humans
2. Avoidance of areas with ticks
3. Personal protection
4. Tick control
5. Rodent control

In enzootic areas, which now includes much of the United States—the eastern seaboard, southeastern states, the Midwest, and the Pacific coast—the possibility of Lyme disease must be kept in mind not only by physicians but equally by persons who live in such areas. Public health departments help to keep the disease in the minds of the citizenry during tick season so that they will seek medical help if the early signs of the disease occur.

Keeping clothing tight at the ankles and wrists as well as using a repellent such as deet helps keep ticks off. Tick inspection, with the help of another person, is essential after a day in the woods.

Ticks in the *Ixodes ricinus* complex are the only known competent vectors. Several other genera of ticks have been found to harbor *Borellia burgdorferi*, but they do not appear to be good vectors. *I. ricinus*-complex ticks require a moist climate since they do not retain water well. They are found under plant litter and in shady areas except when they are questing. Control requires ingenuity to develop methods that reach the ticks in their hiding places.

A product called Daminex is effective in reducing populations of ticks. The product consists of acaricide-soaked cotton placed in tubes where *Peromyscus* will find it and take it back to their burrows for nesting material. Their ticks are killed and thus the population of adult ticks, which are the hazard to human health, are eliminated. It has been reported that guinea fowl are especially fond of eating ixodid ticks and that they may be able to keep the population down. If true, this would be an excellent biological control method in some localities.

Rodent control around houses can keep ticks to a low level, but it is difficult to maintain a low population of rodents since as soon as some are taken out, others immigrate.

HUMAN GRANULOCYTIC EHRLICHIOSIS

Human granulocuytic ehrlichiosis (HGE) is caused by an *Ehrlichia equi*-like rickettsial agent. This potentially fatal disease is vectored by the deer tick, *I. scapularis,* and occurs widespread in the United States.

FAMILY ARGASIDAE—THE SOFT TICKS

The argasids are leathery and lack the scutum seen in the hard ticks; the mouthparts cannot be seen from above. There are some differences between the life cycles of the hard and soft ticks. The hypostome is usually not well developed. The soft ticks have a number of nymphal stages, usually three, but sometimes more. The females feed more than once and they lay several batches of eggs, sometimes over a period of many months (Fig. 51.19).

Name of Organism and Disease Associations

Argas persicus, the fowl tick or blue bug. This tick is the vector of *Borellia anserina* (syn. *B. gallinarum*), the cause of fowl spirochetosis.

Hosts and Host Range

The chicken is the principal host, but the tick has been taken from all kinds of birds including members of the orders Galliformes, Anseriformes, Passeriformes, and Falconiformes. It also occasionally feeds on rabbits, rodents, and humans.

Geographic Distribution and Importance

Cosmopolitan in temperate and tropical climates. It causes production losses and sometimes death in poultry, as well as being the vector of fowl spirochetosis.

Morphology

These ticks are yellowish-brown when unfed and slate blue when engorged with blood. The males are 3 by 4.5 mm and the females are 5.5 by 8.5 mm although both are occasionally larger. A distinct sutural line separates the dorsal from ventral part of the body (Fig. 51.20); this line can be seen even when the tick is engorged.

Life Cycle

The life cycle of *A. persicus* is typical of argasid ticks (Fig. 51.19). The larvae seek hosts and remain attached for 2 to 10 days. They drop off and molt in 4 to 16 days, and the nymphs seek hosts and feed rapidly. They usually engorge within 30 minutes. There are three or more nymphal stages that feed and molt. The adults feed at night and usually engorge in 20 to 45 minutes. The pattern in the females is to feed, lay eggs, and feed again. The female may feed daily and deposit eggs every day. The number of eggs is high early and tends to decline as the female ages; as many as 274 eggs can be laid in the first clutches, and as few as 25 in the later ones. Eggs hatch in 10 to 28 days.

Diagnosis

Since the larvae remain attached for several days, they may be found under the wings or near the vent. The larvae are extremely irritating and the area where they feed may be inflamed. The nymphs and adults feed at night and it may be necessary to examine birds at that time in order to find the ticks.

Host–Parasite Interactions

The fowl tick takes a large amount of blood and causes production losses because of decreased weight

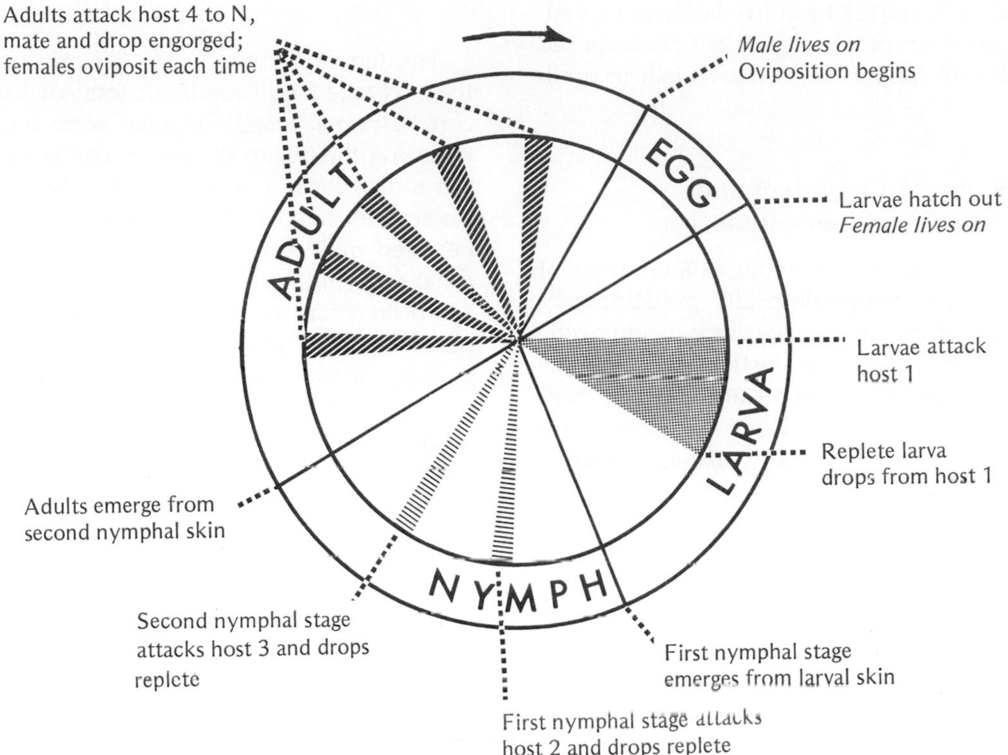

FIGURE 51.19 The life cycle and feeding pattern of a soft tick.

gains and lowered egg production. Heavy infestations can cause the death of the host through anemia. Tick paralysis (discussed later) sometimes occurs in chickens, ducks, and geese infested with *A. persicus.*

Epidemiology and Control

Treatment usually entails the use of a second-generation acaricide on the birds and their houses. If birds have roosts in a building where they spend the night, the legs of the perch can be placed in cups of oil to prevent the nymphs and adults from reaching their objective.

A. persicus represents almost the ultimate in patience and survival. Even the larvae have been found to survive as long as 246 days, more than eight months, without feeding, and an unfed female was reported to survive for five years. With such a long survival time, active steps must be taken to kill the stages in the environment. Not much can be done to control the

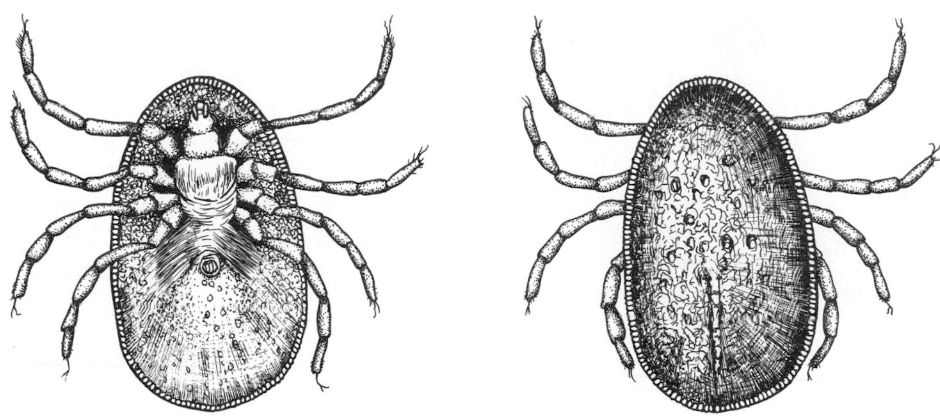

FIGURE 51.20 Adult of *Argas persicus*, the blue bug. The left side is a ventral view and the right side is a dorsal view. [Redrawn from Cooley, R. A, and Kohls, G. M., 1944.]

organisms that are outside of poultry houses. Surveillance of birds must be continual so that ticks acquired out of doors do not have time to reestablish in poultry houses.

Name of Organism and Disease Associations

Ornithodoros moubata is a member of a complex of four species that are morphologically indistinguishable. The species of greatest importance on domestic animals is known as *O. moubata*. The tick not only sucks blood but also serves as the vector of relapsing fever caused by *Borellia duttoni*. Others in the "*moubata*" complex are *O. porcinus* in Africa, and *O. tholozani* and *O. erraticus* in the Middle East.

Hosts and Host Range

The original host of this tick was most likely African warthogs, *Phacochoerus* spp., but they have transferred to domestic swine and then to humans.

Geographic Distribution and Importance

O. moubata (in the narrow sense) is found in arid or semiarid areas of Africa from South Africa northward to Kenya. It takes blood and vectors *Borellia duttoni.*

Morphology

This is a leathery, wrinkled tick with a mammilated exoskeleton (Fig. 51.21). It lacks eyes, unlike *O. savignyi*, which has two pairs of eyes. Adults average 6.5 by 8 mm with engorged individuals reaching a length of 11 mm.

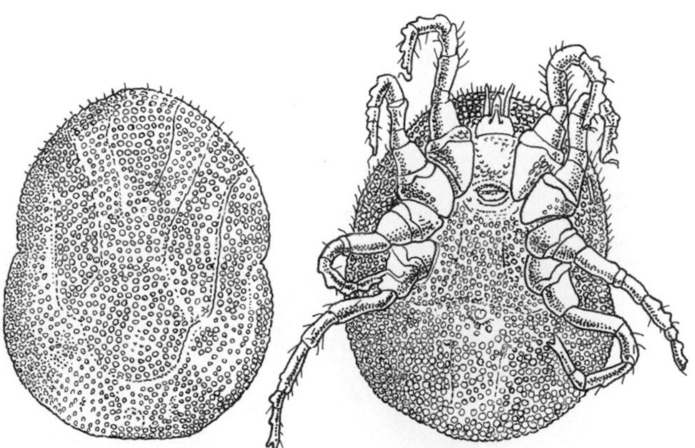

FIGURE 51.21 Adult of *Ornithodoros moubata*. The left side shows the dorsal surface and the right side shows the ventral surface.

Life Cycle

The female oviposits the 0.5 mm eggs in batches that average 247; they lay a total of 1926 eggs in 7.8 clutches, on average. Eggs hatch in eight days at 30°C releasing the hexapod larvae. The larvae do not feed, but molt within a short period of time to the nymph. There are three or more nymphal stages ,which feed between molts. About four months are required for the organism to go from egg to adult. An activity that has been interpreted as "brooding" of eggs has been observed in *O. moubata,* since females remain in the vicinity of the eggs and sometimes have been seen with nymphs clinging to them. However, eggs, nymphs, and adults are all in the same habitat in the house or burrow, so it may be only that they are present in such large numbers that they are seen on top of one another.

Host–Parasite Interactions

Swine can be killed by infestations with *O. moubata* and these ticks are significant pests of humans when they move into huts and feed on people. Its greater importance, however, lies in its role as a vector of *Borellia duttoni,* the cause of tick-borne relapsing fever.

Epidemiology and Control

Control of *O. moubata* is directed mostly toward preventing transmission of relapsing fever. In central Africa, the ticks move into houses and feed on people at night. Houses in villages and small towns are largely made of mud, and the ticks crawl into cracks in the walls to spend the day. Control involves decreasing resting sites by plastering the insides of dwellings to make them smooth and crack-free. The house is then treated with a second-generation acaricide.

Related Organisms

The genus *Ornithodoros* contains perhaps 90 species that are found mostly in relatively dry habitats and are associated with rodents and other small mammals. In the western United States, *O. hermsi* is associated with rodents such as squirrels and it serves as a vector of relapsing fever (discussed later). A number of other species are also found in the Western Hemisphere including *O. turicata, O. parkeri, O. talajae,* and *O. savignyi.*

TICK-BORNE RELAPSING FEVER

Relapsing fever, caused by the spirillar bacteria *Borellia recurrentis, B. duttoni,* and probably other species of *Borellia*, occurs widely throughout the world, and strains of the organisms, are either tick adapted or louse adapted (Chapter 44). In North America, tick-borne relapsing fever is most often contracted when a person enters a nidus where the agent is cycling in rodents and soft ticks. Individual cases often occur in campers who sleep on the ground near rodent burrows.

A classic outbreak occurred in 1973 in Grand Canyon National Park when 62 people contracted relapsing fever at a resort lodge. The disease occurred in those persons who stayed in rustic log cabins as opposed to those who stayed in a large, central lodge. Investigation showed that the cabins had large amounts of rodent nesting material both under the floors and in the attics. The cabins were rather old and not constructed to keep rodents out, so rodents had moved in and brought their ectoparasites with them. It was also observed that rodent populations were at a low point during that summer; there probably had been a die-off of rodents during the previous year. The vector, *O. hermsi*, did not have its usual rodent hosts to feed on and moved to the human inhabitants in the cabins instead.

Control of the outbreak consisted of removing the nesting materials from the cabins (3000 kg were removed) and then the cabins were sprayed with an acaricide. Rodent-proofing of the cabins was also undertaken to prevent recolonization in subsequent years. Inquiries during the following year revealed that no additional cases of relapsing fever had occurred.

The disease results in fever and prostration followed by a period when the person feels relatively normal. The course of the disease may run over several months with the patient never feeling entirely well, but that is interspersed with fever and prostraton. The bacterium changes it antigenic composition frequently thus allowing it to survive and multiply, it seems, almost endlessly. Broad spectrum antibiotics are usually effective in treating the disease.

Name of Organism and Disease Associations

Otobius megnini, the spinose ear tick.

Hosts and Host Range

The ticks are found principally on cattle, but they have only a low degree of host specificity and are found on other domestic animals, wild ruminants, carnivores, and humans.

Geographic Distribution and Importance

Cosmopolitan in warm climates. They are sometimes found in temperate climates, but probably do not complete the life cycle there.

Life Cycle

Only the larvae and nymphs of *O. megnini* are parasitic (Fig. 51.22). The larvae seek hosts and move to the ears where they feed in the ear (auditory) canal. They molt in the ear and the nymphs remain on the same host. Once having reached a host, the larvae and nymphs remain on it for seven months or sometimes longer. The nymphs drop from the host and molt to the adult stage; copulation takes place off of the host. The adults are free living.

Host–Parasite Interactions

When large numbers of ticks are present in the ear canal, it becomes plugged with ticks, their shed skeletons, ear wax, and other debris. This causes cattle considerable distress and may also lead to secondary bacterial infections of the ears.

It is generally stated that the spinose ear tick is occasionally found in the ears of humans; however,

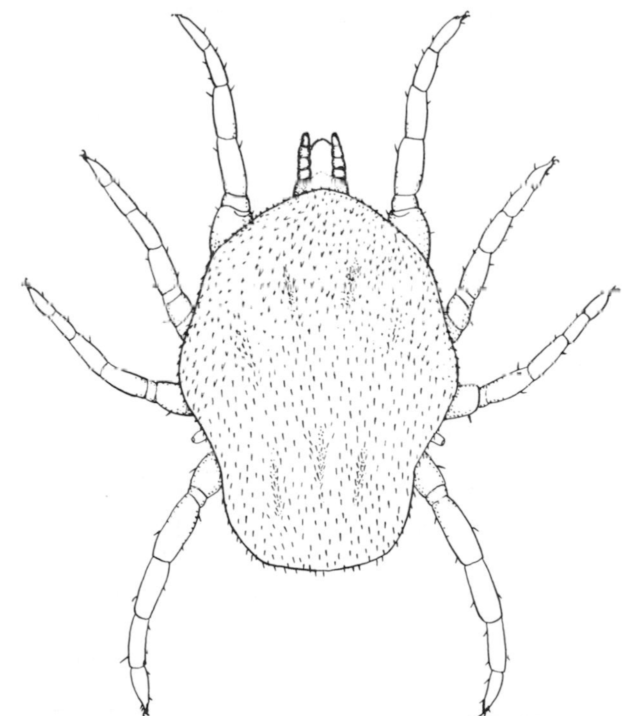

FIGURE 51.22 Nymph of *Otobius megnini*, the ear tick of cattle. Cattle are the usual hosts of *O. megnini*, but many other hosts including human can be infected.

humans may be parasitized more often than indicated in the literature. Data from an investigator at the Centers for Disease Control showed that 12 individuals in 1978 in New Mexico had spinose ear ticks. We were brought a tick by a practicing physician who had removed it from the ear of a woman who had not lived in an enzootic area for a year. Not only can one have the discomfort of a tick in the auditory canal for many months, but the ticks can penetrate the tympanic membrane and also somehow cause a unilateral facial paralysis.

Epidemiology and Control

In warm climates, the spinose ear tick can be a continuing hazard in livestock, and frequent inspection and treatment is the best approach to control. Treatment is by second-generation acaricide and one method of administration is to put the liquid in a pump-type oil can that can be inserted a little way into the auditory canal and administration given directly to the ticks.

In humans, the ticks are usually removed from the auditory canal by grasping them with forceps and pulling them out. Additional symptomatic treatment may be required.

TICK PARALYSIS

Tick paralysis is an acute, ascending paralysis of vertebrates that results when one or more ticks attach to engorge. Mammals are most frequently affected, and cattle, bison, sheep, dogs, cats, poultry, and humans are among the common hosts susceptible to tick paralysis.

The disease usually develops when ticks embed at the base of the skull. Within a day or two of attachment in humans, the host begins to lose coordination and sensation in the hands and feet. The paralysis progresses centrally and the legs and arms become useless.

Ticky Dogs

Families living in suburban, and rural areas often keep dogs, and where there are no leash laws, or where properties are large, dogs roam. Among the two- and three-host ticks discussed in this chapter, all can have dogs as their hosts. Most often the dog serves as a host for the adult stages of a particular tick species, but they can harbor the larvae and nymphs of some species as well. An infestation of the family dog with ticks is hazardous because (1) anemia can be caused, (2) tick paralysis can occur in the dog, (3) the dog can suffer from a tick-borne disease, and (4) members of the family can be exposed to ticks or certain tick-borne agents.

In North America, several species of ticks parasitize dogs, depending upon the geographic location (Fig. 51.8). In addition to those shown in the figure, *Dermacentor andersoni, D. variabilis, Amblyomma americanum,* the lone star tick, the other ticks found on the dog are *Rhipicephalus sanguineus,* the brown dog tick, *Ixodes scapularis,* the deer tick, and *Haemaphysalis leporispalustris,* the rabbit tick.

R. sanguineus is a warm climate tick, not usually found in areas where there are cold winters. Nevertheless, this tick is seen on dogs in cold climates, because it can move into houses and complete its life cycle there.

Tick paralysis is seen in dogs, and especially in those with long hair; it may not be easy to find the ticks at the base of the skull without careful inspection.

Several tick-borne apicomplexan and rickettsial diseases are seen in dogs in North America. *Babesia canis* is a cosmopolitan infection of dogs in both warm and temperate climates. Its principal vector is *R. sanguineus,* but other genera of ticks are also vectors in various parts of the world. *B. gibsoni* occurs in North America but is uncommon; *R. sanguineus* is the vector.

Haemobartonella canis is a rickettsial organism that is on the surface of red blood cells. Experimentally, the vector is *R. sanguineus* in which there may be both transtadial and transovarial transmission, but other arthropods have not been ruled out as vectors.

Mark Twain is quoted as saying that, "A few fleas are good for a dog, it keeps him from forgetting that he is a dog." Perhaps. But ticks present hazards that should remind owners of their responsibilities to their dogs.

If the ticks remain attached, the host is likely to die when the paralysis reaches the breathing center of the brain. If the ticks are found and removed, recovery begins almost immediately and a person or animal that had been helpless will be up and around within a day. Within a few days to a week, all signs of paralysis are usually gone.

Not all ticks and not all populations of a species are likely to cause tick paralysis. Some of the species that have been implicated in tick paralysis are listed in Table 51.3.

The incidence of tick paralysis is erratic. *Dermacentor andersoni* may cause paralysis in humans or domestic animals all through its range, but the more northerly populations, such as that in British Columbia, are more likely to cause the disease. Smaller or younger hosts are more likely to show paralysis; thus children are more susceptible than adults. However, mature, large ruminants such as cattle and bison have been killed by tick paralysis.

The toxin causing tick paralysis is a part of the salivary fluid that the tick injects while feeding. It acts at the myoneural junction, preventing normal control of muscle and resulting in incoordination. The observation that tick paralysis is usually associated with ticks attached near the base of the skull and the rapid recovery when they are removed lead to the conclusion that the toxin acts locally and that it breaks down rapidly or is rapidly neutralized.

Tick paralysis is so sporadic that the principal obstacle to overcome in diagnosis is becoming aware that ticks might be the cause of an ascending paralysis.

TABLE 51.3 Some Ticks Known to Cause Tick Paralysis

Tick	Locality
Dermacentor andersoni	North America
Dermacentor variabilis	United States
Amblyomma maculatum	South America
Ixodes homocyclus	Australia
Ixodes ricinus	Britain and Continental Europe
Ixodes rubicundus	South Africa
Rhipicephalus evertsi	South Africa
Argas persicus	Cosmopolitan

Children, dogs, cats, livestock, and birds are all likely candidates, and the vague early signs or symptoms are likely to be insufficient to elicit a search for ticks. Once the decision has been made that tick paralysis is a possibility and they have been found, removal of them is all that is needed.

Readings

Azad, A. F., and Beard, C. B. (1998). Rickettsial pathogens and their arthropod vectors. *Emerg. Infect. Dis.* **4,** 179–186.

Boyer, K. M., Munford, R. S., Maupin, G. O., *et al.* (1977). Tick-borne relapsing fever: An interstate outbreak originating at Grand Canyon National Park. *Am. J. Epidemiol.* **105,** 469–479.

Cooley, R. A., and Kohls, G. M. (1944, June). The Argasidae of North America, Central America and Cuba. *Am. Midl. Nat. Monogr. Ser.* **1.**

Daniels, T. J., Falco, R. C., Schwartz, I., Varde, S., and Robbins, R. G. (1997). Deer tick (*Ixodes scapularis*) and the agents of Lyme disease and human granulocytic ehrlichiosis in a New York City park. *Emerg. Infect. Dis.* **3,** 353–355.

De Castro, J. J., and Nelson, R. M. (1993). Host resistance in cattle tick control. *Parasitol. Today* **9,** 13–17.

Glines, M. V., and Samuel, W. M. (1989). Effect of *Dermacentor albipictus* (Acari: Ixodidae) on blood composition, weight gain and hair coat of moose, *Alces alces. Exp. Appl. Acarol.* **6,** 197–213.

Hamilton, J. G. C. 1992. The role of pheromones in tick biology. *Parasitol. Today.* **8,** 130–133.

Jaenson, T. G. T. (1991). The epidemiology of Lyme borreliosis. *Parasitol. Today* **7,** 39–45.

Piesman, J., and Gage, K. L. (1996). Ticks and mites and the agents they transmit. In *The Biology of Disease Vectors* (B. J. Beaty and W. C. Marquardt, Eds.). Univ. Press of Colorado, Niwot.

Samuel, W. M. (1988). The use of age classes of winter ticks on moose to determine the time of death. *Can. Soc. Forensic Sci. J.* **21,** 54–59.

Samuel, W. M. (1991). Grooming by moose (*Alces alces*) with the winter tick, *Dermacentor albipictus* (Acari): A mechanism for premature loss of winter hair. *Can. J. Zool.* **69,** 1255–1260.

Sonnenshine, D. E. (1993). *Biology of Ticks.* Oxford Univ. Press, New York.

Sonnenshine, D. E., and Mather, T. N. (1994). *Ecological Dynamics of Tick-Borne Zoonoses.* Oxford Univ. Press, New York.

Varde, S., Beckley, D. J., and Schwartz, I. (1998). Prevalence of tick-borne pathogens in *Ixodes scapularis* in a rural New Jersey county. *Emerg. Infect. Dis* **4,** 97–99.

Walker, D. H. (Ed.) (1991). *Biology of Rickettsial Diseases.* CRC Press, Boca Raton, FL.

Wikel, S. K. (1996). Immunologic control of vectors. In *The Biology of Disease Vectors* (B. J. Beaty and W. C. Marquardt, Eds.). Univ. Press of Colorado, Niwot.

Willadsen, P., Bird, P., Cobon, G. S., and Hungerford, J. (1995). Commercialisation of a recombinant vaccine against *Boophilus microplus. Parasitology* **110,** 543–550.

Glossary

acanthella Acanthocephalan larva following the acanthor and prior to the cystacanth; reproductive system is not fully developed.

acanthor Acanthocephalan larva with bladelike hooks; develops inside the egg capsules.

acetabulum Ventral sucker or holdfast of digenetic trematodes; a sucker on a tapeworm scolex.

acoelomate A condition in which a body cavity is lacking, as in the members of the phylum Platyhelminthes where the organs lie embedded in parenchyma.

ala (-ae) Winglike projection such as the cuticular expansions in certain nematodes.

alb A root meaning white.

allergy See hypersensitivity.

alveolus (-i) A small cavity; the air sac in the lung where gaseous exchange takes place.

amastigote Round to oval body with internal flagellum seen in some euglenotistans such as *Trypanosoma spp.* and *Leishmania spp.*

ametabolous A type of metamorphosis in insects in which there is no external change as they proceed through a series of molts to the adult. Ametabola refers to the taxonomic group.

amphid Anterior sensory structures of nematodes (see also phasmid).

anaphylaxis An extraordinarily strong hypersensitive reaction in which the individual may collapse, stop breathing, and die; each species of animal has its own peculiar syndrome of signs and symptoms.

anapolysis The process in which terminal gravid proglottids are not shed in certain tapeworms (ant. apolysis).

anisogamete Male and female gametes which are morphologically different.

anterior station Protistan development in the anterior part of an insect vector. For example, Salivaria of the genus *Trypanosoma;* transmission takes place by biting.

anthelmintic A chemical used to remove worms usually from the intestinal tract of a vertebrate host, a vermifuge.

antibiotic A chemical produced by a microorganism and which is used to treat infectious diseases.

antibody Serum protein (immunoglobulin) synthesized by lymphoid cells in response to an antigenic stimulus.

antigen Any substance, but usually a protein, which stimulates an immune response.

antigenic mimicry Acquisition of or production of host antigens by a parasite so that it is not recognized as nonself, as in *Schistosoma.*

apical complex Organelles characteristic of members of the phylum Apicomplexa: polar rings, subpellicular microtubules, conoid, rhoptries, and micronemes.

apolysis The process in which terminal, gravid proglottids are detached and shed by certain tapeworms (ant. anapolysis).

areole Round or polygonal areas on nematomorphan cuticle; function unknown.

autogeny The ability of some bloodsucking arthropods to lay eggs without having had a blood meal (adj. autogenous).

autoinfection A process in which the progeny of a parasite reinfect the host without passing out of it, for example, *Hymenolepis nana.*

axostyle A longitudinal rodlike or tubelike structure in members of the protistan order Trichomonadida; probably serves as a cytoskeleton.

biramous Divided into two branches; typical of the terminal segments of the legs of Crustacea.

bladderworm See cysticercus.

bothridium (-ia) Muscular, leaflike sucking structure on the scolex of tapeworms of the order Tetraphyllidea.

bothrium (-ia) Shallow, sucking groove on the scolex of tapeworms of the order Pseudophyllidea.

brachy A root meaning short.

bradyzoite Slow-growing zoite or meront in the pseudocyst of *Toxoplasma* and related Apicomplexa.

bug An insect of the order Hemiptera; something that has legs and cannot be identified as anything else.

bulla A structure seen in some female symbiotic copepods that serves to anchor the maxillae; elaborated by head and maxillary glands.

bursa (copulatory bursa) A muscular copulatory structure at the posterior end of males of the order Strongylida; useful in taxonomy and identification.

cadre Chitinous ring surrounding the mouth of members of the phylum Pentastomida.

calotte Light-colored anterior end of members of the phylum Nematomorpha

campestral An adjective referring to a plain (see sylvatic).

capitulum The part of a tick which bears the mouthparts; also called the gnathosoma.

cellular immunity A specific response to an antigen in which lymphoid cells are the primary effectors.

cephalo A root meaning head.

cercomer Tail-like appendage, which often retains the hooks of the hexacanth embryo, on procercoid and cysticercoid metacestodes of certain tapeworms.

chalimus Specialized copepodid larva of certain members of the class Copepoda; larvae attach to their hosts by a filament secreted by the frontal gland.

chemoprophylaxis Use of a chemical that acts to prevent the invasion or development of a parasitic agent.

chemotherapy Use of a chemical that has a specific action in removing or killing a parasitic agent.

chromatoidal bar Rod-like masses of RNA in cysts and occasionally trophozoites of *Entamoeba spp.*

coenurus Fluid-filled metacestode of the tapeworm family Taeniidae; has a nonlaminated wall which produces protoscolices; no brood chambers.

commensalism Symbiosis in which there is no discernible damage to the host.

concomitant immunity A form of acquired immunity in which an established infection persists long after resistance has developed against a challenge infection.

conjugation A temporary union of two ciliated protistans for the exchange of nuclear material.

conoid Spirally coiled filaments in the anterior tip of the zoite of certain apicomplexans.

coracidium Free-swimming, Ciliated embryophore of tapeworms of the order Pseudophyllidea.

costa A striated, rodlike structure that lies just under the recurrent flagellum of certain members of the order Trichomonadida; composed of carbohydrate and protein.

cryptozoite Exoerythrocytic meront of malaria.

cuticle A secreted surface covering, generally considered to be nonliving.

cypris A parasitic, postnaupliar larva of symbiotic members of the order Copepoda.

cyst A general term used when an organism has a membrane surrounding it, whether the covering is of its making or of host origin; a resistant stage in protists.

cystacanth A juvenile acanthocephalan that is surrounded by a capsule of host origin.

cysticercoid A tapeworm metacestode in which the scolex is surrounded by solid tissues; characteristic of many cyclophyllidean families such as Hymenolepididae, Dilepididae or Anoplocephalidae.

cysticercus A tapeworm metacestode in which the scolex develops in an inverted form and which has a fluid-filled bladder surrounding it; one of the bladder worms; characteristic of the cyclophyllidean family Taeniidae.

definitive host Host in which the sexually mature form of a symbiont is found.

diarrhea Frequent passage of fecal material containing an abnormally high proportion of water (see dysentery).

didelphic Having two ovaries and a uterus with two horns: usually applied to nematodes.

dioecious Separate sexes (ant. monoecious).

direct life cycle A life cycle in which only a single host is required for its completion.

disease Abnormal performance of physiologic functions as a result of injury to cells performing those functions.

domiciliated (domiciliation) The condition in which an unwanted animal associates with humans, usually by moving into houses; cockroaches, house flies, and house mice are examples.

dysentery A form of diarrhea in which blood and mucus originating in the intestinal tract are passed (see diarrhea).

ecdysis See molt.

-ectomy A suffix meaning to remove, usually by surgery.

ectoparasite A parasite that lives on the external surface or in the integument of a host.

edema (Br. **oedema)** Abnormal accumulation of fluid in cells, tissues, or tissue spaces resulting in swelling.

egg The germ cell of a female, an ovum, the term egg is usually reserved for the ovum plus its outer coverings such as a shell or capsule.

-emia (Br. **-aemia)** A root referring to blood.

endemic A disease or disease agent that occurs in a human community at all times (see also enzootic).

endodyogeny A special form of merogony in which two daughter cells are formed each with its own pellicle, while still in the mother cell; occurs in certain apicomplexans such as *Toxoplasma.*

endopodite The inner or medial branch of a biramous appendage.

entero- A root that means cavity but usually in reference to the digestive tract.

enteritis Inflammation of the intestinal tract.

entomo- A root that refers to insects, as in *entomology,* the study of insects, or *entomophagous,* eating of insects.

enzootic A disease or disease agent that occurs in an animal population at all times (see also endemic)

epidemic A disease or disease agent that spreads rapidly through a human population (see also epizootic)

epidemiology The study of the causes of disease; the complex of factors that lead to disease outbreaks; usually reserved for diseases in humans, *epizootiology* is used for diseases in other animals.

epizootic A disease or disease agent that spreads rapidly through an animal population (see also epidemic).

erratic parasite Parasite normal to a particular host, but in an abnormal location.

euryxenous Having a broad host range

eutely Having a constant number of cells and usually nuclei.

exflagellation Process of formation of microgametes in certain apicomplexans such as *Plasmodium.*

exopodite The outer branch of a biramous appendage.

facultative parasite An organism that is normally free-living but can become symbiotic when the proper conditions are presented.

falx Densely ciliated margin on the anterior of certain members of the protistan phylum Opalozoa.

feral Wild; a feral cycle of a parasitic agent is one that takes place in the wild as opposed to an urban site.

flame cell (=protonephridium) The terminal cell of the excretory system in members of the phylum Platyhelminthes; a tuft of cilia in the cavity of the cell beats to move fluid along the tubule; the beating of the cilia give the impression of a flickering flame.

flotation In parasitology, the term is used for techniques of fecal examination in which eggs or cysts are concentrated by suspending them in a medium of high specific gravity so that they will rise to the top of the liquid.

fomite An inanimate object that is involved in the transmission of an infectious agent.

gamogony (=gametogony) Formation of gametes

glochidium (-ia) Larva of members of freshwater mussels of the family Unionidae.

gonotyl A muscular sucker, often with spines, surrounding the genital pore in certain digenetic trematodes such as *Heterophyes.*

granuloma (-ata) A swelling composed of leukocytes, fluid, and connective tissue, often a foreign-body reaction.

gubernaculum A sclerotized plate located on the dorsal surface of the cloaca of certain male nematodes; serves as a guide when the copulatory spicules are protruded.

gynecophoral canal The longitudinal groove on the ventral surface of male schistosomes in which the female worm lies.

helminth A worm

hema- (Br. **haema-)** A prefix meaning blood

hematophagous Bloodsucking; usually refers to the feeding habits of various insects and acarines such as mosquitoes and ticks.

hematuria Blood in the urine; a condition seen in some persons infected with *Plasmodium falciparum.*

hemimetabolous A type of development in insects in which there is a gradual change in the external structure as development proceeds to the adult stage; Hemimetabola is the name of the taxonomic group.

hemorrhage Escape of blood from vessels.

hepato- A root referring to the liver.

heterogonic Reproduction in which sexual and asexual generations alternate, as in the nematode *Strongyloides.*

heteroxenous Having more than one host required to complete a life cycle, such as in the digenetic trematodes (see homoxenous).

hexacanth embryo See oncosphere

holometabolous A type of development in insects in which there is a distinct change in the morphology of the stages; the cycle usually includes several larval stages, a pupa, and the adult; Holometabola is the name of the taxonomic group.

homoxenous An adjective referring to a parasite that has a direct life cycle, or one in which only a single host is required for its completion.

horizontal transmission Transmission of a parasitic agent among members of a group (see vertical transmission).

host range The number of species of hosts in which a parasitic agent can develop (see euryxenous and stenoxenous).

humoral immunity A specific response to an antigen in which the principal effectors are antibodies that circulate in the blood.

hydatid cyst Laminated, fluid-filled cyst in *Echinococcus* which produces many protoscolices.

hyper- A prefix meaning more or greater than normal, (ant. hypo-).

hyperemia (Br. **hyperaemia)** An abnormally large amount of blood in a tissue.

hyperplasia An abnormally high number of cells in a tissue.

hypersensitivity (=allergy) A condition in which a mammal is sensitized to a particular substance and has an abnormally strong reaction when the substance is contacted again; hay fever is an example.

hypertrophy An abnormal increase in the size of a tissue

hypnozoite Dormant exoerythrocytic stage seen in some species of malaria.

hypo- A prefix meaning less than normal, under or below (ant hyper-).

-iasis A suffix meaning to be infected with, as in helminthiasis (see -osis).

imago The adult stage of an insect.

immunity A specific response in vertebrates to a foreign protein in which cells respond by producing humoral and/or cellular antibodies.

immunopathology An immune response that is damaging in itself.

incidence (of infection) The proportion of a population infected or showing disease over a particular time period; in public health, the incidence of measles, for example, would be given as 23/100,000 persons per year.

incidental parasite Parasite found in a host other than its usual one.

incubation period The period of time between infection and the appearance of clinical signs or symptoms (see prepatent period).

indirect life cycle A life cycle in which more than one host is required for its completion (see heteroxenous).

inflammation A response by a vertebrate to physical or chemical insult in which there is pain, reddening, increased temperature, and swelling at the site (see -itis).

instar A stage in the life cycle of an insect, such as a larval or nymphal instar.

intermediate host Host in which a parasite is not sexually mature.

-itis A suffix meaning inflammation.

juvenile An organism similar to the adult of the species, but which is sexually immature.

kentrogen The undifferentiated cell mass injected into a host by larvae of certain parasitic barnacles (Class Cirripedia).

kinetoplast An organelle characteristic of protists in the order Kinetoplastida; actually a mitochondrial compartment packed with minicircles and maxicircles of DNA.

kinety A longitudinal row of ciliary basal bodies and their connecting fibrils which extend anteriorly from each basal body.

lacunar system A system of fluid-filled canals in the tegument of members of the phylum Acanthocephala, apparently serves as a circulatory and hydraulic system.

larva An embryo that becomes self-sustaining and independent before it has developed the characteristic features of the adult form; a larva is anatomically different from the adult.

larviparous Giving birth to larvae.

Laurer's canal A tubule, usually blind-ended, which arises near the junction of the oviduct and vitelline duct in many digenetic trematodes; probably represents a vestigial vagina.

lemniscus (-i) One of a pair of lateral, fluid-filled sacs at the base of the proboscis in members of the phylum Acanthocephala.

LM Light microscope.

lumen (-ina) The central cavity of an organ such as the lumen of the intestine.

lycophore The ten-hooked or decacanth larva that develops within the egg capsules of tapeworms of the cohort Gyrocotyliidea.

mammillated Having many small nipplelike protrusions.

mastigont apparatus A group of structures in members of the protistan order Trichomonadida: flagella, parabasal body, costa, axostyle, pelta.

-megaly A suffix meaning to be enlarged beyond normal size.

Mehlis' gland Secretory cells surrounding the ootype of certain platyhelminths; serous and mucous cells are present.

merogony A type of asexual reproduction in which there is nuclear replication without plasmotomy and then two to many merozoites or daughter cells are produced simultaneously, a type or schizogony in which merozoites are formed; examples are found in many apicomplexans such as *Eimeria* and *Plasmodium* (see schizogony).

merozoite Product of merogony; usually an elongate organism that infects another host cell to undergo either merogony again or gamogony.

meta- A prefix meaning many, after, changed or behind.

metacestode Tapeworm stage following the oncosphere, but one not yet sexually mature.

metamerism Segmental repetition of homologous parts; in each metamere or segment there are identical structures such as muscles, neural ganglia, and nephridia.

metraterm Muscular, terminal portion of the uterus of certain digenetic trematodes; a diagnostic feature not present in all species.

microneme Slender, chordlike bodies in the anterior of zoites of certain members of the phylum Apicomplexa.

microtriches (sing. **microthrix**) Surface projections from the tegument of tapeworms; resemble microvilli of vertebrate intestinal epithelial cells, but have characteristic dense caps; function to increase surface area.

molt (=ecdysis) Shedding of an external covering such as integument or exoskeleton; in arthropods and nematodes, shedding the external covering is integral to growth.

monoecious Both male and female sex organs in one individual; hermaphroditic (ant. dioecious).

monoxenous Having a single host in the life cycle (see heteroxenous).

monozoic Refers to a condition in tapeworms in which the body consists of a single unit (ant. polyzoic).

morbi- A root meaning disease.

mort- A root meaning death.

mucous membrane Any of several moist surfaces in the body of vertebrates in which there are mucus secreting or goblet cells; examples are the orbit of the eye, nasal passages, inside the mouth.

mucron An organelle of certain gregarines which anchors the organism to its host cell; formed from elements of the apical complex.

multivoltine Having a number of generations in a year.

mutualism Symbiosis in which both partners benefit.

naiad The preadult stage of an insect, which has hemimetabolic development in an aquatic environment (see nymph).

neoteny A condition in which an individual which still has larval characteristics becomes sexually mature.

nephro- A root referring to the kidney.

nymph The preadult stage of an insect, which has hemimetabolic development in a terrestrial environment (see naiad).

obligate parasite A parasite that requires a host for the completion of its life cycle.

-oma A root meaning tumor or swelling.

oncomiracidium A free-swimming, ciliated larva of members of the subclass Monogenea.

oncosphere The six-hooked embryo that is contained in the egg membranes of members of the Eucestoda; hexacanth embryo.

oocyst A stage in the life cycle of certain apicomplexans in which the zygote secretes a wall around itself; often highly resistant to environmental conditions.

ookinete The zygote in the life cycle of certain members or the phylum Apicomplexa following syngamy of macro and microgametes; the term most often refers to the motile stage of *Plasmodium* which is seen in the midgut of the mosquito shortly after syngamy.

opisthaptor The highly specialized, posterior holdfast of members of the subclass Monogenea; sometimes also refers to the ventral adhesive disk of members of the class Aspidobothrea.

-osis A suffix meaning diseased, as in helminthosis

-otomy A suffix meaning to cut.

oviparous Egg laying; producing eggs that hatch after leaving the body of the mother.

ovoviviparous Producing eggs with persistent membranes through which the young escape while still within the body of the mother.

ovum (-a) The female germ cell.

papilla (-ae) A nipplelike structure

parabasal body An organelle that is part or the mastigont apparatus of certain members of the protistan order Trichomonadida; has the function of the Golgi of metazoan cells.

parasitism An association between the populations of two species in which the smaller (parasite) is physiologically dependent on the larger (host), the prevalence of the parasites and the intensity of the infection are non random and the parasite species has a higher reproductive potential than the host species; the parasite has the potential of harming the host.

parasitophorous vacuole A clear space between an intracellular parasite and the host cell cytoplasm.

paratenic host (=transport host) A host in which a parasite resides but does not develop and which is not physiologically essential for the completion of the life cycle.

parenchyma A reticulum of cells between the organs of an animal; also, the cells that perform the principal functions of the organ.

paroxysm A sudden intensification or recurrence of symptoms of a disease.

parthenogenesis Development of an organism from an unfertilized egg; common in insects such as aphids and in some nematodes such as *Strongyloides*.

patent period The period during an infection when the causative agent can be found by some means.

pellicle A double external membrane.

peritoneum A thin membrane of mesodermal origin that lines the body cavity of vertebrates (and some other higher metazoans) and supports the organs of the body cavity.

peritrophic membrane A covering that forms around the blood meal of a hematophagous insect; digestion usually takes place within the membrane; the membrane sometimes serves as a barrier to a parasitic agent moving from the blood to the tissues of the host.

petechia (-iae) Pinpoint hemorrhage in a tissue or organ.

phago- A root meaning to eat.

phasmid Sensory pit located on the posterior part of nematodes of the class Secernentea (see amphid).

-philia A root meaning affinity for or an excess of.

plasma The fluid portion of the blood (see serum).

plasmodium (-ia) An organism that is multinucleate but has a single outer limiting membrane.

plasmotomy Fission of a multinucleated protist into two or more multinucleated daughter cells without direct relationship to nuclear division.

plerocercoid A metacestode developing from a procercoid in the life cycle of tapeworms of the orders Proteocephala and Pseudophyllidea; this type of tapeworm larva is solid (as opposed to hollow) and has a rudimentary holdfast at the anterior end.

pleura- A root meaning *at the rib;* refers to the lining of the thorax.

polar filament A coiled filament in the spore of myxozoans, the filament is extruded when the spore is ingested by a host and anchors the spore to the hosts intestinal epithelium.

polar tube Hollow elastic tube of microsporans which is extruded into host tissue, and through which the parasite sporoplasm enters the host cell.

polyembryony A process in which a zygote gives rise to more than one embryo.

polyzoic Consisting of more than one zooid or animal or proglottid.

posterior station Development of a parasite in the posterior portion of the gut of insects; transmission is by fecal contamination.

premunition A type of immunity in which the continued presence of the parasite in the body of the host is necessary for the maintenance of effective immunity.

prepatent period That time after infection but before the causative agent can be found by usual diagnostic techniques.

procercoid A metacestode that develops from the hexacanth; it has no sex organ development; found in members of the tapeworm orders Proteocephala and Pseudophyllidea; this type of larva is solid (as opposed to hollow).

proglottid A body segment of a tapeworm containing a complete set of reproductive organs.

prohaptor The anterior holdfast of members of the subclass Monogenea.

prophylaxis Prevention; procedures that are carried out to prevent the transmission of the parasitic agent or the occurrence of disease.

protandry The condition in which the male matures before the female

protoscolex (protoscolices) A holdfast of tapeworms of the order Cyclophyllidea which forms from a germinal epithelium in a coenurus, hydatid, or alveolar cyst.

pseudocoelom A body cavity of a metazoan that is not completely lined with mesoderm.

pter- A root meaning *wing.*

quarantine Limitation in the freedom of movement of humans or animals in order to contain the spread of a disease; the length of time is slightly longer than the longest known incubation period of the disease agent in question.

recrudescence The recurrence of signs or symptoms of a disease after an abatement of days or weeks (see relapse).

relapse The recurrence of signs or symptoms of a disease after an abatement of weeks or months; in malaria, the term is used for the reappearance of clinical disease after successful meronticidal treatment.

renal Of or near the kidney.

reportable disease A disease that, by law, must be reported to a health authority such as a state department of health or the office of the state veterinarian; in general, such diseases are of special concern to the health of the human or animal population; examples in the United States are malaria, rabies, and tuberculosis.

reservoir host Any organism in which a parasitic agent normally lives and multiplies and from which those hosts important to humans can become infected.

retrofection A process of infection in which the parasite leaves the body of the host and then almost immediately penetrates the skin; an example is *Strongyloicles,* a common nematode of humans and dogs.

rhoptry (-ies) Saclike, electron-dense structure in the anterior portion of a zoite of a member of the phylum Apicomplexa; involved in the penetration of host cells.

Romaña's sign Periorbital swelling characteristic of the early stages of infection with *Trypanosoma cruzi,* the cause of Chagas' disease.

Romanowsky stain Any of a number of blood or tissue stains that contain eosin and methylene blue; examples are Wright and Giemsa stains.

rostellum A prominence on the anterior end of the scolex, usually fitted with hooks, of certain tapeworms of the order Cyclophyllidea.

Saefftigen's pouch A muscular, fluid-filled sac in the posterior end of male acanthocephalans that helps to evert the copulatory bursa.

schizogony A type of asexual reproduction in which there are multiple nuclear divisions and then plasmotomy takes place giving rise to a large number of daughter cells; occurs in many members of the phylum Apicomplexa and some other protists; merogony, sporogony, and microgametogony are types of schizogony

scolex (scolices) The holdfast or organ by which a tapeworm attaches to the intestine of its host.

scutellum A shield.

SEM Scanning electron microscope.

sequela (-ae) A diseased condition resulting from a previous disease.

serum The fluid part of vertebrate blood after the fibrin has been removed.

sign Any objective evidence of disease; fever, diarrhea, and skin rash are examples (see symptom).

sparganum A plerocercoid, usually of the order Pseudophyllidea, of unknown specific identity.

spicule (=copulatory spicule) An elongate, sclerotized structure of male nematodes used in holding open the vulva of the female during copulation and transfer of sperm.

spleno- A root referring to the spleen.

spore A resistant stage that is formed internally by the mother cell (see cyst).

sporogony Schizogony in which the product is the sporozoite.

sporozoite The infective or transfer stage in members of the phylum Apicomplexa.

stenoxenous Having a narrow host range (see euryxenous).

stichosome A column of large, rectangular cells (stichocytes) posterior to the short, muscular esophagus of members of the nematode order Trichurida.

strobila A chain of tapeworm proglottids or segments.

swimmer's itch (=cercarial dermatitis) A skin reaction to the penetration or cercariae or certain members of the trematode family Schistosomatidae; actually a hypersensitivity to the cercariae and their secretions.

sylvatic Refers to forest or a wooded area; used as an adjective to describe the location of a disease cycle in the wild, but often used imprecisely, such as in referring to sylvatic plague when the more correct term is *campestral plague*.

symbiosis An intimate association of two organisms of different species.

symptom usually reserved for subjective indicators of a disease condition such as pain, dizziness, nausea (see sign).

symptomatic treatment Nonspecific therapy of a disease that is designed to reduce the symptoms or the effects.

syzygy End-to-end joining of two or more gamonts of members of the classes Gregarinea and Coccidea.

tachyzoite Rapidly growing meront or zoites characteristic of the early stage of infection with *Toxoplasma* and related organisms of the phylum Apicomplexa.

TEM Transmission electron microscope.

temporary parasite A parasite that visits a host at intervals and only for relatively short period; examples are mosquitoes and ticks.

transport host See paratenic host.

trochophore larva A free-swimming larval form of some marine annelids and mollusks.

trophozoite The growing, feeding stage of a protistan, also called the *vegetative stage*.

uniramous Having one branch.

univoltine Having one generation per year.

uterine bell A funnel-shaped structure in female acanthocephalans that serves as a sorting device for eggs.

vector An arthropod, mollusk, or other invertebrate that serves to transmit an infective agent to a vertebrate host. A mechanical vector is one in which the parasite neither multiplies nor develops; a biological vector is one in which the parasite either multiplies or develops; some vectors are intermediate hosts, such as snails in the life cycles of digenetic trematodes; some vectors are definitive hosts, such as mosquitoes in transmitting the causative agent of malaria.

vertical transmission Transmission of a parasite from one generation to the next through the egg or in utero.

virulence The ability of a parasite to produce pathogenic effects or to invade.

Winterbottom's sign Enlargement of the cervical lymph nodes early in the course of African trypanosomsis in humans.

worm An organism without legs that creeps or crawls and is not obviously anything else.

xenodiagnosis A diagnostic method in which the natural vector of the suspected organism is allowed to feed on the host and later the organism is looked for in the tissues of the vector; used almost exclusively for the diagnosis for Chagas' disease in humans.

zoonosis (-es) A disease common to humans and other animals.

zoonotic agent An organism that causes a zoonosis.

Index

D

E

Q

R